THE
MERCK
MANUAL

★

EIGHTH EDITION

THE MERCK MANUAL is dedicated
to the Doctor of Medicine
and to his colleagues and aides
in the allied professions.

THE
MERCK
MANUAL

OF

DIAGNOSIS AND THERAPY

A SOURCE OF READY REFERENCE
FOR THE PHYSICIAN

Published by

MERCK & CO., Inc.

RAHWAY, N. J., U.S.A.

Export Subsidiary: MERCK (NORTH AMERICA) Inc.
In Canada: MERCK & CO. LIMITED, MONTREAL

1950

Printed in the U. S. A.

FOREWORD

THE MERCK MANUAL is intended to supply the physician with accurate, condensed, readily available medical information. Emphasis is laid upon diagnosis and treatment, but care has been taken to include certain basic physiologic, pathologic, and other facts essential to effective therapy. Surgical procedures, where indicated, have been mentioned but not described.

The Eighth Edition is a completely new handbook, not a revision of previous editions. More than 100 outstanding clinicians throughout the United States have served as authors or consultants, and assisted the Editorial Board and staff of 12 physicians. The advice of noted clinicians has ensured that the facts presented are as complete, authentic, and up-to-the-minute as possible. Thus, the phenomenal advances in medical research and practice of the past few years have been reflected in the broadened scope of THE MERCK MANUAL.

Part I, which is devoted to diseases and major symptoms, has been enlarged to contain 338 chapters, as compared with 256 in the last edition. Important among the new or expanded chapters are those on nutritional deficiencies, drug addiction, prenatal and postnatal care and the care of premature infants, dental emergencies the physician may have to treat, tropical and other exotic diseases of increasing significance, and summaries of anticoagulant, sulfonamide, and antibiotic therapy and of treatment with adrenocortical steroids or substances of related action.

Part II presents completely new chapters on routine immunization measures, clinical and bedside procedures, laboratory tests practicable for the doctor's office, suggested items for the physician's bag, an outline of preoperative and postoperative care, a section on diets, and helpful ready reference data and conversion tables.

In general, the prescriptions call for drugs included in the Thirteenth Edition of *The United States Pharmacopœia*, the Eighth Edition of *The National Formulary*, and *New and Non-official Remedies*, 1949. However, a number of products which carry proprietary names have been specified by our authors and included for that reason. The mention of any preparation does not imply, therefore, any editorial preference or that it is the only product of its kind available. Its inclusion under a given designation is not to be regarded as the publisher's opinion that such word or name is or is not a descriptive term, nor as to whether or not it is subject to proprietary rights. A convenient dose table of Alternative Proprietary Preparations is provided.

On the next page a few "Suggestions for Readers" have been included, aimed at facilitating the use of this reference volume in its new form.

SUGGESTIONS
FOR
READERS

1. The Table of Contents, opposite, shows the sections into which chapters have been grouped.

2. A list of chapters and, where necessary, of subchapters, is placed at the beginning of each section.

3. A time-saving Index, greatly expanded and liberally cross titled, is provided. It should be consulted whenever possible. Chapters are generously supplied with plainly indicated textual cross references.

4. Prescriptions are grouped into categories according to therapeutic action, and appear at the end of each section. Their numerical designations correspond to those of the ℞ symbols in the chapters. Dosage is in metric quantities throughout, with apothecaries' equivalents whenever appropriate. Unless otherwise specified, the doses suggested are for the average adult.

5. In the text, names of proprietary preparations are capitalized; among the prescriptions, they appear within quotation marks.

6. Each page heading indicates the page number, the section title and the subject matter on that page.

7. A list of standard and special Abbreviations, as employed throughout, appears in the front of the book.

8. Many chapters contain helpful tables, those on Cardiac Arrhythmias and Cardiac Blocks are illustrated by typical ECG tracings, and a useful miscellany will be found at the end of Part II.

9. Medical Emergencies, such as Drowning, Burns, Poisoning, Venomous Bites, Electric Shock, Infusion Reactions, and the like, with appropriate therapy of each, are dealt with in chapters bearing these titles, contained in the Physical and Chemical section.

THE EDITOR

CONTENTS

PART I

ABBREVIATIONS AND SYMBOLS

B.M.R.	basal metabolic rate	N.N.R.	New and Nonofficial Remedies
BUN	blood urea nitrogen		
C.	Centigrade	NPN	nonprotein nitrogen
cc.	cubic centimeter(s)	O_2	oxygen
cm.	centimeter(s)	oz.	ounce(s)
C.N.S.	central nervous system	PSP	phenolsulfon-phthalein (test)
CO_2	carbon dioxide	pt.	pint(s)
cu.	cubic	q.s. ad	quantity sufficient to make
ECG	electrocardiogram		
EEG	electroencephalo-gram	qt.	quart(s)
		q.v.	which see
E.S.R.	erythrocyte sedi-mentation rate	sat.	saturated
		sol.	solution
F.	Fahrenheit	sp. gr.	specific gravity
Fr.	French (size)	sq.	square
ft.	foot, feet	subcut.	subcutaneous(ly)
Gm.	gram(s)	tbsp.	tablespoon(s)
gr.	grain(s)	tsp.	teaspoon(s)
hr.	hour(s)	u.	unit(s)
I.M.	intramuscular(ly)	U.S.P.	United States Pharmacopœia
in.	inch(es)		
I.U.	International Units	wt.	weight
I.V.	intravenous(ly)	ℨ	dram(s)
Kg.	kilogram	℥	ounce(s)
L.	liter(s)	♏	minim(s)
lb.	pound(s)	μ	micron(s)
mcg.	microgram(s)	%	per cent
mEq.	milliequivalent(s)	℞	Take
mg.	milligram(s)	<	less than
mm.	millimeter(s)	>	more than
min.	minute(s)	āā	equal parts
N.F.	National Formulary	°	degree(s)

ALLERGY

ALLERGY: GENERAL CONSIDERATIONS

Allergy connotes an altered reaction of the tissues in certain individuals on exposure to agents which, in similar amounts, are innocuous to other persons. **Anaphylaxis** now is more often used to describe sensitivity reactions occurring in laboratory animals. **Sensitivity** is a term closely interrelated to allergy and anaphylaxis, the lines of demarcation between the three often being indistinct.

In many of the manifestations of allergy a familial tendency is conspicuous. The exciting agents, known as allergens or antigens, are specific substances which stimulate the production of correspondingly specific antibodies within a sensitive organism. Antibodies may be free in the blood stream, or attached to tissue cells (i.e., sessile). It is the interaction of the antigen with sessile antibodies that produces symptoms. That the release of histamine (or a histamine-like substance) from injured cells plays a role in producing allergic reactions is a widely held theory. Considerable evidence supports it (e.g., the success of treatment with "antihistaminic" drugs), but definite proof is lacking.

The chief manifestations of allergy are "hay fever," asthma, gastrointestinal disturbances, urticaria, angioneurotic edema, and serum sickness (an anaphylactic-like reaction). Migraine (q.v.), which some tentatively attribute to allergy, is discussed elsewhere. The term "hay fever" is a misnomer, since the symptoms are not necessarily related to hay nor is fever present. The symptoms result from inhalation of certain pollens, so that the syndrome is more accurately called pollinosis. Because of popular usage, however, it will be called hay fever throughout this text.

An allergic individual may be sensitive to only one allergen, but multiple sensitivities are the rule. Substances capable of acting as allergens are innumerable; they may be generally classified as follows:

Inhalants: These constitute the most important allergens causing symptoms in the respiratory tract. They include pollens, fungi, other vegetable or animal epithelial emanations, various dusts, vapors (such as tobacco smoke and train smoke), cosmetics, perfumes, and sundry strong odors.

Foods: Food allergy as a major or minor cause of symptoms is relatively frequent and often is overlooked as a complicating factor in patients sensitive principally to inhalants. Although any food may be responsible for allergic symptoms, the most common offenders are wheat, eggs, milk, cottonseed, fish, nuts, chocolate, pork, and strawberries.

Drugs: Any drug may act as an allergen, but aspirin probably does so most frequently.

Infectious agents: Bacteria, fungi, parasites, and viruses are capable of producing tissue sensitivity (e.g., tubercles, gummas, and other granulomas), but the exact part they play in producing allergic symptoms (e.g., bronchial asthma, urticaria) remains obscure.

Contactants: These act upon the skin (also the mucous membranes), causing contact dermatitis (q.v.) or other phenomena. They include plants and flowers, various dyestuffs, rubber, flameproofing and waterproofing chemicals, insecticides, furs, leather, jewelry, and cosmetics, as well as a wide variety of industrially important chemicals.

Physical agents: The chief physical causes are heat, cold, light (and other radiations), and pressure. The allergic reactions usually occur in the skin.

Other agents: Mental allergy, in which an emotional stimulus acts as an allergen, has been described. Vaccines and serums used in immunization and therapy may produce allergic reactions, occasionally severe, in previously sensitized individuals.

Diagnostic Procedures

History: A careful history is of paramount importance. The time of attacks (month and year), character of onset (acute or insidious), frequency of the episodes, and probable precipitating factors should be determined. Often, the means by which a patient obtains relief will give a clue to the cause: for example, cardiac asthma, which is not due to allergy, often is relieved by sitting up in bed, while outdoor exercise or fresh air will relieve the patient with allergic rhinitis due to house dust. Hot drinks help allay allergy to cold, while cold drinks exacerbate it and alleviate allergy to heat. Inquiry into the effect of change in the patient's occupation or location should be made. Any food believed to produce symptoms or which is intensely disliked should be noted. The dislikes of children frequently are protective and should not be considered mere whims until so proved. Questions should be designed to elicit from the patient any effects of contact with inhalants in his environment; for example, he should be asked if fluffing a pillow causes sneezing or smarting of the eyes. He also should be asked if symptoms have occurred on exposure to dusts at home, outdoors, at work, on trains or buses, or exposure to hay, animal feeds, or fertilizer. Most allergic people are unfavorably affected by fatigue, excitement, anxiety, overheating, chilling, overexertion, getting wet, and pressure, as from tight garments.

Skin tests: Skin tests have their greatest usefulness in allergy caused by contactants and inhalants, but are becoming increasingly important in the field of diagnosis and in regulating the treatment of various systemic diseases, such as systemic fungus infections (q.v.). The wheal is the characteristic positive response, appearing within 5 to 15 minutes in specific allergic disorders, or developing slowly over a period of 24 to 72 hours in certain systemic sensitivity tests (e.g., tuberculin). The size of the wheal usually is directly related to the degree of sensitivity. (1) Scratch tests are usually performed in two rows on the patient's back or forearm. They should be about 1 cm. in length and 2.5 cm. apart. The skin surface should be torn rather than cut, and without drawing blood. An allergen then should be applied to each scratch. (2) For intracutaneous tests a tuberculin syringe is fitted with a short-bevel 26- or 27-gauge needle. A separate syringe and needle must be used for each test substance. Not more than 0.02 cc. should be injected. (3) Indirect skin testing (passive transfer) may be done when direct skin testing is not feasible (as in dermographism, ichthyosis, eczema). Blood (5 to 10 cc.) is drawn from the patient and centrifuged. Using the 7th cervical vertebra as a landmark, the back of a nonallergic adult is marked off in checkerboard fashion and 0.1 cc. of the allergic patient's plasma is introduced at each test site. These sensitized areas may be skin tested with the suspected allergens 2 to 4 days later, the contralateral side of the back being used as a control. (4) For patch tests, the suspected material is placed on a paper, gauze or linen patch, applied to the skin by means of adhesive tape, and allowed to remain in place for 24 or 48 hours, unless it unduly irritates the skin, in which case it is removed at once. (5) Mucosal tests are not widely employed at present, being resorted to only when skin tests to specific antigens remain negative, despite definite clinical evidence to the contrary. A small amount of antigen may be applied directly to the conjunctival sac or inferior turbinates, or by aerosol to the bronchial mucosa. In sensitive individuals, symptoms appear instantly, and may be terminated by the local use of 1:2,000 to 1:4,000 epinephrine.

(CAUTION! Severe reactions may occur from the administration of an allergen by aerosol to a hypersensitive individual.)

Most allergens used in testing are available as commercial preparations and instructions regarding concentration or dilution accompany the package. In preparing autogenous skin test and desensitization material, experience in selecting the proper strength and amount of the preparation to be used is essential.

Eosinophilia: The blood eosinophile count usually is high during allergic attacks, but the finding of large numbers of eosinophiles in the smears of nasal, ophthalmic, or bronchial exudates is of greater diagnostic significance.

Food diaries and food-elimination diets: Food sensitivities are often not recognized unless recourse is made to food diaries or trial diets. Food diaries should be kept on columnar paper, the foods eaten being listed at the left of the sheet. The adjacent columns should be dated, and a check mark placed opposite each food on the day it is eaten. The dates on which symptoms appear are listed on another page. Thus, the offending foodstuffs may be detected. Food-elimination diets consist of sharply restricted lists of foods (*see* ELIMINATION DIETS). If the patient does not obtain relief or improve on a strict elimination diet, it may be assumed that he is eating an offending food, or that his allergy is not to any food. If he is allergic to any of the foods in this diet his symptoms will become worse by reason of the concentrated exposure, and the omission of each food successively will, in many cases, identify the cause.

Treatment

1. Avoidance: When possible, elimination of the allergen from the patient's environment is the treatment of choice. This may require a change of diet, occupation or residence, or getting rid of a household pet or certain articles of furniture or clothing. Some geographic areas are free of many allergens that are common in others, and thus serve as havens for afflicted individuals. When complete avoidance is impossible, as in the case of pollens, exposure may be reduced by the use of air filters, by keeping windows and doors closed, and by avoidance of trips to rural areas. Any drug the patient may use must be discontinued if found to cause reactions.

2. Desensitization (hyposensitization): Where avoidance of the allergen is not feasible, desensitization should be attempted by injecting an extract of the causative allergen in a series of gradually increasing doses. The same principle applies in attempting desensitization of patients having serum or vaccine sensitivities and in measures aimed at overcoming systemic sensitivity produced by various diseases (e.g., *see* SYSTEMIC FUNGUS INFECTIONS: General Therapeutic Principles, for details of desensitization in various mycoses). Suitable preparations of such agents as pollens, spores, dusts, vaccines, and serums can be obtained from various manufacturers. The dosage will vary with the preparation used, but it must always be adjusted to the degree of sensitivity exhibited by each patient to a given allergen. The rate of increase will depend on the reaction, if any, to the previous dose. After a severe reaction, the next dose must be reduced.

There are three generally employed methods of desensitization: coseasonal, preseasonal, and perennial.

The **coseasonal** method, which probably is the least effective, is employed when a hay fever patient is first seen during the pollen season. Small doses of pollen extract are injected into or under the skin: Of a 1:5,000 dilution, 0.1 cc. (20 noon or pollen u.) initially is tolerated by 95% of patients. Many allergists favor the simultaneous injection of epinephrine hydrochloride (R 13), approximately 0.3 cc. of a 1:1,000 solution. If the patient is relieved by the 20 noon u., he is instructed to return for a similar dose when symptoms recur. If not benefited by the second dose, he is given 40 noon u. the next day. He continues to return until a dose is reached that abates the symptoms (usually about 100 noon u.). The optimum dose having thus been determined, the patient returns every 5 to 7 days for a maintenance injection throughout the remainder of the pollen season.

The **preseasonal** method is employed when the patient is seen 8 weeks or more before the expected onset of symptoms. It affords relief in about 80% of patients. Concomitant non-pollen factors (e.g., foods, animal danders) should not be overlooked. The injections are given subcut. twice weekly in gradually increasing dosage, so that the patient is receiving 1 cc. of a 1:50 extract (20,000 noon u.) just prior to the season. The physician then administers 0.2 cc. of 1:50 extract (4,000 noon u.) every 2 weeks throughout the season. If time is short, the dosage may be increased more rapidly or the injections given 3 times a week, provided no evidence of overdosage appears.

The **perennial** method, which probably is the best, consists in maintaining the antibody titer built up by preseasonal treatment. Doses of 0.2 cc. of 1:50 extract (4,000 noon u.) are injected subcut. every 2 weeks. However, the dose again is built up gradually to 1 cc. of 1:50 extract (20,000 noon u.) just before the expected onset of symptoms.

House dust is perhaps the most important cause of perennial allergy. Its complete avoidance is impossible, but exposure should be reduced by removal of all unessential items from the room most frequented by the patient, such as rugs, drapes, and curtains. The patient's mattress and pillows should be encased in dustproof coverings. Clothing should not be stored in his room and all animal pets should be removed from his environment. The patient should remain away from the house while it is being cleaned. He should avoid handling dusty, stored objects such as books, boxes, or clothing. Desensitization can be started at any time, because the exposure is continuous. If ordinary dust extracts are used, 0.1 cc. of a 1:100 or 1:1,000 strength is given subcut. and the dose gradually increased as tolerated. If refined dust extracts are employed, 1:200,000 or 1:400,000 strength should be used initially.

If the patient has multiple sensitivities, the various antigens found in his vicinity are sometimes combined in one solution, but it is better practice to have separate solutions and employ a separate syringe for each substance. This makes for simplicity and more accurate evaluation of reactions. On those rare occasions when patients are treated with more than 3 or 4 antigens, it is best to give them on different days.

Rapid desensitization in cases of serum sensitivity may be attempted in emergencies where it is necessary to administer immune or antiserum as therapeutic agents (e.g., see DIPHTHERIA). In desensitization procedures used against an infectious agent, diluted antigen or vaccine is injected at 1- to 3-day intervals as determined by the individual case; the dosage being increased and regulated in the same manner as for hay fever desensitization.

Untoward reactions: Desensitization must be carried out with great caution, especially when the antigen is highly potent or the patient extremely sensitive. It is advisable to have a syringe loaded with epinephrine always at hand for emergencies. Severe reactions may result from overdosage, too rapid increase in dosage, or accidental introduction of the extract into a vein. The symptoms may be local or systemic.

The **local** reaction is a swelling at the site of injection which appears within a few hours. It may be ignored if it does not exceed 2.5 cm. in diameter. Although resembling an inflammation (swelling, redness, pain, warmth), it represents a specific interaction of antigen and antibody. When large enough to cause discomfort, the swelling is treated with cold (never hot) compresses and an antihistaminic drug, such as Neo-Antergan (R 1), orally. A local reaction whose diameter exceeds 2.5 cm. indicates that the level of tolerance is being approached and a smaller dose should be given, or at least no further increase made at that time.

The **generalized** (systemic) reaction varies from malaise, sometimes with slight fever, to severe anaphylactic (allergic) shock and death. One of the most frequent signs, and usually the earliest, is urticaria. The more severe reactions simulate one or more of the clinical allergic entities. Thus, respiratory distress with wheezing and cough will occur if the bronchiole is the shock organ. Similarly, conjunctivitis, rhinitis, laryngitis, or tracheitis may appear, or nausea, vomiting, diarrhea, and abdominal cramps. Contractions of the uterus and slight bleeding may occur; abortions have sometimes resulted.

Many of these reactions are preventable. Double checking of the label on the bottle will guard against using the wrong extract. When old extracts are replaced, the initial dose of the new preparation should be reduced. When giving an injection, care always should be taken to avoid intravascular penetration. If, when the plunger is pulled upon, blood appears in the syringe, the needle should be withdrawn, reinserted, and similarly checked before the dose is injected. Epinephrine 0.3 to 0.5 cc. (℞ 13) may be given with the antigen. It is a good precaution to keep the patient in the office 15 to 20 minutes after each injection, especially if he has previously had a reaction. If a systemic reaction begins, a tourniquet should be applied at once, proximal to the site of injection. An antihistaminic, such as Neo-Antergan (℞ 1), should be given by mouth and 0.5 cc. of epinephrine 1:1,000 (℞ 13) injected into the opposite arm. When the symptoms subside, the tourniquet can be loosened but then reapplied and more epinephrine given if symptoms recur. It is advisable to reduce the next injection to half the dose previously given and to make further increases cautiously.

3. Antihistaminics: Although the role of histamine in producing allergic reactions remains uncertain, treatment with antihistaminic drugs such as Neo-Antergan (℞ 1) has met with widespread success. The adult dosage is 25 to 100 mg. by mouth 3 or 4 times daily, after meals and at bedtime; for infants and children, 2 to 3 mg./lb. body wt. divided over a 24-hour period. Antihistaminics can be obtained in either tablet or elixir form. Most of the preparations currently available may produce side reactions of somnolence, nausea, or vertigo in some patients. When these are unduly prominent with one preparation another may be substituted, since different products affect individual patients differently. However, the sedative action is advantageous at bedtime and in those patients who have insomnia due to hyperemic nasal obstruction.

4. Symptomatic Therapy: This is aimed at the relief of allergic manifestations by means other than avoidance, desensitization or antihistaminic drugs. These will be discussed in the treatment section of each allergic disease entity (below).

ALLERGIC RHINITIS
(Hay fever; Perennial rhinitis)

A symptom complex characterized by seasonal or perennial sneezing, rhinorrhea, nasal congestion, and often conjunctivitis and pharyngitis.

HAY FEVER
(Pollinosis)

Hay fever, the seasonal form of allergic rhinitis, is generally induced by wind-borne pollens or fungi. The spring type is almost always due to tree pollens (e.g., oak, elm, maple, pecan, birch, cottonwood). The summer type is usually caused by grass pollens (e.g., Bermuda, timothy, sweet vernal, orchard, Johnson) or fungus spores (e.g., *Alternaria helminthosporium, Hormodendrum,* wheat and corn rusts, and smuts). The fall type is due to pollens of the ragweed family in the Eastern and Central states of the U.S., and to pollens of the chenopod-amaranth family in the Western states.

Symptoms and Signs

These appear abruptly after exposure. Intense itching of the nose, roof of the mouth, pharynx and eyes soon occurs, accompanied or shortly followed by lacrimation, photophobia, profuse clear, watery nasal discharge, and violent sneezing. There also may be frontal headache, irritability, anorexia, insomnia and gastric disturbances. Examination reveals injected conjunctivae and pale, boggy nasal mucous membranes. Angioneurotic edema, urticaria, or asthma may be associated phenomena.

Diagnosis

The patient frequently makes his own diagnosis. The finding of numerous eosinophils in a nasal smear helps differentiate hay fever from other chronic rhinitides. The specific allergen responsible is to be identified by means of history and skin or mucosal tests (*see* ALLERGY: Diagnostic Procedures).

Treatment

Therapy includes avoidance of the allergen, specific desensitization (*see* p. 4), antihistaminics, symptomatic care, and more recently cortisone or ACTH. An antihistaminic drug such as Neo-Antergan (℞ 1) will control the symptoms in 70 to 95% of cases. When indicated, nose drops and inhalants (℞ 2 to 7) are sometimes helpful, but their prolonged use may cause the nasal mucous membranes to become chronically edematous. Sympathomimetic drugs may be administered orally (℞ 8, 9, 16) to clear the nasal passages; usually, fewer side reactions (tremor, palpitation, apprehension) occur with propadrine (℞ 8) or Neo-Synephrine (℞ 9) than with ephedrine (℞ 16). Atropine (℞ 10) at times will control rhinorrhea remarkably well; it should be given to the point where manifestations of mild overdosage appear (dryness of mouth, blurring of vision, tachycardia, flushing of face) before it is judged ineffective in any particular case. Tincture of belladonna (℞ 11) or tincture of hyoscyamus (℞ 12) may be similarly employed.

PERENNIAL RHINITIS

(Vasomotor rhinitis, Hyperesthetic rhinitis)

This syndrome differs from hay fever in that it is not seasonal, but runs a continuous course with variations in severity. The etiologic factors are more numerous, but house dust, animal danders, and foods are the chief offenders. Vapors and dusts encountered in industry are often responsible. Pollens may play a part. Chronic nasal infection, sinusitis, nasal malformations and polyps are contributory factors. In a certain proportion of cases, although an allergic etiology cannot be demonstrated, it probably exists nevertheless.

Symptoms are similar to, but usually less severe than, those of hay fever. Sneezing may be the only manifestation. Nasal blockage is a prominent feature. The discharge is thin and watery, and often extremely profuse. Besides the characteristic history and clinical picture, a high percentage of eosinophiles in the discharge is diagnostic. The specific irritant frequently can be identified by the skin test; when this is negative, an inhalation test may be helpful (*see* ALLERGY: Diagnostic Procedures).

Treatment

Provided the etiologic factor(s) can be discovered, therapy follows the same principles as for hay fever (above). Otherwise, purely symptomatic treatment is indicated.

ALLERGIC CONJUNCTIVITIS

Conjunctivitis of an acute or chronic catarrhal form usually is part of a larger allergic syndrome, such as hay fever (q.v.). An acute conjunctivitis often is associated with contact dermatitis of the eyelids, which may be caused by various drugs used for ophthalmic medication or conveyed to the eyes by the fingers (e.g., antibiotics, by drug handlers), or by face powder or hair dyes. The conjunctivitis may, however, occur alone through direct contact with air-borne substances such as pollen, spores of fungi, various dusts, or animal danders. Food allergy has been demonstrated as an occasional cause.

Symptoms, Signs, and Diagnosis

Itching is a prominent symptom. Cases associated with hay fever generally are of the acute edematous type with pronounced injection of the conjunctivae. Those occurring without other manifestations of allergy usually are of the recurrent irritative type and often are accompanied by a mild palpebral folliculitis. Diagnosis is made by scratch or intradermal test. The conjunctivitis associated with contact dermatitis is best diagnosed by the patch test. If skin tests prove repeatedly negative, an ophthalmic test, cautiously applied, should be tried: a small quantity of the suspected antigen is placed on the conjunctiva of the lower lid of one eye. A reaction is characterized by burning and smarting, followed by itching. The conjunctiva becomes injected and the vessels are engorged. Edema usually follows.

The eye then should be washed out with isotonic saline solution, after which a drop of epinephrine is instilled.

Treatment

Removal from exposure to the causative irritant is primary. Where this cannot be accomplished, the therapeutic measures described under ALLERGY: Treatment, are applied. Eye washes (R 48, 50, 51) are soothing. When itching is intense, ice compresses, or solutions containing Pontocaine (R 49) or another suitable anesthetic agent, may be employed.

BRONCHIAL ASTHMA

A condition manifested by recurrent paroxysms of dyspnea of a characteristic wheezing type, due to narrowing of the lumens of the smaller bronchi and bronchioles.

Etiology

Bronchial asthma usually is found in individuals with a hereditarily allergic constitution. The exciting agent may be an extrinsic substance (e.g., pollen, dust, food, or drug) or an infection within the respiratory tract. The infective type of asthma may be precipitated by a common cold or acute bronchitis. Frequently, the bronchitis, and hence the asthma, is secondary to a chronic infection in the upper respiratory passages (sinuses, tonsils, adenoids). The frequency and severity of asthmatic attacks are greatly influenced by secondary factors such as fatigue, endocrine changes (pregnancy and menstruation), and psychic disturbances.

Pathology and Pathologic Physiology

During the asthmatic attack, the mucosa of the bronchi is thickened and the epithelial cells are distended with mucus, while the smooth muscle of the bronchial wall is contracted. This results in narrowing of the lumen, which is further obstructed by excessive secretion of thick tenacious mucus. Both phases of respiration are hampered by narrowing of the air passages. Expiration, the passive phase, is prolonged and often incomplete because of air being trapped in distended alveoli; while inspiration, which causes dilatation of the narrowed air passages and involves active muscular contraction, is accomplished with relative ease. As a result of incomplete expiration, the lungs become distended with air during the acute attack and repeated attacks may produce chronic emphysema with permanent reduction of vital capacity, loss of pulmonary elasticity, and eventual deformity of the chest (barrel chest).

Asthmatic attacks—wheezing dyspnea due to narrowing of bronchial and bronchiolar lumens—also may occur in various other conditions, such as heart failure (cardiac asthma), chronic bronchitis, obstructive emphysema, endobronchial tuberculosis, and bronchial carcinoma. Where the disease process is thus localized, the diffuse asthma is due to generalized reflex bronchial spasm.

Symptoms and Signs

Asthma may develop gradually during bronchitis or begin abruptly after exposure to an allergen. The attack is manifested by a sense of tightness in the chest with dyspnea and wheezing, usually audible to the unaided ear. Symptoms may subside in an hour or less, continue for several hours, or persist as status asthmaticus for many days. The wheezing may or may not be associated with cough or sputum until termination of the attack, which is usually heralded by coughing with expectoration of thick, tenacious sputum. This is followed immediately by a sensation of relief and "clearing" of the air passages.

The physical signs during an asthmatic attack are suppression of normal breath sounds, prolongation of expiration, and the presence of sonorous and sibilant rales throughout the chest. Uniform distribution of signs is typical, and persistent localization in one area suggests some other bronchial or pulmonary disease. During severe attacks, the chest is conspicuously distended and the patient may become cyanotic. Between attacks abnormal signs may not be detectable on quiet breathing, but forced expiration often will bring out sonorous or sibilant rales.

Diagnosis

Bronchial asthma must be differentiated from asthma due to other diseases and the etiologic agent must be determined. Usually, differential diagnosis is easily made from the history of recurrent attacks, physical signs during the paroxysm, and a family or personal history of allergy. In addition, eosinophiles and Curschmann's spirals may be demonstrated in the sputum, or eosinophilia in the blood. X-ray of the chest will rule out many other causes of bronchial obstruction and dyspnea, such as tumor, aortic aneurysm, and silicosis. Occasionally, bronchoscopy is necessary to exclude foreign bodies or tumors in the bronchi.

The etiologic diagnosis is more difficult. In general, cases are classified for treatment as either extrinsic or infective. However, many patients are affected by both external allergens and infective factors, so that each must be studied for both sensitization and infection. Asthma originating during infancy often is due to foods. Asthma beginning between the ages of 10 and 30 usually is due to inhalants, whereas cases beginning after 45 are most frequently due to infections. Attacks occurring only in the summer are commonly due to pollens or mold spores; those occurring only in winter, to infections. Association of attacks with certain houses or places of business suggests such extrinsic allergens as dust, vapors, or animal danders. The presence of infection in the paranasal sinuses, tonsils, and adenoids should be noted. Foci of infection outside the respiratory system are rarely etiologic.

The results of tests for sensitivity to extrinsic allergens must be judged by correlation with the patient's history. Definite reactions to inhalants usually are important, but in adults reactions to foods are only suggestive. When both infection and skin reactions to inhalant allergens are demonstrated, the relative importance of these factors may be determined by the effect of placing the patient for 3 or 4 days in a dust-free hospital room.

Treatment

1. **Treatment of the acute attack:** There are three main drugs for the relief of asthma—ephedrine, epinephrine, and aminophylline. For relatively mild attacks, ephedrine orally (R 16) is quickly effective in doses of 25 mg. (gr. ⅜); for children, a 3% aqueous solution may be administered in doses of 3 to 10 drops (6 to 20 mg.) according to age. Because of the stimulating effects of ephedrine, combination with a mild sedative such as phenobarbital (R 18) often is desirable, especially at night.

Epinephrine is indicated for severe attacks. It is administered subcut. in a dose of 0.3 to 0.5 cc. of the 1:1,000 solution (R 13), repeated after 15 to 30 minutes if necessary. This drug should be used cautiously in patients with severe hypertension, hyperthyroidism, heart disease, or sensitivity to epinephrine. When repeated injections are needed, the injection I.M. of epinephrine (1:500) in oil (R 14) provides therapeutic effects usually lasting 6 to 10 hours, and thus reduces the number of injections needed. Relief sometimes is obtained from inhaling the vapor of epinephrine 1:100 (R 15) from a nebulizer capable of producing an adequate volume of fine vapor. The patient must use the nebulizer promptly at the onset of an attack while reasonably deep inhalations can still be made. Usually, 4 or 5 deep inhalations suffice, but the patient must learn by experience to adjust the dose. Several derivatives of ephedrine or epinephrine are available and may be tried in individual cases. Of these newer drugs, aludrine (R 17) appears to be promising; it may be administered either sublingually (10 or 15 mg.) or by inhalation (4 to 10 breaths of nebulized 1:200 solution); oral or subcut. administration is not recommended.

For attacks that do not respond to epinephrine the most effective substitute is aminophylline. The quickest results are obtained by I.V. injection of 0.25 to 0.5 Gm. (gr. iv to viiss) (R 19). For self-administration, suppositories (R 20) or a 3% aqueous solution (R 21) may be used per rectum. Large doses of aminophylline are poorly tolerated by mouth, but doses of 0.1 to 0.2 Gm. (gr. iss to iii) (R 22) may relieve mild attacks and, when given at bedtime in entcric coated tablets, may prevent attacks during the night. Combinations of aminophylline with ephedrine and a sedative (℞ 23) are useful oral preparations for mild asthma.

An antihistaminic drug, such as Neo-Antergan (℞ 1), sometimes is effective in mild asthma, but usually is less reliable than ephedrine.

Atropine rarely is helpful in asthma, its bronchodilating action being outweighed by its tendency to dry the already tenacious sputum. Asthma powders, consisting of dried stramonium and Lobelia leaves combined with potassium nitrate (℞ 24), an old remedy of some merit, now are largely replaced by modern drugs. The powder is burned on a suitable dish and the fumes are inhaled.

Gratifying relief has been reported during therapy employing the adrenocortical hormone, cortisone (Compound E), or the adrenocorticotropic hormone (ACTH); final evaluation of these or similar agents, however, must await further studies.

In severe and prolonged asthma, especially attacks that have resisted drugs, or where drug tolerance has developed, oxygen inhalation often is helpful, and sometimes lifesaving. It also is indicated as a last resort in any case of severe dyspnea unrelieved by other measures, and particularly when cyanosis is pronounced. A nasal catheter properly adjusted with an inflow of humidified O_2 at 4 to 6 liters/minute will provide the equivalent of about 35 to 40% O_2 in the inspired air. Higher percentages of O_2, up to 70 or 80%, are obtained through the use of BLB or similar masks, the concentration being adjusted by the gauges with which the masks are equipped. The oxygen tent is sometimes much more comfortable for extremely ill patients, as the air is cooled, and the face and mouth are unencumbered. Most tents, however, cannot provide higher than 50% concentration of O_2.

The use of positive pressure inhalation therapy often is an added advantage, since this will dilate the bronchi. The simplest form is positive pressure expiration, in which the patient exhales against a slight resistance (1 to 6 cm. of water). Special expiratory valves attached to oxygen masks now are standard equipment. More elaborate apparatus giving positive pressure in both inspiration and expiration may be preferable in special cases.

In the most extreme forms of status asthmaticus, helium and O_2 mixtures (80% He, 20% O_2) are sometimes employed, usually combined with positive pressure. This replacement of atmospheric nitrogen by the lighter and less dense helium gas enables the mixture to pass in and out of narrowed bronchi more easily. Owing to the tendency of this light gas to leak out of ordinary apparatus, special equipment and usually a specially trained technician are required for adequate helium therapy.

Sedatives are of definite value in the control of asthmatic attacks. Barbiturates such as phenobarbital (℞ 31), and codeine subcut. or by mouth (℞ 32) are adequate for mild sedation. Should these prove inadequate in severe cases, Demerol (℞ 33) may be given I.M. in a dose of 50 mg. as needed or regularly 3 or 4 times a day.

Morphine (℞ 34) is a two-edged sword. For the restless, apprehensive patient in severe asthmatic distress, an injection of 10 mg. (gr. ⅙) often will provide relief when no other drug will. However, repeated doses may depress the respiration and cough reflex and lead to pulmonary congestion, pulmonary edema, progressive respiratory failure, and even death. It is a good general rule in severe status asthmaticus never to give morphine or morphine derivatives more frequently than every 8 hours, and preferably every 12 hours.

Careful judgment in controlling the cough is important, since a cough reflex is necessary to raise sputum, yet excessive coughing exhausts the patient and aggravates the asthma. Codeine by mouth is useful, either alone (℞ 32) or combined with elixir of terpin hydrate (℞ 35). Expectorants (℞ 38 to 41), especially if given with a sedative (℞ 31, 32), are also beneficial. In the treatment of associated bronchitis (q.v.), inhalation of steam with tincture of benzoin (℞ 38) often is of value.

In prolonged or frequent attacks expectorants are indicated. The saturated solution of potassium iodide (℞ 39), in doses of 10 drops 3 times daily, is the most effective, but when this is not tolerated, ammonium chloride (℞ 40) may be given. Syrup of ipecac (℞ 41) often is useful, especially in children; the dose required usually is that which will induce nausea.

Various nonspecific measures may help to interrupt prolonged status asthmaticus. Typhoid vaccine I.V., in doses sufficient to produce a temperature of approximately 103° F., often is effective. The first dose should be small (30 million organisms) with subsequent doses increased daily until the desired degree of fever is reached. This treatment is not advisable for aged or debilitated patients. Ether in oil by rectum (℞ 36), or paraldehyde (℞ 37), may produce enough relaxation to break a series of attacks.

In protracted attacks of asthma, especially in elderly patients or those who have had the disease severely for a long time, the physician should watch closely for possible development of acute heart failure. The important signs are increase in heart size, peripheral edema, liver enlargement, and gallop rhythm. Treatment is that of acute congestive heart failure (q.v.).

   2. Treatment of asthma due to extrinsic allergens: When extrinsic allergens are found to be of etiologic importance, they should be avoided as far as possible. If this is not feasible, an attempt at specific desensitization is indicated. Treatment with an antihistaminic such as Neo-Antergan (℞ 1) has been successful in some cases of asthma (20 to 30%). In adults, skin reactions to foods are only occasionally significant, and patients should not be kept on severely restricted diets for indefinite periods unless such skin reactions to specific foods are confirmed by clinical trial (see ELIMINATION DIETS). In severe status asthmaticus, if there are many possible food sensitivities all food may be withheld for 3 or 4 days and the patient nourished I.V. with amino acids solution and glucose. If definite improvement does not result, it will be evident that other allergens, or infections, are of more etiologic importance than foods.

3. Treatment of infective asthma: Acute exacerbations of infective asthma are best treated by antibacterial therapy. Ideally, this is preceded by culturing the sputum or nasopharyngeal excretions and determining the sensitivity of the predominant organisms to penicillin, the sulfonamides, and streptomycin. When cultures are not obtainable, penicillin (R 25, 26) is the preferable drug. Penicillin aerosols (R 27) are widely used for inhalation treatment of infective asthma, but in general are less effective than systemic administration. The initial dosage for inhalation should be 5,000 u. in 1 cc. of water and, if tolerated, this may be rapidly increased to 50,000 u. in 1 cc. every 4 hours. The solution may be vaporized in the nebulizers used for epinephrine aerosols, but since a large volume must be vaporized, spraying by hand is rather laborious and it is more convenient to remove the rubber bulb and attach the nebulizer to a source of O_2 or of compressed air. Inhalation of penicillin may cause irritation in the air passages; therefore, an increase of dyspnea after treatment is a contraindication to its further use.

When penicillin is not effective, sulfadiazine (R 30) or streptomycin (R 28, 29) may be indicated (see ANTIBIOTIC THERAPY; SULFONAMIDE THERAPY). A period of 5 to 7 days usually provides adequate trial of these agents in infective asthma; longer use only increases the danger of toxic reactions. Chemotherapy may abolish the existing infection and relieve the attack of asthma, but there is a strong tendency to recurrences if new respiratory infections occur.

When infective asthma is associated with sinusitis (q.v.), local treatment of the sinuses is helpful. Removal of nasal polyps and submucous resection are effective in asthma only if they relieve nasal obstruction and facilitate drainage of the sinuses. Tonsillectomy and adenoidectomy may be of value in children, and more occasionally in adults, who have infective asthma associated with chronically infected tonsils and adenoids. If adenoidectomy has been followed by the regrowth of considerable lymphoid tissue in the nasopharynx, expert radiation of the nasopharynx with X-ray or radium may be effective in reducing susceptibility to the upper respiratory infections, which often precipitate attacks of asthma.

When recurring infective asthma is associated with chronic sinusitis, an operation on the sinuses may be considered. However, there is considerable difference of opinion as to the efficacy of such procedures. The best results have followed radical operations designed to remove as completely as possible the infected sinus membrane, e.g., the Caldwell-Luc operation on the antrums, the exenteration of the ethmoids and sphenoids. More conservative procedures such as simple antrotomy, or antral "windows" rarely are effective. The advisability of a radical sinus operation must be carefully considered in each case, taking into account the severity of the asthma, the efficacy of other methods of treatment, the evidences of sinus infection, the degree of irreversible pulmonary emphysema, and the presence or absence of sensitivity to extrinsic allergens. Operation should be undertaken only after all sensitivities to known extrinsic allergens have been controlled. Penicillin (℞ 25, 26) should be administered before and after operation, and an adequate period of convalescence allowed.

The use of vaccines often is helpful in chronic infective asthma. Combined catarrhal vaccines (℞ 52) may be employed but, since asthmatic patients sometimes are unusually sensitive to them, the first dose should not exceed 0.1 cc. of a 1:100 dilution of the standard vaccine (1 to 2 million organisms/cc.). In the average patient, subsequent injections may be made subcut. at weekly intervals, each dose being increased by 50 to 100% until 0.2 cc. of the full-strength vaccine is reached. This dose then may be repeated at intervals of 1 to 4 weeks according to the condition of the patient. Autogenous vaccines can be prepared from cultures of the sputum, the nasopharyngeal secretions, antral irrigations, or tissues removed during operations on the nose and throat. These may be injected at weekly intervals following a schedule of dosage similar to that accompanying stock catarrhal vaccines. A logical procedure is to use a combination of equal parts of autogenous and stock vaccine, in an attempt to protect against not only those bacteria known to be present, but also those commonly acquired with respiratory infections. With any vaccine treatment, overdosages may produce an exacerbation of the infective asthma, and careful observation, with regulation of the dose according to the individual reaction, is essential. From 2 to 3 months' treatment is required before the efficacy of such treatment can be judged.

4. **General measures:** In the care of the asthmatic patient, it is important to maintain general health and nutrition. During the acute attack or in prolonged status asthmaticus, the diet should be light and easily digested, composed chiefly of liquids and semisolids (*see* Diets), since overfilling the stomach hampers respiration, particularly at night. If the patient is unable to take adequate nourishment, or if he is on a stringent elimination diet, supplements of protein hydrolysates, glucose, and vitamin concentrates should be given. However, obesity must be avoided, as it throws a greater burden on the cardiorespiratory mechanism; weight should be controlled by regulating the caloric intake.

Exposure to nonspecific irritants (e.g., smoke, fumes of paint and turpentine, cold, damp, and dust), which often precipitate asthmatic attacks, must be avoided. Tobacco smoking may be restricted during the acute stage, but permanent prohibition is rarely necessary. Adequate rest is essential, especially in debilitated patients with chronic infective asthma.

The patient must endeavor to avoid colds and other respiratory infections and the early symptoms of such infections should be treated with even greater care than in nonasthmatic persons.

A change of climate may greatly benefit some patients with infective asthma. They improve in warm, dry regions like the southwestern United States. The response to a warm, moist climate is uncertain.

Suitable breathing exercises are of value in children and young adults, as they help prevent the development of chronic emphysema and chest deformity. Every morning and evening they should exhale 10 to 20 times as slowly and completely as possible. The efficiency of expiration may be measured roughly by blowing a feather, light ball, or bit of paper across a table. The patient may assist complete exhalation by pressing inward on his lower anterior ribs with both hands. The intervening inhalation should be of normal depth, rather than forced.

Many forms of nonspecific treatment have been advised for asthma, such as ascorbic acid (℞ 54), calcium (℞ 42) and histamine (℞ 61). None of these has yet proved so effective as the measures previously mentioned.

Operations on, or infiltration injections of, the sympathetic nerves or the posterior pulmonary plexus have been performed for the control of intractable asthma, but still are in the experimental stage.

Recognition and consideration of psychosomatic factors are important in the management of asthmatic patients. Often, such factors precipitate attacks and considerably increase the disability. Psychosomatic mechanisms, however, are secondary and do not exclude the need to treat primary causes. Removal of the sources of emotional strain often is helpful, but prolonged psychoanalysis and psychotherapy are rarely warranted.

Education of the patient and his family concerning the nature of asthma and inculcation of a proper attitude toward it will contribute greatly to successful treatment. An acute attack, especially at night, is at first a terrifying experience to all concerned. The knowledge that uncomplicated acute asthma is practically never fatal, and having at hand effective remedies for self-medication, such as ephedrine capsules (℞ 16), epinephrine vaporizer (℞ 15), aminophylline rectal suppositories (℞ 20), and aludrine (℞ 17), will do much to allay the panic that tends to aggravate the paroxysms. If the attacks are not controlled by oral or rectal medication, it is often advisable to teach the patient, or a member of his family, to administer epinephrine (℞ 13) subcut., so as to give a sense of security if medical attention is not quickly obtainable. On the other hand, the patient should realize that asthma is a chronic disease and that prolonged medical treatment and supervision are necessary. Even under the most careful management, occasional attacks may occur as a result of common colds or unusual exposures, and these are not to be considered evidence of failure of the regimen. Parents should be told that only a small minority of children can be expected to outgrow asthma spontaneously and a considerably larger percentage will become worse unless systematically treated. The results of treatment are in general better during childhood than in adult life. However, although some children may recover completely, they also are more likely to develop new sensitizations with the passage of time.

GASTROINTESTINAL ALLERGY

A symptom complex manifested by nausea, vomiting, abdominal pain, and diarrhea.

Etiology

Although ordinarily due to ingestion of specific food antigens, gastrointestinal allergy may result from drugs taken by mouth and also from drugs, vaccines, or serums administered parenterally.

Symptoms and Signs

In persons hypersensitive to foods, symptoms appear shortly after the specific food is eaten. The severe acute reaction, which is rare, is characterized by nausea, vomiting, diarrhea, violent pains, circulatory collapse, and sometimes death. Urticaria is a frequent accompaniment in some patients. Much more common than the acute attack just described are subacute and chronic symptoms. The following conditions may at times be solely or partially caused by food allergy: cheilitis, herpes labialis, aphthous ulcers, allergic rhinitis, asthma, nausea, vomiting, pylorospasm, diarrhea, spastic constipation, mucous colitis, pruritus ani and perianal eczema. Henoch's purpura, a symptom complex of acute abdominal pain, blood in the stools, and usually purpura, sometimes is due to food allergy.

Diagnosis

The diagnosis of gastrointestinal allergy usually is difficult. Careful history, physical examination, and elimination diets (*see* DIETS) will assist in establishing a diagnosis. Skin tests usually are not of much value in food allergy. The regular occurrence of symptoms following the ingestion of a particular food is of the greatest diagnostic importance (*see* ALLERGY: Diagnostic

Procedures). It is important to remember, however, that the presence of allergy does not exclude organic disease of the gastrointestinal tract.

Treatment

Aside from elimination of the offending foodstuffs (*see* ELIMINATION DIETS) there is no specific treatment. Sensitivity to one or more foods may disappear spontaneously during a patient's lifetime and develop as regards single or multiple other foods. Parenteral desensitization is tedious and usually unsuccessful. Oral desensitization by first eliminating the offending food for a time and then giving small, daily increased amounts is advocated by some authorities. However, in the case of extreme sensitivity or with notably potent allergens such as fish, eggs, nuts, buckwheat, and cottonseed, this method is not without danger. Sufficiently minute quantities are impossible to obtain in the case of many of the stronger allergens, and fatal reactions have been recorded. The consensus is that abstinence, when it can be accomplished, is preferable. Epinephrine (℞ 13) is helpful in acute episodes. Antihistaminic drugs such as Neo-Antergan (℞ 1) have not been extensively tried in gastrointestinal allergy, but have sometimes proved effective in the relief of abdominal pain due to smooth muscle spasm.

URTICARIA; ANGIONEUROTIC EDEMA

(Hives; Giant urticaria)

Urticaria: *Local allergic wheals arising in the dermis.* **Angioneurotic edema:** *A similar eruption, but the areas of edema are larger and more deeply disposed, involving the subcutaneous structures as well as the dermis.* No really sound basis exists, however, for regarding the two as essentially different entities.

Etiology

Hereditary angioneurotic edema has been described, but most patients with urticaria and angioneurotic edema show only the same familial incidence as is noted in other allergic disorders. Food is the most important specific factor. In acute urticaria, seasonal fruits and vegetables, shell-fish, and nuts often are responsible; frequent offenders in chronic urticaria are eggs, wheat, milk, pork, and onions. Drugs are extremely important in causing chronic urticaria, particularly aspirin, barbiturates, phenolphthalein, bromides, and acetophenetidin. Injectants, among them foreign serums, endocrines (e.g., liver, insulin, pituitrin), and insect bites, also cause hives. Inhalants, such as dusts and pollens, and bacterial antigens sometimes are causative. Angioneurotic edema and urticaria, especially in the chronic form, sometimes are due to psychogenic factors. Physical allergy (q.v.) may manifest itself as hives.

Pathology

The wheal is a swelling made up of exuded serum together with eosinophiles and other white blood cells. The local lymphatic and blood vessels are distended. It is likely that a histamine-like substance produces the dilatation and consequent edema.

Symptoms and Signs

Pruritus, which is generally the first symptom, is followed shortly by urticarial lesions varying considerably in appearance from small pinhead spots to areas as large as a dinner plate. Ordinarily, crops of hives come and go, the lesions remaining in one site for several hours, then disappearing, but only to reappear elsewhere. Rarely, there are bullous or hemorrhagic lesions. The mucous membranes, especially those of the respiratory and gastrointestinal tracts, may be affected, with acute symptoms referable to those systems. Edema of the glottis may cause severe and sometimes fatal respiratory embarrassment.

Diagnosis

The diagnosis usually is obvious, though nonallergenic insect bites may closely simulate the eruptions, and scabies and Hodgkin's disease (q.v.) must be differentiated. The physician needs only to discover the responsible agent, but this may present considerable difficulty in view of the wide variety of possible causes. Skin tests do not have so much value in urticaria as in other allergic conditions.

Treatment

Acute urticaria is a self-limited condition generally subsiding in 1 to 2 weeks; hence, treatment is chiefly palliative. Since the sensitizing agent may be present in the gastrointestinal tract, it will usually be advisable to give an effective cathartic (℞ 53). Etiologic agents must be avoided or eliminated. Fluids should be forced and any medication not essential to the patient's life should be omitted until the acute allergic state has subsided. Antihistaminic drugs such as Neo-Antergan (℞ 1), or calcium gluconate (℞ 42), or epinephrine (℞ 13) have proved effective in relieving itching and reducing the swelling. Colloid baths (see BEDSIDE PROC.) and antipruritic lotions and powders (℞ 43 to 47) also are helpful.

In chronic urticaria, autochemotherapy, by the removal of 20 cc. of blood from the antecubital vein and immediate reinjection into the buttocks, sometimes helps. Thyroid extract (℞ 55) has proved of benefit in a small number of cases. Any suspected drug, especially headache remedies, sedatives, and soporifics, should be eliminated.

SERUM SICKNESS

*A reaction, usually appearing 8 to 12 days after the adminis-
tration of a foreign serum, and characterized by fever, articular
pains, dermal eruptions, and lymphadenopathy.* An immediate, severe, frequently fatal form occasionally occurs and is
known as **anaphylactic** (or allergic) **shock.**

Etiology and Incidence

The incidence of serum disease is from 5 to 90% of the individuals receiving foreign serums, depending on the kind and
amount given and the route of administration. A large dose
(above 100 cc.) is more likely than a small one to produce a reaction; the most severe types follow I.V. administration, and
the incidence is greater with intraspinal than with subcut. or
I.M. injections. Horse serum apparently causes reactions more
frequently than do other types, although this may be at least
partially due to its more widespread use and the fact that more
persons harbor a sensitivity to this agent. It is thought that the
injected foreign serum, whatever its origin, stimulates the production of specific antibodies (precipitins) which react, after a
sufficient concentration has been reached, with the remaining
circulating antigen.

Pathology

In autopsies following fatal serum reactions, the most conspicuous observations have been mural endocarditis and myocarditis, as well as vascular changes similar to or identical with
those of periarteritis nodosa, and to some extent simulating
rheumatoid arthritis, lupus erythematosus disseminatus, and
dermatomyositis (q.v.).

Symptoms and Signs

Urticaria is the usual skin manifestation; less frequently the
rash is multiform or morbilliform; rarely, it may simulate scarlatina, purpura, or erythema nodosum. Fever, which occurs in
33% of patients, either precedes or is coincident with the eruption. It usually is mild and lasts but a day or two; in more
severe cases the temperature may reach 105° F. and last 7 to 10
days. Adenopathy is constant in the region draining the injection site, and may become generalized. Splenomegaly sometimes is present. Mild to severe polyarthritis occurs in about
40 to 60% of patients. Not uncommonly, wheals form in the
intestine, larynx, and bronchi, with resultant local symptoms.
Rarely, neurologic complications have been reported. Eosinophilia is occasionally found.

Anaphylactic Shock: This (better referred to as allergic
shock) is an extreme form of serum sickness, generally fatal but
fortunately rare. It is a primary or atopic serum reaction usually occurring in "horse asthmatics," since horse serum is most
commonly used. Almost before the needle is withdrawn, local

itching begins and is rapidly followed by generalized urticaria, sneezing, coughing, asthma, and apprehension. The patient is in a state of shock; convulsions and death may supervene within 10 minutes. If the patient survives, the symptoms become those of ordinary serum sickness.

Diagnosis

A history of serum injection, plus the classical signs and symptoms, usually make the diagnosis of serum sickness plain. However, differentiation of the scarlatiniform variety from scarlet fever sometimes may be difficult.

Prophylaxis

It is important to identify patients who may become victims of the rare allergic shock. Differentiation between primary (natural or atopic) allergy and the acquired type (serum sickness) often can be made from the history alone. A history of coryza or asthma occurring after contact with horses, or of previous serum injections, with or without untoward reactions, should make the physician extremely cautious. Verification then can be obtained by skin and ophthalmic tests, which generally yield extremely positive reactions even with high dilutions (see ALLERGY: Diagnostic Procedures). If the history and results of the skin and ophthalmic tests are negative, serum usually can be administered safely by any route. If the history is positive and the sensitivity tests negative, it probably will be safe to give the serum in divided doses; in such cases, epinephrine (℞ 13) as well as antihistaminic preparations such as Neo-Antergan (℞ 1) should be in readiness for emergency use. The same applies if the history is negative for allergy and the cutaneous reaction moderately positive. If both the history and sensitivity tests are positive, serum should be given only if mandatory. If a sensitivity test produces a generalized reaction with symptoms involving the respiratory tract, *that serum must not be given*. In such cases reliance cannot be placed on desensitization. However, when serum therapy is likely to be lifesaving, serum from another species of animal may be given if preliminary tests have shown it to be non-antigenic for that particular patient. In any case, epinephrine (℞ 13), ephedrine (℞ 16) and an antihistaminic drug (℞ 1) are valuable in preventing or modifying serum reactions.

Treatment

Once symptoms appear, they run a self-limited course and treatment is purely symptomatic. Itching is controlled by the use of an antihistaminic such as Neo-Antergan (℞ 1), or ephedrine (℞ 16), epinephrine (℞ 13) or calcium gluconate (℞ 42); antipruritic lotions (℞ 43 to 47) and colloid baths (see BEDSIDE PROC.) also are useful. Procaine (℞ 57) may be given I.V. to alleviate the itching and arthralgia. Salicylates (℞ 58, 59) often relieve the articular pains. Ascorbic acid (℞ 54) may be beneficial. Cortisone and ACTH have both shown encouraging results.

PHYSICAL ALLERGY

A sensitivity to one of the various physical agents (e.g., light, heat, cold, mechanical irritation), contact with which produces one of the allergic disorders.

Etiology

Sensitiveness to physical agents may be secondary to food or bacterial allergy. Photosensitivity may be induced by certain drugs (e.g., the sulfonamides). Acute febrile disorders often are followed by physical allergy, as are cerebral injuries and cardiac or vascular diseases. No immunologic mechanism, however, has been demonstrated, so that physical allergy may not be a true allergy.

Symptoms and Signs

Mechanical irritation usually leads only to urticaria in dermographic skins; swelling at pressure sites often results (e.g., under belts or girdles, or on the buttocks or soles). Cold allergy is manifested chiefly by urticaria or angioneurotic edema, but it may cause pronounced lacrimation, sneezing, cough, or bronchial asthma. Exposure to sunlight gives rise to urticaria solaris or eczema-like polymorphic skin eruptions. Hydroa estivale, pellagra, lupus erythematosus, and other conditions not caused primarily by sunlight are exacerbated by it. Heat sensitiveness produces pruritus and urticaria.

Treatment

The adrenergic drugs (℞ 13, 16) and an antihistaminic such as Neo-Antergan (℞ 1) give symptomatic relief. The treatment of persons sensitive to light consists in shielding the skin with protective clothing, veils, and dark gloves, plus the avoidance of photosensitizing drugs and such cosmetic preparations as perfume containing oil of bergamot. Protective cosmetics have been devised (℞ 60). Cold-sensitive persons should live in a warm climate if possible and avoid cold in the form of drinks, foods, and baths. The symptoms, including asthma, may be relieved by heat in any form, from external sources or produced by exercise. Histamine desensitization (℞ 61) is generally unsatisfactory. In the treatment of persons sensitive to heat, effort should be made to expose them to gradually increasing temperatures. For this purpose tub baths, diathermy, and infrared lamps may be employed. Typhoid vaccine I.V. has some advocates.

PRESCRIPTIONS

(Wherever a prescribed "proprietary" is representative of a class of therapeutic agents, alternative proprietary preparations will be found listed in Part II.)

Antihistaminics

1. ℞ "Neo-Antergan Maleate" . . . 25   mg.

    1 to 4 tablets 3 or 4 times daily, preferably after meals and at bedtime.

Nose Drops and Inhalants

2. ℞ Ephedrine sulfate, 1% solution . 30.0   cc.   (℥ i)

    3 or 4 drops in each nostril every 3 or 4 hours if necessary.

3. ℞ "Neo-Synephrine Hydrochloride," 1% solution . . . . . 30.0   cc.   (℥ i)

    3 or 4 drops in each nostril every 3 to 4 hours if necessary.

4. ℞ "Privine Hydrochloride," 0.05 to 0.1% solution . . . 30.0   cc.   (℥ i)

    3 or 4 drops in each nostril every 4 to 6 hours if necessary.

5. ℞ Propadrine hydrochloride, 1% solution . . . . 30.0   cc.   (℥ i)

    3 or 4 drops in each nostril every 4 to 6 hours if necessary.

6. ℞ Amphetamine sulfate . . . . . 0.25   Gm. (gr. iv)
        Light Liquid Petrolatum U.S.P. . 30.0   cc.   (℥ i)

    Use as a nasal spray 3 or 4 times daily. (Caution! Oily nose drops should never be instilled in children.)

7. ℞ Nasal inhaler

    (Various vasoconstrictor type inhalers are commercially available.)

    Inhale vapor once through each nostril, not more frequently than every 2 hours.

Autonomic Drugs

8. ℞ Propadrine hydrochloride . . . 25   mg. (gr. ⅜)

    1 capsule every 2 to 4 hours if necessary.

9. ℞ "Neo-Synephrine Hydrochloride" 25   mg. (gr. ⅜)

    1 capsule every 4 hours if necessary.

10. ℞ Atropine sulfate . . . . 0.2   mg. (gr. ⅟₃₀₀)

    1 tablet every hour until symptomatic relief or evidence of overdosage appears. (Thirst, blurring of vision, tachycardia, flushing.)

11. ℞ Belladonna Tincture U.S.P.. . . 15.0   cc. (℥ ss)

> 10 to 15 drops in water every hour until symptomatic relief or evidence of overdosage occurs.

12. ℞ Hyoscyamus Tincture U.S.P. . . 15.0   cc. (℥ ss)

> 20 to 30 drops in water every hour until symptomatic relief or evidence of overdosage occurs.

13. ℞ Epinephrine hydrochloride,
>   1:1,000 solution   (ampul)

> 0.3 to 0.5 cc. (♏ v to viii) subcut., repeated as indicated.

14. ℞ Epinephrine hydrochloride,
>   1:500 in oil   (ampul)

> 1 cc. I.M. every 8 hours if necessary.

15. ℞ Epinephrine hydrochloride,
>   1:100 solution . . . . 5.0   cc.

> Inhale deeply, 4 or 5 times, the vapor from a nebulizer; repeat when necessary.

16. ℞ Ephedrine sulfate. 25   mg. (gr. ⅜)

> 1 capsule every 3 hours if necessary.

17. ℞ Aludrine. 10   mg.

> 1 or 2 tablets sublingually, or 4 to 10 inhalations of a 1:200 solution, for relief of asthma.

18. ℞ Ephedrine sulfate. 25   mg. (gr. ⅜)
>   Phenobarbital 15   mg. (gr. ¼)

> 1 capsule every 3 or 4 hours if necessary. (Any suitable barbiturate may be substituted for phenobarbital.)

19. ℞ Aminophylline   (ampul)

> 0.25 to 0.5 Gm. (gr. iv to viiss) I.V., injected slowly, for relief of asthma.

20. ℞ Aminophylline (suppositories). . . 0.5   Gm. (gr. viiss)

> 1 per rectum every 4 to 6 hours for relief of asthma.

21. ℞ Aminophylline, 3% solution

> 10 to 20 cc. per rectum for relief of asthma.

22. ℞ Aminophylline (enteric coated) . . 0.1   Gm. (gr. iss)

> 1 or 2 tablets every 4 to 8 hours for asthma.

23. ℞ Ephedrine sulfate. . . . . 0.025 Gm. (gr. ⅜)
>   Aminophylline . . . . 0.12   Gm. (gr. ii)
>   Phenobarbital . . . . 0.015 Gm. (gr. ¼)

> 1 capsule every 3 hours for asthma.

24. ℞ Stramonium . . . . 2.0 Gm. (ʒ ss)
    Lobelia . . . . 1.0 Gm. (gr. xv)
    Potassium nitrate . . . . 2.0 Gm. (ʒ ss)
    For asthma: Burn a small amount of the powder and inhale the fumes.

Antimicrobial Agents

25. ℞ Penicillin (vial)
    30,000 to 50,000 u. I.M. every 3 hours, or 300,000 u. every 12 hours.

26. ℞ Procaine penicillin (vial)
    300,000 u. I.M. daily.

27. ℞ Penicillin
    Dissolve 100,000 u. in 2 to 20 cc. of distilled water and inhale the nebulized vapor of 1 cc. every 4 hours.

28. ℞ Streptomycin (vial)
    0.5 Gm. I.M. every 6 hours.

29. ℞ Streptomycin (vial)
    Dissolve 1 Gm. in 10 cc. of distilled water and inhale the nebulized vapor of 1 cc. every 4 hours.

30. ℞ Sulfadiazine . . . . 0.5 Gm. (gr. viiss)
    4 tablets initially followed by 2 tablets every 4 hours.

Sedatives and Antitussive Agents

31. ℞ Phenobarbital . . . . 15 mg. (gr. ¼)
    1 or 2 tablets every 3 hours, if necessary.

32. ℞ Codeine phosphate (hypodermic tablet) . . . . 30 mg. (gr. ss)
    1 tablet orally or subcut. every 3 or 4 hours for cough.

33. ℞ "Demerol Hydrochloride" (ampul)
    50 mg. I.M. every 6 to 8 hours for cough.

34. ℞ Morphine sulfate
    10 mg. (gr. ⅙) subcut. for asthma (cautiously used), not more often than every 8 hours.

35. ℞ Codeine phosphate . . . . 0.5 Gm. (gr. viiss)
    Terpin Hydrate Elixir N.F.
                           q.s. ad 120.0 cc. (ʒ iv)
    1 teaspoon every 3 hours.

36. ℞ Ether
     Olive Oil . . . . āā   120.0   cc.   (℥ iv)
         Administer slowly, per rectum.

37. ℞ Paraldehyde . . . . 30.0   cc.   (℥ i)
         2 teaspoons in iced fruit juice, repeated once
         if necessary.

Expectorants

38. ℞ Compound Benzoin Tincture
     U.S.P. . . . . 30.0   cc.   (℥ i)
         Add ½ teaspoon to 1 quart of boiling water
         and inhale steam.

39. ℞ Saturated Potassium Iodide
     Solution N.F. . . . . 30.0   cc.   (℥ i)
         10 drops in water, 3 times daily, after meals.

40. ℞ Ammonium chloride (enteric
     coated) . . . . 0.3   Gm.   (gr. v)
         1 or 2 tablets 3 times daily.

41. ℞ Ipecac Syrup U.S.P.   . . . . 30.0   cc.   (℥ i)
         1 teaspoon every 30 minutes until nausea
         appears.

Antipruritics

42. ℞ Calcium gluconate, 10% solution
     (ampul) . . . . 1.0   Gm.
         Contents of 1 ampul I.V., injected slowly.

43. ℞ Camphor . . . . 4.0   Gm.   (℥ i)
     Menthol . . . . 0.5   Gm.   (gr. viiss)
     Bentonite . . . . 10.0   Gm.   (℥ iiss)
     Zinc oxide
     Talc . . . . āā q.s. ad 120.0   Gm.   (℥ iv)
         Dust on every 2 or 3 hours to allay itching.

44. ℞ Coal Tar Solution N.F. . . . . 15.0   cc.   (℥ ss)
     Black Lotion N.F.
     Olive oil . . . . . . āā q.s. ad 240.0   cc.   (℥ viii)
         Shake well and apply as necessary to relieve
         itching.

45. ℞ Phenol . . . . 1.5   Gm.   (gr. xxii)
     Calamine Lotion U.S.P. q.s. ad   120.0   cc.   (℥ iv)
         Shake well and apply to relieve itching.

46. ℞ Phenol . . . . 2.0   Gm.   (℥ ss)
     Menthol . . . . 0.3   Gm.   (gr. v)
     Calamine . . . . 16.0   Gm.   (℥ iv)
     Zinc oxide . . . . 16.0   Gm.   (℥ iv)
     Glycerin
     Witch hazel . . . . āā q.s. ad 120.0   cc.   (℥ iv)
         Shake well and apply to itching areas.

47. ℞ Coal Tar Solution N.F. . . . . . 2.0   cc.   (℥ ss)
    Compound Benzoin Tincture
      U.S.P. . . . . 15.0   cc.   (℥ ss)
    Camphor Spirit N.F. . . . . . 2.0   cc.   (℥ ss)
    Glycerin. . . . . 15.0   cc.   (℥ ss)
    Witch hazel . . . . . q.s. ad 120.0   cc.   (℥ iv)
      Apply as needed to allay itching.

Eye

48. ℞ Boric acid
      Dissolve 4 teaspoons of boric acid in 1 quart
      of water, store in ice box, and use as an eye-
      wash every 4 hours.

49. ℞ Tetracaine hydrochloride
    ("Pontocaine"). . . . . 0.06   Gm.   (gr. i)
    Epinephrine hydrochloride,
      1:1,000 solution . . . . 0.6   cc.   (℔ x)
    Distilled water. . . . . q.s. ad 30.0   cc.   (℥ i)
      1 drop in each eye when necessary for itching.

50. ℞ Zinc sulfate, 0.25% solution . . 30.0   cc.   (℥ i)
      1 or 2 drops in each eye every 3 hours for itch-
      ing.

51. ℞ Lehrfeld's Solution
    Monohydrated sodium carbonate 0.3   Gm.   (gr. v)
    Distilled water . . . . q.s. ad 30.0   cc.   (℥ i)
      3 or 4 drops in each eye 4 times daily.   The
      eyes should be bathed with cold boric acid
      solution 7 times daily.

Miscellaneous

52. ℞ Combined catarrhal vaccine
    (vial)
      This vaccine is available from several manu-
      facturers and should be administered accord-
      ing to directions given in the text and in the
      manufacturer's package insert.

53. ℞ Magnesium sulfate
      1 to 4 teaspoons for catharsis.

54. ℞ Ascorbic acid. . . . . 0.1   Gm.
      1 tablet 3 times daily.

55. ℞ Thyroid U.S.P.. 15   mg.   (gr. ¼)
      1 tablet 3 times daily.

56. ℞ Menadione. 2   mg.
      1 or 2 capsules or tablets daily.

57. ℞ Procaine hydrochloride   (ampul)

Dissolve 1 Gm. of procaine in 500 cc. of Sterile Isotonic Sodium Chloride Solution for Parenteral Use U.S.P. and administer I.V. at the rate of 4 cc./minute.

58. ℞ Sodium salicylate. . . . . 0.3   Gm. (gr. v)

2 or 3 tablets every 4 hours.

59. ℞ Acetylsalicylic acid . . . . 0.3   Gm. (gr. v)

2 or 3 tablets every 4 hours.

60. ℞ Red ferric oxide. . . . . 6.0   Gm. (℥ iss)
     Yellow ferric oxide . . . . 8.0   Gm. (℥ ii)
     Titanium oxide. . . . . 86.0   Gm. (℥ iii)

Apply to exposed areas of skin.   (*Note:* These ingredients may also be dispensed as a 15 to 25% lotion, paste, ointment, or cream.)

61. ℞ Histamine diphosphate, 1:1,000 solution   (vial)

Administer gradually increasing doses subcut. twice a week, until benefit is received or histamine overdosage (flushing, headache) is evident. Beginning with 0.1 cc., progressively increase each succeeding injection by 0.1 cc. until a maximum dose of 1.0 cc. is administered. When a maintenance level is reached give this quantity every week.

BLOOD AND LYMPHATIC

ANEMIA

A condition in which the circulating red blood cells are deficient in number or in total hemoglobin content.

Classification and Terminology

The anemias may be classified etiologically, morphologically, or clinically. The following functional approach combines the three possibilities. Although not an exhaustive classification, it should serve as a useful guide to the subsequent presentation.

I. Anemias of blood loss
    A. Acute posthemorrhagic anemia
    B. Anemia of chronic blood loss (*see* III B.)
II. Hemolytic anemias
    A. Primary hemolytic anemias
        Congenital hemolytic jaundice
        Sickle cell anemia
    B. Secondary hemolytic anemias
        (due to chemical agents, bacterial toxins, hemolysins of
        immune bodies)
III. Defective or decreased blood formation
    A. Macrocytic anemias
        Pernicious anemia
        Other macrocytic anemias (as in sprue, steatorrhea, liver
        disease, gastrointestinal disorders)
    B. Hypochromic microcytic anemias
        Anemia of chronic blood loss; "nutritional" anemia; hypo-
        chromic anemias of pregnancy and childhood
    C. Anemias of decreased blood formation
        Primary refractory anemia
        Myelophthisic anemia

The chief abnormal finding in anemia usually is a reduction in the number of circulating red blood cells (erythrocytes). The normal number for men is between 4,500,000 and 5,500,000/cu. mm., and for women between 4,000,000 and 5,000,000. Newborn infants average about 5,000,000 cells, but by the second week of life their count drops to 4,500,000 and then gradually approaches adult levels during childhood and adolescence.

Morphologically, the anemias may be classified according to the size of the red cells and their hemoglobin content. The anemia may be microcytic, normocytic, or macrocytic if the cells are, respectively, smaller, equal to, or larger than normal. Normal red blood cells average about 7.5 μ in diameter. The size of the cells may be measured directly with a micrometer eyepiece in the microscope. Abnormally small cells (micro-cytes) average less than 5 μ in diameter; abnormally large cells (macrocytes) average greater than 10 μ. The size of the eryth-rocytes can be determined indirectly by calculating the mean corpuscular volume (MCV) from the volume of packed red cells and the red blood cell count (*see* LAB. PROC. for details on this and other tests). The volume of normal red cells as determined in this manner is between 80 and 94 cu. μ. An approximation of corpuscular size may be arrived at by calculating the volume index, which relates the mean volume of the cells being exam-ined to the mean volume of cells in normal blood. A volume index greater than 1 is indicative of a macrocytic anemia, and less than 1 of a microcytic anemia.

The anemia may be hypochromic or "hyperchromic" if the individual cells contain less or more than the normal amount of hemoglobin. The term "hyperchromic" is a misnomer, since the cells so described do not contain a higher concentration of hemoglobin but rather are larger than normal (macrocytes), hence contain a greater volume of hemoglobin. The normal hemoglobin content of the blood ranges from a lower limit of 12 or 13 Gm./100 cc. to 18 Gm./100 cc. The depth of color of the erythrocytes on stained blood smears is indicative of the concentration of hemoglobin in the corpuscles. Hypochromic cells have large pale centers; "hyperchromic" cells are more or less solidly stained. The amount of hemoglobin in 100 cc. of blood may be determined by using a Sahli or other suitable hemoglobinometer. The mean corpuscular hemoglobin (MCH), an expression of the average weight of hemoglobin in a red cell, may be calculated from the hemoglobin in 100 cc. of blood and the red cell count. The normal range is 27 to 32 micromicrograms/cell. The mean corpuscular hemoglobin concentration (MCHC), the amount of hemoglobin/100 cc. of blood as compared to the volume of packed red cells in 100 cc. of blood, is an extremely useful determination. This gives the average concentration of hemoglobin in the red cells as expressed in per cent. The normal values are from 32 to 38%. The color index is an expression which compares the quantity of hemoglobin in the red corpuscles being examined to an arbitrary normal. If it is greater than 1 the red cells are well filled macrocytes; if less than 1 they are hypochromic.

In addition to abnormalities in size and hemoglobin content, abnormalities in the shape of the red cells and number of immature erythrocytes may be evident upon examination of a stained blood smear. Variation in cell size is called anisocytosis. Poikilocytes are abnormally shaped cells. They may appear oval, saddle-shaped, pear-shaped, or caudate (tailed). Polychromatophilic cells are characterized by a greater affinity for basic stains, hence are bluer with Wright's stain. "Basophilic stippling" refers to abnormal cells containing irregular blue-staining granules. The presence of erythroblasts, megaloblasts, normoblasts, and excessive numbers of reticulocytes also is abnormal.

General Symptoms and Signs

Certain symptoms and signs are characteristic of anemia regardless of its etiology. Any severe anemia will cause these manifestations because of a reduction in the oxygen-carrying capacity of the blood, or a decrease in the total blood volume. Skin and mucous membrane pallor is the most striking sign. It is most obvious in the palms of the hands, the lips, nailbeds, and mucous membranes of the mouth, pharynx, and palpebral conjunctiva. Common subjective symptoms generally associated with severe anemia are faintness, vertigo, headache, roaring in the ears, tinnitus, spots before the eyes, easy fatigability, drowsiness, and irritability.

Dyspnea and tachycardia result from attempts of the respiratory and circulatory systems to compensate for the anemic anoxia. Palpitation is a frequent complaint. Heart murmurs (q.v.) are common in severe anemia, and cardiac dilatation and congestive heart failure not infrequent.

Gastrointestinal complaints are varied and frequent. Anorexia, nausea, vomiting, diarrhea, constipation, and flatulence may be present. Miscellaneous symptoms include amenorrhea in the female, loss of libido in the male, mild fever, and increased B.M.R.

Specific symptoms and signs such as jaundice or splenomegaly occur only in certain types of anemia and are discussed in appropriate parts of this chapter.

General Principles of Treatment

Therapy of the anemias consists of symptomatic or general treatment, plus specific procedures for particular forms of anemia. Symptomatic treatment includes a diet adequate in essential blood building materials, especially proteins; sufficient rest, particularly if cardiac and respiratory symptoms are present; a digitalis preparation for cardiac failure, if present; sedation for the relief of C.N.S. symptoms; and blood transfusions when indicated. Blood transfusions should not be given indiscriminately. In chronic anemias they are rarely indicated unless the blood count falls below 1,000,000, or the hemoglobin below 6 Gm.

Specific treatment includes iron for anemias due to iron deficiency; preparations which stimulate erythrocyte maturation, such as liver, vitamin B_{12} and folic acid, for megaloblastic anemias; and splenectomy for congenital hemolytic jaundice. These measures will be discussed in detail under the various specific anemias.

"Shotgun" treatment is mentioned only to be condemned. Multiple-content preparations seldom produce a good therapeutic response because they usually contain too little of each specific medicament per dose to be of value. Even when a favorable result is observed, the physician cannot tell which drug was responsible. Treatment of this sort is not justified as a therapeutic diagnostic test.

I. ANEMIAS OF BLOOD LOSS

A. ACUTE POSTHEMORRHAGIC ANEMIA

An anemia caused by the rapid loss of a large amount of blood.

Etiology and Pathogenesis

Massive hemorrhage resulting in posthemorrhagic anemia may be due to traumatic rupture of a large blood vessel, erosion of an artery by lesions such as peptic ulcer or a tuberculous process, spontaneous rupture of aneurysms or varices, or the hemorrhagic diatheses. The immediate effects of the hemorrhage depend upon the rapidity and amount of blood loss. Sudden loss of ⅓ of the blood volume may prove fatal, but as much as ⅔ may be lost over a 24-hour period without fatal outcome. Symptoms are due both to a sudden decrease of blood volume and to the consequent decrease in oxygen carrying capacity of the blood.

Symptoms and Signs

Characteristic symptoms of acute blood loss are faintness and dizziness, thirst, sweating, weak rapid pulse, and rapid respiration, at first deep then shallow. The blood pressure may at first rise slightly because of reflex arteriolar constriction, and then gradually fall. If bleeding continues, the blood pressure may fall to shock levels and death from acute circulatory collapse may ensue.

Laboratory Findings

During and immediately after hemorrhage the red blood cell count, hemoglobin and hematocrit are deceptively high because of a concurrent decrease of plasma volume and vasoconstriction. Within a few hours fluid enters the circulation from the tissues, resulting in hemodilution and a drop in the red count and hemoglobin proportional to the severity of the bleeding. The resultant anemia is normocytic with a color index near 1 since there is a parallel drop in both red count and hemoglobin. Polymorphonuclear leukocytosis as high as 35,000, and a rise in the platelet count to as high as 1,000,000 may take place within the first few hours. Evidence of blood regeneration becomes apparent several days after the bleeding has ceased. Examination of blood smears at this time may reveal polychromatophilia, reticulocytosis, slight macrocytosis, and occasional normoblasts. A transient hypochromia often occurs if the red cells are replaced faster than hemoglobin is manufactured.

Treatment

Immediate treatment consists of measures for stopping the bleeding, restoring the blood volume, and combating shock. Blood transfusion is the only reliable means of restoring blood volume and is indicated for severe bleeding with threatening vascular collapse. Plasma is a satisfactory temporary substitute for blood. Infusions of saline or glucose have only transient beneficial effect. Absolute rest, opiates, fluids by mouth as tolerated, and other standard measures for treatment of shock (q.v.) are indicated.

The subsequent treatment of the posthemorrhagic anemia is simple. A high protein diet supplemented with vitamins (*see* DIETS) usually is sufficient. Iron therapy (℞ 1 to 6) is indicated only if the iron stores of the body have been depleted by repeated hemorrhages or inadequate dietary intake.

B. ANEMIA OF CHRONIC BLOOD LOSS

A hypochromic microcytic anemia caused by prolonged moderate blood loss, as from a chronically bleeding peptic ulcer, menometrorrhagia, or bleeding hemorrhoids. The clinical features and treatment of this condition are discussed in the section on the hypochromic microcytic iron deficiency anemias (q.v.).

II. HEMOLYTIC ANEMIAS

A. PRIMARY HEMOLYTIC ANEMIAS

CONGENITAL HEMOLYTIC JAUNDICE

(Chronic familial icterus, Chronic acholuric jaundice,
Spherocytic anemia)

*An inherited chronic disease characterized by hemolysis of
spherical red blood cells, anemia, jaundice, and splenomegaly.*

Etiology and Pathogenesis

The cause of this disease is thought to be a congenital defect
which results in the formation of spheroidal erythrocytes. These
spherocytes are fragile and rupture in the blood stream or are
destroyed in the spleen. Hemolysis of large numbers of these
cells results in anemia and acholuric jaundice.

Symptoms and Signs

Moderate jaundice and the usual symptoms of anemia may
be present if the anemia is severe. Hemolytic crises characterized by fever, abdominal pain, and rapidly increasing jaundice
and anemia occur. These attacks may be precipitated by
trauma, infections, or pregnancy. Splenomegaly is an almost
invariable finding and may be so great as to cause abdominal
discomfort. Hepatomegaly occasionally occurs. Leg ulcers and
bone changes as seen in sickle cell anemia (q.v.) may be present. Cholelithiasis is a common accompaniment of this disease. Congenital skeletal abnormalities such as tower-shaped
skull and polydactylism are occasionally associated.

Laboratory Findings

The anemia varies greatly in degree. Usually, the red cell
count is between 3,000,000 and 4,000,000, but during a hemolytic
crisis it may fall below 1,000,000. The hemoglobin drops proportionately with the cell count, so that the color index approximates 1. Since the red cells are spheroidal, even though the
mean corpuscular diameter is somewhat below normal, the mean
corpuscular volume is within normal limits. Anisocytosis is
striking. Reticulocytosis of 15 to 30% is a common finding, and
during a hemolytic crisis it may reach as high as 90%. Leukocytosis usually occurs during a hemolytic crisis.

The fragility of the red cells to hypotonic saline solutions is
characteristically increased. Hemolysis of the spherocytes usually begins with a concentration of saline between 0.51 and
0.72%. Control blood (which always should be used) begins to
show hemolysis at about 0.46% saline.

The icterus index usually is between 15 and 20, but may be as
high as 100. Increased amounts of urobilinogen are found in
the blood and stool. The bone marrow is hyperplastic and
normoblastic in character.

Prognosis

The prognosis for life generally is good. It is more serious when the symptoms begin in childhood. Death may occur during a hemolytic crisis.

Treatment

Splenectomy is the only treatment of value. In the vast majority of cases it is followed by abatement of symptoms and a rise in the red count. However, spherocytosis and increased erythrocyte fragility usually are unaffected by such surgery. Blood transfusions may be necessary following a hemolytic crisis; transfusion reactions are common, however, and may occur despite careful preliminary cross matching.

SICKLE CELL ANEMIA
(Drepanocytic anemia, Meniscocytosis)

A chronic hemolytic anemia occurring almost exclusively in the Negro race and characterized by sickle-shaped red blood cells.

Etiology, Incidence, and Pathogenesis

The sickle cell trait is an inherited congenital defect. Approximately 7% of Negroes have these abnormal cells, but only about 1 in 40 of these develops sickle cell anemia. It is not known why one individual will have sickle cells without anemia (sicklemia) and another be anemic.

Many of the clinical manifestations of sickle cell anemia are thought to be due to thrombosis in the arterioles and capillaries as a result of impaction of the misshapen cells. The anemia is a result of excessive red cell destruction.

Symptoms and Signs

The usual symptoms of a severe anemia often are present. Many of the patients are moderately jaundiced. Episodes of severe abdominal pain with vomiting may simulate a surgical condition of the abdomen. Arthralgia with fever may occur. Chronic punched-out ulcers are common about the ankles. Hemiplegia, cranial nerve palsies, and other neurologic disturbances may result from cerebral thromboses.

These individuals usually are poorly developed and often have a relatively long trunk with short extremities. A tower-shaped skull may be noted. The long bones frequently show cortical thickening, irregular density, and evidence of new bone formation within the medullary canal. Splenomegaly and hepatomegaly are common findings. The heart usually is enlarged to both right and left with prominence of the pulmonary conus. Heart murmurs simulating rheumatic or congenital heart disease may be present.

Laboratory Findings

The anemia usually is normocytic and severe in degree with the red count between 1,000,000 and 2,000,000 and the hemo-

globin reduced proportionally. The pathognomonic laboratory
finding is sickling in an unstained drop of blood which has been
prevented from drying (*see* LAB. PROC.): the red cells appear
crescentic in shape, often with elongated or pointed ends. Dry,
stained smears may show little or no sickling.

Normoblasts frequently are seen in the peripheral blood and
a reticulocytosis of 10 to 40% or more is common. Leukocytosis
as high as 25,000 with a shift to the left often occurs. The platelets usually are increased in number. The bone marrow is hyperplastic with normoblasts predominating.

The serum bilirubin usually is elevated; an icterus index between 15 and 25 is not uncommon. Fecal and urinary urobilinogen values are high.

Prognosis

Very few with this disorder live beyond the age of 40. The
majority die during the first few years of life. Intercurrent infection, especially tuberculosis, or thrombosis of a vessel supplying a vital area frequently is the cause of death.

Treatment

No specific measures are available and treatment must be
purely symptomatic. Iontophoresis with Mecholyl (℞ 61) is
of use in the treatment of leg ulcers (*see* CLIN. PROC.). Splenectomy and liver and iron preparations are not indicated.

B. SECONDARY HEMOLYTIC ANEMIAS

*A group of hemolytic anemias caused by certain chemical
agents, vegetable and animal poisons, bacterial toxins, and blood
parasites.* Erythroblastosis fetalis and transfusion reactions
(q.v.) are conditions in which hemolytic anemia is caused by
hemolysins.

Etiology

Phenylhydrazine, saponin, methyl chloride, and large doses
of colloidal silver have a primary hemolytic effect. Other such
substances include benzene and the amino and nitro compounds
of phenol, benzol and toluol. Hemolytic anemia due to an
idiosyncrasy to such drugs as acetanilid, phenacetin, the sulfonamides, and certain of the sulfones, occurs occasionally.
Favism is a severe hemolytic anemia due to the ingestion of the
fava bean by a hypersensitive individual. Snake venom is a
powerful hemolytic agent. Bacterial toxins produced by *Cl.
welchii*, *Str. hemolyticus* and *Str. viridans* act similarly. The
plasmodia of malaria and the *Bartonella bacilliformis* of Oroya
fever cause hemolytic anemia by actually destroying the red
cells.

Symptoms and Signs

The severity of the clinical manifestations is proportional to
the rapidity and degree of hemolysis. Rapid blood destruction
is accompanied by aching pains in the extremities, back and ab-

domen, malaise, chills and fever. Massive hemolysis may result in prostration and shock, hemoglobinuria, and oliguria or
anuria. Jaundice develops rapidly.

The more chronic secondary hemolytic anemias are characterized by the usual symptoms of anemia and moderate jaundice.

Laboratory Findings

The degree of anemia is proportional to the rapidity, amount,
and duration of the hemolysis. It usually is normocytic but
may become somewhat macrocytic if red cell regeneration is
especially active. Active hemopoiesis also is manifested by
reticulocytosis (as high as 60% in acute cases), anisocytosis,
polychromatophilia, and the presence of numerous normoblasts
in the peripheral blood. Leukocytosis with a shift to the left
usually occurs.

Hemoglobinemia and bilirubinemia with a high icterus index
and positive indirect van den Bergh are the rule. The urine
contains large amounts of urobilin and urobilinogen but no bile.

Prognosis

The prognosis depends upon the primary cause of the hemolytic anemia, its severity, the condition of the patient, and the
promptness and adequacy of treatment. In the severe hemolytic anemias due to transfusion reaction, snake venom poisoning, erythroblastosis fetalis, and infections, the prognosis should
be guarded.

Treatment

Treatment should be directed toward eliminating the hemolytic agent (e.g., chemical or bacterial toxin, blood parasite),
and maintaining renal function and fluid balance, with specific
measures for combating the severe anemia, in addition to general supportive therapy.

Treatment of the hemolytic anemias of transfusion reaction,
erythroblastosis fetalis, and snake venom poisoning are described elsewhere (q.v.).

For massive hemolysis, alkalinization of the urine by parenteral administration of sterile solutions of sodium bicarbonate,
sodium lactate, or Ringer's solution is indicated (see INFUSION
REACTIONS; ACID-BASE AND ALLIED DISORDERS). Glucose 5%
in water I.V. may aid in preventing renal shut-down. If vascular collapse occurs measures for the treatment of shock (q.v.)
are indicated. Blood transfusions may be used if the anemia is
severe, or to combat shock, but only with great care since additional hemolysis resulting from a transfusion may overtax the
kidneys. A stimulant such as caffeine sodium benzoate (℞ 60)
may be of value.

For the more chronic secondary hemolytic anemias, the above
mentioned treatment usually is unnecessary. Of primary importance is the elimination of the hemolytic agent. Blood transfusions may be given with caution if the anemia is severe. Iron

and liver preparations usually are unnecessary but may be used if a depletion of the body stores of these substances is suspected. A high protein diet supplemented with vitamins is of value (*see* Diets).

III. DEFECTIVE OR DECREASED BLOOD FORMATION

A. MACROCYTIC ANEMIAS

PERNICIOUS ANEMIA
(Addisonian anemia, Biermer's anemia)

A chronic macrocytic anemia characterized by achlorhydria and certain other gastrointestinal and neurologic disturbances, occurring almost exclusively in the white race, but rarely before the age of 30.

Pathogenesis

The permanent deficiency of an unidentified "intrinsic" factor normally present in the gastric juice appears to be the fundamental defect. It is associated with atrophy of the gastric mucosa and achlorhydria. The "intrinsic" factor produced by the normal stomach mucosa promotes the absorption of "extrinsic" factor present in various foods; after absorption in the gastrointestinal tract the extrinsic factor is stored in the liver and is presumably identical with the erythrocyte maturation factor. This substance is essential for normal bone marrow erythropoietic activity. In the absence of the erythrocyte maturation factor, as in pernicious anemia, red cell maturation progresses abnormally and is arrested at a megaloblast stage of development. Hemolysis also contributes to the anemia.

Pathology

The bone marrow is red and of a jelly-like consistency. Microscopically, it appears hyperplastic, with megaloblasts predominating. A considerable portion of the usually yellow marrow of the long bones may be so involved. Areas of extramedullary hemopoiesis may occur in the spleen and occasionally in the liver and kidneys. These organs frequently contain large quantities of iron. The mucosa of the stomach and tongue usually is atrophic, and a chronic gastritis or enteritis may be present.

Subacute combined degeneration of the spinal cord (posterolateral sclerosis) is a common finding in pernicious anemia. It is characterized by myelin degeneration of the posterior and pyramidal tracts. Similar degeneration may occur in the peripheral nerves, plexuses of the gastrointestinal tract, and the subcortical areas in the motor region of the brain.

Symptoms and Signs

Onset usually is insidious, the symptoms not becoming severe until the anemia is well advanced. General symptoms of anemia such as weakness, shortness of breath, and palpitations are usual. Soreness of the tongue and paresthesias of the hands and feet are common initial complaints. Gastrointestinal symptoms include anorexia, nausea, vomiting, diarrhea, and attacks of abdominal pain. Considerable weight loss is common, and the skin frequently takes on a lemon yellow tint. The tongue usually is smooth as a result of papillary atrophy, and of a beefy red color. The spleen and liver may be moderately enlarged. If the anemia is very severe, signs of cardiac failure may appear.

Complaints referable to degenerative changes in the nervous system are noted in about 80% of the patients. Paresthesias resulting from peripheral nerve degeneration are common. Difficulty in walking, especially in the dark, weakness and stiffness in the extremities, and mental disturbances are characteristic. Loss of the vibratory sense in the lower extremities (revealed by using a tuning fork with a frequency of about 128 vibrations/sec.) is the outstanding sign of degenerative changes in the posterior columns. A positive Romberg sign, incoordination, and loss of position sense also are indicative of posterior column damage. Exaggerated tendon reflexes, hypertonicity, and pathologic reflexes such as the Babinski sign occur if the lateral tracts are involved. Absence of tendon reflexes and hypotonicity may be found if the damage is mainly in the vicinity of the posterior columns.

Laboratory Findings

Macrocytosis is the characteristic finding in the stained blood smear. The cells usually are well filled with hemoglobin, but may be hypochromic if an iron deficiency is coexistent. In severe pernicious anemia, anisocytosis, poikilocytosis, polychromatophilia, punctate basophilia, and nucleated red cells are prominent features. Smears of the bone marrow obtained by sternal puncture (*see* CLIN. PROC.) reveal increased numbers of red blood cells with megaloblasts predominating.

The anemia may be extremely severe, with the red cell count often below 1,000,000. The hemoglobin usually is not reduced proportionally. The mean corpuscular volume and the mean corpuscular hemoglobin usually are increased, but the mean corpuscular hemoglobin concentration is characteristically normal.

A decrease in the total white cell count to between 3,000 and 5,000, with a relative lymphocytosis, is common. The polymorphonuclear leukocytes usually are large and may be hypersegmented. Myelocytes may be present if the anemia is severe. The platelet count is low.

The absence of free hydrochloric acid in the gastric juice after an injection of histamine (*see* LAB. PROC.) is a constant finding. The icterus index and the fecal and urinary urobilinogen usually are increased.

Diagnosis

The characteristic sore red tongue, asthenia, achlorhydria, C.N.S. symptoms and signs, and the typical blood smear make the diagnosis a simple matter in the average case. The diagnosis in doubtful cases is facilitated if a reticulocyte response follows the administration of a potent liver extract.

Course and Prognosis

The term "pernicious" no longer is applicable to this disease. Except in patients with serious complications such as severe intercurrent infections and far advanced C.N.S. damage, the outlook is excellent. Adequate therapy can be expected to result in complete relief of the anemia and in the prevention, arrest, or lessening of the neurologic manifestations.

Treatment

The aim of treatment is to restore the red blood count to normal and to prevent or arrest neurologic manifestations. This is accomplished by the administration of substances containing the erythrocyte maturation factor, or antianemic principle. Purified liver extract, pteroylglutamic acid, and crystalline vitamin B_{12}, such as Cobione, are potent hemopoietic agents. These substances are used to bring about and maintain remission of the anemia. The amounts of antianemic principle necessary for those purposes vary considerably from patient to patient.

Purified liver extract (R 10) by the parenteral route is the most commonly used treatment. It is effective in bringing about a rise in the red count and in preventing or arresting the neurologic manifestations. In the average case, 30 U.S.P. u. I.M., repeated after 3 or 4 days is adequate initial therapy and usually produces a maximal reticulocyte response. Weekly doses of 30 to 40 u. then should be given until the anemia is completely overcome. For maintenance, about 1 u./day is required. This may be given as 15 u. every 2 weeks or 30 u. once a month. Patients with severe anemia, those in the older age groups, and those with infections may require larger amounts of liver extract. When subacute combined degeneration of the spinal cord is present even more intensive treatment with purified liver extract is indicated.

Crystalline vitamin B_{12} is a highly potent antianemic substance effective against neurologic as well as hematologic manifestations, which may be used without ill effects in patients hypersensitive to liver extract. The minimum effective dose of crystalline vitamin B_{12} (R 32) is about 1 microgram (mcg.) I.M. or subcut. daily; hence 1 mcg. is approximately equivalent to 1 U.S.P. unit of liver extract. Crystalline vitamin B_{12} may therefore be given on a dosage schedule similar to that of liver extract by substituting mcg. of vitamin B_{12} for units of liver.

Pteroylglutamic (folic) acid is an erythrocyte maturation agent active orally as well as parenterally. A daily dose of 5 mg.

by mouth (℞ 13) usually produces a maximal reticulocyte response and satisfactory increases in red cell counts and hemoglobin. However, the value of this substance in pernicious anemia is limited since it is ineffective against the neurologic manifestations.

Iron (℞ 1 to 6) is rarely needed, but is indicated if the hemoglobin values do not increase in proportion to the increase in red cell count.

The gastrointestinal symptoms usually disappear following treatment with the antianemic principle. If they persist, 4 to 8 cc. of dilute hydrochloric acid (℞ 59) in half a glass of water sipped through a glass straw during the meal may be of value.

Blood transfusion usually is unnecessary because of the prompt response that follows the parenteral administration of antianemic preparations. It is needed only if the anemia is so severe that circulatory collapse threatens.

Bed rest is indicated during the period of severe anemia. A high protein diet supplemented with vitamins is of value (*see* DIETS).

OTHER MACROCYTIC ANEMIAS

Those that occur in a variety of conditions leading to inadequate production, absorption, storage, or utilization of the erythrocyte maturation factor.

Etiology and Pathogenesis

In sprue, idiopathic steatorrhea, celiac disease, and chronic intestinal inflammatory disease, the anemia is thought to be a result of inadequate intestinal absorption of the antianemic principle. Lack of the extrinsic factor in the diet may cause a nutritional macrocytic anemia. The intrinsic factor may be lacking in extensive gastric neoplastic disease or, rarely, following total gastrectomy. Macrocytic anemia may be associated with severe liver disease, especially cirrhosis. The etiology of the macrocytic anemias of pregnancy and infestation by the fish tapeworm is obscure.

Symptoms and Signs

The major symptoms and signs usually are those of the primary condition. Since the anemia is characteristically mild or moderate, its general manifestations usually are mild. Fatigue, pallor, and other symptoms of anemia may be present. Glossitis is frequent. Subacute combined degeneration of the spinal cord rarely if ever occurs in these macrocytic anemias. Achlorhydria is an inconstant finding.

Laboratory Findings

Morphologically, the anemia is identical with pernicious anemia (q.v.). The red blood count rarely drops below 2,000,000. The hemoglobin, though decreased, is not reduced in proportion to the red cell count, so that a high color index results.

The mean corpuscular volume and hemoglobin are usually increased.

Diagnosis

The finding of a macrocytic anemia without achlorhydria or C.N.S. changes suggests the presence of one of the conditions mentioned in the discussion of etiology.

Treatment

The administration of liver extract (℞ 10), pteroylglutamic acid (℞ 13), or crystalline vitamin B_{12}, such as Cobione (℞ 32), as outlined for the treatment of pernicious anemia (q.v.) usually is specific for these macrocytic anemias. Larger amounts of these substances may be necessary for the treatment of sprue than are needed for pernicious anemia. The macrocytic anemia of pregnancy may not respond to parenteral liver preparations or crystalline vitamin B_{12}. Large oral doses of crude liver extract (℞ 11), desiccated hog's stomach (℞ 12), or yeast (℞ 33) may be effective if parenteral preparations fail.

B. HYPOCHROMIC MICROCYTIC ANEMIAS

(Anemia of chronic blood loss, Iron deficiency anemia, "Nutritional" hypochromic anemia, Chlorosis, Hypochromic anemia of pregnancy, infancy, and childhood)

Chronic anemias characterized by small, pale, red blood cells.

Etiology and Pathogenesis

The basic etiologic factor in all the hypochromic anemias is a depletion of the body's iron stores. Chronic blood loss is the most frequent cause of this type of anemia. Disorders of the alimentary tract such as achlorhydria, chronic diarrhea, and hookworm infestation may cause a deficient absorption of iron. The hypochromic anemia of pregnancy results from the increased iron requirements due to the presence of the fetus. Hypochromic anemia due to inadequate intake of iron and protein, the so-called "nutritional" anemia, is rare.

Symptoms and Signs

The clinical manifestations are insidious in onset. The usual symptoms of anemia include weakness, easy fatigability, irritability, and a variety of nonspecific complaints. Gastrointestinal symptoms such as heartburn, flatulence, vague abdominal pains, and anorexia or capricious appetite suggesting a neurosis, are common. Dysphagia occasionally occurs with glossitis and hypochromic anemia; this is the so-called Plummer-Vinson syndrome. Vasomotor disturbances, neuralgic pains, numbness, and tingling in the extremities, palpitations, and menstrual irregularities are common.

The skin and mucous membranes are pallid. The sclera appears blue or pearly white. The nails often are brittle, ridged longitudinally, flat or even concave (spoon nails). Papillary atrophy of the tongue often is present, but is not as severe as in pernicious anemia. Fissures may occur at the corners of the mouth. Systolic hemic murmurs are common, and slight cardiac enlargement due to dilatation may be found. Splenomegaly is present in about ⅓ of the cases; the liver is occasionally enlarged.

Laboratory Findings

The characteristic finding is a deficiency of hemoglobin in the individual blood cells. The cells have large, pale centers and often appear to be mere rings of hemoglobin. They are smaller than normal, averaging between 6.2 to 6.8 μ in diameter. The hemoglobin/100 cc. of blood is usually reduced to between 6 to 10 Gm. The red cell count is characteristically not reduced proportionally. It usually is between 3,000,000 and 5,000,000. The mean corpuscular volume, hemoglobin, and hemoglobin concentration are all low, as are the volume and color indices. There are no consistent abnormalities in the fragility of the red cells, the number or type of leukocytes, or in the platelets.

Achlorhydria as manifested by failure to demonstrate hydrochloric acid in the gastric juice following an injection of histamine (see LAB. PROC.) is a common but not constant finding. A hyperplastic bone marrow with normoblasts predominating is typical.

Prognosis

The prognosis is excellent following treatment with iron and control of the underlying etiologic factor such as chronic blood loss.

Treatment

Iron is specific for the treatment of the hypochromic microcytic anemias. In adequate dosage a maximal reticulocyte response usually occurs from the 5th to the 10th day after the beginning of treatment. There are many iron preparations which may satisfactorily be given by mouth. In general, the ferrous preparations are more easily absorbed than the ferric. Ferrous sulfate (℞ 2), ferrous gluconate (℞ 3), and ferrous carbonate (℞ 4) usually are well tolerated by mouth. However, the iron preparations occasionally cause abdominal discomfort and diarrhea. This may be avoided by giving the medication after meals, and starting treatment with small doses. For infants and children, iron is best administered as liquid preparations containing ferrous sulfate (℞ 6) or ferrous chloride (℞ 5). Iron therapy should be continued for at least one month after the hemoglobin reaches normal levels so that the depleted body iron stores may be replenished.

Adequate vitamin supplementation and a high protein diet (see DIETS) aid in hemoglobin production. Factors contributing to the anemia such as hookworm infestation, chronic blood loss, and infections should be eliminated whenever possible.

C. ANEMIAS OF DECREASED BLOOD FORMATION

PRIMARY REFRACTORY ANEMIA
(Aplastic anemia)

A normochromic normocytic anemia usually with associated leukopenia and thrombopenia, resistant to treatment, and almost always fatal.

Etiology and Pathogenesis

Certain chemical and physical agents cause refractory anemia by toxic depression of blood formation. The chief toxic agents are benzol, gold, arsenic, dinitrophenol, trinitrotoluol, radium, and X-rays (*see* RADIATION SICKNESS). Not infrequently an idiopathic form of refractory anemia occurs, in which there has been no apparent exposure to toxic agents.

The bone marrow in refractory anemia is typically atrophic (aplastic), consisting chiefly of fat and fibrous tissue. In some cases, the marrow may appear normal or even hyperplastic; in these cases it is functionally inadequate. The bone marrow hypofunction usually results in anemia, granulocytopenia and thrombopenia.

Symptoms and Signs

The onset usually is insidious and often delayed for weeks or months following exposure to the toxic agent. In occasional cases, however, the onset is explosive. The clinical manifestations vary with the severity of the pancytopenia. The general symptoms of anemia (q.v.) usually are severe. A waxy pallor of the skin and mucous membranes is characteristic. Chronic cases may show considerable brown pigmentation of the skin. If severe thrombopenia is present, blood may be extravasated into the mucous membranes and skin. Hemorrhages into the ocular fundi are frequent. Granulocytopenia may be manifested by the development of agranulocytic angina (*see* AGRANULOCYTOSIS). Splenomegaly is rare.

Laboratory Findings

The anemia is striking, the red cell count usually between 1,000,000 and 2,000,000. Hemoglobin is reduced in proportion to the red cell count (normochromic anemia). The red cells appear normal in size and shape except in rare instances of macrocytosis. A white cell count of 1,000 or lower is common, the reduction occurring chiefly in the granulocytes. The platelets are likewise severely reduced. Reticulocytes are rare. The aspirated bone marrow usually appears acellular, but occasionally normal or even hyperplastic. There is no evidence of hemolysis in this anemia, and no characteristic alteration of gastric acidity.

Diagnosis

The diagnosis is readily apparent in the presence of a normo-chromic anemia, granulocytopenia, thrombopenia, and an aplas-tic bone marrow, especially if a history of exposure to a toxic substance is obtained. An "aleukemic" leukemia may produce a peripheral blood picture similar to that occurring in a pri-mary refractory anemia. The bone marrow is hyperplastic with young cells predominating, and splenomegaly and lymphaden-opathy frequently are present. A pancytopenia, secondary to the replacement of bone marrow hemopoietic tissue by neoplas-tic tissue, may rarely simulate an aplastic anemia.

Prognosis

The prognosis generally is extremely poor; the majority of patients die despite repeated blood transfusions. Survival after the development of anemia usually is less than 6 months.

Treatment

Whole blood transfusion is the only treatment of value. Other measures include avoidance of contact with the toxic causative agent if identified, avoidance of medicaments generally believed to be toxic to bone marrow, bed rest if the anemia is severe, and iron (R 1 to 6) if an iron deficiency occurs because of bleeding. A high protein diet and vitamin supplements may be of value (see DIETS).

MYELOPHTHISIC ANEMIA
(Osteosclerotic anemia, Leuko-erythroblastic anemia)

An anemia, usually normocytic, associated with space-occupy-ing lesions of the bone marrow.

Etiology and Pathogenesis

Replacement of the bone marrow with neoplastic tissue or fibrosing or sclerosing lesions causes myelophthisic anemia by decreasing the amount of functioning hemopoietic tissue. Car-cinoma metastasizing to the bone marrow from primary tumors, most often located in the breast, prostate, lung, adrenal, or thy-roid is the most common cause. Multiple myeloma, leukemia, Hodgkin's disease, myelosclerosis, marble bone disease of Albers-Schönberg, and various other congenital bone diseases are less common causes.

Symptoms and Signs

The general symptoms and signs of anemia are present in a degree proportional to the severity of the anemia. Symptoms referable to the underlying disease also may be present. There is nothing clinically characteristic of this anemia. Splenomegaly may occur.

Laboratory Findings

The anemia usually is only slight or moderate. Normal blood counts or even a tendency to polycythemia are not uncommon.

Most often the anemia is normocytic but may be macrocytic on occasion. The outstanding feature is an unusual number of nucleated red blood cells, mostly normoblasts. Polychromatophilia and reticulocytosis often are present. The white count may be normal, reduced or increased. The platelet count often is low.

Treatment

Treatment is that of the underlying disorder. Blood transfusions may be of temporary benefit.

POLYCYTHEMIA

An increase in the number of circulating red blood cells, whether relative or absolute. This may occur as a symptom secondary to a mechanism interfering with blood oxygenation, or as the chief manifestation of the clinical entity, **polycythemia vera.**

RELATIVE POLYCYTHEMIA

A relative increase in the number of erythrocytes occurs in hemoconcentration. It may be a result of abnormally low fluid intake, or loss of body fluids as in severe sweating, vomiting, or diarrhea. The shift of plasma fluids into the extracellular compartment in shock, severe burns, and adrenal cortical insufficiency also will cause relative polycythemia.

ERYTHROCYTOSIS

(Symptomatic polycythemia, Secondary polycythemia)

Erythrocytosis usually occurs as a result of deficient oxygenation of arterial blood. High red cell counts are found in those exposed to chronic anoxia by prolonged residence at high altitudes. Pulmonary fibrosis and emphysema, silicosis, Ayerza's disease, congenital heart disease with partial shunting of blood past the pulmonary circulation, and acquired heart disease, especially mitral stenosis, cause anoxemia and associated polycythemia. Abnormal hemoglobin pigments such as methemoglobin and carboxyhemoglobin caused by poisoning with coal tar derivatives and carbon monoxide, respectively, by diminishing the oxygen-carrying power of the blood, resulting in erythrocytosis. The treatment of erythrocytosis is directed at correcting the anoxia-producing mechanism.

POLYCYTHEMIA VERA

(Erythremia; Polycythemia rubra vera; Polycythemia rubra; Splenomegalic polycythemia; Vaquez's disease; Osler's disease)

A chronic, slowly progressive disease characterized by an absolute increase in the total number of red blood cells, an increase in the blood viscosity and the total blood volume, splenomegaly, a tendency to thrombosis and hemorrhage, and a variety of vasomotor and neurologic complaints.

Etiology and Incidence

The cause is unknown. In several families a high incidence of the disease has been reported, but in the usual case no familial tendency can be demonstrated. Polycythemia vera is a disease of middle and late life. It affects twice as many males as females, is relatively more frequent among Jewish people, and rarely occurs in Negroes.

Pathology

All organs show profound hyperemia. This accounts for the splenomegaly and the frequent enlargement of the liver. Infarcts commonly occur in the spleen and other organs. Varices may be present in the esophagus, intestines, and elsewhere. Arteriosclerosis often is severe, and vascular thrombosis is not uncommon. The bone marrow shows hyperemia, increased megakaryocytes and pronounced erythroblastic hyperplasia with little increase in megaloblasts. Occasionally, immature myeloid elements may be much increased. The fatty marrow of the long bones is replaced by red marrow.

Symptoms and Signs

Onset is gradual. The patient complains of headache, weakness, prostration, vertigo, abdominal pains, irregularly distributed neuritic pains, and a variety of vague symptoms. Ménière's syndrome may be present. Erythromelalgia (q.v.) may be a distressing symptom. The occurrence of thrombosis gives symptoms referable to the part of the body involved. Cerebrovascular thromboses, with a tendency to rapid recovery, occur frequently. Hemorrhages into the skin and mucous membranes are common. Massive gastrointestinal hemorrhage, usually from associated peptic ulcer, may occur. This event may, by reducing the blood count and blood volume, bring about a remission of symptoms. Often, the color of the skin is striking and quite characteristic, due to the engorgement of the skin capillaries. There is a deep red flush which may be dusky and cyanotic, particularly in cold weather when peripheral circulation is retarded. In a number of cases the color of the skin is normal, and rarely there may be actual pallor. The spleen is almost invariably enlarged, occasionally extends down to the level of the iliac crests, is hard and smooth, and may be painful and tender when infarcts are present. Nodular lesions of the skin may occur. The disease has a definite relationship to myeloid leukemia. Cases which initially show all the features of polycythemia vera may gradually change to leukemia.

Laboratory Findings

Except after treatment or hemorrhage, the red blood cell count is increased. Counts as high as 13,000,000/cu. mm. have been reported, the average being about 9,000,000. There is an increase in the hemoglobin, but the color index usually is less than 1. In the majority of cases the white blood cell and platelet counts also are increased. A few immature cells of the red and white series are commonly seen. There is a pronounced increase in the hematocrit reading and the blood volume. Sedimentation rate is delayed, and the viscosity of the blood is 5 to 8 times above normal. Bleeding and clotting times are normal, but clot retraction is slow. The blood uric acid may be elevated. There often is an increase in the basal metabolic rate.

Diagnosis

Polycythemia vera must be differentiated from secondary polycythemias. On occasion, the diagnosis of these conditions is not obvious. If an arterial O_2 saturation can be obtained, the diagnosis can almost always be made, as the saturation in polycythemia will be 90% or above, and in secondary polycythemia below this value. Secondary polycythemia also differs from polycythemia vera in that immature cells of the red and white series are not found in the peripheral blood. Occasionally, in the early stages of chronic myeloid leukemia, the red count and hemoglobin may be increased. This condition should be suspected if the white count is over 30,000 and particularly if many immature white cells are found in the peripheral blood.

Prognosis

Polycythemia vera is a chronic disease which may persist for 10 to 20 years. Death usually is due to some complication, such as thrombosis (cerebral, mesenteric, coronary) or occasionally the development of myelogenous leukemia.

Treatment

Repeated venesections are of great value in reducing the blood volume to normal levels. An average regimen is a phlebotomy of 500 cc. or 600 cc. every month or two. Some patients will tolerate removal of large amounts, up to 1,000 cc., if their blood counts are very high.

Spray X-radiation, carefully controlled, causes a remission in the majority of cases which may last up to two years or more. Occasionally, severe granulocytopenia or thrombopenia may be produced.

Radioactive phosphorus (P^{32}) provides a most effective method of treatment. A sterile, isotonic solution of sodium acid-phosphate containing 5 to 10 millicuries of the substance in 1 to 20 cc. is given I.V. Remissions lasting 6 months to 5 years result in the majority of cases. If the effect is not satisfactory the dose may be repeated in 3 months. Radioactive phosphorus is available only from special sources. There is some indication that leukopenic myeloid leukemia occurs more frequently with this treatment and with spray X-ray treatment than it does in patients receiving other forms of therapy.

Mechlorethamine (nitrogen mustard) also will produce prolonged remissions and is a valuable therapeutic agent (℞ 19) for this disease (see HODGKIN'S DISEASE).

Phenylhydrazine hydrochloride (℞ 17) may be given in daily oral doses of 0.1 to 0.2 Gm. with a maximum total dose of 1 Gm. This produces an initial leukocytosis followed by a fall in red cell count which continues for 7 to 10 days after the drug is withdrawn. Vomiting, diarrhea, slight jaundice, and an increase in the tendency to thrombosis may occur. Death may result from a severe hemolytic crisis. Acetyl-phenylhydrazine (℞ 18) given in the same dosage also may be used. The therapy may be repeated after 10 days.

Fowler's solution (℞ 21) has been used but is of little value. The use of benzol is to be condemned.

ERYTHROBLASTOSIS FETALIS

(Erythroblastosis neonatorum)

A condition in the newborn, originating before birth, characterized chiefly by a hemolytic anemia, and accompanied by a compensatory increase in erythropoiesis. It is caused by the passive transfer of hemolytic antibodies from the maternal circulation to the fetus.

Etiology

The Rh factor is present in the blood cells of about 87% of the white population of the United States. Such individuals are referred to as "Rh-positive." The remaining 13% are known as "Rh-negative." Immunization of an Rh-negative mother to the Rh factor is the usual cause. In rare instances immunization to the Hr factor or hyperimmunization to A or B antigens has been reported as the responsible agent; this accounts for the rare appearance of erythroblastosis in the newborn of an Rh-positive mother. Immunization to the Rh antigen may be produced in an Rh-negative woman by the introduction of Rh-positive blood into her circulation by transfusion or through the placenta in pregnancy. The almost invariable failure of the first child to be affected unless the mother has been transfused previously or has had an abortion leads to the conclusion that immunization is probably initiated prior to the pregnancy in which an affected child is born. Immunization is believed to result from the passage of fetal Rh-positive cells (or fragments of cells which carry the Rh component) into the maternal circulation through the placenta during the course of pregnancy or delivery. It appears that immunization to the Rh factor can be accomplished by the direct introduction of Rh-positive blood cells into the circulation in only about half of all individuals in whom such an attempt is made. A much smaller percentage of women than this become immunized during pregnancy. The exact reason is unknown although it is presumed by some investigators that the escape of fetal cells into the maternal circulation is an abnormal condition and that only when it occurs does immunization take place. If a woman has been immunized by transfusions or by fetal cells introduced into her circulation during pregnancy, the Rh antibodies pass through the placenta into the fetal circulation and, if the fetus is Rh-positive, exert a hemolytic action on the fetal blood cells. Immunization once produced is permanent and all Rh-positive infants conceived by an immunized woman will be affected.

Rh is a general term and includes 3 principal subgroups. These are called Rh' or C, Rh_0 or D, or Rh'' or E. They are uncommonly present alone but more often are found in the combination Rh_0 and Rh' (called Rh_1); or Rh_0 and Rh'' (called Rh_2); or Rh_0, Rh' and Rh'' (called $Rh_1 Rh_2$). Rh_0 is the most common and is present alone or in combination with one or both of the others in almost 87% of all individuals. It also appears to be more strongly antigenic than Rh' or Rh''.

In the absence of any one or more of 3 Rh subgroups a corresponding Hr' or c, Hr_0 or d, or Hr'' or e is present in its stead. Since all traits are governed by the presence of a pair of genes all individuals must be homozygous or heterozygous for C or c, D or d, and E or e.

Pathology

In severe cases, there are extensive areas of hemopoiesis in the liver, spleen, kidneys, and occasionally in other tissues. The bone marrow often is hyperplastic. As a result of hemolysis, there often is widespread hemosiderosis of the tissues. The basal ganglia and other portions of the brain may be icteric (kernicterus). If the fetus is hydropic the placenta also is edematous and is consequently enlarged.

Symptoms, Signs, and Types

Three forms of erythroblastosis are recognized: Hydrops fetalis, Icterus gravis, and Congenital anemia of the newborn.

1. Hydrops Fetalis: Birth usually is premature. There is generalized edema, anasarca, and hydramnios. The amniotic fluid and the vernix caseosa are occasionally light yellow. The liver and spleen are markedly enlarged. The infant is either stillborn or dies shortly after birth.

2. Icterus Gravis: Vernix caseosa and amniotic fluid are biled stained. Jaundice appears soon after birth. If the child lives, the jaundice deepens and is accompanied by progressive anemia and, occasionally, hemorrhages and purpura. The bleeding time may be prolonged. Hepatomegaly and splenomegaly often are prominent but in mild cases no enlargement of either the spleen or the liver may be demonstrable. Edema usually is absent. Muscular twitching or even convulsions may result from C.N.S. irritation. In surviving children, the jaundice fades over a period of a few days to several weeks and the anemia lessens. Rarely, such infants may show some mental retardation or choreoathetosis.

3. Congenital Anemia of the Newborn: Anemia is present at birth or shortly after. The spleen and liver are rarely enlarged. Jaundice usually is mild or may be absent; edema is almost never present. Recovery is usual in these cases.

Laboratory Findings

Anemia is present, with various numbers of nucleated red cells present in the blood smear, depending on the severity of the hemolytic reaction. Reticulocytosis is usually depressed in the early stages and often remains abnormally low for a considerable period of time. The number of leukocytes is extremely variable.

Diagnosis

The most important diagnostic criteria are evidence of hemolytic anemia and jaundice in the infant and the presence in the mother's serum of antibodies specific for the variety of Rh or Hr factor existing in the infant's red blood cells. If antibodies can be shown in the blood or attached to the cells of an Rh-positive infant the diagnosis is almost certain. If either infantile anemia or evidence of maternal immunization to an Rh or Hr blood factor is lacking, the diagnosis is almost never warranted. Jaundice often is the first symptom to be discovered and any infant who becomes icteric in the first 24 hours of life should be thoroughly studied.

Prognosis

Hydrops fetalis is almost invariably fatal and results either in stillbirth or death within the first few hours of life. In icterus gravis the outlook for infants varies with the severity of the anemia present. Some will die regardless of treatment, others will survive only if properly treated, others will survive and be normal without treatment. About 10% of those with severe prolonged jaundice who survive will have permanent brain damage. The remaining infants are normal after abnormal blood destruction ceases early in the newborn period except for the occasional presence of blue or green discolorations of the deciduous teeth. Infants almost never need further treatment after 2 months of age.

Prophylaxis

When maternal immunization is once established it is permanent and all subsequently conceived Rh-positive fetuses will be affected by erythroblastosis. With succeeding pregnancies the symptoms commonly become more severe. Consequently,

all Rh-negative females of all ages should be transfused only
with Rh-negative blood. The giving of I.M. and intraperitoneal
blood to infants is not recommended. If parents are heterozygous, an Rh-negative offspring is possible and a second pregnancy may be allowed after one offspring with erythroblastosis
is born. If erythroblastosis occurs a second time, pregnancy
is to be avoided. However, successful artificial insemination
with sperm of an Rh-negative donor will yield an Rh-negative
child who will be unaffected by maternal Rh antibodies.

(Preliminary results indicate that the administration of Rh
hapten to either sensitized mothers or erythroblastotic infants
will inactivate Rh antibodies; however, additional studies will
be necessary before the full value of hapten is determined.)

Treatment

Transfusion: The essential treatment is the I.V. administration of blood to combat the anemia. The hemoglobin level and
erythrocyte count should be checked at least every 12 hours
during the first few days because sudden decreases occasionally
occur. Transfusion is indicated if blood values fall below 12
Gm. hemoglobin or 3,500,000 or 3,000,000 erythrocytes during
the next 5 to 10 days. After this, levels may be permitted to
fall slightly lower without ill effect. Rh-negative blood (from
a donor who has never received Rh-positive blood) is believed
preferable to Rh-positive blood by almost all investigators, inasmuch as it provides cells which are ordinarily unaffected by
Rh antibodies present in the infant's circulation. Blood should
be of the same type as the infant's and, for the safety of the
recipient, is best obtained from a female donor. Group O (universal donor) blood is to be used only in an emergency. The
mother's whole blood must never be used, since it obviously
contains Rh antibodies. Blood may be given in several ways:

**1. Exchange or exsanguination transfusion using the
umbilical vein:** If the diagnosis can be established within the
first 12 hours of life, exchange transfusion through the umbilical vein may be used. Subsequent transfusions are rarely
needed. A fine, plastic catheter is introduced into the umbilical
vein through the stump of the umbilical cord into the liver.
The opposite end is fitted over a 17- or 19-gauge needle which
in turn is attached by rubber tubing to two 3-way stopcocks
which are fitted together. The outlet of one stopcock is connected by tubing with the flask holding the blood to be transfused, the outlet of the other is connected with a rubber tube
through which the blood withdrawn from the baby is discarded, and the end of the joined stopcocks, opposite to the
one receiving the tube leading from the umbilicus, is attached
to a 25 cc. syringe. By this single system blood can be withdrawn from the baby into the syringe and discarded; fresh
blood can be drawn into the syringe and injected into the
baby. The amounts injected and withdrawn at each time

are about 20 cc. and a total of at least 500 cc. of blood should be used. In order to avert clotting, care must be taken to prevent the infant's blood from standing in the tubing. Citrate solution should be drawn through syringes and tubing between at least each second exchange. The administration of 10 cc. of a 10% solution of calcium gluconate (℞ 22) immediately after the transfusion is recommended as a precautionary measure to prevent possible ill effects from the citrate solutions.

2. Exchange transfusion using other vessels: Blood can be easily introduced into any of several superficial blood vessels. Withdrawing blood, however, is difficult because of clotting. Withdrawing blood from one of the cerebral sinuses, from the femoral or another artery following surgical exposure, or from a deep vein after the administration of heparin to temporarily prevent coagulation has been recommended.

3. Transfusion of concentrated cells: Removal of part or all of the serum from the blood with resuspension of the cells in small amounts of saline has been recommended. If the only source of Rh-negative blood is the mother, her cells may be washed free of plasma and resuspended in saline. Cells without serum in many instances seem to give a more satisfactory elevation of erythrocyte levels than whole blood and evidence is accumulating which seems to show that the introduction of adult plasma often accelerates the destruction of the infant's cells by enhancing the antigen-antibody reaction. Amounts equivalent to 25 to 30 cc. of packed cells are ordinarily given at each transfusion.

4. Transfusion with whole blood: The amount given at one time should be small and should not exceed 10 cc./Kg. body wt. Any of the available superficial vessels may be used. The blood should be Rh-negative and of a compatible type. However, if Rh-negative blood is not available, it then is permissible to administer Rh-positive cells rather than to withhold transfusion entirely.

Supportive measures: The infant must be kept warm; food and fluid intake must be adequate. If respiratory distress is present, O_2 may be administered, preferably by introduction into a closed incubator. The infant should be disturbed as little as possible.

Medication: The administration of crude liver extract and iron has been recommended although there seems to be little basis for their use since infants with erythroblastosis do not lack iron or the antianemic principle found in liver. The anemia is usually hyperchromic in character and except for a temporary reduction in reticulocytes normal numbers are almost always present. If liver is given, 1 unit of crude liver injection (℞ 9) may be administered I.M. once or twice a week. Syrup of ferrous sulfate (℞ 7) 20 drops 3 times a day is well tolerated by infants. Elixir of ferrous gluconate (℞ 8), 15 drops daily, also is satisfactory.

HEMORRHAGIC DISEASES

Conditions in which an abnormal tendency to bleed is a prominent symptom.

Physiology and Classification

Three elements are concerned in the process of blood coagulation: the vascular endothelium, the blood platelets, and the blood plasma. The intact endothelium is conducive to the maintenance of the fluidity of the blood; when traumatized, thromboplastin is liberated and coagulation is initiated. Blood platelets serve 3 functions: they maintain normal capillary integrity by plugging up potential lacunae in the capillary walls; liberate thromboplastin after injury; and are necessary for the production of a firm clot. Plasma contains prothrombin, calcium, and fibrinogen, which enter into the process of coagulation; substances (e.g., heparin) also may be present which prevent coagulation *in vivo*. The process of coagulation may be summarized as follows:

1. Thromboplastin + calcium + prothrombin → thrombin.
2. Thrombin + fibrinogen → fibrin (clot).

All these substances are required for blood coagulation, and a hemorrhagic diathesis may occur whenever any of them is diminished or absent.

Classification of the hemorrhagic disorders may therefore be made according to a defect of platelets; plasma; or vascular factors.

Laboratory Tests

Those laboratory studies that are of particular importance in the study of hemorrhagic disorders may be grouped as follows (*for details see* LAB. PROC.):

Platelet tests: (1) Platelet number: Normal is 250,000 (direct methods of counting), or 500,000/cu. mm. (indirect methods of counting). Qualitative examination of a well-spread stained blood smear is an excellent method of noting the number of blood platelets. (2) Clot retraction: The normal clot begins to retract within an hour after it has formed, and is completely retracted within 18 to 24 hours. If the platelets are markedly reduced, clot retraction is delayed or absent. (3) Bleeding time and tourniquet tests are determinations of capillary permeability but, since capillary integrity depends partly on platelets, these tests also give abnormal results when the platelets are reduced.

Plasma tests: (1) Coagulation (clotting) time: Venous blood placed in small glass test tubes normally becomes coagulated in 5 to 15 minutes. Coagulation time is prolonged when the plasma factors are abnormal. (2) Prothrombin time: Normal oxalated plasma, to which optimum amounts of calcium and thromboplastin have been added, coagulates in approximately 10 to 15 seconds under standard conditions

(Quick test). When the plasma prothrombin is diminished, the time required for coagulation (prothrombin time) becomes increased. (3) Plasma fibrinogen: Normal plasma contains about 0.25 Gm. of fibrinogen/100 cc.

Vascular tests: (1) Bleeding time: When the earlobe is punctured sharply, it normally bleeds for 1 to 3 minutes, and then spontaneously stops bleeding. In both vascular and platelet defects, but particularly in the latter, bleeding may continue for many minutes and even hours. (2) Tourniquet test: When pressure is applied to the upper arm under standard conditions (midway between systolic and diastolic, 5 to 15 minutes), few or no petechiae appear at the forearm. The appearance of over 10 petechiae in a standard circle (2.5 cm. diameter) is presumptive evidence of vascular or platelet defects.

PLATELET DISORDERS

A reduction in the quality of platelets (thrombasthenic purpura) is very rare. Reduction in the number of platelets (thrombocytopenia) is common, and may be idiopathic or secondary in nature.

IDIOPATHIC THROMBOCYTOPENIC PURPURA

(Primary thrombocytopenic purpura, Splenic thrombocytopenic purpura, Werlhof's disease)

A hemorrhagic disorder due to a reduction in blood platelets which has not been traced to any demonstrable underlying cause, and which usually is cured by splenectomy.

Pathogenesis

The disorder may be a form of hypersplenism, in which an abnormally active spleen causes a reduction in the number of blood platelets, possibly by producing a substance which inhibits the production of platelets from the megakaryocytes within the bone marrow. According to some, the spleen exerts its effect largely by withdrawing circulating platelets from the blood. Increased numbers of megakaryocytes are present within the marrow, but virtually no platelet formation occurs. After splenectomy, the megakaryocytes show active platelet formation.

Symptoms and Signs

A previously well individual, usually a young woman, begins to bleed from the mouth and into the skin following slight trauma. Bleeding also may occur from the body orifices or into the brain; it may be chronic and low grade, or acute and fulminating. In severe cases, there may be complaints secondary to the loss of blood, but blood loss usually leads to only slight anemia and correspondingly slight symptomatology. Examination shows only petechiae and ecchymoses, plus bleeding points at the gums and skin. Enlargement of the spleen is uncommon. Pallor is rare. In fulminating cases, there may be collapse.

Diagnosis

Examination of the blood shows a diminution in platelets, slight or no anemia, and slight polymorphonuclear leukocytosis. As in all thrombocytopenias, the bleeding time is increased, the tourniquet test is positive, clot retractility is poor, and the coagulation time is normal. It is essential to examine the bone marrow, which, in cases of idiopathic thrombocytopenia, shows increased numbers of megakaryocytes but little platelet formation (maturation arrest of megakaryocytes). Other clinical causes of petechiae and ecchymoses (e.g., various types of vascular purpura, including meningococcus infection and scurvy) are readily ruled out by simple inspection of a blood smear for platelets. Secondary thrombocytopenic purpuras can be differentiated by the blood and marrow pictures (see below).

Treatment

The first essential is accurate diagnosis. When the diagnosis of idiopathic thrombocytopenia is established, splenectomy must be seriously considered. It is almost always advisable to give 2 or 3 transfusions of fresh whole blood preoperatively over a period of 3 or 4 days. Some patients, especially children, may begin to show a remission during this therapy; if this occurs splenectomy may be postponed. If bleeding continues, and especially in cases of fulminating thrombocytopenia, splenectomy should be undertaken promptly. This operation is followed by 1 of 3 responses: (1) Dramatic cessation of all bleeding, usually with return of the platelets to normal or higher than normal values; (2) gradual cessation of bleeding with a gradual increase in platelet count over a period of a few weeks to as long as a year; and (3) no response. Groups (1) and (2) constitute 70 to 80% of cases.

In patients who show little or no response, and in those for whom splenectomy is contraindicated because of coexisting disease elsewhere (e.g., severe heart disease), the following measures may then be tried: Blood transfusions; injections of moccasin snake venom in an attempt to "increase capillary strength" (R 23); administration of parathyroid hormone (R 24). Little can be expected of these measures, however.

General measures—bed rest, sedation—and local measures at the sites of bleeding (see vascular types of purpuras, below) are indicated.

SECONDARY OR SYMPTOMATIC THROMBOCYTOPENIC PURPURAS

Conditions in which reduction of platelets occurs due to involvement of the bone marrow by infiltration with foreign cells or tissues (leukemia, sarcoma, carcinoma, fibrosis), or by hypoplasia or complete aplasia.

3

Pathogenesis

Platelets are formed from the megakaryocytes within the bone marrow. Infiltration of the marrow results in a crowding out of these megakaryocytes; aplasia, in a nonproduction of the megakaryocytes. In either case, since there are few megakaryocytes, few platelets are formed and thrombocytopenia results.

Symptoms and Signs

Bleeding occurs from any of the body orifices and into the skin. In severe cases, there may be rectal bleeding, gum bleeding, ecchymoses, intracranial hemorrhages. In milder cases, there may be only petechiae, ecchymoses, and slight bleeding from the gums. Usually, weakness and fatigue are also present, due to the underlying disease. Physical examination may show severe pallor (anemia), hepatosplenomegaly (leukemia), lymphadenopathy (leukemia or lymphoma), and bleeding points in the gums and skin due to the thrombocytopenia. In acute leukemia—a common cause of secondary thrombocytopenic purpura—no findings except pallor and bleeding may occur.

Diagnosis

The combination of petechiae and ecchymoses is characteristic of thrombocytopenia. If pallor (anemia) also is present, it may be suspected that the thrombocytopenia is secondary, since anemia is uncommon in primary thrombocytopenic purpura. Enlargement of the spleen, liver, or lymph nodes suggests some form of leukemia. Examination of the blood and marrow usually establishes the diagnosis: the blood shows thrombocytopenia, considerable anemia, and leukopenia or leukocytosis with abnormal cells in the blood. The marrow shows infiltration with leukemic cells (leukemia) or malignant cells (sarcoma, carcinoma, myeloma); or it may show fibrosis (myelofibrosis) or aplasia (aplastic anemia). The megakaryocytes of the marrow are much reduced in number. As in all thrombocytopenic states, the tests for platelets and platelet function are abnormal: i.e., the platelets are low in number, the bleeding time is prolonged, the tourniquet test is positive, and the retractility of the clot is poor. The coagulation time, being a test of the plasma constituents, is normal.

Treatment

Treatment consists in correct diagnosis and therapy of the underlying disease. Except in certain instances of hypoplastic and aplastic anemia, the prognosis is extremely grave. Therapy is of a supportive nature, repeated transfusions of fresh whole blood being of greatest value. Splenectomy may be beneficial in certain hypoplastic cases. In chronic leukemias, the usual means of therapy (especially X-ray) may afford temporary relief. Local treatment of bleeding sites may be temporarily efficacious (see below).

PLASMA DISORDERS

Deficiency in calcium does not result in hemorrhagic disease. Deficiency or absence of fibrinogen is exceedingly rare, but may occur in children born of consanguinity, with a heredofamilial history. The disorder is characterized by incoagulable or markedly hypocoagulable blood. Rarely, hypofibrinogenemia may complicate severe liver disease. The two important "plasma" syndromes are hypoprothrombinemia and hemophilia.

HYPOPROTHROMBINEMIA

Prothrombin deficiency may be due to a deficiency in vitamin K (q.v.), severe liver disease (q.v.), and dicumarolization (*see* ANTICOAGULANT THERAPY). All cases of hypoprothrombinemia show a tendency to bleed spontaneously from the nose, mouth, skin, kidneys, and gastrointestinal tract. The coagulation time may be increased, but the pathognomonic finding is an increased prothrombin time (normal, 10 to 15 seconds—Quick test). Treatment consists of immediate oral or parenteral administration of any of the products having vitamin K activity (℞ 37, 38), plus the treatment of the underlying cause. Bile salts are useful as an adjuvant in obstructive jaundice.

HEMOPHILIA

A hereditary disorder affecting only males and transmitted through females, the immediate cause of which probably is a deficiency in the plasma of some normal globulin substance ("antihemophilic globulin"), which is present in normal individuals. (Some investigators believe, however, that it is due to an excess of antithromboplastin in the plasma.)

Symptoms and Signs

As a result of the coagulation defect, the individual bleeds severely after slight trauma, severe exercise, or even spontaneously, because of an inability of his blood to coagulate in normal time. Hemorrhage often occurs into joints and causes ankylosis.

Diagnosis

This depends upon the finding of an increased coagulation time not otherwise explicable: i.e., the prothrombin time is normal, and the fibrinogen level is normal. The platelet count and clot retraction are normal, as are the bleeding time and the tourniquet tests. A history of bleeding in other male members of the family is significant.

Treatment

Local treatment at the site of bleeding aims to cause prompt local coagulation. Pressure pledgets are used at accessible sites of bleeding (cuts, tooth sockets). These may consist of plain gauze, or pledgets soaked in 1:1,000 epinephrine (℞ 25). Various coagulants have been incorporated into pledgets for local use: topical thrombin (℞ 27), fibrin foam (℞ 28), gelatin sponge (℞ 29), oxidized cellulose (℞ 30). These materials cannot be used if bleeding is not accessible.

Supportive therapy (as for swollen joints, swollen eyes, subcutaneous hematomas) consists of bed rest, rest of the part involved, and the use of warm local applications to aid absorption of blood.

Systemic therapy aims to remedy the plasma defect which is the cause of the bleeding. This consists of prompt transfusion with whole blood or fresh plasma, 1 to 3 pints of blood (or corresponding units of plasma) being given over 1 or 2 days. Recently, an active antihemophilic fraction of normal plasma globulin has been used parenterally with good results, but it is not yet commercially available.

Prophylactic treatment is highly important: such patients must be warned to avoid trauma, including strenuous exercise, and to receive prompt medical care if bleeding does occur.

HYPERHEPARINEMIA

The excessive use of heparin in the treatment of vascular diseases (*see* ANTICOAGULANT THERAPY) occasionally results in bleeding from the skin, gastrointestinal tract, or kidneys. In a patient who is receiving heparin, the occurrence of such bleeding should lead to prompt cessation of heparin therapy, estimation of the coagulation time, and administration of whole blood or of protamine (℞ 31).

VASCULAR DISORDERS

In all the vascular purpuras, the capillaries are exceedingly fragile, so that blood oozes out into the perivascular spaces and through the body surfaces. The cause of the excessive fragility is different for each group. In general, the platelet and "plasma" tests are always negative; the vascular tests usually are positive.

PURPURA OF ACUTE INFECTIONS

The cause of the increased capillary permeability is either actual inflammation of the capillary walls or injury by a "toxic" material. The exanthems, typhus fever, and typhoid fever, all show petechial eruption due to inflammatory changes in the capillaries. Acute meningococcal meningitis is especially important here, in that the vascular damage may be aggravated by adrenal hemorrhage (loss of cortin, necessary for capillary tonus), and generalized hemorrhages and shock may lead to death (Waterhouse-Friderichsen syndrome). In these conditions, all the hemorrhagic tests are negative except the tourniquet test, which sometimes is positive. Once the diagnosis is made, therapy is directed to the underlying disease process.

SCURVY

Lack of ascorbic acid, which is necessary for the integrity of the capillary wall, may result in petechiae and easy bleeding (*see* VITAMIN C DEFICIENCY). Frank scurvy today is rare; but the occurrence of petechiae, spongy gums, and tendency to bleed, usually in association with other evidences of nutritional deficiencies, suggests the possibility of scorbutic purpura. Determination of the plasma ascorbic acid level (normal about 1.5 mg./100 cc.) usually establishes the existence of the deficiency. Treatment consists in administration of ascorbic acid, 50 to 300 mg. daily (Ŗ 36). Since multiple deficiencies usually are present in such a patient, a high vitamin, high calorie diet with the use of multivitamin preparations is usually indicated.

PURPURA SIMPLEX

(Devil's pinches, Vascular purpura, Nonthrombocytopenic purpura)

Many individuals, especially young women with soft skin, tend to bruise easily for no obvious cause. In some cases, they also bleed slightly from the gums. Physical findings are limited to evidences of skin ecchymoses. Laboratory tests are negative, except for the tourniquet test, which sometimes is positive. The main consideration with this disorder, which is apparently due to fragile capillaries, is to rule out other causes for the symptoms, such as the thrombocytopenic purpuras.

Treatment is of little avail for the skin manifestations, although control of bleeding from the gums may sometimes be aided. Local massage to the gums, plus the empiric use of ascorbic acid (Ŗ 36), rutin (Ŗ 26), and sometimes snake venom injections (Ŗ 23), may help.

SCHÖNLEIN-HENOCH PURPURA

This is a presumably allergic purpura occurring chiefly about the joints and within the abdomen, especially in children. There is no specific treatment. If infected tonsils or teeth are found, their removal is justified.

PSEUDOHEMOPHILIA

This term should be restricted to a bleeding tendency affecting both males and females, often familial in occurrence, and characterized by an increased bleeding time despite the presence of a normal number of platelets. The condition apparently is due to an inability of the injured capillaries to contract properly after trauma, with resultant persistent bleeding, which may occur from cuts, gums, tooth sockets, the gastrointestinal tract, and the uterus.

Diagnosis is made by the findings of abnormal vascular tests (marked increase in bleeding time) coexisting with normal platelet tests (normal count, normal retraction of the clot). The coagulation time is normal. Treatment, though not entirely satisfactory, consists in the use of thrombin and fibrin foam for accessible bleeding (℞ 27, 28), and rest and symptomatic care for inaccessible bleeding. Rutin (℞ 26) also may be tried.

HEREDITARY HEMORRHAGIC TELANGIECTASIS
(Osler-Weber-Rendu disease)

A congenital, hereditary dilatation and thinning out of the walls of certain small blood vessels renders them liable to easy spontaneous rupture and bleeding which may occur from the nose, into the skin, and from the gastrointestinal tract. Telangiectatic dilatation of the small vessels in the skin of the cheeks, in and on the nose, at the lips, on the tongue, and beneath the fingernails is pathognomonic of the condition. Diagnosis is based upon the physical abnormalities. The hemorrhagic tests usually are negative, although the tourniquet test may be positive. Treatment is local in character, and consists of pressure packing of the bleeding site, if accessible, in the usual manner (℞ 25, 27 to 30). Rutin may be used in daily doses of 60 to 300 mg. (℞ 26), but this drug still is in the process of evaluation.

General Considerations of Therapy In All Hemorrhagic Disorders

Local measures: Accessible bleeding, whatever its cause, may be combated by the same mechanisms: pressure packing with or without the use of certain adjunct chemicals. Of the latter, the most important are epinephrine (℞ 25), thrombin (℞ 27), fibrin foam (℞ 28), gelatin sponge (℞ 29) and oxidized cellulose (℞ 30).

Systemic measures: (1) Whole blood or plasma transfusions combat hemorrhagic diathesis by supplying those plasma substances that are lacking in the patient, and are specifically of value in hemophilia, severe hypoprothrombinemia, and hypofibrinogenemia. (2) Transfusions of whole blood are used to supply platelets in cases of idiopathic thrombocytopenic purpura. However, if 1 or 2 transfusions are not followed by remission, splenectomy should be done in these cases. (3) Splenectomy is indicated only in patients with idiopathic thrombocytopenic purpura, and is curative in most such cases. It is contraindicated in the bleeding of leukemia, polycythemia, and vascular and plasma defects. (4) X-ray is used to relieve the bleeding of secondary thrombocytopenic purpura, when leukemia is the underlying cause. Its effect on the bleeding is indirect: when the underlying disorder is relieved, the platelet count rises, and bleeding ceases. X-ray is occasionally applied over the spleen in cases of idiopathic thrombocytopenic purpura where operation cannot be done, but is rarely beneficial.

Drugs: (1) Moccasin snake venom (℞ 23) increases the capillary resistance in some cases of vascular purpura. It is given in doses of 0.25 to 2.0 cc. (increasing doses) subcut., once or twice a week, in courses of 3 to 4 weeks. (2) Ascorbic acid, 50 to 300 mg./day (R 36) is effective in scorbutic purpura. It also is used empirically in unexplained vascular purpuras. (3) Rutin, 60 to 300 or more mg./day (R 26), is being used in various vascular purpuras to strengthen the vascular wall. Its exact effect is yet undetermined. (4) Vitamin K substances (R 37, 38) are of specific value in hypoprothrombinemic conditions due to dietary lack of vitamin K and to nonabsorption of vitamin K from the small intestine. They are of no value in the therapy of the other hemorrhagic conditions. (5) Parathyroid hormone (R 24) has been used in patients with idiopathic thrombocytopenic purpura in whom splenectomy has proved valueless; its value is questionable. (6) Liver extract has no place in the therapy of hemorrhagic disorders.

Adjuvant measures: Supportive measures include the use of blood transfusions, rest, and the prophylactic avoidance of injuries. Iron medication (R 1 to 6) may be of use for the hypochromic anemia following chronic bleeding, whatever its cause.

AGRANULOCYTOSIS

(Neutropenia, Granulocytopenia, Agranulocytic angina, Malignant neutropenia)

A term reserved for an acute illness, due usually to drug hypersensitivity, and characterized by extreme neutropenia, the presence of necrotic infected ulcerations of the mucous membranes of the mouth, and constitutional symptoms including high fever and marked weakness. **Neutropenia:** *A diminution in the number of polymorphonuclear neutrophils (granulocytes) in the blood stream.*

Etiology

Although some cases of agranulocytosis are idiopathic, a definite etiologic agent, usually a drug or chemical, can be discovered in most cases. These agents, in certain circumstances and in susceptible individuals, may have a selective effect on the granulocytes within the bone marrow. This effect may be direct or mediated through a hypersensitivity (allergic) reaction. The following are the most important agents which have been known to produce the disorder; aminopyrine; the sulfonamides; thiourea, thiouracil; radium and X-rays; nitrogen mustards; and gold.

Pathology

The prominent finding is first a maturation arrest, then a disappearance of granulocytes from the bone marrow, and thus from the blood, with relatively little change in the other hematologic elements. Granulocytes, the first barrier to infection, are lacking at the areas of ulceration in the mucous membranes (mouth, gastrointestinal tract, uterus, vagina, skin), which show numerous bacteria. Myeloblasts may be present within the bone marrow, but there are few or no myelocytes, metamyelocytes, or polymorphonuclear granulocytes. Megakaryocytes and erythrocytes are normal. In terminal cases, the marrow shows little more than lymphocytic or plasma cell tissue.

Symptoms and Signs

The acute disease is quite typical. The patient, who has usually become sensitized to one of the known etiologic agents, suddenly develops malaise, chilliness, chills, fever, sore throat, dysphagia, and ulcers of the oral mucosa. Physical examination discloses an acutely ill individual with necrotizing ulcerations of the pharyngeal and buccal mucosae. There may be regional enlargement of the lymph nodes, but no enlargement of other nodes, liver, or spleen. Fever and tachycardia are regularly present.

Blood Findings

The blood shows a leukopenia (500 to 3,000) with an extreme reduction in polymorphonuclear cells (0 to 2%). There is little or no anemia and no thrombocytopenia. The severity of the reduction in granulocytes is virtually pathognomonic. There are no pathologic leukocytes in the blood stream.

The bone marrow shows normal megakaryocytes and normal red cells, but white cells are virtually lacking except in the earliest phases of the disease and in beginning recovery. In both these phases, granulocytic elements may be present in normal numbers, but with little tendency to the formation of mature granulocytes.

Diagnosis

The presence of any oral ulceration should suggest the possibility that the ulceration may be secondary to a neutropenia in the blood, and appropriate blood studies should be made accordingly. If leukopenia and neutropenia are found, it is of prime importance to ascertain their cause, and specifically to determine whether they are the result of leukemia, aplastic anemia, or hypersplenism. Leukemia may be suggested on clinical grounds by splenomegaly, lymphadenopathy, and pallor; on hematologic grounds by a reduction in all the elements of the blood (pancytopenia), not merely in the neutrophils; and on examination of the bone marrow by the proliferation of lymphocytes (lymphatic leukemia), granulocytes (myelogenous leukemia), monocytes (monocytic leukemia), or blasts (acute leukemias). Aplastic anemia shows a reduction in red cells and platelets, as well as white cells, and shows a marked diminution in all bone marrow elements (marrow aplasia). In hypersplenism, splenomegaly is invariably present and the marrow shows normal or increased production of granulocytes, despite their diminution in the peripheral blood.

If all these causes for neutropenia (agranulocytosis) can be ruled out, the form of agranulocytosis here discussed may be diagnosed. A history of exposure to aminopyrine, nitrogen mustard, X-ray, the sulfonamides, gold, or thiourea derivatives supports the diagnosis. The finding in the bone marrow of a specific disappearance of all granulocytes beyond the primitive (myeloblast) stage establishes the diagnosis.

Prophylaxis and Treatment

The principles of treatment are based on the fact that acute agranulocytosis is usually, if not always, the end result of the action of some toxic agent upon the granulocytes in the body, and that symptoms are secondary to the infectious state which develops when marked granulocytopenia is present. For this reason, prophylactic avoidance of nonessential toxic medications such as aminopyrine should be observed whenever possible. When incriminated agents must be used (e.g., the sulfonamides, thiourea derivatives, nitrogen mustards, X-ray), periodic blood studies should be made, so that any tendency to a leukopenia may be detected early enough to prevent serious granulocyte damage by discontinuance of the medication. White cell and differential counts at least once weekly should be performed on each patient receiving these agents over a period of time. However, there is no evidence that giving so-called bone marrow stimulants (liver, folic acid) prophylactically, together with the offending drugs, is of any help.

Once acute agranulocytosis is established, treatment aims to prevent severe infection and to tide the patient over until the toxic effect has disappeared, thus allowing the bone marrow the possibilities of again becoming normal. When the underlying responsible agent can be ascertained, its use should be stopped immediately. If this discovery is not possible, all medication which may produce neutropenia should be discontinued, with the occasional exception of the sulfonamides (see below).

Antibiotics should be given to combat secondary infection, thus allowing the marrow to return to normal. The drug of choice is penicillin (R 39); however, if penicillin therapy is not possible, sulfadiazine (R 40) or sulfamerazine (R 41) may be employed, provided that the disease itself does not seem to have been due to sensitivity to the sulfonamides. Whichever drug is used is continued until the patient and the blood count are well on the way to normal.

Local measures: Careful oral hygiene to prevent or care for oral ulcerations is very important (see STOMATITIS). Ulcerated areas may be sprayed with potassium chlorate (R 56). Gargles of plain warm saline (R 57), hydrogen peroxide (R 54), or sodium perborate (R 55) help to relieve the sore throat. Anesthetic lozenges (R 58) help relieve pharyngeal pain.

General measures: The patient should be put on bed rest and given a high vitamin, high calorie diet consisting, if necessary (because of soreness of the mouth), of semisolid and liquid foods (*see* DIETS). Codeine (℞ 43) or Demerol (℞ 44, 45) may be given for pain; rest and sleep may be encouraged by a barbiturate (℞ 48, 49). Clinical results with cortisone or ACTH have proved encouraging.

Measures of less or doubtful value: These include (1) blood transfusions, intended to supply granulocytes and thus tide the patient over the acute stage; (2) injections of liver extract, 15 to 30 u. daily (℞ 10), used in the hope of "stimulating" the bone marrow; (3) "white cell stimulants," such as pentnucleotide (℞ 15), adenine sulfate (℞ 16), and folic acid (℞ 13, 14); (4) bone marrow transfusions; (5) injection of leukocyte cream or buffy coat; and (6) injections of yellow bone marrow extract. Small so-called "stimulating" doses of X-ray are definitely contraindicated.

LEUKEMIA
(Leukosis)

A term to include various generalized malignant diseases of the leukocyte-producing tissues, in which neoplastic proliferation occurs throughout the entire white cell tissue involved, following which the proliferated cells pass to all portions of the body.

Etiology

The reason for the disturbance in cell growth is unknown. Excessive exposure to X-rays or radioactive materials or to such chemicals as arsenic, the tars, or benzene may be a factor. Although there is no general agreement upon the concept of leukemia as a tumor, the disease is obviously a disordered growth of the blood cell, and clinically behaves like a malignant tumor.

Classification

Any of the blood cells may be involved in the proliferative process, including the red cell (erythroblastoma; red cell leukemia) and the megakaryocyte (megakaryocytic leukemia; megakaryocytoma). However, it is customary to consider leukemia as a proliferation of the white cells only. The disorder that corresponds to each cell is named as follows:

Earliest recognizable white cell (histiocyte, stem cell; reticulum cell)............................reticulum-cell leukemia

Primitive white cell..........................acute myeloblastic leukemia
acute lymphoblastic leukemia

Granulocyte..........................myelocytic (myelogenous) leukemia
  neutrophil........................myelocytic (myelogenous) leukemia
  eosinophil....................................eosinophilic leukemia
  basophil.......................................basophilic leukemia

Monocyte......................................monocytic leukemia

Lymphocyte.......................lymphocytic (lymphatic) leukemia

Each of these generalized leukocytic proliferations has growth potentialities which differ from case to case; the ones with slowest proliferative activity and greatest differentiation are called "chronic"; those with most rapid growth and least differentiation are called "acute." Intermediate forms ("subacute") also are discriminated.

Pathologic Physiology

It is convenient to consider leukemia as beginning idiopathically as a proliferation of a particular group of cells, either in the bone marrow (where granulocytes are formed), in the lymphoid tissue (where lymphocytes are produced), or in the reticulo-endothelial system (where monocytes are formed). Such proliferation ordinarily rapidly overgrows its bounds, so that the involved cells pour out into the blood stream and thence into distant organs. During the stage before the blood stream is invaded—and, in those cases in which, for unknown reasons, the blood stream is never invaded—the disease is spoken of as "aleukemic," "subleukemic," or "leukopenic" leukemia. In such cases the leukocyte count is normal or low. Ultimately, in most instances, the abnormal cells pour out into the blood stream, so that the leukocyte count rises ("leukemic" leukemia).

The signs and symptoms are a consequence of the great leukocytic proliferation and infiltration in various organs. Proliferation locally causes hyperplasia (of lymph nodes, spleen, liver). The proliferated white cells in the marrow crowd out other elements, leading to anemia and thrombocytopenia. Weakness, pallor, fatigue, and weight loss occur and symptoms referable to various organs develop as they are progressively involved. The main forms of the disease will be discussed separately:

CHRONIC MYELOCYTIC LEUKEMIA

A malignant and relatively slow proliferation of one of the bone marrow white cell elements.

Pathology

An idiopathic hyperplasia of the granulocytes occurs first within the bone marrow and later throughout the body. The marrow therefore shows an increase in granulocytic forms at all stages of maturity which ultimately crowd out the megakaryocytes and erythrocytes (resulting in thrombocytopenia and anemia). The cells pour out into the tissues and the circulating blood, and the blood smear reveals young granulocytes (cells which ordinarily do not appear outside the bone marrow: metamyelocytes, myelocytes, promyelocytes, myeloblasts). Infiltration or proliferation (or both) of granulocytes at other areas—liver, spleen, tissues—causes enlargement of these organs.

Certain aberrant forms of the disease are not uncommon. In the aleukemic form, the abnormal cells do not appear in the blood stream in any appreciable number, although they are numerous throughout the tissues. In the splenic form of the disease, the proliferation is largely restricted to the spleen, so that the patient shows the blood picture of myelocytic leukemia, a large spleen, but a marrow devoid of abnormal cells.

Symptoms and Signs

Anemia is regularly present and results in weakness, fatigue, pallor and weight loss. The patient appears drawn and haggard, and often has a low grade fever. Thrombocytopenia occurs as a late manifestation and produces a bleeding tendency, which may be manifested as petechiae and ecchymoses, as excessive bleeding after cuts and injuries, or as spontaneous hemorrhages from the body orifices. The spleen is enlarged, and often the liver. Lymphadenopathy is rare.

Laboratory Findings

Typically, the circulating blood shows abnormalities in the white cells, red cells, and platelets. The white cells are increased in number (25,000 to 500,000). All the granulocytes that occur in the marrow are found in the circulating blood: mature neutrophils, band forms, metamyelocytes, myelocytes, promyelocytes, and a few myeoblasts. A few lymphocytes and monocytes are present, as normally. The red cells are reduced in number (normochromic anemia). The platelets are at first numerous, but eventually become reduced. The bone marrow shows hypercellularity, with a predominance of granulocytic forms, especially early forms. In early stages, the number of megakaryocytes and erythroid elements is normal or even increased, but ultimately becomes much reduced.

Diagnosis

Myelocytic leukemia should be suspected clinically whenever debilitating symptoms occur in association with splenomegaly. All cases of chronic normochromic anemia with unexplained hepatosplenomegaly should be suspect. The diagnosis is established by the findings of leukocytosis and of immature granulocytes in the blood, myeloid hyperplasia in the marrow, and the clinical picture of a chronic illness, pallor, and hepatosplenomegaly.

In the typical case, the diagnosis will be quite evident. Occasionally, other causes for leukocytosis (infections, hemolysis) or leukopenia (marrow aplasia, toxic granulocytopenia) may require differentiation.

Prognosis

The course is invariably progressive and ultimately fatal, death being due to chronic debilitation and anemia over an average period of about 3 years from the date of diagnosis. Rarely, patients live for 8 to 15 years. Patients with the disease may live a normal productive life for one to several years, depending largely upon how well they react to treatment. For the first 1 to 3 years of treatment remissions, as obtained with X-ray or urethane or both, are prolonged. Later, relapses become more frequent until finally therapy becomes completely ineffective. The cases in which "cure" is obtained probably are "leukemoid reactions" rather than true leukemia. Just before death the peripheral blood often shows an increase of immature granulocytes, especially myeloblasts ("myeloblast crisis"); their appearance in a patient with chronic myelocytic leukemia suggests an impending acceleration of the disease. For this reason, a moderate number of blasts in the blood smear often is regarded as indicating "subacute" myelocytic leukemia, and if present when a patient is first seen he is considered to have subacute rather than chronic leukemia and his prognosis is correspondingly more grave.

Treatment

Therapy is directed chiefly toward control of symptoms; best results are obtained when the leukocyte count is lowered to 20,000 or less. Radiation therapy is the chief means of palliating the symptoms of myelocytic leukemia.

X-ray: This may be given in small doses as a "spray" over the entire body, or repeatedly over the spleen, administered by a competent radiologist. X-radiation aims to destroy the proliferating cells, and thereby to reduce the size of enlarged, infiltrated organs (liver, spleen). Destruction of abnormal cells in the bone marrow allows normal production of red cells, so that the anemia is relieved. Another course is given when symptoms recur or the leukocyte count rises above 50,000. The nausea and malaise associated with X-radiation may be minimized by administration of pyridoxine (℞ 34, 35) immediately before each treatment. X-ray therapy is contraindicated when leukopenia or severe thrombocytopenia is present.

Radioactive phosphorus (P^{32}) has similar effects and may be substituted for X-ray, but is not now generally available and its handling requires special precautions.

Urethane (ethyl carbamate) produces effects similar to those of radiation, i.e., destruction or inhibition of growth of white blood cells, especially immature granulocytes. It can be given orally (℞ 20) in doses of 2 to 4 Gm. daily. Alleviation of symptoms and a drop in the leukocyte count indicate the effectiveness of treatment. There usually is no reduction of platelets. When the white count has fallen to about 20,000, the dosage can be reduced and the patient followed clinically. A maintenance dose of 0.5 to 3.0 Gm. daily usually suffices. The effect of urethane, however, is not always predictable, and if no improvement is noted after 3 to 4 weeks, X-ray should be substituted. Best effects in prolonging and maintaining a remission often are achieved by the judicious use of urethane combined with X-ray therapy.

Arsenic: If X-ray and urethane are not available, potassium arsenite (Fowler's solution) may be administered, often with good results. An initial dosage of 5 drops 3 times a day is given, each dose being increased by 1 drop every 2 days until signs of arsenical toxicity (q.v.) appear (℞ 21). The medication is withheld for 3 to 5 days, then continued in subtoxic doses until clinical symptoms and blood count show improvement. Arsenic is not recommended, however, except when other methods are not available, for it causes severe toxic side effects.

Other drugs: Benzol should not be used. Thiouracil has no effect on leukemia. The nitrogen mustards (*see* HODGKIN'S DISEASE) sometimes are beneficial, but less so than the treatment outlined above.

Adjuvant measures: Rest in bed is indicated during the stages of severe malaise and high fever. Transfusions of whole blood (300 to 500 cc.) are given for severe anemia. Sedatives (℞ 48, 49), and anodynes (℞ 42 to 47) are used for mental rest and relief of pain. Oral hygiene (℞ 54, 55) is indicated for involvement of the buccal cavity. Splenectomy is generally contraindicated since it hastens death. If a greatly enlarged spleen is mechanically troublesome, splenectomy may (rarely) afford temporary symptomatic relief.

In leukopenic cases, X-ray and urethane cannot be used; only blood transfusions can be employed for relief.

OTHER VARIETIES OF CHRONIC MYELOCYTIC LEUKEMIA

Eosinophilic leukemia is a form of chronic myelocytic leukemia in which the proliferation consists largely of eosinophilic granulocytes. It is extremely rare, and is treated in the same way as chronic myelocytic leukemia.

Basophilic leukemia is a form in which a large number of basophilic granulocytes occur in the blood and bone marrow. This also is extremely rare, and probably represents merely chronic myelocytic leukemia in which there is a terminal basophilia. Treatment is that of chronic myelocytic leukemia.

CHRONIC LYMPHOCYTIC LEUKEMIA

(Chronic lymphatic leukemia; Chronic lymphoid leukemia)

An idiopathic, relatively slow hyperplasia of the lymphoid tissue throughout the body, manifested first by lymphocytic proliferation at the site of production (lymph nodes, spleen), and later by pouring out of the lymphocytes into the blood stream with infiltration into all body organs. The lymph nodes show a proliferation of lymphocytes and the blood shows a lymphocytic leukocytosis. Lymphocytic infiltration of spleen, liver, lungs, and bone marrow occurs.

Symptoms and Signs

The onset is insidious, with increasing weakness, fatigue, anorexia, debility, and lymphadenopathy. The patient may lose much weight before he consults a physician. Physical examination reveals generalized lymphadenopathy, slight to moderate splenomegaly and hepatomegaly, pallor, and (in cases of severe thrombocytopenia) petechiae and ecchymoses. Nodular infiltrations of the skin may occur. In elderly persons, the disease may produce no symptoms and be found only by accident during routine hematologic studies.

Laboratory Findings

The leukocyte count is elevated (10,000 to 300,000), and most of the white cells (80 to 95%) are mature lymphocytes. There is a normochromic normocytic anemia, and a reduction in platelets. The bone marrow shows infiltration with lymphocytes, which may form from 20 to 80% of the marrow cells (normally 0 to 10%). Granulocytes, erythrocytes, and megakaryocytes are reduced.

Diagnosis

Lymphatic leukemia should be suspected whenever generalized lymphadenopathy and chronic debilitation coexist. The diagnosis usually can be established by blood counts and smears. In "aleukemic" (leukopenic) cases, demonstration of lymphocytic infiltration in the bone marrow gives the diagnosis. Biopsy of a lymph node will help rule out Hodgkin's disease, reticulum cell sarcoma, and other lymphomatous disorders. Acute infections that give rise to pronounced lymphocytic leukocytosis are rare (pertussis, infectious mononucleosis), and can be differentiated by the history, physical findings, and the absence of anemia, thrombocytopenia, and bone marrow infiltration.

Prognosis

The course is progressive, and death usually occurs within 3 to 4 years after a diagnosis is possible. Occasionally, patients live for 10 or more years. Death results from chronic cachexia, intercurrent infections, and sometimes hemorrhages.

Treatment

In general, treatment is the same as for chronic myelocytic leukemia (*see* above). The most important measure is X-ray, administered successively to involved areas of the body and to the spleen. Radioactive phosphorus (P^{32}) usually is not very effective in lymphatic leukemia, and urethane (R 20) is much less beneficial than in myelocytic leukemia. Arsenic (R 21) may be used when X-ray is unavailable. The usual sympto-

matic measures—especially blood transfusions for anemia—
make the patient more comfortable.

THE ACUTE LEUKEMIAS

Rapidly proliferative and therefore fatal forms of all varieties
of leukemia occur. The term "acute" is clinical, and these patients usually die in 1 week to 3 months after the onset. The
characteristic blood cell is the "blast" (myeloblast in acute
myelocytic leukemia, lymphoblast in acute lymphatic leukemia).
Since the differentiation between myeloblast and lymphoblast
always is difficult and sometimes impossible and, in these patients, quite academic, both forms of the disease may be considered under the single heading of "acute leukemia."

Pathology

A fulminating overgrowth of primitive white cells (myeloblasts or lymphoblasts) is present throughout the body, resulting in obliteration of the normal structures in the lymph nodes,
spleen, liver, and bone marrow. The marrow infiltration results
in profound anemia and thrombocytopenia. The cells in the
peripheral blood are almost exclusively blast forms, with virtually no mature cells.

Symptoms and Signs

Acute leukemia at first resembles an overwhelming infection.
The patient rapidly becomes extremely ill and has constant
high fever. Because of the profound thrombocytopenia, free
bleeding—from the gums, kidneys, bowel, and into the skin and
brain—is common. Secondary infection, especially of the mouth
and throat, often occurs. Physical examination characteristically shows an appearance of severe illness, extreme pallor,
petechiae, ecchymoses, and frank bleeding. Enlargement of the
spleen, liver, and lymph nodes sometimes is present, but never
striking.

Laboratory Findings

The white cell count usually is high (10,000 to 50,000), but
sometimes subnormal (1,000 to 4,000). The smear shows blasts
almost exclusively. There is pronounced anemia, and platelets
are virtually lacking. The bone marrow shows an extreme and
uniform proliferation of blast cells, which replace all other elements.

Diagnosis

Examination of the blood usually establishes the diagnosis.
In cases of doubt, a marrow puncture, revealing largely primitive
white cells is conclusive. Patients with chronic myelocytic leukemia often have a terminal myeloblast crisis, in which the
bulk of the peripheral white blood cells are blasts, so that the
picture resembles acute leukemia. Differentiation is made by
the chronicity of the illness and the finding of a large, hard
spleen.

Prognosis

The disease always is fatal, often within a few days, but usually within 3 months. Death is due to hemorrhage into the brain or from the gastrointestinal tract, or to severe anemia. Occasionally, there is a remission of symptoms to a subacute or chronic form and the patient's clinical status improves temporarily.

Treatment

The trial of almost any form of treatment is justified in such a highly fatal disease. X-ray therapy, however, is contraindicated because it may hasten death. The best standby is whole blood transfusion, which should be given as often as economically possible, in the hope that it may produce remission. Oral hygiene (℞ 54, 55) and sedation (℞ 48, 49) are important. Remissions have been reported after treatment with a variety of drugs (the sulfonamides, penicillin, colchicine, tyrosinase, derivatives of pteroyltriglutamic acid, and more recently, cortisone and the adrenocorticotropic hormone, ACTH).

MONOCYTIC LEUKEMIA

A malignant, rapidly progressive proliferative disorder of the monocytes.

Pathology

The monocyte is probably produced in the reticulo-endothelial system throughout the body. Circulating monocytes normally constitute some 4 to 10% of the white cells (200 to 1,000/cu. mm.). In monocytic leukemia, there is an abundant overflow of monocytes into the blood stream, corresponding to an increase of monocytes and their precursors (histiocytes) in the lymph nodes, spleen, and bone marrow.

Symptoms and Signs

The symptoms are those of the other acute leukemias: pallor, weakness, debility, lymphadenopathy, hepatosplenomegaly, bleeding tendency. Extensive hyperplasia of the gingival tissue is a common finding.

Laboratory Findings

The leukocyte count is elevated, and monocytes predominate in the blood smear. A normochromic anemia is present, as well as thrombocytopenia. The bone marrow shows an increase in histiocytes and monocytes. When the marrow is myeloid and the blood picture resembles that of monocytic leukemia, the probability is that the "monocytes" are being incorrectly identified and that they are myelocytes; therefore the disease is really myelocytic leukemia.

Treatment

This is the same as for the myelocytic leukemias. Especial attention must be given to the mouth, where extreme gingival hyperplasia with bleeding may occur. Mouthwashes (℞ 54, 55) and sedatives (℞ 48, 49) may help to relieve the oral symptoms.

LYMPHOMA

A group of tumors of varying malignancy derived from the lymphocytes, in any one of their developmental stages or from the reticulum cells of lymphatic structures. These tumors include the **lymphosarcomas,** which may be classified as lymphoblastomas, lymphocytomas, and reticulum cell sarcomas, depending upon their degree of cell differentiation and type of cell from which they arise. **Hodgkin's disease** often is included in the lymphoma group of neoplastic diseases, though many believe it to be an infectious granuloma.

LYMPHOSARCOMA

A malignant tumor arising in the lymph nodes or mucosal lymphatic tissue, especially of the gastrointestinal tract, characterized by lymphadenopathy, infiltration of surrounding tissues, and regional lymphatic spread.

Symptoms and Signs

The complaints and physical findings vary with the location of the lesions. Nonspecific complaints of fever, sweating, loss of weight, and asthenia are common in the late stages of the disease. Large, hard lymph nodes matted together and adherent to the skin may be evident in the cervical, axillary, or inguinal regions. Mediastinal and retroperitoneal lymphadenopathy may cause symptoms of pressure on various organs. Gastric and intestinal lymphosarcoma may simulate gastrointestinal carcinoma. The tonsils are not uncommon sites of origin. The spleen, liver, and bone marrow are occasionally involved. Blood findings usually are nonspecific. However, with bone marrow involvement, a myelophthisic anemia (q.v.) may develop. Most patients die within 1 or 2 years, but some may survive 5 years or longer.

Diagnosis

A definitive diagnosis of the disease can be made only by histologic study of excised tissue. It must be differentiated from Hodgkin's disease, the leukemias, tuberculosis (especially primary tuberculosis with hilar adenopathy, and tuberculous adenitis), and other causes of lymphadenopathy (q.v.).

Treatment

The treatment is similar to that of Hodgkin's disease (q.v.).

HODGKIN'S DISEASE
(Lymphadenoma)

A chronic advancing fatal disease of unknown etiology, manifested by painless and progressive enlargement of the lymph nodes and frequently of the spleen and liver. In the later stages, fever, anemia, and cachexia are prominent.

Etiology and Incidence

The cause is unknown. Many investigators consider it a malignant neoplastic entity; others, an infectious granuloma. Various organisms have been suspected, such as the tubercle bacillus, the *Brucella* organism, and a filtrable virus.

Hodgkin's disease is more prevalent among males than females, in the ratio of 7:3. It may occur at any age but its greatest incidence is in the 3rd and 4th decades of life. The disease has little racial predilection.

Pathology

Hodgkin's disease is a hyperplastic process which involves the reticulo-endothelial system, and tends to become generalized. The lymph nodes, spleen, liver, and bone marrow are chiefly involved.

The enlarged lymph nodes are firm, rubbery, and discrete until the later stages, when they may be matted together. The capsule of the nodes and the surrounding tissues are rarely invaded. However, the enlarged nodes may envelop an adjacent structure, such as a ureter or a bronchus. The spleen is enlarged in about 50% of the cases, and contains scattered foci of whitish "Hodgkin's tissue" which are in marked contrast to the red background. The liver is frequently enlarged. The vertebrae and other bones often are involved in the hyperplastic process; fracture is rare but collapse of a vertebra is not uncommon. The lung may present the first evidence of Hodgkin's disease.

Microscopically, the lesions are similar in all tissues in which the disease is found. Striking hyperplasia of the reticulo-endothelial cells is observed, with replacement and eventual disappearance of lymphoid tissue. Multinucleated (Reed-Sternberg) cells are characteristic. In many cases, eosinophils are prominent. As the disease progresses, areas of necrosis may develop, particularly in the spleen, and accompanying fibrotic changes replace the cellular constituents. The early cellular stage usually responds to radiation; the fibrotic phase is radioresistant.

Symptoms and Signs

In most cases, the disease begins with a painless superficial lymphadenopathy and pursues a fairly typical clinical course. However, the symptoms may vary, depending upon the region of the body chiefly involved in the hyperplastic process. Pruritus may appear early and may be severe and persistent; this sometimes precedes by months the first complaints of glandular enlargement.

As regards lymphadenopathy, the cervical lymph nodes, first on one side and then the other, frequently are the first to manifest the disease. Less commonly, those in the axillary or inguinal regions are initially involved. The nodes are discrete, painless, nontender, and increase in size progressively without evident constitutional symptoms. Enlargement of the nodes usually spreads from the initial group to involve the superficial and deep nodes elsewhere.

Splenomegaly is evident in about half the cases, and the liver frequently is palpable. Sometimes hepatic and splenic enlargement constitute the only abnormal physical signs. Still more rarely, the disease is confined to the retroperitoneal lymph nodes (abdominal Hodgkin's). Involvement of the bone marrow may produce pain, disability, rarefaction, compression of a vertebra, and rarely fracture. Involvement of the C.N.S. by pressure from extradural granulomatous infiltrations and from involved bony structures may result in paraplegia. Infiltration of the lung parenchyma may simulate lobar consolidation.

Enlarged regional lymph nodes may compress adjacent structures and produce secondary symptoms. Pressure on the bronchi and trachea may lead to cyanosis and dyspnea. Horner's syndrome and laryngeal paralysis may result from pressure on the cervical sympathetic and recurrent laryngeal nerve. Neuritic pains follow compression of nerve roots of the brachial, lumbar, or sacral plexuses. Obstruction of the bile duct produces jaundice; edema of the legs may follow pressure on the vena cava. Involvement of the ureter may interfere with urinary flow. A frequent phenomenon in the later stages is recurring accumulation of fluid in the chest or abdomen, secondary to lymphatic obstruction.

Systemic intoxication develops progressively as the disease advances, and is evidenced by fever, pruritus, elevated white blood cell count, eosinophilia, anemia, and cachexia. Fever is present at some time during the course of the disease and is most common when the mediastinal and abdominal nodes are involved. The fever may be of almost any type and degree but usually is irregular. It may be of the Pel-Ebstein type—a regularly recurring cycle: a few days of high fever succeeded by a few days, or even 2 or 3 weeks, of normal temperature. In highly toxic stages, continuous fever of 104° or 105° F. may persist for weeks. High fever usually indicates an early fatal termination. A peculiar bronze pigmentation of the skin may appear as a late manifestation. Herpes zoster is unusually frequent during Hodgkin's disease. Lymphocytosis may appear early in the disease, to be replaced later by a polymorphonuclear leukocytosis. The eosinophil count sometimes is elevated, rarely to 60 or 80%.

Anemia, usually of normocytic type (*see* MYELOPHTHISIC ANEMIA), rarely is present in the first stages but may become pronounced as the marrow is progressively involved. Cachexia and continued weight loss appear as the disease advances.

Diagnosis

The symptom complex of unexplained fever, lymph node enlargement, especially cervical, and pruritus should suggest Hodgkin's disease. The diagnosis can be established only by histologic examination. When available, an entire lymph node should be removed for biopsy. It is best not to use an inguinal lymph node, since such tissues are likely to have had their structure altered by past infections due to other causes.

When no enlarged lymph nodes are present in the peripheral node-bearing area, roentgenographic studies, especially of the chest, may reveal mediastinal or hilar adenopathy. Occasionally, aspiration biopsy of a lung lesion or of the spleen has permitted diagnosis.

A three-way check on diagnosis (i.e., lymph node biopsy, sternal or iliac crest bone marrow aspiration, and peripheral blood cell count) is ideal. However, to the experienced pathologist, aspiration biopsy of lymph nodes may be a satisfactory substitute where the available material is unsuitable for surgical biopsy.

Diagnostic X-ray therapy sometimes is resorted to, since Hodgkin's disease in its early stages is relatively radiosensitive, but such evidence is of limited value as other lymphogenous conditions also are radiosensitive.

Even after biopsy material has been obtained, exact differentiation of Hodgkin's disease from lymphosarcoma and leukemia sometimes is difficult. Hodgkin's disease may be simulated closely by bronchogenic cancer, and only bronchoscopy, aspiration biopsy, or aspirated sputum studies may differentiate them. Sarcoidosis (q.v.) may be very difficult to differentiate, but if present, the classical bone changes, skin eruption, and blood chemical alterations are significant. Tuberculosis (q.v.) may imitate Hodgkin's disease very closely, and vice versa. Metastatic cancer must be ruled out as a cause of lymphadenopathy. When splenomegaly is the outstanding feature of the disease, all other causes of splenomegaly (q.v.) must be excluded, such as leukemia, lymphosarcoma, polycythemia vera, thrombocytopenic purpura, Banti's syndrome, Gaucher's disease, amyloidosis, syphilis, malaria, endocarditis, typhoid fever, brucellosis, hepatic disorders with portal hypertension, and the rickettsial diseases. In many cases, the diagnosis of these conditions will be obvious from clinical and laboratory findings. Plasma cell myeloma may be differentiated by characteristic bone changes visualized by X-ray, hyperglobulinemia, and sternal bone marrow studies. Here, too, bone marrow biopsy is the most reliable diagnostic measure.

Prognosis

Untreated Hodgkin's disease tends to run a progressively declining course, death usually occurring within 2 to 3 years due to cachexia or mechanical compression of a vital structure. With treatment, about 20% of patients survive for 5 years, rarely longer.

Treatment

At present, there is no cure for Hodgkin's disease. Therapy is palliative and symptomatic, aimed at making the patient's life more tolerable. In some instances, life also may be prolonged, as with cortisone or ACTH. Surgical excision of the chain of enlarged nodes in the early "localized" form of Hodgkin's disease may possibly effect a cure.

General measures consist of good nourishment with a diet high in protein and vitamins (*see* DIETS). Iron (℞ 1 to 6) and antipruritics (℞ 50 to 53) are beneficial. Blood transfusions are useful when indicated. However, extreme caution is necessary since patients with Hodgkin's are prone to develop transfusion reactions (q.v.).

During the early stages there usually are few manifestations other than pruritus and the discovery of the presence of enlarged nodes. As the disease progresses, there will be increasing weakness and cachexia, pains from pressure or neurological involvement which may be extreme, or obstructive manifestations in the trachea, bronchi, or elsewhere. Suitable analgesics and narcotics (℞ 42 to 47) will be required in increasing amounts.

Surgical excision of a tumor mass is indicated only when the disease appears to be limited to one group of lymph nodes or where relief from mechanical obstruction is necessary.

High voltage X-ray therapy, administered by one experienced in its use, is of great value in ameliorating symptoms and prolonging life. Pruritus, pain, and tumor size may be lessened by X-radiation. The sensitivity of lymphatic tissue to the rays makes possible the use of small frequent doses of radiation. This so-called fractional method allows exposure of the patient to the largest permissible total dose of X-ray. Until fibrosis in the terminal stage renders the nodes radioresistant, radiation reduces the size of the nodes from 30 to 100%. Abdominal lesions are least affected. Nausea and vomiting due to radiation sickness (q.v.) may be relieved by pyridoxine (℞ 34, 35), avoidance of oral feeding, and the use of parenteral fluids and alimentation. As the disease progresses, the favorable response to this form of treatment lessens until a point is reached where X-ray therapy is ineffective. The use of radioactive isotopes has offered no advantage over the above.

Nitrogen mustard therapy is indicated where X-ray therapy is not available or has become ineffective, or where extensive systemic involvement makes radiation impractical. Temporary remissions may sometimes be induced in 7 to 10 days by the use of mechlorethamine (℞ 19), which produces regression of lymphadenopathy, splenomegaly, and fever. However, such remissions are of shorter duration than those following X-ray therapy, so that treatment must be given more frequently. The dose is 0.1 mg./Kg. body wt., administered rapidly I.V. once or twice daily for 4 to 6 doses. Adequate nitrogen mustard therapy regularly depresses the hemopoietic system within 3 weeks, so that a marked leukopenia may occur. Should the white cell count fall below 1,000, the patient should be treated for agranulocytosis (q.v.). Thrombocytopenia, with or without purpura, is not uncommon. Therapy may be repeated as necessary, provided the blood picture is or has returned to normal. Nausea and vomiting frequently occur an hour or longer after an injection of nitrogen mustard, and may last several hours. These symptoms may often be allayed by the routine use of 100 mg. pyridoxine (R 35) given 30 minutes after (never before) the nitrogen mustard. Daily blood studies are necessary both during and 3 to 4 weeks after treatment with either X-ray or nitrogen mustard therapy.

SPLENIC DISORDERS

The spleen is an organ weighing 75 to 100 Gm. which is composed of supporting connective tissue, lymphoid and reticulo-endothelial tissue, and a large amount of vascular tissue, and which has several functions: (1) It stores a varying amount of blood (reservoir function). (2) It produces blood cells. The lymphatic tissue of the spleen gives rise to lymphocytes. The reticulo-endothelial tissue of the spleen produces monocytes. In the fetus, the reticulo-endothelial tissue also produces red cells, granulocytes, and megakaryocytes; and it is probable that, under conditions in which the bone marrow in the adult loses its ability to produce blood cells, the splenic reticulo-endothelial tissue reverts to its fetal function ("extramedullary hemopoiesis" or "myeloid metaplasia" of the spleen). (3) It destroys aged red cells. It is possible that the spleen also destroys aged white cells and platelets. (4) It regulates to some extent, probably by hormones, the production and delivery of red cells, granulocytes, and platelets at the bone marrow. (5) It probably has other less clear functions.

The normal spleen is not necessary to life, but the diseased spleen often threatens health and life.

In most instances, disorders which involve the spleen are widespread, and the splenic involvement is merely part of a generalized disorder of the lymphatic or reticulo-endothelial tissues of the body. In general, therefore, diffuse disorders of the lymphatic tissue such as lymphosarcoma, and of the reticulo-endothelial tissue (e.g., Hodgkin's disease, Gaucher's disease) also involve the spleen. Less commonly, a disorder of the spleen occurs because of a localized disease in the neighborhood—portal vein hypertension, carcinoma of the tail of the pancreas.

PHYSIOLOGIC DISORDERS OF THE SPLEEN

Physiologic derangement of splenic function, with or without splenomegaly, is of great clinical importance. The underlying mechanism of this dysfunction is not established. One view considers increased phagocytosis of the cellular elements of the blood to be responsible. More recently, various splenic syndromes have been explained on the basis of "hypersplenism," a term denoting an exaggerated inhibitory effect of the spleen on the bone marrow with or without increased phagocytosis by the spleen. Although not accepted by all workers, the theory of hypersplenism lends itself well to the discussion of splenic disorders and so will be employed in the ensuing chapters. Anatomic enlargement of the spleen, which may be due to a variety of causes, will be considered later.

HYPERSPLENISM

A term applied to a number of conditions in which there is presumably overactivity of the "normal" functions of the spleen in regulating the numbers of blood cells in the circulation.

Etiology

Hypersplenism may occur with idiopathic splenomegaly ("primary hypersplenism") or with a variety of splenopathies ("secondary hypersplenism")—e.g., Gaucher's disease, rheumatoid arthritis, or cirrhosis of the liver. The occurrence, therefore, of splenomegaly with leukopenia, thrombocytopenia, or pancytopenia does not give a clue to the anatomic basis for the enlargement of the spleen.

Pathogenesis

The normal spleen probably regulates the production and delivery of red cells, granulocytes, and platelets at the bone marrow; it also destroys old red cells and, perhaps, white cells and platelets. When any of these functions becomes exaggerated, a definite hematologic syndrome follows, characterized by numerical reduction, in the blood stream, of the blood cell involved, despite excellent production of that cell in the marrow. The important clinical syndromes are as follows: exaggeration of effect on platelets—splenic thrombocytopenia; exaggeration of effect on granulocytes—splenic neutropenia; exaggeration of effect on platelets, granulocytes, and erythrocytes—splenic pancytopenia. In actual practice, these forms of hypersplenism are almost always associated with enlargement of the spleen, except in splenic thrombocytopenia. Conversely, almost any splenomegaly may give rise to hypersplenism.

Symptoms and Signs

In general, anemia produces weakness, pallor, and sometimes jaundice, if hemolysis is present. Neutropenia results in weakness, fatigue, polyarthralgia, and a tendency to recurrent and lingering infections in the lungs, pharynx, skin. Thrombocytopenia gives rise to petechiae, ecchymoses, and sometimes a frank hemorrhagic diathesis.

Splenomegaly is almost always present. If there is an underlying disease, the other symptoms and signs of that disorder also are present.

Treatment

As a rule, splenectomy results in a return of the abnormal blood values to normal, while other forms of treatment do not.

PRIMARY SPLENIC THROMBOCYTOPENIA
(Idiopathic thrombocytopenic purpura)

A form of hypersplenism which occurs when overactivity of the spleen hampers production of platelets at the bone marrow. As a result, although many megakaryocytes are present in the marrow, there are few platelets, and thrombocytopenia and purpura follow.

The disease is better known as **idiopathic thrombocytopenic purpura** and is described in the chapter on Hemorrhagic Diseases (q.v.). Splenectomy is curative in more than 85% of cases.

PRIMARY SPLENIC NEUTROPENIA

A variety of hypersplenism that occurs when overactivity of the spleen hampers delivery of granulocytes from the bone marrow. Some workers believe there also is destruction of granulocytes by the overactive spleen. As a result, there is damming back of the marrow granulocytes in the marrow (granulocytic hyperplasia) and a paucity of neutrophils in the blood stream. The etiology is unknown, but probably due to chronic infections of the spleen resulting in splenomegaly.

Symptoms and Signs

The patient becomes chronically ill, with vague symptoms such as malaise, fatigability, and polyarthralgia. Numerous mild or severe infections develop. Physical examination reveals only splenomegaly, usually of 1 to 3 fingerbreadths' extent.

Blood Findings

The red cell count and platelets are normal, but there is a marked leukopenia, 1,000 to 3,000 cells, and a neutropenia of 10 to 30%. There are no pathologic white cells in the blood smear. The bone marrow shows normal red cells and megakaryocytes and, despite the few white cells in the blood, normal or even increased numbers of mature granulocytes. In other words, there is a "block" between the marrow and blood.

Diagnosis

The disease should be suspected whenever idiopathic splenomegaly and neutropenia coexist. Diagnosis depends upon the elimination of other causes of neutropenia: e.g., leukemias, lymphomas, agranulocytosis. Chronic myelocytic leukemia usually can be ruled out by the absence, in splenic neutropenia, of anemia and thrombocytopenia; and by examination of the marrow which, in leukemia, shows reduction in megakaryocytes and disarrangement of granulocytic maturation with many early forms present. Lymphoma causes fever, high sedimentation rate, and usually pancytopenia with abnormal leukocytes in the marrow. Lymphatic leukemia shows lymphocytic infiltration of the marrow. In acute agranulocytosis (q.v.), there often is a history of exposure to a known toxic drug, and the marrow shows an absence of granulocytes—the opposite of splenic neutropenia.

Treatment

Medical therapy is of no avail: liver extract, yellow bone marrow, pentnucleotide, do not affect the neutropenia. When the diagnosis has been established, the patient may be observed for a period of weeks to months. However, remissions rarely if ever occur, and splenectomy must be done. Return of the blood values to normal and relief of symptoms may be expected in almost every case.

FELTY'S SYNDROME

A form of hypersplenism due to overactivity of the enlarged spleen in rheumatoid arthritis (q.v.).

Pathogenesis

The cause for the splenomegaly which occurs in many patients with rheumatoid arthritis is unknown. However, when the spleen does enlarge, it may—like any enlarged spleen—result in leukopenia, thrombocytopenia, or pancytopenia by its inhibitory effects on the marrow and its destructive effects on blood cells. Neutropenia may occur alone; but usually neutropenia plus thrombocytopenia, or even pancytopenia, are present. Anemia alone is a frequent manifestation of rheumatoid arthritis.

Diagnosis

In a patient with rheumatoid arthritis and splenomegaly, the occurrence of cytopenia (e.g., neutropenia) not due to medication (e.g., gold) suggests Felty's syndrome. The demonstration that the marrow production of the involved cells is normal establishes the diagnosis.

Treatment

Splenectomy is indicated for the symptoms due to the blood changes. It probably has no effect on the rheumatoid arthritis itself.

BANTI'S DISEASE

(Congestive splenomegaly with hypersplenism; Banti's syndrome; Splenic anemia)

A disorder characterized by splenomegaly, hypersplenism (leukopenia, anemia, thrombocytopenia), and cirrhosis of the liver. The term "splenic anemia" is a poor one.

According to Banti, the splenomegaly preceded the other changes and was directly responsible for them; but most investigators today doubt that this is true, or that there is a specific entity such as he described. It is probable that these cases are merely instances of splenomegaly due to congestion which is secondary to early cirrhosis of the liver or, less often, to portal or splenic vein occlusion; the reduction in the blood elements is merely the usual result of hypersplenism.

Pathogenesis

Since any splenomegaly may be followed by hypersplenism, there is no longer any justification for placing "congestive splenomegaly" in a separate category. The spleen enlarged by congestion has distant inhibitory effects upon the bone marrow, resulting in neutropenia, anemia, and thrombocytopenia, in the same manner as any enlarged spleen.

Symptoms and Signs

In the early stages, weakness, fatigue, and splenomegaly are noted. With progression, the anemia becomes severe and is aggravated by bleeding from esophageal varices that produces hematemesis and melena. Ultimately, the usual signs of hepatic cirrhosis (q.v.)—hepatomegaly itself often is present for a long time—supervene. In general, the clinical course is similar to that of cirrhosis of the liver, except that the degree of splenic enlargement is unusually great, and the symptomatology attributable to hypersplenism correspondingly more marked.

Blood Findings

Neutropenia, anemia, and thrombocytopenia—usually but not necessarily all together—are present. The anemia often is hypochromic, probably because of the additional factor of bleeding from the varices of the esophagus. The bone marrow shows normal production of red cells, granulocytes, and megakaryocytes.

Diagnosis

The diagnosis of hypersplenism can be made when cytopenia and splenomegaly coexist in the presence of normal marrow production of the involved cells, provided that other causes, especially leukemia, can be ruled out by blood and marrow studies. There are many causes for hypersplenism, and the specific diagnosis of "congestive splenomegaly" can be made only if there is evidence of cirrhosis of the liver or other causes of portal hypertension.

Treatment

When the diagnosis of congestive splenomegaly with hypersplenism has been made, splenectomy is indicated and usually is followed by a return of the blood values toward normal. The decision to operate depends largely on the medical condition of the patient. Splenectomy has no effect on the hepatic cirrhosis, which must be treated separately. Nor does it have any beneficial effect on the esophageal varices, which must be treated by other surgical procedures.

OTHER HYPERSPLENIC SYNDROMES

Hypersplenism often is seen with Gaucher's disease, splenic sarcoidosis, sarcoma of the spleen, and a variety of other splenomegalic states. If the blood abnormality causes symptoms, splenectomy may be undertaken, provided that the general condition of the patient and the nature of the disease causing the splenomegaly do not contraindicate the operation. As a general rule, one does not remove the spleen which is enlarged by leukemia, Hodgkin's disease, or other lymphomatous processes.

ANATOMIC DISORDERS OF THE SPLEEN

Enlargement of the spleen usually is an indication of a more basic, widespread disease. Because treatment of splenomegaly is the treatment of the underlying disorder, it is of prime importance to diagnose the cause correctly before attempting therapy. The several causes of splenomegaly are discussed below.

INFECTIONS

1. Acute infections: Typhoid fever, malaria, infectious mononucleosis, subacute bacterial endocarditis, secondary syphilis, lymphohematogenous tuberculosis, kala-azar, measles, brucellosis. The splenomegaly in these conditions needs no treatment, and in most cases disappears after the acute infection has subsided. Treatment is directed at the underlying disease.

2. Chronic infections: Tuberculosis, syphilis, leishmaniasis, schistosomiasis, malaria. In these cases, too, treatment must be directed at the basic disorder, for the splenomegaly is not of fundamental importance. Occasionally, hypersplenism complicates the splenomegaly and results in symptoms (e.g., severe neutropenia with weakness; thrombocytopenia with bleeding; hemolytic anemia), and in such cases splenectomy may be expected to relieve the corresponding hematologic abnormalities. Each case, however, must be individualized before operation is undertaken.

3. Infection-like states: Rheumatoid arthritis and Boeck's sarcoid frequently result in splenomegaly. No treatment is indicated for the spleen, however, except in certain instances in which complicating hypersplenism occurs. Splenic amyloidosis may complicate any chronic infection.

CONGESTIVE SPLENOMEGALY

Chronic splenic congestion occurs in cirrhosis of the liver, and in thrombosis of the portal or splenic veins. In general, no treatment directed at the spleen is indicated, unless hypersplenism produces symptoms.

RETICULO-ENDOTHELIAL INFILTRATION

Deposition of lipid material within the cells of the reticulo-endothelial system results in enlargement of liver and especially spleen. This type of disorder includes Gaucher's disease (kerasin within the cells), Niemann-Pick's disease (sphingomyelin), and Hand-Schüller-Christian's disease (cholesterol). In all these conditions, there is involvement of reticulo-endothelial cells throughout the body, and the splenomegaly is incidental to a widespread disease. No treatment of these splenomegalies is indicated. In occasional cases of Gaucher's disease, splenectomy may be done for either (1) hypersplenism or (2) mechanical difficulties due to the tremendous bulk. Splenectomy has no effect on the underlying disease process.

EXCESSIVE DESTRUCTION OF BLOOD CELLS
(Hemolytic anemia)

Since red cells are destroyed within the reticulo-endothelial system, and since the spleen constitutes a large portion of the reticulo-endothelial system, anything which causes an excessive number of red cells to be destroyed usually results in splenomegaly. This is true for the various familial hemolytic anemias —familial spherocytic hemolytic anemia, Mediterranean anemia, sickle cell anemia—and for the various acquired hemolytic anemias.

In general, the spleen is not the fundamental cause of these disorders. In Mediterranean and sickle cell anemias, for example, there are developmental defects of the red cells which may render them more easily destroyed than normally. Splenectomy, although it reduces the amount of hemolysis through removal of a large part of the reticulo-endothelial system, does not affect the character of the red cells, and therefore has no effect on the other symptoms and signs of these disorders.

In familial spherocytosis (congenital hemolytic anemia, congenital acholuric jaundice), however, splenectomy, by eliminating virtually all signs of blood destruction, results in clinical and hematologic "cure," although the spherocytosis persists. In acquired hemolytic anemias, splenectomy cures about 60% of the patients. In the special form of acquired hemolytic anemia which seems to be due to excessive destruction of normal red cells by a hyperactive spleen (hypersplenic hemolytic anemia), splenectomy is curative in some 80% of the cases.

EXCESSIVE PROLIFERATION OF CELLS

Splenomegaly occurs in acute and chronic leukemias and in the lymphomas, such as giant follicle lymphoma, lymphosarcoma, Hodgkin's disease. In all these disorders, the enlargement of the spleen merely is an incident in a widespread disease. The diagnosis of the particular type of disorder present often depends ultimately upon histologic study of an enlarged lymph node, or of the spleen itself. In general, treatment consists of radiotherapy: the spleen shrinks because the malignant cells are preferentially destroyed by irradiation. As a rule, no other therapy directed at the spleen itself is indicated.

EXCESSIVE PRODUCTION OF CELLS

When the marrow becomes fibrotic or sclerotic, the spleen may take up the function of producing the various blood cells, and in so doing become enlarged. This extramedullary hemopoiesis is called "myeloid metaplasia" of the spleen, and is a contraindication to any form of therapy including X-ray or surgery directed at the organ, for the bulk of hemopoiesis goes on in these diseases.

In polycythemia vera (q.v.), enlargement of the spleen is common, at first perhaps because of congestion, but ultimately because of extramedullary hemopoiesis. Again, splenectomy is not indicated; but treatment of the polycythemia vera by phlebotomies, radioactive phosphorus, nitrogen mustard, and spray X-ray, may result in diminution of spleen size.

SPLENIC TUMORS

True tumors of the spleen are very rare, and range from cysts to localized malignant processes. The diagnosis may be considered when splenomegaly is completely unexplained after blood and marrow studies. Splenectomy is indicated if the diagnosis is made.

Diagnosis in Splenomegaly

The diagnosis is based upon the combination of history, physical examination, and laboratory studies; and sometimes depends upon the course during observation of the patient.

Familial splenomegaly occurs in congenital spherocytic anemia and in Gaucher's disease. A history of rheumatoid arthritis, cirrhosis of the liver, malaria, or granulomatous infection may suggest the etiology. On physical examination, the combination of splenomegaly with lymphadenopathy should suggest a malignant process, such as leukemia, Hodgkin's disease, or giant follicle lymphoma. Splenomegaly with an enlarged liver occurs in some of these lymphomas, but also in cirrhosis of the liver. Splenomegaly alone follows old malaria, occurs in Gaucher's disease and in Boeck's sarcoid, and is found in true splenic tumors, but sometimes may occur in the lymphomatous processes. It often is unexplained.

Studies of the blood and marrow may give a clue to the cause of the splenomegaly, as in leukemia, or in Gaucher's disease. On the other hand, the enlarged spleen itself may result in the changes associated with hypersplenism.

If these measures have not led to a diagnosis, the patient often can be followed for a period of time. Sometimes lymphadenopathy occurs, and biopsy is diagnostic. Shrinkage of the spleen following therapeutic trial with X-ray suggests a lymphomatous process. Occasionally, because of severe hypersplenism, splenectomy becomes necessary, and the diagnosis is made from the surgical specimen.

Treatment of Splenic Disease

Irradiation, supervised by someone experienced in the procedure, is indicated in malignant splenopathies: leukemia, lymphosarcoma, Hodgkin's disease, giant follicle lymphoma. Irradiation is aimed at the entire disease process, not merely the splenic involvement. Forms of irradiation other than X-ray, such as radioactive phosphorus (P^{32}), are sometimes used. Mechlorethamine, a nitrogen mustard, is especially effective in Hodgkin's disease (q.v.).

Splenectomy is indicated in various splenopathies. It is mandatory and urgent if traumatic splenic rupture has occurred. It is urgent, and should be done with little delay, in idiopathic thrombocytopenic purpura and in acute hemolytic crises. It is less urgent, but essential, in familial spherocytic anemia, primary splenic neutropenia or pancytopenia, splenic cysts, splenic tumors, splenic abscesses, and the splenomegalies of secondary hypersplenism (rheumatoid arthritis, Gaucher's disease, Boeck's sarcoid). It is of little value, but not contraindicated, in Mediterranean anemia, sickle cell anemia, and in some very bulky spleens. It is contraindicated in myeloid metaplasia of the spleen, in most instances of leukemia, lymphomas, and infectious splenomegalies.

The patient in whom splenomegaly is accidentally discovered and who, after a thorough investigation, is found to have no demonstrable cause of splenomegaly, may be followed indefinitely without therapy. Intervention is unnecessary unless complicating hypersplenic states occur.

PRESCRIPTIONS

(Wherever a prescribed "proprietary" is representative of a class of therapeutic agents, alternative proprietary preparations will be found listed in Part II.)

Hematinics

1. ℞ Iron and ammonium citrate . .30.0   Gm. (ℨ i)
       Distilled water q.s. ad. . . . 120.0   cc. (ℨ iv)
        2 teaspoons 3 times daily after meals.

2. ℞ Ferrous sulfate . . . . 0.2   Gm. (gr. iii)
        1 to 3 tablets 3 times daily after meals.

3. ℞ Ferrous gluconate. . . . . . . 0.3   Gm. (gr. v)
        1 capsule 3 times daily after meals.

4. ℞ Ferrous carbonate . . . . 0.3   Gm. (gr. v)
        1 or 2 capsules 3 times daily after meals.

5. ℞ Ferrous chloride . . . . 6.0   Gm.   (ℨ iss)
     Syrup U.S.P. . . . . .30.0   cc.   (ℨ i)
     Chloroform Water N.F. q.s. ad 120.0   cc.   (ℨ iv)
       1 teaspoon in milk 3 times daily after meals.

6. ℞ Ferrous sulfate . . . . 3.0   Gm.   (gr. xlv)
     Dextrose. . . . . 30.0   Gm.   (ℨ i)
     Chloroform Water N.F. q.s. ad 120.0   cc.   (ℨ iv)
       1 teaspoon 3 times daily after meals.

7. ℞ Ferrous Sulfate Syrup N.F. . 60.0   cc.   (ℨ ii)
       Infants: 15 to 30 drops 2 or 3 times a day
       after meals.

8. ℞ Ferrous gluconate, 5% elixir . 60.0   cc.   (ℨ ii)
       Infants: 15 drops daily after meals.

9. ℞ Liver Injection (Crude) U.S.P.
     (vial)
       Administer I.M. according to schedule given
       in text.

10. ℞ Liver Injection U.S.P. (vial)
       Administer I.M. according to schedule given
       in text.

11. ℞ Liver Solution U.S.P.
       1 or more U.S.P. u. daily by mouth.

12. ℞ Powdered Stomach U.S.P.
     (bulk powder)
       1 or more U.S.P. u. daily by mouth.

13. ℞ Pteroylglutamic (folic) acid. . . 5   mg.
       1 tablet daily.

14. ℞ Pteroylglutamic (folic) acid
     (vial)
       15 to 40 mg. I.M. daily.

15. ℞ Pentnucleotide (vial)
       10 to 20 cc. I.M. twice daily for 4 or 5 days.

16. ℞ Adenine sulfate (sterile powder)
       Dissolve 1 Gm. in 30 cc. of Sterile Isotonic
       Sodium Chloride Solution for Parenteral Use
       U.S.P. and administer I.V. 3 times daily for
       3 days.

Antihemic Agents

17. ℞ Phenylhydrazine hydrochloride . 0.1   Gm.   (gr. iss)
       1 or 2 capsules daily. (Maximum total dose
       is 10 capsules.)

18. ℞ Acetyl-phenylhydrazine . . . . 0.1   Gm.   (gr. iss)

    1 or 2 capsules daily. (Maximum total dose is 10 capsules.)

19. ℞ Mechlorethamine hydrochloride
    (Nitrogen mustard)   (vial)

    0.1 mg./Kg. body wt. administered rapidly I.V. once or twice daily for 4 to 6 doses.

20. ℞ Urethane (Ethyl carbamate) . . 0.5   Gm.   (gr. viiss)

    2 to 4 capsules 3 times daily; maintenance dose is 1 to 6 capsules daily.

21. ℞ Potassium Arsenite Solution
    U.S.P. (Fowler's Solution) . 120.0   cc.   (℥ iv)

    5 drops in water 3 times daily, the dose being gradually increased as directed for the treatment of leukemia (q.v.).

Hemostatics

22. ℞ Calcium gluconate, 10% solution
    (ampul) . . . . 1.0   Gm.   (gr. xv)

    Contents of 1 ampul I.V. to combat any effects due to excessive citrate injection.

23. ℞ Moccasin snake venom   (vial)

    0.25 cc. (♏ iv) subcut. once or twice weekly, gradually increasing the dose (if tolerated) to 2 cc. in courses of 3 to 4 weeks, repeated after a similar period of rest.

24. ℞ Parathyroid Injection U.S.P.
    (vial)

    100 to 300 u. subcut. or I.M. twice a week.

25. ℞ Epinephrine hydrochloride, 1:1,000
    solution

    Soak pledget of gauze or cotton in solution and apply with pressure to local bleeding point.

26. ℞ Rutin 20   mg.

    3 to 15 tablets daily.

27. ℞ Thrombin, topical   (ampul)

    Apply to the bleeding site as the dry powder or in sterile saline solution containing 20 to 100 u./cc. (CAUTION! Thrombin must never be injected.)

28. ℞ Fibrin Foam N.N.R.

    Moisten the necessary amount of fibrin foam in a sterile solution of thrombin containing 20 to 100 u./cc. (℞ 27) and apply to bleeding site.

29. ℞ Absorbable Gelatin Sponge N.N.R.

> Saturate the gelatin sponge in a sterile thrombin solution containing 20 to 100 u./cc. (℞ 27) and apply to bleeding site.

30. ℞ Oxidized Cellulose N.N.R.

> Apply with pressure to site of bleeding.

31. ℞ Protamine sulfate, 1% solution
    (ampul)

> 5 to 10 cc. (50 to 100 mg.) I.V., administered in 500 cc. of Sterile Isotonic Sodium Chloride Solution for Parenteral Use U.S.P.

Vitamins

32. ℞ "Cobione" (Crystalline Vitamin B_{12})   (ampul)

> Administer subcut. or I.M., according to schedule given in text. (*See* Pernicious Anemia.)

33. ℞ Dried Yeast U.S.P. . . . . . . 0.5   Gm. (gr. viiss)

> 1 or 2 tablets 3 times daily.

34. ℞ Pyridoxine hydrochloride
    (Vitamin B_6) 25   mg.

> 4 to 8 tablets immediately before radiation therapy.

35. ℞ Pyridoxine hydrochloride
    (Vitamin B_6)   (ampul)

> 100 mg. I.V. or I.M. immediately before radiation therapy; when used in conjunction with mechlorethamine (nitrogen mustard) (℞ 19), it is given after, never before, the drug.

36. ℞ Ascorbic acid 25   mg.

> 2 to 12 tablets daily.

37. ℞ Menadione 2   mg.

> 2 to 6 tablets daily.

38. ℞ Menadione sodium bisulfite
    (ampul)

> 2 to 5 mg. I.M. daily.

Antimicrobial Agents

39. ℞ Penicillin   (vial)

> 50,000 u. or more I.M. every 3 hours.

40. ℞ Sulfadiazine . . . . 0.5   Gm. (gr. viiss)

> 2 tablets every 4 hours.

41. ℞ Sulfamerazine . . . . 0.5   Gm. (gr. viiss)

> 2 tablets every 6 to 8 hours.

Analgesics and Sedatives

42. ℞ Acetylsalicylic acid . . . . . . 0.3   Gm. (gr. v)
      2 tablets every 4 hours for pain.

43. ℞ Codeine phosphate (hypodermic
      tablet). 30   mg.   (gr. ss)
      1 tablet orally or subcut. every 4 to 6 hours
      for pain.

44. ℞ "Demerol Hydrochloride" . .   50   mg.
      1 tablet every 6 hours for pain.

45. ℞ "Demerol Hydrochloride"
      (ampul)
      50 mg. I.M. every 4 hours for pain.

46. ℞ Methadone Hydrochloride
      N.N.R. 5   mg.
      1 tablet every 4 hours for pain.

47. ℞ Morphine sulfate
      15 mg. (gr. ¼) subcut., every 4 hours for pain.

48. ℞ Phenobarbital 15   mg.   (gr. ¼)
      1 or 2 tablets 3 times daily.

49. ℞ Phenobarbital sodium   (ampul)
      60 to 100 mg. (gr. i to iss) I.M. at bedtime.

Antipruritics

50. ℞ Menthol. . . . . 0.3   Gm. (gr. v)
      Phenol. . . . . 1.0   Gm. (gr. xv)
      Zinc oxide . . . . 20.0   Gm. (℥ v)
      Talc. . . . . 20.0   Gm. (℥ v)
      Glycerin. . . . . 15.0   cc.   (℥ ss)
      Ethyl alcohol, 50% q.s. ad 120.0   cc.   (℥ iv)
      Apply to pruritic areas as necessary.

51. ℞ Menthol. . . . . 0.3   Gm. (gr. v)
      Benzocaine. . . . . 6.0   Gm. (℥ iss)
      Solution of Coal Tar N.F. . . 12.0   cc.   (℥ iii)
      Zinc oxide . . . . 20.0   Gm. (℥ v)
      Talc. . . . . 20.0   Gm. (℥ v)
      Glycerin. . . . . 15.0   cc.   (℥ ss)
      Water. . . . . q.s. ad 120.0   cc.   (℥ iv)
      Apply to pruritic areas as necessary.

52. ℞ Benzocaine, 5% ointment . . 60.0   Gm. (℥ ii)
      Apply to pruritic areas as necessary.

53. ℞ Menthol. . . . . 0.2   Gm. (gr. iii)
    Phenol. . . . . 0.3   Gm. (gr. v)
    Solution of Coal Tar N.F. . . . 6.0   cc.   (℥ iss)
    Hydrophilic Ointment
      U.S.P. . . . . . . q.s. ad 60.0   Gm. (℥ ii)
        Apply to pruritic areas as necessary.

Oral Antiseptics and Anesthetics

54. ℞ Hydrogen Peroxide Solution
     U.S.P.
      Dilute with an equal volume of water and use
      as a mouthwash 3 times daily.

55. ℞ Sodium perborate, 2%
     solution . . . . 1,000.0   cc.   (℥ xxxii)
      Use as a mouthwash 3 times daily.

56. ℞ Potassium chlorate, 2%
     solution. . . . . 120.0   cc.   (℥ iv)
      Spray or apply to oral lesions twice daily.

57. ℞ Sodium chloride . . . . 4.0   Gm. (℥ i)
    Warm water. . . . . q.s. ad 240.0   cc.   (℥ viii)
      Use as a mouthwash as necessary.

58. ℞ Benzocaine (lozenges)
      Dissolve 1 lozenge on the tongue every 3 or
      4 hours.

Miscellaneous

59. ℞ Diluted Hydrochloric Acid
     U.S.P. . . . . 180.0   cc.   (℥ vi)
      1 or 2 teaspoons in ½ glass of water with each
      meal; should be sipped through a glass straw
      during meals.

60. ℞ Caffeine and Sodium Benzoate
     Injection U.S.P. (ampul) . . 0.5   Gm. (gr. viiss)
      Contents of 1 ampul I.M.; repeat in 1 hour if
      necessary.

61. ℞ "Mecholyl Bromide"
      Administer by iontophoresis (see CLIN. PROC.)
      as a 0.2 to 0.5% solution in distilled water.

CARDIOVASCULAR

CONGENITAL ANOMALIES

Anomalies of the circulation due to embryonic defects in development during the period when the heart and great vessels are formed from the primitive vascular tube. Accordingly, any one or combination of anomalous defects is possible, depending on the stage at which normal development was altered.

A simple classification of congenital anomalies appears below, but only the more common anomalies will be discussed in this chapter.

A. **Cyanotic group**
1. Without pulmonary hypertension
   Tetralogy of Fallot.
   Tricuspid stenosis.
   Single ventricle with pulmonary stenosis.
2. With pulmonary hypertension
   Eisenmenger's complex.
   Transposition of great vessels.
   Truncus arteriosus.

B. **Acyanotic group**
1. Coarctation of the aorta.
2. Patent ductus arteriosus.
3. Subaortic stenosis.
4. Vascular rings.

C. **Tardive cyanosis group**
1. Interventricular septal defect.
2. Interauricular septal defect.

Diagnosis

The principal clinical diagnostic methods are physical examination, fluoroscopy and X-ray, and ECG. The physiologic tests include catheterization of the chambers of the heart and angiocardiography (X-ray following I.V. injection of a radiopaque substance).

Principles of Management and Medical Treatment

The clinical course and prognosis in congenital heart disease will vary, depending on the location and extent of the lesion or lesions, from that of individuals who live a full span of years with no symptoms to that of infants who survive only a few hours or days. In general, cases with cyanosis have a much poorer prognosis than those without cyanosis.

In **acyanotic** individuals, those with interventricular septal defects, small interauricular defects, or a small patent ductus arteriosus are frequently without symptoms. When the lesions are more extensive, the earliest sign in childhood often is a retardation of growth and development, perhaps coupled with easy fatigue and slight exertional dyspnea. Such children should be protected from overstrain and should receive special dietary care. Definite symptoms, such as palpitation, dyspnea, and weakness may be present early in life, and these will become more severe in later years. As symptoms increase, activity must be further restricted, with treatment for congestive heart failure (q.v.) if the latter supervenes.

In **cyanotic** patients, early symptoms will be similar, with the addition of cyanosis. The anoxia in such cases may lead to periods of unconsciousness. General treatment is the same as for the acyanotic group. In advanced stages O_2 therapy may be tried, but marked relief cannot be expected since the chief defect is due to shunting of venous blood directly to the arterial side, and not to failure of aeration of that blood which does pass through the lungs. In cases with increased pulmonary blood flow and true pulmonary congestion, on the other hand, O_2 therapy may be helpful. If polycythemia and increased blood volume are prominent features, phlebotomy may be beneficial for adults or grown children; 500 to 750 cc. every month or two. This procedure usually does not help in infants, and may cause collapse. Fluid intake is extremely important if polycythemia is present; dehydration of a mild degree may precipitate cerebral thromboses.

TETRALOGY OF FALLOT

A not uncommon congenital cardiac anomaly in which the malformation consists of pulmonic stenosis, ventricular septal defect just below the aorta, an aorta which overrides both right and left ventricles, and hypertrophy of the right ventricle.

Pathologic Physiology

The low O_2 saturation of the arterial blood and the cyanosis in this condition are the result of intracardiac admixture of venous blood of low O_2 saturation with pulmonary vein blood of high O_2 saturation. Insufficient gas exchange through the lung, or a decrease in pulmonary blood flow alone is not responsible for the anoxemia. Catheterization of the heart reveals an elevation of the right ventricular blood pressure and a relative decrease in the pulmonary arterial pressure. The blood flow through the pulmonary artery is reduced, the overall direction of the intracardiac shunt is from right to left.

Symptoms and Signs

Cyanosis of varying intensity and clubbing of the fingers and toes are usually present from early infancy. Physical development is frequently retarded. By far the majority of these persons die at puberty. The cyanosis is generally most marked in the lips, the mucous membranes, and the nail beds. There is advanced polycythemia, with red blood cell counts up to 10,000,000; blood volume is also greatly increased. History discloses some decrease in exercise tolerance and, in severe cases, spells of unconsciousness brought about by cerebral anoxemia.

The rough systolic murmur and thrill of pulmonic stenosis is noted over the 3rd and 4th interspaces to the left of the sternum. The ECG shows right axis deviation. On fluoroscopic examination the pulmonary conus is seen to be absent in the anterior-posterior position. Pulsations in the lung field are absent.

Treatment

An artificial ductus is constructed surgically between one of the pulmonary and one of the subclavian arteries to increase the flow of blood through the lung. The optimal age for this operation ranges from 4 to 12 years. The reported operative mortality ranges from 12 to 18%.

EISENMENGER'S COMPLEX

A congenital cardiac anomaly in which the malformation is identical with that present in the tetralogy of Fallot, except that pulmonic stenosis is absent.

Pathologic Physiology

In contrast to tetralogy of Fallot, intracardiac catheterization reveals hypertension in the pulmonary artery as well as in the right ventricle. As in the tetralogy of Fallot, the cyanosis and anoxemia encountered in Eisenmenger's complex are the result of intracardiac admixture (right to left) of unsaturated with fully oxygenated blood.

Symptoms and Signs

The history and symptoms are similar to those described in patients with tetralogy of Fallot. However, cyanosis develops later in life, often after the age of 10, and the life expectancy is much longer, usually to the 4th decade. In some cases, the history reveals hemoptyses resulting from pulmonary hypertension. A systolic murmur is heard over the entire precordium. The ECG shows right axis deviation. The X-ray and fluoroscopic findings demonstrate enlargement of the pulmonary artery and vascular pulsations in the lung fields. Definitive diagnosis of this condition is often impossible without physiologic diagnostic procedures.

Treatment

There is no surgical or specific medical treatment for Eisenmenger's complex.

COARCTATION OF THE AORTA

A localized constriction of the aorta occurring at or below the entrance of the obliterated ductus arteriosus, usually just distal to the origin of the left subclavian artery.

Pathologic Physiology

The cardiac output is normal. There is marked elevation of the systolic pressure and slight rise in the diastolic pressure in the arm. The systolic pressure in the leg is reduced but the diastolic pressure in that extremity is only slightly decreased. The blood flow through the leg is less than the flow through the arm. There is extensive collateral circulation to the lower extremities originating primarily from branches of the subclavian artery.

Symptoms and Signs

The history may reveal persistent headaches which are the result of the arterial hypertension. The age of onset of symptoms depends upon the severity of the aortic constriction and the ability of the patient to develop good collateral circulation. In individuals with severe coarctation and insufficient circulation, numbness and weakness in the legs are observed. Most of the clinical signs result from the collateral circulation. The retinal arteries are markedly tortuous. There are pulsations in the interscapular region, at the angle of the scapula, and in the supraclavicular fossa. Murmurs are audible in the interscapular region and over the abdomen. Notching or "scalloping" under the lower edges of the ribs, as revealed by X-ray, results from the increased size, elongation, and tortuosity of the intercostal arteries. Under the fluoroscope, enlargement of the left ventricle is observed. In the left anterior oblique position the shadow cast by the ascending aorta is particularly wide. In contrast, the descending aorta is difficult to visualize. Of greatest diagnostic importance, however, is the inequality of the pulses and of the pressures between the upper and lower extremities.

Treatment

Surgical treatment of this condition is imperative in most cases since 75% of the patients with coarctation die before the age of 40. The procedure consists of an excision of the stenosed area and an end to end anastomosis between the proximal and distal aortic stumps. The over-all mortality of this operation is reported as being less than 10%.

PATENT DUCTUS ARTERIOSUS

A persistent communication between the aorta and the pulmonary artery. Normally, this communication undergoes obliteration shortly after birth, but patent ductus arteriosus is one of the more common congenital heart lesions.

Pathologic Physiology

Blood under high aortic pressure is forced with each systole through the patent ductus into the relatively low pressure pulmonary arterial system. The output of the left ventricle exceeds that of the right.

Symptoms and Signs

A continuous "machinery" murmur, during both systole and diastole, best heard to the left of the cardiac border, is characteristic. The second pulmonic sound is loud. The difference between the arterial systolic and diastolic pressures is usually greater than normal. Fluoroscopic examination reveals an accentuation of the pulmonary conus as well as marked pulsating vascular lung markings. The main complications of this malformation are cardiac failure and subacute bacterial endocarditis, the vegetations usually being limited to the patent ductus itself.

Treatment

Ligation and excision of the ductus represent the treatment of choice. The optimal age for the operation ranges from 4 to 10 years. A complicating subacute bacterial endocarditis (q.v.) should receive appropriate therapy both before and after surgery.

VENTRICULAR SEPTAL DEFECT
(Maladie de Roger)

The most common congenital circulatory anomaly, the defect in the interventricular septum being usually near the apex of the heart, and either large or small in size.

Pathologic Physiology

Oxygenated blood from the left ventricle is forced into the right ventricle during systole. As a result, pulmonary blood flow is greater than systemic blood flow. In occasional instances, the pressure in the right ventricle may become high enough so that right ventricular (venous) blood passes during systole into the left ventricle. Cyanosis then occurs (tardive cyanosis).

Symptoms and Signs

Symptoms occur only if the lesion is severe, as indicated in general considerations above. The characteristic physical sign is a loud blowing systolic murmur heard all over the precordium, maximal over the center of the heart. The second pulmonic sound is increased. The right ventricle is enlarged and the pulmonary conus is prominent by fluoroscopy. Hilar shadows are increased and may pulsate visibly (hilar dance) if pulmonary hypertension is present. Ordinarily the fluoroscopic examination is normal. The ECG is not diagnostic.

Treatment

There is no treatment, but the life expectancy is normal, unless pulmonary hypertension develops.

AURICULAR SEPTAL DEFECT

A defect, usually quite large, which is a true congenital failure of development of the interauricular septum, and not a patent foramen ovale.

Pathologic Physiology

There is a large flow of blood from the left auricle into the right auricle, causing a greatly increased blood flow through the pulmonary circulation as compared with the systemic circuit. A mild or moderate cyanosis due to some backflow of blood, from right to left, during part of the cardiac cycle, also is not uncommon in this condition. Pulmonary congestion may contribute to the cyanosis.

Symptoms and Signs

There may be no symptoms, but palpitation and dyspnea are more common than in ventricular septal defect. There usually is a fairly loud blowing systolic murmur over the base of the heart. The second pulmonic sound is increased. In advanced cases this may be followed by the diastolic murmur of pulmonic valvular insufficiency (Graham Steell murmur). The right ventricle and pulmonary conus are markedly enlarged. The pulmonary arteries also are apt to be very large, sometimes with true aneurysmal dilatations. Hilar dance is striking. The ECG may show high P waves and there usually is right axis deviation.

Increased pulmonary blood flow may lead to pulmonary congestion, with rales at lung bases, cough, and chronic bronchitis. Polycythemia and increased blood volume are not infrequent; phlebotomy may help such patients. Digitalis is indicated for decompensation and paroxysmal auricular tachycardia, the latter being a not uncommon complication.

OTHER VASCULAR ANOMALIES

The aorta may arise from the right primitive arch instead of the left. The descending aorta may be on either the right or left. If the aorta is entirely on the right, as is found in about 25% of tetralogy of Fallot cases, there are no symptoms. However, in cases in which the aorta courses posteriorly to the esophagus and trachea and descends on the left, a syndrome known as dysphagia lusoria is often seen. In these cases stridor, dysphagia and persistent cough are prominent symptoms and are caused by compression of the esophagus and trachea. The constriction actually is due to a small anterior left aortic arch, a patent ductus arteriosus, or ligamentum arteriosum, or an anomalous subclavian artery. Diagnosis is made by means of fluoroscopic and bronchoscopic examination. Complete relief may be obtained by surgical division of the constricting structure. If symptoms develop in infancy, surgical intervention is imperative, because of the danger of pulmonary complications.

CORONARY ARTERY DISEASE .

Narrowing or occlusion of the coronary arteries, usually due to arteriosclerosis, resulting in myocardial ischemia with subsequent myocardial damage and impairment of cardiac function.

Etiology

Arteriosclerosis (q.v.) is the most common cause of coronary artery disease. The exact cause of the arteriosclerosis is unknown, although it appears to be related to hypertensive vascular disease, diabetes mellitus, old age and vasomotor instability. Coronary arteriosclerosis may be localized in the coronaries or be part of a general arteriosclerosis. Less common causes of coronary artery disease are syphilitic and rheumatic arteritis, and coronary ostial obstruction associated with aortitis; embolism; periarteritis nodosa; and congenital cardiovascular anomalies.

Incidence

Coronary artery disease is essentially a disease of middle and old age. It is more than 3 times as frequent in males as in females and has a definite familial tendency. Approximately 90% of the cases occur in the 6th to 8th decades of life. However, the disease is being recognized with increasing frequency in the younger age groups. As many as 2% of the cases occur before the age of 30. Coronary occlusive disease is found occasionally in infants and children.

Pathogenesis

Coronary artery disease in itself does not necessarily produce clinical manifestations. It is only when the damage becomes severe enough to cause a critical deficit of blood supply in proportion to myocardial demand that symptoms occur. Such a disproportion can come about through either a diminution in blood supply below a critical level, or an increase in demand rising above that level. The clinical syndrome that develops depends upon the size and location of the myocardial region inadequately supplied with blood, the severity of the deficiency, its rate of development and its duration. Angina pectoris (q.v.) results from a short period of relatively mild ischemia. Myocardial infarction (q.v.) results from severe and prolonged ischemia in a more localized portion of the myocardium—often from occlusion of one of the larger coronary arteries.

ANGINA PECTORIS
(Anginal syndrome)

A characteristic thoracic pain, usually substernal, precipitated chiefly by exercise or emotion, relieved by vasodilator drugs and a few minutes' rest, and resulting from a moderate inadequacy of the coronary circulation.

Acute coronary insufficiency or **coronary failure** are terms often used to describe a syndrome characterized by prolonged substernal pain, usually not relieved by vasodilators or a short period of rest, and due to a more severe inadequacy of the coronary circulation. The symptoms in this condition are more intense and prolonged than in angina pectoris, but abnormal ECG and other laboratory findings associated with myocardial infarctions (q.v.) are absent.

Etiology and Pathogenesis

The anginal syndrome is caused by a temporary inability of the coronary arteries to supply sufficient oxygenated blood to the heart muscle. An adequate blood supply to the myocardium is needed to provide the materials used in producing the chemical energy which is converted into contractile myocardial stress. Although this conversion may occur under anaerobic conditions, new material to supply subsequent chemical energy is continually reformed during cardiac diastole through an oxidative process. An adequate flow of blood through the myocardium is needed, therefore, to supply oxygen (O_2) for the oxidative process and to carry away the products of combustion.

The pain of angina pectoris is thought to be due to stimulation of afferent nerve endings in the myocardium by the accumulation of unoxidized metabolic products resulting from myocardial anoxia.

Coronary insufficiency is a relative state and may be induced by any factor that increases the O_2 demand of the heart or decreases the coronary blood flow. A restricted circulation due to arteriosclerotic coronary narrowing, plus a slight increase in O_2 demand on mild exertion may precipitate an anginal attack. Conversely, a large increase in O_2 demand due to severe exertion in the presence of mild coronary artery disease also may precipitate an attack. Spasmodic contraction of the coronary arteries on a neurogenic basis may be responsible, especially if the work of the heart is increased. Other underlying factors causing reduced coronary blood flow include aortic insufficiency resulting in incomplete coronary filling as a consequence of low diastolic pressure, and lesions of the first portion of the aorta which obstruct the entrance of blood into the coronary ostia. A relative myocardial ischemia may result from increased O_2 demand (as during extreme exertion, hyperthyroidism, or a bout of paroxysmal tachycardia); or from cardiac hypertrophy and increased work of the heart without parallel increase in the coronary circulation (as in hypertensive and valvular heart disease). In the presence of severe anemia or in a rarefied atmosphere, the coronary circulation may be unable to maintain the necessary O_2 tension in the myocardial tissue.

A patient with chronic coronary insufficiency due to any of the above causes may be asymptomatic because his coronary blood flow is not sufficiently embarrassed to cause myocardial anoxia; however, in such an individual an anginal attack may be precipitated by any condition that places additional strain on the heart, e.g., physical exertion as in ascending stairs or walking against the wind, coitus, excitement, or ingesting a heavy meal. Cessation of the activity usually relieves the pain through reducing the O_2 demand of the myocardium. Attacks sometimes occur, however, during rest or sleep (angina decubitus).

Pathology

The characteristic findings are twofold: diseased coronary arteries and resultant myocardial damage. Atheromatous narrowing, or an old complete occlusion of one of the major coronary arteries is usual. Arteriosclerotic, syphilitic, or rheumatic lesions of the first portion of the aorta involving the coronary ostia may be present. In rare instances no abnormalities of the coronary arteries are to be found. The pathologic myocardial changes usually, but not invariably, present are caused by partial anoxemia and ischemia. Scattered areas of myocardial fibrosis and cardiac dilatation and hypertrophy are due to the impaired myocardial nutrition. Not infrequently, myocardial changes are absent on postmortem examination.

Symptoms and Signs

Pain in the chest is the outstanding clinical manifestation. Its location, distribution, type, and duration, and its relation to increased cardiac work are characteristic. The distress is usually localized behind the sternum, and only rarely in the apical region or left anterior axillary line. Occasionally it is located in the neck, shoulder, or epigastrium. It frequently radiates to the left shoulder, thence down the left arm to the elbow, or even as far as the finger tips—uncommonly, to the right shoulder and arm.

The pain may be called more appropriately a feeling of oppression or distress, and is usually described as a squeezing, crushing, or viselike sensation, rather than as sharp or knifelike in character. The intensity varies from mild substernal discomfort to severe and incapacitating distress. The typical seizure lasts only a few minutes. Exceptionally, an attack may persist as long as 30 to 60 minutes, and if accompanied by circulatory collapse it is highly suggestive of myocardial infarction (q.v.). The patient usually relates the attack to exertion, overeating, or an emotional upset, and notes that it disappears with rest. Other symptoms at times associated are palpitation, faintness and dizziness, dyspnea and digestive disturbances.

There are no physical findings typical of angina pectoris. The objective signs vary with the nature of the underlying disorder. Hypertension, cardiac enlargement, valvular heart disease, cardiac arrhythmias, and peripheral arteriosclerosis are not uncommon. In as many as 25% of the cases, however, no cardiovascular abnormalities can be detected on physical examination.

Clinical Course and Complications

The frequency and duration of the attacks are extremely variable. The clinical course depends upon the degree of coronary insufficiency, the development of a collateral coronary circulation, the response to treatment and the occurrence of complications. The attacks may vary in frequency from several daily to occasional seizures separated by symptom-free intervals of weeks, months, or years. The attacks may increase in frequency and severity to a fatal outcome, or may gradually decrease or disappear entirely if an adequate collateral coronary circulation develops. Also, if congestive heart failure supervenes, the anginal attacks tend to disappear.

The complications in angina pectoris result either from prolonged myocardial anoxia, or directly from the underlying etiologic disorder. Cardiac dilatation with subsequent congestive heart failure may be caused by myocardial fibrosis. Myocardial infarction following thrombosis in a sclerotic coronary artery also is a common complication. Cerebral and renal complications of associated hypertensive vascular disease or generalized arteriosclerosis, and congestive heart failure in associated valvular heart disease are frequent terminal events.

Laboratory Findings

The laboratory workup often is of little or no aid in establishing a diagnosis of coronary insufficiency. Chest X-ray may reveal an enlarged heart, chiefly to the left, especially when hypertension is coexistent. Widening and tortuosity of the aorta, and calcification of the aortic knob also may be seen. The ECG may appear normal, but often evidence interpreted as indicating myocardial damage is present. The most frequent significant ECG changes are flattening or inversion of the T waves, low voltage in the QRS complexes, and various degrees of AV and bundle branch block (q.v.).

Diagnosis

Since angina pectoris is essentially a symptom, the history is of major diagnostic importance. The typical exertion-pain-rest-relief pattern of symptoms is the main diagnostic point. The relief of pain following administration of nitrites (R 8, 9) is so striking as to warrant their employment as a diagnostic test. Abnormal physical and laboratory findings, when present, are only confirmatory. The discovery of an etiologic factor which may cause myocardial anoxia or ischemia further aids in establishing the diagnosis.

A severe and prolonged anginal attack must be differentiated from the pain of an acute myocardial infarct (q.v.). The following conditions are among those that may cause pain resembling that of angina pectoris: neurocirculatory asthenia, cardiospasm, hiatus hernia, gastritis, gallbladder disease, myositis and intercostal neuralgia or neuritis.

Prognosis

The average life expectancy for patients with angina pectoris is approximately 5 years from the onset. However, death may occur during the first attack, or a patient may live longer than 20 years. The prognosis depends largely upon the underlying disorder. For example, anginal pain complicating myocardial anoxia secondary to paroxysmal tachycardia or to coronary vasospasm carries an excellent prognosis if these conditions are relieved. Anginal pain resulting from severe coronary sclerosis or from interference with the entrance of blood into the coronary ostia has a rather poor prognosis. Other factors adversely affecting the prognosis are anginal pain occurring at rest, the presence of heart block or pulsus alternans, severe hypertensive vascular disease, a history of coronary occlusion and the development of congestive heart failure.

Treatment

Physical rest and avoidance of excitement are essential. In relatively mild cases, limited activity may be allowed provided the patient works slowly and avoids fatigue, overexertion, and exposure to cold and stormy weather. In severe cases, a period of bed rest followed by a gradual return to restricted activity may give considerable relief. Mental relaxation is almost as important as physical. Worry should be avoided as far as possible. Psychotherapeutic orientation of the patient to a life of restricted activity should be attempted. Gradual reduction in weight may be beneficial in obese patients. Overeating, especially if hurried, may bring on an attack. Generally, no special diet is necessary, but a low fat diet may have some value when hypercholesteremia is thought to contribute to the coronary atherosclerosis. A mild cathartic (℞ 81) should be given daily if needed. Smoking should be discouraged.

Drugs that increase coronary blood flow by dilating the coronary arteries, and sedatives, are both valuable in treating angina pectoris. They may be used to terminate an anginal attack, or prophylactically beforehand. For an attack unrelieved by rest, amyl nitrite is the most immediately effective of the vasodilators. Inhalation of the contents of 0.2 cc. (♏ iii) amyl nitrite (℞ 8) usually brings relief within ½ to 1 minute. A hypodermic tablet of nitroglycerin, 0.3 mg. (gr. 1/200) (℞ 9) sublingually also is effective, but takes 2 to 3 minutes to act. Both of these rapid-acting vasodilators, especially amyl nitrite, may cause severe headache, dizziness and even syncope. Reduction of the dosage to tolerated levels therefore becomes necessary. If prompt relief is not obtained from rest and administration of nitrites, morphine in a dose of 10 or 15 mg. (gr. ⅙ or ¼) subcut. (℞ 57) may be required.

The slower-acting, longer-lasting vasodilators are valuable prophylactically and are especially helpful in hypertensive patients. Erythrol tetranitrate (℞ 10), mannitol hexanitrate (℞ 11), or sodium nitrite (℞ 12) taken several times daily may decrease the number of attacks or abolish them entirely. Amyl nitrite (℞ 8) or nitroglycerin (℞ 9) may prevent symptoms if taken immediately before an activity known to provoke an attack. Other prophylactic vasodilator drugs are aminophylline (℞ 13), theobromine and sodium acetate (℞ 16) and papaverine (℞ 17). The moderate use of alcoholic beverages is frequently helpful, since alcohol is a vasodilator.

Sedation is extremely valuable in reducing anxiety during an attack and producing the mental and physical relaxation so important in preventing attacks. Chloral hydrate (℞ 43) or phenobarbital (℞ 44) may be given several times daily.

The administration of cobra venom (℞ 89) has increased exercise tolerance and produced clinical improvement in some patients. Thiouracil (℞ 88) may give relief by depressing an elevated B.M.R. and thus decreasing the work of the heart.

If the above means of control are unsuccessful, and the attacks frequent and severe, paravertebral sympathetic block with alcohol may give relief. Cervical and dorsal sympathectomy, total thyroidectomy, and implantation of muscle or omentum into the pericardium are occasionally of benefit.

MYOCARDIAL INFARCTION

Damage to a portion of the heart muscle by myocardial ischemia usually resulting from occlusion of a coronary artery, and characterized by severe substernal oppression, shock, cardiac dysfunction, and often sudden death.

Coronary occlusion and **coronary thrombosis** are terms frequently used as synonyms for myocardial infarction. Often, however, they are used incorrectly, since myocardial infarction may occur without coronary occlusion or thrombosis; conversely, coronary occlusion or thrombosis frequently occurs without resultant myocardial infarction.

Etiology and Pathogenesis

Myocardial infarction usually is produced by thrombotic occlusion of one of the larger branches of the coronary arteries. The thrombus most commonly occurs in a sclerotic vessel with a narrow lumen; often in the bed of an atheromatous ulcer or on a calcified plaque. The clot may form gradually, or in some cases rapidly. The left anterior descending branch of the left coronary artery is perhaps most often affected, but frequently the posterior descending branch of the right coronary is involved; less often the lesion is in the posterior descending branch of the left coronary, and still more rarely the left circumflex. Generally, occlusion of the left anterior descending branch causes the "anterior" type of infarct, in which the apex of the heart, the anterior wall of the left ventricle and the adjacent portion of the interventricular septum are the chief regions involved. The "posterior" is usually associated with thrombosis of one of the large posterior descending branches, and involves mainly the posterior portion of the interventricular septum and the diaphragmatic and posterior portions of the right and left ventricles. Occlusion of any of the above-named branches may take place gradually, or even suddenly, without causing myocardial infarction. This is not infrequent in patients who have an efficient collateral coronary circulation.

Less common causes of coronary obstruction leading to infarction are: embolism from left auricular mural thrombi in mitral stenosis or from the auricular appendages in auricular fibrillation; embolism from vegetations or thrombotic masses in bacterial endocarditis or arteriosclerotic valvular disease; occlusion of a coronary ostium by pedunculated thrombotic vegetations of the aortic valve; scarring in the ostial region due to syphilitic aortitis; and simple gradual sclerotic occlusion of a vessel without thrombosis.

Myocardial infarction may occur without coronary occlusion. For example, a coronary circulation which is moderately insufficient but still adequate for maintaining normal myocardial activity may become inadequate when faced with increased myocardial demands due to unusual exertion, so that relative ischemia with subsequent infarction results.

Pathology

In cases of sudden death following coronary occlusion, no morphologic changes in the myocardium may be demonstrable. If the patient survives, the usual results of ischemia secondary to arterial occlusion, i.e., infarction and anemic necrosis, will follow. After a few hours, the involved muscle fibers become eosinophilic and stain more deeply; the area may become hemorrhagic. Fragmentation of the muscle fibers and pyknosis of their nuclei become apparent within 24 hours, and polymorphonuclear leukocytes begin to appear at the periphery of the necrotic area. This process increases for 4 to 5 days. At about the 4th day, fibroblasts appear and gradually replace the leukocytes; granulation tissue begins to grow in. Scar tissue forms about 10 to 12 days after the occlusion and becomes extensive in 3 weeks. After 3 months, dense scar tissue remains.

If the necrosis involves the epicardial surface, a fibrinous exudate is formed on it causing the pericardial friction rub often heard on auscultation. A mural thrombus may develop on the endocardium of either the right or left side of the heart, depending upon the site of the infarction; it may give rise to emboli which pass to the pulmonary or systemic circulation. Other pathologic sequelae are aneurysmal dilatation in the region of the infarct and rupture of the heart. Rupture may occur during the 1st week when the infarcted area still is necrotic, or later as a complication of aneurysmal dilatation.

Pathologic Physiology

Cardiac dysfunction, with infarction and fibrosis of the myocardium, may arise whenever the nutritional requirements of the heart muscle exceed the ability of the coronary arteries to supply the nutriments. Myocardial ischemia causes the characteristic pain of angina pectoris (q.v.), and is directly responsible for the various pathophysiologic conditions occurring in that disease. Sudden death almost immediately following a coronary occlusion, before actual infarction and necrosis can take place, often results from the functional derangement of an ischemic myocardium. The myocardium so affected frequently serves as an irritative focus for the establishment of a variety of arrhythmias, and may cause death from ventricular fibrillation or asystole.

Myocardial damage also impairs the efficiency of the cardiac musculature, hence the force of the cardiac thrust is diminished and cardiac output decreases. Two different pathophysiologic consequences of reduced cardiac output and resultant slowing of the circulation may occur. In one, the heart is unable to deliver as much blood as it receives via the venous return. Increased venous pressure and congestive heart failure then develop. Acute left ventricular failure with pulmonary edema is not infrequently produced by this mechanism. The other consequence, often seen, is severe peripheral vascular collapse. If the cardiac output falls low enough, the slowing of the circulation may produce anoxemia with resulting tissue anoxia and increased permeability of the capillary bed. Loss of fluid into the tissue spaces, fall in blood volume, hemoconcentration and decreased venous return all contribute to establish the state of shock commonly seen in myocardial infarction. Loss of fluid due to the profuse sweating and the nausea and vomiting common in these patients also helps to precipitate peripheral vascular collapse.

Symptoms and Signs

An attack of acute myocardial infarction, especially when due to coronary thrombosis, is usually preceded by a history of angina pectoris or hypertensive vascular disease. Many patients, however, have had no history of cardiovascular complaints. The symptoms may come on while the patient is at rest, asleep, or during or immediately after unaccustomed exertion. The most characteristic complaint is severe substernal oppression, often described as a squeezing, pressing, or constricting sensation. Its location and distribution are similar to those of angina pectoris, but its overwhelming nature, failure of relief with nitrites, and persistence for hours or days show it to be a different and more serious condition. Dyspnea commonly accompanies the severe substernal oppression; the patient complains that the crushing pressure on his chest prevents him from breathing properly. Dyspnea without pain may be the chief symptom. Nausea, vomiting, hiccups, and abdominal distention sometimes occur. Extreme weakness and fear of impending death usually are present.

The patient appears to be in acute distress. The skin often is pale, cold, and moist, with some degree of cyanosis. After 24 to 48 hours moderate fever (rarely exceeding 102° F.) generally develops. At first the respirations may be rapid and shallow, or of Cheyne-Stokes type. If acute left ventricular failure occurs, the respirations may be noisy, with coarse rales heard throughout the lung fields, and a frothy sputum may be produced. The blood pressure usually falls within a few hours after onset of the attack. In hypertensive patients it may drop to normal or hypotensive levels; sometimes shock levels are reached. The pulse may be weak and thready, and the rate usually exceeds 100/minute, but may be slow during the first few hours. The heart sounds generally are feeble, but occasionally loud and sharp; there is often a gallop rhythm. Arrhythmias (q.v.) are common and range from premature systoles, auricular flutter or fibrillation and ventricular tachycardia to AV block. The arrhythmia may be transitory or permanent. Murmurs are not characteristic, but a systolic murmur is frequently audible at the apex. A pericardial friction rub often is heard on about the 4th or 5th day of illness.

Signs of congestive failure, such as dyspnea, orthopnea, enlarged liver, dependent edema and evidence of increased venous pressure, may develop.

Clinical Course and Complications

The clinical course following myocardial infarction is highly variable. It may be insignificant; it may cause sudden and apparently painless death; or it may be prolonged, hazardous and complicated, terminating in recovery or death. Some patients succumb to shock or to acute congestive heart failure soon after the acute episode. The majority survive the first 2 or 3 days, with gradually diminishing symptoms, but then either slowly decline or improve, depending upon the ability of the collateral coronary blood flow to supply the infarcted area. The 2nd and 3rd weeks following the infarction are an extremely critical period. The complication most to be feared during this period is a suddenly fatal embolism arising from thrombi in the heart or in the veins of the leg and pelvis. Mural thrombi may form over the endocardium lining the necrotic infarcted area of myocardium. Thrombi in the right heart may cause pulmonary embolism; thrombi in the left heart may cause embolism to the brain, kidneys, spleen, or other site in the distribution of the systemic circulation. If auricular fibrillation is present, cardiac thrombi may form in the auricular appendages and embolize as indicated above. Massive pulmonary embolism occurs more often from the femoral and iliac veins. Thrombosis is encouraged in these veins by an increased circulation time and the physical inactivity of these patients.

Cardiac arrhythmias may develop at any time during this period. Frequent ventricular extrasystoles are common and may be forerunners of ventricular tachycardia, which often degenerates into fatal ventricular fibrillation if untreated. Congestive failure also is likely to develop at any time within this stage, and may be acute and rapidly fatal or become chronic, or disappear almost entirely.

Ventricular rupture through the softened necrotic area before the scar has formed is a rare complication. Ventricular aneurysm may result from thinning of the scar; rupture of such an aneurysm occasionally occurs.

The usual clinical course is uneventful, following a gradual diminution of pain during the first few days. If the patient survives the first 3 weeks, he is well on his way to a convalescence relatively free from hazard. In the average case, healing is complete in 6 weeks, the ECG has returned to normal, and gradually increasing activity can be tolerated.

Laboratory Findings

Leukocytosis and increased E.S.R. accompany the characteristic fever and usually appear after 24 to 48 hours. They are roughly proportional to the degree of myocardial necrosis. (The fever rarely goes above 102° F. and generally subsides within a week.) The leukocyte count may reach 25,000, but usually is between 12,500 and 17,500 with a marked shift to the left. It drops to normal in 7 to 10 days, unless a pneumonia or other complication develops. The E.S.R. is perhaps the most sensitive of these tests, and may remain elevated for 4 to 6 weeks until healing is well established.

The ECG findings, while often characteristic, frequently are atypical or inconclusive. When typical, they are extremely valuable in confirming the diagnosis of infarction, but myocardial infarction can occur without producing diagnostic ECG changes. These changes usually become apparent within 24 to 36 hours, but may take as long as 72 to 96 hours. In general, in anterior wall infarcts (Q_1-T_1 type), early changes are elevation of the S-T segments of leads I and IV, with Q waves and inverted T waves also present in these leads. This is followed by a gradual depression of the S-T segments in leads I and IV to the isoelectric level with cove plane inversion of the T waves in these leads. In posterior wall infarcts (Q_3-T_3 type), the early changes consist of elevation of the S-T segments in leads II and III, with Q waves and inverted T waves also present in these leads. Cove plane inversion of these T waves develops subsequently as in the anterior wall infarctions. A combination of the above ECG configurations may occur if the infarct is atypically situated.

Diagnosis

The location, severity, and duration of the characteristic pain, with its attendant manifestations as described under Symptoms and Signs, usually is sufficient to make a diagnosis of myocardial infarction highly probable. The development of fever, leukocytosis, increased E.S.R. and typical ECG changes confirms it. Symptoms due to severe coronary insufficiency without infarction may closely imitate those of myocardial infarction, but confirmatory laboratory evidence of necrosis is then absent. Angina pectoris usually is easy to differentiate from myocardial infarction. In angina the pain usually appears during exertion, it is relieved by rest or nitrite therapy, is not so overwhelming as in infarction, and is not accompanied by circulatory collapse. Myocardial infarction also must be differentiated from dissecting aneurysm of the aorta, pneumonia, mediastinal emphysema, mediastinitis, pleurodynia, pleurisy, spontaneous pneumothorax, perforated peptic ulcer, acute pancreatitis, acute cholecystitis, subphrenic abscess and other acute abdominal conditions.

Prognosis

Sudden death at any time during the first month is not unusual. In general, 80% of the patients survive the initial attack. The majority of these die within 3 to 5 years from another infarction or from cardiac failure. A few patients may live as long as 10 to 20 years or even more. Complications developing in the first few weeks following the attack, such as acute congestive failure, embolic phenomena, cardiac arrhythmias, and pneumonia, make the prognosis much graver.

The recent routine use of anticoagulant therapy (q.v.) following myocardial infarction has strikingly reduced the mortality rate by lowering the incidence of thromboembolic complications. As much as a 50% decrease in the immediate mortality rate has been reported following the use of dicumarol in the first few weeks of illness.

Treatment

The treatment of myocardial infarction should include: (1) emergency measures for relief of pain, and for the treatment of vascular collapse and acute pulmonary edema; (2) provisions for relative rest of the injured heart; (3) measures for the prevention and treatment of complications such as thromboembolic disease, cardiac arrhythmias, and congestive failure; and (4) adequate after-care to rehabilitate the convalescing patient.

The immediate aim is to secure complete physical and mental rest for the patient as rapidly as possible. Pain and apprehension should be relieved promptly by morphine ($\math773$ 57) in doses of 15 or 30 mg. (gr. $\frac{1}{4}$ or $\frac{1}{2}$), subcut. or I.V., repeated in $\frac{1}{2}$ hour if necessary, and as often thereafter as needed. Dilaudid ($\math773$ 54) or Demerol ($\math773$ 55) may be used instead of morphine. The antispasmodics help relieve pain and increase blood flow to the infarcted area by overcoming reflex spasm of the coronary arteries. The following drugs, alone or in combination, are useful for this purpose: papaverine ($\math773$ 18) 0.1 Gm. (gr. iss) I.V. every 4 hours; atropine ($\math773$ 19) 0.5 to 1 mg. I.V., or aminophylline ($\math773$ 14) 0.5 Gm. (gr. viiss) slowly injected I.V. every 4 to 6 hours until pain is relieved. Increasing the O_2 saturation of the blood by continuous administration of 100% O_2 (using face mask, tent, or the less efficient nasal catheter) may give prompt relief.

If the patient is in shock, the opiates (℞ 54, 57) or Demerol (℞ 55) are indicated, as suggested above, to relieve anxiety and secure sedation. Oxygen should be administered continuously to combat tissue anoxia—the usual consequence of peripheral circulatory failure and also a major factor in perpetuating the state of shock. If the shock is profound, with a systolic blood pressure below 60, a cold and clammy skin and rapid pulse, the administration of plasma I.V. is of value in combating hemoconcentration, fall in blood volume and deficient venous return. No more plasma should be given than is necessary to boost the systolic pressure to 90 or 100. Approximately 250 cc. injected I.V. during 1 hour usually is sufficient. Care must be taken not to overload the circulation with fluid because this is likely to induce pulmonary edema.

If the infarction is extensive, pulmonary edema may develop suddenly soon after its onset. This complication is treated by O_2 under positive pressure (*see* CLIN. PROC.), rapid digitalization, aminophylline I.V., and phlebotomy, as described under Congestive Heart Failure.

Congestive heart failure may develop at any time during the course of the disease, and should be treated in the usual way. Digitalization by one of the accepted methods is indicated.

Special care must be taken to avoid digitalis intoxication, which is likely to increase the irritability of an already irritable myocardium and produce dangerous arrhythmias.

Cardiac arrhythmias often occur, and may or may not require treatment. Auricular flutter and fibrillation usually are transient and can be ignored, but if persistent should be treated in the usual way, with digitalis or quinidine (*see* CARDIAC ARRHYTHMIAS). Frequent premature ventricular systoles, and especially paroxysmal ventricular tachycardia, should be actively treated with quinidine because they may lead to ventricular fibrillation.

Thromboembolic complications can be significantly reduced by the routine administration of dicumarol (℞ 62) for the first 3 to 4 weeks. The dosage is governed by the prothrombin activity of the plasma, which must be carefully watched. Before beginning dicumarol the prothrombin time should be determined to establish the patient's "normal" (usually between 12 and 14 seconds). Further determinations must be made daily during treatment, and for several days afterward. The dosage of dicumarol is 300 mg. by mouth on the 1st day, 200 mg. on the 2nd day, and 100 to 200 mg. daily thereafter as necessary to maintain the prothrombin time between 30 and 35 seconds. If the time rises above 35 seconds during therapy, dicumarol should be discontinued until it drops below 35 seconds. A prothrombin determination must be carried out daily (for additional information *see* ANTICOAGULANT THERAPY).

Anticoagulants have been used with encouraging results for

the prevention of subsequent attacks of coronary thrombosis in patients with a history of one or more occlusions. A dose of 75 mg. daily for months may be given to such patients to maintain their prothrombin times between 25 and 30 seconds. During the first few weeks of such therapy, daily estimations of prothrombin time should be done to avoid overdosage. After a satisfactory maintenance dose has thus been established, the estimations can be less frequent, so that after 6 months one every 2 weeks should be sufficient.

A period of absolute bed rest is necessary to keep the work of the heart at a minimum. Up to 6 weeks or more of bed rest and restricted activity are indicated depending upon the extent of the infarction. During the 1st week of the acute illness, bed rest should be absolute. The patient should lie relatively supine, or with the head and shoulders moderately elevated if more comfortable, and should exert no muscular effort. Phenobarbital (R 44) or chloral hydrate (R 43) should be given for sedation during the day, and to ensure sleep at night. An attendant should feed the patient; the daily bed bath and change of linen can be temporarily omitted. Bowel movements are best discouraged in the first few days, and then facilitated by mineral oil (R 81). During the 2nd week if convalescence is proceeding smoothly, the patient's legs should be massaged 2 or 3 times daily to stimulate venous return and protect against venous thrombosis. During the 3rd and 4th weeks, the patient's activity in bed is begun by passive leg raising 10 to 20 times, 2 or 3 times daily, and gradually increased to active movements of the extremities. He may be allowed to feed himself by the end of the 3rd week. At the end of the 4th week, sometimes earlier, he is allowed to sit up in a chair once a day for a few minutes, gradually increased to an hour or longer twice daily. Walking and other activities are allowed thereafter as tolerated. The optimal level of activity is usually reached in about 3 to 6 months.

The diet should be light, bland, and of low caloric value. During the first few days, when symptoms usually are severe, fluids alone are sufficient. During the latter part of the 1st week, a diet of about 800 calories may be begun, and increased gradually in convalescence to 1,200 to 1,500 calories or more. Salt should be restricted (see LOW SALT DIET) until there is no danger of congestive failure.

The continued oral use of aminophylline or theophylline during convalescence may hasten recovery through dilation of the coronaries. Aminophylline (R 13) 0.1 to 0.2 Gm., or theophylline (R 20) 0.2 to 0.3 Gm., is given 3 or 4 times daily.

Following a favorable course most patients feel able to resume normal activity. However, they should be warned to live at a slower pace, avoid overexertion, smoking and excesses of any kind. Some patients are never able to become normally active and so remain chronic invalids.

CONGESTIVE HEART FAILURE

A syndrome caused by a failing heart, with congestion in either the pulmonary or systemic circulations, or both. The manifestations of pulmonary vascular engorgement are commonly referred to as **left heart failure** and those of systemic venous and capillary engorgement as **right heart failure.**

Etiology

Heart failure from any cause, if it persists, usually leads to the development of the congestive state. The more common forms of heart disease, and their respective types of congestive failure follow.

In the group of arteriosclerotic heart diseases left ventricular failure tends to develop. The designation in these conditions usually is that of the most prominent abnormality of each, such as hypertensive heart disease, arteriosclerotic heart disease with hypertrophy and fibrosis of the myocardium, coronary arteriosclerosis, and myocardial infarction.

Of the rheumatic valvular diseases, aortic insufficiency, aortic stenosis, and mitral insufficiency lead to left ventricular failure. The left-sided congestion of pure mitral stenosis originates from the damming of blood in the left auricle; this form tends also to the early development of right ventricular hypertrophy.

Syphilitic aortic valvular disease causes left ventricular failure.

The most common type of primary right heart failure is encountered in cor pulmonale, that is, right ventricular failure secondary to chronic pulmonary disease with hypertension in the pulmonary artery. Other causes of purely right heart failure are constrictive pericarditis, tricuspid insufficiency and congenital pulmonic stenosis.

Most cases of left heart failure, as they progress, become eventually both left and right heart failure. Conditions that often develop the double failure early are thyroid heart disease, idiopathic (Fiedler's) myocarditis, diphtheritic myocarditis, severe anemia with heart failure, beriberi heart disease and active rheumatic carditis.

Pathology

The pathologic lesions in the heart in congestive failure are extremely variable, as indicated in the preceding section. There are certain features, however, which all failing hearts tend to have in common.

A failing myocardium is one that does not adequately empty one or more of the chambers of the heart (the ventricles being the most important) during systole; that is, the amount of blood in the affected ventricle at the end of systole is greater than normal. This leads to progressive dilatation, which may extend to involve most or all of the cardiac chambers as the congestive state becomes both right and left sided. A valvular stenosis will result in dilatation of the chamber behind it—an insufficiency dilatation of the chambers both in front and behind.

The degree of hypertrophy of the cardiac muscle wall is extremely variable. In general, it can be said, first, that it tends to increase with the chronicity of the cardiac failure; and second, that in conditions in which the myocardium itself is not diseased, the amount of hypertrophy increases with the additional work which that chamber performs. This increased work consists of increased cardiac output, for example in thyroid heart disease, or increased systolic pressure in arterial hypertension (hypertrophied left ventricle), mitral stenosis (hypertrophied left auricle), and cor pulmonale (hypertrophied right ventricle).

In intrinsic myocardial disease, the hypertrophy may be great, as in rheumatic heart disease with failure, or in some hypertensive arteriosclerotic hearts; but in other arteriosclerotic forms, the myocardium may be flabby, not much thickened, or even thinned out with scar tissue.

Since, in the body tissues generally, congestive heart failure is reflected by circulatory stasis, the pathologic changes outside the heart are those resulting from congestion. If the congestive process has been severe and of sufficient duration, changes may be noted in all organs; however, the principal changes are seen in the lungs and liver.

In acute congestion the lung is heavy and of doughy consistency. Edema is marked, especially in the dependent portions, and fluid runs from the cut surface. The alveoli are distended with fluid and blood. Chronic congestion produces a heavy, tough, brown lung (brown induration). The pulmonary capillaries are distended with blood. The alveoli contain red cells and large hemosiderin-filled phagocytes (heart failure cells). In acute congestion the liver is enlarged, with a tight capsule. Central veins and sinusoids are distended with blood, making the lobular divisions appear indistinct. Persistence of venous distention results in mottling of the surface (nutmeg liver). There may be some increase in the amount of liver parenchyma due to pressure atrophy of the liver cells. Fatty degeneration occurs in the cells at the periphery of the lobule where congestion is less pronounced.

Pathologic Physiology

The classic approach to the pathogenesis of the congestive state has been to assume that failure of the efficiency of the heart as a mechanical pump to maintain effectively the normal hemodynamic relationships was solely to blame. A somewhat more recent view holds that the congestive state develops primarily as a result of decreased renal blood flow subsequent to a reduced cardiac output. According to proponents of this theory, the decrease in renal blood flow leads to decreased glomerular filtration, retention of salt and water, increased blood volume, and hence increased venous pressure so causing the congestive state. It seems probable, however, that a combination of cardiac and extracardiac factors is responsible for the production of congestive heart failure.

In cardiac failure the basic fault is in the heart muscle itself. Either a diseased myocardium is unable to meet normal circulatory demands, or an intrinsically normal and previously adequate myocardium is no longer capable of the increased effort necessitated by a physical defect (such as valvular disease), or by an excessive circulatory stimulus (as in hyperthyroidism).

As failure begins, the heart chamber in its systolic contraction fails to eject its full quota of blood, and the chamber becomes dilated. With dilatation, however, comes a compensatory increase in the next systolic output, because stretched muscle (if not overstretched) contracts more forcibly (Starling's law). Thus, cardiac output may be for a time maintained, but at the cost of dilatation. Increased heart rate, if not excessive, also will tend to increase cardiac output. As dilatation increases, the pressure of blood in the distended chamber begins to build up during diastole, and this extends backward to the auricles and the venous inflow, to produce the congestive state, or congestive failure.

The systolic contraction sooner or later weakens, and cardiac output or total blood flow is diminished.

There are thus these two vital and essential elements in cardiac failure: excessive (diastolic) pressures in the heart and venous vessels, i.e., congestive failure (or "backward failure"); and insufficient cardiac output, i.e., failure of blood flow (or "forward failure"). These may be present in different degrees, in any given state of cardiac failure; but both factors are usually involved.

Incipient heart failure, or **decreased cardiac reserve:** As the heart begins to lose its normal vigor, it has been demonstrated both that cardiac output shows less than a normal increase under conditions of severe exercise, and that the pressures in the pulmonary artery then are increased (early pulmonary congestion). The decreased blood flow through the tissues causes increased acidity and this in turn produces an excessive hyperpnea. The latter may be further increased reflexly by the pulmonary hypertension. This abnormally increased respiration is the chief cause of increased exertional dyspnea in early heart failure. Vital capacity and breathing capacity are not decreased.

Left heart failure: Failure of the left side of the heart is for the most part left ventricular failure. An important exception is mitral stenosis, where the congestion is chiefly in the left auricle. Since, however, in mitral valvular disease, there usually is insufficiency as well as stenosis, a left ventricular element is present here also.

As the diastolic pressure rises in the failing left ventricle or left auricle, the congestive state extends backward to involve the entire pulmonary circulation. Pulmonary arterial pressure (systolic) may increase from the normal of 20 to 25 mm. of mercury to 100 mm. or higher in extreme pulmonary congestion.

The unfavorable effects of pulmonary congestion are numerous: the engorged pulmonary vascular bed stiffens the lung, and its expansibility or vital capacity is much reduced, sometimes to 1,200 cc. or less. This is an important factor in the later stages of cardiac dyspnea. Congested capillaries leak fluid into interstitial and alveolar spaces, with development of pulmonary edema. This, if it develops gradually leads to chronic pulmonary congestion, cough, and increased difficulty in breathing. If the condition is advanced there may be interference with blood oxygenation in the lungs, increasing the cyanosis which may already be present due to stagnant cutaneous blood flow.

Orthopnea, or dyspnea in recumbency is due largely to increase in pulmonary congestion in this position. It has been shown that vital capacity is about 300 cc. less than in the standing or sitting position. If pulmonary congestion develops acutely, it may precipitate an attack of acute pulmonary edema, with large amounts of fluid exuding into the alveoli and being coughed up as frothy pinkish or blood-tinged sputum. The obstructive breathing in so-called cardiac asthma probably is a manifestation of pulmonary congestion.

In attacks of dyspnea at night, the so-called paroxysmal nocturnal dyspnea, there are several factors involved. One is orthopnea. Another is the fact that total blood volume is increased at night. A period of hyperpnea in Cheyne-Stokes respiration occurring in the semiconscious state, may set off a paroxysmal attack. Anxiety and fear may precipitate, aggravate and prolong these attacks.

Right heart failure: This is almost always right ventricular failure. The only important exception is constrictive pericarditis, where the constriction prevents complete and adequate filling of right auricle and ventricle but does not prevent their emptying.

Right ventricular failure occurs most commonly as an event secondary to failure of the left side of the heart. Obviously, pulmonary congestion and pulmonary hypertension demand increased right ventricular work. If the condition comes on gradually the right ventricular muscle may hypertrophy to a considerable degree, as in some cases of mitral stenosis, and remain compensated for many years. In other cases, left ventricular failure may be quickly followed by right ventricular failure.

The progression from a compensated right ventricular hypertrophy to a state of decompensation or failure takes place in the same manner as already described for the left ventricle— inadequate systolic emptying with consequent increased diastolic pressure, causing in turn increased auricular and peripheral venous pressures.

The same sequence occurs also where primary pulmonary hypertension of emphysema or chronic fibrotic pulmonary disease, with right ventricular hypertrophy (cor pulmonale), progresses to right-sided congestive failure.

The consequences of the increased venous pressure and tissue congestion of right heart failure are:

Congestion of viscera: Liver enlargement usually occurs even with moderate increase in venous pressure; often extending to the umbilicus if venous pressure reaches high levels (over 200 mm. H$_2$O) over a number of days. After long-standing passive congestion, liver enlargement may persist even after venous pressure has been brought back to normal, due to chronic pathologic change (cardiac cirrhosis).

Renal congestion often is associated with moderate albuminuria, sometimes with casts and moderate nitrogen retention. The most significant effect is salt and water retention (see below, under EDEMA).

Congestion of the gastrointestinal tract may cause such functional disturbances as epigastric distress, anorexia, constipation, or intestinal distention.

Edema is the most important manifestation of right heart failure. It is known that early in the congestive state there is an increase in plasma and blood volume. The increased exudation of fluid from capillaries to tissues is due in part to increased venous and capillary pressure. Anoxia of capillaries from stagnant and sluggish blood flow may be a factor. Decreased plasma protein may play a part in chronic cases with malnutrition. Endocrine and other metabolic disturbances also are probably concerned in the sodium and water retention and in capillary permeability.

Peripheral edema begins in dependent parts, ankles and pretibial regions, extending to the knees and thighs, and sometimes almost all subcutaneous tissues (anasarca). With advancing congestion, hydrothorax often develops, more commonly on the right; and, less frequently, ascites. With successful treatment diuresis occurs, followed by venous pressure fall and progressive disappearance of edema. Sometimes some edema will persist even with normal venous pressure, probably due to the increased permeability of anoxic capillaries.

Low cardiac output: This is not strictly a feature of the congestive state as such, but it is an integral part of cardiac failure. Inadequate blood circulation to the tissues is responsible for the weakness and easy fatigue of cardiac patients. Retarded blood flow is a chief cause of Cheyne-Stokes breathing.

In its more advanced stages, secondary cerebral anoxia leads to insomnia, poor mental function, delirium, and coma. Stagnation of the circulation in the skin is the chief cause of chronic cardiac cyanosis. This may be due to local circulatory stasis with congestion but often is a manifestation of general decrease in blood flow. The possible importance of decreased blood flow in causing edema has been mentioned.

Arteriosclerotic heart disease and rheumatic heart disease are most likely to show an early decrease in cardiac output, as cardiac failure develops. The arrhythmias, especially auricular fibrillation, will regularly cause a further drop in cardiac output.

There is an important group of conditions known as "high-output failure," in which congestive failure develops (often right heart and left heart failure simultaneously), while a cardiac output greater than normal is maintained. This group includes hyperthyroid heart failure, anemic heart failure, and beriberi heart failure. A similar condition, though showing right-sided failure only, is cor pulmonale. All these cases, however, have during failure a relative decrease in cardiac output: when compensated, the cardiac outputs are even higher, due to the greatly increased circulatory stimulus. The primary treatment of such conditions is obviously to remove this excessive stimulus.

Symptoms and Signs

The clinical features of congestive heart failure vary considerably depending upon the acuteness or chronicity of the process. In addition, the pattern of the acute form will be determined by the heart chamber which fails first, i.e., right ventricle or left ventricle, as explained in the preceding pages. In some instances, both ventricles fail simultaneously, producing a syndrome embodying features of each.

Precipitating factors: Congestive failure may result from factors which directly or indirectly reduce the functional capacity of the heart itself (intrinsic factors), or from factors which increase the demands on a heart of limited reserve (extrinsic factors).

Intrinsic factors include myocardial disease such as progressive coronary artery disease, myocardial infarction, rheumatic fever with carditis, infectious or toxic myocarditis; disorders of rhythm, especially auricular fibrillation or paroxysmal tachycardia; subacute bacterial endocarditis, dissecting aneurysm, beriberi, pericarditis, rupture of valve cusp or other mechanical accident, and congenital cardiac abnormalities.

Extrinsic factors include acute arterial hypertension from any cause, pregnancy, respiratory infections, asthma, anoxic states, uremia, thyrotoxicosis, anemia, physical exertion, long-standing overstrain and fatigue, and anxiety.

The onset of failure may be insidious, or sudden. Frequently the patient will have noticed gradual loss of energy, over months or years, with increasing exertional dyspnea, perhaps some tendency to ankle edema; then an episode of acute failure following one of the precipitating factors mentioned above may occur (*see* Etiology). An acute myocardial infarction, or abrupt onset of paroxysmal auricular fibrillation may send a patient into acute failure without preceding symptoms.

Acute left heart failure: Because of pulmonary congestion which results from left ventricular failure, the characteristic manifestations are respiratory in nature. The chief and earliest complaint usually is dyspnea. This may be noted on exertion or may occur in paroxysmal attacks, frequently at night (paroxysmal nocturnal dyspnea). Occasionally the attacks of dyspnea are accompanied by wheezing (cardiac asthma). As failure progresses the dyspnea becomes more intractable and persists even at rest. Often the dyspnea is accompanied by severe coughing, with the raising of sputum when the congestion is severe. Orthopnea, or difficulty in breathing while recumbent, is usually associated with dyspnea and may be the first symptom of congestive heart failure in sedentary individuals. A frequent initial sign is respiratory discomfort while lying flat at night, relieved by the use of two or more pillows. By the time that fatigue, muscular weakness, prostration, and cerebral symptoms develop, decreased cardiac output and inadequate circulation to the tissues are well established.

On physical examination, the patient in moderate to severe left heart failure will be found sitting up, or occasionally standing and leaning forward on some support. There is labored breathing, and the obviously uncomfortable patient is restless, anxious, often coughing, sometimes sweating, and, in the severer stages, more or less cyanotic.

The size and shape of the heart and the presence or absence of murmurs will depend on the type of heart disease present. Important signs often associated with the failing heart are: tachycardia, arrhythmias, faint or slurred heart sounds, embryonal (tic-tac) rhythm, gallop rhythm, and pulsus alternans.

Left ventricular failure is accompanied by signs of alveolar congestion and engorgement of the pulmonary vessels. The congestion is indicated by the presence of fine rales in the dependent portions of the lungs, by diminution in vital capacity, by an accentuation of the pulmonic second sound and by the typical X-ray appearance of the engorged pulmonary vessels. The circulation time through the lungs is prolonged, and the degree of alveolar congestion varies widely from a few basal rales to severe pulmonary edema with the production of frothy blood-tinged sputum. In early congestive failure dyspnea may precede development of rales. Sibilant rales are heard in those patients who wheeze.

Acute right heart failure: Dependent edema which pits on pressure often is the first evidence of right ventricular failure. In the ambulatory patient, ankle swelling will be noted initially during the day and disappear overnight, but as failure continues it becomes more persistent and extends upward to involve the legs and thighs. Less commonly it extends to the buttocks and abdomen, resulting finally in generalized edema or anasarca. Shortly before, or coincidental with the appearance of peripheral edema, the patient may become conscious of discomfort or tenderness in the epigastrium or right hypochondrium due to distention of the capsule of the liver resulting from swelling of that organ. Hepatomegaly may become marked. Congestion of stomach and other abdominal viscera may lead to complaints of anorexia, indigestion, and constipation.

The edema is associated with an increase in peripheral venous pressure which is manifested by distention of the jugular and peripheral veins at levels well above the heart. As water and salt are retained by the body in the form of edema, urinary output decreases. As a further manifestation of systemic circulatory stasis, fluid may collect in the pleural cavity (hydrothorax) or abdomen (ascites). The hydrothorax usually occurs first on the right side. Fluid accumulation in the pleural space may become so massive as to cause respiratory embarrassment and necessitate emergency removal.

Acute combined right and left heart failure: This is not usual, as an initial episode of heart failure, but it may take place when both ventricles are affected by a diffuse pathologic process. It is seen in such conditions as fulminating rheumatic carditis, Fiedler's myocarditis, severe acute nephritis with heart failure, and thyrotoxicosis with heart failure.

Combined right and left heart failure also is likely to ensue in the generally weakened heart after several attacks of acute left ventricular failure. As would be expected, the clinical features represent a combination of those symptoms and signs which already have been described for right- and left-sided failure, together with manifestations of forward failure. Both ventricles dilate with resulting congestion in both the pulmonary circulation and systemic veins. Respiratory symptoms, edema, increased venous pressure, and accumulation of fluid in the serous cavities may then occur simultaneously. In the advanced stage there is considerable dilatation of both heart chambers with feeble and distant heart sounds, a low pulse pressure, and sometimes pulsus paradoxus when respiration is very labored.

Chronic congestive failure: This usually develops by a sequence of events beginning with repeated bouts of acute left ventricular failure and progressing through a period of combined right and left ventricular failure which then becomes chronic. Chronic right-sided failure may develop in patients suffering from mitral stenosis; less commonly in cases of cor pulmonale. Tricuspid insufficiency, when present, usually is relative, due to dilatation of the valvular ring. In chronic right-sided failure, persistent elevation of the venous pressure, and edema, are prominent.

With continuing heart failure, the effects of decreased cardiac output and chronically inadequate circulation to the tissues become more manifest. The cardiac output usually becomes progressively diminished and additional symptoms develop. These include weakness, chronic gastrointestinal disturbances, loss of weight; insomnia, loss of mental vigor, judgment and memory, and even psychotic manifestations (cardiac psychosis); chronic Cheyne-Stokes respiration; persisting edema with elevated or even with normal venous pressures, in part due to inadequate renal blood flow; occasionally moderately elevated blood nitrogen figures; and especially in chronic right-sided failure, chronically enlarged liver, eventually with the so-called cardiac cirrhosis of the liver.

Diagnosis

The differential diagnosis of congestive failure is concerned primarily with the evaluation of the mechanisms of the more prominent symptoms and signs. Since dyspnea is so frequently a presenting complaint in heart failure, its evaluation is of prime importance. The dyspnea of chronic pulmonary disease with the greatly restricted ventilatory capacity of advanced pulmonary fibrosis, or the obstructive dyspnea of emphysema and asthma, may be mistaken for cardiac dyspnea. Careful physical examination and X-ray of the chest usually will establish the diagnosis in these diseases. It should be noted that chronic pulmonary disease and heart disease with failure frequently occur together in the same patient. Effort syndrome, respiratory neuroses, and anxiety states with symptoms of dyspnea are frequently confused with true cardiac failure. Other causes of dyspnea are severe anemia; acidosis, especially diabetic ketosis; pulmonary tumors, embolism, and tuberculosis; pneumonia; asthma; pulmonary fibrosis and emphysema; and certain of the pneumoconioses.

Laboratory findings such as X-ray evidence of pulmonary congestion or cardiac disease, measurement of peripheral venous pressure, changes in the circulation time, and ECG abnormalities are helpful when the diagnosis is in doubt.

Course and Prognosis

Few other disease states are as variable in course and prognosis. For this reason proper diagnosis and evaluation of precipitating factors are essential in order that therapy may be rationally planned. Important points which must be considered are the cardiac reserve, the ability to eradicate or control the precipitating factors, the nature and severity of the underlying organic heart disease, number of previous attacks, age of the patient, complications of failure, and the type of response to therapy.

A knowledge of the usual clinical course of the various primary heart disorders offers much prognostic assistance. Experience has shown that patients with heart failure resulting from mitral stenosis or persistent hypertension respond well to therapy, and the heart may compensate satisfactorily. While the outlook is less bright when failure results from syphilitic disease of the aortic valve, many cases will recover compensation, and with properly regulated lives some may live for 5 or even 10 years. Failure following myocardial infarction carries a guarded prognosis; however, if the infarct heals, and is not too massive in extent, prognosis for recovery from failure is excellent.

Treatment

First will be described the general management of the patient:

1. **Incipient heart failure, or diminished cardiac reserve:** This is the patient with increased exertional dyspnea, with or without palpitation and heart consciousness, fatigue, and some loss of energy, and perhaps edema of the ankles at the end of the day. The management of the patient resolves itself into proper attention to the underlying disease or precipitating factors, such as hypertension (q.v.) and the regulation of the patient's activities so these will not exceed his cardiac reserve. Physical activity must be reduced below the level which will cause dyspnea or fatigue. Psychological factors are most important. The patient's disease, its course and treatment must be reviewed with him carefully. Causes of anxiety and emotional strain must be searched out and removed or relieved so far as possible. The patient must take regular and sufficiently long and relaxing vacations. Sometimes, long, quiet week ends, or one day resting at home in the middle of the week will be of benefit. A low salt regimen (*see* DIETS) may be helpful, especially in hypertensive states, if the patient is willing to cooperate. Digitalis or other cardiac drugs are not required unless there is a specific indication such as rapid auricular fibrillation. A mild sedative (R 44) during the day or at bedtime may be desirable.

2. **Relatively mild congestive heart failure:** In this group are those with increased symptoms of dyspnea, including attacks of orthopnea or dyspnea at night; some peripheral edema may persist through the night. Such patients may be put to bed for a few days to a week. Manifestations of failure will usually subside readily in response to the general management described under (1) above; but if symptoms of failure return, the management becomes more that of the ambulatory cardiac considered in the succeeding paragraphs of this section.

3. **Moderate and severe congestive heart failure:** These patients present clinical emergencies that demand prompt, vigorous, and comprehensive treatment.

Special nursing care will be needed for the more severe cases. Particular attention should be given to making the patient as comfortable as possible in his bed. The ordinary bed, provided with back rest and extra pillows, will be satisfactory for some, but most patients prefer a hospital (Gatch) bed with head end raised, which also is preferable for nursing purposes. Occasionally, an elderly cardiac patient, in the acute dyspneic phase, will do better sitting in a chair.

The bedpan and urinal often are very difficult to use, especially for the elderly patient. Here, constant nursing assistance is most important. It often is actually less effort for the patient to be assisted to the standing position to void, or to be lifted onto a commode at the bedside, than to struggle with a bedpan.

Restlessness, dyspnea, anxiety, and pain require sedation. A barbiturate (R 44, 45) plus codeine (R 52) or Demerol (R 55, 56) may suffice but the opiates are more effective (R 54, 57, 59). These may be repeated if necessary. For cough and dyspnea, codeine (R 51, 52) or morphine (R 57) is indicated.

Diet should be light, soft, with frequent feedings, and strictly low-sodium (*see* DIETS). Water need be limited only if the low sodium regimen cannot be strictly maintained. The patient should be weighed at least every other day, to measure fluid loss. Bowels should be regulated with mild cathartics or enemas as needed (*see* BEDSIDE PROC.).

For the severely dyspneic subject, other measures must be considered: removal of chest fluid if it is present in considerable amount; tourniquets on limbs or actual phlebotomy if pulmonary edema is present; O_2 therapy. These are described further below.

Cardiac medication, particularly digitalis and diuretics, should be started promptly (*see* below). If there is fever, leukocytosis, pyuria, signs of pneumonia, thrombophlebitis, or other infection, appropriate measures should be taken.

With vigorous treatment most patients in moderate to severe congestive failure begin to respond in from 2 to 24 hours. As the acute symptoms subside and the action of the heart improves, the decision must be made when to get the patient out of bed and how much to increase his activity.

Cases with active myocardial disease, especially acute rheumatic fever (q.v.) or diphtheritic myocarditis (q.v.) require prolonged bed rest. Myocardial infarction (q.v.) is a special problem. With these exceptions, the criteria for getting the patient up are: the heart rate, character of sounds, decrease in heart size, ECG improvement; the disappearance of peripheral edema; and the subsidence of dyspnea. The patient should be allowed out of bed at least an hour or two a day, as soon as the heart can tolerate it, as there is then less likelihood of developing phlebothrombosis or thrombophlebitis, urinary tract infections, or hypostatic pneumonia.

As the patient reaches the ambulatory stage, his condition must be followed closely to determine how much his activity will have to be restricted to keep within his tolerance, and how much medication he will need. A maintenance dose of digitalis should be continued if failure develops without medication during a period of limited activity. The low sodium diet should also be continued. Some cases will benefit by a weekly injection of a mercurial diuretic. For obese patients systematic weight reduction is indicated (*see* DIETS).

Diet and fluids: In patients with edema resulting from congestive failure, the use of a diet low in sodium is a definite aid in mobilizing excess extracellular fluid and as prophylaxis against further fluid collection. The average normal daily diet contains from 6 to 15 Gm. of salt. The low sodium diet should contain no more than 1 Gm. or at the most 2 Gm. of sodium daily (*see* DIETS).

While the strict low sodium diet is best managed in a hospital, it can be maintained in the home, with sufficient instruction and dietary supervision. The patient's cooperation also is essential, but often difficult to obtain. Potassium chloride and other salt substitutes may be helpful. It must be remembered that all drugs containing significant amounts of sodium must be withheld, such as sodium bicarbonate, sodium citrate, or the sodium salt of sulfonamides. The "rice diet" (*see* DIETS) may be tried in patients with hypertension.

With strict low sodium diet, water can be given as desired. Forcing fluids may help in some instances to increase sodium excretion from the body. If low sodium diet cannot be strictly maintained, total fluid should be restricted to about 1,500 cc. in moderate or severe failure. Body weight is the best index of fluid retention in ambulatory cases.

Diuretics: The use of diuretics is one of the most effective means of treating congestive heart failure. Mercurial and xanthine derivatives are most commonly employed; these drugs are thought to exert a primary action on the renal tubules and glomeruli, respectively.

It is important to remember that diuretics are effective even in the absence of obvious peripheral edema, if tissue fluids are at all increased. By their action extracellular fluid accumulations are mobilized and blood volume is decreased both in lungs and periphery so that respiratory manifestations (e.g., dyspnea) as well as peripheral edema may respond to diuretic therapy.

1. Mercurial diuretics: Most effective in their diuretic action are the organic mercurial compounds which act by depressing tubular resorption of water in the kidney. Mercury in combination with theophylline (R 34) may be administered I.V. or I.M., in an initial dose of 0.5 to 2 cc. of the 10% solution. If necessary it may be repeated at intervals of 1 to 5 days; some authorities give it daily for a week or more. In many patients with chronic congestive failure, the repeated use of mercurials is necessary, once or twice a week over periods of months. Other mercurial preparations which may be employed similarly are Salyrgan-Theophylline (R 35) and Mercuhydrin (R 36).

I.V. administration is more rapid and more effective than the I.M. route. The use of these drugs is contraindicated in acute glomerulonephritis and other ailments associated with marked renal insufficiency.

2. Xanthine diuretics: Theobromine, in combination with sodium salicylate (℞ 37), calcium salicylate (℞ 38), or theophylline (℞ 20), and its derivative, aminophylline (℞ 13), occasionally may produce a satisfactory diuresis although of much less degree than the mercurials. Diuresis is thought to occur as a result of renal vasodilatation. The theobromine salts should be administered in average doses of 0.5 Gm., 3 times daily as enteric coated tablets. Theophylline or aminophylline may be given 3 times a day in oral doses of 0.1 to 0.2 Gm. and also are available in 0.5 Gm. rectal suppositories (℞ 15). Toxic symptoms are nausea and vomiting. If no signs of toxicity develop, they may be continued as long as necessary.

3. Urea: Urea (℞ 39) may be used for diuretic purposes, but is inferior to mercurial compounds. The dose is 20 Gm. 2 to 5 times daily, preferably in fruit juices because of its disagreeable taste. Minor elevations of nonprotein nitrogen do not preclude its use, but if renal insufficiency is severe it should not be employed.

4. Acid-forming salts: The acidifying diuretics, ammonium chloride (℞ 40), ammonium nitrate (℞ 42), and potassium nitrate (℞ 41), are employed as adjuvants to the mercurial diuretics. By producing acidosis these salts cause excessive excretion of sodium which carries water with it. Enteric coated tablets should be used for administering these salts in divided doses of from 4 to 12 Gm. daily at mealtime, best given in intermittent courses of a week or two. Nausea and vomiting from gastric irritation may occur. The danger of producing severe acidosis precludes their use in patients with poor renal function.

Digitalis: This drug should be administered to all patients with congestive heart failure, except in cases of specific contraindication (*see* below).

The chief actions of digitalis (℞ 1) are: (1) The cardiac muscle fibers are shortened, and the systolic contraction is more rapid and more powerful. Cardiac dilatation is thus diminished, and systolic emptying and cardiac output increased. (2) The refractory period of the muscle is prolonged, thus delaying the "circus movement" in auricular fibrillation. (3) Conduction of impulses through the heart muscle and conduction system is prolonged, by both a direct muscle and an indirect vagus nerve effect. (4) The irritability of the heart muscle is increased. (5) Peripheral arterioles are constricted, tending to increase arterial blood pressure.

The standard digitalis preparation still is the dried leaf, but a number of purified glycosides now are available, which have special properties, and which are coming into use also for maintenance dosage because of effectiveness and constancy of action (*see* accompanying table, CARDIAC GLYCOSIDES).

The significant differences between them concern chiefly dosages, relative speed of action on the heart, and degree of absorbability from the gastrointestinal tract. Thus ouabain (strophanthin) when given I.V. exerts its maximum action in 15 minutes to 1 hour, digoxin 1 to 4 hours, digitoxin 4 to 8 hours. Most digitalis preparations are about 20% absorbed from the gastrointestinal tract; digitoxin is 100% absorbed; ouabain is not absorbed by mouth. Digoxin is eliminated more promptly than digitoxin.

CARDIAC GLYCOSIDES

Glycoside	Digitalization Oral	Digitalization I.V. (only in emergency)	Maintenance Oral
Ouabain (G Strophanthin)	. . . .	0.7–1.0 mg.	. . . . . .
Digitoxin	1.2 mg.	1.25 mg.	0.1–0.3 mg.
Digoxin	2–5 mg.	0.75–1.0 mg.	0.5–0.75 mg.
Lanatoside C	7 mg. in 24 hr. 16 mg. in 72 hr.	1.6 mg.	0.5–1.0 mg.
Strophanthin K	. . . .	0.7–1.0 mg.	

For full digitalization a safe dosage rule is 0.1 Gm. of digitalis leaf/10 lb. of body wt. The rate at which the patient should be digitalized depends on the acuteness and severity of his condition.

In the ordinary case, a satisfactory procedure is as follows: First determine whether the patient has had any digitalis within the past 2 weeks, or whether he has any known sensitivity or idiosyncrasy to the drug. If not, on the 1st day give half the digitalizing dose, in divided portions at 4-hour intervals. On succeeding days, give 2 to 4 times the maintenance dose, in divided portions, continuing until the full digitalizing dose has been administered or until satisfactory clinical response is achieved. For maintenance, 0.1 to 0.2 Gm. (gr. iss to iii) of digitalis leaf orally, once a day, is generally adequate.

In severe decompensation, more rapid digitalization is required. For extreme emergency, digitoxin (℞ 3) or lanatoside C (℞ 4) may be given I.V. In most instances, digitoxin acts sufficiently rapidly. An I.V. dose of 1 mg. of digitoxin may be given, or if there is a question about previously administered digitalis, 0.5 mg. repeated once or twice at 4- to 8-hour intervals according to clinical response.

Satisfactory clinical response consists in a slowing of the heart to a rate of between 68 and 80/minute, relief of dyspnea, fall in venous pressure, decrease in circulation time, diuresis, decrease in heart size. The ECG shows flattening or inversion of T waves, often also depression of ST segments.

Cardiac conditions that respond best to digitalis are arteriosclerotic heart disease in failure, and chronic rheumatic heart disease in failure; this is especially true when auricular fibrillation is present, but also applies to regular sinus rhythm. In general, the more chronic the failure and the more deteriorated the heart muscle, the less will be the response. Thyroid heart disease, active rheumatic carditis, and so-called "toxic" conditions with tachycardia are apt to respond poorly to digitalis; syphilitic heart cases sometimes do quite well, sometimes not. Myocardial infarction with acute congestive failure also is variable in response; some cases, however, show dramatic improvement.

The question of maintenance of digitalis therapy when the patient is ambulatory depends on the cardiac reserve. If there are any symptoms of congestive failure, or if the patient apparently develops such symptoms, even mildly, under physical stress, digitalis should be continued.

Toxic effects of digitalis are: (1) systemic effects: anorexia, nausea, vomiting, diarrhea, malaise, mental depression, blurred or (rarely) colored vision; (2) conduction abnormalities: prolonged P-R interval, partial or complete heart block; (3) muscle irritability effects: premature contractions, ventricular tachycardia. Most toxic effects subside within a day or two after discontinuing the drug, but some, such as complete heart block, may persist for 2 or 3 weeks.

Contraindications to the clinical use of digitalis are chiefly those under (2) and (3) above. With diminished dosage toxic effects usually disappear, but sometimes, especially if there is a tendency to ventricular tachycardia, digitalis may have to be discontinued.

Mechanical measures: Fluid accumulates rapidly in the pleural cavity in some cases of congestive heart failure. When the vital capacity has been lowered by pulmonary congestion, free fluid in the thorax may cause severe respiratory embarrassment. Thoracentesis, therefore, may be indicated as an emergency procedure, and is attended by dramatic relief of the distressed patient. Very rarely, fluid may collect in the pericardial sac and emergency removal is necessary. Abdominal paracentesis may be helpful when the pressure of ascites contributes to the heart failure.

In acute left ventricular failure, venesection may be helpful, for it produces a temporary reduction in the output of the right ventricle, allowing the pulmonary pressure and associated congestion to diminish. This may best be accomplished by the rapid removal of 300 to 500 cc. of blood from the antecubital vein. The method of so-called "bloodless phlebotomy" may be employed by placing tourniquets about the proximial portions of all extremities in order to pool blood in the peripheral veins. This latter measure is more effective when the venous pressure is relatively low, for when it is high the veins are already filled to capacity. The tourniquet pressure should be slightly below that required to eliminate the peripheral pulses.

Sedation: The selection of a proper sedative is a prime consideration in the initial management of congestive heart failure. In acute failure, when respiratory discomfort is prominent, prompt administration of a narcotic, such as morphine sulfate (℞ 57) subcut. is highly desirable. Its chief value rests in its anxiety-reducing action and its tendency to depress the respiratory reflexes. Alleviation of apprehension is rapid, and respiratory distress is often speedily relieved by this measure alone. Acute dyspnea, restlessness, or pain, is the primary indication for the use of morphine in cardiac patients. In delirium, anoxemia with marked cyanosis, and chronic congestive failure, narcotics should be avoided if possible.

When situations arise wherein narcotics cannot be used, the drug of choice is paraldehyde (℞ 46). Employed in doses of 3 to 6 cc. I.M., it is singularly effective in the management of cardiac patients in delirium. In chronic failure it may be used repeatedly without fear of addiction. Other sedative drugs of value in congestive failure are chloral hydrate (℞ 43) and the barbiturates (℞ 44, 45, 47).

Aminophylline (theophylline ethylene-diamine): This drug already has been mentioned for its diuretic properties. Other therapeutic attributes ascribed to it necessitate further consideration. It is said to be a coronary dilator and, as such, may be indicated in congestive heart failure. Its chief value, however, is in relieving bronchial spasm in those patients who have an asthmatic component to their dyspnea or have an associated obstructive emphysema. In patients with chronic failure, aminophylline is generally successful in relieving Cheyne-Stokes respiration. The most effective and efficient means of administration is I.V., in dosage of 0.24 Gm. (℞ 14). (CAUTION! The drug should be injected very slowly in any severely decompensated patient.) Sudden cardiac arrest has been known to follow too rapid injection. Administration I.M. of 0.5 Gm. produces a less pronounced but more prolonged effect. Oral administration is relatively ineffective. An aminophylline rectal suppository (0.5 Gm.) nightly may be an effective prophylactic against attacks of paroxysmal dyspnea (℞ 15).

Oxygen: One of the most important therapeutic measures in severe heart failure is the administration of O_2. In severe cardiac decompensation the O_2 saturation of the blood may be considerably reduced, due in part to pulmonary congestion which prevents normal oxygenation, and in part to stagnant anoxia. Cyanosis and severe unrelieved dyspnea are the criteria for the emergency administration of O_2. The concentration given should be adjusted to the amount necessary to relieve cyanosis. Selection of the method of administration will depend upon the equipment available, the desired O_2 concentration, the patient's ability to cooperate, and the presence or absence of coughing or vomiting. Breathing of O_2 under positive pressure, with due caution (*see* CLIN. PROC.) is indicated in the management of pulmonary edema (q.v.).

EDEMA

An abnormal accumulation of fluid in the body tissues. Clinically, edema denotes an excess of extracellular fluid in the interstitial spaces and in the serous cavities. It may be localized or general. Severe generalized edema is referred to as **anasarca.** The accumulation of serous fluid in the peritoneal cavity is called **ascites;** in the pleural cavity, **hydrothorax;** in the pericardial space, **hydropericardium.**

Etiology

Edema is caused by disturbance of one or more of the mechanisms of fluid exchange between the blood plasma and the tissue fluids. The chief types of disturbance and typical conditions that may be responsible for them are: (1) alteration of the normal osmotic pressure relationship of the plasma and tissue fluids, such as occurs with changes in protein concentration; (2) increase in capillary blood pressure, as in cardiac failure or venous obstruction; (3) increased capillary permeability resulting from damage to the capillary wall by local anoxia or toxins; (4) obstruction of lymphatic drainage by neoplasm, parasites, or inflammation. Other factors that influence fluid balance are the sodium ion concentration of the plasma and tissue fluids (*see* ACID-BASE and ALLIED DISORDERS); the amount of fluid and sodium ingested, and the amount excreted via the kidneys, lungs, skin and gastrointestinal tract.

Clinical Types

1. **Cardiac edema** occurs when heart failure causes sufficient slowing of the peripheral blood flow to produce a rise in capillary pressure. This tends to increase the exodus of fluid from the capillaries into the tissue spaces as well as to prevent the return of tissue fluids to the plasma. Capillary membrane damage due to insufficient oxygen (stagnant type of anoxia) may cause greater capillary permeability and thereby increase the quantity of fluid leaving the plasma. Plasma proteins lost into the tissue fluids, and reduced renal efficiency with lessened output of fluid and sodium both tend to disturb the balance still further toward edema formation.

During cardiac decompensation (*see* CONGESTIVE HEART FAILURE), the preponderance of manifestations may point to a left-sided heart failure that produces pulmonary edema (q.v.), or a right-sided heart failure affecting the peripheral circulation. Edema due to "right heart" failure is most severe in the dependent parts of the body where, due to gravity, the venous capillary hydrostatic pressures are greatest. Pitting, i.e., a temporary indentation in the skin following pressure, occurs with this type, and hydrothorax or ascites frequently develops. Edema is diagnosed as being of cardiac origin when there are symptoms and signs indicative of heart disease plus pulmonary edema or peripheral edema with an elevated venous pressure (above 12 cm. of water).

2. **Renal edema** occurs in patients with chronic glomerulonephritis and the nephrotic syndrome (q.v.). The edema is primarily due to loss of plasma proteins from the body (hypoalbuminemia), resulting from long-continued or severe albuminuria. Ascites and hydrothorax may be present as well as edema of the subcutaneous tissues. Anasarca (formerly known as "dropsy") is frequently encountered. With acute nephritis (q.v.), the capillary walls are damaged and their increased permeability permits plasma proteins to escape into the interstitial fluids. Thus, there is a relatively high protein concentration in the edema fluid. The edema is not necessarily dependent in distribution, but appears first in the looser tissues (e.g., eyelids). With both acute and chronic renal disease, cardiac failure may be associated, leading to increased venous pressure and additional impairment of renal excretion of sodium and water.

3. In **cirrhosis of the liver** (q.v.) edema is predominantly peritoneal (ascites), but also may involve the subcutaneous tissues. Portal (venous) obstruction and hypoalbuminemia both contribute to this edema.

4. In **malnutrition,** edema is traceable to prolonged improperly balanced diet, insufficient food intake (as in "war edema"), or poor absorption of nutriment. Subsistence on diets deficient in proteins and vitamins results in hypoproteinemia and capillary wall damage (e.g., in wet beriberi and scurvy, q.v.).

5. **Inflammatory edema** develops as a result of locally increased capillary pressure from dilatation of the blood vessels, slowing of the blood stream and blockage of returning veins and lymphatics. Capillary walls are damaged by bacterial or other toxic agents and a fluid high in protein escapes from the vessels.

6. **Angioneurotic (giant) edema** (q.v.) arises from a localized increase in capillary permeability due to allergy. It appears most frequently about the face, hands, genitalia, and larynx and is characterized by its rapid appearance and disappearance within a few hours. It may be associated with generalized urticaria (hives) which is quantitatively different, but represents essentially the same mechanism.

7. **Traumatic edema** is likewise due to localized capillary damage. It may result from mechanical trauma, heat, or cold. On occasion prolonged exposure to excessive heat causes generalized vasomotor changes (*see* HEAT DISORDERS) which ultimately produce increased capillary blood pressure and edema.

8. **Toxic edema,** localized or general, may develop from contact with or absorption of substances such as arsenic, salts of heavy metals (e.g., lead, antimony, gold, mercury), and the toxins of certain infections (e.g., diphtheria, scarlet fever).

9. **Venous obstruction** produces edema which may be uni-

lateral and not confined to the dependent parts. Any portion of the venous system may be involved. Obstruction of the superior or inferior vena cava by tumor, constrictive pericarditis, or fibrous tissue growth, or obstruction of the smaller veins by thrombophlebitis, may be responsible. The edema results from increased hydrostatic pressure in the capillaries, developing in the same manner as in congestive heart failure. With infectious thrombophlebitis, an additional factor tending to increase capillary permeability is damage to the capillary membrane by bacterial toxins.

10. **Lymphedema** results from obstruction of lymphatic drainage (e.g., by neoplasms, inflammation, filarial parasites). It usually is unilateral and accompanied by regional lymphadenopathy, but without evidence of venous obstruction such as distended surface veins, discoloration, or lowered skin temperature.

11. **Myxedema** is a form of hypothyroidism (q.v.) in which the edema is produced by subcutaneous deposition of protein and fluid. It affects chiefly the hands and face, does not pit readily, and clears under thyroid therapy.

Course and Prognosis

As seen from the foregoing, edema is a symptom rather than a disease. Its nature, extent, and distribution are important aids in the diagnosis and prognosis of the primary disorder. Edema may appear and disappear rapidly or persist for months to years according to the underlying cause. In long-standing edema, local changes may occur, such as discoloration of overlying skin, or formation of fibrous tissue deposits in the affected part. Edematous tissue is particularly susceptible to infection, acute or chronic, which may result in cellulitis, superficial or deep ulcerations, or occasionally gangrene.

Treatment

Obviously, the underlying disease must be given appropriate therapy. General measures in the treatment of edema are extremely important and include the following:

1. **Rest** and elevation of lower extremities should be prescribed for any patient with persistent edema of the lungs or of the dependent portions of the body. The hydrostatic pressure in the veins and capillaries is thereby reduced and absorption of fluid from the interstitial spaces facilitated.

2. **Digitalization** (see CONGESTIVE HEART FAILURE) is absolutely essential for any patient in whom cardiac failure contributes to the edema to even a minor extent. By increasing cardiac output and improving circulation digitalization alone may produce a diuresis, and when combined with other diuretic measures will potentiate their action.

3. **Diet** should be well balanced and contain all the essential food factors. Absence of thiamine (vitamin B_1) may

result in heart failure and increased edema. A high protein intake (90 to 125 Gm./day for the average-sized adult) is essential when hypoalbuminemia is present. Casein or lactalbumin drinks are useful to supplement the ordinary high protein foods (meat, milk products, and eggs), especially when sodium chloride intake must be severely restricted.

4. **Colloid infusions** I.V. are beneficial for mobilization of edema fluid when peripheral vascular collapse and diminished colloid osmotic pressure due to hypoalbuminemia are etiologic factors. (a) Concentrated human serum albumin is the most effective of these, especially preparations having a reduced sodium chloride content. The dose is 25 to 75 Gm./day. (b) Human plasma and (c) whole blood are more readily available and are given in amounts of 500 cc. or more as needed. Reactions are less likely to occur from plasma, but many anemic patients benefit from the addition of erythrocytes.

5. **Pressure bandages** may prevent the accumulation of edema in such conditions as thrombophlebitis of an extremity, trauma, or burns.

6. **Surgical removal,** if possible, of lesions producing venous obstruction (e.g., tumors, abscesses, calcified pericardium).

Specific measures in the treatment of edema are as follows:

1. **Restriction of sodium intake** which is important in treating most forms of edema, applies not only to sodium chloride but also to other sodium salts such as sodium bicarbonate, sodium lactate, and sodium sulfadiazine. Ordinary diets cooked without salt contain approximately 2 to 4 Gm. of sodium chloride, and are adequate in mild and moderate cases (*see* DIETS). For patients with severe edema or anasarca, sodium intake must be less than 1 Gm./day, and special foods such as salt-free bread and dialyzed milk are necessary. However, sodium intake should not be restricted in salt-depleted patients, i.e., those who have lost sodium through the kidneys or by vomiting, and whose edema is due to failure of internal exchanges ("dehydration with edema") or to primary water retention.

2. **Restriction of water,** which should be resorted to only in cases of anuria (complete suppression of urine), need not be limited beyond the amount of insensible water loss (800 to 1,500 cc./day in an average afebrile adult). Patients with other types of edema, such as in cardiac disease, may drink water freely if their sodium intake is being strictly limited.

3. **Administration of diuretics:** (a) Organic mercurials and drugs of the xanthine group act by specific inhibition, within the kidney, of the tubular reabsorption of sodium, and hence of water. The mercurials are the more potent, and may be given I.V. or I.M. A test dose of 0.5 cc. of Mercuhydrin (℞ 36), Mercuzanthin (℞ 34), or Salyrgan-Theophylline (℞ 35) should be given first; if no evidence of sensitivity appears (viz.,

albuminuria, diarrhea, circulatory collapse), a full dose of 2 cc. may be administered several times/week. (CAUTION! Overuse may lead to sodium depletion and dehydration, and if no diuresis takes place renal tubular cells may be damaged.) Inadequate renal blood flow for any reason, hemoconcentration (an indication of diminished plasma volume), and severe renal insufficiency are contraindications. Mercurials are therefore most useful in treating the edemas of heart disease and cirrhosis of the liver. Their diuretic effect may be enhanced by the simultaneous administration of an acidifying salt such as ammonium chloride (*see* below). Cardiac patients should always be digitalized before mercurials are given. (CAUTION! Diuretics liberate digitalis from the tissues and overdigitalization of the heart may result. Therefore, during administration of diuretics the dosage of digitalis must be carefully regulated.) *(b)* Xanthine diuretics are both less effective and less toxic than mercurials, but may be given to patients with renal disease. These drugs include theobromine salts (℞ 37, 38) 2 to 5 Gm./day; theophylline (℞ 20) 1 Gm./day; aminophylline (℞ 13) 0.4 to 1.0 Gm./day. Aminophylline in 0.5 Gm. doses also may be given I.V. (℞ 14) or as a suppository (℞ 15). The suppository is particularly useful in treating patients with cardiac disease associated with paroxysmal nocturnal dyspnea. *(c)* Acidifying salts such as calcium chloride and ammonium chloride are diuretics. As the calcium in calcium chloride is excreted in the intestinal tract and the ammonia in ammonium chloride is converted to urea, the remaining chloride produces an acidosis; as a result the kidney excretes chloride and some sodium, and hence water. Ammonium chloride (℞ 40) is given orally as enteric coated tablets in doses of 4 to 6 Gm./day. Prolonged administration of acidifying salts may result in severe acidosis, and as soon as this development is suspected, the drug should be stopped. *(d)* Salts such as potassium nitrate (℞ 41) are diuretic because of their rapid excretion. They may be given orally in doses of 4 to 6 Gm./day and are most effective if water is restricted. *(e)* Urea (℞ 39) is one of the most useful diuretics because it is harmless to patients with renal disease. Urea in the glomerular filtrate is reabsorbed only by back-diffusion; increasing the urea content therefore inhibits the reabsorption of water and a diuresis results. For patients with intractable edema of heart disease or portal cirrhosis, the use of urea may prolong the periods between injections of mercurial compounds. Urea also may be used for patients suffering from the nephrotic stage of chronic glomerulonephritis, without azotemia, since with azotemia (NPN above 60 mg./100 cc.) a maximum diuretic stimulus from this mechanism already has been obtained.

4. **Mechanical removal of fluid** from serous cavities should be done whenever indicated; thoracentesis may give tremendous relief to a dyspneic patient. The first withdrawal

of fluid should be limited to 500 cc. lest some mediastinal shift occur, with respiratory embarrassment or even pulmonary edema. Paracentesis also should be done in cases of ascites not responding to other treatment. Abdominal support must be given to avoid splanchnic dilatation and syncope. These two procedures should not be resorted to when the fluid can be delivered through the kidneys, as there is less depletion of protein by the latter route. Direct incision and drainage of subcutaneous edema through Southey's tubes is a drastic measure and seldom of lasting benefit.

5. **Antihistaminic drugs** have proved useful for angioneurotic edema (*see* ALLERGY).

Purgation is not advisable in edema for fear of salt depletion and consequent circulatory collapse.

SHOCK

A state of collapse caused by acute peripheral circulatory failure, which may occur in such conditions as severe trauma, major surgery, massive hemorrhage, dehydration, overwhelming infections, and drug toxicity. (N.B.! To be distinguished from emotional "shock," insulin shock, therapeutic electric shock, and other less definite conditions for which the term is loosely used.) Anaphylactic (allergic) shock (q.v.) is dealt with under ALLERGY.

Etiology

Many types of injury or disease may result in shock or shocklike states, mild or severe. While all forms have similarities and differences, there are a few well defined patterns of peripheral circulatory failure that may lead to shock. In such conditions as syncope (fainting), hemorrhage and wound shock, thermal burns, dehydration shock, "toxic" or "septic" vasomotor collapse, each has its special pattern of disordered physiology. The pathologic physiology of the more important types of shock, their clinical aspects, and treatment will be described.

Pathologic Physiology

The circulatory system consists of a set of branching elastic vessels, through which blood is propelled by the pumping action of the heart. The pressure maintained in any part of the system depends upon the amount of blood flowing and the degree of constriction (tone) of the vessels in that region. This relation, for the circulation as a whole, is termed "peripheral resistance," which is actually calculated as the mean arterial blood pressure divided by the cardiac output. In shock, the normal relation of blood pressure to blood flow is disturbed.

Syncope, or fainting, is perhaps the simplest form of shock.

As it develops, there is usually an increase in pulse rate, with a decrease in systolic and an increase in diastolic arterial pressure. Cardiac output and venous pressure are but little altered. Then comes an abrupt change: pulse rate is slowed, arterial blood pressure drops sharply due to sudden arteriolar dilatation, especially of the arterioles in muscle tissues. With the drop in arterial pressure, cerebral blood flow decreases and faintness or complete loss of consciousness (syncope) ensues. Even in this phase, cardiac output is not diminished.

Traumatic or **wound shock** is divided into "primary" shock, the initial stunning effect of injury, which is similar in many respects to syncope; and "secondary" shock, the progressively developing peripheral circulatory failure. In most traumatic injuries the chief circulatory damage is massive loss of whole blood, either externally or into the tissues; hence, this secondary phase of traumatic shock closely resembles shock due to hemorrhage. In severe traumatic shock, about 40% of the total blood volume may be lost, and this results in diminished return of blood to the right side of the heart, lowered central venous pressure and decreased cardiac output. Vasomotor tone is increased, the blood vessels becoming constricted in compensation for the decreased blood volume. Arteriolar constriction tends to maintain arterial blood pressure, but this compensation is not complete and the arterial pressure falls. This compensatory vasoconstriction also is selective, being more intense in tissues not needed for immediate survival, such as the extremities and the kidneys. The increased vasoconstriction in the kidneys often results in temporary anuria.

As the state of shock continues, other progressive changes occur. Tissue fluid enters the blood stream from uninjured tissues, tending to restore blood volume slightly; also causing some hemodilution. The diminished blood flow to the tissues results in tissue anoxia, increased lactic acid, and acidosis. In long continued shock acidosis may become severe, with serum pH at 7.1 or even lower. The phenomenon of blood "sludging" may occur and further disrupt capillary blood flow and gas exchange.

If the injury is not too severe and shock is treated promptly by replacement of blood loss with whole blood and plasma transfusions, the cardiac output and arterial and venous pressure will immediately increase and acidosis will disappear within a few hours. Renal function will be resumed, but may not return to normal for 12 to 24 hours.

A state of irreversible shock may supervene under certain circumstances: i.e., after massive injuries, or when treatment is delayed for many hours; or when, after the injured patient has responded favorably to shock therapy, he suffers a reaction to subsequent operative procedures or to a progressing infection. In irreversible shock, the arteriolar and capillary vasomotor tone is lost and despite massive transfusions the circulation gradually fails, arterial blood pressure cannot be sustained, and the patient dies.

Shock in thermal burns (q.v.) also may be primary or secondary. In overwhelmingly extensive and severe burns, the patient may go into shock and die in a few minutes to an hour or two after injury. Pulmonary edema or aspiration of vomitus may be the terminal event. Secondary shock in burns is due mainly to loss of large quantities of fluid into the lesions and into the underlying tissues (edema). This fluid loss begins immediately after the burn, accelerates from about the 4th to 12th hour, and slows down 24 to 36 hours following injury. A total of 10 to 15 liters may thus pass into injured tissues, profoundly depleting the plasma volume and also the body stores of water and sodium chloride. Electrolyte imbalance results from the loss of sodium, which is the essential cation in extracellular fluid.

The circulation in burn shock is characterized by decreased blood volume, chiefly of the plasma; pronounced hemoconcentration, and decreased cardiac output. Despite these factors, arterial blood pressure is usually maintained temporarily, due to increased viscosity of the blood together with active vasoconstriction. Acidosis develops progressively as in wound shock. In the treatment of burn shock large volumes of fluid replacement are essential during the first 2 days after injury and should consist of plasma, some whole blood, and abundant sodium supplied by sodium chloride, bicarbonate, or lactate solutions.

Abdominal injuries produce a special form of traumatic shock, in that the peritoneal irritation and infection lead to extensive loss of fluid into the peritoneal cavity. With such injuries there is almost always hemoconcentration in these injuries rather than hemodilution. Similarly, loss of fluid into the damaged tissues may occur in crush injuries. Dehydration shock, and that following prolonged exposure may complicate traumatic shock, especially if the injured patient has remained for many hours untreated.

Shock is encountered in various **medical conditions.** It may be due to dehydration, as in cholera or diabetic acidosis. Another form occurs in sepsis, severe infections, and certain poisonings—the so-called "toxic" or "septic" shock. In this, blood volume is normal, but arterial pressure low because of loss of arteriolar or capillary tone, with vasodilatation. Cardiac output is usually decreased, and tissues thus suffer from anoxia. "Sludging" of blood in capillaries adds to the disorganization of blood flow.

Operative and **postoperative shock** may be due to a variety of causes, among which the most common are vasomotor collapse from anesthesia (especially spinal anesthesia) or from traumatic surgical manipulation; dehydration; and blood loss. The main aspects of circulatory dysfunction are summarized in the table, CIRCULATION: IN HEALTH AND IN VARIOUS FORMS OF SHOCK, with average figures for each of the measurements in the above described conditions:

THE CIRCULATION: IN HEALTH AND IN VARIOUS FORMS OF SHOCK

(Figures in parentheses represent typical values)

	Cardiac Output	Blood Volume	Hematocrit	Vasomotor Tone (B.P.)
In Health	Normal (5.4 liters per minute)	Normal (6.0 liters)	Normal (45%)	Normal (120/80)
Syncope	Normal	Normal	Normal	Low (70/50)
Wound Shock Hemorrhage	Low (3.5 L./min.)	Low (3.1 L./min.)	Low (32%)	Low (70/40)
Burns	Low (3.0 L./min.)	Low (3.2 L./min.)	High (55%)	Variable, often no change (114/70)
Abdominal Injury Dehydration	Low (3.2 L./min.)	Low (4.0 L./min.)	High (52%)	Moderately low (80/50)
Medical (toxic) Shock	Low (3.5 L./min.)	Normal	Normal	Low (70/50)

SYNCOPE
(Fainting)

Temporary loss of consciousness due to cerebral anemia. Predisposing factors include fatigue, prolonged standing, getting up after protracted bed rest, nausea, pain, surgical instrumentation, emotional disturbances, anemia, dehydration, infection, heart disease, hypertension, arteriosclerosis (especially cerebral) and other states causing vasomotor instability.

Symptoms and Signs

Fainting may occur suddenly but, except for cases that follow a physical blow or other abrupt trauma, there usually are premonitory symptoms. The patient feels uncomfortable, weak, squeamish, giddy, faint, and begins to sweat. This is the stage of rapid pulse rate and diminishing pulse pressure. If unrelieved, the condition progresses and, with the vasovagal reaction, blood pressure falls and true syncope supervenes. Physical signs are sudden and include increasing pallor, sweating, thin rapid pulse, followed by abrupt slowing of pulse rate, fall in blood pressure, and loss of consciousness. If the condition persists for more than a few minutes, there may be clonic muscular contractions; even involuntary micturition and defecation may occur.

Diagnosis

In the diagnosis of simple syncope it is necessary to rule out organic disease. In an individual who has suddenly lost consciousness, the manifestations of such disease must be looked for, even though adequate immediate cause for the syncope seems apparent. In addition to the predisposing factors previously mentioned the following may be listed: head injury, brain tumor, cerebral hemorrhage, meningitis, arterial hypertension, heart failure (especially when due to coronary thrombosis, cardiac arrhythmias, or Adams-Stokes seizures), carotid sinus reflex, gastrointestinal hemorrhage, sudden onset of an acute illness of any kind, and drug poisoning.

Treatment

In the premonitory state, with mild symptoms of faintness, it may be sufficient to seat the patient and instruct him to lower his head between his knees for a minute or two until the acute cerebral anoxia is relieved. The cause of the fainting episode should then be sought and, if possible, corrected.

If a patient has lost consciousness, he should be placed in the supine position, either horizontally or with feet elevated. Clothing should be loosened. If consciousness is not promptly regained, simple vasomotor stimulants may be used, such as inhalation of aromatic spirit of ammonia or cold water to the face. After consciousness returns, the patient should remain recumbent for 10 to 30 minutes and then be allowed up gradually. With prolonged syncope, especially if associated with convulsions, more drastic circulatory stimulants may be needed: Neo-Synephrine (℞ 21), ephedrine (℞ 23), epinephrine (℞ 24), or Metrazol (℞ 26). In extreme cases, I.V. administration of fluid may become necessary. Artificial respiration (see RESUSCITATION METHODS) is not indicated unless the fainting attack is marked by respiratory failure. If the patient is breathing normally and is not cyanotic, artificial respiration is not indicated no matter how long the duration of unconsciousness.

TRAUMATIC AND HEMORRHAGIC SHOCK

Shock following injury, or loss of blood, or both.

Symptoms and Signs

Evidence of injury may or may not be readily apparent. Usually, the patient is conscious and able to answer questions, but appears benumbed and is apathetic. The most frequent complaint is thirst. Pain may be severe, mild, or absent. Restlessness is common; anxiety, fear or panic relatively uncommon unless there is much pain. In deep shock consciousness may be lost. Pallor and sweating occur; cyanosis rarely is severe except with chest injuries. Vomiting is not infrequent. The pulse is soft, faint, and rapid; blood pressure usually is low, though very early after injury it may be normal or even elevated. Respirations are usually increased, sometimes sighing, but true dyspnea suggests either chest injury or the "air hunger" of rapid and continued blood loss. Renal output is greatly reduced or shut down entirely in severe shock.

Diagnosis

In traumatic shock, the cause generally is evident, but if there are no external signs of injury, other conditions may be suspected, such as coronary thrombosis, perforated viscus, or acute pancreatitis.

Treatment

The severity of shock and the amount of treatment required to restore the circulation depend chiefly on the extent of the injury and the time that has elapsed before treatment is started. The level of arterial blood pressure still is the best index to the degree of shock. Persons in shock are in danger of sudden death and must be closely and continuously watched until the circulation is restored.

The patient should lie supine, except with certain chest and head injuries, when head and chest may have to be raised. If shock is profound or rapidly progressing, the feet should be elevated above the head; about 12 inches usually is sufficient; occasionally up to 24 inches is necessary. The body should be kept warm, but external heat is applied only if there has been exposure to cold, and then cautiously. It is better if the extremities remain cool. The patient should not be moved about, nor his injuries manipulated, until at least some fluid replacement has been effected.

Adequate sedation must be given promptly, with dosage dependent upon symptoms. In most cases a single dose of morphine (℞ 57) 15 mg. (gr. ¼) will be sufficient to control restlessness and pain, but for severe pain or anxiety larger or repeated doses are required. If shock is profound and the circulation extremely poor, the initial dose should be given I.V. Because of the faulty circulation in such patients, subcutaneous doses are not advisable, because they are slowly absorbed and, if repeated, may have a cumulative toxic effect which appears as the circulation is restored.

Patients often complain of thirst. In mild shock, water, or preferably saline solution, may be given as tolerated. In severe shock water is allowed only in sips, if at all.

In deep shock, vomiting often occurs and is a grave danger to the patient. Aspiration of vomitus, resulting in sudden death is a frequent occurrence in such cases. The patient should lie with his head turned to one side and if he vomits, the oral and air passages must be cleared quickly. A suction apparatus should be kept constantly available.

While drug treatment of shock has been generally ineffective, preliminary reports on cortisone or ACTH therapy appear encouraging. Cardiocirculatory stimulants such as Metrazol (Ŗ 26), Coramine (Ŗ 27), caffeine (Ŗ 28), or epinephrine (Ŗ 24) may improve the circulation momentarily but cannot be relied upon for lasting benefit. Digitalis is contraindicated. Ephedrine and other sympathomimetic amines may cause transient rise in blood pressure, but often further decrease cardiac output.

The definitive treatment of traumatic and hemorrhagic shock is by fluid replacement given immediately I.V. to restore circulating blood and tissue-fluid volumes. Whole blood is the fluid of choice. Plasma, or less desirably, saline, may serve as a substitute if whole blood is not immediately available. For small or moderate injuries with mild shock, treated early, 500 cc. initially usually will suffice; for massive injuries or deep shock, or injuries treated late, 1,000 cc. or more may be required. It should be infused as rapidly as possible, 500 cc. in 5 to 10 minutes. If the patient is *in extremis*, fluids should be injected under forced pressure or stripped down the infusion tubing, to fill the empty right heart. Danger of running this initial fluid in too rapidly exists only in chest injuries, where pulmonary edema (q.v.) must be avoided.

A rapid and remarkable improvement in the circulation almost always results from the first infusion, but more fluid must be given to sustain it. The initial response lasts longer after blood or plasma than after saline. In moderately severe injury with shock there is an average deficit of 2 liters in the circulating blood and an equal or greater deficit of fluid in the tissues generally. The tissue-fluid deficiency will be accentuated if the condition has remained untreated for several hours, or in extensive crush injury with serous effusion into tissues. Severe acidosis develops progressively in untreated shock. A good plan of therapy is (1) to attempt to restore the blood volume by transfusion of whole blood, or whole blood and plasma, within the first 12 to 24 hours; (2) supplement this by at least an equal volume of saline, or of ⅙ molar sodium lactate solution, given by continuous I.V. drip; and (3) continue the saline infusion until a good urinary volume (1,000 to 1,500 cc. daily) has been established. (CAUTION! Care must be taken to avoid overhydration during the period of oliguria or anuria.) As the patient improves, oral administration of fluids can be substituted for the infusions. Subsequent blood transfusions will depend upon the general surgical situation.

Sometimes the patient's circulation, after an initial response, will fail progressively, despite vigorous fluid replacement. This usually means either an irreversible state of shock due to massive injuries or a continued progressive blood loss from internal hemorrhage, and it often is most difficult to determine which condition is responsible. The only recourse is to pour in whole blood until indications justify operative search for a bleeding source.

Oxygen therapy, by mask or tent, is indicated in most cases of chest injury. It can be expected to aid to a limited extent, if at all, in the treatment of shock due to other forms of injury.

THERMAL BURNS
(For the clinical aspects and treatment of shock due to burns, *see* chapter on BURNS.)

ABDOMINAL INJURIES

The treatment of shock in abdominal injuries is essentially the same as in traumatic shock, as given above. The frequent occurrence of hemoconcentration in abdominal injuries indicates a greater relative loss of plasma than of red cells from the blood, but there is a large deficit of both, and whole blood or whole blood and plasma, still constitute the optimum initial replacement therapy. In later treatment a greater proportion of saline may be needed to restore and maintain normal body fluid volumes.

DEHYDRATION SHOCK

A careful history is important, as physical signs may be unreliable in evaluating the amount of fluid loss. The duration of symptoms, and the severity of such underlying conditions as exposure, fever, diarrhea, vomiting, and diabetic acidosis, should be determined if possible. General symptoms are weakness and thirst, with special symptoms according to the underlying disease. Physical signs are similar to those in other forms of shock, plus the specific signs of dehydration: dry, loose skin, soft eyeballs, dry tongue, hemoconcentration (as shown by hematocrit reading). The chief difficulties in diagnosis lie in evaluating the degree of dehydration and, sometimes, in identifying the underlying disease.

Treatment

The general approach is the same as in traumatic shock. Since the body is deficient chiefly in water and electrolytes, rather than blood or plasma, fluid replacement should consist mainly of saline solutions. In mild shock these can be started at once by vein or by clysis; in profound shock it is best to give whole blood or plasma I.V. as the initial treatment.

The optimum form of electrolyte solution to use depends on the electrolytes lost and the presence or absence of acidosis. In most cases there is severe acidosis, and I.V. fluid used at first should be combinations of isotonic salt solution and 5% sodium bicarbonate solution, or isotonic salt solution and $\frac{1}{6}$ molar sodium lactate solution. Blood CO_2 determinations will be helpful in determining the degree of acidosis and its response to therapy. Occasionally, if vomiting has been excessive, alkalosis may be present, with high blood CO_2 values (*see* ACID-BASE AND ALLIED DISORDERS).

Large amounts of I.V. and subcut. fluids are needed in severe dehydration. Often, 5 to 10 liters must be administered over a 24- to 48-hour period to restore body fluids. The restoration of a normal urinary volume usually is a reliable index of body fluid adequacy. As soon as possible, oral administration of fluids should be started and, if tolerated, can progressively replace the parenteral method. It is particularly important to give by mouth such electrolytes as potassium, calcium, and phosphates, either in fluids or in food, as these often are lost in large amounts and cannot easily be administered parenterally. This is especially true in diabetic acidosis (q.v.).

MEDICAL (TOXIC) SHOCK

That due to overwhelming infection or poisoning.

Etiology, Symptoms, and Signs

Peripheral circulatory failure is not infrequent in the late stages of severe infections, such as pneumonia, meningitis, or various forms of septicemia. Apparently, the primary defect in such cases is a loss of function in the smaller blood vessels, resulting in vasomotor collapse. The symptoms and signs are those of a progressively failing circulation: i.e., rapid pulse, becoming first soft, then thready; low blood pressure; rapid, weak heart sounds; usually pallor, sweating, and cold extremities; great weakness and prostration; often delirium, stupor or coma.

In some forms of poisoning, vasomotor collapse appears so abruptly, that it may be mistaken for ordinary syncope.

Diagnosis

In a patient with an overwhelming infection the chief difficulty is to evaluate the relative importance of the many factors present, especially heart failure, dehydration, and peripheral vasomotor collapse. Very rapid heart rate and weak heart sounds do not necessarily indicate primary myocardial weakness. Embryonal (tic-tac) rhythm is suggestive and gallop rhythm strongly indicative of early heart failure, as are other cardiac arrhythmias (q.v.), or increase in heart size. Rise in venous pressure also is suggestive, if it is not due to pulmonary causes. Acute pulmonary edema, when it occurs, most often results from left-sided heart failure. The ECG may be of great aid in evaluating the cardiac factor. Signs of dehydration have already been discussed.

Treatment

The failing circulation in overwhelming infection usually is of a complex nature, as indicated above, and must be treated with great caution as well as skill. True shock or collapse usually will respond, at least temporarily, to a transfusion (500 cc. of blood or plasma) or an infusion (500 to 1,000 cc. of saline or glucose and saline), but all fluids must be given carefully, the lungs watched for pulmonary edema, the pulse for irregularity, the heart for gallop rhythm, other arrhythmias, or acute enlargement, and the circulation for undue rise in venous pressure. Sometimes an enlarged or tender liver will be the first sign of venous circulatory congestion. If a small transfusion or infusion is well tolerated, it may be repeated as indicated.

Cardiocirculatory stimulants may be of help in temporarily improving the circulation in the vasomotor forms of toxic medical shock. Available drugs include caffeine (R 28) 0.5 Gm., I.M. or I.V.; Metrazol (R 26) 0.1 to 0.3 Gm., I.M. or I.V.; Coramine (R 27) 1.5 to 5.0 cc., I.M. or I.V.; Neo-Synephrine (R 21) 3 to 5 mg., I.M. or I.V.; and epinephrine (R 24) 0.5 to 1.0 cc., subcut.; or aminophylline (R 14) 0.25 Gm., I.V. given very slowly. (The pulse and heart action should be observed very closely for unfavorable effects with the latter two medicaments.)

All treatment in this type of medical shock should be looked upon only as a temporary expedient, used in an endeavor to sustain the circulation until the infection itself can be brought under control.

In poisoning, with shock due to vasomotor collapse—when the diagnosis and clinical state have been established—treatment should be more vigorous, with transfusions and I.V. fluids. In such cases the circulation usually will respond promptly and favorably.

SHOCK OR SHOCKLIKE STATES IN OTHER CONDITIONS

Complex states manifested by shock or shocklike symptoms occur in such conditions (q.v.) as coronary thrombosis with myocardial infarction, the Waterhouse-Friderichsen syndrome (adrenal hemorrhage) in meningitis, or the acute circulatory failure of addisonian crisis.

HEART MURMURS

Adventitious sounds, due to vibrations produced by motion of blood within the heart or adjacent great vessels, and heard in the region of the heart during systole or diastole, or both.

When heart murmurs are encountered they must not be regarded as entities divorced from other conditions, but should be carefully related to the history of the patients; to the physical findings, reinforced by X-ray, fluoroscopic, ECG, circulation time and further laboratory or other examinations as necessary; and to the condition of the whole circulatory system in terms of observed normal or disturbed dynamics. The importance of the murmur in the diagnosis and prognosis of cardiovascular disease, if any, can then be evaluated.

Many patients, upon learning that they have a heart murmur, become unduly apprehensive, voluntarily restrict their normal activities and curtail their pleasures to the point of becoming neurotic semi-invalids. A physician owes it to his patient to prevent or dissipate such fears by a reassuring explanation of what a murmur is and what, if anything, this murmur means to the patient's future.

The more commonly encountered heart murmurs, together with symptoms and signs likely to be associated with their causal conditions are described below. The reader will find additional details concerning the etiology, diagnosis, prophylaxis, and treatment of cardiovascular disease of which valvular lesions are only one part, in the several chapters of the Cardiovascular Section. Further information about etiology and prophylaxis is contained in the chapters on RHEUMATIC FEVER, SCARLET FEVER, SYDENHAM'S CHOREA, and SYPHILIS.

Pathologic Physiology

Most commonly, a murmur is caused either by forward flow of blood through a narrowed orifice, as in aortic or mitral stenosis, or by reflux of blood backward through an incompetent valve, as in aortic insufficiency. Blood flow past valvular or great vessel irregularities as in sclerotic valves or aorta, or the outflow of blood into enlarged chambers as in aortic aneurysm also can set up vibrations which are heard as murmurs. Physiologic and hemic murmurs (q.v.) may, however, be audible in the absence of any demonstrable structural abnormality of the heart. Furthermore, even though of organic origin, the loudness or intensity of a murmur is not necessarily a criterion of the heart's functional capacity and may prove to be of minor prognostic significance.

Types, With Related Symptoms and Signs

1. Physiologic: A short, soft systolic murmur at the apex, or a short systolic murmur heard over the precordium or at the base over the pulmonic valve, occurs rather frequently in normal hearts. A similarly nonorganic systolic murmur may accompany the acute stage of various febrile illnesses in some patients. A physiologic murmur in the precordium usually is soft, whereas at the base it may be soft, rough, or even scratchy. Such a basal murmur will sometimes disappear with a change of bodily position, or temporarily following exercise, or when breathing is halted momentarily in deep inspiration. The so-called 3rd heart sound, a faint, short, low-pitched sound occasionally heard in mid-diastole in hearts with slow rate, may be mistaken for a mid-diastolic mitral murmur.

2. Hemic: The accelerated blood flow in anemia often is associated with a heart murmur. Most commonly this is a blowing systolic sound, maximal at the apex and heard also over the precordium. In severe anemia with cardiac dilatation, the systolic apical murmur probably is due, at least in part, to mitral valvular dilatation and relative mitral insufficiency. A systolic basal or aortic murmur occasionally is heard in anemia. Presystolic mitral murmurs in extremely severe anemia have been reported; an aortic diastolic murmur due to this cause, if it ever occurs, is exceedingly rare.

3. Mitral valvular murmurs: Although lesions of the mitral valve are predominantly rheumatic in origin, relative insufficiency also may result from stretching of the mitral ring due to left ventricular dilatation, as in various forms of myocardial damage, acute or chronic, or in long-continued arteriosclerosis and hypertensive vascular disease.

The characteristic murmur of mitral valvular insufficiency is a blowing systolic sound, which may be short, medium, or long. It is maximal at the apex and transmitted toward the axilla. This murmur is caused by reflux of blood backward through the mitral valve during systole.

The murmur of mitral stenosis, in the typical form as heard in the presence of a greatly narrowed "keyhole" mitral opening, is a long rumbling sound starting early in diastole, with a crescendo just before the 1st heart sound (due to acceleration of blood flow produced by auricular systole). It is usually best heard over the precordium, in the axilla, and in the back. With lesser degrees of valvular stenosis, the sounds become shorter and softer and late diastolic or presystolic in timing. In some cases of definite and well established mitral valvular disease, even in the presence of heart failure, the presystolic murmur may be extremely difficult or impossible to detect. It is best brought out by having the patient exercise briefly or lie well over on his left side. A short presystolic murmur sometimes is hard to differentiate from a presystolic gallop rhythm. The 2nd pulmonic heart sound is regularly accentuated ("snapping") in mitral valvular disease as long as compensation is maintained.

When auricular fibrillation supervenes, the murmur of mitral stenosis is heard in mid-diastole. The absence of auricular systole explains the lack of any presystolic crescendo element.

In patients with mitral disease, particularly the slowly progressive forms of mitral stenosis, the heart tends to remain relatively well compensated for a surprisingly long time. Some mitral lesions are almost purely stenotic, others are mainly regurgitant, many are both. In any event, some degree of valvular incompetence usually develops sooner or later as the condition progresses. When symptoms do appear in persons with mitral disease, they are characteristically due to venous stasis and are first referred to the pulmonary system, with cough, dyspnea on moderate or slight exertion, moderate to severe cyanosis, and often hemoptysis. Palpitation, lassitude, anorexia, indigestion, and frequent respiratory infections are commonly encountered. Precordial pain, seldom truly anginal, is not unusual.

Examination of the heart shows enlargement to both sides of the sternum in insufficiency, with the apex beat rather diffuse and displaced outward; in stenosis the main enlargement is to the right. (These findings can be confirmed by X-ray or fluoroscopic examination.) An apical systolic thrill may be felt in cases of insufficiency, but in mitral stenosis a presystolic thrill, located in the left 4th or 5th interspaces close to the nipple line, is pathognomonic. This frequently ends in a systolic shock synchronous with the apex beat.

The pulse is hardly characteristic. In insufficiency it may be regular and full until decompensation renders it irregular and of poor tension. In stenosis the pulse is small, often slow, and frequently irregular, becoming completely irregular with the onset of auricular fibrillation. The blood pressure tends to be low or normal in most patients with mitral lesions.

In patients with decompensation the usually easily demonstrable findings are pulmonary congestion, an enlarged tender liver, edema of the feet and ankles, and cardiac irregularity.

4. Aortic valvular murmurs: Syphilis, rheumatic fever, a bicuspid valve, and subacute bacterial endocarditis are the common causes of aortic insufficiency, while rheumatic fever and calcific aortic disease of arteriosclerotic origin are mainly responsible for aortic stenosis. Occasionally, aortic insufficiency occurs in a hypertensive arteriosclerotic heart.

With a large aortic valvular defect such as occurs with the shortened, rolled-up valve leaflets of syphilitic aortic disease, the typical murmurs are the long, low-pitched "falling-away" diastolic murmur of aortic insufficiency, heard along the left sternal border from the base downward; and a blowing, often somewhat rough, aortic systolic murmur. Two other (accessory) murmurs, either or both of which may be present or absent, are an apical systolic murmur due to relative mitral insufficiency and a presystolic "Austin-Flint" murmur at or inside the apex due to fluttering of the mitral cusps in the current of regurgitated blood.

When the aortic valvular insufficiency is less extensive, the accessory murmurs usually are absent, and the characteristic aortic diastolic murmur becomes softer and fainter. It may be short or long, high or low pitched. It is best heard with the Bowles stethoscope, or with the unaided ear applied directly to the chest, with the chest in maximal expiration and the patient either lying flat or sitting upright.

The heart is found to be enlarged to the left and downward; the apex beat is forcible, heaving, and often as low as the 6th or 7th interspace and as far laterally as the midaxillary line. Visible pulsation of the abdominal aorta, the carotids and other large arteries, and of the retinal arteries, should be looked for. A capillary pulse may be elicited in the rubbed forehead, the nail beds, and the moistened lip pressed upon by a glass slide. The pulse strikes the examining finger with great force, then fades away to nothing in a collapsing or "water-hammer" fashion (Corrigan pulse). In the radial artery this can be exaggerated by encircling the patient's wrist with the fingers while holding it aloft over his head. The systolic blood pressure is ordinarily increased, sometimes reaching 180 or higher, while the diastolic pressure is low and may even be difficult to determine. A high pulse pressure is the obvious result. In the lower limbs the systolic pressure may be considerably higher than in the arms. Over the larger arteries, and most easily detectable over the femoral, a to-and-fro murmur (Duroziez's sign) can be elicited under moderate stethoscope pressure, together with a local systolic shock—the so-called "pistol-shot" sound. The arteries themselves are apt to be hard and tortuous, indicative of arteriosclerotic changes generally, where arteriosclerosis is the cause of the aortic valvular involvement.

Patients with aortic insufficiency often are anemic and may appear pallid. Some, however, have a ruddy complexion. They may remain fairly comfortable for several years, but are more likely to complain of throbbing headaches, vertigo, head noises, faintness on rising or on stooping over, flashes of light, precordial pain that may be truly anginal, dyspnea (even syncope) on exertion, spells of palpitation, irritability and restlessness coupled with faulty memory, insomnia, and disturbing dreams. Some of these individuals nevertheless remain capable of great exertion, taking part in athletics or heavy labor with few or no symptoms prior to the onset of decompensation. After the first break in compensation the former cardiac reserve is rarely if ever regained. Decompensated patients with aortic insufficiency rapidly experience nocturnal dyspnea and orthopnea, edema of the feet and ankles, cough and hemoptysis, mental disturbances and, if they survive long enough, generalized edema. Sudden death is common—more so than with any other form of chronic valvular disease.

Aortic stenosis without some degree of regurgitation probably does not occur. The murmur of aortic stenosis is a harsh blowing systolic sound, maximal over the aortic valve and transmitted to the neck, particularly the right side. As a rule, it is associated with a palpable thrill in the same regions. The 2nd aortic sound is usually diminished and often absent. Ordinarily there is only moderate left-sided cardiac enlargement, with the apex beat shifted slightly downward and to the left. The pulse is characteristically slow and small, and it persists under the examining finger as a deliberate, prolonged impulse. The blood pressure shows a lowering of systolic value and a rise in diastolic, with resultant low pulse pressure.

In patients with aortic stenosis the symptoms frequently are mild, indefinite, and delayed. When they do appear, they tend to resemble those described for aortic insufficiency but are less severe. When and if congestive heart failure develops, the symptoms and signs are those of decompensation.

In some patients with a murmur at first thought to be characteristic of aortic stenosis, further investigation reveals that instead of having a narrowed valve orifice opening into a normal aorta, they have a relatively normal orifice opening into a dilated aorta. Thus, in syphilitic aneurysm of the aorta, there sometimes is a loud aortic systolic murmur, occasionally accompanied by a thrill, even though no true aortic stenosis is present. Here it is thought that the blood eddying into the aneurysmal sac produces the murmur. In such instances, however, the 2nd aortic sound is usually accentuated, and the pulse is not that of aortic stenosis.

5. Pulmonic valvular murmurs: Involvement of the pulmonic valve occurs very rarely in rheumatic disease; it can result in a systolic or a diastolic murmur over the pulmonic valve area. Relative dilatation of the pulmonic ring secondary to enlargement of the pulmonary conus, with a diastolic murmur that comes and goes, is the mechanism of the so-called Graham Steell murmur. It is found occasionally in mitral disease, and sometimes in other conditions, such as interauricular septal defect, which also cause a major enlargement of the conus. Thus, except in purely congenital pulmonic stenotic lesions, the symptoms and signs are those related to the underlying cardiac disease and to the degree of heart failure present.

6. Tricuspid valvular murmurs: Relative tricuspid insufficiency, with a dilated tricuspid ring, is quite common in dilated rheumatic hearts. It also may occur in prolonged obstruction of the pulmonary circulation, as in chronic pulmonary diseases. There may or may not be the typical systolic murmur heard along the right border of the lower portion of the sternum. When this murmur is due, as it often is, to organic disease of the tricuspid valve, the cause is almost always rheumatic disease. Tricuspid stenosis is rare and seldom diagnosed when present. Almost invariably it is secondary to rheumatic involvement and mitral stenosis is present.

Patients with tricuspid valvular lesions usually will present the characteristic history, symptoms and signs of the causal rheumatic heart disease as described earlier with respect to other valves. A venous pulse, especially in the veins of the neck, can be demonstrated in insufficiency. Evidence of hepatic enlargement and pulsation, pulmonary congestion, and other signs of congestive heart failure are to be expected as the course continues.

7. Congenital heart murmurs: For a description of these, *see* chapter on CONGENITAL CARDIOVASCULAR ANOMALIES.

CARDIAC ARRHYTHMIAS

Rhythm changes of the heart caused by disturbances, either physiologic or pathologic, of the regular automaticity of the cardiac impulse, or by changes of the conductance pattern of the cardiac impulse.

Normally, the impulse which stimulates the auricles and ventricles originates in the sinoauricular (SA) node. It then spreads over both auricles in a fanlike fashion to reach the auriculoventricular (AV) node. This produces the initial upward (positive) deflection of the electrocardiogram (ECG) arbitrarily identified as the P wave. The impulse passes from the AV node through the AV bundle (common bundle or bundle of His) which divides into right and left bundle branches. These branches terminate in the network of Purkinje, the main portions of which come in contact with the muscular fibers of the

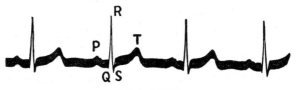

Normal ECG

ventricles. The impulse is retarded somewhat in the AV node and bundle and in this period no electrical impulse is inscribed on the ECG. On reaching the bundle branches and the network of Purkinje, the impulse is conducted rapidly to the endocardial surface of each ventricle, from whence it spreads to the epicardial surfaces. This phase produces the QRS deflections of the ECG. During the period of recovery of the ventricles from contraction, a T wave is inscribed on the ECG and is believed to be due to the repolarization of the cellular membranes of the ventricular fibers. Although the inscriptions of the P and QRS deflections precede the actual muscular contraction of the respective portions of the heart, the ECG serves to identify chronologically the several phases of the heartbeat and to a certain extent furnishes information concerning the character of the heartbeat.

The SA node is the cardiac structure which normally has the highest automaticity and, as the pacemaker, regularly initiates impulses which produce normal sinus rhythm. Rate changes and rhythm changes are caused by variations in the amount of stimulation of the SA node by the vagus nerve, or by relative decrease in automaticity of the SA node below that of some other part of the heart. When another part of the heart acquires a higher automaticity it assumes the role of pacemaker.

Only those that are of most frequent occurrence or are of significant clinical importance will be described here.

Occasionally, the patient is not aware of the existence of an arrhythmia and it may be detected only by careful physical examination. Certain arrhythmias can be identified by observing their effect on the pulse rate or rhythm, or by cardiac auscultation. Others can be discovered and identified only by means of the ECG. While the use of the ECG is definitely limited in diagnostic and prognostic value in many forms of heart disease, it is of especial usefulness in demonstrating and identifying rhythm disturbances. However, the prognosis can be determined only by careful history and physical examination, by evaluation of the clinical manifestations present, and by adequate follow-up.

SINUS BRADYCARDIA

A slow sinus rhythm, less than 50 beats/minute.

Etiology and Incidence

Most cases of sinus bradycardia probably are due to an increase in vagal tone. Meningitis and increase in intracranial pressure (as by intracranial tumor or hemorrhage) produce sinus bradycardia by irritation of the vagus center. Vagal tone also may be increased reflexly, by pressure on the carotid sinus or the eyeballs, or by irritation of the mucosa of the upper

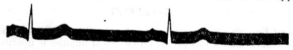

Sinus Bradycardia (*rate 40 / min.*)

respiratory tract. In persons with a hypersensitive carotid sinus, a slight and temporary pressure (e.g., tight collar) may lead to severe sinus bradycardia or even cardiac standstill. Profuse hemorrhage giving rise to prolonged hypotension may cause sinus bradycardia after an initial stage of tachycardia. Sinus bradycardia often occurs normally during rest and sleep. It is common in athletes, and frequently develops in patients convalescing from infectious diseases and in patients with jaundice. Inhalation anesthesia has been reported occasionally to lead to sinus bradycardia, and even sinus standstill and death, by reflex stimulation of the vagus.

Symptoms and Signs

Uncomplicated sinus bradycardia (e.g., sinus bradycardia without orthostatic hypotension) does not produce any symptoms unless it is extreme, in which case it may lead to syncope and convulsions. The pulse rate and, on auscultation, the heart rate are slow, below 50 beats/minute. Hyperthermia, exercise and emotion accelerate the cardiac rate in sinus bradycardia.

Treatment

Sinus bradycardia usually requires no treatment. If a patient has recurrent fainting spells due to episodes of pronounced sinus bradycardia, he should avoid the conditions that bring about the bradycardia (such as standing immobile, wearing tight clothing about the neck). He must be cautioned to lie down if faintness or vertigo occurs, so as to combat cerebral ischemia and prevent possible injury from a fall. Atropine (R 19) seldom is useful in preventing such fainting spells, but should be tried in cases of hypersensitive carotid sinus.

SINUS TACHYCARDIA

A sinus rhythm greater than 100 beats/minute.

Etiology

Any agent or condition that abolishes or decreases vagal tone or stimulates the sympathetic accelerator nerve, or does both, may lead to sinus tachycardia. Emotion, exercise, thyrotoxicosis, hypotension, anoxia, hyperthermia, anemia, hemorrhage, infections, certain neuroses, and neurocirculatory asthenia are frequent causes. Cardiac failure and many diseases of the pericardium, myocardium or endocardium often are accompanied by sinus tachycardia. Certain drugs such as atropine, epinephrine, and nicotine may produce the condition by various mechanisms.

Symptoms and Signs

Sinus tachycardia does not of itself give rise to severe symptoms although the patient may be aware of the fast rate or

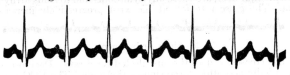

Sinus Tachycardia (*rate 150/min.*)

forceful action of the heart, especially when due to hyperthyroidism, muscular exercise, or neurocirculatory asthenia. Evidence of cardiac insufficiency may appear in patients with low cardiac reserve. It is of clinical importance to remember that, unlike paroxysmal tachycardia, sinus tachycardia usually does not start and stop suddenly, but comes on gradually and tapers off when the cause is removed. In sinus tachycardia, the ventricular rate and the pulse rate are equal. The ECG shows 100 or more P-QRS-T complexes/minute. Maneuvers that increase the vagal tone (such as carotid sinus pressure or pressure on the eyeballs) slow the heart rate somewhat, but as soon as pressure is released the previous rate is resumed. Such maneuvers never stop sinus tachycardia.

Prognosis

The prognosis depends entirely on the cause of the sinus tachycardia and on the condition of the heart. It may have no clinical significance whatever, since it is a normal reaction of the heart in many instances, such as in anemia, hemorrhage, or exercise. It is, however, of great clinical significance if due to active rheumatic carditis, in which case the prognosis is that of rheumatic fever (q.v.). Furthermore, severe and prolonged sinus tachycardia, whatever its cause, may lead to secondary cardiac failure, especially in hearts with low reserve.

Treatment

The therapy of sinus tachycardia is directed at the cause. If the patient is aware of forceful and rapid heart action, sedation should be used (Ŗ 44). If secondary cardiac failure develops, it must be treated in the same manner as congestive heart failure (q.v.) from any other cause.

SINUS ARRHYTHMIA

A condition common in children and the aged, wherein the heart rate alternately increases and decreases. It probably is the result of changes in vagal tone and not indicative of any disease process. The increased rate usually occurs with respiratory inspiration, and the decreased rate with expiration, but occasionally these phasic changes are not associated with respiration.

Symptoms and Signs

Seldom, if ever, are there any symptoms due to sinus arrhythmia. The pulse rate felt at the wrist progressively increases,

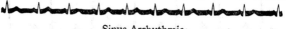

Sinus Arrhythmia

then decreases, as does the auscultated heart rate. Deep breathing usually accentuates the sinus arrhythmia. The ECG shows normal P-QRS-T complexes with a progressively shortening then lengthening diastole.

Treatment

Agents that abolish the tone of the vagi abolish sinus arrhythmia. Drugs having this effect include atropine (Ŗ 19), and barbiturates, such as phenobarbital (Ŗ 44). Since sinus arrhythmia is neither a disease nor a sign of one, treatment is rarely necessary.

WANDERING PACEMAKER

A term limited to the progressive shift of the pacemaker, from beat to beat, from the SA node to areas closer and closer to the AV node, and even to the AV node itself—and vice versa. It is not used to designate isolated shifts from the SA node to

the auricle or the AV node, giving rise to premature auricular
or AV nodal contractions.

Etiology

Wandering pacemaker is generally associated with pronounced
sinus arrhythmia and is most often due to phasic variations in
vagal tone.

Symptoms and Signs

Most persons with wandering pacemaker also have sinus arrhythmia (q.v.). They will have a progressively increasing and
decreasing heart rate and pulse rate, especially on deep, slow
breathing. The ECG shows progressively shortening and lengthening cardiac cycles as in sinus arrhythmia. Furthermore, the
P-R interval progressively, from beat to beat, decreases then

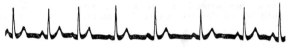

Wandering Pacemaker and Sinus Arrhythmia

increases and the P waves change in appearance. If the pacemaker shifts to the lower part of the AV node, the P waves may
even occur after the QRS complex. Since the impulse that activates the ventricles is of supraventricular origin, the QRS complex is normal.

Treatment

This is identical with that of sinus arrhythmia (q.v.).

PREMATURE CONTRACTIONS

*Contractions occurring when the automaticity of the normal
cardiac pacemaker (the SA node), or of any portion of the
auricles or ventricles, is altered in such a way that one of these
structures releases prematurely an impulse which spreads to the
whole heart or to part of it.* Such a beat is called a premature
beat and, depending on its site of origin, can be a premature
sinus, auricular, nodal, or ventricular contraction.

Etiology

Premature contractions may be caused by many conditions,
such as arteriosclerotic heart disease, myocardial infarction,
hypertension, acute and chronic rheumatic heart disease, syphilitic heart disease, cardiac failure from any cause, hyperthyroidism, and myocardial ischemia. It also may be caused by
digitalis and digitalis-like agents, nicotine, tobacco, coffee, calcium, barium, and many other drugs or combination of drugs
such as chloroform-epinephrine and cyclopropane-epinephrine.
Mechanical stimulation may be responsible for extrasystoles
during operations on the heart, such as pericardectomy. Con-

stipation often is the only abnormality found in persons with numerous premature ventricular contractions. Often no abnormality, cardiac or otherwise, can be detected.

Symptoms and Signs

The patient complains of feeling something turning over in his chest, a shock in the chest, a skipped heart beat, or a choking

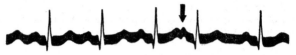

Premature Auricular Contraction

sensation. Such symptoms are annoying chiefly when premature beats first make their appearance. Later, the patient apparently becomes accustomed to them and may take little notice

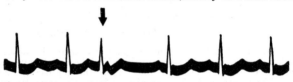

Premature Nodal Contraction

even though they increase in frequency. Occasionally, a cough or hiccup accompanies each extrasystole. Many patients, however, remain unaware of the abnormal beats.

On auscultation a premature beat may be heard which differs little, if at all, from the normal heart sounds, although certain

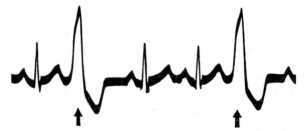

Premature Ventricular Contractions

premature contractions of ventricular origin may sound distinctly different from normal. Some of the premature contractions are sufficiently strong to yield a palpable pulsation of the radial artery.

Diagnosis of the site of origin of premature contractions can be made accurately only by ECG. This is accomplished by determining the time relationship of the abnormal or premature contraction to the rhythm on which it is superimposed, and by identifying the abnormal P-QRS-T complex by its peculiar characteristics, which vary according to the site of origin (e.g., nodal, auricular, ventricular).

Extrasystoles do not seem to affect the circulation appreciably except when they become numerous. The significance of extrasystoles depends on the underlying disease. The appearance

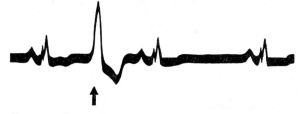

Premature Contraction, Interpolated in Regular Sinus Rhythm

of auricular extrasystoles in hyperthyroidism or chronic rheumatic heart disease often precedes the onset of auricular flutter or fibrillation (q.v.).

Treatment

When possible, treatment is directed at the cause. However, if extrasystoles persist and cause discomfort, the patient should be reassured and sedated. Phenobarbital (℞ 44), 30 mg. (gr. ss) 3 times a day, will be of help. A hypnotic may be administered if the patient cannot sleep because of being disturbed by the arrhythmia, which may be especially noticeable when he is lying quietly in bed. Pentobarbital sodium (℞ 47), 0.1 Gm. (gr. iss) repeated once in the 1st hour if necessary, often suffices. If sedation does not give relief, an attempt can be made to depress the irritability of the ectopic cardiac focus by administering quinidine sulfate (℞ 6) provided there are no contraindications to its use. A test dose of 0.2 Gm. (gr. iii) should be given by mouth, and, if no sign of idiosyncrasy appears (i.e., tinnitus, deafness, urticaria, rash, diarrhea, fall in blood pressure) within 3 to 4 hours, rapid and maximal therapeutic effects can be obtained by giving 0.8 Gm. (gr. xii) by mouth, followed in 4 hours by 0.2 Gm. (gr. iii) every 4 hours for 3 or 4 doses. The dosage then has to be adjusted according to the results obtained. However, such doses of quinidine are seldom needed in the treatment of extrasystoles, except when there is acute myocardial infarction; or when the premature contractions are of ventricular origin, especially if they are numerous and multifocal in origin and ventricular fibrillation is feared. (CAUTION! If the patient is in, or on the verge of, cardiac failure, quinidine in these doses may depress an already jeopardized myocardium.)

To prevent troublesome premature contractions over long periods of time when no emergency treatment is necessary, 0.2 to 0.4 Gm. (gr. iii to vi) of quinidine sulfate 3 times a day is recommended. When patients are receiving quinidine, they should be observed carefully for any signs of idiosyncrasy. The blood pressure and heart rate should be checked and an ECG (if available) made at frequent intervals (every 4 to 7 days for the first 2 weeks) especially if the doses given are large. If there is a fall in blood pressure, an abrupt change in heart rate (either increase or decrease), or the development of any kind of cardiac block (q.v.) further administration of quinidine should be carried out with great caution.

PULSUS BIGEMINUS
(Coupling, Bigeminy)

A condition in which each normal beat of sinoauricular origin is followed immediately by a premature ventricular contraction. The cause, manifestations, significance, and treatment are identical with those of premature contractions (q.v.).

NODAL ESCAPE

Occasionally, when the SA node is slow in originating an impulse, as in sinus bradycardia, sinus arrhythmia or sinus standstill, the auriculoventricular node may release an impulse which

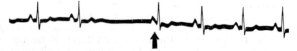

Sinoauricular Block (*Sinus Standstill*) and Nodal Escape

then is conducted to the ventricles and backward to the auricles. The signs and symptoms are essentially the same as those of a premature contraction. The ECG is similar to that produced by a nodal contraction; the abnormal beat, however, is not premature but, on the contrary, delayed.

Treatment

Nodal escape generally requires no therapy unless, as seldom occurs, it is frequent and bothersome. Sedation or correction of the sinus bradycardia and sinus arrhythmia with atropine rarely is necessary. When nodal escape occurs after sinus standstill due to accidental compression of a hypersensitive carotid sinus, the nodal escape is a fortunate occurrence as the AV node then takes over the function of the inhibited SA node.

PAROXYSMAL TACHYCARDIA

A condition in which the heart rate suddenly increases to 100 or more/minute when the role of the normal pacemaker (the SA

*node) is suddenly taken over by an ectopic focus in the auricles,
in the AV node, or in the ventricles.* According to the location
of the new pacemaker, the arrhythmia is termed paroxysmal
auricular, nodal, or ventricular tachycardia. An attack may last
for minutes, hours, or even days, ending as abruptly as it began.

Etiology

The cause of paroxysmal tachycardia probably is essentially
similar to that of the premature contractions (q.v.), since the
paroxysm is essentially an uninterrupted series of auricular,
nodal, or ventricular extrasystoles.

Symptoms, Signs, and Diagnosis

Paroxysmal tachycardia starts suddenly, although it may be
heralded by a few isolated premature contractions of the same

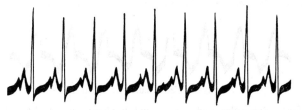

Paroxysmal Auricular Tachycardia

type. The patient is almost always aware of the onset, since
it is accompanied by the subjective sensations described for
premature contractions (q.v.). He also may have symptoms of
weakness, nausea, eructations, and fainting.

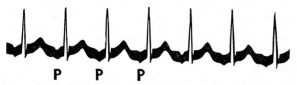

Paroxysmal Nodal Tachycardia

Occasionally, no symptoms accompany the paroxysm, but frequently the patient has a fluttering sensation in the chest and
feels weak and faint. The arterial blood pressure may fall and
the clinical manifestations be similar to those of secondary surgical shock (*see* Shock), or cardiac failure may develop with or
without signs of shock. The danger of such complications increases with the rapidity of the heart rate, and is greater with
ventricular tachycardia than with supraventricular tachycardias

of the same rate. During an attack, some patients complain of precordial discomfort or even anginal pain.

Auscultation reveals a rapid regular heart rate, but is of no help in differentiating the types of tachycardia. The patient's history is important in distinguishing sinus tachycardia from paroxysmal tachycardias. Maneuvers designed to interrupt the tachycardia are useful for diagnosis as well as for treatment. These include (1) expiration against a closed glottis, (2) attempted inspiration with the glottis closed, (3) lying down with feet in the air, (4) bending over, (5) emesis, induced mechanically or with warm soda bicarbonate or mustard solution orally, or with apomorphine hypodermically, (6) pressure on the eyeballs, or (7) compression of one or both carotid sinuses. The last named probably is the easiest and most effective maneuver. It stops auricular tachycardia and nodal tachycardia. Both can recur, however, soon after the compression ceases. It does not

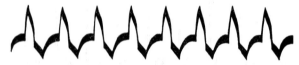

Paroxysmal Ventricular Tachycardia

affect ventricular tachycardia and it slows sinus tachycardia only slightly and only as long as the sinuses are compressed, at least in patients who have no hypersensitivity of the carotid sinus. During the time it is applied, carotid sinus compression also slows the ventricular rate in auricular flutter and fibrillation, without appreciably modifying the flutter or the fibrillation itself. Paroxysmal auricular or nodal tachycardia is common in relatively young individuals without attendant heart disease, although it may be associated with organic heart disease or be part of the Wolff-Parkinson-White syndrome. The ECG shows an uninterrupted series of beats similar to the ones in auricular, nodal, or ventricular premature contractions.

Treatment

The patient should be reassured and given a sedative (℞ 44, 45). Then carotid sinus compression or one or more of the other maneuvers mentioned above should be applied to stop the paroxysm. If these are not successful, Mecholyl (℞ 7) may be tried subcut. in doses of about 20 to 30 mg. If the carotid sinuses are compressed when the effect of Mecholyl is at its height, the results may be successful. Mecholyl is contraindicated in asthmatic patients and it should be given carefully to hypertensive individuals. When receiving this drug, the patient should be recumbent because of the possibility of fainting from the accompanying fall in blood pressure. Atropine (℞ 19) 0.6

or 0.8 mg. (gr. 1/100 or 1/75) should be at hand ready for subcut. injection in case too extreme a sinus bradycardia or even a cardiac standstill supervenes. If carotid sinus compression, or Mecholyl, or both, fail, quinidine (B 6) should be tried. A test dose of 0.2 Gm. (gr. iii) is given by mouth, and if no idiosyncrasy (tinnitus, deafness, urticaria, rash, diarrhea, drop in blood pressure) is revealed within 3 to 4 hours, a therapeutic dosage of 0.8 Gm. (gr. xii) followed every 2 hours by 0.2 to 0.4 Gm. (gr. iii to vi) for 3 or 4 doses may be given. This often will stop the paroxysms of tachycardia. While the patient is receiving quinidine, he should remain in bed; his blood pressure should be taken every hour, especially if idiosyncrasy or overdosage is suspected. Where possible, an ECG should be taken, since it may reveal an unsuspected block, either sinoauricular, auriculoventricular, or intraventricular; or premature ventricular contractions (q.v.). Another schedule, more frequently used, for the administration of quinidine is 0.4 Gm. (gr. vi) every 4 hrs. for 4 doses on the 1st day; if no result is obtained, 0.4 Gm. (gr. vi) 5 times on the 2nd day, and if necessary 0.4 Gm. (gr. vi) 6 times on the 3rd day. Once the auricular or nodal tachycardia has been stopped, a maintenance dose of 0.2 Gm. (gr. iii) 3 to 4 times a day for a few days is recommended. If the patient under care has few attacks, the protracted use of quinidine to prevent the attacks is not advisable. Such prevention should be attempted only when the attacks are frequent or when the patient's cardiac reserve is low, in which case 0.2 to 0.4 Gm. (gr. iii to vi) 3 to 4 times a day is the recommended dose.

Even in the absence of any cardiac failure or heart disease, digitalization (particularly rapid parenteral digitalization) has been used with success in auricular and nodal tachycardia. For oral administration, a purified cardiac glycoside, such as digitoxin (B 2) in an initial dose of 1 to 1.5 mg., should be used. This may be given as a single dose if the patient has not previously received digitalis. (CAUTION! If digitalis has been administered within 3 weeks, the dosage must be adjusted accordingly.) For parenteral digitalization, 1 mg. digitoxin (B 3) or lanatoside C, 1.5 mg. (B 4) administered slowly I.V., will be most effective in stopping paroxysmal auricular or nodal tachycardia. During the injection, auscultation should be done constantly, in order to detect immediately any ventricular extrasystoles, which are indications for slowing down the rate of administration. Compression of the carotid sinus, unsuccessful before digitalization, may become effective thereafter. It is questionable whether the maintenance of digitalization will prevent the recurrence of auricular or nodal tachycardia.

Digitalization should always be employed to stop a paroxysmal supraventricular tachycardia when the patient has cardiac failure or a low cardiac reserve. If rapid digitalization in a patient with heart failure does not relieve the tachycardia, quinidine sulfate should be tried, with or without a maintenance dose of digitalis. The danger of giving digitalis and quinidine simultaneously is greater when the doses of each drug are much larger than those recommended here. However, it probably is safer to give the maintenance dose of digitalis orally rather than I.V.

In the treatment of ventricular tachycardia, the dosage and administration of quinidine sulfate (℞ 6) are the same as described above. Much larger doses, up to 3 and 4 Gm./day, often are required to stop ventricular tachycardia but they may lead to cardiac standstill, ventricular fibrillation, or both. If the patient is in cardiac failure and has not responded to the quinidine sulfate, it may become advisable to digitalize him before giving further quinidine, but this must be done cautiously because of the possibility of inducing ventricular fibrillation. A suitable preparation of digitalis should be given orally; parenteral administration is contraindicated. Preparations having a wide margin of safety should be used, e.g., digitoxin, 1 to 1.5 mg. (℞ 2), given in fractionated doses over a 24-hour period. Quinidine therapy then is resumed. By cautious administration of these drugs and careful observation of their effects, dangerous complications may be avoided.

If the paroxysms of ventricular tachycardia recur often enough to be disturbing or even dangerous, and especially if the cardiac reserve is low, prophylactic administration of quinidine in the doses mentioned for prevention of supraventricular tachycardia (q.v.) should be attempted.

NODAL RHYTHM

An abnormal rhythm that occurs when the rhythmicity of the SA node is depressed and falls below that of the AV node, which then becomes the pacemaker. In nodal rhythm the rate

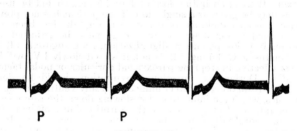

P   P

Nodal Rhythm

falls to between 30 and 50 beats/minute. **Nodal tachycardia,** a type of nodal rhythm, is due to an increase in the rhythmicity of the AV node above that of the SA node. The cause of nodal rhythm is often difficult to determine clinically, but arteriosclerotic heart disease, and medication with digitalis, are capable of inducing it. The symptoms are those of the causative disease and often, if the heart is well compensated, there are no symptoms. The ECG shows an uninterrupted series of typical nodal beats, occurring at the rate of 30 to 50/minute.

Treatment

Treatment is only that of combating the causative agent, although occasionally, if the heart rate is very slow, atropine (℞ 19) may restore the cardiac mechanism to regular sinus rhythm.

AURICULAR FLUTTER AND AURICULAR FIBRILLATION

Characteristic arrhythmias that result from the aberrant spread of the cardiac impulse through the tissues of the auricles, usually as a result of disease or injury, each type depending upon the respective nature of the pathway taken by the impulse. With auricular flutter the auricles contract regularly, at a rate above 200 beats/minute; the ventricular rate is equal, or ½, but may be ⅓, ¼, or ⅕ that of the auricles. In fibrillation, the rate is higher than in auricular flutter, but the ventricles respond irregularly.

Etiology and Pathogenesis

The causes of fibrillation and flutter include arteriosclerotic heart disease, myocardial infarction, acute and chronic rheumatic heart disease, hyperthyroidism, infiltration of the auricles by neoplasm, intrathoracic operations, especially on the esophagus and in pericardotomy. In some patients, auricular flutter and fibrillation occur in paroxysms without known cause. Such cases are said to be neurogenic in origin.

In auricular flutter and fibrillation, the spread of the impulse throughout the auricles is abnormal. Instead of originating in the sinus node, spreading through the auricles and dying out, the

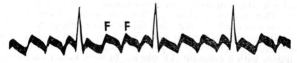

F F

Auricular Flutter

impulse keeps traveling around the auricles continuously. In auricular flutter it always follows the same pathways, whereas in fibrillation it travels in a haphazard fashion. In flutter there is a definite order in which the auricular fibers are stimulated, and each time the impulse travels around the auricles the ECG shows a deflection, designated as an F wave, whose outline may resemble rather closely a normal P wave. In fibrillation, however, there is no order in the spread of impulse, and the ECG waves (in this instance called f waves) are extremely variable in shape and frequency. In cases of paroxysmal auricular fibrillation and in most cases of auricular fibrillation of recent onset, the f waves are quite tall and show some constancy in shape. Sometimes, the f waves are so big and so regular that it is difficult to differentiate flutter from fibrillation. In both flutter and fibrillation, many impulses of supraventricular origin try to

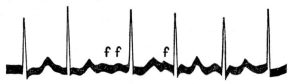

Auricular Fibrillation, Uncontrolled.

reach and activate the ventricles, but only a certain number of them are conducted to the ventricles. The QRS complexes are normal, but are unevenly spaced, except in some cases of flutter wherein each supraventricular impulse, or every 2nd, 3rd, 4th,

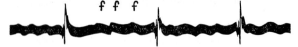

Auricular Fibrillation, After Digitalis Therapy

5th, or more does reach the ventricle. In cases of flutter, the ratio between the number of f waves and the number of QRS complexes is noted and reported as 1:1, 2:1, 3:1, 4:1, 5:1, and so forth.

Symptoms and Signs

At onset of flutter or fibrillation the symptoms may be very similar to those of paroxysmal tachycardia (palpitations, fainting, pallor, nausea, weakness). Sometimes the patient may go into shock or cardiac failure, but this is rather infrequent, except when the cardiac reserve is low. The beats of the radial pulse are irregularly spaced and uneven in amplitude, except in cases of flutter with a constant AV block. In both flutter and fibrillation the heart rate is rapid, but, when the conduction in the bundle of His is poor because of disease or of medication as with digitalis, the ventricular rate slows down. When this rate is rapid, some beats expel little or no blood into the aorta and are not felt at the radial pulse. The difference between the number of apical beats and those felt at the pulse is known as the pulse deficit.

Course and Prognosis

Both auricular flutter and fibrillation tend to occur in paroxysms before becoming constant. Persisting auricular flutter almost always converts to fibrillation. With permanent fibrillation, mural thrombi usually form and may lead to embolic phenomena which in turn may cause death.

Treatment

In flutter, full digitalization (℞ 2; and *see* CONGESTIVE HEART FAILURE) will slow down the conduction in the bundle of His and decrease the ventricular rate. It may convert flutter into regular sinus rhythm, or occasionally into auricular fibrillation and then into sinus rhythm. Quinidine usually is of little value. However, when fibrillation has been induced by digitalization for auricular flutter, quinidine (℞ 6) may be used in an attempt to establish sinus rhythm.

Treatment of auricular fibrillation is less clearly delineated. Whatever the cause of acute or paroxysmal auricular fibrillation, if the arrhythmia is not accompanied by cardiac failure and if the cardiac reserve is not too low, quinidine therapy (℞ 6) as outlined for the treatment of the paroxysmal tachycardias (q.v.) probably is the treatment of choice. When the paroxysm of auricular fibrillation has been stopped by quinidine, a maintenance dose should be continued for a few days. If the condition recurs often or if it is thought that, because of the existing heart disease, the patient may go into permanent auricular fibrillation, quinidine should be used continuously as a preventive. Although quinidine is the usual therapy, such cases also respond well to rapid digitalization. Administration I.V. of 1 to 1.6 mg. digitoxin (℞ 2) or 1.5 mg. of lanatoside C (℞ 4) stops practically all paroxysms of auricular fibrillation. However, digitalization does not seem to prevent their recurrence as quinidine does.

If paroxysmal auricular fibrillation occurs in the presence of cardiac failure, the safest procedure is to digitalize the patient, slowly or rapidly as the situation requires, then, concurrently with a maintenance dose of digitalis, to give quinidine in the doses mentioned before. If conversion to regular sinus rhythm does not occur, digitalization should be maintained and quinidine discontinued. Although controversy exists over the question of whether to stop digitalis before giving quinidine, it must be emphasized that if the patient's heart has been fibrillating for some time, especially if embolic phenomena have occurred, or if he is in chronic cardiac failure, or if heart block is present, digitalization alone should be used and quinidine avoided.

VENTRICULAR FIBRILLATION

A completely haphazard spread of the cardiac impulse over the ventricular conduction network, causing disorganized and inefficient contractions of the ventricles, with resulting circulatory failure and death.

Etiology

Ventricular fibrillation may be due to coronary occlusion or to overdosage with digitalis, quinidine, procaine, potassium chloride, barium chloride, papaverine, or emetine, or with a combination of such drugs. It may occur during chloroform or cyclopropane anesthesia, particularly if epinephrine is used. In electrocution, ventricular fibrillation may be the cause of death. It occasionally occurs during surgical procedures on the heart or pericardium.

Symptoms and Signs

Ventricular fibrillation produces sudden death; the blood pressure falls to zero and the heart sounds become inaudible. At the inception of fibrillation an ECG will show 5 or 6 deflections similar to those produced by ventricular extrasystoles, but occurring very close together, then the deflections become lower

Ventricular Fibrillation

in height and more erratic in frequency and shape. Within a short time, variable from patient to patient, no electrical activity traceable to the ventricle is recorded, as the fibrillation is followed by ventricular standstill.

Treatment

This is mostly preventive and consists of using every precaution when administering drugs that can induce fibrillation. The use of quinidine (℞ 6) to prevent ventricular fibrillation after coronary occlusion must be considered. Before cardiac operations, the heart should be made more resistant to external stimuli by administration of quinidine (*see* Treatment, Premature Contractions) and by the topical application of procaine. If fibrillation begins, an electric countershock applied to the ventricles may save the patient's life. Artificial respiration and massage (manual compression) of the heart also should be used during the attempts to stop fibrillation.

PULSUS ALTERNANS

A pulse that is characterized by a strong pulsation alternating with a weak one, due to alternate contractions, vigorous and less vigorous, of the ventricles. Although pulsus alternans is not truly a cardiac arrhythmia, it usually is included in that category.

Etiology

The mechanical alternation probably indicates a relative insufficiency of the ventricles resulting from disease or toxicity, or from too great a load on their efficiency. The condition is seen chiefly in hypertensive cardiovascular disease, arteriosclerotic heart disease, and acute rheumatic and diphtheritic myocarditis. Tachycardia, especially ventricular, may lead to mechanical alternation.

Symptoms and Signs

The manifestations of ventricular alternation are those of the disease or intoxication causing it. The alternate strong and weak beats can be palpated at the radial pulse, if the difference in amplitude between them is not too slight. Alternation may be revealed by sphygmomanometer, the pressure cuff being placed on the arm and inflated above the systolic pressure of the strongest beat, then slowly deflated. At first, only the stronger beat is heard. As the pressure cuff is further deflated, the weaker sound joins in and the difference can be detected. The ECG may be completely normal although, depending on the cause of the alternation, it may show signs of hypertensive cardiovascular disease, arteriosclerotic heart disease, or tachycardia of any type. Sometimes there is only electrical alternation without any evidence of mechanical alternation.

Prognosis

Whether the patient has mechanical alternation, or electrical alternation, or both, the prognosis is the same. If the heart rate is high (as in paroxysmal tachycardia, especially of ventricular origin), such tachycardia, even in an otherwise normal heart, may lead to cardiac failure. But if the heart rate is not above 120/minute and the patient has alternation, it means that such a heart is in bad condition. Whether recovery is possible depends on the cause of the alternation. Few patients live more than 5 years after they develop alternation due to hypertensive cardiovascular disease or arteriosclerotic heart disease.

Treatment

There is no treatment for pulsus alternans other than that of its cause and of the cardiac failure that often accompanies it.

CARDIAC BLOCKS

Conditions in which the cardiac impulse is slowed or interrupted in a portion of the pathway over which it is usually conducted. Symptoms depend on the localization of the block and its degree of intensity. The different types are described as sinoauricular, auriculoventricular, and bundle branch block.

SINOAURICULAR (SA) BLOCK

A type of heart block in which an occasional, normally discharged impulse is prevented from leaving the region of the sinoauricular (SA) node because the latter is surrounded by a temporary barrier, or block, which the impulse cannot traverse. Therefore, the auricles and ventricles, deprived of the stimulus, do not contract. The next contraction that occurs is in response to the next normal SA impulse that is not blocked. Occasionally, when a sinoauricular impulse is blocked, the AV node takes over the role of pacemaker for one beat, a phenomenon known as nodal escape (q.v.).

Etiology

SA block (or standstill) may occur in arteriosclerotic heart disease and chronic rheumatic disease, but is most commonly encountered as a result of intoxication by digitalis, potassium salts, or quinidine. It also may be produced by vagal stimulation. Hypersensitivity of the carotid sinus leads to a sinus bradycardia and standstill rather than to SA block.

Symptoms and Signs

When SA block occurs at infrequent intervals, it usually produces no symptoms; when it is frequent and persistent, it may lead to dizziness, fainting spells, or even convulsions. On precordial auscultation the missing beats can be detected. The ECG

Sinoauricular Block

shows omission of an entire P-QRS-T complex, and the distance from the normal beat preceding to the one following the SA block is equal to 2 normal cardiac cycles.

Prognosis and Treatment

Prognosis depends on the cause of the block and its frequency. SA block generally requires no therapy. Overdosage with the drugs that can induce it should be avoided. When symptoms do appear, a sedative (℞ 44), atropine (℞ 19), ephedrine (℞ 22), or amphetamine sulfate (℞ 29) may be tried.

AURICULOVENTRICULAR (AV) BLOCK

A type of heart block in which an occasional impulse or several or all impulses coming from the SA node are delayed or blocked in the AV node and bundle.

Etiology

AV block usually is due to acute or chronic rheumatic heart disease, diphtheria, syphilis, myocardial infarction, or arteriosclerotic heart disease, and occasionally to congenital cardiac anomalies. Several drugs may produce this block, but most often digitalis or quinidine is responsible. Stimulation of the vagi and the action of parasympathomimetic drugs such as Mecholyl also can produce it.

Two main types occur. **First degree AV block** is caused by retardation of the impulse as it travels from the SA node to the AV node. As a result, the P-R interval on the ECG is prolonged and the ventricular contraction delayed. A P-R interval of 0.21 second or longer is a 1st degree AV block.

Second degree AV block is distinguished by failure of the impulse to reach the ventricle, and the ventricular contraction

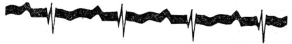

Auriculoventricular Block, 1st degree (*P-R interval =
0.28 sec.*)

therefore does not occur (dropped beat). Several patterns of 2nd degree AV block exist: (1) Various degrees of block in the passage of impulses from auricles to ventricles resulting in 2 or

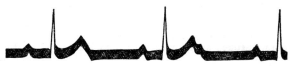

Auriculoventricular Block, 1st and 2nd degree (*P-R
interval = 0.26 sec.; 2:1 AV Block*)

more auricular beats for each ventricular contraction—expressed as 2:1, 3:1, 4:1, and so on, to complete AV block. (2) The Wenckebach phenomenon, in which the AV conduction time as

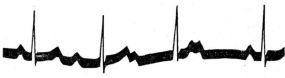

Auriculoventricular Block (*Wenckebach*)

represented by the P-R interval is prolonged progressively from beat to beat until one ventricular contraction is blocked, and the cycle begins again. (3) Complete AV block, in which the

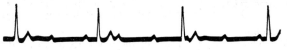

Auriculoventricular Block, complete

SA node sets the pace of the auricles and a focus in the ventricles quite independently regulates the slower rhythm of the ventricles.

It is not unusual for 1st and 2nd degree AV blocks to coexist, and almost any combination of degrees and patterns may be observed.

Symptoms and Signs

Clinical manifestations of AV block are variable. They depend both on the variety of AV block present and on the type and gravity of the accompanying heart disease. Many patients may have a complete AV block without any symptoms. First degree block itself produces no symptoms, but if it is caused by a disease such as acute rheumatic myocarditis with cardiac failure, signs and symptoms of that condition will be present. At the onset of 2nd degree block, the patient may feel faint and dizzy, or may actually collapse if there are many dropped ventricular beats. Most patients, however, have no symptoms other than palpitation and chest sensations similar to those due to premature contractions (q.v.). With complete AV block, many patients are symptomless, while others have vertigo, syncope, or even convulsions.

Adams-Stokes syndrome: This term is reserved for those patients who have fainting spells and convulsions, usually due to an AV block. Such symptoms occur at the onset of complete block and most often in patients whose heart reserve is exhausted. An otherwise normal heart is able to compensate and assure a normal output even in complete AV block with a slow ventricular rate, whereas a heart with low reserve is unable to do so. Adams-Stokes syndrome also is seen when, in complete AV block, the automaticity of the ventricular pacemaker suddenly decreases, usually for no demonstrable reason.

Diagnosis

Many times the existence of an AV block is first revealed by the ECG, although the various patterns producing an irregularly dropped beat can be determined by auscultation or palpation of the pulse. A 1st degree block, a regularly occurring 2:1, 3:1, or other incomplete block, or a complete block with the slow but usually regular independent ventricular rhythm, cannot be recognized definitely by ordinary clinical methods. An ECG is essential to establish the existence of and to identify an AV block. This is accomplished by measuring the P-R time interval (over 0.21 second indicates 1st degree AV block), and by recognizing the time relationship between the auricular contractions (P waves) and the ventricular contractions (QRS complexes).

Prognosis

This depends on the cause of the block, its degree, and the type and gravity of the concomitant cardiac disease, especially the presence or absence of cardiac failure. The prognosis is better in 1st degree block than in complete block, which may lead to prolonged cerebral ischemia, and because 1st degree block indicates a lesser degree of injury to the conducting system. Most cases of AV block due to acute myocardial infarction, even when complete, disappear or become less severe after a few days. So do those due to acute rheumatic carditis or to diphtheria once the acute episode is past. Complete block caused by chronic arteriosclerotic heart disease without recent coronary occlusion is much more persistent and in fact, usually permanent.

Treatment

If the patient complains of palpitation because of the dropped beats, phenobarbital (℞ 44) 15 to 30 mg. (gr. ¼ to ss) 3 times a day will be of help. A 1st degree block due to digitalis does not call for discontinuance of that drug if its use is necessary to control cardiac failure. It is only when frequent dropped beats occur that digitalis should be stopped; after 1 or 2 days it should be resumed in slightly smaller doses. Generally, it is possible to give sufficient digitalis to obtain the full benefit of digitalization without producing a dangerous degree of AV block. Whatever the degree of block, however, if cardiac failure exists, digitalis should be given (see CONGESTIVE HEART FAILURE). If the Adams-Stokes syndrome appears, the patient's bed should be placed on shock blocks to prevent cerebral ischemia as far as possible. If a patient subject to the Adams-Stokes syndrome is ambulatory, he should avoid situations in which he may injure himself or others (e.g., climbing ladders, swimming, or driving a car). During these seizures, oxygen therapy is indicated during the acute episode (see CLIN. PROC.). Atropine (℞ 19) should be given to prevent dangerous degrees of block, but therapeutically it seems to be helpful only when the block is of functional origin, as in overdigitalization or overdosage with Mecholyl. Depending on the urgency of the situation, it can be given I.V., subcut. or even orally. Epinephrine (℞ 24) should be administered during seizures, and also prophylactically to patients subject to frequent episodes, as in acute rheumatic carditis and arteriosclerotic heart disease. Epinephrine also is helpful in the acute attack. If ventricular standstill is present, a smaller dose (0.3 to 0.5 cc.) may be given intracardially. Epinephrine, 2 mg. in oil (℞ 25), I.M. also may be used during or after an attack to prevent recurrence. In cases of Adams-Stokes syndrome due to complete AV block after recent coronary occlusion, epinephrine should be given with great caution. Ephedrine (℞ 22), 50 mg. (gr. ¾) 3 to 6 times a day orally, also is helpful in preventing Adams-Stokes seizures. It must be emphasized, however, that control of the heart failure with adequate digitalization probably is the best way to prevent the attacks.

BUNDLE BRANCH BLOCK

A type of heart block in which the cardiac impulse originating in the SA node follows a normal pathway until it reaches the bifurcation of the common bundle into its two branches, beyond which point it is slowed or blocked in one or the other of the bundle branches. The spread of impulse within the ventricles supplied by the defective bundle branch becomes abnormal in pattern.

Etiology

Bundle branch block usually indicates severe myocardial damage; rarely, it is without significance. It usually is due to arteriosclerotic heart disease. Less frequently it occurs in acute

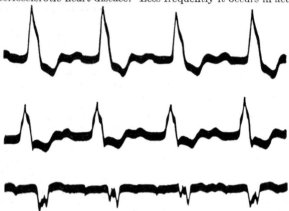

Left Bundle Branch Block (*leads I, II and III*)

myocardial infarction, acute and chronic rheumatic myocarditis, syphilitic heart disease, diphtheria, tumor of the heart, and acute and chronic myocarditis of unknown etiology such as Fiedler's myocarditis. It may be congenital. Overdosage with quinidine, digitalis, and papaverine also may produce bundle branch block.

Symptoms and Signs

There are no constant or pathognomonic signs. In some cases, a split 1st or 2nd heart sound, or both, may be heard. There may be a gallop rhythm, but this is more likely to be due to the underlying heart disease.

Diagnosis

Diagnosis can be made only by ECG studies which also will reveal whether the bundle branch block is left or right, determined by the direction of the main deflection of the QRS complex in the 3 limb leads. This latter differentiation, however, is unimportant clinically since damage usually is present in both bundle branches, though more extensive in one than the other.

Prognosis

A few cases of bundle branch block are only temporary. However, the prognosis is uncertain, being more related to the gravity of the underlying cardiac condition than dependent on the

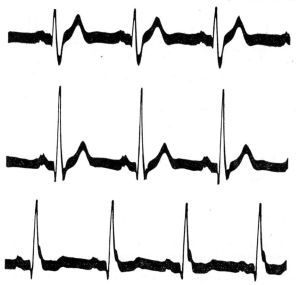

Right Bundle Branch Block (*leads I, II and III*)

presence or absence of block. The outlook is definitely worse when the patient exhibits gross cardiac enlargement or well developed cardiac failure.

Treatment

There is no treatment for bundle branch block; the cause must be eliminated when possible.

FALSE BUNDLE BRANCH BLOCK
(Wolff-Parkinson-White syndrome)

An anomaly of congenital origin demonstrable by ECG, and which consists in the coexistence of a short P-R interval and a QRS complex which is too wide and notched. Persons with such an anomaly are prone to have paroxysmal tachycardia, mostly auricular or nodal, but occasionally ventricular in origin;

they rarely have paroxysmal auricular fibrillation or flutter. The only significance of a Wolff-Parkinson-White syndrome is that it indicates a predisposition to paroxysmal tachycardia

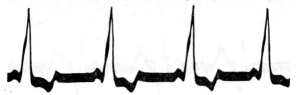

False Bundle Branch Block (*Wolff-Parkinson-White Syndrome*)

(q.v.), and when diagnosed enables the physician to take preventive measures against such seizures.

NEUROCIRCULATORY ASTHENIA

(Soldier's heart, Irritable heart, Effort syndrome, Cardiac neurosis)

A symptom complex characterized by breathlessness, giddiness, fatigue, precordial pain, and palpitation.

Etiology

Neurocirculatory asthenia is a hypochondriac-like expression of neurasthenia (q.v.), wherein cardiac symptoms are dominant. It is a so-called "cardiac" neurosis which rarely occurs before the age of 20 or after the age of 40, and is common in either sex. Operating in a predisposed personality, some stress (e.g., worry, pregnancy, acute illness, protracted convalescence) expresses itself in imbalance of the autonomic nervous system, which accounts for the symptoms. The type of temperament often associated with the asthenic physique (i.e., tall, slender, with narrow costal angle, low diaphragm and small heart) may predispose to the disorder.

Symptoms, Signs, and Diagnosis

Symptoms such as flushing, tremor, faintness, or rapid sighing respirations—all primarily related to systems other than circulatory—usually are present. These aid in making the diagnosis when symptoms of palpitation, tachycardia, precordial pain, or of functional arrhythmia are present without objective evidence of organic heart disease. Sometimes there are gastrointestinal symptoms. The customary shortness of breath with minor exertion prompted the name "effort syndrome." A true dyspnea may not exist, but rather a consciousness of respiratory effort; sometimes, however, a distinct increase in breathing rate is encountered. A tendency to sigh is frequent, and this is not usual in organic heart conditions. Substernal pain rarely occurs, but ordinarily discomfort is experienced as a dull ache in the region of the left breast, which usually does not radiate, and perhaps lasts for several hours. Occasionally, there may be attacks of stabbing pain lasting for a few seconds. The exhaustion after slight effort often is unrelieved by rest, but the pulse rate generally returns to normal after 1 or 2 hours of sleep. Cold, moist, cyanotic extremities and cyanosis of the nailbeds are characteristic. ECG and fluoroscopic findings usually are normal, also the blood pressure; however, the latter may be slightly elevated. Functional tests of the heart based on exercise tolerance or vital capacity frequently are subnormal and of little aid in ruling out the possibility of an organic cardiac condition. At times patients with organic heart disease show evidences of neurocirculatory asthenia as well.

Prognosis and Treatment

The course is usually protracted unless measures are taken early to correct the psychogenic factors which form the background of this disorder. Subsequently a plan of life must be worked out whereby the patient will spare himself such strain as may produce a relapse. Some clinicians believe that usually a degree of so-called constitutional inadequacy coexists; in any event, the patient's physical state must not be neglected. Asthenic or other malnourished individuals may profit greatly from an improved diet, especially one containing adequate vitamins and minerals. Palliatively, phenobarbital 30 mg. (gr. ss) 3 times daily (℞ 44) may allay nervousness.

MYOCARDITIS

An acute, sometimes chronic, inflammation of the heart muscle, in contrast to myocardosis which is a noninflammatory degeneration such as accompanies coronary insufficiency. Myocarditis may be focal or diffuse and interstitial or parenchymal (or both), depending on the cause. Healing is by fibrosis.

Etiology and Incidence

The incidence of myocarditis is unknown, since it is seldom diagnosed during life. It is most common in children and young adults, and probably always is secondary to other diseases, principally acute infections and particularly diphtheria, typhoid, scarlet fever, and septicemia. Bacterial toxins or chemical poisons may sometimes be responsible. Idiopathic (Fiedler's) myocarditis is not infrequent.

The myocardial lesions of rheumatic fever and beriberi are considered in separate chapters (q.v.). Parasitic disease (e.g., trichinosis, cysticercosis) occasionally invades the myocardium.

Symptoms, Signs, and Diagnosis

Onset of symptoms usually occurs during or immediately after the primary illness, but may occasionally be delayed for several weeks. It is seldom recognized because of the more prominent manifestations of the underlying disease (q.v.). Myocarditis produces no characteristic symptoms or signs, but must be suspected in all patients who, during the illnesses named, suddenly develop circulatory disturbances such as precordial oppression, dyspnea or cyanosis otherwise unexplained, cardiac arrhythmias or dilatation, electrocardiographic changes, murmurs, peripheral vascular failure, or heart failure.

Prognosis

The prognosis always must be guarded since the severity of the myocardial lesion is not always reflected by the clinical manifestations. Depending on the cause and the degree of involvement, acute myocarditis may be followed by complete recovery or by some degree of functional impairment, or may become chronic. Death occurs not infrequently with diphtheritic or septic myocarditis. Idiopathic myocarditis usually carries a fatal prognosis.

Treatment

Prophylaxis requires thorough treatment of any disease (q.v.) likely to cause myocarditis, with emphasis on continued bed rest until all evidence of active disease has disappeared.

Once myocarditis is suspected or apparent, maximal rest for the heart is secured by complete bed rest and sedation, in addition to continued therapy of the underlying disease. Phenobarbital (R 44) in doses of 30 to 60 mg. (gr. ss to i) may be given as needed for restlessness or insomnia. O_2 is indicated and is perhaps the most useful agent in cardiac failure. Digitalis is contraindicated in many cases, as it may increase cardiac irritability and aggravate arrhythmias. However, if there is marked dilatation with frank congestive failure (q.v.) digitalis may be tried cautiously. Caffeine (R 28), 0.5 Gm. subcut. is a useful cardiac stimulant. Peripheral vascular failure (shock) usually is an indication of profound cardiac weakness, for which little can be done. If, however, the shock is due to a general toxemia, I.V. fluid or plasma or blood transfusion may be given.

Rest must be continued until all evidence of circulatory disturbance has disappeared. Normal activity must be resumed very gradually, over a period of several months.

BACTERIAL ENDOCARDITIS

Infection of the endocardium by bacteria, characterized by the symptoms of infectious disease, embolic phenomena, and the presence of vegetations on the endocardium. The course may be acute, but the subacute form is much more frequent.

Etiology

The organisms chiefly concerned in the production of endocarditis are the streptococcus, staphylococcus, pneumococcus, gonococcus, and *H. influenzae.* The cardiac infection uniformly follows a bacteremia, which may in itself be transient and asymptomatic. The subacute form is due to *Str. viridans* in about 95% of cases. In susceptible persons it frequently follows the temporary bacteremia that occurs after tooth extraction. Heart valves congenitally deformed or damaged by previous disease are predisposed to infection; whether normal valves also become infected is unknown.

Pathology

The fundamental lesion of bacterial endocarditis is a vegetation, composed largely of fibrin masses and mesh, in which entrapped red cells, polymorphonuclear leukocytes, and bacteria are generally abundant. Foci of necrosis are common. While the valve is the usual primary site, vegetations also may extend to the mural endocardium. The leaflet shows signs of acute or subacute inflammation in the neighborhood of the vegetation. In the subacute form, along with the evidence of bacterial action and the deposition of fibrin, there are evidences of repair. Signs of preexisting disease or malfunction of the valve can almost always be demonstrated.

Symptoms and Signs

In **subacute bacterial endocarditis,** onset usually is insidious and may for a time mimic that of many general systemic diseases, with no signs of cardiac involvement. Fever usually is remittent but may be irregular or sustained, a daily peak of 103.6° F. being common. There are occasional chills or chilly sensations. A progressive anemia often exacerbates the lassitude and anorexia caused by the infection. A moderate leukocytosis is usual. Petechiae and embolic phenomena are common. Crops of tiny red spots appear in the skin and mucous membranes, and splinter hemorrhages occur under the nails. Tender nodules 2 to 5 mm. in diameter frequently develop about the terminal digital joints and tips of the fingers and toes. Infarcts of the spleen are common, with resultant acute left upper quadrant pain, often of pleuritic type, and increase in fever and leukocytosis. Microscopic or gross hematuria, due to the presence of petechial lesions or frank infarcts in the kidneys, is frequent. If the mitral or aortic valves are involved, massive peripheral embolization may result.

The cardiac signs of the infection may be obscured at first by evidences of preexisting valvulitis. Later, the murmurs change in character, presumably as a result of the severe infection and growth of vegetations on the valvular surface. Such change occurring rapidly may give the first clue to the true nature of the disease. As a rule new murmurs, particularly in diastole, are heard where none was before, and murmurs previously noted become louder and harsher. As the disease progresses, signs of congestive failure may appear. The most consistent and most important single finding is bacteremia. In most cases moderate to large numbers of bacteria are demonstrable in the circulating blood, but in some they can be detected only by repeated cultures. As the infection continues, the anemia increases and the patient progressively loses weight and strength. Death may result directly from the infection, or from anemia, cerebral or pulmonary embolism or cardiac failure.

In the acute form the symptoms and signs are similar but the course is more severe. The endocarditis may occur as a complication of a frank staphylococcal or pneumococcal infection, its onset heralded simply by a sudden worsening in the patient's condition, with increased fever and leukocytosis, hematuria, petechial or papular eruptions, and increased signs of intoxication. Or it may complicate some seemingly inconsequential focal infection and the apparently well person will be suddenly taken with chill, fever, and the general symptoms of systemic infection. In either case, the symptoms and signs of bacteremia (q.v.) appear. The bacteremia is apt to be sustained at a much higher level than in the subacute form. There usually is an eruption, its character depending on the nature of the invading organism. There often will be evidences of infarction in the viscera, and a greatly elevated leukocyte count (10,-000 to 25,000). As in the subacute form, changing murmurs in the heart direct attention to this organ as the primary seat of the infection.

Diagnosis

The diagnosis of bacterial endocarditis is based upon the presence of symptoms of an infectious disease, the evidence of valvular heart disease with changing murmurs, the demonstration of petechiae and embolic phenomena, and the presence of bacteremia. Endocarditis in its early stages is easily confused with other infectious diseases, especially in the aged, in whom a low grade continued fever is apt to be ascribed to urinary or respiratory tract infection. However, most of the endocarditis patients are between 20 and 40 years of age, and the presence of fever not attributable to other causes, particularly in a patient in this age group with heart disease, should suggest bacterial endocarditis. Frequent blood cultures, even when the source of infection seems to be known, will prevent many diagnostic errors.

Prognosis

The prognosis of untreated bacterial endocarditis is dismal. A few recoveries are reported but the mortality rate probably is 99% or more. With the advent of antibiotic therapy this rate

rhagic), or fibroid (chronic adhesive, constrictive, synechia cordis, concretio cordis). Effects vary with the character of the inflammation, but all cases may be generally classified as either acute fibrinous pericarditis, pericarditis with effusion, or chronic constrictive pericarditis.

Etiology

Pericarditis is most frequently secondary to rheumatic fever, pulmonary tuberculosis, or pneumococcal infections. Other common causes are thoracic wounds, myocardial infarction, and uremia. Less common are gonorrhea, influenza, tularemia, meningococcemia, undulant fever, and various obscure infections, probably viral. Pericarditis is frequent in disseminated lupus erythematosus, and relatively so in rheumatoid arthritis. Malignant metastases and hemorrhagic states are occasional causes. Primary disease of the pericardium is rare.

ACUTE FIBRINOUS PERICARDITIS

Inflammation of the pericardium characterized by fibrinous exudation. An outpouring of fibrin occurs on the pericardial surfaces. This may remain relatively dry or fibrinous in character as in pericarditis associated with myocardial infarction and uremia, or may become serous (serofibrinous pericarditis) or purulent, producing pericardial effusion, as often is the case in pericarditis due to bacterial infections.

Symptoms and Signs

The constitutional symptomatology is influenced by the primary disease. Usually, acute pericarditis is painless, but severe precordial pain may occur, especially when nearby pleural surfaces are involved. Pain is absent in uremic pericarditis but occasionally is severe in cases of bacterial origin. The most important and often the sole physical finding is a precordial to-and-fro friction rub. It may be audible as a soft scratchy sound barely heard with a stethoscope, or as a low grating noise heard a few inches from the precordium by the ear alone. The rub disappears if a fluid exudate develops and separates the visceral and parietal layers of the pericardium, but may be audible anteriorly with a considerable fluid collection laterally and posteriorly.

Diagnosis

Changes in the ECG usually occur early in pericarditis and are thought to be due to subjacent myocarditis. Characteristically there is an initial elevation of the R-S-T segments in all the limb leads and often in the precordial leads. Early, the T waves are upright but as the disease progresses they diminish in amplitude and become negative or diphasic. The reciprocal elevation and depression of the R-S-T segments in limb leads I and III, respectively, and the development of Q waves in the precordial leads seen in myocardial infarction do not occur in pericarditis. Pleuropericardial rubs may be differentiated by requesting the patient to hold his breath. The bubbling, crunching sounds of mediastinal emphysema may be recognized by their peculiar acoustics.

Prognosis

The prognosis is dependent upon the nature of the underlying disease.

Treatment

General: Bed rest; force fluids (for infectious types); regulate bowels (℞ 79, 80, 81). For relief of pain, give acetylsalicylic acid, codeine or morphine, depending upon the intensity (℞ 48, 52, 57). An ice bag over the precordium occasionally affords relief. To combat insomnia or nervousness, barbiturates (℞ 44, 45) may be useful.

Specific: Penicillin (℞ 70) should be administered parenterally in pericarditis due to gram-positive cocci, gonococci or meningococci, and streptomycin (℞ 71) in cases due to susceptible gram-negative or acid-fast organisms. If purulent effusion occurs, the appropriate antibiotic also should be given directly into the pericardial cavity after aspiration of the fluid by needle or surgical drainage (*see* Pericarditis with Effusion). For pericarditis due to rheumatic fever (q.v.) salicylates (℞ 49) may be administered. If gallop rhythm and signs of heart failure develop, salt and fluids may have to be restricted and the patient digitalized (*see* CONGESTIVE HEART FAILURE).

PERICARDITIS WITH EFFUSION

A type of pericarditis secondary to inflammation of the pericardium, which is characterized by the exudation of fluid within the pericardial cavity. It most often occurs in pyogenic infections, tuberculosis, and rheumatic fever.

Pathologic Physiology

Pericardial effusion of magnitude sufficient to produce clinical symptoms does so by causing cardiac tamponade, which impedes the entrance of blood from the great veins into the heart. The cardiac output consequently diminishes, venous pressure rises, arterial blood pressure and pulse pressure decrease, the velocity of blood flow diminishes, the excursion of the heart borders is reduced, and during inspiration the pulse becomes weak or imperceptible (pulsus paradoxus).

Symptoms and Signs

Onset usually is insidious, the severity of the constitutional symptoms such as malaise and fever depending upon the underlying disease. Dyspnea and orthopnea are present with large effusions, and precordial pain or substernal oppression occurs occasionally.

Examination reveals distention of the veins of the neck and

upper extremities. The apical impulse vanishes. On percussion there is increased precordial dullness, which may shift with change of body position from upright to horizontal. The heart sounds usually are distant and feeble. Disturbances of rhythm, or murmurs, are common. At the angle of the left scapula, bronchial breathing and pectoriloquy may be present due to compression of the lung by the distended pericardium (Ewart's sign). A paradoxical pulse usually is noted.

Diagnosis

With as much as 300 cc. of fluid within the pericardium, X-ray examination reveals a slight bulging of the inferior margin of the cardiac silhouette. With large effusion the normal curves of the heart disappear and the bulging inferior borders and widened area at the base produce a pear-shaped silhouette characteristic of pericardial effusion. With fluoroscopic examination the pulsations of the heart are seen to be decreased.

Diagnostic puncture: The proof of pericardial effusion may be established by aspiration of fluid from the pericardium (see Treatment, below). Examination of this fluid should include determination of specific gravity, protein content, cytology, and culture. If tuberculosis is suspected, guinea pig inoculation as well as culture should be performed.

Treatment

If sufficient fluid has accumulated within the pericardial cavity to produce symptoms and signs, needle aspiration and withdrawal of fluid is indicated. When the causative agent is susceptible to chemotherapy, the appropriate antibiotic should be given not only parenterally but also directly into the pericardial cavity (℞ 70). In cases of purulent pericarditis with thick pus due to bacteria other than the tubercle bacillus, surgical drainage by rib resection is indicated. Pericardial effusion associated with acute rheumatic fever usually subsides spontaneously and rarely requires aspiration. In such cases salicylate therapy is indicated (℞ 49). In tuberculous pericarditis frequent aspiration may be required. Since the prognosis in tuberculous cases is grave, streptomycin should be given both systemically and locally (℞ 71).

Technic of pericardial aspiration: Numerous approaches to the pericardial sac for the purpose of aspiration have been recommended. The most favored sites are either the 5th left interspace at the outer border of percussion dullness, or via the epigastrium. If the latter route is chosen, the needle is inserted just below the lower border of the ensiform cartilage and the bevel kept close to the under surface of the sternum while it is pushed upward to enter the pericardial cavity above the diaphragm. A three-way stopcock attached to a 50 cc. syringe facilitates removal of the fluid. As much as 100 cc. may be aspirated in large effusions but the procedure should be discon-

tinued if the cardiac contractions become palpable beating
against the needle. It should be emphasized that pericardial
aspiration is dangerous unless carefully performed, as a coronary
artery may be torn or the ventricles lacerated; sudden death
from cardiac arrest occurs occasionally during the procedure.

CHRONIC CONSTRICTIVE AND OTHER FORMS
OF ADHESIVE PERICARDITIS

*Conditions resulting from adhesions between the visceral and
parietal layers of the pericardium, or occasionally between the
parietal pericardium and various intrathoracic structures.*

Pathologic Physiology

Adherent pericardium resulting from antecedent acute fibrinous pericarditis handicaps the heart only when extreme thickening of the pericardium, producing a dense envelope of scar tissue,
prevents normal dilatation during diastole and proper filling,
or when torsion or angulation of the heart is caused by dense
adhesions binding the heart to various intrathoracic structures.
Deposits of calcium in the fibrous inflammatory tissue may
occur and produce the conditions termed concretio cordis.

Symptoms and Signs

In **chronic constrictive pericarditis,** characterized by enlargement of the abdomen, prominence of the veins of the neck,
and frequently edema of the legs, the systolic blood pressure is
low, and the pulse and pulse pressure small. A decrease or disappearance of the pulse during inspiration (pulsus paradoxus)
is common. Heart sounds are distant. A systolic apical murmur may be present. Rhythm usually is regular, but premature
contractions or even auricular fibrillation may occur. Pleural
effusion is common and ascites with enlargement of the liver is
regularly encountered in advanced cases.

In **external pericardial adhesions** (mediastinopericarditis),
unless the symptoms of myocardial insufficiency are present, no
symptoms occur. The most important physical signs are systolic retraction at the apex and systolic retraction posteriorly
at the left side between the 11th and 12th ribs (Broadbent's
sign). It should be noted that this sign also is seen in cardiac
enlargement without pericardial adhesions. Only when complicating hypertension or valvular disease is present does one
encounter the pronounced enlargement of the heart described
in older textbooks.

Diagnosis

In chronic constrictive pericarditis, the actual heart size is
normal or small. However, due to the thickness of the pericardium the silhouette may appear slightly enlarged by X-ray.
Fluoroscopy shows reduction in the amplitude of the pulsations.
The electrocardiogram shows low voltage of the QRS complexes
and the T waves are of low amplitude or inverted.

Chronic constrictive pericarditis must be differentiated from cirrhosis of the liver and from rheumatic and arteriosclerotic heart diseases with predominant right-sided failure.

Treatment

Chronic constrictive pericarditis may be relieved by resection of the pericardium. Medical treatment is palliative and consists of the administration of mercurial diuretics (Ɓ 34, 35, 36) and of a diet low in sodium chloride. Digitalis is contraindicated.

Adherent pericardium: With adhesions, resection of several ribs and costal cartilages overlying the pericardium has been advocated in an effort to permit the heart to pull against yielding rather than rigid structures. The value of this operation has not been established.

ARTERIOSCLEROSIS

A chronic vascular disease, characterized by thickening, hardening, and loss of elasticity of the arterial walls, with inflammatory, degenerative, or hyperplastic changes. These changes may be generalized or prominent in certain locations, such as the brain, heart, kidneys, or extremities.

Etiology and Incidence

The cause of arteriosclerosis is unknown. It has been variously attributed to abnormal metabolism of fats; exogenous toxins, such as lead; and endogenous toxins and infection. There is clear-cut evidence that heredity plays a large part in its development. Long-established hypertension appears to be a predisposing factor. The disease is most common in obese individuals and in males. The onset usually occurs during the 4th or 5th decade of life.

Pathology and Pathologic Physiology

The earliest changes are generally found in the media of the arteries. There is loss of normal structure, with degeneration of muscular layers and replacement by various products of fat metabolism, especially lipids. As the disease progresses, calcium may be deposited in this abnormal tissue and may be visualized by X-ray. Calcified lesions frequently are found in the aorta, the coronary vessels, and the peripheral arteries especially of the lower extremities. The degenerative process often extends to the intima. In the earliest stages there is simply roughening of the usual smooth surface, followed by depositions of lipids. Some of these may become calcified and form "plaques." Elsewhere the roughened areas form ideal locations for the attachment of platelets and the formation of thrombi, which tend to occlude the lumens. Normal function of the tissues supplied by these diseased vessels becomes altered and various symptoms develop, depending on the location of the vessels involved.

Symptoms and Signs

Subjective evidence of arteriosclerosis usually precedes objective changes by many months. Loss of memory for recent events, repetitious statements, dizziness, headache, and tinnitus are evidence of cerebral arteriosclerosis; shortness of breath, palpitation and anginal pain indicate coronary sclerosis; blurring and haziness of vision occur with retinal sclerosis, and intermittent claudication with impairment of arterial circulation in the legs. Gangrene of the leg may develop if the arteries become rapidly occluded.

Thickened peripheral vessels or even beading of the most superficial arteries may sometimes be palpated. Tortuosity and narrowing of the retinal arterial vessels ("silver wire" appearance) with pressure on the veins sometimes occurs before the patient complains of visual disturbance. Later, edema of the disks or hemorrhages along the vessels may develop. Abnormalities of the ECG readings usually appear late and consist of changes in conduction, arrhythmias, alterations of the T wave and the S-T segment, and the appearance of abnormal Q waves. X-ray of the extremities may show calcium deposits in the peripheral arteries before paresthesias or claudication occur. Failure of the kidneys to concentrate, as shown by the concentration and dilution tests (see LAB. PROC.) or the pituitrin test, is one of the earliest evidences of renal arteriosclerosis. Edema of the liver, lungs, or legs develops with cardiac failure.

Diagnosis

Long before definite symptoms are complained of, arteriosclerosis may be suspected in patients over 45 who present the following appearance: prematurely gray hair, poor growth or roughening of the finger and toe nails, loss of the normal healthy appearance of the skin and a loss of substance in the muscles, especially of the legs. Diagnosis requires the following procedures: (1) A careful history, including the patient's subjective symptoms and whether any of his family have died of cerebral accidents, or coronary occlusion, or have had renal disease or gangrene of the extremities. (2) Estimation of the patient's mental status. (3) Careful physical examination including the eye grounds; palpation of the temporal, radial, ulnar, brachial, femoral, posterior tibial and dorsalis pedis arteries; inspection of the skin, hair, and nails; and a thorough cardiac examination. (4) Laboratory procedures, such as ECG, X-ray of the heart, aorta and of the extremities for calcification of the arteries; renal function studies including BUN and NPN (and their ratio); blood cholesterol and urine concentration tests, together with examination of urine for albumin and urinary solids, for casts, and their type.

Oscillometric studies of the pulses in the extremities may show early signs of impaired circulation in localized areas. However, in using the oscillometer care must be taken always to apply the cuff in the same manner and over similar locations, to see that the extremities are at heart level and that the patient is not subjected to sudden changes of temperature or emotional upsets while being examined.

Prognosis

With generalized arteriosclerosis the patient may live to an advanced age, but when a particular organ is severely affected, death may occur in early middle life, with cerebral thrombosis or hemorrhage or coronary occlusion as the immediate cause. Thrombus formation may lead to dry gangrene of the extremities.

Treatment

There is no known method of prevention or cure for arteriosclerosis. All treatment is therefore directed toward secondary symptoms.

General: The patient must be instructed to alter his mode of life so as to lessen both physical and emotional strains on his vascular system. He must be warned, without causing undue alarm, of the serious results that may follow further vascular damage. It has been frequently noted that if a patient survives an acute episode of arterial closure, adequate collateral circulation will develop to maintain life for many years.

Diet: Eating too rapidly and overeating must be avoided. Because of the frequent finding of high blood cholesterol in arteriosclerotic patients and the fact that many investigators believe the disease is due to faulty metabolism of fats, these substances should be kept at a minimum in the diet. Since vascular accidents occur more frequently in the obese, weight reduction often is indicated (*see* OBESITY). In patients with subnormal metabolism, thyroid extract (℞ 85) may be of value in reducing the blood cholesterol.

Medication: Iodides (℞ 90) have long been used in treating arteriosclerosis, and although their effect is questionable they should not yet be discarded. The tension associated with hypertension or present in persons who lead a "high pressure" life may be relieved by judicious use of sedatives (℞ 43, 44, 47). If doses are kept small and the patient remains under observation they may be safely given over long periods of time. Vasodilators release the spasm in undamaged collateral vessels and thus frequently relieve annoying symptoms. The xanthines and the slow-acting nitrites (℞ 8 to 13) are indicated. In coronary thrombosis, large doses of opiates (℞ 54, 57, 59) together with atropine sulfate (℞ 19) are imperative. In peripheral lesions the generally-acting vasodilators seem to have little effect. However, whisky (℞ 32) together with acetylsalicylic acid (℞ 48) often relieves rest pain as effectively as any other medication.

Papaverine (℞ 17, 18) given frequently in large doses (even intra-arterially to the affected extremity) is of value as emergency treatment in acute arterial occlusion.

Anticoagulants (℞ 60, 61, 62) often are indicated in the treatment of acute thromboses occurring in arteriosclerotic vessels (*see* ANTICOAGULANT THERAPY). Heparin should be given for 48 hours, preferably by continuous infusion or in a slowly absorbing menstruum, in a dosage adequate to keep the clotting time of the blood increased 100 to 200%. This should be checked every hour or two during administration. If the blood plasma prothrombin time can be determined accurately, dicumarol may be started with the heparin and, 48 hours later, after its effect becomes manifest, heparin may be discontinued. Adequate dosage to increase the prothrombin time to at least double is indicated. It should be continued long enough to eliminate the likelihood of further thrombosis.

Tobacco, ergot, and epinephrine have a highly vasospastic action and must be avoided or used with utmost caution in arteriosclerotic patients. They may cause so much spasm in collateral vessels as to produce a serious shutdown in arterial flow to vital tissues.

HYPERTENSIVE VASCULAR DISEASE

(Essential hypertension, Hyperpiesia)

A disorder in which the arterioles exhibit abnormal resistance to the flow of blood, usually associated with an abnormal increase in systolic, diastolic and mean arterial pressures.

Etiology

The etiology of hypertensive vascular disease is obscure. Elevation of blood pressure has been induced in animals through central, neurogenic, renal and other mechanisms as well as by administration of certain drugs and sterols. Constriction of the renal arteries of experimental animals produces hypertension through a humoral mechanism which closely resembles hypertensive vascular disease in man.

Although renal humoral and autonomic nervous system factors may play a part, it is difficult to ascribe the entire disorder to a single cause. While there is some evidence of adrenal cortical dysfunction or disturbed sodium chloride metabolism, perhaps mediated through the kidneys or through altered reactivity of vessels, conclusive proof is lacking.

Incidence

About 5% of the adult population of the United States is affected. Hypertensive vascular disease is said to be less prevalent among primitive peoples but is observed in a high per-

centage of those transferred to more civilized environments.
Heredity is an important factor. Obesity, short and stocky body
configuration, and hyperkinetic bodily reactions appear to be
frequently associated with hypertension. Characteristic psychological types have been described. The disease is somewhat
more common among women. Although symptoms usually do
not bring the patient to the doctor until long after the establishment of the disease, the first signs can be detected in early
adult life in the majority of instances.

Pathology

There may be no pathologic changes, the increased peripheral resistance being due initially to functional spasm. In the
majority of instances, hypertensive vascular disease becomes
more than casually associated with arteriosclerotic lesions.
The arterioles involved include primarily those of the kidneys,
pancreas, liver, and periadrenal tissues. Development of arteriosclerosis does not parallel the duration of hypertension or the
level of blood pressure.

In the rapidly progressive (malignant) phase of the disease,
necrosis, more advanced hyalinization, and petechial hemorrhages also may be present, particularly in the kidneys and
retinas.

Cardiac hypertrophy, beginning with the left ventricle, may
or may not be present. No multiplication of capillaries or
demonstrable alteration in vascular tissue accompanies the enlargement, which is primarily cellular and which cannot be correlated with the intensity or duration of the disease.

Although arteriosclerosis is frequently encountered in similar
age groups, the frequency of coincident coronary artery disease,
cerebral vascular accidents, and peripheral vascular changes
makes it probable that hypertensive vascular disease accelerates
this degenerative process.

Physiology

In uncomplicated hypertensive vascular disease there is no
appreciable change in cardiac output, blood volume or viscosity,
pulse rate or venous pressure. The peripheral resistance, with
the exception of the pulmonary circulation, is increased fairly
uniformly throughout the body. Blood flow is unaffected because of the concomitant increase in arterial blood pressure.

In the early stages of the disease, kidney function may be
normal, but diminution in effective renal blood flow and to a
lesser extent impairment in maximal tubular excretory capacity
are generally observed in the course of time and in variable
degrees.

Different degrees of vasomotor lability, differences in response
to sympathectomy, transient vascular spasms, all suggest that
some patients possess an autonomic imbalance in addition to
the sustained increase in peripheral resistance.

Lability of blood pressure recordings is characteristic of the early hypertensive state. The systolic blood pressure usually is increased, but may at times be normal. In many hypertensive subjects tension drops to normal with rest or relaxation, fever, or following a myocardial infarction or cerebral vascular accident.

Symptoms and Signs

Hypertensive vascular disease may be present for many years without symptoms or signs other than an elevated blood pressure, but most patients complain of fatigue, nervousness, dizziness, palpitation, insomnia, weakness, and headaches at some time in the course of the disorder. These symptoms are common and therefore should not be attributed routinely to the hypertensive state.

Retinal abnormalities, secondary to sclerotic vascular changes, include arteriovenous compression, hemorrhages, exudates, or papilledema. Acute recurrent attacks of convulsions, severe headaches, vomiting, mental changes, and transitory paralyses occur infrequently. These manifestations are termed "hypertensive encephalopathy," and are probably due to cerebral anoxia secondary to areas of vascular spasm.

Cardiac hypertrophy is common, and ECG changes—left axis deviation, so-called left ventricular strain patterns, and evidence of myocardial damage—may appear. Cardiac pain and myocardial infarction due to coronary artery disease are frequent complications of hypertensive vascular disease, while congestive failure may occur as a result of coronary insufficiency or of hypertrophy of the heart, or both.

Cerebral vascular accidents may take place as a result of arteriosclerotic thrombosis or hemorrhage. Nosebleeds and menorrhagia are not uncommon but hemorrhage from other internal sites is rare.

Polyuria, nocturia, diminished ability of the kidney to concentrate urine, albuminuria, hematuria, cylindruria, and nitrogen retention may develop as a result of arteriolar nephrosclerosis.

Diagnosis

Hypertension should be suspected if the diastolic blood pressure occasionally rises above 90 mm. of mercury. The diagnosis becomes increasingly probable the more often this value is exceeded. The diagnosis of hypertensive vascular disease rests on repeated finding of hypertension when other causes of diastolic blood pressure elevation are excluded.

Epinephrine-producing pheochromocytomas may cause a curable hypertension clinically indistinguishable from essential hypertensive vascular disease. The test with Benodaine, an adrenolytic drug, will aid in differentiating hypertension due to pheochromocytoma (q.v.).

Other causes of hypertension include: many congenital and

acquired primary disorders of the renal parenchyma or circulation, particularly acute and chronic glomerulonephritis, polycystic kidneys, pyelonephritis, and urinary tract obstruction; coarctation of the aorta; hyperthyroidism (mild hypertension); toxemia of pregnancy; adrenal tumors; lupus erythematosus disseminatus; and periarteritis nodosa.

Prognosis

The course of hypertensive vascular disease is extremely variable. Average life expectancy probably is at least 15 years from onset, with extremes of several years and many decades. In general, the disease runs a more favorable course in women. Long survival is not a rarity. Rapidly progressive (malignant) disease occurs in a small percentage of cases, frequently among patients who have previously exhibited a mild and static course.

The initial level or the maintained height of the blood pressure, symptoms such as palpitation or headache, signs of cardiac enlargement or retinal arteriovenous compression, are unassociated with the rate of progression or the development of complications. On the other hand, a steadily rising blood pressure, retinitis, progressive renal damage, and coronary or arteriosclerotic vascular complications usually indicate a relatively short life expectancy.

Death results from congestive failure in about 50% of cases; myocardial infarction and cerebral hemorrhage are each responsible for about 15 to 20%, and uremia for about 5%.

Treatment

There is no treatment now known that consistently and completely reverses the course of hypertensive vascular disease. It is of prime importance to reassure the patient and not to limit his activities unnecessarily. An optimistic attitude on the part of the physician is both psychologically sound and justified by the natural history of the disease.

In this day of periodic health examinations, it may be wise to tell the patient he has high blood pressure, although in most cases the exact readings are best withheld. Reassurance and planning for situations and fears before they arise must be constantly practiced. An annual or semiannual medical examination prevents the apprehension caused by frequent visits to the doctor and yet provides opportunity for observing the course of the disease and for allaying any fears that may have arisen in the interval. The hypertensive patient without symptoms or complications does not require limitation of activity, but peaks of unusual physical exertion or emotional stress are undesirable; the subject should be taught to "act his age." The regular use of alcohol in small amounts, for those who find it palatable, is advantageous rather than detrimental. Tea, coffee, and tobacco need not be restricted unless some form of sensitivity is demonstrable. Weight reduction in the obese is beneficial. Hypertension increases the hazards during pregnancy and the rate of fetal mortality. Careful supervision, and induction of labor as soon as the fetus is viable, are generally recommended unless the hypertensive state is clearly aggravated, in which case pregnancy should be terminated by the simplest procedure feasible.

Many of the symptoms of uncomplicated hypertension respond to the combination of reassurance and time. Symptoms should always be considered in the light of causes other than hypertension. The short-term use of periods of rest, change of environment, and the judicious use of mild sedatives such as phenobarbital (℞ 44) 30 mg. twice a day, or chloral hydrate (℞ 43) 0.3 Gm. 2 or 3 times a day, may give dramatic results.

The use of strong sedatives, nitrites and nitrates (℞ 8, 10, 11, 12), thiocyanates (℞ 30), such pyrogens as typhoid vaccine (℞ 84) 10,000,000 to 20,000,000 organisms I.V., or phlebotomies (400 to 600 cc.) may lower the blood pressure for transitory periods. These are not curative but subjective improvement may follow their use, possibly through a psychotherapeutic component. Thiocyanate therapy, which appears to exert a hypotensive effect in some patients, should be used only by those experienced in this form of therapy and when facilities for repeated estimations of the blood levels of the drug are available. Even so, toxic manifestations are not infrequent and deaths have been reported in the absence of abnormally high blood concentration values. The therapeutic level is 6 to 12 mg./100 cc. Toxic effects usually develop when the level rises above 14 mg. Thiocyanates may be given as the sodium or potassium salt in doses of 0.3 Gm. daily (℞ 30). Such measures, together with lumbar puncture, hypertonic I.V. solutions, and magnesium sulfate, may be of limited value in the treatment of encephalopathy.

The use of veratrum viride (℞ 31) in lowering the blood pressure is receiving renewed interest. The dose is initially 2 tablets (each containing 10 Craw units) daily in divided doses, being increased at weekly intervals by 1 tablet daily until a therapeutic response or toxic manifestation (nausea or vomiting) is evident.

It is particularly effective when used to combat encephalopathy since its hypotensive effect is most striking when used only for relatively short periods. For encephalopathy, the dose is 1 tablet every 2 hours until the blood pressure is reduced.

Many new vasodilator and blood pressure-lowering drugs, such as tetraethylammonium compounds, are under investigation, but their status is not yet defined.

Headaches are variable in their frequency, intensity, and duration, so that time and psychotherapy should be enlisted. Often the use of simple analgesics such as acetylsalicylic acid 0.3 Gm. (℞ 48), acetophenetidin 0.3 Gm. (℞ 50) or strong coffee or tea on arising is sufficient. Blocks placed under the head of the bed should be tried. In rare instances, phlebotomy or lumbar puncture may deserve trial. Sympathectomy has much to offer the patient with intractable headache, but should be resorted to only after sufficient time has elapsed to be sure that other devices are ineffective. It must always be remembered that headaches bear little, if any, relationship to blood pressure levels and that their continuation or ultimate disappearance is unpredictable.

If congestive failure appears, its treatment is that of heart failure (q.v.) from any cause. Similarly, the arteriosclerotic complications (q.v.) associated with hypertension are no different from those seen in normotensive individuals. Treatment is identical, except that factors introduced by virtue of lowered cardiac or renal reserve must be considered. Therapy of arteriolar nephrosclerosis is that of chronic glomerulonephritis (q.v.).

The rigid dietary restriction of sodium chloride to less than 1 Gm./24 hours has some influence on resting blood pressure levels, but the resultant nutritional deprivations often exceed the benefits. Excess salt should be avoided, but the clinical value of drastic salt restriction is doubtful, though it may be given a therapeutic trial. Pepper, mustard, and lemon may be used for flavoring, and glutamic acid serves as a satisfactory and safe salt substitute. Similarly, the old idea that proteins (e.g., red meats) should be rigidly avoided is no longer valid, although moderation in this as in other dietary essentials is recommended.

A special form of dietary therapy is the "rice diet" (see DIETS) in which both the sodium content and the protein content of the diet are kept at a minimal level. Some patients with severe hypertension are reported to be symptomatically improved as long as they continue on the regimen, with systolic and diastolic blood pressures possibly lowered. If the diet is to be tried it should be continued for at least 2 to 5 months.

It is clearly established that bilateral lumbodorsal sympathectomy may lower the blood pressure for at least a short period in a small but perhaps significant percentage of cases, and that symptomatic improvement may ensue even without fall in blood pressure. It would appear that the progression of malignant hypertension may be altered by sympathectomy. Improvement in angiospastic retinal changes and cardiac and renal functions has been reported.

Determination of the value of surgical procedures must await further data. There is some evidence that there is a diminishing return of favorable results the longer the patients are followed. Although operative mortality has been reduced to 2% or less, the procedure requires long hospitalization, may produce considerable early disability, and postoperative complications may occur.

Consideration of sympathectomy seems justified only in malignant hypertension, in hypertensive vascular disease where a definite progressive tendency has become evident, and in patients with long-sustained and severe headaches in whom an adequate trial of medical treatment has failed to bring relief. It remains to be seen whether the natural history of hypertension will be modified by this procedure.

ANEURYSM; AORTITIS

Aneurysm: *A localized dilatation of a blood vessel, particularly an artery.* **Aortitis:** *Inflammation of the aorta.*

Etiology

True aneurysms result from focal weakness and distention of an arterial wall, the majority occurring secondary to syphilitic aortitis, and hence most often in the thoracic portion of the aorta, occasionally in its abdominal portion. Arteriosclerosis and hypertension commonly produce diffuse dilatation of the aorta, but rarely an aneurysm. However, while dissecting aortic aneurysms do occur from arteriosclerosis such usually are due to cystic necrosis of the media—a process of undetermined etiology. In these latter, hypertension is almost invariably a factor also. Bacterial infection (mycotic aneurysm), trauma, or congenital wall hypoplasia are the usual causes in aneurysmal dilatation of peripheral arteries. Trauma of penetrating nature, as from bullet or knife, may result in an arteriovenous aneurysm, particularly in the iliac, femoral, brachial, or carotid regions where artery and vein are sheathed proximately. Congenital arteriovenous aneurysms vary from vascular nevi called "port wine stains" to the huge networks of vessels known as "circoid" or "racemose" aneurysms, and which usually affect the head, tongue, or cheek.

Certain factors that predispose to aneurysm have been demonstrated: Middle or advanced age; heavy manual work; males 10 times more susceptible than females; in Negroes, an incidence 6 to 8 times that in the white race. Some of these factors perhaps have their origin in economic and social differences, as reflected in necessary habits of work and in the care accorded syphilitic infections.

Pathology and Pathologic Physiology

Mycotic aneurysms are more common in smaller arteries; otherwise, aneurysms are more apt to involve the larger vessels. Except for the aorta, aneurysmal dilatation is more common in the cerebral vessels, and syphilis is rarely the cause of these. Congenital wall hypoplasia is responsible for most aneurysms of the circle of Willis.

Arteriosclerotic changes begin in the intima of an artery, while syphilis involves the medial coat. The location and extent of the syphilitic mesaortitis (inflammation of the media) determine the clinical manifestations of aortitis in individual cases. Since the ascending portion of the aorta is most frequently involved, this is the most common site of aneurysms in the body. The aneurysms may produce little symptomatology unless there is associated encroachment upon coronary orifices (coronary ostial stenosis), or aortic valvular insufficiency. Otherwise, symptoms usually will depend on the pressure of the expanding mass upon nerves, the respiratory structures, esophagus, and bone. The erosion of bone usually causes severe pain. If rupture occurs there is apt to be a sudden fatal exsanguinating hemorrhage, or a subsequent fatal compression of vital organs adjacent to the sac.

Cystic necrosis of the media often extends along the aorta from its intrapericardial to its abdominal portion, thus predisposing to dissecting aneurysm.

Consequently these aneurysms may cause cerebral (carotid), upper extremity, renal, or lower extremity symptoms through secondary blocking and closure of vessels. Rupture into the pericardium is most commonly the terminal event, but rupture into chest or abdomen may occur. Occasionally, a dissecting aneurysm canalizes effectively and the patient continues to live for months or years.

Symptoms and Signs

Syphilitic aortitis (a rheumatic form also is described) may produce no symptoms. Encroachment on the aortic valves and the orifices of the coronary arteries often accounts for the symptoms which are listed as those of aortitis. These are substernal oppression and pain, dyspnea, palpitation, orthopnea, cough, and edema. A hollow, amphoric, bell-like second aortic sound is suggestive of aortitis, as is a widened area of dullness at the base of the heart, especially to the right of the sternum.

The symptoms produced by an aneurysm will depend upon its location, as will the physical signs. With **intrathoracic aneurysm,** the common symptoms are cough, hoarseness (paralysis of recurrent laryngeal nerve), dyspnea, dysphagia, and pain which may be constant or anginal. The diagnosis may be suggested by a Horner's syndrome, deviation of the trachea, a tracheal tug, or inequality of the blood pressure in the arms (usually not a reliable sign). Consolidation of lung tissue from bronchial compression is not unusual.

By causing erosion of the lumbar vertebrae, an **abdominal aortic aneurysm** may produce excruciating, boring abdominal pain. The blood pressure in the legs may be reduced so that it is equal to or lower than that in the arms.

Dissecting aortic aneurysm usually begins acutely with severe pain and sometimes shock. Such extreme symptoms occasionally are lacking, however. **Intracranial aneurysms** at the base of the brain may evoke no symptoms, or may rupture spontaneously and lead to death. There may be signs of mild cerebral hemorrhage or of fulminating apoplexy owing to rupture into the ventricles. The perforation may be so small that there is only slow oozing into the subarachnoid space, with red blood cells in the spinal fluid, increased protein, or xanthochromia. If it occurs periodically such oozing may give rise to a syndrome resembling that of pachymeningitis hemorrhagica. Rupture may follow trauma, exercise, coitus, fear, or any other condition which elevates blood pressure.

In **arteriovenous aneurysm** there usually is some hypertrophy of the limb involved, with marked dilatation of its superficial veins, those near to the aneurysm perhaps pulsating. Sometimes a thrill is felt and a bruit is heard in both directions. In an arteriovenous carotid aneurysm, the patient usually is cognizant of a disagreeable rhythmic, swishing noise with each heart beat.

Diagnosis

The pain with aortitis usually is easily differentiated from that of angina pectoris. At times substernal, it is more often to the right of the upper sternum, and is customarily a prolonged ache.

A pulsating tumor may prove to be an inflammatory or neoplastic mass adjacent to a large artery. However, it is safer to consider a pulsating tumor an aneurysm until identified otherwise. If the aneurysm presents as a subcutaneous mass, the diagnosis usually can be made. In other locations this may be difficult, as in abdominal and cerebral aneurysms. The latter may defy diagnosis during life, but a history of a number of attacks of meningeal irritation is suggestive, especially if fluid changes were accompaniments. Diagnosis of an intrathoracic aneurysm usually is possible by X-ray or fluoroscopic, sometimes by physical, examination. Surgical exploration may be necessary to exclude such intrathoracic tumors as retrosternal goiter, thymoma, lipoma, neurofibroma, teratoma, or bronchogenic carcinoma. The technics for outlining the heart and great vessels by Diodrast or Thorotrast represent an important diagnostic development.

A Wassermann test on the blood and spinal fluid should always be performed, since the blood test will be positive with 80 to 90% of syphilitic aneurysms.

Prognosis

In syphilitic aneurysm the prognosis depends upon its location and the progression of the syphilitic process. Persons with coronary ostial stenosis or aortic insufficiency who suffer from cardiac symptoms are said to have a life expectancy of less than 2 years. At times, however, patients with relatively stabilized luetic lesions live 8 or 10 years with aortic insufficiency and recurring cardiac symptoms. With aneurysms in other locations, the prognosis depends upon the pressure or other disturbances produced locally.

An individual with a dissecting aneurysm is in a precarious state, and usually suffers a fatal episode within a year or two.

The prognosis in congenital aneurysm of a cerebral artery is extremely variable. Sudden death from cerebral hemorrhage may occur in childhood or any time thereafter, or the lesion may remain unruptured and never cause symptoms.

Treatment

Adequate treatment of early syphilis (q.v.) usually will forestall the occurrence of cardiovascular involvement and aneurysm.

In order to avoid a possible fatal Herxheimer reaction, a patient with syphilitic aneurysm who has received no previous antiluetic therapy must be carefully prepared with iodides, and mercury or bismuth, prior to being given arsenicals (*see* accompanying schedule of treatment). Whether the same preparation is necessary before penicillin therapy is debatable. Alternate plans for penicillin therapy therefore are outlined. The second, which dispenses with such preparation, is included in a note at the end of this chapter.

If there is congestive heart failure, this should be treated appropriately (q.v.). Occasionally, bronchial or tracheal compression will cause a brassy cough which is constant and severe. Cough is controlled, if possible, by the usual measures (R 51, 52). Intractable pain, if not relieved by methadone, Demerol, or morphine (R 53, 55, 57), may require sympathectomy or paravertebral alcohol injections. Further surgical procedures, which occasionally are successful, include wiring of the aneurysmal sac, endoaneurysmorrhaphy, and ligation or excision of the sac.

Treatment of Syphilitic Aneurysm Where No Previous Antiluetic Therapy Has Been Given

1. Iodides: Give saturated solution of potassium iodide (R 90), 1 cc. (℩ xv) 3 times a day for 5 days of the week, in conjunction with mercury (R 75) or bismuth (R 76) injections. Watch for symptoms or signs of iodism, e.g., rash, salivation, gastrointestinal upset.

2. Mercury: Start with deep I.M. injections of mercury succinimide (R 75), 5 mg. at weekly intervals. After 1 month increase to 10 mg. weekly, and continue for another 2 months.

3. Bismuth: (May be given in place of mercury.) Start with bismuth subsalicylate (R 76), 50 mg. by deep I.M. injections at weekly intervals. Increase dose gradually to 0.2 Gm. at the end of a month. Continue 0.2 Gm. weekly for another 2 months.

4. Penicillin (R 70): (Give only after 3 months of preparation as above.) To be given as I.M. injections every 2 hours as follows:

First 24 hours:	500 u./dose
Second 24 hours:	1,000 u./dose
Third 24 hours:	5,000 u./dose

Fourth and subsequent days 40,000 u./dose, to a total of 6 million u. or more, as indicated.

5. Arsenic: Mapharsen (℞ 77) should be given only after 3 months of preparation as above. It may be used instead of penicillin and is to be administered slowly, I.V., every 5 to 7 days as follows:

First 4 to 6 weeks 20 mg./dose, then increase to 40 mg./dose and continue for 10 to 12 weeks. Then return to bismuth, or mercury and iodides, for 3 months. (*See* above.) Then alternate between the use of arsenoxide and mercury-bismuth iodide for 15 to 18 months of continuous treatment.

Note: The use of penicillin in cardiovascular syphilis, either alone or in conjunction with heavy metals, is not yet completely evaluated. However, it has been suggested that treatment with penicillin alone, without earlier preparation with iodides and mercury or bismuth, entails no great danger. Penicillin, 50,000 u. every 3 hours for 15 days (6 million u. total), has been recommended. (CAUTION! Because of the danger inherent in the treatment of syphilitic aneurysms, it is essential that the treatment be supervised by both internist and cardiologist, and individualized in every instance.)

VENOUS THROMBOSIS

(Phlebothrombosis, Thrombophlebitis, Bland thrombosis, Phlebitis, Milk leg, Phlegmasia alba dolens)

The presence of a thrombus in a superficial or deep vein. There are two main types of venous thrombosis: **phlebothrombosis,** in which the thrombus is associated with little or no inflammatory reaction, and **thrombophlebitis,** in which there is marked inflammation in the wall of the affected vein.

Etiology

The basic causes of venous thrombosis are not known. Predisposing factors include venous stasis, particularly that associated with bed rest; tissue destruction anywhere in the body whether surgical, neoplastic or traumatic; cardiac insufficiency; senility; debility; obesity; varicosities; infection; and hemoconcentration.

Pathology

Deep venous thrombosis of the lower extremities starts with the formation of a clot in the veins of the calf or foot. This thrombus propagates proximally as a "tail" waving freely in the larger veins, often reaching a length of over 12 inches. As this "tail" increases in diameter it obstructs the larger veins. Part or all of the clot may break loose and be transported by the blood stream to become a pulmonary embolus. A secondary inflammatory response may occur locally, followed by invasion by fibroblasts and fixation of this portion of the thrombus to the vein wall. Eventually, the processes of inflammation and fixation overtake the proximal growth of the clot and the whole thrombus becomes fixed. Recanalization and the development of collateral circulation then proceed over a period of many months. Infrequently, cases of acute thrombophlebitis start as an inflammation of the vein wall itself, with secondary thrombus formation.

Symptoms and Signs

Noninflammatory venous thrombosis (phlebothrombosis) may be completely asymptomatic, although careful examination made early will often reveal a feeling of fullness, and sometimes tenderness, on palpation of the affected calf. Strong passive dorsiflexion of the foot frequently causes pain in the calf (Homan's sign). As the inflammatory process spreads, tenderness becomes more marked and may extend into the popliteal space and the femoral canal. The superficial veins may appear unusually prominent. The patient usually complains of a feeling of heaviness in the affected limb. Obstruction of the larger veins may cause swelling of the leg, which can best be determined by daily palpation and measurements. Low grade fever, mild leukocytosis, and elevated erythrocyte sedimentation rate may or may not be present.

In some cases of acute thrombophlebitis the inflammatory response in the vein wall and lymphatics is intense. These patients have severe pain, extreme tenderness, and moderate to severe swelling, with increased local temperature. Fever, leukocytosis, and elevated sedimentation rate are usual. There may be reflex vasospasm, causing a cold, pale, cyanotic extremity with diminished or absent peripheral pulse. When the inflammatory reaction subsides, the only remaining symptom is edema from venous or lymphatic obstruction, or both; this may be massive but often is minimal or absent. As collateral circulation develops, the edema usually subsides slowly, but occasionally persists indefinitely.

Since the symptoms and signs of venous thrombosis are caused by obstruction and inflammation, they give no indication as to the size of the waving "tail" of the thrombus. Thus, massive pulmonary emboli may arise from a phlebothrombosis of the leg veins without any local evidence of their presence. However, thrombi usually break off before pronounced inflammatory changes occur, so that embolism is somewhat less likely in the presence of severe local tenderness and pain.

Diagnosis

The diagnosis of venous thrombosis requires that its possibility be considered in all patients with symptoms referable to the lower extremities. It may be confused with a strained muscle or, more infrequently, with a sciatic neuritis.

Prognosis

Previous to the use of anticoagulants or venous ligation therapy, pulmonary embolism occurred in about 20% and fatal embolism in 6% of all cases. Hospital stay was usually prolonged to 5 or 6 weeks, with postphlebitic symptoms almost the rule. Cases with subsequent thrombosis ran as high as 15%.

With anticoagulant therapy, pulmonary embolus occurs in approximately 1.5% and fatal embolus in approximately 0.3% of all cases. The hospital stay is about 2 weeks. When the process remains confined to the calf, no sequelae result. If there is involvement at the iliofemoral level, swelling may persist for 4 to 5 months, then disappear completely or become minimal. Recurrent thrombosis appears in 1.1% of cases.

With surgical therapy, pulmonary embolus occurs in about 5% and fatal embolus in less than 1%. Hospital stay averages 8 days. Ankle edema persists in less than half the cases treated by femoral vein ligation.

Prophylaxis

Early ambulation by itself is not sufficient prophylaxis against thromboembolism, although it is advisable to avoid unnecessarily prolonged bed rest. Instruction of the patient as to the necessity of frequent movements of toes and lower extremity while still at bed rest is essential. Specific measures (either anticoagulants or vein ligation) are indicated in selected individuals with those clinical disturbances in which the incidence of thromboembolism is significantly higher than usual (*see* Etiology).

Treatment

The primary objective of treatment is the prevention of pulmonary emboli. Once a definite or presumptive diagnosis of deep venous thrombosis is established, the patient should be immediately placed at complete bed rest and instructed to avoid unnecessary activity or strain. This is continued for a minimum of 6 days. Venous return is facilitated by slight elevation of the lower extremities, while a cradle over the foot of the bed removes the weight of bed clothes. The local application of heat or cold often relieves pain.

Anticoagulant therapy should be instituted immediately, using heparin alone, or combined heparin and dicumarol (*see* ANTICOAGULANT THERAPY).

If anticoagulant therapy is complicated by a hemorrhage of such severity that further such treatment seems inadvisable, a decision must be made at once concerning the patient's management. When adequate anticoagulant therapy has been maintained for more than 8 days, a period of observation may be indicated. If, however, the treatment has been too brief, ligation of the peripheral venous system at the appropriate level should be performed as soon as major bleeding is controlled.

If vasospasm, severe pain, or extensive edema is present, the following measures may be employed: papaverine (℞ 17, 18) may aid in relaxing the venospasm; pain may be relieved with codeine (℞ 52), Demerol (℞ 55) or morphine sulfate (℞ 57); whisky (℞ 32) may help to relax vasospasm; mercurial diuretics (℞ 34, 35, 36) may be effective in decreasing the edema of an extremity that resists other treatment. In acute deep thrombophlebitis with severe pain, edema, or vasospasm, lumbar sympathetic block gives relief. Ten to 15 cc. of a 1% solution of procaine is injected into the region of lumbar ganglia 1 through 4 on the affected side. One effective block relieves 90% of cases, and the rest require a 2nd or 3rd injection at 24-hour intervals.

If after 6 days of bed rest signs of active phlebitis have subsided and the patient's general condition warrants it, he may be ambulated progressively. Anticoagulant therapy should be continued during this period, preferably until the patient is fully ambulatory, which usually takes 6 days. If the clinical situation then is satisfactory, anticoagulants may be discontinued. Firm support for both legs (e.g., elastic bandage or stocking) should be maintained whenever the patient is out of bed, and discarded only when edema fails to recur without it.

Surgical management: The surgical management of venous thrombosis entails ligation of the main venous channel proximal to a thrombus. Since the deep veins of the calf usually are affected, bilateral ligation of the superficial femoral vein generally is the procedure of choice.

As compared with phlebothrombosis, acute iliofemoral thrombophlebitis less frequently causes emboli, and therefore ligation of the vein is rarely necessary. For iliofemoral venous thrombosis giving off repeated emboli, inferior vena cava ligation may be indicated whether or not the superficial femoral vein has previously been ligated. This is a major operation requiring general anesthesia and is not recommended unless anticoagulant therapy is impossible or has failed to control embolic phenomena.

In suppurative thrombophlebitis, vein ligation is mandatory to prevent discharge of septic emboli. In suppurative pelvic involvement, ligation of the inferior vena cava plus both ovarian or spermatic veins is necessary.

VARICOSE VEINS

Abnormally lengthened, dilated, sacculated superficial veins. Frequently their valves are incompetent. They are found almost exclusively in the lower extremities and in the lower abdominal wall.

Etiology

Varicose veins develop spontaneously, presumably because of a hereditary weakness in the structure of the vein wall and possibly also of the valves. Because of these weaknesses the veins dilate when subjected to increased pressure from within, or because of a decreased support from the surrounding tissues. Increased pressure within the veins may result from mechanical obstruction, such as by a tumor within the pelvis, or phlebitis. Varicose veins frequently become evident or are exaggerated during pregnancy. Man's upright position, particularly when associated with physical effort, increases the venous pressure considerably. With aging and with obesity the support afforded by the tissues to the superficial veins is lessened.

Pathologic Physiology

The essential pathologic changes in varicose veins are (1) dilatation or increase in the transverse diameter and circumference; (2) elongation and tortuosity; (3) loss of elasticity from increase in fibrous connective tissue; (4) variations in the thickness of the wall, and (5) disappearance or atrophy of valves.

The long saphenous is involved most frequently, but incompetence of the communicating veins is not uncommon. In the upright position there is stasis of the venous blood in the dilated veins and, in some cases, there is reverse flow of blood.

Symptoms and Signs

In many persons extensive varicose veins may not cause any symptoms in the absence of swelling of the legs. In others, particularly after a long period on their feet, there may be increased fatigability of the leg muscles, muscle cramps, an annoying sensation of tension and soreness in the popliteal space and in the region of the veins. Ankle swelling, when present, tends to disappear during the night.

Many women notice an increase in the severity of symptoms during the menses. Itching and localized or generalized eczematoid dermatitis may develop (stasis dermatitis). Pigmentation may appear, particularly if there is injury to the skin. In emotional or nervously exhausted patients the number and severity of symptoms in uncomplicated varicose veins are increased.

The complications of varicose veins include chronic venous insufficiency with its various manifestations such as edema, ulceration, and thrombophlebitis.

Diagnosis

A complete history should be taken and a general physical examination made. It is important in all instances to determine the state of the cardiovascular and renal systems. Evidence of an abdominal tumor, of previous thrombophlebitis, or of cellulitis in the tissues should be sought. Inspection and palpation of the veins should be carried out in a good light, with the patient in a standing position.

It is important to test for the competency of the valves of the long and the short saphenous veins by the Trendelenburg test. This test consists of two parts, the constriction and the release. With the patient lying down, the extremity is elevated and the veins emptied by stroking the leg toward the thigh. A tourniquet is applied around the upper thigh tightly enough to constrict the superficial veins, but not the femoral artery or vein. The patient then is told to stand. If the veins remain empty or fill very slowly (20 to 30 seconds) this (constrictive) part of the test is considered negative. If the veins fill rapidly (5 to 15 seconds) the constriction test is positive. This means either that the valves of the communicating veins are inadequate or else that the deep venous system (femoral) is not patent. The other important part of the test is concerned with observations after release of the tourniquet as soon as the patient stands. If a column of blood is observed to fall downward and fill the varicose veins rapidly after release of the tourniquet, incompetency of the valves in the upper saphenous system is present and the test is positive. On the other hand, if release of the tourniquet is followed by slow filling, at least some of the major valves of the upper portion of the saphenous vein are competent and the test is negative.

Another test useful in estimating the patency of the deep circulation and the adequacy of the valves of the communicating veins has been described by Perthes. A tourniquet is placed around the thigh above the varicosities just tight enough to prevent reflux of blood down the saphenous trunk. The patient then is instructed to walk vigorously for a minute or two. If the communicating and deep veins are patent and functioning normally, the saphenous varicosity will become emptied because exercise has forced the blood into the deep system and into the general circulation.

The competency of the deep veins can be assumed if there is no edema of the legs. If edema is present, the patient should be put to bed long enough for it to disappear, in order to determine whether or not a good pressure bandage applied from the toes to below the knee is well tolerated. If it is, the competency of the deep veins is confirmed. It is important to test the arterial circulation and to determine the presence or absence of arthritis (q.v.), particularly of the knee joint. Such conditions frequently are responsible for the symptoms complained of by persons with varicose veins. The presence of chronic venous insufficiency is evidenced by the presence of static edema, eczema, indurated cellulitis, or ulceration.

Treatment

The treatment of varicose veins includes a variety of measures. The method to be employed in a particular case is dependent on many factors. To avoid aggravation of symptoms, rest, elevation of the extremity, and the use of some form of external support such as elastic bandages or elastic stockings will serve. Elastic stockings should be made to measure. They should extend from the toes to below the knee, preferably with the heel included.

Elastic supports or Unna's paste boot (℞ 82) is recommended for persons in the advanced age group, during pregnancy, in the presence of debilitating diseases, and in the presence of severe impairment to the arterial supply, previous or coexistent phlebitis, and tumors of the pelvis.

Application of Unna's paste boot: With a 2-inch (5 cm.) brush, or with the hand, the softened paste is applied from the knee to the toes. The leg then is wrapped with ordinary cotton gauze bandage. The physician should exercise care, so that no ridges of bandage remain over the tibia remain. Over this bandage then is applied a layer of Unna's paste, which is thoroughly rubbed into the bandage. If a large ulcer is present a reinforcement is made by dipping a large square of gauze into the Unna's paste and placing it over the area. Another layer of gauze then is applied from the knee to the toes, to incorporate the reinforcement of gauze into the cast. After this second layer of gauze has been applied, another application of the Unna's paste is thoroughly rubbed into this gauze and the whole cast then is allowed to cool. In the course of about 10 minutes the paste has become "set" and the patient can continue with normal activity. If 4 to 6 layers of gauze have been used, the "boot" will give support for from 3 to 4 weeks before it wrinkles and becomes uncomfortable. It is important to avoid the occurrence of wrinkles in the bandage, particularly over the tibia or over the foot, and it is desirable to place the gauze layers evenly and smoothly and to employ a well mixed solution, which should be rubbed thoroughly into the bandage. In hot summer weather it is advisable to increase slightly the content of gelatin, whereas in cold weather the gelatin content may be decreased somewhat.

The injection treatment is permissible for the treatment of smaller varicosities below the knee. Various solutions, such as hypertonic glucose (℞ 65), hypertonic saline (℞ 66), sodium salicylate 20% (℞ 67), quinine and urethane (℞ 68), and 5% sodium morrhuate (℞ 69), are employed. The latter solution now is most generally used because it has been proved by experience to be associated with fewer complications. A test dose of 0.5 cc. is recommended to discover the occasional patient sensitive to this drug. If no such contraindication exists, 2 to 3 cc. of the solution may be injected 2 or 3 times weekly, provided there is no significant degree of reaction in the tissues from previous injections.

In choosing the site for the injection, it is preferable to inject from above downward. A needle with a medium-long bevel and a 5 cc. syringe is used. The patient is placed preferably in an upright position, but with the arms supported on a rest. The injection also may be made with the patient sitting with legs over the side of a table. The varix is emptied and occluded above and below and care is taken to avoid infiltration of the tissues. After the injection is completed, a small pressure bandage should be worn for several hours. The patient is kept ambulant.

With larger veins, particularly those above the knee, the injection treatment is followed by too rapid recurrence. Consequently, operative treatment alone or operative treatment plus the injection of a sclerosing solution into the distal segment at the time of the high ligation of the saphenous vein becomes necessary. High ligation of the saphenous vein together with the ligation of all the important communicating veins with incompetent valves between the deep and superficial systems is desirable before the use of sclerosing solutions. After such a procedure, a sclerosing solution may be used to eliminate small residual varices.

Ligation of the saphenous vein near its termination, together with the excision of lengths of varicosed veins above and below the knee, is regarded as the method of choice by many. Hospitalization for 7 to 10 days is required. Pulmonary embolism following the treatment of varicose veins is a rare complication. It is prevented by the same procedures as are used in the postoperative period following any surgical procedure.

The various types of eczema which occur in association with chronic venous insufficiency are the result of nutritional disturbances in the skin, irritation of sensory nerves, scratching, and the reaction to irritating applications. A local hypersensitiveness to many drugs and foods exists in the regions affected by venous insufficiency. The hypersensitiveness may be present in other parts of the body as well. Treatment consists in the correction of the venous insufficiency by elevation of the leg and elastic support and in the use of bland and nonirritating applications. The local use of sulfonamide ointments should be avoided.

Treatment of Varicose Ulcers

Varicose ulcers are best treated by rest in bed with elevation of the foot of the bed 3 to 4 inches when edema is present. The ulcerated areas should be cleansed daily with soap and water. Warm saline packs help in the cleansing process and also improve the blood flow, thus making the healing more rapid. The administration of penicillin (℞ 70) will aid in eliminating the infection which is almost always present. By the above procedures most varicose ulcers can be healed in 3 to 8 weeks. After this has been accomplished, elastic stockings or bandages should be worn indefinitely to lessen the likelihood of a return of the ulceration.

Whenever the ulcers are large, and particularly if they have occurred repeatedly, it often is desirable to skin graft the area involved, using a split thickness graft. The skin of the grafted area is thicker and more resistant to trauma than is the skin which gradually covers such areas by growing in from the margins.

Many smaller, less chronic ulcers can be treated with the patient ambulatory. The ulcerated area is cleansed and just enough of a bland ointment, such as zinc oxide (R 83), is applied to keep a fine mesh gauze bandage from sticking. Then, an elastic pressure bandage of one type or another is worn for 1 to 3 weeks depending on the amount of exudate. Most ulcers will yield to such treatment in 4 to 12 weeks. Good results often are obtained in chronic varicose ulcers by the frequent application of red blood cell powder or paste, or of the patient's whole blood.

Very occasionally malignant degeneration occurs in the margin of large chronic varicose ulcers. This is recognized by the piling up of the cells lining the ulcers to above the level of the surrounding skin. A proper biopsy will establish the diagnosis. If positive, such ulcer margins should be excised adequately and the ulcer covered with a split thickness skin graft. The inguinal lymph nodes should not be excised unless evidently involved in the malignant process. Spread of such a cancer is slow and usually remains local. Amputation therefore is necessary only rarely.

PERIPHERAL VASCULAR DISORDERS

Disorders affecting the blood supply to the extremities, which may be either organic or functional in origin.

ORGANIC DISEASES

ARTERIOSCLEROSIS (q.v.)

THROMBO-ANGIITIS OBLITERANS
(Buerger's disease)

A disease involving the peripheral arteries, veins and nerves, and characterized by structural changes in the vessels, with associated venous and arterial thromboses frequently leading to gangrene.

Etiology

The cause of Buerger's disease is unknown. The condition occurs in young males, usually under 45 years of age, and rarely is seen in women. In the nonsmoker, its occurrence is most unusual. Excessive cigarette smoking, trauma, exposure to extremes of temperature, the use of ergot or epinephrine, and infection (general or local) may be precipitating factors of acute episodes.

Pathology and Pathologic Physiology

In the walls of the arteries and veins structural change associated with a perivascular reaction of round and giant cells may be seen. The intima of the vessels becomes roughened and thrombosis results. Fibrotic incorporation of the artery, vein, and nerve accompanies the healing process. Recanalization of the vessels usually is slight and the thrombophlebitic element may be predominant. In all cases, reflex vasospasm involving the normal arteries further reduces the blood supply.

Symptoms and Signs

Onset may be gradual or acute, with rapid development of gangrene.

The patient may complain of coldness, numbness, tingling or burning before objective evidence of the disease is present. Intermittent claudication in the involved extremity, usually the leg, is characterized by a sensation of weakness or tightening, which occurs only after muscular exertion. Rapid relief follows a brief period of rest. Symptoms occur more quickly with strenuous than with mild exercise. Pain is experienced late in the disease and is noted at rest as well as with activity. It occurs in the pregangrenous stage and is severe in the ulcerated or gangrenous condition.

Rubor of the toes and foot in the dependent position, and pallor in the same areas with the extremity elevated above heart level are cardinal signs of arterial insufficiency. Coldness of the involved extremity is typical. Trophic changes in the nails and skin may occur quite early in the disease. Migratory phlebitis is found in 30 to 40% of the cases. Diminution or absence of arterial pulsation, as determined by palpation of the arteries or by the oscillometer, is always noted, except in the earliest stages of the disease. Ulceration and gangrene involving the skin and deeper tissues, starting as a rule in the distal parts, are common findings in the long-standing, untreated case and in the acute malignant form of the disease.

Prophylaxis and Treatment

Since no specific therapy is available, supportive treatment should be directed toward removal of all factors which reduce blood supply, and application of all possible means to increase blood supply.

Factors to be eliminated include: (1) Tobacco in any form. Even after the disease has been controlled the resumption of smoking may cause an exacerbation. (2) Exposure to very low or very high temperatures. (3) Trauma, especially that resulting from poorly fitted footwear or careless chiropody. Injury to the tisues by chemical substances such as iodine, carbolic or salicylic acids or any other strong chemicals must be avoided. (4) The use of vasospastic drugs such as ergot or epinephrine.

(5) Excessive use of the involved extremity. (The patient should be cautioned against forced walking when the symptoms of intermittent claudication are present.) (6) Fungus infections.

The following means should be used singly or together in an attempt to increase the arterial inflow: (1) Complete bed rest when gangrene, ulceration or rest pain is present. When these symptoms are absent, frequent use of the involved extremity is advisable, but not to the extent that claudication will result. (2) Maintaining the involved extremity well protected by soft padding at about room temperature to aid reduction of the metabolic demands of the tissues; and application of contact, radiant or electrical heat to the trunk to promote reflex vaso-dilatation. (3) The use of gravity to fill and drain the affected vessels of the extremity. The patient should sleep with the feet at a lower level than the heart. Buerger's exercises can be carried out frequently during the day in the following manner: The extremity should be elevated actively or passively until the tips of the digits begin to pale, and then lowered until a fair degree of rubor has developed. The 3rd phase of the cycle is a minute's rest with the extremity horizontal. An oscillating bed, so adjusted that the above vascular changes take place within each cycle, provides an excellent means of continuing this treatment in a passive manner for an extended period of time. (4) Suction and pressure to fill and empty the arteries can be accomplished by use of a "boot" into which the extremity fits. Excessive periods of ischemia or rubor must be avoided by proper attention to the degrees of suction and pressure, and the duration of application. (5) Promotion of a reflex inflow of arterial blood through use of venous constriction by cuff pressure. (6) The release of arterial spasm by I.V. or I.M. injection of foreign protein. Typhoid vaccine (℞ 84) is the agent of choice and should be given I.V. in doses adequate to produce a slight temperature rise without a chill. It usually is best to begin with a small dose, 3,000,000 to 5,000,000 organisms I.V., increasing to 50,000,000 or 100,000,000 organisms, according to tolerance. In some cases this form of therapy is not successful. (7) The release of arterial spasm by the blocking of the sympathetic nervous system by procaine, paravertebrally injected; by I.V. administration of tetraethylammonium bromide (℞ 91); by the local application of Mecholyl (℞ 33) by galvanic current (iontophoresis; see CLIN. PROC.) in superficial lesions; by relief of pain through the administration of papaverine (℞ 17, 18), with secondary release of vascular spasm; by severance of the sympathetic nervous system (sympathectomy). For severe pain opiates (℞ 54, 57, 59) should be used only in the acute period, since addiction may result. Acetylsalicylic acid (℞ 48) with an ounce of whisky every 4 hours often will relieve pain and act as a mild vasodilator as well. (8) Anticoagulants (℞ 60, 61, 62) also may be used (see ANTICOAGULANT THERAPY) to combat the progressive thrombosis which frequently results in arterial occlusion so severe as to necessitate amputation (*see* ARTERIOSCLEROSIS).

FROSTBITE
(Chilblain, Pernio, Immersion foot)

A condition characterized by destruction of superficial tissues resulting from exposure to cold, with secondary structural and functional disturbances of the smaller surface blood vessels.

Etiology

Exposure to cold, especially moist cold. Contributing factors may be tight clothing, moisture and long periods of inactivity of the extremities involved. Individuals with underlying vascular disease or other systemic disorders are the most readily affected. The very young and, especially, the old may likewise be affected.

Pathology

Crystallization of the fluids in the superficial tissue cells, together with vascular stagnation, edema, and thrombosis, produces structural changes resulting in disordered function of the vascular system, which is characterized primarily by spasm of the arterioles.

Diagnosis

Blanching or erythema of the affected area is prominent initially. In the early stages the erythema blanches with pressure. Later, edema and superficial blisters develop, and may break down and form superficial ulcers or gangrene. Secondary local infection may occur, which in turn may be complicated by general sepsis. Severe pain together with various paresthesias usually leads to the development of a causalgia-like state.

Prophylaxis

It is important to look for and correct, if possible, any underlying metabolic or circulatory disease, such as anemia, nutritional deficiency, and hypothyroidism, by the use of iron (℞ 86), vitamins, and thyroid extract (℞ 85). The extremities should be protected with light but well-fitting woolen clothes. Tight clothing is to be avoided, as are long periods of sitting or standing, especially when the clothing is wet.

Treatment

This consists of 3 principal approaches: (1) Maintain a low environmental temperature, in order to reduce the metabolism of the superficial tissues so that the available blood supply may be adequate, if possible, to keep the tissues alive. By covering the involved extremities with a cradle, to avoid pressure on the sensitive tissues, and by surrounding the cradle with ice bags, a low air temperature can be maintained within it. As circulation improves, this environmental temperature may be slowly raised. (2) Maintain maximal circulation by the relief of vasospasm and the avoidance of thromboses. Heparin (℞ 60, 61) administered prior to intravascular clotting will reduce the frequency and degree of gangrene and permit a more normal return of circulation. It may be given by continuous infusion at the rate of 30 to 60 mg./hour (approximately 250 mg. in all) or I.M. 100 mg. 4 times a day, so that the clotting time is at least 15 to 20 minutes. To maintain increased clotting time dicumarol (℞ 62) should be administered during and after the initial heparinization. This should be maintained until all acute symptoms have disappeared. Vasospasm may be treated by keeping the uninvolved parts of the body warm, thus producing reflex vasodilation; by the use of an ounce of whisky (℞ 32), plus acetylsalicylic acid (℞ 48), every 3 hours; by I.V. administration of tetraethylammonium bromide (℞ 91); or with daily paravertebral nerve blocks to the extremity involved. Papaverine (℞ 17, 18) every 4 hours is of value in producing vasodilatation. Tobacco should be eliminated to avoid the vasospasm associated with its use, and a sedative (℞ 44) prescribed for the relief of the nervousness coincident with the discomfort of frostbite. Analgesics (℞ 54, 57, 59) may be necessary for the relief of pain in the acute stage of the disease, but they should not be administered for the paresthesias which occur in the healing stage. (3) Prevent secondary infection by the use of soft nonirritating sterile dressings and the application of an antiseptic ointment such as Furacin (℞ 78). If infection ensues, penicillin (℞ 70) or a sulfonamide (℞ 72) is indicated. In mild cases with the skin unbroken, the application of a camphor and phenol ointment (℞ 87) is soothing.

In late cases with residual paresthesias or indolent ulcers, the daily use of Mecholyl (℞ 33) by iontophoresis (*see* CLIN. PROC.) will promote healing and frequently relieve discomfort. In cases with a severe residual paresthesia, sympathectomy may be of value.

ARTERIAL EMBOLISM AND THROMBOSIS

Either of these conditions may cause a sudden closure of one or more arterial channels. Arterial embolism results from lodgment of part or all of a thrombus, bacterial vegetation, fat globule, gas bubble, or other matter foreign to the artery. An embolus may originate from a thrombus in one of the veins of the pelvis or lower extremity, formed in the course of thrombophlebitis, which is an occasional sequel to prolonged postoperative bed rest. Such an embolus usually passes through the right heart and comes to rest in one of the pulmonary arteries. In rare instances it may traverse a congenital septal defect and occlude one of the systemic arteries. Myocardial infarction, mitral stenosis or auricular fibrillation may be responsible for the formation of a mural thrombus, from which emboli break off and pass to either the pulmonary or systemic circulation. In cases of bacterial endocarditis, emboli consisting of bacterial vegetations from involved heart valves (usually mitral and aortic) are disseminated, as a rule, to the systemic circulation. Clumps of bacteria may enter the blood stream during the course of an infection and, after lodgment, cause small abscess and septic infarcts. Often, as a result of bone fracture or severe trauma to fat depots, fat globules enter the blood stream and occlude the smaller arterioles and capillaries. Gas bubbles may occur in the circulatory system through accidental injection; injury to chest and lungs; or, as in caisson disease (q.v.), through change in environmental atmospheric pressure. They may lodge in the brain, lung, or coronary arteries, or in other, less important arteries, where they have the same obstructive effect as fat globules.

Thrombi often form in the small blood vessels of the lungs during congestive heart failure. Arteriosclerotic changes, syphilitic involvement, or an acute or chronic inflammatory reaction in and around the blood vessel not infrequently cause thrombosis. The most common forms of arterial thrombosis are cerebral, pulmonary and coronary (q.v.).

Pathology

The sudden occlusion of a systemic artery by a thrombus or an embolus causes an immediate ischemia of the tissues in the area supplied, and a secondary vasospasm of the arteries in the involved region or extremity, further reducing the blood supply.

Symptoms, Signs, and Diagnosis

Sudden coldness, numbness, tingling, and the rapid development of severe pain in an extremity are the characteristic symptoms. The finding of a cold extremity, usually blanched or mottled with a cyanotic patchiness, together with absent arterial pulsations and absent or diminished oscillometric readings, confirms the diagnosis. Sometimes the embolus can be localized by the presence of arterial pulsation proximal to it, but reflex spasm may diminish the pulsation above the clot, the vasoconstriction even occurring at times in the opposite extremity. The known presence of a potential source of the embolus is of further assistance in diagnosis.

Treatment

If the embolus or thrombus is large, involving a major vessel high in the extremity, embolectomy is indicated. It must be done within 12 hours after the episode if reopening of the vessel below the point of blockage is to be expected. Good results with this procedure are more probable if the involved vessel is a healthy one. Surgery should be done under spinal anesthesia to facilitate maximum dilatation of the collateral vessels. When local anesthesia is used it should be followed by a paravertebral block of the sympathetic system supplying the involved extremity. Anticoagulants (R 60, 61, 62) should be used following embolectomy until there is no further danger of clotting at the operative site (*see* ANTICOAGULANT THERAPY).

In cases where embolectomy is not possible, where diseased arteries are present, or where the blockage is distal, immediate and intensive medical treatment is indicated. Pain should be relieved by analgesics (R 54, 57, 59). Vasodilatation can be achieved by paravertebral blocks, papaverine I.V. or intra-arterially (R 18) in doses of 30 or 60 mg., whisky (R 32) and acetylsalicylic acid (R 48), reflex heat and complete bed rest. The involved extremity should be protected by soft, loosely applied padding, and its environmental temperature kept low (*see* Frostbite). If infection occurs locally, penicillin (R 70) or a sulfonamide (R 72) should be administered systemically.

In cases progressing to massive gangrene, amputation should be done as soon as demarcation is clear.

FUNCTIONAL DISORDERS

These vascular disorders may result from disturbances in the sympathetic innervation of the blood vessels, or may be secondary to organic vascular disease. However, after the primary functional form has been present for some time, secondary organic changes in the vessels appear.

RAYNAUD'S DISEASE OR SYNDROME

A condition, secondary to many factors, manifested by an abnormal degree of vascular spasm of the superficial vessels, especially those in the digits.

Etiology

This syndrome may be idiopathic. It may be associated with primary vascular disease or secondary to disease of the endocrines, the C.N.S., arthritis of the spine, scleroderma, sensitivity to certain substances such as ergot, arsenic and tobacco, to neuroses, and to certain types of trauma, especially vibration. It may be precipitated by emotional upsets or overexposure to cold.

Pathology and Pathologic Physiology

Due to an abnormal reaction of the sympathetic nervous system, any of the above mentioned stimuli may produce marked vasospasm, which may be severe enough to produce trophic changes in the skin and nails of the extremities, and in extreme cases gangrene limited to the superficial tissues. Attacks of vasospasm may last for minutes to hours. This rarely is severe enough to cause the loss of any amount of tissue. The small trophic ulcers occurring, however, may be very painful and slow to heal. Late organic changes include marked dilatation of the skin capillaries in the involved areas.

Symptoms and Signs

The criteria for diagnosis are: Intermittent attacks of blanching of the digits alternating with a stage of rubor; bilateral or quadrilateral involvement (onset may be unilateral). For idiopathic Raynaud's disease, the absence of a primary vascular or systemic disease; limitation of gangrene, if present, to the superficial tissues; existence of the syndrome for at least 2 years.

Treatment

Treatment of the secondary forms of Raynaud's disease depends on recognition of the primary disease and attention to its treatment. However, once the autonomic nervous system has established this peculiar type of activity, removal of the cause does not always eliminate the syndrome.

In the idiopathic form, no type of therapy has been entirely satisfactory, although some excellent results have been noted following psychiatric therapy. Many patients improve if they are removed from the precipitating factor, such as trauma or cold. In severe forms with active gangrene, the maintenance of an even, warm environmental atmosphere is necessary for healing. From the surgical standpoint, sympathectomy should offer complete relief and in many cases it does. However, this usually requires a quadrilateral operation and it does not always provide permanent relief from the syndrome. To be successful, this surgery must be preganglionic with all fibers supplying the extremities being severed and the associated ganglia being removed.

Drug therapy has been of very little value. The use of mild sedatives such as one of the barbiturates (℞ 44) will reduce the severity of the attacks. So-called vasodilator drugs taken by mouth or by hypodermic injection have little or no effect.

In endocrine deficiencies an attempt should be made to replace the lack of the specific glandular function. Acetylsalicylic acid (℞ 48) will relieve the ache and pain. Opiates should be used with extreme caution because of the chronicity of the disease.

ERYTHROMELALGIA

A state of permanent vasodilation of the capillaries of the extremities accompanied by severe burning and dryness. The etiology is unknown, but the condition is a manifestation of a disturbance of the sympathetic nervous system. There is a complete paralysis of the vasomotor tone of the smaller arteries that supply the superficial tissues of the extremities. This results in a constant high pressure in the capillary loops with marked dilatation of these vessels. These lesions are symmetrical and usually quadrilateral. The extremities are hot, red, and usually dry. Diagnosis is made on the basis of these findings and the patient's complaints as above outlined.

Treatment

There is no known treatment for this disease. Symptoms may sometimes be relieved by salicylates (℞ 48) or small, frequent doses of barbiturates (℞ 44).

CAUSALGIA

A syndrome arising as a result of irritation or injury of a peripheral nerve and characterized by persistent, diffuse burning pain, subject to exacerbations from almost any stimulus, even contact with air or drying of the skin. The excruciating pain is accompanied by vasomotor and dystrophic changes and may cause extreme alteration in the emotional status. Signs of localized autonomic dysfunction noted in examination of the hyperalgesic skin are discoloration, hyperhidrosis, and coldness. Vasospasm often is so severe that the major pulses of the involved extremity are greatly reduced. Disuse atrophy of the muscles in the affected limb occurs as a result of the patient's continuous protective immobilization of the extremity.

Treatment

The most promising results have been obtained in severe cases with sympathectomy. In milder types paravertebral nerve blocks with procaine are beneficial. Occasionally, relief can be obtained by local infiltration with procaine, Mecholyl iontophoresis (*see* CLIN. PROC.), or warm, wet dressings. Tetraethylammonium bromide (℞ 91) administered I.V. 1 to 3 times weekly has been tried with encouraging results.

ANTICOAGULANT THERAPY

Anticoagulant therapy with heparin or dicumarol, or both, is effective in preventing or inhibiting intravascular clotting. The action of these drugs is to impair the clotting mechanism to an extent sufficient that pathologic clotting will not occur. Experimental evidence has been presented recently to show that these agents actually do have some further effect which brings about partial dissolution of early thrombus material *in vivo*. During treatment, careful supervision of the patient and frequent testing of the clotting mechanism are necessary to avoid the hemorrhagic complications which sometimes occur.

Pharmacology

Except for their anticoagulant effects, both heparin and dicumarol are relatively nontoxic. Each possesses certain advantages and disadvantages. Heparin acts antagonistically to thrombin, prothrombin, and thromboplastin, and by decreasing the adhesiveness of the formed elements. Heparin therapy should be controlled by determination of the venous clotting time (*see* Lab. Proc.). Following a single I.V. or subcut. injection of sodium heparin in saline solution, the anticoagulant effect is almost immediate, but it lasts a relatively brief period, often as short as 1 to 3 hours. With another preparation—heparin in Pitkin's menstruum—administered deep subcutaneously, the effect is more prolonged but pain and induration at the site of injection are fairly frequent. Furthermore, heparin in either form is expensive and can be given only by injection.

Dicumarol depresses prothrombin formation by the liver, producing hypoprothrombinemia, thereby prolonging the prothrombin time. Dicumarol also acts as an antithrombin, possesses an antithromboplastic action, and diminishes the adhesiveness of the cellular elements of the blood. Dicumarol must be administered for 1 or 2 days, or longer, before an anticoagulant effect is evident; and its activity persists for 1 to 7 days after its use is discontinued. It is inexpensive and is given orally.

Indications

Anticoagulants are employed in the treatment of venous thrombosis or pulmonary embolism, myocardial infarction, and acute arterial embolism of the extremities (q.v.). Their use is being studied and evaluated in the treatment of frostbite, cerebral thrombosis, and multiple sclerosis, and in the prophylaxis of coronary occlusion in patients with a history of 1 or more attacks. Further study is being carried out in attempts to prevent venous thromboembolic disease and embolic phenomena from intracardiac thrombi.

Contraindications

Anticoagulant therapy is contraindicated in patients with recent or current gastrointestinal bleeding, and in individuals who have, within the preceding week, undergone operation on the central nervous system. It should be used with more than average caution during the last month of pregnancy, and in individuals with purpura, open wounds, operative drains, and renal and hepatic insufficiency.

If surgery is indicated in a patient receiving anticoagulant therapy, the clotting mechanism ideally should be restored to normal by appropriate methods (*see* below) before operation; postoperatively, anticoagulant therapy may be resumed as early as 24 hours after operation.

Dosage and Administration

When indicated, anticoagulant therapy should be instituted immediately, using heparin alone, or combined heparin and dicumarol.

Heparin Alone: The administration of heparin is guided by the venous clotting time of whole blood (*see* Lab. Proc.). Any of the following methods may be employed:

1. Continuous I.V. infusion: 100 mg. of the sodium salt of heparin (℞ 60) is placed in 1,000 cc. of physiologic saline or 5% glucose. The rate of flow is 25 drops/minute. The blood clotting time is determined after 2 hours and the rate of flow adjusted to maintain the clotting time at 20 to 40 minutes (normal range: 5 to 12 minutes). Further clotting times should be taken as indicated, usually twice daily.

2. Intermittent I.V. injection: Heparin (sodium salt) is injected I.V. every 4 hours (average dose 50 mg.). The clotting time, determined twice daily 3½ to 4 hours after an injection, may be normal but should not be longer than 20 minutes.

3. Intermittent subcut. injections: Immediately following an initial I.V. dose of 25 mg., 50 mg. of heparin is given by deep subcut. injection. Three hours later, average maintenance doses of 30 mg. every 3 hours are started. Clotting time is determined 2½ to 3 hours after the 3rd dose of heparin and twice daily thereafter. The dosage is adjusted to maintain the clotting time at 20 to 40 minutes.

4. Heparin/Pitkin menstruum: This preparation consists of heparin in a water-soluble menstruum which releases the drug gradually over a prolonged period. Heparin/Pitkin 300 mg. (℞ 61), by deep subcut. injection, is the average dose required to prolong the clotting time adequately for 36 to 48 hours. As with the other methods, the venous clotting time should be determined once or twice daily and maintained at 20 to 40 minutes. Other repository forms of heparin now are becoming available.

Heparin and Dicumarol Combined: Since the anticoagulant effect of dicumarol does not become evident for 24 to 48 hours after administration, heparin, which acts promptly, is given during the first 24 to 48 hours of combined therapy until adequate prothrombin deficiency can be produced by the dicumarol. It is administered in the dosage and manner described above. Heparin also may be given at any subsequent time if the anticoagulant effect of dicumarol becomes unsatisfactory.

Dicumarol (℞ 62) is given orally in 1 dose daily. The amount depends on a daily prothrombin time determination on whole plasma by the Quick 1-stage prothrombin test. Because of the varied potency of thromboplastins used in this test, a control also should be run, using undiluted normal plasma. The initial dose of dicumarol ranges from 200 to 300 mg.; the next, 100 to 200 mg. Thereafter, dosage is gauged by the daily prothrombin test. The aim of dicumarol therapy is to increase the prothrombin time (normal, 10 to 15 seconds—Quick test) to between 30 and 35 seconds. After the initial dose, 200 mg. should be given daily until the prothrombin time reaches 30 seconds. As long as the prothrombin time reaches 30 to 35 seconds, 50 to 100 mg. should be given daily. If the prothrombin time exceeds 35 seconds, dicumarol should be withheld until it drops below 30 seconds. The results of the daily prothrombin determinations also may be expressed in per cent of normal prothrombin activity. The corresponding values for per cent of prothrombin activity and seconds vary with the thromboplastin preparation used in various laboratories. When dicumarol is discontinued, the prothrombin activity may not return to normal for 1 to 7 days.

Complications

Even with controlled supervision, bleeding occurs in up to 5% of all cases treated with anticoagulants, particularly dicumarol. It is severe in 1 to 2% of patients but rarely is fatal. Therapy may be continued cautiously in the presence of mild epistaxis, ecchymosis, or hematuria. Major bleeding from operative wounds, into the gastrointestinal tract, or around drainage tubes, is an indication for discontinuing anticoagulant therapy and instituting appropriate measures to vitiate the anticoagulant effect. Reappraisal of all factors should precede possible resumption of anticoagulant therapy.

With a heparinized patient, transfusion of 500 cc. of relatively fresh whole blood, repeated as necessary, returns the clotting time toward normal. A 1% solution of protamine sulfate (R̥ 63), 5 to 10 cc. (50 to 100 mg.) I.V., will immediately restore the clotting time to normal. Toluidine blue also appears to be effective in combating hyperheparinemia, but is not yet generally available.

When major bleeding complicates dicumarol therapy, a large dose of menadione (vitamin K), 70 to 100 mg. I.V. (R̥ 64), may restore the prothrombin time to a safe range within 12 to 48 hours. If necessary, the dose should be repeated in 12 or 24 hours. (Recent investigations suggest that vitamin K_1 is more effective for this purpose.) If massive bleeding occurs, 500 cc. of whole fresh blood or of reconstituted lyophilized plasma should be given in addition to vitamin K. Such transfusions will immediately produce a safe prothrombin time, but only for about 6 hours; hence, they should be repeated as clinically indicated, as frequently as every 6 hours until major bleeding ceases.

PRESCRIPTIONS

(Wherever a prescribed "proprietary" is representative of a class of therapeutic agents, alternative proprietary preparations will be found listed in Part II.)

Cardiovascular Agents

1. R̥ Digitalis

> Several digitalis preparations are currently available which differ in dosage and speed of therapeutic effect; for details, *see* CONGESTIVE HEART FAILURE.

2. ℞ Digitoxin . . . . 0.1 mg.

For digitalization, 10 to 16 tablets as a single dose or in divided doses during the first 24 hours, then 1 or 2 tablets daily for maintenance.

3. ℞ Digitoxin (ampul)

1 mg. I.V., slowly for digitalization.

4. ℞ Lanatoside C (ampul)

1.5 mg. I.V. for digitalization (*see* ℞ 5).

5. ℞ Lanatoside C . . . . 0.5 mg.

2 tablets daily for maintenance, following digitalization with ℞ 4.

6. ℞ Quinidine sulfate . . . . . 0.2 Gm. (gr. iii)

1 tablet initially as a test dose. If there are no signs of idiosyncrasy within 3 or 4 hours give 4 tablets followed by 1 tablet every 4 hours for 3 or 4 doses. For maintenance give 1 or 2 tablets 3 times a day. Alternative schedules of administration are given in the text; *see* CARDIAC ARRHYTHMIAS. (CAUTION! A fall in blood pressure, an abrupt increase or decrease in the cardiac rate, or the development of any degree of heart block [q. v.] is an indication for extreme caution in administering further quinidine.)

7. ℞ "Mecholyl Chloride" (ampul)

20 to 30 mg. (gr. ⅓ to ss) subcut.

8. ℞ Amyl nitrite (ampul). . . . 0.2 cc. (♍ iii)

Crush 1 ampul in handkerchief and inhale as necessary.

9. ℞ Nitroglycerin (hypodermic tablet). . . . . 0.3 mg. (gr. 1/200)

1 or 2 tablets sublingually as necessary.

10. ℞ Erythrol tetranitrate . . . . 15 mg. (gr. ¼)

1 or 2 tablets 3 times daily.

11. ℞ Mannitol hexanitrate . . . . 30 mg. (gr. ss)

1 or 2 tablets 3 times daily.

12. ℞ Sodium nitrite . . . . 30 mg. (gr. ss)

1 or 2 tablets 3 times daily.

13. ℞ Aminophylline (enteric coated) 0.1 Gm. (gr. iss)

1 or 2 tablets 3 to 5 times daily.

14. ℞ Aminophylline   (ampul)

    0.24 to 0.5 Gm. (gr. iv to viiss) I.V. *slowly,* or
    I.M. every 4 to 6 hours as necessary.

15. ℞ Aminophylline   (suppository)   0.5   Gm.   (gr. viiss)

    For rectal administration 1 to 3 times a day.

16. ℞ Theobromine and Sodium Acetate
    U.S.P. . . . .   0.5   Gm.   (gr. viiss)

    1 or 2 tablets 3 times daily after meals.

17. ℞ Papaverine hydrochloride . .   0.1   Gm.   (gr. iss)

    1 tablet 3 times daily.

18. ℞ Papaverine hydrochloride
    (ampul)

    0.03 to 0.1 Gm. (gr. ss to iss) I.M., I.V., or
    intra-arterially every 4 hours as necessary.

19. ℞ Atropine sulfate   (hypodermic
    tablet)

    0.5 mg. (gr. 1/120) orally, or subcut.
    To combat Mecholyl overdosage, 0.6 to 0.8
    mg. (gr. 1/100 to 1/75) may be administered
    subcut. or even I.V. if necessary.

20. ℞ Theophylline. . . . .   0.1   Gm.   (gr. iss)

    1 to 3 tablets 3 or 4 times daily.

21. ℞ "Neo-Synephrine Hydrochloride"
    (ampul)

    3 to 5 mg. subcut., I.M. or I.V., repeated in
    20 minutes if necessary.

22. ℞ Ephedrine sulfate.   25   mg.   (gr. 3/8)

    1 or 2 tablets or capsules 3 to 6 times daily.

23. ℞ Ephedrine sulfate   (ampul)

    25 mg. (gr. 3/8) subcut.

24. ℞ Epinephrine hydrochloride,
    1 : 1,000 solution   (ampul)

    0.2 to 1 cc. (♏ iii to xv) subcut.

25. ℞ Epinephrine hydrochloride, 1 : 500
    in oil   (ampul)

    1 cc. (♏ xv) I.M., once a day.

26. ℞ "Metrazol"   (ampul)

    0.1 to 0.3 Gm. (gr. iss to v) I.M. or I.V.

27. ℞ "Coramine"   (ampul)
       1.5 to 5 cc. I.M. or I.V.

28. ℞ Caffeine and Sodium Benzoate
       Injection U.S.P.   (ampul)
       0.2 to 0.5 Gm. (gr. iii to viiss) subcut. or I.V.

29. ℞ Amphetamine sulfate   5   mg.
       1 tablet 3 times daily.

30. ℞ Potassium thiocyanate. . . .   0.3   Gm. (gr. v)
       1 tablet daily for 4 to 7 days, or until the
       blood level is 6 to 12 mg./100 cc.   This level
       is then maintained by adequate intermittent
       dosage.

31. ℞ Veratrum viride (tablets contain-
       ing 10 Craw units each)
       2 tablets daily after meals, initially, increas-
       ing the dose at weekly intervals by 1 tablet
       daily until a therapeutic or toxic (nausea,
       vomiting) response appears.

32. ℞ Whisky
       1 to 2 ounces every 4 to 8 hours for vaso-
       spasm.

33. ℞ "Mecholyl Chloride"   (bulk
       powder) . . . .   1.0   Gm. (gr. xv)
       Make a 0.5% solution (1 Gm. to 200 cc. of
       distilled water) to be applied as a compress
       under the positive electrode of a galvanic ap-
       paratus.

Diuretics

34. ℞ "Mercuzanthin"   (ampul)
       0.5 cc. initially, followed by 1 to 2 cc. I.M. or
       I.V., repeated as necessary.

35. ℞ "Salyrgan-Theophylline"
       (ampul)
       0.5 cc. initially, followed by 1 to 2 cc. I.M.
       or I.V., repeated as necessary.

36. ℞ "Mercuhydrin"   (ampul)
       0.5 cc. initially, followed by 1 to 2 cc. I.M.
       or I.V. as necessary.

37. ℞ Theobromine and Sodium Sal-
       icylate N.F. . . . .   0.5   Gm. (gr. viiss)
       1 or 2 tablets 3 times daily after meals.

38. ℞ Theobromine calcium salicylate 0.5   Gm. (gr. viiss)
       1 or 2 tablets 3 times daily after meals.

39. ℞ Urea
    5 teaspoons in fruit juice 2 to 5 times daily.

40. ℞ Ammonium chloride (enteric coated) . . . . 0.5   Gm. (gr. viiss)
    8 to 24 tablets daily in divided doses.

41. ℞ Potassium nitrate (enteric coated) . . . . 0.5   Gm. (gr. viiss)
    8 to 24 tablets daily in divided doses.

42. ℞ Ammonium nitrate (enteric coated) . . . . 0.5   Gm. (gr. viiss)
    8 to 24 tablets daily in divided doses.

Sedatives and Analgesics

43. ℞ Chloral hydrate. . . . . . . 0.3   Gm. (gr. v)
    1 to 3 capsules 3 times daily.

44. ℞ Phenobarbital 15   mg. (gr. ¼)
    1 to 4 tablets 3 or 4 times daily.

45. ℞ Phenobarbital sodium   (ampul)
    0.1 to 0.3 Gm. (gr. iss to v) subcut. for restlessness or anxiety.

46. ℞ Paraldehyde
    3 to 6 cc. I.M. for delirium.

47. ℞ Pentobarbital sodium . . . . 0.1   Gm. (gr. iss)
    1 or 2 capsules as necessary for sleep.

48. ℞ Acetylsalicylic acid . . . . . 0.3   Gm. (gr. v)
    1 or 2 tablets as needed.

49. ℞ Sodium salicylate (enteric coated) . . . . 0.3   Gm. (gr. v)
    3 tablets every 4 hours initially, increasing the dose to 4 or 5 tablets every 4 hours if no toxic reactions occur (tinnitus, skin rash or gastrointestinal disturbances).

50. ℞ Acetophenetidin . . . . . . 0.3   Gm. (gr. v)
    1 or 2 tablets 3 times a day.

51. ℞ Terpin Hydrate and Codeine Elixir N.F . . . . 90.0   cc.   (℥ iii)
    2 teaspoons every 3 hours as required for cough.

52. ℞ Codeine sulfate. 30   mg. (gr. ss)
    1 or 2 tablets every 4 hours for pain.

53. ℞ Methadone Hydrochloride
      N.N.R. 5   mg.
      1 or 2 tablets every 4 hours.

54. ℞ "Dilaudid Hydrochloride"
      (ampul)
      2 mg. (gr. 1/30) subcut. Repeat as neces-
      sary.

55. ℞ "Demerol Hydrochloride"
      (ampul)
      50 to 100 mg. I.M. every 4 hours for pain and
      restlessness.

56. ℞ "Demerol Hydrochloride" . . 50   mg.
      1 or 2 tablets every 4 hours for pain and rest-
      lessness.

57. ℞ Morphine sulfate
      10 to 30 mg. (gr. ⅙ to ½) subcut. or, if
      necessary, I.V. every 4 hours for pain and
      restlessness.

58. ℞ Morphine sulfate . . . . . . 15.0   mg.   (gr. ¼)
      Atropine sulfate . . . . . . 0.4   mg.   (gr. 1/150)
      Subcut. every 4 hours for pain and restless-
      ness.

59. ℞ "Pantopon"   (ampul)
      20 mg. (gr. ⅓) subcut. every 4 hours for pain
      and restlessness.

Agents Affecting Blood Coagulation

60. ℞ Heparin Sodium N.N.R.   (ampul)
      I.V. or subcut. according to directions given
      in text (see ANTICOAGULANT THERAPY).

61. ℞ Heparin/Pitkin menstruum
      (ampul)
      300 mg. deep subcut. every 48 hours.

62. ℞ Dicumarol. 50   mg.
      Administer according to directions given in
      text (see ANTICOAGULANT THERAPY).

63. ℞ Protamine sulfate, 1% solution
      (ampul)
      5 to 10 cc. (50 to 100 mg.) I.V.

64. ℞ Menadione sodium bisulfite
      (ampul)
      70 to 100 mg. I.V. for major bleeding asso-
      ciated with dicumarol therapy.

Sclerosing Agents

65. ℞ Dextrose, 30 to 50% solution (ampul)

    Inject up to 20 cc. at a single site.

66. ℞ Sodium chloride, 20% solution (ampul)

    Inject up to 20 cc. at a single site.

67. ℞ Sodium salicylate, 20% solution (ampul)

    Inject 2 to 5 cc. at a single site.

68. ℞ Quinine and Urethane Injection U.S.P. (ampul)

    Inject 1 to 2 cc. at a single site.

69. ℞ Sodium morrhuate, 5% solution (ampul)

    Inject 1 to 2 cc. at a single site.

Antimicrobial Agents

70. ℞ Penicillin (vial)

    200,000 to 1,600,000 u. or more I.M. daily, according to schedule given in text. In the treatment of bacterial endocarditis, the minimal daily dose is 500,000 u. For intrapericardial injection, administer 20,000 to 50,000 u. in saline (1,000 u./cc.) after first aspirating an equal volume of pericardial fluid.

71. ℞ Streptomycin (vial)

    0.5 Gm. I.M. every 3 to 12 hrs. for the treatment of bacterial endocarditis or pericarditis. For intrapericardial injection, administer 0.2 Gm. in 20 cc. saline after first aspirating an equal volume of pericardial fluid.

72. ℞ Sulfadiazine . . . . 0.5 Gm. (gr. viiss)

    8 tablets initially, then 2 tablets every 4 hours.

73. ℞ Aureomycin (capsules). . . . 0.25 Gm.

    25 to 100 mg./Kg. body wt./day, divided into 4 to 8 equal doses. Reduction of dosage is permissible following the acute phase of the disease. Minimum duration of therapy should be 3 weeks.

74. ℞ "Chloromycetin" (capsules). . 0.25 Gm.

    Administer as for ℞ 73, above.

75. ℞ Mercury succinimide (ampul)

    5 mg. (gr. 1/12) deep I.M. once weekly. Increase dose as per schedule given in text (*see* ANEURYSM; AORTITIS).

76. ℞ Bismuth Subsalicylate Injection
   U.S.P.   (vial)

> Give equivalent of 50 mg. bismuth subsalicylate deep I.M. once weekly. Increase dosage to 0.2 Gm. as per schedule given in text (see ANEURYSM; AORTITIS).

77. ℞ "Mapharsen"   (ampul)

> Administer I.V. as directed in text (see ANEURYSM; AORTITIS).

78. ℞ "Furacin" . . . . 60.0   Gm. (℥ ii)

> Apply ointment locally to affected areas.

Laxatives

79. ℞ Cascara Sagrada Extract Tablets
   U.S.P. . . . . 0.13   Gm. (gr. ii)

> 1 or 2 tablets at bedtime.

80. ℞ Milk of Magnesia U.S.P.

> 2 tablespoons at bedtime.

81. ℞ Liquid Petrolatum U.S.P.

> 1 to 2 tablespoons as necessary.

Miscellaneous

82. ℞ Unna's paste boot

Zinc oxide	30 parts
Phenol	2 parts
Gelatin	30 parts
Glycerin	50 parts
Water	90 parts

> The gelatin is dissolved in boiling water in the upper part of a double boiler or in a water bath. The glycerin and zinc oxide are mixed together, so that an even, homogeneous mass is obtained; it is then added to the solution of gelatin and the whole mixture is carefully stirred for complete and even mixture. When it is thoroughly mixed it is allowed to cool until it has the form of a semisolid mass. When the paste is needed, the container is warmed in a pan of hot water, to soften it. It should be applied only when it is warm, not hot.

83. ℞ Zinc oxide, 10% ointment . 120.0   Gm. (℥ iv)

> Apply to ulcer.

84. ℞ Typhoid vaccine

> Dilute appropriately with sterile saline and administer 3 to 5 million organisms I.V., increasing each succeeding dose by 50 to 100% to produce a temperature rise of 1° to 2° F.; to be given every 2nd or 3rd day.

85. ℞ Thyroid U.S.P. 30   mg.   (gr. ss)
    1 or more tablets daily as indicated.

86. ℞ Ferrous carbonate. . . . . .   0.3   Gm.   (gr. v)
    1 to 3 pills after each meal.

87. ℞ Phenol. . . . .   0.6   Gm.   (gr. x)
    Camphor . . . .   1.3   Gm.   (gr. xx)
    Lanolin U.S.P. . . . . . .   16.0   Gm.   (℥ iv)
    Apply as directed to affected areas.

88. ℞ Thiouracil . . . .   0.2   Gm.   (gr. iii)
    1 tablet 3 times daily for 2 weeks, then 1
    tablet daily.

89. ℞ Cobra venom (ampul containing
       10 mouse u./cc.)
    1st day, 3 I.M. injections of 1 cc. each; 2nd
    to 7th day, 1 cc. I.M. daily.   Thereafter, 1
    cc. twice a week.

90. ℞ Saturated Potassium Iodide
       Solution N.F. . . . . . .   60.0   cc.   (℥ ii)
    3 to 5 drops in water after each meal.

91. ℞ Tetraethylammonium bromide
       (ampul)
    100 to 500 mg. I.V. every 1 to 7 days.

DEFICIENCY AND METABOLIC

NUTRITIONAL DEFICIENCIES

The term "deficiency disease" indicates a physiologic dysfunction due to an insufficiency of one or more nutritional factors necessary for normal health and well-being.

Etiology

Primary deficiency is due to inadequate intake of nutrients by reason of poor eating habits or economic or regional factors. **Secondary (conditioned) deficiency** results from failure of absorption or utilization of nutrients, increased requirements, or excessive excretion. Impaired digestion and absorption may occur through poor mastication of food and gastrointestinal disease. Utilization and storage may be interfered with in cases of thyroid dysfunction and advanced disease of the kidney, liver, or pancreas. Nutritional requirements are increased during growth, pregnancy, lactation, febrile disease, metabolic disease, surgical procedures, and convalescence.

General Principles of Treatment

Nutritional deficiencies usually are multiple in that more than one essential nutrient is lacking. All such deficiencies, evident or suspected, must be treated at one time. Detailed dietary instruction is necessary for each patient; it is not sufficient merely to prescribe a "balanced diet." (See DIETS.)

When a patient will not or cannot eat a satisfactory diet, because of allergy, gastrointestinal disease, dietary fads, business preoccupation, or other conditions, certain nutritional supplements are indicated.

Vitamin deficiencies (q.v.) may be corrected by the oral or parenteral administration of necessary individual or polyvitamin supplements. Therapeutic and maintenance doses may be found in the Vitamin Table (q.v.). A practical therapeutic preparation, available through several manufacturers, contains 25,000 u. of vitamin A, 1,000 u. of vitamin D, 5 mg. of thiamine, 150 mg. of niacinamide, 150 mg. of ascorbic acid, and 5 mg. of folic acid. Two capsules are given daily for 7 to 10 days, then 1 a day for maintenance. The significance of pantothenic acid, pyridoxine, pyridoxal and inositol in human nutrition is uncertain and requires further study. Recent studies strongly suggest that vitamin B_{12} may act as a significant growth factor in some undernourished children.

For patients with increased protein requirements (see PROTEIN DEFICIENCY), ingestion of appropriate foods is the method of choice, provided the digestive tract is normal. An additional 15 to 20 Gm. of protein may be supplied by one of the following: 2 glasses of milk, 3 oz. of cottage cheese, 1 average portion of meat, 3 egg whites, or 1½ oz. of dried skimmed milk powder. Also available are several commercial products consisting chiefly of milk protein, combined with carbohydrate for palatability. These can be added to food and drink the patient already is receiving. When the patient cannot consume, digest, or absorb protein in food due to surgical procedures, infection, diarrhea, or absence of proteolytic enzymes, protein hydrolysates or mixtures of amino acids are indicated to prevent depletion. These are unpalatable but patients can be induced to take them if the taste is disguised as advised in the printed directions accompanying the products. Sometimes it is necessary to give such oral preparations by stomach tube or by drip through a nasal catheter. When oral ingestion is contraindicated, or complete gastrointestinal rest is indicated, a suitable amino acid preparation can be given I.V. to correct or prevent protein depletion. Usually one, but sometimes two, 50 Gm. infusions within a 24-hour period will be sufficient.

Mineral deficiencies usually are restricted to iron, calcium, phosphorus, and iodine. Magnesium, copper, and zinc are essential but clinically unimportant. The minimum daily requirements of minerals for adults are calcium 0.7 Gm., phosphorus 1.3 Gm., and iron 0.015 Gm. Numerous calcium-phosphorus supplements are obtainable commercially. Iodine may be administered as iodized salt, or 1 drop weekly of Lugol's solution.

Salient Facts about
THE PRINCIPAL VITAMINS

VITAMIN	PRINCIPAL SOURCES	PROPERTIES	PHYSIOLOGIC EFFECTS	DEFICIENCY SYMPTOMS	DAILY ALLOWANCES	THERAPEUTIC DOSAGE

Vitamin A	Fish liver oils, liver, eggs, milk, butter, green leafy or yellow vegetables	Oil-soluble; susceptible to oxidation, especially at high temperatures; nontoxic in recommended doses	Promotes bony growth; essential to normal function of epithelial cells and visual purple	Night blindness Xerophthalmia Hyperkeratosis of skin	Children units under 1 1,500
					  1–3 2,000
					  4–6 2,500
					  7–9 3,500
					  10–12 4,500
					  13–20 5,000
					Boys units
					  13–15 5,000
					  16–20 6,000
					Women 5,000
					  Preg. 6,000
					  Lact. 8,000
					Men 5,000
						Up to 100,000 u./day

Vitamin B$_1$ (Thiamine)	Yeast; whole grains; meat, especially pork, liver; nuts, eggs, legumes, most vegetables	Stable to heat, unstable to alkali; nontoxic in recommended doses	Carbohydrate metabolism; nerve function; promotes growth	Beriberi Peripheral neuritis Cardiac disease	Children mg.
					  under 1 0.4
					  1–3 0.6
					  4–6 0.8
					  7–9 1.0
					  10–12 1.2
					Girls
					  13–15 1.4
					  16–20 1.2
					Boys mg.
					  13–15 1.6
					  16–20 2.0
					Women 1.2–1.8
					  Preg. 1.8
					  Lact. 2.3
					Men 1.5–2.3
						10–100 mg./day

Vitamin B$_2$ (Riboflavin) (Vitamin G)	Milk and cheese, plus the sources of B$_1$	Slightly water-soluble; unstable to light and alkali; nontoxic in recommended doses	Promotes growth, general health; essential to cellular oxidation	Cheilosis Keratitis Glossitis Photophobia Follicular keratosis	Children mg.
					  under 1 0.6
					  1–3 0.9
					  4–6 1.2
					  7–9 1.5
					  10–12 1.8
					Girls
					  13–15 2.0
					  16–20 1.8
					Boys mg.
					  13–15 2.4
					  16–20 3.0
					Women 1.8–2.7
					  Preg. 2.5
					  Lact. 3.0
					Men 2.2–3.3
						5–15 mg./day

For Vitamin B$_{12}$ and Pteroylglutamic (folic) acid, *see* chapters on PERNICIOUS ANEMIA and SPRUE.

	Sources	Properties	Essential for / Function	Deficiency	Requirements	Therapeutic dose
Nicotinic Acid (Niacin)	Same sources as for both B₁ and B₂	Water-soluble; stable; produces intolerance flushing, burning, itching (rare with Niacinamide)	Essential for health, tissue respiration, growth, gastro-intestinal function, and normal skin	Pellagra: (Dermatitis, glossitis, gastro-intestinal disturbance, nervous system dysfunction)	Children mg. — under 1 4.0; 1–3 6.0; 4–6 8.0; 7–9 10.0; 10–12 12.0; Girls 13–15 14.0; 16–20 12.0. Boys mg. — 13–15 16.0; 16–20 20.0; Women 12.0–18.0; Preg. 18.0; Lact. 23.0; Men 15.0–23.0	50–500 mg./day
Vitamin C (Ascorbic acid)	Citrus fruits, potatoes, cabbage, tomatoes, green pepper	Water-soluble; stable in dry state but oxidized by heat and light; nontoxic in recommended doses	Essential to osteoid tissue, collagen formation, vascular function, and tissue respiration	Scurvy: (Hemorrhages), loose teeth, gingivitis	Children mg. — under 1 30.0; 1–3 35.0; 4–6 50.0; 7–9 60.0; 10–12 75.0; Girls 13–20 80.0. Boys mg. — 13–15 90.0; 16–20 100.0; Women 70.0; Preg. 100.0; Lact. 150.0; Men 75.0	100–1,000 mg./day
Vitamin D — D₂ (Calciferol) D₃ (Activated cholesterol)	Fish liver oils, eggs, milk, butter, sunlight and irradiation	Oil-soluble; in large doses may cause hypercalcemia	Metabolism of calcium and phosphorus	Infantile rickets, Infantile tetany, Osteomalacia	units — Infants 800–1,200; Prematurity 5,000–10,000; Children 400; Pregnancy 800; Lactation 800	Up to 300,000 u./day
Vitamin K (activity)	Intestinal bacterial synthesis and a normal diet		Prothrombin formation; normal blood coagulation	Hemorrhage, Prolonged pro-thrombin time	Undetermined	
Menadione		Oil-soluble, slightly soluble in water; unstable to light; nontoxic in recommended doses				2–5 mg. (or more)/day (with bile salts when indicated)
Menadione sodium bisulfite		Freely soluble in water; unstable with alkalis; nontoxic in recommended doses				2–5 mg. (or more)/day (bile salts not necessary)
Vitamin K₁		Oily liquid; unstable to heat and light; insoluble in water				Oral: 4–10 mg./day I.V. (in dextrose solution): Adult, 5 mg./day; Newborn, 0.25 mg./day

Deficiencies or excesses of the chief bodily electrolytes—sodium, chloride, potassium, bicarbonate—occur in various metabolic, circulatory, and endocrine dysfunctions (q.v.).

VITAMIN DEFICIENCIES

VITAMIN A DEFICIENCY

Vitamin A is essential to endochondral bone growth; to vision, since it is a component of visual purple (rhodopsin); and to maintenance of the normal vitality of epithelial tissues. The plant pigment, carotene, is converted into vitamin A in the body. The daily allowances of this vitamin for normal health are given in the Vitamin Table. Inadequate intake or utilization results in deficiency disease affecting growth in the young, acuity of vision, and the integrity of the epithelial structures, especially of the conjunctiva, trachea, hair follicles, and renal pelvis. It also increases susceptibility to pyogenic infections.

Etiology

Primary vitamin A deficiency disease is caused by inadequate intake of the vitamin or of carotene. Secondary (conditioned) deficiency results (1) from failure to absorb the vitamin, as in chronic diarrhea, celiac disease, sprue, pancreatic fibrosis, impaired biliary cycle, the excessive use of mineral oil, the removal by surgery of a major portion of the bowel, and (2) from failure to convert carotene into Vitamin A, as in diabetes mellitus, idiopathic carotenemia, and advanced liver disease.

Symptoms and Signs

In children the most common clinical sign is retarded growth. In both children and adults there is increased susceptibility to infections. Night blindness is an early and constant symptom. Renal stones and renal pelvis infections are frequent presenting conditions. Dermal changes are characterized by follicular hyperkeratoses, appearing first on the lateral surface of the arm and the extensor surface of the thigh. In advanced conditions the entire body may be affected. Associated with these follicular lesions is a keratoderma of the palms and soles with thickening, drying, and an accentuation of normal markings. If the deficiency is well advanced the eyes show Bitot's spots, with dry, wrinkled and lusterless conjunctivae, and scaly blepharitis with canthal fissures. These symptoms constitute the syndrome of xerophthalmia.

Diagnosis

Various instruments to measure light adaptation are useful. Consistent low blood levels of vitamin A, below 20 micrograms/100 cc., indicate little recent vitamin A intake or storage.

Low levels of carotene are indicative only of poor intake or absorption of carotene.

To be distinguished from vitamin A deficiency are the follicular lesions of acne vulgaris, adolescent folliculosis, dirt and chemical folliculitis, folliculosis of ascorbic acid deficiency, and many skin lesions of unknown etiology included in the terms follicular hyperkeratosis, keratosis pilaris, keratosis follicularis, and lichen spinulosus.

Treatment

Treatment consists of correcting the cause of the deficiency, immediate administration of vitamin A in therapeutic doses, and subsequent maintenance of the required intake. In infants and young children, 10,000 to 20,000 u. of vitamin A daily for 7 to 10 days is sufficient; in older children, 25,000 to 50,000 u. daily; in adults, 50,000 to 100,000 u. daily.

In conditioned vitamin A deficiency treat first the disease or condition responsible (*see* Etiology). When due to mineral oil ingestion, stop the mineral oil and treat as a primary deficiency. Control of diarrheal diseases generally permits therapy as in a primary deficiency. Inability to correct the cause of the deficiency is an indication for deep I.M. injection of vitamin A, in maximal doses of 100,000 u. daily for 7 to 10 days, followed by 50,000 u. once or twice a week.

Where evidence suggests that dietary fat is not being properly absorbed by the intestine, absorption of the oil-soluble vitamins may be aided by the use of a wetting agent, such as the polyoxyethylene derivative of sorbitan monooleate, given as 1.5 Gm. doses with each meal (℞ 49).

VITAMIN C DEFICIENCY
(Scurvy, Scorbutus)

The function of vitamin C is to maintain intracellular substances of mesenchymal derivation, such as connective tissue, osteoid tissue of the bones, and dentine of the teeth. Severe deficiency results in scurvy, an acute or chronic disease characterized by hemorrhagic manifestations and abnormal osteoid and dentine formation. The daily allowances of vitamin C for the maintenance of health are given in the Vitamin Table.

Etiology

In infants, primary deficiency is most commonly due to lack of preventive supplementation of the diet with vitamin C. In adults, it usually is due to food idiosyncrasies or inability to obtain a proper diet. Secondary deficiencies occur in gastrointestinal disease, especially when the patient is on an "ulcer diet," consisting chiefly of milk, cream, cereals, and eggs. Infections increase the physiologic requirement for vitamin C and, in persons with poor dietary habits, they are likely to precipitate the appearance of symptoms.

Pathology

Defective formation of intercellular cement substances is seen in connective tissues, bones, and dentine. This results in two significant changes: a weakening of the capillaries with subsequent hemorrhage, and defects in the bone and related structures. The hemorrhages are avascularly organized so that wounds heal poorly and easily break open. The bone lesions result from cessation of endochondral bone growth (*see also* VITAMIN D DEFICIENCY) owing to a failure of the osteoblasts to form osteoid tissue. Instead, a fibrous union is formed between the diaphysis and the epiphysis, with resulting enlargements of the costochondral junctions. Embedded in this fibrous tissue are densely calcified fragments of cartilage, giving the "white line" visualized by X-ray. Complicating these lesions are hemorrhages, either small ecchymotic ones within or along the bone, or large subperiosteal ones due to small fractures in the shaft just shaftward of the white line.

Symptoms and Signs

Infantile scurvy usually occurs between the 6th and 12th months. Early symptoms are irritability, failing appetite, and failure to gain weight. The child screams when moved and sometimes fails to move one or both legs. If the deficiency is well developed, examination discloses angular enlargements of the costochondral junctions of the ribs (scorbutic rosary), swelling of the extremities over the ends of the long bones (especially lower end of the femur), and a tendency to hemorrhage as shown by swollen hemorrhagic gums surrounding erupting teeth, ecchymoses, and petechiae. X-ray findings are characteristic. The ends of the long bones show a transverse thickening and increased density—the white line. The epiphyses exhibit a "halo." Immediately shaftward of the white line is a localized area of rarefaction, first evident at the lateral margins, and appearing in the X-ray as a small fracture or nick. The trabecular markings of the shaft become indistinct, giving the shaft a "ground glass" appearance, and the cortex becomes thinner. As a rule, subperiosteal hemorrhages do not cast a shadow because of the lack of osteoblastic activity. After therapy for 7 to 10 days some calcification results so that the X-ray shows a clublike swelling extending from the white line to the middle of the shaft (never into the joint). As treatment proceeds the hemorrhage is reabsorbed and the bone resumes its normal shape. In less severe cases, the gingival, bony, or hemorrhagic manifestations may be present alone. Fever, increased pulse and respiration rates, and hypochromic anemia are common in scorbutic infants. Death results unless the condition is treated.

Adult scurvy remains latent for 3 months to a year under severe vitamin C deficiency. Manifest scorbutic symptoms are preceded by lassitude, weakness, irritability, vague muscle aches and pains, and weight loss. Bleeding gums, gingivitis, and loosening of the teeth occur early. During this period, metabolic stress such as infection is apt to precipitate the clinical syndrome. Here hemorrhagic manifestations predominate, and can occur at sites of even slight pressure or trauma. Large muscle hemorrhages are common as are petechial and purpuric skin manifestations. The capillary fragility test, with use of tourniquet, is positive. Perifollicular congestion is frequent. Rapidly developing gingival hemorrhages give the appearance of bags of blood. They rupture and bleed on slight pressure. Epistaxis, conjunctival, retinal, cerebral, gastrointestinal, and genitourinary bleeding may occur in extremely severe cases. Bone lesions are absent except for subperiosteal hemorrhages due to trauma.

Laboratory Findings

In manifest scurvy the plasma ascorbic acid content usually is zero to a trace, but this is not always diagnostic, as similarly low levels may sometimes be found in nonscorbutic persons. Ascorbic acid levels in the white cell–platelet layer of centrifuged blood are more significant; levels below 0.1 mg./100 cc. are closely correlated with scurvy. When storage of vitamin C is depleted, very little ascorbic acid appears in the urine following a test dose. This test again is not diagnostic, but indicates only depletion of reserves. Increased capillary fragility is an almost constant finding in scurvy, though negative tests may occur in scorbutic patients, and positive tests in the nonscorbutic. The slow decolorization of the dye 2, 6-dichlorphenol indophenol, when injected intracutaneously, is indicative only of tissue depletion of ascorbic acid. Hypochromic anemia, not due to blood loss, is a common finding. Bleeding, coagulation and prothrombin times usually are normal.

Diagnosis

Infantile scurvy must be differentiated from rickets, poliomyelitis, rheumatic fever, and various other diseases with hemorrhagic manifestations, such as blood dyscrasias, severe anemias and allergic purpuras. Rickets most commonly occurs before the 5th month and scurvy almost never before the 6th. There are no hemorrhagic manifestations in rickets. The costochondral junctions are enlarged in both rickets and scurvy, but in scurvy the swellings are angular while in rickets they tend to be rounded. Poliomyelitis often is considered because the baby frequently does not move one or both legs and cries on being moved. The absence of neurologic changes, the presence of hemorrhagic manifestations, and the bone changes in scurvy distinguish between them. The changes about the joints may suggest rheumatic fever, but this disease is practically unknown in patients under 2 years of age. In scurvy, the bone swellings never extend into the joint, which is diagnostically significant.

The various diseases causing hemorrhagic manifestations usually can be excluded by their own characteristic tests. In doubtful cases, a therapeutic test can be tried by giving 300 to 500 mg. of ascorbic acid by mouth. In infantile scurvy, pain will subside within 24 to 48 hours and swelling of the gums and hemorrhagic manifestations will decrease within 72 hours.

Adult scurvy must be differentiated from arthritis, hemorrhagic diseases and acute or chronic gingivitis. In adult scurvy the joint symptoms are due to hemorrhages around or sometimes into the joint. Presence of hemorrhagic manifestations elsewhere, and blood studies, may aid in the diagnosis. Acute gingival symptoms in scurvy will show obvious improvement within 72 hours or less on a therapeutic test with vitamin C. In chronic scorbutic gingivitis, superimposed infection and calcareous deposits prevent rapid response and ascorbic acid brings only slow improvement.

In both infantile and adult scurvy, ruling out of other causes for hemorrhagic manifestations and the presence of very low or absent ascorbic acid levels in plasma or white cell-platelet layer are important diagnostic aids.

Prophylaxis

Vitamin C deficiency can be prevented by a diet containing or supplemented by adequate amounts of this vitamin (*see* Vitamin Table). Infants should be given orange juice daily, beginning with 1 teaspoonful in the 2nd to 4th week of life and progressively increasing the amount until at 5 months the intake is 2 to 3 oz. If tomato juice is used, 3 times as much should be given. If the infant reacts unfavorably, 25 to 30 mg. of ascorbic acid should be administered daily up to the age of 3 months, and 50 to 75 mg. thereafter.

Treatment

The specific treatment is administration of vitamin C. In infantile scurvy, 300 mg. daily by mouth usually will result in a rapid cure. This dose can be halved within a week, and after a month ordinary preventive doses can be used. It also is advisable to give preventive amounts of orange or tomato juice. Vitamin C may be given in the form of orange or tomato juice alone, using daily 4 to 8 oz. of freshly prepared orange juice or 12 to 24 oz. of tomato juice. These doses can be halved within 1 or 2 weeks and after a month preventive amounts can be used. When parenteral administration of ascorbic acid is indicated, as in vomiting or diarrhea, give half the recommended oral doses I.V. or I.M.

For adult scurvy, 1,000 mg. of ascorbic acid daily in divided doses for 1 week is recommended, then half as much is given until all signs have disappeared. The usual preventive doses can then be given. When daily parenteral therapy is required, use half the oral dosage. When combined oral and parenteral therapy is indicated, the oral dosage outlined above should be supplemented, I.V. or I.M., by 100 mg. of vitamin C, 2 or 3 times daily until the disease is under control. In chronic scurvy with gingivitis, repeated hemorrhagic manifestations, or joint symptoms, 300 to 500 mg. of ascorbic acid daily in divided doses is advisable. This must be continued for several months.

VITAMIN D DEFICIENCY
(Rickets; Osteomalacia)

At least 10 compounds having vitamin D activity are known but only 2 have practical importance. These are vitamin D_2, or calciferol, which is the chief form of vitamin D found in viosterol, irradiated yeast and "metabolized" or yeast milk; and vitamin D_3, or activated 7-dehydrocholesterol, the chief form found in fish oils, eggs, and irradiated milk. Both have been isolated in crystalline form.

All the known functions of vitamin D are believed to result from its effect on the calcium and phosphorus content of the body fluids, which it exerts primarily by regulating the "net absorption" of these minerals from the intestinal tract, thus obtaining concentrations ideal for the maintenance of normal bone metabolism. In the presence of vitamin D deficiency, with any calcium-phosphorus ratio ingested, the absolute amounts in the serum increase proportionately with the intake. When vitamin D and sufficient absolute amounts of calcium and phosphorus are available in the diet the blood serum values tend to become normal regardless of their ratio in the diet. In vitamin D deficiency there is an increased excretion of both calcium and phosphorus in the feces. This is accompanied either by decreasing intestinal absorption or by increasing intestinal reexcretion, or both. The result is a decrease in the net absorption. Vitamin D administration increases the net absorption of both calcium and phosphorus chiefly by decreasing the fecal excretion so that the balance becomes positive. Thus the main function of vitamin D is to control the net absorption of calcium and phosphorus so that the concentration of Ca^{++} and $(PO_4)^{---}$ in the body fluids is ideal for maintaining normal bone metabolism.

The daily dietary requirements of added vitamin D are extremely variable, depending upon the amount of vitamin D formed in the skin as the result of ultraviolet radiation and upon the efficiency with which the body can metabolize calcium and phosphorus. Few infants can metabolize calcium and phosphorus without added vitamin D, but as age increases, the ability to do so progressively increases. Vitamin D requirements are met in infancy, childhood and adolescence by 400 u. daily, and in prematurity, pregnancy and lactation by double that amount (see Vitamin Table). For adults 400 u. daily probably is satisfactory. In the colored races, because of the interference of the skin pigment with synthesis of vitamin D by ultraviolet rays, the daily requirement for added vitamin D should be considered 50% greater in all categories.

Vitamin D deficiency causes a disturbance of calcium and phosphorus metabolism, which results in rickets (English disease) in infancy and childhood and osteomalacia in adult life. Other symptoms are spasmophilia and tetany.

Etiology

Vitamin D deficiency basically results from a lack of exposure to ultraviolet rays, but under usual living conditions in temperate climates it is most frequently due to inadequate intake of added vitamin D. Conditioned deficiencies are caused by failure to absorb the vitamin, as in the chronic steatorrheas.

Pathology

The pathologic changes in children consist essentially of defective calcification of the growing bone, due to the absence of lime salts, and hypertrophy of the epiphyseal cartilages. The first anatomical evidence of vitamin D deficiency is a cessation of the normal degeneration of epiphyseal cartilage cells which occurs in the process of bone formation; nevertheless, new cartilage continues to form, so that the epiphyseal cartilage becomes greatly but irregularly increased in width. Calcification ceases and osteoid material accumulates around the capillaries of the diaphysis. In long-continued vitamin D deficiency there may be resorption of the cancellous bone of the diaphysis and of cortical bone. After adequate vitamin treatment, the first histologic evidence of repair is degeneration of the cartilage cells within 24 hours and penetration by a vascular network within 48 hours which permits the deposition of lime salts. The formation of osteoid material at the diaphyseal side ceases, and normal endochondral production of new bone is resumed. In adults, the metabolic features are the same except that, since there is no endochondral formation of new bone, only a disappearance of cancellous bone of the diaphysis and resorption of cortical bone are noted.

Symptoms and Signs

Infants with early deficiency (rickets) are restless and sleep poorly; constant movement on the pillow denudes the head of occipital hair. Such infants do not sit, crawl, or walk early and there is a delay in closing of the fontanels. Craniotabes probably is the earliest physical sign and is followed by enlargements of the epiphyseal cartilages of the long bones. These are particularly noticeable at the costochondral junctions of the ribs ("rachitic rosary") and at the lower ends of the radius, ulna, tibia, and fibula. Weight-bearing bends the bones and causes characteristic deformities such as bowlegs and pigeon breast.

Roentgenographic changes precede clinical signs, becoming evident in the 3rd or 4th month of life, and sometimes as early as the 2nd month or even at birth if the mother is deficient in vitamin D. Bone changes are most evident at the lower ends of the radius and ulna. The diaphyseal ends lose their sharp clear outline, are cup-shaped, and show a spotty or fringy rarefaction. Later, the distance between the ends of the radius and ulna and the metacarpal bones appears increased because the true ends are invisible due to failure of calcification. The shadows cast by the shaft decrease in density and the network formed by laminas becomes coarse. Characteristic deformities are produced by bending of the bones at the cartilage-shaft junction and in the substance of the shaft. As healing begins, a thin line of calcification appears at the epiphysis, first as a thin white line but denser and thicker as calcification proceeds. Later, lime salts are deposited beneath the periosteum, the shaft casts a denser shadow, and the lamellas disappear.

In adult deficiency demineralization (osteomalacia) occurs, particularly in the spine, pelvis, and lower extremities, so that the fibrous lamellas become visible on the roentgenogram, while incomplete fissure-like fractures appear in the cortex of the bone. As the bones soften, weight causes bowing of the long bones, vertical shortening of the vertebrae, and flattening of the pelvic bones, which alters the pelvic outlet.

Rachitic tetany is caused by low calcium blood levels. It may accompany either infantile or adult vitamin D deficiency. In the latent form there are no obvious symptoms, but hyper-irritability of the nervous system may be elicited by applying galvanic current to the peripheral nerves (Erb's phenomenon) or by eliciting Chvostek's sign or Trousseau's phenomenon (*see* TETANY). At this time the serum calcium levels are below 8.5 mg./100 cc. and usually between 6.5 and 8.0 mg. In manifest tetany there are carpopedal spasms, the characteristic "tetany facies," laryngospasm, and convulsive seizures. At this time the serum calcium levels usually are between 5.0 and 6.5 mg./100 cc.

Laboratory Findings

The most important laboratory findings are the roentgeno-graphic changes. After these become apparent the serum calcium is found to be lowered, and may fall as low as 5.0 mg./100 cc. in manifest tetany. Simultaneously the serum phosphorus usually becomes lowered (below 5.0 mg./100 cc. in infants and 3.0 mg. in adults).

It has been claimed that if the concentration of calcium be multiplied by that of phosphorus, each being expressed as mg./100 cc. of blood serum, a product is obtained which in the normal child is above 40; when below 30 rickets usually is present; when above 40 rickets is either absent or healing. This is a practical formula, though exceptions occur.

Diagnosis

In advanced cases of rickets, when all signs and symptoms are present, the total picture readily gives the diagnosis. Early cases, however, may present a problem, since many of the separate symptoms are common to other diseases. A history of deficient vitamin D intake is strongly suggestive of rickets, and helps to distinguish it from infantile scurvy (q.v.) and other conditions. Congenital syphilis can be identified by the serologic reactions and other evidences of syphilis (q.v.). Chondrodystrophy is seldom manifest before the age of 6 months and can be distinguished by the patient's large head, short extremities, and thick bones. Other conditions such as osteogenesis imperfecta, cretinism, congenital dislocation of the hips, hydrocephalus and poliomyelitis may occasionally be confused with rickets but should be readily distinguishable. Manifest tetany in infantile rickets must be differentiated from convulsions due to other causes (*see* Tetany). Normal serum calcium determinations rule out rachitic tetany.

Osteomalacia is to be differentiated from several diseases characterized by widespread bone decalcification, such as hyperparathyroidism, senile osteoporosis, the osteoporosis of hyperthyroidism, basophilic adenoma of the pituitary, suprarenal cortical tumor, multiple myeloma, and atrophy of disuse. Other signs of these diseases, serum calcium-phosphorus and alkaline phosphatase determinations, and the characteristic X-ray pictures determine the diagnosis.

Prophylaxis

Full term infants should be given vitamin D, beginning in the 3rd or 4th week of life with 200 u. daily and increasing the amount by 200 u./week up to 800 to 1,200 u. This level should be maintained until the child is 2 years old, after which 400 u. daily usually will be sufficient. Premature infants require approximately 10 times these amounts.

Treatment

Uncomplicated infantile rickets, in the presence of adequate calcium-phosphorus intake, can be cured, though slowly, by ordinary preventive doses of vitamin D (*see* Vitamin Table), using any suitable commercial preparation. Larger doses (about 1,200 u. daily) are more rapidly effective. The first evidence of improvement (a rise in serum phosphorus) will occur in about 10 days, followed in the 3rd week by deposition of lime salts in the osseous tissues. After about a month the dosage can be gradually reduced to preventive levels. If tetany is a complication, this treatment should be supplemented during the first week by calcium I.V., but never subcut. or I.M. (*see* Tetany).

Refractory cases are occasionally encountered in children over 3 years old. Before instituting heroic vitamin D therapy, refractory rickets must be differentiated from the rare cases of renal rickets (renal hyperparathyroidism) and endogenous rickets characterized by glycosuria with normal blood sugar, neither of which responds to vitamin D. For refractory rickets the dosage of vitamin D should be increased by 10,000-u. jumps at 3-week intervals until an effect is produced. As most cases respond to 50,000 or 60,000 u. daily, some physicians go immediately to that level. Cases have been reported that require 1,000,000 to 1,500,000 u. daily to induce healing, and from 150,-000 to 300,000 u. daily as a maintenance dose. When large doses (20,000 u. daily in infants and prematurity, 50,000 u. daily in children) of vitamin D are employed in the treatment of rickets, the physician should be on guard for signs of toxicity. Renal insufficiency increases the possibility of toxicity. The rule probably holds that toxic manifestations do not occur as long as the rickets remains entirely unaffected, so the physician should watch for the first sign of healing, indicated by an increase in phosphorus in the blood and the beginning deposition of lime salts, as visualized by X-ray. In ordinary cases (50,000 to 100,000 u. daily) these examinations should be made at weekly or fortnightly intervals; if the dose is extremely large (100,000 u. daily), at weekly or semiweekly intervals. These signs of healing do not necessarily mean that the dose of vitamin D should be immediately lowered but indicate that toxic signs now are possible. If the dose of vitamin D is not immediately lowered as is ordinarily advisable, semiweekly serum calcium-phosphorus determinations should be made, and the urine checked for calcium casts (these will not occur if the urine is kept acid). If the serum calcium exceeds 11.5 or 12.0 mg./100 cc. or if calcium casts appear, stop vitamin D immediately, and keep the urine acid. There is no other treatment for the toxic manifestations of vitamin D.

Occasionally, it is important to effect a rapid cure of rickets, as when weakness of the thorax menaces life. In these instances 50,000 u. of vitamin D should be given daily, and the dosage reduced to 1,200 u. daily the instant healing is evidenced by a rise in serum phosphorus or by X-ray. In the steatorrheas, cod liver oil is contraindicated. Here one may use either concentrated fish oils or viosterol in oil in 30,000 to 50,000 u. doses or give it as viosterol in propylene glycol or as crystalline D. There are preparations of crystalline vitamin D suitable for parenteral use.

The treatment of adult osteomalacia is the same as for infantile rickets.

VITAMIN K DEFICIENCY

In this chapter the term "vitamin K" signifies vitamin K activity. Vitamins K_1 and K_2 occur naturally and are fat-soluble. Several synthetic naphthoquinone derivatives exerting vitamin K activity have been synthesized. These vitamin K analogues include menadione (fat-soluble), and menadione sodium bisulfite (water-soluble). Physiologically, vitamin K is necessary for normal blood coagulation, which occurs through two consecutive reactions: (1) the inter-reaction of calcium and thromboplastin (thrombokinase, from tissue platelets) on prothrombin to form thrombin and (2) the inter-reaction of thrombin and fibrinogen to form fibrin. Vitamin K is essential for the formation of prothrombin by the liver. Its deficiency causes hypoprothrombinemia and is manifested by defective coagulation of the blood and a hemorrhagic diathesis. The human requirements of vitamin K have not been ascertained although it is known that 1 or 2 mg., if properly absorbed and utilized, usually will correct temporarily a vitamin K deficiency.

Etiology

Vitamin K is derived both from the diet and from intestinal bacterial synthesis, the latter being the most important source. The occurrence of vitamin K deficiency from inadequate intake alone is unlikely. Since the intestinal tract is sterile in the newborn, absence of intestinal bacterial synthesis probably explains the "physiologic" hypoprothrombinemia observed during the first 3 to 5 days of life. The hypoprothrombinemia which sometimes occurs during therapy with nonabsorbable sulfonamide drugs or oral streptomycin also is explainable by the striking reduction in intestinal flora caused by these drugs.

Most vitamin K deficiencies are conditioned by the lack of bile salts, which are necessary for the absorption of bacterially synthesized vitamin K. Therefore, vitamin K deficiency is most commonly secondary to external biliary fistulas or to obstructive jaundice from any cause. Inadequate absorption has been encountered in a number of other gastrointestinal conditions, including chronic ulcerative colitis, regional enteritis, gastrocolic fistula, entero-anastomosis, ileac enterostomy, intestinal polyposis, and the steatorrheas. Excessive amounts of mineral oil may prevent absorption of vitamin K. Severe liver disease frequently causes hypoprothrombinemia because the liver fails to make prothrombin. Overtreatment with dicumarol (*see* ANTICOAGULANT THERAPY) may produce hypoprothrombinemia by inhibiting its formation by the liver.

Symptoms and Signs

The symptoms of vitamin K deficiency are those of hypoprothrombinemia superimposed upon the conditioning disease. Hemorrhages may occur in any organ or tissue. In obstructive jaundice, hemorrhage usually begins by the 1st to 5th day. It may begin as a slow ooze from an operative wound, the gums, nose, or gastrointestinal tract, or as a massive hemorrhage into the gastrointestinal tract. In severe liver disease with hypoprothrombinemia, oozing from the gums or nose and large ecchymotic areas around venipunctures are commonly the first clinical manifestations. In the newborn, many of the intra-cranial hemorrhages of birth and hemorrhagic diatheses may be explained by the "physiologic" hypoprothrombinemia of the first 5 days of life.

Laboratory Findings

Alteration in blood prothrombin is the most important laboratory finding. It is usually expressed as prothrombin time (normal 10 to 15 seconds) or as quantitative prothrombin in terms of per cent of normal (normal 100%).

Reduction of the quantitative prothrombin to 80% of normal or below is considered abnormal, and a reduction to 20% of normal or less is associated with an increasing incidence of active bleeding. Bleeding time and coagulation time are as a rule little altered until the prothrombin level has fallen below 20% of normal.

Diagnosis

Diagnosis of vitamin K deficiency is not difficult if it is remembered that hypoprothrombinemia may result from failure to absorb vitamin K or from severe liver damage. In the presence of hypoprothrombinemia the liver factor probably can be ruled out if 2 to 5 mg. of a water-soluble synthetic K, given I.V., produces a significant increase in prothrombin levels within 2 to 6 hours. Many diseases such as scurvy, allergic purpura, anemia, leukemia and thrombocytopenia give hemorrhagic manifestations without hypoprothrombinemia.

Treatment

Treatment with vitamin K is indicated in subjects having prothrombin levels below 80% of normal and in patients with diseases (*see* Etiology) likely to cause hypoprothrombinemia, who must undergo surgery.

The dose and route of administration vary with the needs of the patient and according to the form of vitamin K selected. Menadione is available for oral administration as tablets or capsules, each containing 1 or 2 mg., and for I.M. injection as an oil solution containing 1 or 2 mg./cc. The average dose is 1 to 2 mg./day, but 5 mg. or more may be required. When administered orally to patients with bile obstruction, 2 to 4 Gm. bile salts should be given with the menadione. Menadione sodium bisulfite is a water-soluble form of vitamin K, available in tablets for oral administration (bile salts not necessary), and in aqueous solution for subcut., I.M., or I.V. injection. The average daily dose is 0.5 to 2 mg., but 5 mg. or more may be necessary as indicated by prothrombin level determinations. Vitamin K_1 also is available for oral or I.V. use. Reports suggest that it has a more prolonged effect than menadione. With this form of the drug, the oral dose is 4 to 10 mg., with or without bile salts, and the I.V. dose for adults may be as much as 10 mg. dispersed in dextrose solution. Newborn infants may be given 0.25 mg. I.V.

Prophylactic administration of vitamin K is advisable for patients who must undergo surgery, whenever a disease exists that is likely to cause hypoprothrombinemia. When the prothrombin levels are between 50 and 80% of normal, give 1 or 2 mg. of synthetic vitamin K daily by mouth for 2 to 5 days preoperatively. If immediate operation is indicated, give 2 to 5 mg. of a water-soluble preparation I.V. as part of the preoperative preparation. Postoperatively, give 2 mg. of a water-soluble form I.V., every other day, until oral medication can be resumed. If prothrombin levels are less than 50% of normal, it is advisable to administer a water-soluble vitamin K product I.V. in 2 to 5 mg. doses daily until prothrombin levels are normal, then continue with prophylactic therapy. As a rule, only one such dose is necessary.

The problem of treating patients with hypoprothrombinemia and active bleeding is more difficult: 2 to 5 mg. of water-soluble vitamin K should be given immediately by vein, and if hemorrhage is considerable, blood transfusion is indicated. The I.V. dose of vitamin K should be repeated daily if necessary until the prothrombin level becomes normal, after which the prophylactic regimen can be instituted.

In severe liver disease with hypoprothrombinemia, some patients may not respond to vitamin K therapy. In such cases, therapy should nevertheless be continued as there is evidence that more of these patients will recover if vitamin K is administered I.V. in doses of 2 to 5 mg. daily or every other day. In addition, whole blood transfusions may be required for symptomatic relief of bleeding.

In the newborn infant, vitamin K may be used to prevent "physiologic" hypoprothrombinemia, to reduce the incidence of intracranial hemorrhage incidental to birth trauma, and prophylactically whenever surgery is contemplated. Several procedures are recommended: (1) Give vitamin K to the mother in prophylactic doses for a week prior to expected confinement; (2) give the mother 2 to 5 mg. (or more if necessary) of water-soluble synthetic vitamin K, I.V., 6 to 24 hours before delivery; (3) give the newborn child 2 mg. of a water-soluble synthetic vitamin K, I.M., immediately after delivery. This also is the procedure when surgery is contemplated in the newborn.

(For the use of vitamin K to counteract effects of dicumarol, *see* ANTICOAGULANT THERAPY.)

RIBOFLAVIN (VITAMIN B$_2$) DEFICIENCY

Riboflavin is a water-soluble vitamin, which is essential for proper growth and tissue function. Estimated normal human allowances are listed in the Vitamin Table (q.v.). Deficiency results in characteristic oral, cutaneous, and corneal lesions.

Etiology

Primary riboflavin deficiency is almost always associated with inadequate milk consumption. Conditioned deficiencies are most common in chronic diarrheas, liver disease, postoperatively when dextrose infusions are given without preventive vitamin therapy, and in chronic alcoholism.

Symptoms and Signs

The symptoms of riboflavin deficiency are most prominent in the lips, mouth, skin and eyes. Cheilosis with angular fissuring is an outstanding symptom. Simple chapping is the most common form of cheilosis, but an atrophic form is frequently seen in adults, in which the exposed mucosa becomes thin and parchment-like. Angular stomatitis manifests itself as a pallor, erythema, or slight maceration of the mucosa in the angles of the mouth. Dermatitis of the adjacent skin follows and fissures appear in the affected areas. In healing, these fissures often leave scars. Perlèche is a grayish white lesion usually caused by secondary infection of the angular fissures with *Monilia albicans*. The "magenta" tongue, as its name implies, is of a purplish color and is frequently associated with riboflavin deficiency.

The cutaneous manifestations are usually described as "dyssebacia," a clinical term embracing a series of disturbances of the sebaceous glands. First there is increased oiliness, then greasy yellowish flaky scales appear, usually in the nasolabial folds but sometimes behind the ears, lateral to the external canthi, or in other sebaceous areas. After the flaking, either filiform excrescences, fissures, or both, develop. The filiform excrescences generally appear first in the nasolabial folds and frequently spread over the midportion of the face and the forehead. In the nasolabial folds they may become so prominent as to resemble warts. Still later, innumerable plugs of inspissated sebum project from the dilated orifices of the sebaceous follicles over the cheeks, nose, and forehead. Their characteristic appearance is denoted by the name "shark skin." Fissures are apt to occur in the body creases and folds and are very painful when around the anus.

In typical eye lesions the cornea becomes vascularized by blood vessels growing into it from the limbic plexus. When sufficiently advanced, circumcorneal injection is grossly evident. Examination with the slit lamp at this time reveals engorged blood vessels invading the cornea. The engorgement causes burning, itching, and photophobia.

Laboratory Findings

There is no satisfactory laboratory test for riboflavin deficiency. Neither the blood levels of riboflavin nor its urinary excretion have been correlated with clinical findings.

Diagnosis

None of the lesions described is specific in diagnosis. Cheilosis may result from chapping due to various causes. Angular stomatitis, dermatitis, and fissures frequently occur in edentulism and from ill-fitting dentures. The dyssebacia may resemble seborrhea, and the ocular lesions may be produced by a great number of conditions. Diagnosis of riboflavin deficiency is therefore dependent upon the history, the presence of suggestive lesions, elimination of other causes, and a controlled therapeutic trial. Under a therapeutic test with riboflavin, engorgement of the corneal blood vessels due to deficiency rapidly disappears. After the engorgement has been eliminated, vestiges of the empty capillaries remain for years, and may become temporarily refilled through minor trauma, such as rubbing the eyes, or smoke, dust and glare.

Treatment

The first principle in relieving riboflavin deficiency is the basic therapy outlined under general therapy. Supplementary riboflavin by mouth, 10 to 20 mg. daily in divided doses, is indicated until a response is obtained, or until the urine becomes highly colored from excess riboflavin. When this happens continue with 2 to 4 mg. daily until recovery. It is seldom necessary to give riboflavin parenterally, though when indicated it can be injected I.M., 5 to 20 mg. daily, in single or divided doses.

THIAMINE (VITAMIN B$_1$) DEFICIENCY

Thiamine is essential for the proper metabolism of carbohydrate and fat, for normal functioning of nervous tissue, and for enzymatic function (cocarboxylase). Human requirements are given in the Vitamin Table (q.v.). Thiamine deficiency may cause neurasthenia and neurologic, cardiac, and gastrointestinal symptoms due to lack of the coenzyme, cocarboxylase (thiamine pyrophosphate). Severe and prolonged deficiency gives rise to beriberi.

Etiology

Primary deficiency in normal persons is due to inadequate intake of thiamine. The most important conditioning factors in this country are: (1) Disorders increasing the vitamin requirement, such as hyperthyroidism, pregnancy, lactation, fever from any cause, and mental disease with increased psychomotor activity; (2) diseases causing impaired absorption, such as long-continued diarrheas, and (3) those causing impaired vitamin utilization, such as liver disease. In alcoholism there is a combination of decreased intake, impaired absorption and utilization, and possibly increased requirement. Glucose requires thiamine for its oxidation, and frequent or long continued glucose infusions, coupled with a low thiamine intake are potent factors in precipitating thiamine deficiency in medical and surgical practice.

Pathology

The most striking and constant findings of vitamin B_1 deficiency arise from incomplete carbohydrate oxidation and pyruvemia, which lead to edema and serous effusions and to anatomic changes in the C.N.S. and heart. In the nervous system the most advanced pathology occurs in the peripheral nerves, particularly, though not exclusively, those of the lower extremities. Degeneration of the myelin sheath is most frequent, and later the axis cylinders become fragmented or atrophied. Changes in the spinal cord are seldom grossly apparent. Degeneration of the medullary sheath has been demonstrated in all tracts of the cord, especially in the posterior columns and in both the anterior and posterior nerve roots. In the brain the lesions are those of hemorrhagic polioencephalitis, but they probably occur only in very severe depletion. The heart in acute beriberi may be dilated and enlarged. Microscopic sections of the heart muscle show swollen, fragmented, and vacuolized muscle bundles, with the interstitial spaces dilated by edema fluid.

Edema and serous effusions in patients with thiamine deficiency may occur either in the absence or the presence of congestive heart failure. The mechanism of the edema in the former is unknown.

Symptoms and Signs

The signs and symptoms can be classified under three headings: neurasthenic, neurologic, and circulatory. A **neurasthenic syndrome** probably is the earliest and most constant symptom of thiamine deficiency. As in neurasthenic syndromes of any origin, the outstanding symptoms are anorexia, fatigability, and sleep disturbances. Other common symptoms are irritability, poor memory, inability to concentrate, precordial pain, heart consciousness, "gas" and other vague abdominal complaints, and constipation.

Neurologic changes seldom occur until after the neurasthenic symptoms have developed, and the most frequent manifestation is polyneuropathy. The peripheral neuropathy of thiamine deficiency is bilateral and symmetrical, involving predominantly the lower extremities. In its mildest form, it is ushered in by paresthesias of the toes, burning of the feet particularly severe at night, and perhaps calf muscle cramps and pains in the legs. Calf muscle tenderness, difficulty in rising from a squatting position, a quantitative diminution in the vibratory sensation in the toes, and plantar dysesthesia are the earliest signs elicited. Combined with a history of inadequate intake or of conditioning factors, these signs are suggestive, and when addition ankle jerks are absent, a diagnosis of mild peripheral neuropathy can be made. Continued deficiency causes loss of knee jerks, loss of vibratory and position sensation in the toes, and atrophy of the calf and thigh muscles. Foot drop and toe drop complete this sequence of events. After the leg signs are well established the upper extremities may become similarly involved. In very advanced or very acute deficiencies ophthalmoplegia may develop, particularly after bouts of severe vomiting, diarrhea, pneumonia, or delirium. Here, the 3rd nerve usually is first affected, with complete ophthalmoplegia soon following.

Circulatory manifestations may be classified as follows: (1) Edema and serous effusions without congestive heart failure, enlarged heart, or other recognized etiologic factor; (2) edema and serous effusions with supporting symptoms of congestive heart failure, usually with definite roentgenographic evidence of cardiac enlargement; (3) sudden circulatory collapse, which may be the first manifestation of circulatory failure or may occur after other signs are well advanced. These circulatory manifestations are more likely to occur in patients with mild neuropathy, who are capable of muscular activity, than in those with advanced neurologic impairment, who are relatively immobile.

In the female, there is some evidence that destruction of circulating estrogen by the liver may be impaired in thiamine deficiency, leading to hyperestrinism and endometrial hyperplasia.

Laboratory Findings

Urinary excretion of thiamine, even after a test dose, is practically nil in acute thiamine depletion. In any case, test doses reflect only the recent dietary intake and reserves, rather than the metabolic thiamine deficiency. The same is true of blood thiamine determinations.

Fasting blood pyruvic acid levels are elevated in metabolic thiamine deficiency but as a rule not significantly so prior to the clinical signs of neuropathy. Abnormal elevations of pyruvic acid following the metabolic stress of 100 Gm. of dextrose, or of exercise, or both, occur in thiamine deficiency before the development of clinical neuropathy, and probably are the most important indices of incipient thiamine deficiency. The pyruvic acid test may be negative in chronic neuropathy, as the metabolic defect may have been corrected without reversal of the anatomic lesion.

Diagnosis

The development of a neurasthenic syndrome in a subject with a previously normal psyche is particularly apt to be due to thiamine deficiency. If of short duration, and if a therapeutic trial of thiamine is successful, the diagnosis probably is thiamine deficiency. If of long duration the neurasthenia may become "fixed" and no amount of therapy will cause early reversal. Neurasthenic syndromes in people with good dietary habits and without conditioning factors can seldom be attributed to thiamine deficiency.

Other forms of bilateral, symmetrical polyneuropathy beginning first in the lower extremities are infrequent. Single-nerve mononeuritides and those beginning elsewhere than in the legs are very unlikely to be due to thiamine deficiency. The following forms of polyneuropathy usually are due to thiamine deficiency: alcoholic, gestational, diabetic, cachectic, and those occurring in pernicious anemia, sprue, and pellagra. A form of polyneuropathy occurs in uncontrolled diabetics which is clinically similar to that of thiamine deficiency but does not respond to thiamine.

In the diagnosis of congestive heart failure it is most important to bear in mind that in beriberi heart disease the circulation time is normal or decreased and in most other forms of congestive heart failure it is increased. A notable exception is in thyroid heart disease. It also must be remembered that edema in beriberi heart disease responds to bed rest alone as well as, or better than, the edema of most other forms of heart disease, but responds poorly to digitalis and mercurial diuretics. Response to a therapeutic trial of thiamine in uncomplicated beriberi heart disease usually is prompt and complete. When complicated by hypertensive, degenerative, or infectious heart disease, the diagnosis often is impossible or at best speculative.

Treatment

The basic therapy outlined in the chapter on treatment of nutritional deficiencies in general is most important. In addition, 10 to 100 mg. of thiamine chloride should be given daily by mouth or parenterally, depending upon the clinical manifestations. In the neurasthenic syndrome and in mild polyneuropathies, 10 to 50 mg. daily in divided doses by mouth is recommended. When parenteral administration is indicated 10 to 20 mg. once a day is adequate. If the neuropathy is moderate or advanced give daily 20 to 100 mg. in divided doses by mouth or 20 to 50 mg. parenterally. In beriberi heart disease and in ophthalmoplegia of Wernicke's syndrome, 50 to 100 mg. by subcut. or I.V. injection twice daily usually is given. These large doses should be continued until a therapeutic response is obtained or saturation of the tissues is indicated by a strong odor of thiamine in the urine. Basic therapy then can be resumed.

Although there is no strictly scientific basis for giving more than 10 to 20 mg. of thiamine daily, experience has shown that the larger doses recommended here are effective in severe cases of thiamine deficiency. They may safely be used since no undesirable side effects have been encountered. A very few deaths (2 or 3 authenticated) due to allergic or anaphylactic reactions following I.V. injection of thiamine have been recorded, but these were unrelated to the size of the dose. The possibility of such reactions must be considered when the vitamin is given I.V., particularly if the patient has received it previously by parenteral injection and an interval has elapsed without treatment.

Use of thiamine in other conditions: Thiamine either alone or in combination with other water-soluble vitamins in dextrose infusions is good preventive therapy against deficiency disease, based upon sound scientific principles and clinical experience. It is recommended in alcoholism (q.v.) and also other conditions in which there is potential thiamine deficiency. Its use in single-nerve mononeuritides, or to relieve pain as in lumbar myositis, trigeminal neuralgias, sciatica, radiculitis with or without herpes, and other neurologic conditions, is empiric without satisfactory evidence of its value.

NIACINAMIDE DEFICIENCY

Severe deficiency of niacin (nicotinic acid) or its amide (niacinamide, nicotinamide) is the cause of pellagra, a disease characterized by mental, neurologic, cutaneous, mucous membrane, and gastrointestinal symptoms. Protein containing tryptophane apparently protects against a low niacinamide intake, and there are indications that tryptophane is a precursor of niacinamide. This may explain the fact that, on the same niacinamide intake, protection against pellagra is afforded by proteins containing tryptophane, such as wheat, milk, or egg protein, while corn protein, which is deficient in tryptophane, gives no such protection. The daily requirements of niacinamide average 5 mg./1,000 calories, but it is probable that diets containing an abundance of tryptophane may require less, and those containing little tryptophane more, than this standard allowance (*see* Vitamin Table).

Etiology

Primary deficiencies of niacinamide usually are associated with a high maize diet, and pellagra is endemic in sections where corn forms a major part of the food consumed. Secondary deficiencies frequently occur in diarrheal disease, cirrhosis of the liver and alcoholism and following liberal use of dextrose infusions postoperatively without preventive vitamin therapy.

Pathology

There is no recognized specific pathology of niacinamide deficiency. The pathology in the skin is a reaction to trauma. In the mucous membranes and gastrointestinal tract the pathology is hyperemia and congestion, with secondary infection and ulceration. Brain lesions are thought by most observers to be nonspecific. Myelin degeneration in the spinal cord and the peripheral neuropathy are believed to be due to thiamine deficiency.

Symptoms and Signs

The complete syndrome of advanced niacinamide deficiency (pellagra), with scarlet stomatitis and glossitis, diarrhea, dermatitis, and mental aberrations, is well known. The several symptoms of deficiency may, however, appear alone or in various combinations.

There are four general types of **cutaneous lesions:** (1) The 1st and most acute consists of erythema followed by vesiculation, bullae, crusting, and desquamation. Secondary infection is common and usually results from exposure to sunlight (actinic trauma). (2) The 2nd type, also acute, is intertrigo, characterized by redness, maceration, abrasion, and secondary infection in the characteristic intertriginous areas. (3) The 3rd is chronic hypertrophy: the skin becomes thickened, inelastic, fissured, and deeply pigmented over pressure points. There is often secondary infection. When healing starts the lesion shows a sharply defined pearly border of regenerating epithelium. (4) The 4th type consists of chronic ichthyotic lesions, with dry, scaly, atrophic, inelastic skin, too large for the part it covers. This usually is seen only in older pellagrins. Distribution of the lesions is more characteristic than their form. They occur at trauma points: sunlight causes butterfly-shaped lesions on the face and affects other exposed parts. The cutaneous lesions are most frequently symmetrical but unilateral lesions are sometimes seen.

Changes in the **mucous membranes** involve chiefly the mouth—sometimes also the vagina, urethra, and conjunctiva. Scarlet glossitis and stomatitis are characteristic of acute niacinamide deficiency. The tip and lateral margins of the tongue and the buccal mucosa around Stenson's ducts are first affected. As the lesion progresses, the entire tongue and oral mucous membranes become a bright scarlet color. Soreness of the mouth, increased salivation, and edema of the tongue are present. Ulcerations may appear anywhere, but are especially common on the undersurface of the tongue, the mucosa of the lower lip, and opposite the molar teeth. They often are covered by a grayish slough containing Vincent's organisms.

Gastrointestinal symptoms are indeterminate in early cases: there may be burning of the mouth, pharynx, and esophagus, and abdominal discomfort and distention; later, nausea, vomiting and diarrhea. Diarrhea is the classic gastrointestinal symptom and is of serious import. It often is bloody because of the gastrointestinal hyperemia and ulceration.

Three types of **C.N.S. involvement** are observed. (1) The 1st and most frequent is a neurasthenic syndrome indistinguishable from that of thiamine deficiency. (2) The 2nd is organic psychosis, usually characterized by memory impairment, disorientation, confusion, and confabulation. In some patients, excitement, depression, mania, and delirium predominate; in others the reaction is paranoid. (3) The 3rd type is the "encephalopathic syndrome." The clinical picture of encephalopathy due to niacinamide deficiency is fairly well defined and is characterized by clouding of consciousness, cogwheel rigidities of the extremities, and uncontrollable sucking and grasping reflexes. This syndrome is most common after a period of delirium or high fever, or postoperatively following a series of dextrose infusions without preventive vitamin therapy. The peripheral neuropathy and signs of spinal tract involvement noted probably result from a simultaneous thiamine deficiency. There is no characteristic or diagnostic laboratory finding.

Diagnosis

Early niacinamide deficiency is to be distinguished from the neurasthenic syndrome; later cases, from the other causes of stomatitis, glossitis, diarrhea, and dementia. When the clinical picture is fully developed, with dermatitis, mouth lesions, diarrhea, delirium, and dementia, the diagnosis is easily made. More frequently, however, the condition is less fully developed; in these cases, history of a diet lacking in foods containing niacin or tryptophane is significant.

Treatment

In no deficiency disease is the basic treatment, outlined in the section on General Principles of Treatment (q.v.), more important. Supplementing this, 300 to 1,000 mg. of niacinamide should be given daily by mouth in divided doses. In most cases 300 to 500 mg. is sufficient. When diarrhea or lack of cooperation precludes oral therapy, 100 to 250 mg. should be injected subcut. 2 or 3 times a day. In encephalopathic states, 1,000 mg. by mouth plus 100 to 250 mg. parenterally is recommended. When the disease is under control, the basic therapy usually is adequate. Niacinamide is preferable to nicotinic acid, since it usually can be given in large doses without causing vasomotor disturbances.

PROTEIN DEFICIENCY

In addition to a simple lack of protein in the diet, protein deficiencies may result from a variety of diseases which cause impaired digestion or absorption, impaired synthesis of plasma proteins, increased catabolism and excessive loss of body protein. In general, two types of protein deficiency may occur, acute and chronic.

Etiology

Acute protein deficiencies: These result from the rapid loss of a large amount of the plasma proteins without their immediate replacement. This may occur in severe hemorrhage, external or internal; extensive burns; copious exudation from wounds; or transudation into body cavities, traumatized tissues, the walls of the intestines in intestinal obstruction, or into the lungs in pneumonia.

Chronic protein deficiencies: A period of negative nitrogen balance (i.e., where more protein is catabolized or lost from the body than is ingested and utilized during a given period) as short as 1 or 2 weeks may result in chronic deficiency. Inadequate dietary intake of protein is the usual cause. Chronic illness (e.g., with fever, elevated B.M.R.) also may produce a negative nitrogen balance by increasing protein catabolism, and resulting in a reduced dietary intake because of anorexia. Other causes include impaired intestinal absorption such as occurs in sprue, steatorrhea and the chronic inflammatory diarrheas; imperfect utilization of ingested protein, as in diseases of the liver; and excessive loss of proteins, as in prolonged albuminuria and draining fistulas.

Pathologic Physiology

The protein requirement necessary to maintain nitrogen balance (i.e., as much protein ingested and utilized as is broken down or lost) averages about 1 Gm./Kg. of body weight/day. If this amount is not ingested or utilized, or if increased catabolism occurs, a cumulative protein deficit ensues. For example, it has been found that as much as 10 to 15 Kg. (20 to 30 lbs.) of tissue protein may be lost by an average-size adult during the course of a severe illness. A sizeable portion of this loss is from the plasma proteins, resulting in hypoproteinemia. The reduced plasma osmotic pressure consequent to the hypoproteinemia may result in "nutritional" edema. In addition, all the vital functions dependent upon proteins are impaired. These include body growth, and repair of injury and normal tissue wear and tear, the production of enzymes, hormones and antibodies, and the formation of fibrinogen for the clotting mechanism.

Symptoms and Signs

The outstanding clinical manifestation of the acute loss of protein (e.g., as occurs in hemorrhage or burns) is pronounced and sudden circulatory collapse.

The manifestations of chronic protein deficiency are varied. Chief among them is the gradual development of edema. This usually begins in the dependent portions of the body, first appearing in the ankles, scrotum, and over the sacrum. It also occurs in the walls of the gastrointestinal tract and may be responsible for severe digestive disturbances. Ascites may de-

9

velop in severe cases. Weight loss is common, except in individuals consuming large amounts of carbohydrate. However, the loss of body tissue may be masked, and the patient actually gain in weight as a result of retained water in the form of nutritional edema.

Anemia, weakness, and anorexia are common. The skin often is dry, shiny, and rather stiff. Decubitus ulcers frequently develop. Faulty wound healing and lowered resistance to infection usually occur.

Diagnosis

Protein deficiency will not be overlooked if the various conditions which may result in a disparity between the intake and loss of protein are kept in mind. The amount of protein foods ingested should be determined. A diet containing less than 0.5 to 1 Gm. of protein/Kg. body wt./day over a prolonged period, especially during an illness, will likely lead to considerable protein deficiency. Of the laboratory methods that may be used for the diagnosis, the most important is the measurement of the plasma proteins, especially the albumin fraction. If the plasma albumin is below 3.5 Gm./100 cc., or the total plasma protein below 6.0 Gm./100 cc., a protein deficiency probably is present. However, the value for the total plasma proteins may be normal despite severe protein deficiency in the presence of hemoconcentration, or an increase in plasma globulin such as occurs in certain infectious diseases. Nitrogen balance studies are practicable only in hospital practice.

Prophylaxis

Acute protein deficiency may be prevented by avoiding unnecessary tissue trauma and blood loss during surgical procedures, by prompt treatment of extensive infections, and by the replacement of protein loss as soon and as completely as possible by whole blood or plasma transfusions. Chronic deficiency may be prevented by assuring adequate protein intake, especially if protein requirements are greater than normal as a result of increased metabolism or protein loss; and by the correction of any primary disease affecting the digestion, absorption or catabolism of protein.

Treatment

Acute deficiency: Whole blood transfusions are the best and quickest way to correct protein deficiency due to blood loss. When only the plasma fraction is lost, injections of plasma are preferable. In general, a fall in the red cell count calls for whole blood; a rise, for plasma.

Chronic deficiency: When possible, oral administration of protein is preferable to the parenteral route. Orally, protein may be taken as whole protein, protein hydrolysates, or an amino acids mixture. Parenterally, protein is administered as whole blood, plasma, concentrated albumin, protein hydrolysates, or amino acids mixture. Of these, blood, plasma, and albumin are expensive and impractical as the sole I.V. sources of protein.

If the patient can take food by mouth, a diet containing at least 150 Gm. of protein daily is indicated. In very severe deficiencies, as much as 300 Gm. of protein daily is required. This may be achieved by a high protein diet (*see* DIETS) supplemented by a palatable high protein drink (R 45), or by one of the commercial protein concentrates or protein hydrolysates. The total caloric intake should exceed 2,000 calories daily, with supplementary vitamins provided. The physician, nurse, and dietitian should work as a team to ensure that the patient both receives and consumes the required diet.

Oral amino acids mixtures and hydrolyzed proteins may be substituted when large amounts of whole proteins orally administered cause such gastrointestinal disturbances as distension and diarrhea. These substances have the further advantage of being easily administered via stomach tube to patients who cannot swallow, or via gastrostomy and jejunostomy tubes. Most of such preparations are not too palatable but, if administered properly, usually can be tolerated fairly easily. A useful method is to dissolve 20 Gm. of the protein hydrolysate powder in a half glass of water, shake thoroughly and swallow in one draught. This is followed immediately by 20 Gm. of carbohydrate similarly prepared. Taken every hour for 12 doses, this provides an intake of 240 Gm. each of protein food and carbohydrate. The disadvantage of preparing and keeping larger volumes is the danger of bacterial growth, since amino acids mixtures are excellent culture media.

Parenteral administration of protein should be used when complete oral feeding is impossible, contraindicated, or difficult, as for example, (1) during inability to take any food by mouth because of intestinal obstruction, vomiting, severe diarrhea, or high intestinal fistula; (2) when gastrointestinal rest is essential, as after certain abdominal operations, peritonitis or severe gastroenteritis; or (3) where supplementary feeding is necessary for certain patients unable to take large amounts of protein by mouth. Adequately hydrolyzed protein is the most physiologic, convenient, and inexpensive preparation for this purpose. Many such preparations are available and must be administered according to directions contained in the manufacturer's package. Nausea and vomiting are frequently produced by those hydrolysates containing aspartic and glutamic acids; removal of these relatively unessential amino acids usually eliminates undesirable side effects and permits more rapid administration. Increased speed of administration is an important factor to facilitate the daily administration of large amounts of protein hydrolysates as 5 to 10% solutions in distilled water, saline, or glucose solution. A representative 24-hour I.V. diet is as follows: Distilled water, alternated with saline, to a total of 3,000 cc. containing 150 to 300 Gm. of glucose and 100 to 150 Gm. of amino acids mixture or hydrolyzed protein. This may be given in the form of 5 or 10% amino acid mixture in 5 or 10% glucose in saline or water. In addition, twice the minimal daily requirement of the various vitamins should be given parenterally (*see* NUTRITIONAL DEFICIENCIES).

Care must be taken to avoid the too rapid administration of fluid I.V., or of too large quantities of water and salt in a patient whose circulation is already embarrassed. As soon as possible, partial and then complete oral feeding should be instituted in order to bring the caloric intake up to normal.

HYPERVITAMINOSIS

A condition produced by quantitative extension of the physiologic action of vitamins into pathologic degrees, induced by excessive vitamin intake.

Generally speaking, the vitamins are nontoxic and relatively nonallergenic. Hypervitaminosis is not to be confused with hypersensitivity (allergic reactions) or with physiologic side reactions (e.g., vasomotor flushes from niacin), both of which may occur with small doses. Hypervitaminosis may result from huge doses of certain vitamins, as has been demonstrated in animal experiments. Toxic symptoms did not appear until 600 to 60,000 times the amounts required for optimal nutrition had been administered. The suggested safe upper limits of daily dosage for the adult human are as follows:

Vitamin K	12 mg.
Vitamin D	80,000 units
Niacin	5,000 mg.
Thiamine	2,500 mg.
Vitamin A	300,000 units
Pyridoxine	6,000 mg.

In treating deficiency disease, these amounts are seldom if ever exceeded or even approached, except in refractory rickets (*see* VITAMIN D DEFICIENCY). It is in vitamin therapy for nondeficiency disease that hypervitaminosis may result, or when overzealous patients take many times the prescribed dose for prevention or treatment of vitamin deficiency. Human instances of hypervitaminosis have been reported with vitamins D and A.

HYPERVITAMINOSIS D

As little as 50,000 u. of vitamin D daily may produce toxicity within 1 to 4 weeks, while two-thirds of the patients taking 300,000 u. daily may show no toxic symptoms under prolonged administration. Serum calcium elevation (11 to 16 mg./100 cc.) is said to be a constant finding when toxic symptoms occur and frequent serum determinations should be made in all patients receiving large doses of vitamin D for nondeficiency disease. The first symptoms are anorexia, nausea and vomiting. These are followed by polyuria, polydipsia, weakness, nervousness, and pruritus. Renal function is impaired, as evidenced early by low specific gravity of the urine, albuminuria and casts, and later by nitrogen retention. Metastatic calcifications, particularly in the kidneys, are being reported with increasing frequency. They represent a real hazard in the use of vitamin D as a drug in large doses. The symptoms sometimes simulate hyperparathyroidism. Localized osteoporosis may occur and simulate metastatic malignancy.

Treatment consists of discontinuing administration of the vitamin and placing the patient on a low calcium diet. If kidney damage or metastatic calcification has occurred, the damage often is irreversible.

HYPERVITAMINOSIS A

This condition is rare and thus far has been described only in young children receiving more than 100,000 u. daily. Sparse coarse hair, disappearance of the eyebrows, and a dry rough skin are early signs. Craving for butter has been noted. A hemorrhagic diathesis sometimes develops, most frequently under the periosteum, causing painful localized swellings. In addition, the bones become decalcified. Hepatomegaly without splenomegaly is frequent.

Laboratory findings include hypoprothrombinemia, accounting for the hemorrhages; high blood levels of vitamin A—over 100 micrograms (300 u.)/100 cc.; and, because of the liver damage, increased serum lipids; and increased serum phosphatase. Signs and symptoms promptly disappear within a week to a month after stopping vitamin A. Excessive ingestion of carotene has not been found to produce hypervitaminosis A, apparently because the carotene is not sufficiently converted into vitamin A. However, the serum content of carotene may become so high as to cause clinical carotinemia, a condition in which the skin takes on a deep yellow color suggestive of jaundice, but which is otherwise symptomless.

Differential diagnosis includes hypervitaminosis D (ruled out by a normal serum calcium) and other diseases causing hepatomegaly and hypoprothrombinemia. Treatment is by ceasing to administer vitamin A and giving vitamin K (℞ 46) if hemorrhagic manifestations are present. Vitamin K is of no value if symptoms are not due to hypoprothrombinemia. The prognosis is excellent.

HYPERPROTEINEMIA

A relative or absolute increase in the amount of plasma protein. Its presence is suggestive of a variety of conditions and is therefore of diagnostic aid. Hyperproteinemia of itself does not cause clinical manifestation.

Dehydration and hemoconcentration will produce a relative increase in both the albumin and globulin fractions of the plasma proteins. Severe diarrhea or vomiting may result in total protein values as high as 10 Gm./100 cc. Pyloric obstruction, intestinal fistulas, heat exhaustion, shock, and burns also cause hyperproteinemia secondary to hemoconcentration.

Hyperproteinemia due to an increase in the plasma globulin occurs commonly in multiple myeloma, sarcoidosis, lymphogranuloma venereum, and in chronic bacterial infections such as subacute bacterial endocarditis, osteomyelitis, empyema and lung abscess. Hyperglobulinemia is not infrequently seen in cirrhosis of the liver, syphilis, tuberculosis, leprosy, malaria, rheumatic fever, rheumatoid arthritis, disseminated lupus erythematosus, periarteritis nodosa, the leukemias, trypanosomiasis, schistosomiasis, filariasis, and kala-azar.

An increase in the albumin fraction alone seldom occurs and is of no clinical significance.

SPRUE

A chronic deficiency disease characterized, when fully developed, by weakness, weight loss, diarrhea with excess fat in the sour, foamy stools, flatulence, glossitis, pigmentation of the skin, impaired absorption of glucose and fat-soluble materials, a low serum carotene value and a macrocytic anemia with megaloblastic arrest of bone marrow. All such findings are not necessarily present in milder cases.

Etiology and Incidence

While sprue is classed as a deficiency disease, it not infrequently develops in only one member of a family, all on the same diet. Microorganisms have apparently been excluded as having a causal role.

Sprue and pernicious anemia exhibit similarities, but the gastrointestinal absorptive defect in sprue, as well as other features, separates the two clinically, and it is concluded that they differ etiologically. When of the same degree, the anemias of the two diseases may be identical, the hematologic response to liver extract, vitamin B_{12} and pteroylglutamic (folic) acid similar, and the bone marrows indistinguishable. Patients with sprue, however, usually do not exhibit achlorhydria, and many retain the intrinsic factor in the gastric juice. (This factor is almost invariably absent in pernicious anemia.) The diet in Puerto Rico, where sprue is common, often is deficient in the extrinsic factor. Thus, patients presumably develop sprue either because of poor gastrointestinal absorption, or inadequate intake of the extrinsic factor, or both.

Sprue occurs sporadically in South America, Africa, Europe, and throughout the United States. It is endemic in many tropical regions.

Symptoms and Signs

The onset usually is insidious, flatulence and loss of appetite being first noted, followed by diarrhea, glossitis, weakness, and loss of weight; however, this sequence of development may vary. The stools characteristically are bulky, frothy, and foul smelling, but even in fully developed cases such stools may be absent. Usually, the abdomen is distended and unduly prominent, since the remainder of the body may become greatly emaciated. Apathy and listlessness are usual.

There often is diffuse brown pigmentation, particularly over the exposed areas of the trunk and extremities. The tongue may be red, "beefy," sore, and tender. Although the patient may be pale from anemia, the lemon tint frequently seen in pernicious anemia is lacking. Purpura of the skin and mucous membrane is seen occasionally, and hemorrhages into the ocular fundi may occur. The blood pressure usually is low, systolic values falling as low as 80.

Paresthesias are not uncommon, but the definite entity, subacute combined degeneration of the cord, so frequently a complication of pernicious anemia, is rarely encountered in sprue.

Laboratory Findings

The absorptive defect in sprue is amply reflected in the laboratory data, when these are characteristic.

The upper limit for normal fecal fat is 20% by dry weight. This is exceeded in sprue when the diet contains ordinary amounts of fat, but less may be found if the diet has been relatively fat-free.

The oral glucose tolerance curve is flat, the maximum rise seldom exceeding 40 mg., while the I.V. glucose tolerance curve is normal. Serum carotene levels usually are low (carotene is the fat-soluble precursor of vitamin A). A flat curve is found after giving vitamin A orally. Often, the serum calcium and phosphorus levels are low and, in severe cases, a vitamin K deficiency (hypoprothrombinemia) has been described.

X-ray examination of the gastrointestinal tract discloses loss of the normal "feathering" of the small intestine, together with clumping or puddling of the barium.

The anemia, a component of the fully developed syndrome, usually is of macrocytic type, but it may be microcytic and hypochromic. When macrocytic, there generally is an associated leukopenia, relative lymphocytosis, and thrombopenia, as in pernicious anemia.

Diagnosis

A trend is noted toward applying the term idiopathic steatorrhea when patients exhibit only the gastrointestinal symptoms found in sprue, the term sprue being reserved for the complete syndrome. No difference seems to exist between sprue as seen tropically and nontropically, and the fully developed disease offers little difficulty in diagnosis. From the laboratory standpoint, anemia, increased fecal fat, flat oral glucose tolerance curve, and a low serum carotene level, are the findings essential for the diagnosis.

The anemia of sprue may closely simulate that of "pernicious anemia of pregnancy," so-called tropical macrocytic anemia, and pernicious anemia. Of these, only sprue has an associated absorptive defect. The achlorhydria in pernicious anemia, plus the usual increase in the icteric index, further aids in differentiation.

In sprue, fat alone is increased in the stools, while in pancreatic disease there is an increase of nitrogen and a loss of the pancreatic enzymes, as well. Celiac disease occurs almost exclusively in children, and is further differentiated by the absence, in most cases, of macrocytic anemia and glossitis. Pigmentation, together with arterial hypotension and weakness, may suggest Addison's disease. However, neither pigmentation of the buccal mucosa nor the serum electrolyte disturbance characteristic of advanced Addison's disease is seen in sprue.

Prognosis

Therapeutic failure most often occurs where only part of the sprue syndrome is present, which raises the question of accurate diagnosis. Conversely, the best results are to be expected when all manifestations of sprue are present. The prognosis also varies with the duration of the disease, being poorest when the condition has existed for a number of years before treatment is begun.

In favorable cases, appetite and weight usually are regained rapidly with adequate treatment, and the diarrhea soon ceases. Early relief of the hematologic abnormalities and glossitis also can be expected. However, improvement of the various absorptive defects occurs slowly, and may not be complete.

Relapses are not infrequent, and the patient tends to respond less well to treatment following each relapse. However, with adequate treatment during acute phases, and full cooperation subsequently as to diet, hygiene, and perhaps a change in climate, most cases may be restored to a reasonably normal existence. Some are completely cured.

Treatment

When the manifestations of the disease are severe, bed care is indicated. The banana diet, found useful in the past, no longer is advocated. Instead, a low fat, high vitamin, high protein diet, rich in lean meats, is given. In the initial phases of treatment, supplemental vitamin therapy is advisable, in particular vitamin D (℞ 48), plus calcium lactate (℞ 23) and phosphate (℞ 24) when the serum levels of calcium and phosphorus are low. The intestinal absorption of dietary fats and of oil-soluble vitamins may be aided by the use of a wetting agent, such as the polyoxyethylene derivative of sorbitan monooleate, given as 1.5 Gm. doses with each meal (R 49).

Liver extract (R 1), pteroylglutamic (folic) acid (R 5, 6), and crystalline vitamin B_{12} are valuable and effective therapeutic agents. In sprue, 15 mg. of pteroylglutamic acid daily by mouth, or the same dosage by I.M. injection, has been shown to bring about complete relief of severe grades of macrocytic anemia, rapid general improvement in the sense of well-being, rapid relief of glossitis and diarrhea, and marked gain in weight. The reticulocyte response in all respects is similar to that seen in pernicious anemia following the administration of liver extract. In commencing therapy, probably both oral and parenteral administration of the pteroylglutamic acid is advisable.

Larger amounts of liver extract (R 1) may be necessary for sprue than are required for the treatment of pernicious anemia. Because of the gastrointestinal absorptive defects, I.M. administration of liver extract is preferable. After an initial injection of 30 to 50 u., the dose is repeated in 3 or 4 days, followed by 30 u. or more given weekly thereafter.

A single subcut. or I.M. injection of 15 to 30 micrograms of crystalline vitamin B_{12}, such as Cobione (R 4), usually is effective in inducing a remission. This dose should be repeated at 15- to 30-day intervals when needed to maintain remission.

Where the anemia is hypochromic, or becomes so during treatment, iron is indicated. Ferrous sulfate (R 7), 0.3 Gm. 3 times daily after meals, usually is effective. Hypoprothrombinemia is combated with menadione (R 46), 2 mg. I.M. daily, until it is corrected. Blood transfusions rarely are required, although in elderly persons, particularly, they may be needed occasionally. Maintenance therapy with liver extract, pteroylglutamic acid, or crystalline vitamin B_{12} usually is necessary in sprue.

CELIAC DISEASE

A chronic intestinal disorder manifesting itself between the ages of 6 months and 6 years and characterized by steatorrhea, anorexia, arrest of growth, and deficiency symptoms.

Etiology and Pathology

The etiology is unknown. In some patients, a deficiency in the vitamin B complex may be responsible. No specific pathology has been established. Pathologic changes which may be found are due to secondary malnutrition or infection.

Symptoms and Signs

The onset is insidious, occurring between the ages of 6 months and 6 years, rarely otherwise. Irritability may be the first clinical manifestation, followed by anorexia, failure to gain weight, and weakness. The abdomen is protuberant, the stools are bulky, loose, pale, frothy, with a very foul odor due to faulty absorption of fat and carbohydrate from the intestine. Occasionally, there may be alternating diarrhea and constipation. Symptoms and signs of secondary nutritional deficiencies (q.v.) may appear. The disease is characterized by remissions and exacerbations.

Laboratory examination of the feces demonstrates increased content of fat and carbohydrate. An oral test dose of vitamin A will be poorly absorbed, as shown by measuring plasma levels 4 to 6 hours after administration. The amount of pancreatic enzymes within the duodenum is normal. The glucose tolerance curve is flat.

DIFFERENTIAL DIAGNOSIS

Celiac Disease	Carbohydrate Intolerance	Pancreatic Deficiency
Age		
6 mos. to 6 yrs.	3 mos. to 1 yr.	Congenital
Abdomen		
Protuberant	Normal or protuberant	Protuberant
Metabolic Dysfunction		
Carbohydrate, fat	Carbohydrate	Starch, fat, protein
Nature of Feces		
Bulky, loose, foul, frothy	Bulky, foul, frothy	Bulky, foul, formed
Fecal Fat		
Elevated	Normal	Elevated
Fecal Starch		
Normal or slightly elevated	Elevated	Elevated
Pancreatic Enzymes		
Normal	Normal or decreased amylase	Absent

Prognosis

With treatment, recovery occurs in most cases after a prolonged period of remissions and exacerbations. Infection and dietary indiscretion tend to precipitate a relapse. From 1 to 2 years may be required for complete recovery, which may be assumed when a patient on a full diet has consistently normal stools. Death from uncomplicated celiac disease is very uncommon.

Treatment

Several dietary regimens have been successfully used in the treatment of celiac disease. Most such diets are high in protein and low in fat. Small amounts of simple sugars also may be given, such as corn syrup, glucose, invert sugar (honey, ripe banana), and levulose. A satisfactory dietary regimen is as follows:

Initially, the patient should receive frequent feedings of dilute protein milk or skimmed milk with added casein. Banana powder may be added to sweeten. When improvement occurs, in a few days or weeks, additional proteins and sugars may be added gradually, including ground lean meat, cottage cheese, egg white, ground raw apple, and puréed vegetables. The speed with which new foods may be allowed depends on the patient's improvement and tolerance to previously added items. After about 6 months of well-being, a full diet is gradually achieved, by adding one new food at a time. Starchy foods are added last (potatoes, rice, macaroni products, bread, puddings).

Throughout therapy, vitamin supplements should be given daily to combat nutritional deficiencies (q.v.). Some patients show a striking response to the use of crude liver extract (R 2), 2 cc. I.M. every other day until improvement occurs, after which an oral preparation (R 3) may be utilized. The intestinal absorption of fat may be aided by the use of a wetting agent, such as the polyoxyethylene derivative of sorbitan monooleate, given as 1.5 Gm. doses with each meal (R 49).

A patient in a severe relapse may require parenteral fluids and alimentation to combat acidosis, dehydration, and starvation.

GOUT

A disturbance in purine metabolism associated with recurrent attacks of acute arthritis, which may become chronic and deforming.

Etiology and Incidence

Gout occurs most often in middle life, but may begin at any age. The ratio of affected males to females is reported to be about 19:1. The disease is of unknown etiology, and has been wrongly ascribed to dietary indiscretions, excessive intake of certain alcoholic beverages, a sedentary existence, or exposure to lead. The incidence is highest among middle-aged men without showing racial or national preference. A hereditary factor may be apparent in some cases.

Pathologic Physiology

Uric acid is the end product of purine metabolism and is excreted in the urine. The nucleoproteins in the body are the principal source of endogenous uric acid, while ingested substances such as liver, kidney, thymus, pancreas, and sardines are the sources of exogenous purine. The level of serum uric acid in gouty patients usually is above 6.0 mg./100 cc. (normal 3 to 5), a level manifested by no other arthritic condition and few other morbid states. Deposition of sodium urate in soft and bony tissue eventually resulting in the formation of tophi, is a distinguishing morphologic feature. Urate deposits are more likely to develop in avascular than vascular tissues. The common sites are cartilage, epiphyseal portions of bone, synovial membrane, bursas, ligaments and tendons. In advanced cases all the articular and periarticular structures of several joints may be riddled by urate tophi, leading to changes suggestive of rheumatoid arthritis or of osteoarthritis.

Symptoms and Signs

Acute Gouty Arthritis: The acute attack may appear without warning or it may be precipitated by minor trauma as from ill-fitting shoes or tight gloves, by overindulgence in food or alcohol, by surgical procedures, infections, or treatment with liver extract, insulin, or mercurial diuretics. Acute articular pain, often of nocturnal onset, usually is the first symptom. The metatarsophalangeal joint of the great toe seems to be the most susceptible, but the instep, ankle, and knee also are common sites. Two or more joints may be affected at the same time. The pain often is moderate at first but soon becomes progressively more excruciating due to effusion into the joint space and edema of the surrounding soft tissues. The joint is swollen and exquisitely tender and the skin tense, hot, shining, and of a red or purplish color. Soft-tissue tophi rarely are the sites of acute symptoms. Systemic reactions to acute gouty arthritis include fever, headache, tachycardia, chills, malaise, anorexia, oliguria, and leukocytosis.

Mild attacks usually last only a few days but, if untreated, may persist with intermissions for several weeks. Proper treatment is the most important limiting factor. Subsidence of the acute arthritis is manifested by regression of local and systemic symptoms. Full function in the affected joints may not return for 2 or 3 weeks. Local desquamation of the skin often follows a prolonged attack.

The asymptomatic intervals between acute attacks vary considerably but tend to become shorter as the disease progresses. Eventually, there may be several attacks each year. Permanent deformity results only after numerous attacks over a period of years.

Chronic Gout: A diagnosis of chronic deforming gout should not be made until irreparable changes are apparent by X-ray as well as by physical examination. There is pronounced limitation of motion, or ankylosis, often involving many joints of the hands or feet, or both. Occasionally, the shoulder, sacroiliac, or sternoclavicular joints are invaded. However, only a small percentage of patients become bed-ridden. In advanced cases, skin sinuses may communicate with urate deposits and discharge chalky material. At any time during the chronic deforming stage, acute articular attacks similar to those that preceded it may occur.

Complications and Associated Diseases

Renal involvement is a frequent and serious extra-articular complication. The pathologic lesion is nonspecific and may give symptoms suggestive of arteriolar nephrosclerosis, chronic glomerulonephritis, or pyelonephritis. Albuminuria and a few formed elements in the centrifuged specimen may be noted early in the disease, with or without a history of renal colic and the passage of urate gravel or stones. The inability to concentrate solids, delayed excretion of phenolsulfonphthalein dye, and poor concentration of a radiopaque dye during pyelography follow. Evidence of renal involvement characteristically may be noted for many years before renal insufficiency ensues. Even then, the nonprotein nitrogen of the serum may be elevated above normal for one or more years before death from uremia occurs. The pathogenesis of the renal lesion in gout is not known. Since the solubility of urate is near the maximum in blood, one explanation presumes that, during resorption of fluid from the glomerular filtrate, the sodium urate is precipitated in the renal tubules causing mechanical damage and acting as a nucleus for urate calculi. Several clinical entities are thought to have some connection with gout; i.e., lead intoxication, diabetes mellitus, obesity, leukemia, polycythemia vera, pernicious anemia, hemolytic jaundice, purpura hemorrhagica, hemophilia, and Paget's disease. The association is infrequent and no satisfactory explanation is apparent except in leukemia and polycythemia vera, conditions in which an increased formation of purine substances may lead to urate deposits in joints and to acute articular attacks.

Diagnosis

Gout may be suspected even before the first attack if two clues are noticed: a family history of gout and the urinary excretion of a urate calculus. The serum uric acid should be determined in any patient who passes such a calculus. Recurring attacks of acute joint pain with asymptomatic intervals in an otherwise healthy person are highly suggestive. An increase of serum urate is significant, but this also may be found in renal insufficiency, leukemia, polycythemia vera, starvation, and certain acute infections such as pneumonia. Since renal insufficiency may develop in a patient with gout, the uric acid level should be cautiously interpreted in patients with joint disease and renal impairment, especially those over 50. The response of an acute gouty joint to colchicine usually is conclusive. Patients suspected of having gout should be given full doses for possible therapeutic benefit as well as for diagnostic information. Nongouty arthritis does not respond to colchicine. Tophi in the ear alae are pathognomonic of gout. Late in the disease, subcutaneous tophi, sometimes as large as a golf ball, may appear about many joints. Chemical identification of the contents of a tophus is recommended. Sodium urate deposits must attain a size of approximately 5 mm. in diameter before they are visible by X-ray, and even then the X-ray shadow is nonspecific. The roentgenograms in rheumatoid arthritis, osteoarthritis, Boeck's sarcoid, multiple gangliomas, multiple myeloma, hyperparathyroidism, Paget's disease, chronic trauma, and syphilis of the bone resemble those of gout in some respects. The presence of demonstrable tophi in bone indicates irreparable joint involvement and usually means that several acute exacerbations have occurred at the site.

An acutely septic joint may be confused with a gouty joint, but the serum content of uric acid should settle the question. Acute rheumatic fever with joint involvement and polyarticular rheumatism may simulate gout, particularly in younger persons. Acute rheumatic fever has a predilection for large joints, gout for the small ones. Joint involvement in rheumatoid arthritis tends to be symmetrical, the duration of a single attack is longer, and the onset is more gradual than in gout. Here again the blood uric acid may be the determining factor. Heberden's nodes of osteoarthritis may resemble gouty tophi but are not associated with acute joint symptoms.

Prognosis

The condition is chronic and progressive, but the rate of progression is an unknown factor, which may be further modified by treatment. The younger the patient, the greater the tendency to anatomic involvement. Advanced polyarticular changes seldom are found in patients whose first attack of acute gout occurred after the age of 50. The prognosis for renal complications is even less definitive. However, since renal lesions are a greater threat to life than the articular ones, careful attention should be given to the efficiency of the kidneys. There appears to be no direct relation between the pathologic changes in the kidney and the severity of the joint disease.

Treatment

Although there is no known cure for gout, proper therapy may control its manifestations. Recently, dramatic and prompt remissions of acute gouty arthritis have been achieved following therapy with the adrenocortical hormone, cortisone, or with the adrenocorticotropic hormone (ACTH); however, final evaluation of these or similar agents must await further studies.

Acute attack: Colchicine (℞ 25) is specific in the treatment of gout and the response to it is dramatic. The dose is 0.5 mg. (gr. $\frac{1}{120}$) by mouth every 1 to 2 hours until complete relief is obtained or until diarrhea or vomiting results. Thereafter most patients learn from experience the proper number of tablets to take in each attack. Severe episodes may require from 8 to 16 tablets; the average is approximately 10. Administration of the required dose should be continuous, even if the patient must be awakened through the night. It is not sufficient to take half of the anticipated effective dose one day and half the next. A sedative (℞ 29) may be given to enable the patient to return to sleep between doses. Subsidence of joint pains usually begins after 12 hours of treatment and should be complete within 24 to 48 hours if sufficient colchicine has been taken. Rarely, an attack is not materially benefited by the first course of colchicine, in which case a second course should be started 2 or 3 days later. If colchicine therapy is repeated earlier, untoward symptoms may develop before enough has been administered to relieve the joint symptoms. When treatment is carried to the point of gastrointestinal distress and then discontinued, camphorated opium tincture (R 30) may be given to alleviate these symptoms. Salicylates (R 28) aid in the excretion of uric acid and have an analgesic effect upon painful joints.

Bed rest, abundant fluid intake, and a soft diet are indicated in addition to specific therapy. The joints should be put at rest under a cradle as early as possible after onset of acute symptoms, but active function should be resumed without undue delay after the attack. Abundant fluid intake serves a dual purpose by combating dehydration and decreasing the precipitation of urate in the kidneys. A soft diet, rich in carbohydrate, is recommended as for other febrile disturbances. Codeine (R 26) or even morphine (R 27) may be given occasionally if the pain is severe and not controllable by other means (CAUTION! Habituation).

Intercritical period: Between attacks attention should be paid to adequate exercise, a liberal intake of food and fluids, proper medication, recognition of premonitory symptoms, and avoidance of precipitating stimuli. A low purine diet is advisable (see DIETS). Minimum fluid output should approximate 2 liters daily. Alcohol (in patients accustomed to it) should be taken in moderation rather than forbidden. The recognition of prodromal symptoms is particularly helpful in certain cases. On their first appearance, one or more colchicine tablets should be taken. An extended course is unnecessary if the attack does not materialize within a few hours. If joint symptoms progress and a full-blown attack seems imminent, colchicine should be continued without interruption until an adequate amount has been taken. The need for continued vigilance should be stressed. A few hours' delay in beginning treatment may increase the severity as well as the duration of an acute episode. All patients having more than one attack of acute gout a year should take some colchicine regularly. The dosage may vary from 1 or 2 of the 0.5 mg. tablets a week to 1 or 2 a day. No untoward effects have been observed from prolonged ingestion of the drug. Tolerance does not develop and, if an acute attack supervenes, the full course seems to be as effective as for patients who have not previously taken colchicine. The gouty person should never be without a supply. Salicylates (R 28) have been recommended in intercritical gout because they possess diuretic properties helpful in the excretion of urates; they should be taken for several days each week. Although cinchophen enjoys wide use, it is neither specific for gout nor more effective than salicylates in promoting the excretion of urate. Since cinchophen in large amounts may be toxic to some patients, its use is condemned by many physicians.

Chronic Deforming Gouty Arthritis: A full course of colchicine therapy is indicated for acute symptoms irrespective of the extent of the chronic deformity. Low grade symptoms may persist at other times despite apparently adequate treatment of the acute episode. Such symptoms are attributed to extensive structural damage rather than to mild incipient acute attacks. One to 3 of the 0.5 mg. colchicine tablets should be taken daily without interruption for this condition. Exercise is desirable if the joints permit. Heat and massage are of little value.

Surgical treatment, which has no place in the acute attack, may be of great help in the rehabilitation of chronically deformed joints. Excision of unsightly tophi for cosmetic reasons presents no problem, and small tophi of the hands or feet that interfere with the wearing of gloves or shoes should be removed. Tophaceous deposits in muscles or tendons that hamper free movement of the fingers and hands should be excised. Any discharging sinus associated with a tophaceous deposit should be repaired. Ankylosis and immobility of the fingers or toes may be ameliorated by radical surgery. Incisions heal remarkably well if carried to the point of normal tissue. Sepsis rarely develops. However, surgery may precipitate a postoperative gouty attack, and colchicine should be given prophylactically. A satisfactory dosage is 3 colchicine tablets (0.5 mg. each) for 2 days before operation and for 3 days after operation. The incidence of postoperative gouty arthritis usually is low with such a regimen.

OBESITY

That physical state in which excessive fat is stored in the body.

Incidence and Etiology

Ordinary obesity is quite common, especially in middle life, and is more frequent in women than in men. Extreme obesity or localized accumulation of body fat is less common and suggests unusual etiologic factors.

Although heredity may play a contributory role, there only is one immediate cause of obesity: a caloric intake persistently exceeding the caloric output. Since the capacity of the body to store protein and carbohydrate is strictly limited, excess food in any form is converted into and stored as fat. Obesity often is divided into exogenous and endogenous types. Actually, all obesity is both exogenous (due to excess food, absolute or relative) and endogenous (since the caloric imbalance results from a disturbed body mechanism, psychologic or physiologic). Thus, even if simple overeating or lack of exercise is the only discoverable cause, some abnormal state, physical or mental, or both, must underlie these aberrations.

Physiologic factors: Digestion and absorption are not more efficient in obese persons; neither is lipophilia (extraordinary ability of the body to retain fat) demonstrable. Local factors may be of importance when the adiposity has a characteristic distribution: in lipomatosis, lipodystrophy, Cushing's syndrome (q.v.).

The total metabolism of obese persons is higher, not lower, than normal. The specific dynamic action of foods is not significantly lowered in obese persons, although it may be somewhat diminished during a weight-gaining phase.

Although endocrine disorders do not primarily cause obesity, they may favor its development by encouraging either an increased food intake or a decreased energy output. Lesions of the hypothalamus may produce obesity. Pituitary disease does not predispose to adiposity unless the hypothalamus also is functionally or organically injured. Severe hypopituitarism does not cause obesity but results in pituitary cachexia (Simmonds' disease). Fröhlich's syndrome and other types of adiposogenital dystrophy characterized by adiposity and hypogonadism apparently are due to hypothalamic disturbance with associated pituitary malfunction and consequent gonadal inadequacy. Hypothyroidism rarely is a cause of obesity. The B.M.R. in the great majority of obese persons is normal. Hyperinsulinism may cause excess hunger, high food intake, and resultant obesity. Cushing's syndrome and hyperadrenocorticism are characterized by obesity. Removal or destructive disease of the gonads favors obesity. Gradual sex failure at the male or female climacteric is a predisposing factor. The localization of fat deposits is at least suggestively characteristic in certain endocrine disorders: in hypothyroidism, about the face, neck, supraclavicular regions, wrists and ankles; in adrenocorticism, face, neck, and trunk; in hypogonadism, buttocks, hips, and thighs.

Limitation of energy output from any cause favors obesity. Factors include laziness due to psychologic factors or organic disease; enforced inactivity during treatment of heart disease, tuberculosis, fractures, poliomyelitis, and the like.

Psychologic factors: Habit, improper childhood training, nervous tensions, frustrations and dissatisfactions may be expressed in increased food intake or decreased physical activity. Pleasure in eating may become a dominant personality trait and may serve as a substitute when social, business, or sexual desires are unsatisfied. Obesity itself may be used as a weapon against undesired contacts or activities and to justify withdrawal from normal pursuits due to loss of physical attractiveness and efficiency. Thus, obesity may result from either defensive or offensive neuroses, and in either case a vicious circle is apt to be established. "Problem children" often become obese and use the condition to demand special attention. In the great majority of cases both physiologic and psychologic abnormalities are present.

Pathology

In obesity, the amount of fat stored in normal sites is excessive, and fat accumulates in abnormal places. In extreme cases subcut. fat may exceed 10 cm. in thickness. Large amounts of fat may be found in retroperitoneal tissues, omentum, mesentery, perirenal tissues, mediastinum, and pericardium. Fatty infiltration may occur in the pancreas and in skeletal and heart muscle. The liver may be enlarged, many hepatic cells containing large fat vacuoles.

Symptoms and Signs

Usually, the first symptoms noted are fatigue and dyspnea. The legs and back ache, the knees and feet hurt. Maceration and infection of the skin may occur beneath rolls of fat. Signs of hypertension, heart failure, arthritis, diabetes, and other conditions to which obesity predisposes are apt to develop later.

Diagnosis

Excessive fat is obvious, but the degree of obesity as compared with normal weight should be ascertained. Etiologic factors should be determined, if possible, since successful therapy depends upon knowing what to treat. History, physical characteristics, family background, and environmental influences must be evaluated. Special laboratory tests often valuable are: skull X-rays (for pituitary disease or hyperostosis), B.M.R., blood cholesterol, serum iodine, sugar tolerance, water and salt balance determinations, ECG and hormone studies. Psychiatric evaluation often is rewarding.

Prognosis

Obesity, if present for many months or years, always causes complications, and statistically it increases the mortality rate and lowers life expectancy. At age 45 to 50, in persons 10 lb. overweight, there is an elevation above the average death rate of 8%; 20 lb., 18%; 30 lb., 28%; 50 lb., 56%. Obese persons succumb to cardiovascular-renal disease about 60% more frequently than persons of normal weight. Corpulence likewise results in higher death rates from diabetes, nephritis, pneumonia, and postsurgical complications. Even death from accidents or suicide is considerably more common in the obese, owing to psychologic factors.

Long-standing adiposity predisposes to diabetes, hypertension and myocardial failure, degenerative arthritis of the back and knees, orthopedic foot troubles, venous varicosities and leg ulcers. Menstrual disorders may occur but usually are secondary to the same endocrinologic or psychologic factors that cause the obesity.

If the etiologic factors can be discovered, proper treatment instituted, and the cooperation of the patient secured, the results are excellent in early obesity but, in cases of long duration, complications may continue despite weight loss.

Prophylaxis and Treatment

Whenever a predisposition to obesity is evident, proper eating habits should be established, and unless there is a contraindication, moderate regular exercise should be encouraged. In mild, uncomplicated cases, a regimen of low caloric diet (q.v.) and exercise is sufficient. In other cases multiple forms of therapy—physical, psychologic, drug, and hormone—often must be employed.

Treatment may be divided into two phases: removal of etiologic factors and elimination of excess fat stores. If hypogonadism is a factor, gonadotropins (B 40) or gonadal hormones (B 36, 38, 39) are helpful. When hypothyroidism (q.v.) is present, desiccated thyroid (B 35) is indicated. In cases of hyperadrenocorticism or pancreatic adenoma, operation may be advisable. When water retention is a factor salt limitation and diuretics should be employed. Psychologic and environmental influences should be analyzed and adjusted. Drugs to decrease appetite (B 47) may prove effective.

Regular exercise, such as walking, swimming and golf, is helpful in increasing caloric output but is even more valuable for improving muscle tone, morale, and general health. The value of exercise in weight reduction is limited, since activity stimulates appetite and it takes a walk of 2½ miles to consume the energy (120 calories) represented by 1 slice of bread.

Amphetamine sulfate (B 47), which will increase psychic and physical activity in many patients, also may increase energy expenditure without elevating the B.M.R. Moreover, when given before meals it diminishes appetite. If given after noon it may cause insomnia. Dinitrophenol accelerates metabolism, but it is a toxic drug and should never be used. Desiccated thyroid gland should be given only in cases of hypothyroidism.

Diet restriction is always necessary, no matter what caused the obesity. Limitation to 10 calories/Kg. of ideal body weight, if the patient is inactive, or 15 to 20 calories/Kg. body wt./day with moderate activity and work usually is successful. Such diets would allow 700, 1,050, and 1,400 calories, respectively, per day for persons with an ideal weight of 150 lbs. The protein allowance should be liberal and fats minimal. Carbohydrate should be supplied chiefly in the low-carbohydrate bulky fruits and vegetables (*see* Low Caloric Diet). Moderate restriction of salt and water is advisable if fluid retention is present. Supplements of vitamins A, D, and B should be prescribed since foods containing these vitamins are restricted.

DIABETES MELLITUS

A chronic disorder of carbohydrate metabolism due to inadequate endogenous production or utilization of insulin and characterized by hyperglycemia, glycosuria, polyuria, polydipsia, polyphagia, pruritus, weakness, and loss of weight.

Etiology and Incidence

Damage of the insulin-producing cells of the islets of Langerhans, by causes as yet unknown, is responsible for most cases of diabetes mellitus. Some experiments have shown that continued hyperglycemia will produce such permanent damage, reducing the endogenous output of insulin. In certain cases the diabetic state results from increased insulin requirement by the tissue cells to maintain normal carbohydrate metabolism.

The simple concept of diabetes as a deficiency of the islet cell secretion can no longer be held. Clinical diabetes is more complex. For example, the diabetes in pancreatectomized dogs can be inhibited by removal of the pituitary, or of both adrenal glands.

Although the exact cause of diabetes has not been found, many contributory factors are known. Excessive consumption of sugar and fat, resulting in most instances in obesity (q.v.), has been indicted. Heredity apparently is important, since there is a familial history of diabetes in 25% of cases. Disorders of endocrine glands other than the pancreas often are associated with the development of diabetes mellitus. Infection is a common precursor to the appearance or exacerbation of the disease, probably making a latent diabetes manifest. Pancreatitis, generalized amyloidosis, infections of the gallbladder and biliary tract, pancreatic tumors, calculi, hemochromatosis, and trauma have each been responsible for occasional cases of diabetes.

The disease is most common in the 5th and 6th decades of life and in prosperous individuals. It is estimated that between 1 and 2% of the U.S. population are diabetics, with males and females equally affected.

Pathology and Pathologic Physiology

Hyaline degeneration, fibrosis, atrophy, and lymphocytic infiltration of the islets of Langerhans, singly or in combination, are found in the majority of diabetic patients at autopsy. Hydropic degeneration, a transient, early and reversible lesion in experimental animals, is an unusual autopsy finding. The liver in uncontrolled diabetes mellitus often is enlarged and fatty. The kidneys, particularly in diabetes of long duration, are likely to show intercapillary glomerulosclerosis. Glycogen deposition in the tubules also is seen. Vascular degeneration is common in those who have been diabetics for 15 or more years, as manifested clinically by the unusually high incidence of arteriosclerotic disease of the heart, retina, kidney, and lower extremities in these patients.

The primary defect in metabolism is a decreased ability to utilize carbohydrates by oxidation, conversion to fat, or storage as glycogen. This is due to diminished output or lowered effectiveness of insulin. While the exact mechanism has not been determined, it is known that insulin increases glycogen storage in the liver, and to a lesser extent in the muscles; it enhances the normal breakdown of glucose to CO_2 and water; it appears to aid indirectly in the synthesis of certain amino acids used in the production of body protein, and by increase of glucose utilization it decreases the loss of nitrogen from the body and the need for mobilization and oxidation of fat.

Because of decreased carbohydrate utilization in diabetes, the blood glucose becomes elevated. When the "renal threshold" of approximately 170 mg./100 cc. is attained, glycosuria ensues. With severe glycosuria there is polyuria and resultant thirst. If the process continues uncorrected, stored fat is made available so that the normal production of ketone bodies by the liver is greatly increased; this stage is known as ketosis (q.v.). With increasing severity of the process, body protein is lost as nitrogenous waste products. With the elevation of blood ketone concentration, acidosis (q.v.) develops, due in part to the loss of sodium and potassium with the acid ketone bodies (β hydroxybutyric and aceto-acetic acid) in the urine. The serum CO_2 content is decreased as a compensatory adjustment and serves as an indication of the severity of the acidosis. The reduction of the total salt concentration causes dehydration because water is excreted to maintain isotonicity in the tissues. Thus the patient is acidotic (due to reduction of the alkali reserve of the blood), hyperpneic, and dehydrated.

Symptoms and Signs

In children or young adults onset may be abrupt, whereas in older patients it usually is so insidious that evidence of diabetes may be discovered only on routine urine examination. When symptoms do exist they are so mild that they do not cause the patient to seek medical advice. Often diabetes mellitus is first discovered when a complication arises.

The major symptoms are polyuria, polydipsia, pruritus, polyphagia, weakness, and loss of weight. Large amounts of urine are passed day and night, resulting in excessive thirst and dryness of the skin. In many instances severe pruritus may be the most prominent symptom.

Diagnosis

The term "diabetes mellitus" signifies passage of sugar in the urine, and persistent glycosuria is presumptive evidence of this disease, though there are, of course, other causes of glycosuria. The diagnosis, therefore, depends on the blood sugar level. If the venous blood sugar, determined 1½ hours after a mixed meal, is greater than 150 mg., or the fasting value greater than 110 mg./100 cc., diabetes mellitus is the presumptive diagnosis. Postprandial values between 130 and 150 mg./100 cc. require further observation. In the absence of clinical symptoms and glycosuria, diabetes should never be diagnosed from a single determination of blood sugar, since a laboratory error or some unrecognized cause for temporary hyperglycemia may be present. The glucose tolerance test is needed only when the findings are equivocal. The diet for the 3 days before the test should include at least 250 Gm. of carbohydrate/day. Factors other than diabetes mellitus that cause a decrease in glucose tolerance include low carbohydrate diet, old age, prolonged bed rest, previous repeated insulin administration in a nondiabetic individual, gallbladder disease, hepatic cirrhosis, severe arteriosclerosis, hyperthyroidism, hyperpituitarism, chronic arthritis, acromegaly, pregnancy, apoplexy, and ulcerative colitis. If the impaired glucose tolerance associated with these conditions is pronounced and of more than temporary duration, the diagnosis of diabetes mellitus usually is justified. In many borderline cases an immediate exact diagnosis may be impossible and observation over months or years may be necessary. Diagnosis of diabetes during pregnancy is complicated by the low renal threshold and the lactosuria that occasionally occurs (renal glycosuria). Other benign meliturias will occasionally be found.

Course and Complications

The course of this chronic disease is extremely variable, but total recovery is rarely if ever seen. However, with improved methods of therapy the life expectancy of diabetic patients is steadily increasing. There now seems to be no reason to believe that adult diabetics cannot, under proper care, live as long as nondiabetics and carry on relatively normal activities. (The life expectancy of child diabetics is less than that of nondiabetic children.) Glucose tolerance usually improves under rigorous control of diabetes of recent onset or exacerbation, and following weight reduction of obese individuals through decreased caloric intake. In well controlled cases (i.e., blood sugar normal or nearly so), there are fewer complications. Serious complications due to the diabetes, other than ketosis and acidosis, usually develop only after several years of illness. The most important complications are the following:

Ketosis, acidosis and coma: The state of ketosis (q.v.) may be rapidly followed by acidosis (q.v.), which is the most serious acute complication of diabetes. It occurs when diabetes is uncontrolled owing to inadequate insulin dosage, acute inter-current infection, or prolonged irregularities of diet. Other, less frequent, precipitating factors are vomiting and diarrhea, trauma, surgical operations, diabetes of acute onset, thyrotoxi-cosis, and pregnancy. The symptoms of diabetic ketosis are lassitude, mental dullness, malaise, decrease in appetite, and heavy glycosuria and ketonuria. Hyperventilation and a fruity (acetone) odor of the breath are evident. If ketosis continues

DIFFERENTIAL DIAGNOSIS: DIABETIC COMA AND INSULIN SHOCK

	Diabetic Coma	Insulin Shock
History		
Food	Excessive	Insufficient
Insulin	Insufficient	Excessive
Onset	Gradual: days	Sudden, except with Protamine Zinc Insulin, 24 to 48 hours
Physical Examination		
Appearance	Extremely ill	Very weak
Skin	Dry and flushed	Moist and pale
Infection	Usually present	Absent
Fever	Frequent	Absent
Gastrointestinal Symptoms		
Mouth	Dry	Drooling
Thirst	Intense	Absent
Hunger	Absent	Intense
Vomiting	Common	Rare
Pain, abdominal	Frequent	Absent
Respiration	Exaggerated, air hunger	Normal or shallow
Breath	Acetone odor, usual	Acetone odor may be present
Blood Pressure	Low	Normal
Pulse	Weak and rapid	Full and bounding
Eyeballs	Soft	Normal
Vision	Dim	Diplopia
Tremor	Absent	Frequent
Convulsions	None	In late stages
Laboratory Findings		
Urine sugar	High	Absent in 2nd specimen
Diacetic acid	High	Absent in 2nd specimen
Blood sugar	Normal or high	Below 60 mg./100 cc.
CO_2 combining power	Below 20 vol./100 cc.	Above 50 vol./100 cc.
Course		
Improvement	Gradual, within 6 to 12 hours following use of insulin	Rapid following carbohydrate administration

unchecked, acidosis develops, causing an exacerbation of existing symptoms and the appearance of nausea, vomiting, polyuria, severe thirst, dizziness, deep breathing, and often coma. The urine contains large amounts of glucose, acetone, and diacetic acid. Leukocytosis and hemoconcentration are the rule. Diagnosis of diabetic coma (*see* table) is based on all these signs and symptoms plus a decrease or loss of consciousness. Coma also may result from such conditions as hypoglycemia (insulin shock), alcohol or drug poisoning, uremia, eclampsia, head trauma, intracranial vascular accident, meningeal infection, and acute pancreatitis with shock (*see* THE UNCONSCIOUS PATIENT).

Vascular complications: Arteriosclerosis appears in most diabetics after 15 years or more. Decreased arterial blood supply to the feet is common and often leads to intermittent claudication, cold feet, paresthesias, slow healing of injuries, local infection, ulceration, and gangrene. Coronary arteriosclerosis is frequent in older diabetic individuals. Punctate retinal hemorrhages and white exudates in the retina and macula may be present (the so-called diabetic retinitis). Clinical evidence of intercapillary glomerulosclerosis also may be seen in diabetes of long duration.

Diabetic neuritis: Early symptoms are numbness and tingling of the hands and feet, and other paresthesias. In severe cases, patellar and Achilles tendon reflexes are decreased or absent. Vibration sense may be diminished or lost. Pain is frequent; it is constant, aching in type, usually worse at night. Spinal fluid findings are not characteristic but the protein often is increased; occasionally there is pleocytosis. (Similar clinical and spinal fluid changes may be seen in patients with neuritis not associated with diabetes.) The autonomic and central nervous systems also may be involved. This complication is rare in well controlled diabetes.

Infections of the skin: These are frequent in diabetics, and patients with recurrent boils or carbuncles always should be examined for diabetes.

Pulmonary tuberculosis: Since this disease is about twice as common in diabetics as in nondiabetics, a chest X-ray of all patients with diabetes is highly advisable.

Cataract: There is no conclusive evidence at this time to indicate that the incidence of lens opacities in diabetic individuals is greater than in nondiabetics; however, the frequency of lens changes appears to increase with the duration of diabetes in the individual.

Treatment

General considerations: The primary objectives are to aid the patient's body mechanisms in the complete metabolism of glucose and to maintain his general health and nutritional status. An important preliminary is determining the concentration of glucose in the blood and urine. The ideal blood glucose values are those maintained by a normal individual on an ordinary diet and under similar conditions; this seldom exceeds 140 mg./100 cc. after meals. In some diabetics this level cannot be achieved without frequent hypoglycemic attacks, and such individuals require a higher blood glucose level.

The most informative determination of blood glucose is that made about 1½ hours after a meal. In unstable or otherwise difficult cases repeated blood glucose determinations and quantitative analyses of all urine voided prior to lunch, supper, bedtime, and on arising in the morning may be necessary to evaluate completely the diabetic status. In pregnant patients and patients with renal disease, determination of the renal threshold during diabetic supervision may be necessary: The patient is requested to void 3 times at 30-minute intervals and a blood sugar specimen is obtained 15 minutes after the second voiding. If sugar is present in the 3rd specimen while the blood glucose concentration is below 170 mg./100 cc., the renal threshold for glucose is considered below normal.

The simplest and most common method of initiating diabetic care is to have the patient's urine analyzed 4 times a day, i.e., before each meal and at bedtime. The competent patient may test these specimens himself, using either Benedict's solution or one of the available pocket kits. In severe cases, the urine should be analyzed on at least 2 days a week; in mild cases, once in 2 weeks is ordinarily sufficient. Through these analyses, the patient may note the effects of his dietary indiscretions. By using a simple diabetic manual, he can learn the important features of his disease and thus make a good adjustment to it. He also may familiarize himself with the essentials of insulin administration, dietotherapy, and proper care of his body.

Therapy of diabetes consists of dietary restriction and administration of insulin. One of the earliest decisions the physician must make is whether diet alone will suffice or whether insulin is needed in addition. Often the obese elderly patient, after weight reduction, can get along with dietary supervision alone. Generally, the younger patients and the older ones with acute diabetes require insulin also.

Dietary measures: The diabetic diet is a regularly ingested "normal diet" with the exception that the more rapidly absorbed carbohydrates and foods containing them in large amounts must be eaten sparingly (*see* DIETS). Nevertheless, a diet maintaining adequate nutrition must be taken regularly. In the diabetic not receiving insulin, regularity helps prevent overloading of the carbohydrate-disposal mechanisms and consequent hyperglycemia. The caloric values should be sufficient to maintain an approximately ideal weight. In general, the diet should contain 0.5 to 0.75 Gm. of protein/lb. ideal body weight/day. The relative amounts of carbohydrate and fat prescribed largely depend upon the eating habits and desires of the patient, and whether he should decrease, maintain, or increase his body weight; the total depends upon the caloric requirement. In general, the fat in the diet of normal-weight diabetic patients varies from 50 to 120 Gm./day, and the carbohydrate from 150 to about 250 Gm. In the absence of rapidly absorbed carbohydrates, most diabetics find that a slight increase in the fat content and isocaloric decrease in the carbohydrate content from the average of the nondiabetic permits a more palatable combination of foods. The daily regimen should include food from each of the following groups: (1) milk and milk products; (2) tomatoes, citrus fruits, raw cabbage, or salad; (3) other vegetables and fruits; (4) meat, poultry, or fish; (5) butter or other vitamin-rich fats; (6) enriched bread and whole grain cereals. Vitamin supplements are not necessary if the diet is properly composed.

The caloric content is adjusted to the physical activity and proper weight of the patient, with attention to the needs for growth in the child and the decreased energy requirements of the aged. Complicated calculations are not necessary. For moderately active adult individuals the following schedule usually will be found satisfactory:

DIETARY ALLOWANCES IN DIABETES

Height	Calories/ day (approx.)	Protein Gm. (1 Gm. = 4 Cal.)	Fat Gm. (1 Gm. = 9 Cal.)	Carbo- hydrate Gm. (1 Gm. = 4 Cal.)
To reduce weight:				
Short	800	60	20	100
Medium	1,000	70	30	110
Tall	1,200	80	40	125
To maintain ideal weight:				
Short	1,800	80	85	180
Medium	2,400	90	115	250
Tall	3,000	100	155	300
To increase weight:				
All heights	3,200 and over	120	170	300

More food may be given patients who are unusually active. The best indications of the effectiveness of the caloric prescription are the weight curve and the degree of diabetic control. During the period of dietary adjustment the patient should be weighed each week. If he does not respond in the usual way to a given regimen, a careful check of actual food ingested should be made. Patients taking large amounts of insulin frequently will be better controlled if the total daily food intake is divided into 4 to 6 feedings. In severe cases, it is desirable to weigh the food to be eaten during the training period and from time to time thereafter to refresh the patient's accuracy in estimating portions. (For further information *see* DIETS.)

Insulin: The patient must be instructed on the self-administration of insulin, with particular care concerning the proper concentrations (usually 40 or 80 u./cc.) and the use of the scale on the insulin syringe, since serious accidents have occurred from ignorance of these matters. The sites of injection should be systematically changed to ensure good absorption and prevent local dystrophies. The amount of insulin necessary to control diabetes varies greatly; usually it depends on the type and time of injections, the carbohydrate content of the diet, high caloric intake, body mass, amount of exercise, the presence of acidosis, fever, infection, or severe trauma, and hypo- or hyperfunction of the thyroid, anterior pituitary, or adrenal cortex. Rarely, there may be marked insulin resistance, sometimes associated with the development of antibodies, which requires the administration of over 1,000 u. daily.

1. **Rapid-acting insulin** includes crystalline insulin (℞ 41) and regular insulin (℞ 42), which have essentially the same action. The maximum effect usually is attained in a few hours, with an appreciable effect lasting for several hours more. The time of maximum depression of blood sugar and duration of effect is increased with larger doses. Insulin usually is given subcut. 20 to 40 minutes before the meal, but may be injected I.M. or I.V. if necessary. Soluble insulin now is seldom used alone except in cases of acidosis, unstable diabetes, during medical and surgical complications, and in some cases during the initial stages of standardization. It is the preferred type where flexibility of regimen is required.

2. **Slow-acting insulins** include protamine zinc insulin, PZI (℞ 43), and globin insulin (℞ 44). The maximum effect of optimal doses of PZI is noted at about 18 to 36 hours and an appreciable effect for approximately another 24 hours. Injections should be given subcut. or I.M., but not I.V. as the prolongation of effect depends upon slow absorption. PZI alone or with one of the soluble insulins is suitable for routine maintenance of most cases of diabetes that require exogenous insulin, injections being given before breakfast. Before use, the precipitated material should be evenly suspended throughout the solution by gentle rolling or turning of the vial. Globin insulin (℞ 44) is a clear slowly absorbed insulin. It is administered subcut. and has a maximum effect at about 8 to 12 hours and a detectable effect continuing for about the same period thereafter.

3. **Mixtures:** The most commonly used mixture is 2 u. of crystalline (or regular) insulin to 1 u. of PZI. Because of the excess of protamine available there is further formation of PZI so that the resultant mixture has more or less the effect of approximately 2 u. of PZI to 1 u. of crystalline insulin. Thus, a fairly rapidly acting component is given along with a slowly acting component in one injection. This method is particularly valuable for patients with abnormal hyperglycemia after meals but approximately normal prebreakfast blood sugar values when receiving PZI alone. Adjustment in the relative dose of the

two insulins may be necessary, and other ratios such as 1:1 often are used to achieve satisfactory control.

Insulin reactions: Hypoglycemia (insulin shock) may occur if too much insulin or too little food is taken. (For diagnosis *see* table under Complications, or chapter on HYPOGLYCEMIA.) It is treated with glucose: by mouth as carbohydrate foods in mild reactions, and by vein as a 25% solution (℞ 15); or 1,000 cc. of a 5% solution (℞ 12) may be given by stomach tube if the patient is unable to swallow. Indoctrination of the patient concerning the symptoms of hypoglycemia and its treatment is important. Sugar or candy should be carried at all times by patients taking insulin, to be eaten immediately if intense hunger is felt. An identification card stating that the patient has diabetes and takes insulin will be helpful in case of an accident.

Other untoward effects: The most common local reaction is urticarial swelling, which often occurs during the first few weeks of PZI injections. In a few patients, local or, rarely, general allergic reactions to PZI and other insulins are severe and persistent. Antihistaminic drugs such as Neo-Antergan (*see* ALLERGY) may be used in such cases with good results, but a type of insulin (beef, pork, or crystalline) to which the patient is not sensitive should be sought. Desensitization may be tried (*see* ALLERGY). Continued injection of insulin at one site may result occasionally in a local fatty tumefaction or in atrophy. Insulin absorption from these areas is poor. Prevention and treatment consists in systematically varying the site of injection.

During the first few weeks of insulin treatment there may be clinically appreciable edema especially apparent in the face. Ammonium chloride (℞ 19) and a low sodium intake may be employed if it becomes severe. Frequently there also are temporary changes in the refractive power of the eyes so that a transient presbyopia appears. Both of these symptoms presumably are due to changes in the electrolyte balance.

Diabetic patients may arbitrarily be divided into the following "therapeutic types":

1. The "obese" diabetic: The majority of adult diabetics are overweight, and if their weight is reduced by decreasing the caloric intake a notable improvement in carbohydrate tolerance usually results.

2. "Mild nonobese" diabetics usually can be controlled without insulin. If this is not possible while they are receiving an adequate diet which maintains ideal weight, insulin should be given. Usually, a dose of 5 to 15 u. of PZI/day is satisfactory.

3. "Severe" diabetics will include most childhood and normal-weight young adult diabetics. The management of these patients usually is best initiated by hospitalization, since all need insulin. For the less severe cases 20 to 40 u. of PZI before breakfast may be sufficient after initial treatment and standardization. During the 1st week considerably more insulin probably will be needed. This may be given as crystalline insulin in 3 preprandial doses (such as 20-10-20) in addition to a basal dose of PZI. With prompt control, decrease in insulin dosage is to be expected. Doses of over 40 to 50 u. of PZI do not usually control postprandial hyperglycemia without hypoglycemic attacks; therefore a mixture of crystalline insulin and PZI (2:1 ratio) given before breakfast should be tried. The total dose necessary varies widely and must be determined by observation. It is generally less than the total dose of PZI plus soluble insulin required as multiple injections. A small noon or evening dose of soluble insulin also may be necessary. Certain patients do better if the insulins are given separately. The diet should contain enough calories to increase or maintain ideal body weight. Food should be eaten from 4 to 6 times/day. Between-meal feedings may consist of such combinations as milk with crackers and peanut butter (especially at night) or fruit (during the day).

4. Relatively severe "brittle" diabetics, particularly children and less often adults, make up a small group unduly responsive to the action of insulin, and who, despite the able and conscientious efforts of all concerned, are extremely difficult or impossible to maintain on what otherwise would appear to be the indicated dosage. Because of the dangers of producing hypoglycemia in such persons, it may be necessary to allow higher levels of blood sugar to exist than would be advisable in other diabetics.

5. The elderly and the incompetent diabetic: In some old or incompetent diabetics, a high blood sugar level may be necessary. Untreated, frequently unrecognized, hypoglycemia is particularly dangerous in this group. Cautious changes in insulin dosage, with ample and repeated indoctrination of the patient, may help.

6. Childhood diabetics usually exhibit a rapid onset and prominent symptoms. Treatment should be instituted promptly because with good control definite improvement in carbohydrate tolerance can be expected. Owing to the wide variations in blood sugar in child diabetics, normal blood sugar levels are all too frequently followed by hypoglycemia. For this reason many children must be considered adequately controlled if there is no ketonuria and the glycosuria in 24 hours is less than 10% of the carbohydrate content of the diet. The diet must allow for growth and be increased at intervals for this purpose. The total caloric requirement may be roughly estimated by the formula 1,000 calories at 1 year, plus 100 to 125 calories for every year thereafter until growth is completed. Approximately 15 to 20% of the calories are derived from protein, 35% from fat, and 45 to 50% from carbohydrates. The maximum carbohydrate intake is 300 Gm./24 hours. The weight and height should frequently be compared with normal standards. Due allowance must be made for familial characteristics.

MANAGEMENT OF COMPLICATING CONDITIONS

Diabetic Acidosis

Treatment of ketosis without acidosis consists of giving additional soluble insulin in small repeated doses and carbohydrate feedings. A search for the cause should be made.

Acidosis is a medical emergency and treatment should be started as soon as a diagnosis has been made. Rapidly acting insulin (℞ 41, 42) in a dose of 25 to 100 u. should be given subcut. and repeated as needed every half hour until the patient is free from all signs of ketosis as proved by laboratory and clinical findings. After treatment with frequent small doses of insulin has been started, the stomach should be gently lavaged with warm water or saline, and a saline enema given. The patient should be kept warm. As soon as it is feasible, fluid, salt, and carbohydrate depletion should be corrected by giving each hour 100 cc. of fluid in the form of grape juice, orange juice, fruit juices enriched with glucose, salty broth, and water. If tolerated, larger amounts may be offered. The patient usually is unable to take sufficient fluids by mouth because of a drowsy or comatose condition or because of nausea and vomiting, so that necessary fluids must be given I.V. as 5% glucose in physiologic saline (℞ 8) or Ringer's solution (℞ 9). The infusion should be run at the rate of 750 to 1,000 cc./hour or more slowly in patients over 40 and those with cardiovascular disease, who should be watched for increased venous pressure. If the acidosis is severe and the CO_2 combining power is below 20 volumes/100 cc., 2,000 cc. of ⅙ molar sodium lactate (℞ 10) or 500 cc. 5% sodium bicarbonate (℞ 11) may be given in the 24 hr. period. When dehydration is corrected, the I.V. administration should be slowed down. As soon as possible, the oral route of administration should be substituted. The foregoing therapy should be continued until the urine is free from acetone and diacetic acid. During this entire period of supervision the physician should be in constant attendance and should test a urine specimen every 1 to 2 hours for sugar, acetone, and diacetic acid. The patient should be catheterized if necessary to obtain a specimen. In the few cases of anuria that occur, therapy should be guided by frequent tests of the CO_2 combining power of the blood. With disappearance of all evidence of acidosis and ketone bodies in the urine, fruit juice should be given and 25 u. of rapidly acting insulin (℞ 41, 42) every 2 hours for at least 4 doses, with urine tests made at each interval.

Loss of potassium may be responsible for increased muscular weakness, irregular breathing in the presence of an increasing serum CO_2 content, ECG changes, and certain hitherto unexplained deaths occurring after apparent "chemical" recovery. Hypopotassemia may be prevented by the administration of meat broths (high in potassium), potassium chloride orally (℞ 20) or 5 Gm. administered I.V. (℞ 13) as a 0.5% solution over a period of 4 hours.

Pregnancy

An increase in insulin requirement usually is found in the 3rd trimester of the well regulated diabetic. Fetal mortality and toxemia of pregnancy have remained high despite fairly adequate supervision. Recent work indicates that abnormally high serum chorionic gonodotropin concentrations associated with decreased excretion of estrin and pregnandiol is a sign of approaching toxemia, and probably preeclamptic fetal death. The use of large doses of estrogenic substances and progesterone has greatly reduced the incidence of preeclampsia and fetal death. This therapy would seem advisable in all patients suspected of possible later development of toxemia.

The diet during pregnancy should contain large amounts of milk and milk products and be high in proteins (0.75 to 1.0 Gm./lb.), with a caloric intake sufficient to permit the normal weight gain of pregnancy. The management of the diabetic during labor is similar to that during surgical operations (q.v.). A definite drop in insulin requirement occurs with delivery but lasts for only a few days. Diabetes, of itself, is not an invariable indication for cesarean section, but delivery about the 37th week is recommended by many authorities. The infant of the diabetic mother is likely to be unduly large and to have congenital defects. To prevent hypoglycemic death of the infant, 20 to 30 cc. of 5% lactose water should be given by medicine dropper every 2 hours for the first few days of life.

Surgical Operations

In the case of patients undergoing surgical procedures, the immediate aim of diabetic therapy should be to prevent ketosis and avoid hypoglycemia. A reasonably well controlled diabetic should receive ⅙ of the previous day's total insulin dose (as crystalline insulin) and ⅙ of the preoperative diet in liquid form at 6 A.M. on the day of operation. Approximately 1 hour before operation 25 Gm. of glucose is given I.V. as a 10% solution in normal saline. After the operation, the previous insulin dose is repeated and 1 liter of 5% glucose in isotonic saline solution (℞ 8) is injected I.V. A total of approximately 150 to 300 Gm. of glucose should be given over the next 24 hours. Crystalline insulin is administered in doses of ⅙ of the total daily requirement at approximately 4-hour intervals. A gradual shift to solid food and a more normal time-dose schedule then is made. Urine specimens should be examined every 4 to 6 hours to aid in the detection of possible ketosis and help prevent hypoglycemia. The absence of glycosuria during the immediate postoperative period is an indication for more glucose or less insulin.

Infections

Control of the infection facilitates control of the diabetes, and vice versa. In the severely ill diabetic a high protein, high carbohydrate diet approximately equal in calories to the pre-illness diet may be given as equicaloric feedings at 4-hour intervals, with crystalline insulin.

Vascular Disease

In diabetic patients, coronary disease should be treated as in the nondiabetic, with particular attention to the prevention of hypoglycemic attacks and ketosis. Moderate hyperglycemia is to be preferred to the dangers of hypoglycemia.

Loss of adequate blood supply to an extremity through arterio-sclerotic occlusive disease is common in diabetics of long standing. For this reason patients should be instructed in proper care of the feet, using a diabetic manual for complete details. Such hygiene is essential to help prevent the minor foot injuries and infections which may become major catastrophes for the arteriosclerotic diabetic patient.

Other Complications

Eye involvement requires the attention of an ophthalmologist. Rigid control of the diabetes is necessary. A high protein diet recently has been proposed as helpful in cases of diabetic retinitis (q.v.). Diabetic neuritis usually develops slowly and lessens with adequate control of the diabetes and a high vitamin intake, especially of the B complex vitamins. Nocturnal diabetic diarrhea, possibly due to visceral neuritis, has responded to injections of liver extract ($\mathbf{R}$ 1).

HYPOGLYCEMIA

An abnormally low blood sugar level.

Etiology

Hypoglycemia may occur spontaneously or it may be induced by an overdose of insulin (*see* DIABETES MELLITUS). Spontaneous hypoglycemia may be due to organic or functional causes.

"Organic" hypoglycemia results from: hyperinsulinism due to islet cell tumors or hyperplasia of the islet cells; hepatic insufficiency from any cause, resulting in glycogen depletion and impaired production of glucose; adrenal cortical deficiency (Addison's disease) due to infection, tumors, amyloidosis or hemorrhage into the gland; hypopituitarism—Simmonds' disease, tumors, atrophy, infection; hypothyroidism, probably due to decreased absorption of glucose; and hypothalamic lesions.

"Functional" hypoglycemia may be due to: oversecretion of insulin by islet cells because of overexcessive response to glucose absorption; muscular exertion; pregnancy and lactation; or anorexia nervosa. Some cases are classed as idiopathic.

Symptoms and Signs

Attacks tend to occur after the patient has gone several hours without food. At the onset, symptoms include sweating, flushing or pallor, numbness, chilliness, hunger, trembling, headache, dizziness, weakness, changes in the pulse rate (usually elevated), increase in blood pressure, cardiac palpitation, apprehension, and syncope. If the hypoglycemia is not relieved, signs of C.N.S. involvement appear. There may be restlessness, incoordination, thick speech, emotional instability, negativism, disorientation and diplopia. This may be followed by tonic and clonic convulsions (often with marked salivation) and subsequently in severe cases by coma and even death. When hypoglycemia develops slowly, as in some cases of overdosage with protamine zinc insulin, the usual symptoms do not appear or are much less severe, often being largely psychological in nature and may appear to be primarily a behavior problem. Diabetic patients may have mild "hypoglycemic" symptoms at relatively high blood glucose concentrations if the rate of fall following insulin administration is too rapid. Patients with hyperinsulinism are not infrequently obese due to frequent eating in response to hypoglycemia.

Diagnosis

Symptoms similar to those of hypoglycemia are commonly seen in anxiety states, neurocirculatory asthenia and after injections of epinephrine, as well as with epinephrine-producing tumors of the chromaffin system. The convulsive and comatose stage of hypoglycemia calls for differential diagnosis from many diseases, including epilepsy, brain tumor, uremia, eclampsia and, in diabetic patients, between insulin coma and diabetic coma. Definitive diagnosis is dependent upon the demonstration of low blood glucose concentrations during an attack. Values less than 50 mg./100 cc. of venous blood may, in general, be considered diagnostic. The dramatic relief of symptoms following the administration of glucose is further evidence of hypoglycemia.

An attack of hypoglycemia usually may be brought on in cases of organic hyperinsulinism and severe hypofunction of the liver, anterior pituitary or adrenal cortex, by a 24-hour fast, possibly supplemented by exercise. Stimulation of islet function by meals or glucose ingestion may precipitate an attack 2 to 5 hours later in both organic and functional hyperinsulinism as well as in severe adrenal and pituitary disease. As a diagnostic aid a 5-hour glucose tolerance test may be performed. A diet containing 350 Gm. of carbohydrate/day should be taken for several days before the test. Blood glucose values below 50 mg./100 cc., particularly if associated with

10

symptoms, may be considered diagnostic. Approximately 70% of all spontaneous hypoglycemia cases are caused by "functional hyperinsulinism." Severe liver disease and organic hyperinsulinism probably account for most of the remainder. The course of organic hyperinsulinism is characteristically a progressive one. The other symptoms associated with severe disease of the liver, anterior pituitary and adrenal cortex as well as with the miscellaneous causes of hypoglycemia usually will indicate the diagnosis or studies needed.

Treatment

An acute episode of hypoglycemia is treated by giving promptly glucose in some form. If the patient can swallow, about 10 to 20 Gm. of glucose or its equivalent in sugar, candy, orange juice, honey, etc., may be given by mouth. The addition of bread or other starch- and protein-containing food will help to prevent a relapse. Response in mild cases should be evident in 3 to 15 minutes. If the patient is unconscious 10 to 20 Gm. glucose is administered by vein as a 25% solution (℞ 15) or by stomach tube as a 5% solution (℞ 12), a concentration which permits rapid gastric emptying. This dose usually is sufficient to raise the blood glucose to normal levels or above. In severe cases, larger amounts may be needed. Repeated doses or the administration by stomach tube of glucose and milk may be necessary in severe cases to prevent relapse. If liver glycogen stores are adequate the subcut. injection of 0.5 cc. to 1.0 cc. epinephrine, 1:1,000 (℞ 37), may be of aid. This should be used only as an emergency measure when glucose therapy cannot be employed. It must be followed by glucose or carbohydrate food. If coma has been present for many hours, clinical response may not occur because of C.N.S. damage. Prompt treatment is imperative.

The definitive treatment of the hypoglycemias depends upon the cause. In cases of **organic hyperinsulinism,** surgical removal of the hypersecreting tissue is indicated. The conditions to be fulfilled before exploration of the pancreas is warranted are: no extra-pancreatic cause for hypoglycemia; abnormally low blood glucose values obtained when symptoms are present and the rapid relief of these by glucose; repeated fasting venous blood glucose values below 50 mg./100 cc. when the patient is receiving an adequate diet; failure to respond to low carbohydrate, high fat, high protein dietary treatment.

Functional hyperinsulinism is best treated by high protein, high fat, low carbohydrate diet. This is given as 7 feedings/24 hours, including a snack on waking and on going to bed. For an adult a satisfactory diet may be composed of 120 to 140 Gm. of protein and 80 to 100 Gm. of carbohydrate with enough fat to maintain ideal body weight. Since autonomic imbalance and emotional disturbances are background features of functional hyperinsulinism psychotherapy is important.

Hepatogenic hypoglycemia should be treated by high protein, high carbohydrate diet with multiple feedings along with other therapeutic efforts directed at the primary liver disease (q.v.). The same is true of hypoglycemic attacks associated with pituitary and adrenal cortical disease (q.v.). All patients subject to hypoglycemic attacks should carry sugar or other rapidly available carbohydrate with them at all times. The occupation and habits of the patient should be revised to prevent injury to himself or others because of an attack and his family should be instructed in recognizing the symptoms and in giving simple emergency treatment for hypoglycemia.

ACID-BASE AND ALLIED DISORDERS

(Acidosis, Ketosis, Dehydration, Alkalosis)

In this chapter are discussed a group of closely related and interdependent conditions in which there is a disturbance of the normal acid-base and water balances.

Acidosis: *A condition characterized by the presence in the body of excess amounts of acid, or diminished amounts of base (i.e., alkali).*

Ketosis: *A condition in which there is in the body an excessive accumulation of ketone bodies, specifically, beta-hydroxybutyric acid, acetoacetic (diacetic) acid, and acetone.* (Since the first two of these are relatively strong acids, ketosis is in most instances also a form of acidosis.)

Dehydration: *A condition marked by excessive loss of fluids from one or all the body compartments (intracellular, extracellular, intravascular).*

Alkalosis: *A condition characterized by excess accumulation of alkali in the body or by a deficiency of acids.*

The body attempts to maintain a state of equilibrium in the composition of its structures both solid and fluid. This is known as homeostasis. It involves among other things the shifting of body water between the intracellular, extracellular and intravascular compartments and alterations in the concentrations of the numerous solutes. Body water is derived either exogenously by ingestion or endogenously (350 cc. daily) from oxidation. Excretion of water constantly occurs through the skin, lungs, gastrointestinal tract, and kidneys. Although all these organs and the adrenals, pituitary and hypothalamus are active in the control of body water levels, the kidneys are the most effective and important organs in the maintenance of both salt and water balance.

Normal body metabolism provides carbon dioxide (CO_2), which combines with water to form carbonic acid (H_2CO_3). Excretion of CO_2 occurs primarily through respiration, the rate and depth of which depend to a considerable extent upon the blood acidity, expressed as pH (the negative logarithm of the hydrogen ion concentration of the blood). Body fluid pH is normally maintained fairly constantly at 7.35 to 7.45, through the action of the dissolved buffers (proteins, carbonic acid, and phosphates), present as weak acids and their sodium and potassium salts. (Sodium is the chief basic ion in extracellular fluids, potassium that in intracellular fluids.) The main action of the buffer substances is to limit (i.e., "buffer") the amount of change in the pH of body fluids. This is accomplished by means of a mechanism that attempts to maintain a constant ratio between the weak acid and its salt, but which can be effective only if the degree of change is not too great. For example, in the case of bicarbonate the ratio, $NaHCO_3:H_2CO_3$, normally is about 20:1. When this value decreases, acidosis develops, while an increase is noted in alkalosis. If the available fixed base is reduced by loss of sodium or by an increase in the stronger acids, the bicarbonate or buffer content of the plasma decreases, the hydrogen ion concentration increases, the pH falls, and acidosis occurs. In the milder forms, bicarbonate falls with but little change in pH. This is known as compensated acidosis. With more severe degrees, pronounced depletion of bicarbonate results in significant change in pH. This is called uncompensated acidosis. Among the stronger acids concerned are the ketone acids, the excess of which in body fluids produces the acidosis of ketosis.

Elevated pH, or alkalosis, results from excess accumulation of base or loss of acid. This may occur through ingestion of large amounts of sodium bicarbonate or other strong basic salt, overventilation and blowing off of CO_2 or loss of chloride due to vomiting.

Mechanisms responsible for correcting alterations in pH are numerous. Minor changes or moment-to-moment alterations are corrected by the varying of respiration, thus increasing or decreasing the amount of CO_2 exhaled. Major changes or day-by-day alterations in the acid-base balance are corrected by the kidneys through: (1) changes in the reaction of the urine, which can vary from the acid pH of 4.8 to the alkaline pH of 8.0, (2) formation of ammonium ions to be substituted for fixed base, which is thus retained while the acid bodies are excreted combined with ammonium ions. Acidosis, whatever its origin, causes diuresis because base and water must be wasted, to varying degrees, in excretion of excessive amounts of acid. Thus dehydration is a frequent concomitant of acidosis.

Acidosis, Ketosis, Dehydration: 1. Gaseous acidosis may occur in the course of serious pulmonary diseases because of interference in the exchange of CO_2 between the blood and outside air through the lungs. The end result is an abnormal accumulation of CO_2. This is of relatively little importance clinically.

2. The excessive ingestion of acid salts such as ammonium chloride frequently produces acidosis, through the following mechanism: The ammonium ion, after being converted to urea by the liver, is excreted in the urine and the remaining chloride ion holds plasma base, the free bicarbonate then being excreted by the lungs as CO_2. The kidney finally excretes large amounts of base and water in order to rid the plasma of the excess chloride. In this way a diuresis also is produced by the ammonium chloride.

3. Excessive muscular exertion, with increased production of lactic acid, causes a transitory acidosis.

4. Ketone bodies are formed from fat by the liver. They are produced in excess amounts when carbohydrate metabolism is reduced or disturbed, and fat and protein metabolism is thus increased. The ketone bodies, beta-hydroxybutyric acid, acetoacetic acid, and acetone, accumulate in the body. The acids hold fixed base at the expense of bicarbonate, producing a state of acidosis. The clinical conditions in which ketosis commonly occurs are referred to below.

5. Disturbances in food intake are common causes of acidosis. In starvation, energy is derived from the metabolism of body protein and fat; in this process ketone body production is accelerated, and ketones in the blood are increased. The ketosis increases as the supplies of carbohydrate decrease. In cases of severe renal glycosuria a similar situation occurs because of depletion in the carbohydrate reserves. Impaired food intake also is a factor contributing to acidosis in childhood diarrhea, Asiatic cholera, recurrent vomiting in children, pernicious vomiting of pregnancy, and overwhelming infections. Rarely, a high fat diet may be responsible for mild acidosis because of excess ketone production.

6. Dehydration of severe degree is usually associated with severe acidosis, since water and base must be wasted in the excretion of acid. Excessive sweating causes loss of water, sodium, and chloride. With less sodium available for combination with carbonic acid, pH decreases and acidosis occurs. Continued loss of sodium and water may ultimately reduce the blood volume to such a degree that renal blood flow is greatly diminished and kidney function is almost nil. Certain severe diarrheas, e.g., diarrheas of childhood and Asiatic cholera, cause acidosis secondary to dehydration and loss of alkaline intestinal fluids. Here again the impaired food intake often is a factor contributing to the acidosis by excess ketone production.

7. Diabetes mellitus (q.v.) is the most important condition in which severe acidosis may occur. Often serious, it is capable of causing coma. The basic derangement is the body's inability to regulate the blood sugar level and to store tissue glycogen because of a relative or absolute deficiency of insulin. The rate of fat metabolism is increased and ketones accumulate in

the blood. Dehydration and hemoconcentration result from the uncontrolled glycosuria with excessive loss of sodium and potassium from the body. The ability of the kidneys to excrete ketone bodies may be diminished and the ketonemia is thus aggravated.

8. Acidosis due to impairment of liver function occurs in hepatitis, during anesthesia, and in the course of fevers. These conditions are characterized by a lack of glucose or glycogen available to the liver leading to overproduction of ketone bodies as a result of excessive breakdown of fat. Fever may cause, in addition, increased carbohydrate demand during a period of deficient intake (starvation), as well as dehydration and occasionally renal damage with acid retention. Von Gierke's disease is a rare condition included in this category because, although there are large stores of liver glycogen, the liver is unable to mobilize them and the result is the same as if glycogen were absent.

9. In advanced renal disease, acidosis often exists and may become extremely severe because of reduced kidney efficiency which is responsible for the loss of excessive amounts of base (sodium) and the accumulation of phosphoric and sulfuric acids. Because of poor food intake and vomiting, ketone production may be increased to contribute further to the acidosis (see UREMIA).

Alkalosis: 1. Loss of acid in excess of base, such as occurs through excessive vomiting, is the most common cause of alkalosis. A similar condition may exist in infants who lose large amounts of acid in severe diarrhea.

2. The administration of strongly alkaline salts often is responsible for alkalosis, especially when renal function is impaired. The disorder results from an intake of alkali greater than the kidney can handle. This condition is most commonly encountered during prolonged or excessive treatment of gastric hyperacidity.

3. Respiratory alkalosis often occurs due to loss of carbonic acid through hyperventilation, in response to a functional or organic disturbance of the respiratory center, or to anoxemia. Hyperthermia, infection, or intoxication (e.g., by sulfonamides, salicylates) are other causes of this derangement.

Symptoms, Signs, and Diagnosis

A developing acidosis may be asymptomatic, but there is usually an abrupt or gradually increasing weakness, dull headache, or general malaise. Abdominal pain, nausea and vomiting are sometimes present. Hyperpnea, frequently manifested by rapid, or sometimes slow, deep (Kussmaul) respirations, is common when the condition becomes severe with plasma CO_2 values below 20 volumes/100 cc., and plasma pH below 7.20. In acidosis due to ketonemia the breath has a fruity odor. Evidence of dehydration including loose skin, soft and sunken eyeballs, and a shrunken dry tongue may be noted. The body temperature is usually depressed due to excessive loss of heat and to circulatory collapse. Stupor, followed by coma, is characteristic of the more severe forms of acidosis. With progression of the acidosis almost all the features of shock become evident.

A patient in prolonged acidosis may lose sufficient cellular potassium to produce the syndrome of potassium deficiency. Potassium excretion is favored by diuresis, dehydration, acidosis, vomiting, or I.V. administration of sodium salts. The patient may exhibit pronounced muscular weakness or paralysis, labored respirations, cardiovascular and electrocardiographic changes, and may die in collapse. The syndrome is related to the low total body potassium level and not merely to the low serum potassium concentration.

Laboratory evidence is extremely helpful in the diagnosis of acidosis. The urine becomes intensely acid and has a high ammonia content. In acidosis due to high ketone concentration in the blood, ketonuria can be demonstrated (see LAB. PROC.). The presence or absence of glucose in the urine will be of aid in determining whether the acidosis is diabetic in origin. It must, however, be kept in mind that a diabetic patient may be acidotic with hypoglycemia and no glucose in the urine, due to excessive insulin administration. This occurs in severely diabetic patients who are sensitive to insulin and whose blood sugar, under insulin administration, may swing rapidly between hyperglycemia and hypoglycemia. An overdose of insulin causes a rapid fall in blood sugar concentration, which tends to deplete the liver of glycogen and will therefore lead to the appearance of ketone bodies in the blood and urine.

Estimation of the CO_2 combining power of the blood by the Van Slyke manometric method is the simplest and most frequently used method of determining the degree of acidosis. In special cases, the plasma sodium and potassium levels, which are low in acidosis and high in alkalosis, should be determined by means of a flame photometer. The classification of all except the gaseous forms of acidosis and alkalosis is usually based upon the CO_2 combining power:

	CO_2 Combining Power in Volumes/100 cc.
Acidosis	
Extreme	Less than 15.0
Severe	15 to 24.9
Moderate	25 to 34.9
Mild	35 to 44.9
Normal	45 to 69.9
Alkalosis	
Extreme	More than 99.9
Severe	90 to 99.9
Moderate	80 to 89.9
Mild	70 to 79.9

During acidosis the leukocyte count may be elevated. The

state of dehydration can be evaluated by determination of the hematocrit, which indicates the degree of hemoconcentration.

Clinically, alkalosis is characterized by increased irritability, restlessness and a neuromuscular hyperexcitability often indistinguishable from that of hypocalcemia. Tetany (q.v.), with positive Chvostek's and Trousseau's signs, tremor and convulsions, is present in the more severe forms. Forceful vomiting is common. Respiration may be shallow in alkali-excess alkalosis, tending to effect retention of CO_2 in the body.

The laboratory examinations necessary for conclusive diagnosis of alkalosis are the same as those for acidosis. Examination of the urine for ketone bodies is indicated since ketosis may exist in the presence of alkalosis. The characteristic findings are alkaline urine, increased bicarbonate content of blood, increased CO_2 combining power of blood, elevated pH, and decreased blood chloride. Blood calcium level should be determined to aid in differentiation from hypocalcemic tetany.

In evaluation of the various disorders that may be responsible for alterations in acid-base balance, a complete investigation of the patient's history and any underlying disorders is essential.

Treatment

Restoration of body fluid and base, and control of the primary disease are the main objectives in the treatment of acidosis. (For treatment of diabetic acidosis, see DIABETES MELLITUS.) In severe acidotic states as much as 80 cc. of normal saline/Kg. body wt. may be necessary to correct the dehydration. The oral ingestion of alkali in the form of sodium bicarbonate (R 21) or sodium lactate (R 22) often is effective in relieving mild acidosis. In the acute stage parenteral administration of alkaline solutions is indicated. Sodium lactate (R 10) is preferred to sodium bicarbonate since it is more easily sterilized, and the lactate ion is useful in providing a source of glycogen to the body. The drug is administered either subcut. or I.V. as a ⅙ molar solution. In patients who have obvious hyperpnea, 25 cc. of solution/Kg. body wt. should be given. Bicarbonate solution (R 11) may be used instead, in a 5% concentration, giving 6 cc./Kg. body wt. Sodium bicarbonate or sodium lactate may be substituted for normal saline in correcting dehydration, only until CO_2 or pH values reach normal. If given beyond this point, serious alkalosis may result. If any evidence of shock is present, a transfusion of 500 cc. of whole blood should be given. Constant observation of the patient, with repeated laboratory examinations, is essential to determine whether normal conditions are being approached. When potassium deficiency is suspected, potassium chloride can be given orally (R 20), I.V. (R 13), or as part of Ringer's solution (R 9). When ketone production is high because of depletion of glycogen stores, administration of glucose 5% is beneficial (℞ 8, 9, 12).

In alkalosis, as in acidosis, correction of the underlying disorder is the prime objective. Alkalosis due to excess alkali ingestion during the treatment of peptic ulcer usually is best treated by substituting aluminum hydroxide gel or resins for the offending alkaline salt. Oral administration of ammonium chloride (℞ 19) in addition is indicated in the more severe states.

Tetany due to hyperventilation is most commonly on a hysterical basis, and may be relieved by reassurance or sedation. Rebreathing into a bag may be effective in raising the blood CO_2 level. In severe alkalotic states in which tetanic convulsive seizures occur, the I.V. administration of hydrochloric acid (℞ 14) diluted with Ringer's solution is helpful in stimulating respiration. Control of convulsions may be accomplished by administering calcium gluconate, 10%, I.V. (℞ 17). Loss of large amounts of intestinal fluid, such as occurs in vomiting or diarrhea, necessitates fluid replacement by means of normal saline. The administration of glucose often is necessary to reduce ketosis and protein destruction when these exist.

AMYLOIDOSIS

A pathologic state characterized by the accumulation in various organs of an abnormal protein complex, amyloid, that has certain starchlike characteristics.

Etiology

The fundamental pathogenic mechanisms of amyloid production and deposition in tissues have not yet been elucidated, but the evidence available points to some disturbance of the endogenous protein metabolism.

Two forms of amyloid disease are recognized. Amyloidosis, when no cause can be discovered clinically or at autopsy, is classified as **primary.** When associated with diseases in which chronic suppuration and tissue necrosis are outstanding features, such as tuberculosis, lung abscess, gummatous syphilis, chronic osteomyelitis, pyelonephritis, and chronically infected burns, amyloidosis is considered **secondary.** It also occurs, rarely, in nonsuppurative diseases. Multiple **myeloma** and rheumatoid arthritis may be inciting factors.

Pathology

Amyloid is a homogeneous, highly refractile substance that has a high affinity for Congo red dye, both in prepared tissues and *in vivo*. In amyloidosis, connective tissues, particularly in and around blood vessels, are distended with intracellular deposits of amyloid.

In **primary amyloidosis** the involvement often is noted in less commonly affected organs such as the heart, lung, skin, tongue, thyroid gland, or the intestinal tract. When the bone marrow is affected, the amyloid substance may almost completely replace its functional elements. Peculiar localized amyloid "tumors" occasionally are found in the upper respiratory tract. Amyloidosis of the myocardium is not necessarily associated with clinical enlargement of the heart.

Secondary amyloidosis shows a predilection for the spleen, liver, kidney, adrenal glands, and lymph nodes. Although no organ system is spared, the C.N.S. seldom is affected. The liver and spleen are uniformly enlarged, firm and inelastic. The kidneys may be normal in size, but usually are enlarged. Cut sections of the spleen show large, translucent, waxy areas where the normal Malpighian bodies are replaced by pale amyloid, producing the "sago" spleen.

Symptoms and Signs

No specific symptoms or signs are characteristic of amyloid disease. Manifestations are general and usually influenced by the organ or system affected. They often are obscured by those of the underlying disease, which may lead to death before secondary amyloidosis is suspected clinically. The most striking manifestation of amyloidosis is the nephrotic syndrome (q.v.) of amyloid nephrosis. In the early stages, albuminuria (slight or massive) may be noted, but later the distinctive symptom complex develops with anasarca, ascites, hypoproteinemia, anemia, and massive albuminuria. Hypertension is rare, and red cells are seldom found in the urinary sediment unless tuberculosis coexists. Anemia is always present, probably due at first to the underlying disease but later representing encroachment on the bone marrow. The anemia often is of a normocytic, normochromic type, refractory to iron or liver therapy, and associated with pallor or weakness. Lymphadenopathy, often generalized, is common. The nodes are firm and nontender. Amyloidosis of the liver (q.v.), i.e., definite extensive involvement, rarely produces hepatic dysfunction, as revealed clinically or by liver function tests. Jaundice is almost never seen. Skin lesions may resemble scleredema when they are of the waxy, translucent type, or dermatitis when they are of the infiltrative type. Purpura may result from amyloidosis of small cutaneous vessels. Evidence of angina pectoris or coronary occlusion, in the presence of hepatosplenomegaly and lymphadenopathy, should suggest the possibility of myocardial amyloidosis. Rarely, a firm symmetrical nontender goiter resembling Hashimoto's or Riedel's struma results from amyloidosis of the thyroid gland.

Diagnosis

As a rule, primary amyloidosis can be diagnosed only by biopsy. A secondary amyloidosis should be suspected in any patient long ill with a chronic suppurative disease, especially when the course is progressively downhill and the common manifestations of amyloidosis such as hepatosplenomegaly and albuminuria also appear. Skin lesions, when present, are not of themselves diagnostic, but together with other findings help to complete the clinical picture. Biopsy of a lymph node (or of the liver by someone experienced in this procedure) may lead to a positive diagnosis. The Congo red absorption test may be of value in detecting amyloidosis. Interpretations are based on the great affinity of amyloid substance for Congo red. When the 1-hour specimen reveals a 60% loss of the dye from the serum, amyloidosis may be suspected. Misinterpretation from false positive tests is minimized when two successive tests show over 90% loss of dye at 1 hour.

Prognosis

The course of generalized secondary amyloidosis is steadily downhill and, if the associated disease is not earlier fatal, leads to death, usually from uremia following renal failure. However, localized amyloid tumors may be removed without recurrence. Myocardial amyloidosis usually causes death in much the same way as does myocardial infarction due to coronary occlusion. In one tuberculosis sanatorium, 25% of autopsies revealed amyloidosis. When the condition was detected in tuberculous patients before death, the maximum duration of life thereafter was 2 years. Despite the generally relentless course of amyloidosis, a few reports indicate that the process is not irreversible. In some instances, it has regressed or disappeared when the underlying disease was cured; e.g., after the arrest of tuberculous empyema by thoracoplasty, and after amputation or successful medical treatment of a part affected with chronic osteomyelitis.

Treatment

Whenever possible, treatment is directed first to the inciting cause. If this can be eliminated, the amyloidosis may possibly be arrested. Therapy of the amyloidosis itself is symptomatic. In the nephrotic stage a high protein, low sodium diet has been used (see Diets), and replacement of serum proteins may be attempted by administration of plasma or sodium-free human serum albumin. (Such therapy may occasionally result in diuresis.) Abdominal paracentesis (see Bedside Proc.) may be employed if reaccumulation of fluid is not too rapid. Antibiotic medication may prevent peritonitis in the nephrotic stage. Since the anemia represents bone marrow replacement, transfusion of whole blood or red blood cells is the only means

of correcting it, but this of course will be of only temporary
value.

TETANY

*A syndrome characterized by neuromuscular hyperexcitabil-
ity, as shown by carpopedal spasm, laryngospasm, or convulsions.* The increased neuromuscular irritability results from a
decreased concentration of ionized calcium in the blood. It is
not uncommon between the ages of 3 months and 2 years, but
is relatively rare during other periods of life. Tetany may be
either **manifest,** with muscular spasm and convulsions, or
latent and demonstrable only by electrical or mechanical stimuli. In a patient with latent tetany, manifest tetany may be
precipitated by an acute infection.

Etiology and Pathologic Physiology

Tetany may be the result of hypocalcemia or alkalosis.

Hypocalcemia is a condition in which there is a deficiency
of ionized calcium in the blood. It may be due to any of the
following systemic disorders: (1) Hypoparathyroidism, congenital or postoperative, in which the decreased elimination of
phosphorus in the urine produces a consequent fall in the serum
calcium level; (2) infantile rickets, characterized by deficient
intake or absorption of calcium; (3) steatorrhea, idiopathic or
secondary to celiac disease, sprue, or pancreatic deficiency, in
which conditions undigested fat combines with ingested calcium to form insoluble soaps, thereby preventing the absorption of calcium; (4) phosphate retention due to renal insufficiency, hypoparathyroidism, or hypervitaminosis D, such retention of phosphorus depressing the calcium level, although
the resulting tetany is seldom severe since the associated acidosis increases the ionization of the serum calcium salts; (5)
nephrosis, wherein the plasma protein lost in the urine carries
off the calcium which is bound to protein; the tetany usually is
mild, since protein-bound calcium is the un-ionized fraction of
blood calcium; and (6) acute pancreatitis, in which digestion
of tissue fat yields fatty acids that combine with calcium ions
to form insoluble soaps.

Alkalosis: The total plasma calcium is within normal limits,
but the ionized fraction is low, due to the decreased ionization
of calcium salts which accompanies alkalosis. It may result
from (1) overmedication with an alkali, such as sodium bicarbonate; (2) loss of chloride ion through excessive vomiting,
gastric lavage, or continuous gastric suction; or (3) hyperventilation associated with hysteria, fever or encephalitis, in
which the elimination of CO_2 leads to alkalosis.

Symptoms and Signs

Carpopedal spasm: The wrists and the metacarpophalangeal joints are flexed, with adduction of the thumbs over the palms. The feet are turned down with marked plantar flexion of the toes. Carpopedal spasm is painful and may persist for hours. It is encountered most frequently in older children, in whom it may be the only symptom.

Laryngospasm: This is usually severe enough to cause some respiratory obstruction, especially in inspiration.

Facial muscle spasm: This is most likely to occur while the patient is crying.

Convulsions may recur as long as the blood calcium is low. They begin abruptly, are generalized, and usually clonic in character. The seizures may last for several minutes. Between attacks, the patient is mentally clear and alert. There is no fever unless a complicating infection is present.

Chvostek's sign is positive. This consists of contractions of the facial muscles when the trunk of the facial nerve is tapped just anterior to the external auditory meatus. It is most easily elicited after a convulsion. Chvostek's sign may normally be present in the newborn and in older children; however, between the ages of 2 months and 2 years, it is almost pathognomonic of tetany. The peroneal sign is obtained, with the knee partially flexed, by striking the peroneal nerve as it passes over the head of the fibula. In tetany, there is dorsiflexion and adduction of the foot. **Trousseau's sign** is a carpal spasm resulting from constriction of the upper arm with a tourniquet. Similar pressure over the leg produces pedal spasm. **Erb's sign,** consisting of a decrease in the electrical stimulus necessary to produce a muscular contraction, is positive in tetany.

Diagnosis

The symptoms and signs of manifest tetany usually are so typical that the diagnosis is seldom difficult. A careful history, physical examination, and laboratory determination of the plasma calcium, phosphorus, and pH will help to identify the underlying cause.

Treatment

Immediate treatment of the convulsive seizure consists in the administration of chloral hydrate, 0.6 to 1.0 Gm. (gr. x to xv) (℞ 31), with or without morphine, 1 mg. (gr. 1/60)/5 Kg. body wt. (℞ 27); the chloral hydrate alone may be repeated in 2 or 3 hours if necessary. Sodium phenobarbital, 60 to 120 mg. (gr. i to ii) subcut., usually is effective within 15 to 30 minutes and may safely be repeated even in infants (℞ 32). Paraldehyde (℞ 33), 1 to 6 cc. I.M., or 30 to 60 cc. in 100 cc. of milk or water as a retention enema, is both safe and useful. In the presence of repeated convulsions, chloroform or ether inhalations are effective, as is tribromoethanol solution rectally,

60 to 80 mg. (gr. i to iss)/Kg. body wt. (℞ 34). The maximum dose of tribromoethanol solution must never exceed 10 Gm. for men or 8 Gm. for women, regardless of body weight. Alternate hot and cold baths are of little, if any, use.

Specific therapy consists of the administration of a soluble calcium salt and control of the underlying disease. Calcium may be slowly injected I.V. as a 10% solution of calcium gluconate (℞ 17) in a dose of 1 Gm. or as a 5% solution of calcium chloride (℞ 16) followed by calcium chloride orally (℞ 18). Alkalosis in general will respond to the I.V. administration of saline. Rebreathing of exhaled air from a paper bag held over the nose and mouth will restore the plasma CO_2 and correct alkalosis due to overbreathing from any cause. The substitution of nonabsorbable alkali (such as magnesium oxide or carbonate) for sodium bicarbonate will prevent subsequent alkalosis due to overmedication. Prevention of further attacks of tetany requires correction or control of the underlying abnormal condition, for details of which the reader should consult the chapter referring to the particular disease.

PRESCRIPTIONS

(Wherever a prescribed "proprietary" is representative of a class of therapeutic agents, alternative proprietary preparations will be found listed in Part II.)

Hematinics

1. ℞ Liver Injection U.S.P. (vial)

   30 to 50 u., I.M., repeated in 3 or 4 days and at weekly intervals thereafter.

2. ℞ Liver Injection (Crude) U.S.P. (vial)

   2 cc. I.M. every other day.

3. ℞ Liver Solution U.S.P.

   1 or more U.S.P. u. daily.

4. ℞ "Cobione" (crystalline Vitamin B_{12}) (ampul)

   15 to 30 or more micrograms subcut. or I.M., repeated every 15 to 30 days until a maximum response is obtained.

5. ℞ Pteroylglutamic (folic) acid   5   mg.

   3 tablets daily until anemia is controlled, followed by 1 tablet daily.

6. ℞ Pteroylglutamic (folic) acid (ampul)

   15 mg. I.M., daily until anemia is controlled.

7. ℞ Ferrous sulfate . . . .   0.3   Gm. (gr. v)

       1 tablet 3 times daily after meals.

Fluids and Electrolytes

8. ℞ Glucose, 5% solution in Sterile Isotonic Sodium Chloride Solution for Parenteral Use U.S.P. (sterile bottle)

       To be given I.V. as indicated.

9. ℞ Glucose, 5% solution in Ringer's Solution for Parenteral Use U.S.P. (sterile bottle)

       To be given I.V., as indicated, in average doses of 50 cc./Kg. body wt.

10. ℞ Sodium lactate, 1/6 molar solution (sterile bottle)

       2,000 cc. subcut. or slowly I.V., to combat acidosis.

11. ℞ Sodium bicarbonate, 5% solution (sterile bottle)

       250 to 500 cc. slowly I.V. to combat acidosis.

12. ℞ Glucose, 5% solution in Water for Injection U.S.P. (sterile bottle)

       1,000 cc. I.V., orally or by stomach tube.

13. ℞ Potassium chloride. . . . .   5.0   Gm. (gr. lxxv)
    Water for Injection U.S.P.
                 q.s. ad 1,000.0   cc.   (℥ xxxii)

       Autoclave solution and administer I.V. over a period of 4 hours.

14. ℞ Hydrochloric acid (concentrated, 14 N). . . . . .   0.75   cc.
    Sterile Ringer's Solution for Parenteral Use U.S.P. .   1,000.0   cc.

       Administer 2 to 3 cc. I.V., once only.

15. ℞ Glucose, 25% solution (ampul)

       25 to 50 cc. I.V., repeated as necessary.

16. ℞ Calcium chloride, 5% solution (ampul)

       5 to 10 cc. I.V., slowly.

17. ℞ Calcium gluconate, 10% solution (ampul)

       10 cc. I.V., slowly.

18. ℞ Calcium chloride (powder)

>   1 teaspoon initially, followed by ¼ teaspoon
>   every 4 to 6 hours; supplement with vitamin
>   D, 10,000 U.S.P. u. daily.

19. ℞ Ammonium chloride (enteric
    coated) . . . . 0.5 Gm. (gr. viiss)

>   2 tablets 3 times a day.

20. ℞ Potassium chloride . . . . . 0.3 Gm. (gr. v)

>   3 tablets every 30 minutes for 4 to 6 doses.

21. ℞ Sodium bicarbonate

>   1 to 5 teaspoons, taken with copious quan-
>   tities of water every hour until acidosis is
>   controlled.

22. ℞ Sodium lactate, 10% solution

>   1 to 3 glasses hourly until acidosis is con-
>   trolled.

23. ℞ Calcium lactate. . . . . . . 0.3 Gm. (gr. v)

>   3 tablets 3 times daily.

24. ℞ Calcium phosphate . . . . . 0.5 Gm. (gr. viiss)

>   2 capsules 3 times daily.

Analgesics and Sedatives

25. ℞ Colchicine . . . . 0.5 mg. (gr. 1/120)

>   1 tablet every 1 or 2 hours until a gouty at-
>   tack is relieved or toxic symptoms occur.

26. ℞ Codeine sulfate. . . . . . 30 mg. (gr. ss)

>   1 or 2 tablets every 4 hours for pain.

27. ℞ Morphine sulfate

>   10 to 15 mg. (gr. ⅙ to ¼) subcut. for pain.
>   For tetany, the dose is 1 mg./5 Kg. body wt.

28. ℞ Sodium salicylate (enteric
    coated) . . . . 0.3 Gm. (gr. v)

>   2 to 4 tablets every 6 hours.

29. ℞ Phenobarbital . . . . . . 30 mg. (gr. ss)

>   2 to 4 tablets to induce sleep.

30. ℞ Camphorated Opium Tincture
    U.S.P. . . . . 30.0 cc. (℥ i)

>   1 teaspoon every 4 hours for gastrointestinal
>   distress.

31. ℞ Chloral hydrate. . . . . . 0.3 Gm. (gr. v)

>   2 or 3 capsules repeated if necessary.

32. ℞ Sodium phenobarbital (ampul)

0.06 to 0.12 Gm. (gr. i to ii) subcut., repeated
in 30 minutes if necessary.

33. ℞ Paraldehyde

1 to 6 cc. I.M. or 30 to 60 cc. in 100 cc. of
milk or water, rectally as a retention enema.

34. ℞ Tribromoethanol Solution
U.S.P.

60 to 80 mg./Kg. body wt., administered
rectally as a 2.5% solution in distilled water.
(CAUTION! Maximum dose, regardless of
body weight, is 10 Gm. for men and 8 Gm.
for women.)

Hormones

35. ℞ Thyroid U.S.P. . . . . 30　　mg.　(gr. ss)

1 or more tablets daily, sufficient to bring
B.M.R. to normal.

36. ℞ Ethinyl estradiol . . . . . . 0.02　mg.

1 or 2 tablets daily.

37. ℞ Epinephrine hydrochloride,
1:1,000 solution

0.5 to 1 cc. (♏ viii to xv) subcut.

38. ℞ Testosterone propionate
(ampul)

25 mg. I.M. 2 to 3 times weekly.

39. ℞ Methyltestosterone . . . . . 10　　mg.

1 tablet orally or sublingually 3 times daily.

40. ℞ Chorionic gonadotropin (vial)

500 to 1,000 u. I.M. 2 to 3 times weekly.

41. ℞ Crystalline Zinc Insulin Injection N.N.R. (vial contain-
ing 40 or 80 u./cc.)

Administer subcut. according to needs (*see*
DIABETES).

42. ℞ Insulin Injection U.S.P. (vial
containing 40 or 80 u./cc.)

Administer subcut. according to needs (*see*
DIABETES).

43. ℞ Protamine Zinc Insulin Injection U.S.P. (vial containing 40 or 80 u./cc.)

Administer subcut. according to needs (*see*
DIABETES).

44. ℞ Globin Insulin with Zinc
N.N.R.   (vial containing 40
or 80 u./cc.)

> Administer subcut. according to needs (*see*
> DIABETES).

Miscellaneous

45. ℞ Whole or skimmed milk . . . 1,000.0 cc. (℥ xxxii)
Skimmed milk powder. . . .   135.0 Gm. (℥ ivss)
Pure casein. . . . .   70.0 Gm. (℥ iiss)
Sugar . . . .   20.0 Gm. (ʒ v)
Cocoa. . . . .   20.0 Gm. (ʒ v)

> *Note:* Each 8-ounce glass of the above pre-
> pared drink will contain 25 Gm. each of pro-
> tein and carbohydrate. Thus, for a mini-
> mum intake of 100 Gm. of protein and car-
> bohydrate, 4 glasses a day are required.

46. ℞ Menadione   (ampul)

> 2 to 5 mg. I.M. daily until hypoprothrom-
> binemia is relieved.

47. ℞ Amphetamine sulfate   5   mg.

> 1 or 2 tablets ½ hour before breakfast and
> lunch daily.

48. ℞ Vitamin D

> 10,000 U.S.P. u. daily.

49. ℞ Sorbitan monooleate, polyoxyethylene derivative. . .   0.5   Gm.

> 3 capsules with each meal. (CAUTION! The
> use of mineral oil during this treatment is
> contraindicated.)

DENTAL AND ORAL

DENTAL DEVELOPMENT

Deciduous* Teeth (20 in number)	No.	Time of** Eruption in Months	Permanent Teeth (32 in number)	No.	Time of** Eruption in Years
Lower central incisors.	2	5– 9	First molars	4	6– 7
Upper central incisors.	2	8–12	Incisors..........	8	7– 8
Upper lateral incisors.	2	10–12	Bicuspids........	8	9–10
Lower lateral incisors.	2	12–15	Canines..........	4	12–14
Anterior molars......	4	12–15	Second molars...	4	12–15
Canines.............	4	18–24	Third molars....	4	17–25
Posterior molars.....	4	24–30			

* An average child should have: 6 teeth at 1 year; 12 teeth at 1½ years; 16 teeth at 2 years; 20 teeth at 2½ years.   ** Varies greatly.

TOOTHACHE
(Odontalgia)

Pain resulting from inflammation of the dental pulp and contiguous structures, particularly the periodontal membrane.

Etiology

Dental caries exposes the pulp of the tooth to painful stimuli, which may be (1) thermal, or mechanical, as caused by heat or cold, food impacted in a cavity, or trauma from malocclusion; (2) chemical, as by sugar, salt, acids; (3) bacterial, as by toxins or, in deep cavities, by the organism's presence. The bacteria most commonly found in deep cavities, in order of frequency, are *Bacillus acidophilus, Streptococcus viridans,* and *Neisseria catarrhalis.*

The dental pulp is a mass of vascular tissue enclosed within the tooth. Inflammation may increase the pressure within the pulp space, with pain due to stimulation of the nerves that enter by way of the root canal. When the nerves become devitalized from an inflammatory process, a superimposed acute inflammation will cause no pain. Either an acute or a chronic infection may extend to the periodontal membrane (periodontitis) through the root canal. The resulting inflammatory exudation may cause abnormal extrusion of the tooth from its socket; hence, a sensation of soreness is experienced on chewing, since the biting surface of the tooth is raised. The infection may spread and cause a dento-alveolar abscess (q.v.). When pulpitis or periodontitis occurs, a cavity or a "leaking" filling generally will be found in the affected tooth.

Diagnosis

Pain arising from pulp inflammation must be distinguished from that due to periodontal inflammation. In typical cases, the pain in pulpitis is sharp, throbbing, shooting, and intermittent. Since it may be referred ipsilaterally to the ear or to an adjacent tooth, the tooth involved is difficult to identify. The pain usually is relieved by cold mouthwashes and intensified by hot ones. A toothache of this nature generally indicates the beginning of an irreversible process that probably will result in a nonvital pulp. In periodontitis, the pain is dull, gnawing, and continuous. It is not affected by heat or cold, although cold may give some relief. The patient accurately locates the affected tooth, which is "tender" to pressure.

Treatment

Pulpitis: Oil of cloves, alone or combined with chlorobutanol (℞ 27, 28), is an effective anodyne. Applied in a moistened cotton pellet, or as a thick paste made by mixing with zinc oxide powder, the medication usually affords prompt relief except when there is frank pulp suppuration. An analgesic occasionally will be required (℞ 30, 31). Frank pulp suppuration generally can be relieved only by extraction or by establishing drainage through a passageway drilled to the pulp space (a dental procedure). For individuals with valvular or congenital heart disease, extraction or surgical drainage should be preceded and followed by large doses of penicillin (℞ 16, 17) administered parenterally. Local application of penicillin, 100,-000 u. in the socket immediately following extraction, is a valuable measure (℞ 18). The patient should consult a dentist as soon as possible.

Periodontitis (*see also* PERIODONTAL DISEASE): An analgesic is necessary in most instances (R 30, 31). An ice bag usually lessens discomfort. A counterirritant (R 32, 33) may be applied to the overlying gum. A dentist should be consulted immediately. He may extract the tooth, or choose root therapy to retain the devitalized tooth. Unless adequate measures are taken a dento-alveolar abscess (q.v.) may ensue. Penicillin (R 16, 17) parenterally is indicated prophylactically.

DENTAL CARIES

(Tooth cavities)

A pathologic process marked by gradual dissolution and disintegration of the enamel, dentine, and eventually the pulp of an affected tooth.

Etiology

According to present knowledge no single agent is responsible for dental caries. The action of the *Lactobacillus acidophilus* and other common oral bacteria on carbohydrate foods results in excessive carbohydrate degradation and consequent acid production. This acid, formed on the surface of the teeth within bacterial plaques, is thought to cause decalcification of the enamel and thus to initiate caries formation. Other predisposing causes implicated are congenital defects in the enamel and dentine; malocclusion, and prosthetic and orthodontic appliances; a diet with insufficient coarseness; malnutrition during periods of tooth formation; and variations in the chemical composition of the saliva that interfere with its neutralizing and antibacterial properties. Systemic conditions play an insignificant role in caries formation. The saying, "For every child a tooth," no longer is tenable; apparently once the permanent teeth are fully formed they are little influenced by the nutritional state or the calcium demands of the body.

Pathology

Dental caries begins as local chalky discoloration of the enamel, which becomes roughened and friable. Bits of enamel break off, exposing the dentine, which then becomes softened and decomposes. Finally, the pulp is included in the process, infection develops, and necrosis occurs. Pain usually begins when the dentine is exposed and becomes more severe the closer the pulp is approached. The infection may progress to include the apical end of the tooth, resulting in an apical abscess or granuloma.

Prophylaxis

The value of the toothbrush and mouthwash in caries control has been greatly overrated. They may be of some value in removing bacterial plaques and are recommended for cosmetic purposes mainly. The proper use of a toothbrush at least twice daily with a warm water solution of salt (R 1) or sodium bicarbonate (R 2), within 15 minutes after eating, will accomplish all that can be expected from a dentifrice. Excessive carbohydrate intake at mealtime and the habit of eating sweets between meals should be avoided. Repeated ingestion of strongly acid foods, such as lemon juice, may result in enamel decalcification.

Recently, the use of fluorides and ammoniated dentifrices has been of some interest. The presence of fluorine in a concentration of 1 part per million in drinking water during the early years of tooth formation appears to be an effective weapon in preventing the future development of caries. Fluorides, when deposited in the organic matrix of the enamel, cause the deposition of its calcium salts, which increase the resistance of the enamel to the formation of caries. The best prophylaxis is to visit the dentist at frequent intervals for prompt correction of factors predisposing to caries.

Treatment

Toothache due to caries may be relieved temporarily by cleaning out the debris, drying the cavity, and inserting a small cotton pellet moistened with oil of clove (R 27, 28) or a cocaine-phenol-collodion mixture (R 29). Carious teeth should be filled by a dentist when possible. If the pulp is infected, root canal therapy may obviate the necessity for extraction. However, in the presence of extensive periapical infection the tooth should be extracted.

———

DENTO-ALVEOLAR ABSCESS

(Suppurative peridentitis)

Acute or chronic abscess formation in the periapical alveolar bone.

ACUTE DENTO-ALVEOLAR ABSCESS

Etiology and Pathogenesis

Infection secondary to pulpitis (*see* TOOTHACHE) extending via the root canal to the periodontal membrane probably is the most common cause. Occasionally, root canal therapy or other instrumentation results in apical abscess formation. The resultant abscess, invading the marrow spaces and destroying the trabeculae, may eventually involve or spread beyond the cortex and periosteum. The organisms most commonly responsible are hemolytic streptococci, *Streptococcus viridans*, and staphylococci.

Symptoms and Signs

The patient complains of a dull, continuous, throbbing pain becoming more intense upon biting or moving the tooth. Identification of the offending tooth is sometimes difficult. Frequently it is loose, carious, and raised, and is the first to occlude. A parulis, or "gumboil," representing direct abscess extension through the periosteum may be seen presenting on the buccal or lingual side of the gum in the vicinity of the involved tooth. A thickened periodontal membrane and a radiolucent area at the root apex usually are visible on roentgen examination.

Edema resulting from the abscess may cause, according to its location, obliteration of the nasolabial fold or angle of the jaw, swelling of the eye, puffed lips, and varying degrees of trismus due to reflex spasm of the masseter and internal pterygoid muscles. Facial cellulitis, abscesses in the floor of the mouth, and osteomyelitis of the mandible may occur.

Differential diagnosis must exclude parotitis (mumps), suppurative infection of the parotid and submaxillary glands, angioneurotic edema, peritonsillar abscess, Vincent's angina, actinomycosis, and neoplasms of the mouth and neck.

Treatment

Successful chemotherapy may be possible, particularly when there is no palpable intra- or extra-oral fluctuation. Since the common causative organisms are penicillin-sensitive, adequate parenteral doses of this drug (℞ 16, 17) are indicated. Analgesics (℞ 30, 31) may be necessary. An ice bag applied to the swollen area for 20 minutes every 2 hours occasionally gives relief. A soft diet (*see* DIETS) will obviate discomfort in mastication. The fluid intake should be moderately increased. Warm, saline mouthwashes or, preferably, oral irrigations with 1 or 2 quarts of warm saline solution every 2 to 4 hours (℞ 3), are helpful. When fluctuation is present, drainage also should be established. For cosmetic reasons, the incision should be intra-oral when possible. If general anesthesia is contraindicated for this procedure, ethyl chloride may be used locally. Drainage should be maintained with a gauze or rubber drain until the infection has subsided.

By special dental procedures the tooth occasionally may be saved; however, extraction usually is necessary. Extraction may effect adequate drainage, provided the abscess has not penetrated to the soft tissues. Edema of itself does not contraindicate extraction. General anesthesia should be used when possible and infiltration anesthesia avoided. Penicillin, 100,-000 u. placed directly into the tooth socket, is useful (℞ 18). Until infection is controlled, parenteral penicillin (℞ 16, 17) should be continued. To minimize hemorrhage, the dentist may prohibit mouthwashes for 24 hours after the extraction.

CHRONIC DENTO-ALVEOLAR ABSCESS

Etiology

The cause of the chronic forms is similar to that of the acute, but a granulomatous reaction in the periodontal membrane allays the immediate infectious invasion of the marrow spaces. A "simple" granuloma, containing leukocytes and plasma cells, may remain small indefinitely, but occasionally increases in size until a large area is involved in a so-called granulating osteitis. An epithelial granuloma, formed from the sheath of Hertwig, may become cystic (radicular cyst) and gradually expand over the root area of several teeth. Any of the three forms may become exacerbated into an acute abscess, or may cause resorption of teeth, condensing osteitis, and hypercementosis, the areas resembling compact bone. Also, they may serve as foci of infection.

Symptoms and Signs

Usually, chronic dento-alveolar abscesses are symptomless, and can be diagnosed only by X-ray.

Treatment

The various dental procedures employed—extraction, root-canal therapy, iontophoresis, and apicoectomy—are designed to eliminate infection and promote replacement of the granulation tissue by normal bone.

PERIODONTAL DISEASE

(Periodontitis, Periodontoclasia,
Pyorrhea alveolaris, Riggs' disease)

An inflammation of the gum margin and dental periosteum, largely due to local irritations, characterized by resorption of the alveolar bone, loosening of the teeth, and often shrinking of the gums.

Etiology

The causes may be local or systemic. Local causes include irregularities in form and position of teeth resulting in food impactions and faulty occlusion; oral sepsis and poor oral hygiene; mechanical irritation by calculus, ill-fitting crowns and bridges, and incorrect tooth brushing. Among systemic predisposing factors are blood dyscrasias, hyperthyroidism, diabetes mellitus, pregnancy, improper diet, vitamin A and C deficiencies, acid-base imbalance, and drug intoxication.

Pathologic Physiology

In pyorrhea alveolaris, a pocket forms between the marginal gingiva and the tooth, an area of low hygiene. Infection produces a break in the external epithelium of the periodontal membrane, which is followed by invasion of exposed connective tissue. Suppuration of infected periodontal structures ensues and causes progressive loosening of the tooth. The role of bacteria in periodontal disease is secondary. They accelerate and complicate the initial lesions. If drainage becomes blocked, suppuration deep within a pocket may result in a periodontal abscess. In traumatogenic occlusion and systemic disease, alveolar atrophy with loosening of teeth may precede pocket formation. Periodontitis consequent to faulty occlusion, in contradistinction to that found in the mouth with poor hygiene but without malocclusion, is more difficult to treat. The pocket usually is narrow and deep, and escapes clinical detection until well advanced. When occlusion is good, the pocket develops before deeper structural changes take place. It is broad and shallow and progresses slowly with evidence of overlying gingivitis. Mobility of teeth occurs late.

Diagnosis

Roentgenographic examination is essential for the early recognition of pyorrhea. It may reveal alveolar bone absorption, widening of the occlusal one-third of the periodontal space, and the presence of periodontal abscesses.

Early local signs of periodontitis may be mobility of teeth, deviation from the normal stippled, pale pink color of the gingival epithelium, injection of capillary vessels of the marginal gingivae, gingival festoons (linear depressions in the marginal gingivae producing festooning of the gum margin), and gingival clefts (vertical cuts or clefts in the gum margin). The advanced disease is easily recognized by the presence of gingival recession with or without gingivitis, severe alveolar bone absorption, deep pockets around the teeth exuding pus, loosening of teeth, and periodontal abscesses.

Prognosis

Early detection and prompt adequate therapy, with the elimination of the etiologic and precipitating factors, most often will result in a favorable prognosis. If elimination of the etiologic factors or obliteration of the gingival pockets proves impossible, the prognosis is hopeless.

Treatment

The treatment is almost entirely a dental matter. In **early cases** in which the gingival involvement is superficial and the gingival pockets are shallow, treatment lies in removing the causes of irritation by correcting malocclusion, removing calculus by mechanical scaling and polishing, and massaging the gums. Subgingival curettage, in which the gingival pocket is cleansed periodically by a caustic, and instrumentation may be necessary to allow tissue repair. Glycerite of tannic acid (℞ 6) or potassium chlorate mouthwash (℞ 4, 8) should be used in the after-treatment. Regular brushing of the teeth with a liquid dentifrice (R 9) and the use of dental floss after every meal are desirable.

In **advanced cases**, or those which do not respond to conservative therapy, radical operative treatment may be necessary. This consists of excising, by knife or cautery, the overlying gingival tissue to the depth of the pocket. Extraction becomes unavoidable in cases of much destruction of alveolar bone or when the subgingival pocket cannot be eliminated.

DENTAL EMERGENCIES

Treatment of the following dental conditions ordinarily belongs in the hands of the skilled dentist or oral surgeon. However, emergency treatment is occasionally required, when dental consultation is not immediately available. Although postoperative complications are rare in proportion to the number of teeth extracted, hemorrhage, pain, swelling, and infection sometimes occur.

HEMORRHAGE

Postextraction bleeding may be arterial or venous in origin but most frequently results from capillary ooze. The bleeding may be due to local or systemic conditions.

Local factors may result in primary hemorrhage immediately after extraction, or secondary hemorrhage 48 to 72 hours later. Primary bleeding may be caused by too early and too violent rinsing of the mouth, constant sucking out and expectoration of blood, or laceration of tissue and bone during operation without proper care immediately after. Secondary bleeding often is caused by a poorly formed lobulated clot or a spongy bulbous exuberant clot in the socket.

In cases of prolonged and uncontrollable hemorrhage, the possibility of blood dyscrasias or other systemic diseases must be considered. Complete blood count and intensive physical work-up are indicated.

Treatment

Primary hemorrhage: Examine postextraction site; cleanse with warm saline solution and dry the area as well as possible to determine the amount and rapidity of the bleeding. Attempt to control the bleeding by pressure. This can be done by folding a 2″ x 2″ sterile gauze pad into a small hard mass, placing it on the extraction site, and having the patient bite and continue firm pressure for 10 to 15 minutes. Then examine the area and watch for several minutes to see if oozing persists. If all is well, dismiss the patient with the admonition to avoid rinsing his mouth and excessive spitting for 24 hours.

If bleeding cannot be stopped by pressure alone, hemostatic

agents should be resorted to. Several mouthfuls of a hydrogen peroxide solution (℞ 37) retained in the region of the bleeding socket, without mechanical rinsing, and followed by compression, may stop the bleeding. Iodoform gauze saturated with epinephrine 1:1,000 (℞ 38), snake venom (℞ 39), thromboplastin (℞ 40), or tannic acid in glycerin (℞ 41) packed firmly into the socket may produce hemostasis. The packing should be left intact for at least 72 hours, and then carefully removed.

Secondary hemorrhage: Therapy is essentially the same as for primary hemorrhage; however, every remnant of the old poorly formed clot must be carefully removed and the socket irrigated with saline (℞ 3) or hydrogen peroxide solution (℞ 37), followed by simple compression or packing with or without hemostatic agents. At times, compression packing is impossible due to severe tissue laceration, and the wound must be sutured to control bleeding. Recently, various forms of absorbable oxidized cotton, gauze, and other coagulating materials have been used with success.

POSTEXTRACTION PAIN

Pain immediately following extraction may be due to infection in the socket or to operative trauma. Delayed pain occurs 2 or 3 days after extraction, becomes increasingly acute after the 3rd day, continues in severe form for about 4 or 5 days, and usually subsides completely by the 10th or 12th day, but may persist for 2 or 3 weeks. Examination of the socket reveals a foul-smelling disintegrating clot with inflammatory reaction in the neighboring tissues. Careful investigative cleansing of the socket with cotton applicators and warm saline irrigation may reveal a portion of the alveolar bone. This condition is called "dry socket," and actually is a local osteitis.

Treatment

Immediate pain may be relieved by frequent cold applications to the face. A painful "dry socket" should be irrigated with warm saline solution (℞ 3) and packed with iodoform gauze saturated with eugenol (℞ 34) or guaiacol with glycerin (℞ 35). Unlike packing for hemorrhage, the gauze is placed lightly into the depth of the socket so that its sedative action will be effective without delaying wound granulation. Systemic analgesics (℞ 30, 31) and a sedative (℞ 36) are indicated for pain and insomnia.

POSTEXTRACTION SWELLING

This usually results from trauma to the soft and osseous tissues and is generally without much pain or tenderness. There may be a slight febrile reaction with little or no malaise.

Treatment

Ice bags are applied externally for one half hour every hour until the swelling decreases. Sedatives such as phenobarbital (℞ 36) are given for nervousness.

POSTEXTRACTION INFECTIONS

Occasionally, a traumatic swelling becomes infected and cellulitis requiring incision and drainage may result. Ludwig's angina (q.v.) is a rare complication. An increase of swelling on the 3rd day suggests infection, and massive doses of penicillin (℞ 16, 17) or a sulfonamide (℞ 21) are indicated. Bed rest in a half-sitting position is essential for good drainage.

A transitory bacteremia usually follows extraction. Patients with congenital heart lesions or a history of rheumatic heart disease should be given penicillin (℞ 17) before and after extraction as a prophylactic against bacterial endocarditis.

OTHER DENTAL EMERGENCIES

In **tooth fractures** that expose the pulp, pain may be relieved (pending definitive dental care) by painting the exposed pulp with eugenol (℞ 34) and covering it with a wax cap.

Fractures of the mandible should be treated by an oral surgeon. Emergency measures consist of manually reducing the fragments, as gently as possible, and maintaining reduction with a four-tail bandage placed over the point of the jaw and fastened securely over the head. Since these fractures usually are compound, penicillin should be given systemically to prevent infection from the oral cavity. It is essential that early and expert management be provided so as to guarantee the best possible occlusal results.

SALIVARY DISORDERS

(Ptyalism, Salivation, Sialorrhea, Mercurialism; Aptyalism, Oligosialia, Xerostomia, Dry Mouth)

PTYALISM

Hypersecretion of saliva, up to 10 quarts/24 hours (normal 2 to 3 pints). **Pseudoptyalism** means drivelling due to paresis of lips, tongue, or pharynx; to coma or anesthesia; to dislocation or fracture of the jaw; or to dysphagia with quinsy or similar situations.

Etiology

The causes of excessive salivation, in order of frequency, include: (1) Drugs or poisons, such as mercury, tobacco, arsenic, bismuth, certain types of mushrooms. (2) Local inflammation, as with stomatitis, pyorrhea, or diseases such as purpura, scurvy, sprue, or the anemias. (3) Local irritation from teething, salivary calculus, jagged teeth, or dental appliances. (4) Infectious diseases, particularly rabies and smallpox. (5) Reflex stimulation from liver, uterus (pregnancy), ovary (sometimes cancer), and stomach. (6) Disturbances of the nervous system, such as car sickness, migraine, hysteria, irritation of chorda tympani (usually with 7th nerve paralysis); in paralysis agitans, encephalitis lethargica, tic douloureux, and tabes. (7) Idiopathic, which may be either intermittent or continuous and may occur in nurslings.

Symptoms and Signs

Disordered taste and thickened speech may ensue; also indigestion and vomiting due to volume of saliva swallowed. In mercurialism, there are enlarged, painful salivary glands and the saliva is irritating to skin and lips. Also noted are a metallic taste; fetid breath; coated, swollen tongue; discoloration of the gums; ulcerations of gums and tongue. Systemically, abdominal pain, diarrhea and asthenia sometimes are encountered.

Treatment

Causal: Treat any underlying disease process, whether local or systemic. With mercurial ptyalism, prevent further ingress of mercury, use saline cathartics, administer sodium thiosulfate (R 42) until BAL (R 43) is obtained.

Restorative: Oral hygiene and dental attention are imperative. Potassium chlorate mouthwash (R 4), especially in mercurialism; or an alkaline mouthwash (R 5), sometimes useful for cleansing action, may be used. Astringent solution (R 6) or mouthwash (R 7) is indicated if gums are swollen. Healing of ulcers is encouraged by silver nitrate solution 5% (R 44) cautiously applied every 1 to 3 days. Vitamins, tonics, stimulants, and penicillin, should be used, as indicated.

Symptomatic: Atropine (R 45) checks ptyalism. In mercurialism its use is probably contraindicated, except in the later stages. X-radiation of the salivary glands, in expert hands, is effective but may cause dry mouth, hence is not usually advisable. Phenobarbital (R 36) is useful to allay nervousness.

APTYALISM

Hyposecretion of saliva.

Etiology

This condition may result from X-ray therapy of facial regions; from certain drugs, as atropine, belladonna, opium, morphine; from dehydration, as with fever, cholera, or kidney disease. A severe form known as xerostomia, seen most frequently in elderly women, usually follows mental shock, but may develop secondary to mumps, typhoid fever, or diabetes. Taste is lost, the teeth may fall out, articulation and deglutition are difficult, and the tongue may eventually resemble crocodile skin. Lacrimal and nasal secretions also may be deficient.

Dryness of all mucous membranes is seen in Sjögren's syndrome.

Treatment

Glycerin as a mouthwash is comforting. In protracted aptyalism, replacing the teeth with well-fitted dentures may help through minimizing respirational drying. Pilocarpine (℞ 46) may be tried. In Sjögren's syndrome, Urecholine (℞ 47) in a few investigational instances has proved helpful.

GLOSSITIS

An acute or chronic inflammatory disturbance of the tongue, which may be either a primary disease of the tongue or a symptom of disease elsewhere.

Classification

The various types of glossitis include: geographical tongue; glossitis rhombica mediana; glossodynia; lingua nigra (black, hairy tongue); Moeller's glossitis (slick tongue, glossy tongue, glazed tongue, glossodynia exfoliativa); transitory benign plaques of the tongue.

Etiology

The causes of glossitis are many and varied, and include:

Local: Infectious agents (monilia, herpes simplex virus, *C. diphtheriae*, streptococci, *Myco. tuberculosis, T. pallidum*); mechanical trauma (jagged teeth, poorly-fitting dentures, mouth breathing, repeated biting during epileptic seizures); primary irritants (excessive use of alcohol, tobacco, hot foods, spices); or sensitization (by tooth paste, mouthwashes, candy dyes, plastic toothbrushes, dentures).

General causes: Avitaminosis (particularly of the B group, as in pellagra), anemia (pernicious anemia, iron deficiency anemia, Plummer-Vinson syndrome with dysphagia), certain generalized skin diseases that frequently have tongue manifestations (lichen planus, erythema multiforme, Behcet's syndrome, pemphigus vulgaris), and certain systemic infections, such as scarlet fever. In addition, there are several primary diseases of unknown etiology which affect the tongue.

Symptoms and Signs

The clinical manifestations vary widely. There often is little correlation between extent or degree of lesions and severity of symptoms. Although some lesions are characteristic, different diseases may be manifested by the same type of glossitis.

Reddened tip and edges of the tongue may indicate excessive smoking, early pellagra, rough lingual surface of a tooth, or anemia. In later stages of pellagra the entire tongue is fiery red, swollen, and often ulcerated. Painful ulcers may indicate herpetic infection, pulmonary tuberculosis with positive sputum, streptococcal infection, Behcet's triple syndrome (uveitis, stomatitis, and genital ulcers), or pemphigus vulgaris. Whitish patches may indicate such conditions as moniliasis, lichen planus, leukoplakia, or mouth breathing. Denuded smooth areas if not painful may indicate "geographical tongue" (superficial excoriations, transitory benign plaques), or if moderately painful might indicate anemia or pellagra, and if very distressing and persistent may be the lesions of Moeller's glossitis. Glossitis rhombica mediana produces a rhomboid-shaped smooth area on the dorsal surface of the middle third of the tongue. Black hairy tongue, often following excessive use of oxygen-liberating mouthwashes, appears as a pigmented profuse overgrowth of the fine papillae beginning at the middle of the posterior third and usually is asymptomatic.

A severe acute glossitis due to local infection, burns, or trauma occasionally is seen and may develop rapidly, producing marked tenderness or pain with swelling sufficient to cause protrusion of the tongue and the danger of obstruction and suffocation. Mastication, swallowing and articulation are painful (sometimes impossible). There may be cervical and sublingual adenitis with evidence of systemic toxicity. Suppuration may occur.

Diagnosis

Since the tongue often serves as a mirror of disease elsewhere, it is most important to investigate thoroughly every patient who shows glossitis. A careful history will reveal possible irritants, contact allergens, drugs to which the patient may be sensitive, deficient diet, or symptoms of disease elsewhere. Other mucosal surfaces should be checked for lesions of erythema multiforme, syphilis, or lichen planus. The skin may reveal evidence of pellagra, syphilis, or erythema multiforme. Pulmonary tuberculosis and sprue should be ruled out. A blood examination for anemia and a serologic test for syphilis should be performed.

Prognosis

The prognosis depends on the cause. When this can be determined and corrected, response is usually prompt. Idiopathic lesions such as Moeller's glossitis, glossitis rhombica mediana, and geographical tongue, tend to persist for long periods. Aphthous ulcers, erythema multiforme, and lingua nigra often recur periodically. The usually painful ulcers associated with pulmonary tuberculosis and with pemphigus vulgaris often indicate a fatal prognosis.

Treatment

General: Treatment should aim to remove the offending agent. Anemia, vitamin deficiencies and systemic infections are treated as indicated. Alcohol, tobacco, spices, hot and irritating drinks are to be avoided. A bland or liquid diet (*see* DIETS), preferably cooled, is given. Good oral hygiene, including proper care of the teeth, should be required. The standard alkaline aromatic solution (R 10) serves as a bland, pleasant-tasting mouthwash. Benzalkonium chloride and cetyl pyridinium chloride mouthwashes (R 11, 12) are most useful because of their detergent action and effectiveness against a wide variety of infectious organisms.

Local: Mouth infections should receive specific therapy (*see* STOMATITIS). Small painful ulcers may be touched with 5% silver nitrate (R 44). Large painful lesions that interfere with eating may be temporarily relieved by rinsing with an anesthetic solution before each meal (R 13). Small pieces of ice held in the mouth may afford some relief, but analgesics containing codeine are occasionally required (R 30, 31).

Moniliasis may be treated by painting the ulcers with 1% gentian violet (R 22). Streptococcal infections respond to penicillin lozenges (R 19) or sulfadiazine tablets used as lozenges (R 21). Systemic administration of these drugs (R 16, 17, 21) may be indicated for severe infections.

Incision and drainage are indicated for suppuration. A tracheotomy may be necessary if obstruction to the airway is threatened by severe edema of the tongue.

In cases of nonspecific or chronic involvement, response may be delayed. Reassurance and encouragement of the patient are important.

STOMATITIS

An inflammatory condition of the mouth, which may occur as a primary disease or as a symptom of systemic disease. **Glossitis** (q.v.) and **gingivitis** (q.v.) are localized forms of stomatitis.

Etiology

A multiplicity of disease agents may produce stomatitis. Locally, pathogens such as the streptococcus, gonococcus, *C. diphtheriae, Candida albicans (Monilia), T. pallidum,* Vincent's fusospirochete, *Myco. tuberculosis,* and the viruses of herpes simplex or measles may attack the mouth. Mechanical trauma from cheek biting, jagged teeth, ill-fitting dentures, nursing bottles with a hard or too long nipple (producing Bednar's apthae), or mouth breathing may produce characteristic lesions. Stomatitis sometimes results from excessive use of irritants such as alcohol, tobacco, hot foods, spices; or from sensitization to substances such as tooth paste, mouthwashes, candy dyes, and plastic toothbrushes or dentures. It also may result from avitaminosis, particularly of the B vitamins as in pellagra or C as in scurvy; or from blood disorders such as pernicious anemia, iron deficiency anemia with dysphagia (Plummer-Vinson syndrome), infectious mononucleosis, agranulocytosis, or leukemia. Certain generalized skin lesions frequently have buccal manifestations: lichen planus, erythema multiforme, lupus erythematosus, Behcet's syndrome, and pemphigus vulgaris; also systemic infections such as scarlet fever, measles, and syphilis. The following drugs not uncommonly produce stomatitis; diphenylhydantoin, iodides, bismuth, mercury, barbiturates, and lead. In addition, there are several types of stomatitis of unknown etiology.

Symptoms and Signs

The clinical manifestations of stomatitis vary widely. The following are the most common entities:

Acute infectious gingivostomatitis occurring as a primary infection with the virus of herpes simplex is common in infants and young children. Frequently, a history of contact with an adult with herpes simplex ("fever blisters") (q.v.) can be obtained. Characteristic symptoms are painful mouth with red, swollen gums which bleed easily, ulcers and whitish plaques of the mucous membrane and often the tonsils, oral fetor, regional adenopathy, fever, and irritability. The disease persists for 10 to 14 days. A mistaken diagnosis of fusospirochetosis may be made.

Ulceromembranous stomatitis (Vincent's fusospirochetal disease, "trench mouth" [q.v.]) may occur as a gingivitis with bluish red, swollen gingival margins which are painful and bleed easily, or it may extend to produce painful ulcers of the mucous membranes. Oral fetor is common. Predisposing factors, such as contact or therapy with heavy metals, blood dyscrasias, vitamin deficiencies, and debilitating diseases, often play a role.

Gangrenous stomatitis (Noma, Cancrum oris) is a rapidly spreading gangrene which occurs in debilitated children 2 to 5 years of age, usually after one of the infectious diseases. A small ulcer covered with gray or black slough begins upon the buccal surface, gums, or inner side of the lip, and the skin over the cheek soon becomes brawny, then red and tense, finally black and necrotic. Gangrene may rapidly destroy one side of the face. Pain and fever are not pronounced. The child is prostrated, and death occurs in 5 to 10 days. The few children who recover are greatly disfigured. Bronchopneumonia, abscess of the lung, and severe diarrhea are complications.

Dermatostomatitis (Ectodermosis pluriorificialis) is a rare disease of children and young people, the worst result of which may be blindness. It is characterized by chill, headache and fever, profuse salivation, conjunctivitis, development of vesicles on the lips, tongue, and cheeks and later erythematous or petechial lesions of the hands.

11

Thrush results from infection with *Monilia* (*Candida albicans*). It is characterized by white, slightly raised patches, which somewhat resemble milk curds and can be removed only with difficulty, then revealing a hyperemic area which may bleed slightly. This mycotic infection usually begins on the tongue and buccal mucosa and may spread to involve the palate, gums, tonsils, pharynx, larynx, gastrointestinal tract, respiratory system, and skin. The mouth usually appears dry. With uncomplicated thrush, the systemic symptoms generally are slight. However, systemic infections, which may be fatal, occasionally occur (*see* MONILIASIS).

Pseudomembranous stomatitis is a type of inflammatory reaction that produces a membrane-like exudate on the mucous membrane. Any membrane resembling that produced by diphtheria should be examined by smear and culture, and proper treatment begun immediately if a diagnosis of diphtheria (q.v.) is made. Other infectious agents such as streptococci, staphylococci, and gonococci, as well as some chemical irritants may produce a pseudomembranous stomatitis. Severe systemic reactions often occur with these conditions.

Ulcerative stomatitis, like other types mentioned, may occur with a variety of systemic diseases. Discrete, small, painful recurrent ulcers called "canker sores" or aphthae (aphthous stomatitis) are very common. Their etiology is in doubt. Some believe they result from ingestion of certain foods, such as chocolate or nuts, while others think the virus of herpes simplex is responsible. Traumatic ulcers and the lesions resulting from severe pulmonary tuberculosis or blood dyscrasias usually are grouped here.

Catarrhal stomatitis is a term used to indicate certain mild superficial lesions of the mouth. The mucous membranes may be red and slightly edematous, and the patient usually complains of tenderness or soreness of the mouth. Irritants (including various allergens and tobacco), B vitamin deficiencies, and anemia should be investigated as possible etiologic agents.

Distinctive forms of stomatitis occur in association with other diseases, the most important of which are the mucous patches of syphilis; the strawberry, then raspberry, tongue of scarlet fever; Koplik's spots of measles; the lacy and reticulate white network of lichen planus; hypertrophic gingivitis from dilantin administration; the ulcers of erythema multiforme, including the Stevens-Johnson syndrome (erythema multiforme bullosum, with involvement of the eye, producing blindness); the triple syndrome of Behcet (stomatitis, uveitis, genital ulcers); and the smooth, fiery red tongue and painful mouth of pellagra.

Diagnosis

Since stomatitis may be of local or systemic origin, discovering its etiology may be difficult. The patient's history may reveal a systemic or degenerative disease, a dietary deficiency, or contact with irritants or allergens. A general physical examination should always be made. This may disclose lesions of other mucous membranes, as in erythema multiforme, moniliasis, or syphilis; or of the skin, as in pellagra, lichen planus, or lupus erythematosus; or the signs of pulmonary tuberculosis, sprue, anemia, or some of the other contributory diseases.

Scrapings from lesions of suspected moniliasis should be cultured and also examined microscopically, in 20% potassium hydroxide, for identification of *Candida albicans*. Other laboratory procedures, such as blood counts, bone marrow examinations, or gastric analysis, may be indicated. Direct smears from the mouth lesions, suitably stained, may reveal etiologic bacteria. Cultures on solid media often are of help, especially when diphtheria is suspected. Penicillin has been so effective in Vincent's disease (q.v.) as almost to constitute a therapeutic test to differentiate the disease from acute herpetic gingivostomatitis. Syphilis must be ruled out, however, before using penicillin in this way. Serologic tests are necessary for suspected syphilis, and darkfield examination of scrapings from the lesions should be performed, with proper precautions to prevent confusion with nonpathogenic spirochetes present in the mouth which may closely resemble the spirochetes of syphilis.

Treatment

Anemia, vitamin deficiencies, and systemic infections, if present, should be appropriately treated. Local infections should receive specific therapy, plus careful oral hygiene. Thrush responds best to gentian violet (℞ 22) applied twice a day; streptococcal, staphylococcal, and gonococcal infection, to penicillin lozenges (℞ 19) or sulfadiazine tablets (℞ 21) held in the mouth until completely dissolved; or to systemic administration of these drugs (℞ 16, 17, 21), or both. Vincent's fusospirochetal disease should be treated with penicillin locally (℞ 19) or, if severe as in gangrenous stomatitis, by parenteral administration (℞ 16, 17). Small, painful ulcers may be touched with 5% silver nitrate (℞ 44) every day. Resistant cases of thrush and ulcerative stomatitis sometimes do well with 1% formalin (℞ 23) applied daily. Large, painful ulcers that prevent eating may be temporarily relieved by rinsing the mouth with a few drops of an anesthetic solution (℞ 13) before each meal. Mouthwashes used carefully may be of distinct benefit in many forms of stomatitis. The quaternary ammonium compounds (℞ 11, 12) make the most useful mouthwashes because of their detergent action and effectiveness against a wide variety of infectious organisms. The standard alkaline aromatic solution (℞ 10) serves as a bland, pleasant-tasting mouthwash. Repeated smallpox vaccination (once

weekly for 8 to 12 weeks) should be tried in the treatment of
recurrent aphthous ulcers of the mouth.

GINGIVITIS

*Inflammation of the gums characterized by congested, red,
and swollen gingivae, which usually are painless and tend to
bleed easily on pressure.* The inflammation may be acute or
chronic and generalized or confined to certain areas. It may
be classified as: (1) **marginal gingivitis**, involvement of the
gum margin alone without enlargement or recession; (2) **hypertrophic gingivitis**, prominent hyperplasia or hypertrophy
of the gum, the free margins of which are thickened and rolled,
with the interdental papillae large and bulbous—usually indicative of a chronic process; (3) **atrophic gingivitis**, characterized by recession of the gum margin.

Etiology

Differentiation of etiology by means of clinical manifestations often is impossible. **Local factors** frequently are the
sole cause. Such include oral sepsis, malocclusion, dental calculus, food impaction, faulty dental restorations, and mouth
breathing.

General causes include hypovitaminosis; blood dyscrasias;
allergic reactions; endocrine disturbances, such as diabetes, or
those of pregnancy and menstruation; drug toxicity, as caused
by diphenylhydantoin, or the heavy metals; and chronic infections, such as tuberculosis and syphilis, or other debilitating
disease. Lowered tissue resistance in systemic disturbances
renders the gingivae more susceptible to local insults. Gingivitis may be the first sign of an underlying systemic disorder.

Symptoms, Signs, and Diagnosis

Simple Inflammatory Gingivitis: A narrow band of bright
red inflamed gum tissue surrounding the neck of a tooth, an
edematous increase in the size of the interdental papillae, comparative freedom from pain, and immediate bleeding on the
slightest injury, are the outstanding signs. The inflammation
usually is acute in onset. It may subside completely or persist
in chronic form.

Diabetic Gingivitis: Characterized by severe gingival disturbances. The rapid accumulation of supragingival calculus
ultimately results in a marginal periodontitis. Diabetic patients
are prone to develop secondary infections superimposed on the
gingivitis. Acute abscesses may be seen on the gums as well
as polyps protruding from the abnormally heavy gingival margin, forcing the gum away from the side of the tooth.

Gingivitis of Pregnancy: Characterized by a mild inflammation of the gingivae in which hypertrophy, especially of the interdental papillae, is prominent. The mucosa may have a purplish color. Pedunculated tumors often form from the gingival papillae (pregnancy tumors). The condition usually arises in the 1st or 2nd month but may persist throughout the pregnancy. Although the tumors usually subside after termination of pregnancy, they often persist. In some cases of dysmenorrhea, a similar gingival condition may appear.

Leukemia Gingivitis: Characterized by engorged, edematous, painful, hypertrophied gums, which are livid in color and bleed readily. They often are secondarily infected with fusospirillary organisms, in which case the gums present the pseudomembranous exudate and necrotic crateriform papillae of Vincent's disease (q.v.). In addition, the entire mouth is inflamed and, in the acute leukemias, the lymph nodes are enlarged and painful. In myelogenous leukemia the hypertrophied gingivae may be of a purplish color, and in lymphatic leukemia they may be yellow or black.

Diphenylhydantoin Gingivitis: Long-continued use of diphenylhydantoin may cause hyperplasia of the gingivae. With enlargement of the interdental papillae initially, the process may progress until the gums are entirely involved. The hypertrophic gingival tissue is firm and not particularly prone to bleed. The hyperplasia may be extensive enough to partially cover and obscure the teeth.

Hypovitaminosis Gingivitis: In scurvy the gingivae are inflamed, hypertrophic, and bleed easily. They are engorged by accumulation of venous blood. Petechial and ecchymotic areas may be seen on the gums as well as elsewhere in the mouth. The color of the gums has been described as gradually changing from normal pink to old rose and finally to dark blue and purple, or even black. Superimposed infections may cause severe destruction of periosteum and periodontal tissue resulting in loosening of teeth.

In pellagra, the gingivae are inflamed, bleed easily, and are subject to secondary infection with Vincent's organisms. The lips are reddened and cracked, the mouth feels as if it were scalded, and the tongue appears smooth and bright red.

Beriberi and rickets present no distinctive oral lesions.

Gingivitis due to heavy metals: Owing to reaction with hydrogen sulfide produced by food decomposition, lead and bismuth may be deposited in the gums as their sulfide salts. While lead and bismuth lines are fairly common, they rarely produce gingivitis. However, a preexisting gingivitis may enhance deposition of the metals.

Vincent's Gingivitis: (*see* VINCENT'S DISEASE).

Prophylaxis

Careful attention to dental hygiene, routine dental prophylaxis at frequent intervals especially during pregnancy, and a diet containing foods requiring thorough mastication will help prevent the occurrence of gingivitis.

Treatment

Dental factors contributing to the development of gingivitis should be eliminated. These include supragingival calculus, malocclusion, and faulty dental restorations. Systemic factors such as drug toxicity, diabetes, and chronic infections should be corrected as far as possible. Ascorbic acid and vitamin B complex are indicated in the treatment of hypovitaminoses (q.v.). In some instances, hypertrophied gums may be excised by the consulting dentist.

Local medication includes mouthwashes containing tincture of iodine (R 14), tincture of myrrh (R 15), or potassium chlorate (R 4), and painting the gums with Talbot's mixture (R 24), or gentian violet (R 22).

VINCENT'S DISEASE

(Trench mouth, Vincent's angina, Fusospirochetal angina, Ulceromembranous stomatitis)

A pseudomembranous ulceration of the mouth, throat, or gums in which the Bacillus fusiformis, *and the* Borrelia vincentii *(a spirillum) predominate.* Poor oral hygiene, absorption of heavy metals (bismuth, lead and mercury), debilitating infections and vitamin deficiencies predispose to this disease. It often occurs in epidemic form in crowded and insanitary environments, especially when contaminated food utensils are shared.

Symptoms and Signs

Onset usually is abrupt and may be accompanied by malaise and a febrile reaction. There often are no constitutional disturbances, the only complaints being pain on swallowing or talking, bleeding and painful gums, salivation, and fetid breath.

The mouth is most often affected. Lesions of the buccal cavity may appear as diffuse superficial ulcerations covered with grayish membranous exudates (pseudomembranes), which are easily removed. The ulcerations frequently have a punched-out appearance, bleed on slight pressure or irritation and are most numerous on the gums.

Vincent's tonsillitis is a common form of the disease. A gray sloughing ulcer is present in one or both tonsils, and fever and malaise are more prominent. Lesions may occur, rarely, in the bronchi, rectum, and vagina. Regional adenitis often accompanies all varieties of the disease.

Diagnosis

Identification of Vincent's organisms in a stained smear from the lesions establishes the diagnosis. Serologic tests for syphilis and bacterial culture of the causative organism also should be performed. Early differentiation from diphtheria is essential, especially when the disease process is restricted to the tonsils. Streptococcal and staphylococcal tonsillitis and pharyngitis, agranulocytosis, syphilis, and aphthous stomatitis also must be considered in the differential diagnosis.

Treatment

Penicillin is the drug of choice. Superficial mucosal lesions can be treated by local application: in the mouth, by penicillin lozenges (℞ 19); in the vagina and rectum, by penicillin suppositories (℞ 20). Deeper infections or those associated with systemic symptoms should receive penicillin I.M. (℞ 16, 17). Local treatment of the gingivae by a dentist is helpful. Effective preparations for daily local applications are Talbot's iodine solution (℞ 24), 10% arsphenamine in glucose solution (℞ 25), and chromic acid 5% (℞ 26). Bismuth injections or any treatment with other heavy metals should be discontinued until the disease is under control. Brushing the teeth usually is painful and frequent mouth cleansing with an oxidizing solution may be substituted (℞ 37). Perhaps the simplest and most effective local treatment that the patient can carry out at home is a hot normal saline solution mouthwash (℞ 3) used for 5 minutes every hour. This serves as a cleansing agent and also as a means of applying moist heat to the affected parts. Each portion of saline solution should be held in the mouth for about 1 minute. Vitamin C (℞ 48) orally has been recommended and should be used if there is a possibility of scurvy. Tobacco or alcohol tends to aggravate the condition during the acute phase and to induce relapse during the recovery period; therefore, both irritants should be firmly prohibited.

LUDWIG'S ANGINA

(Angina ludovici, Submaxillary cellulitis)

An acute, deep infection of the tissues forming the floor of the mouth, caused by streptococci or, occasionally, staphylococci. The organisms usually gain entrance through a mucosal abrasion or an infected tooth socket; frequently the condition is secondary to a tonsil or throat infection. A widespread cellulitis, which may be purulent or gangrenous, develops in the submaxillary region and spreads along the fascial planes of the neck without tendency to localization or fluctuation. Local swelling, pain, and dysphagia are characteristic symptoms. The patient appears toxic and may have a variable degree of fever. Pressure on the larynx or edema of the glottis frequently produces dyspnea and cyanosis. The tongue is pushed forward and upward by the swelling of the floor of the mouth. Trismus (spasm of the jaw muscles) frequently occurs. Differentiation must be made from submaxillary salivary duct calculus, intrinsic submaxillary glandular disease, and dental abscess.

Treatment

Eradication of any existing primary infection is indicated. Penicillin (℞ 16, 17) or a sulfonamide (℞ 21), or both, should be given until the condition has completely resolved. The patient should be kept in bed and placed on a highly nutritious liquid or soft diet (*see* DIETS). Pain may be controlled by analgesics (℞ 30, 31). If obstruction of the respiratory passage occurs, tracheotomy (q.v.) should be instituted. External incision and drainage of the submaxillary region often are necessary even with full courses of chemotherapy.

PRESCRIPTIONS

(Wherever a prescribed "proprietary" is representative of a class of therapeutic agents, alternative proprietary preparations will be found listed in Part II.)

Mouthwashes and Dentifrices

1. ℞ Sodium chloride

> 1 teaspoon in a glass of warm water, used as a dentifrice, 15 minutes after eating. For Vincent's disease, use hourly.

2. ℞ Sodium bicarbonate

> Use in similar manner as sodium chloride (℞ 1).

3. ℞ Sodium chloride . . . . . .   15.0   Gm. (℥ ss)
   Water . . . . . . q.s. ad 1,000.0 cc. (℥ xxxii)

> Warm to point of comfortable tolerance and use as a mouthwash or for irrigation of oral cavity.

4 ℞ Potassium chlorate. . . . . 120.0   Gm. (℥ iv)

> 1 teaspoon in half a glass of warm water, used as a mouthwash after meals.

5. ℞ Sodium borate . . . .   8.0   Gm. (℥ ii)
   Myrrh Tincture U.S.P. . .   4.0   cc.   (℥ i)
   Water . . . . q.s. ad 180.0 cc.   (℥ vi)

> Dilute with an equal volume of water and use as a mouthwash after meals.

6. ℞ Tannic Acid Glycerite U.S.P.   30.0   cc.   (℥ i)

> 3 to 5 drops in half a glass of warm water, used as a mouthwash after meals.

7. ℞ Boric acid. . . . .   2.0   Gm. (℥ ss)
       Tannic acid. . . . .   2.0   Gm. (℥ ss)
       Honey of rose. . . . . .   8.0   cc. (℥ ii)
       Water . . . . . . .q.s. ad   120.0   cc. (℥ iv)
          Use as a mouthwash.

8. ℞ Potassium chlorate. . . . .   30.0   Gm. (℥ i)
       Glycerin. . . . .   30.0   cc. (℥ i)
       Phenol. . . . .   6.0   Gm. (℥ iss)
       Water . . . . . . q.s. ad 1,000.0   cc. (℥ xxxii)
          Use as a mouthwash after meals.

9. ℞ Menthol . . . .   0.6   Gm. (gr. x)
       Saccharin. . . . .   0.6   Gm. (gr. x)
       Calcium oxide. . . . . . .   12.0   Gm. (℥ iii)
       Methyl salicylate . . . . .   2.0   cc. (℥ ss)
       Sodium chloride . . . . .   500.0   Gm. (℥ xvi)
          ⅓ teaspoon in a glass of water, used as a
          liquid dentifrice.

10. ℞ Alkaline Aromatic Solution
          N.F. . . . .   240.0   cc. (℥ viii)
          Use as a mouthwash after meals and at bed-
          time.

11. ℞ Benzalkonium chloride . . .   1.0   Gm. (gr. xv)
       Water . . . . . . q.s. ad 1,000.0   cc. (℥ xxxii)
          Use as a mouthwash after meals and at bed-
          time.

12. ℞ Cetyl Pyridinium Chloride
          N.N.R. . . . .   0.25 Gm. (gr. iv)
       Water . . . . . . q.s. ad 1,000.0   cc. (℥ xxxii)
          Use as a mouthwash after meals and at bed-
          time.

13. ℞ Benzocaine . . . .   5.0   Gm. (gr. lxxv)
       Emulsion of sweet almonds .   2.0   cc. (℥ ss)
       Tragacanth, powdered . . .   2.0   Gm. (℥ ss)
       Water . . . . . . .q.s. ad   100.0   cc. (℥ iiiss)
          Use a few drops as an anesthetic mouth rinse
          before meals.

14. ℞ Iodine Tincture U.S.P. . . .   15.0   cc. (℥ ss)
          5 drops in half a glass of water, used as a
          mouthwash every 2 or 3 hours.

15. ℞ Myrrh Tincture U.S.P. . . .   30.0   cc. (℥ i)
          10 drops in half a glass of water, used as a
          mouthwash every 2 or 3 hours.

Antimicrobial Agents

16. ℞ Penicillin   (vial)

> 30,000 to 50,000 u. I.M. every 4 hours
> or
> 300,000 u. I.M. every 12 hours.

17. ℞ Procaine penicillin   (vial)

> 300,000 u. I.M. every 24 hours.

18. ℞ Penicillin   (dental cone)

> Place 100,000 u. in tooth socket following extraction.

19. ℞ Penicillin (lozenges). . . . 1,000   u.

> Retain 1 in mouth, until dissolved, 4 times daily.

20. ℞ Penicillin (suppositories) . 5,000   u.

> Insert 1 into the rectum or vagina 1 or 2 times daily.

21. ℞ Sulfadiazine. . . . . 0.5   Gm. (gr. viiss)

> 4 tablets initially, followed by 2 tablets every 4 hours. For local effect, 1 tablet may be retained in the mouth, until dissolved, every 2 to 4 hours.

22. ℞ Gentian violet, 1% solution . 30.0   cc.   (℥ i)

> Paint oral lesions twice daily.

23. ℞ Formalin, 1% solution . . . 30.0   cc.   (℥ i)

> Apply to mouth daily with swabs.

24. ℞ Talbot's iodine solution

> | | | | |
> |---|---|---|---|
> | Zinc iodide . . . . | 5.0 | Gm. | (gr. lxxv) |
> | Iodine crystals. . . . . . | 4.0 | Gm. | (℥ i) |
> | Glycerin . . . . | 60.0 | cc. | (℥ ii) |
> | Distilled water. . . . . . | 75.0 | cc. | (℥ iiss) |

> Apply with a swab to affected gums daily, holding the lips and cheeks away until the iodine has dried.

25. ℞ Arsphenamine-glucose solution (ampul containing 10% arsphenamine base). . . . . 3.0   cc.   (♏ xlv)

> Apply daily to affected gums.

26. ℞ Chromic acid, 5% solution. . 4.0   cc.   (℥ i)

> Apply to ulcerated areas daily.

Anodynes, Analgesics, and Sedatives

27. ℞ Clove Oil U.S.P. . . . . . 15.0   cc.   (℥ ss)

> Apply to aching tooth with a cotton pellet or as a thick paste made with zinc oxide powder.

28. ℞ Chlorobutanol. . . . . . . 4.0 Gm. (℥ i)
    Clove Oil U.S.P. . . .q.s. ad 15.0 cc. (℥ ss)
      Use in same manner as ℞ 27.

29. ℞ Cocaine (alkaloid) . . . . . 0.2 Gm. (gr. iii)
    Phenol . . . . 4.0 Gm. (℥ i)
    Collodion. . . . . 4.0 cc. (℥ i)
      Moisten cotton pellet and insert into dried
      cavity of the painful tooth.

30. ℞ Codeine sulfate . . . . . . 15 mg. (gr. ¼)
      1 to 4 tablets every 4 hours for pain.

31. ℞ Codeine sulfate . . . . . . 0.03 Gm. (gr. ss)
    Acetylsalicylic acid. . . . . 0.6 Gm. (gr. x)
      1 capsule every 3 or 4 hours for pain.

32. ℞ Aconite Fluidextract N.F. . 4.0 cc. (℥ i)
    Ethyl alcohol, 70%. . . . . 4.0 cc. (℥ i)
      Paint on buccal and lingual gum surfaces over
      the root of the affected tooth.

33. ℞ Iodine, 10% tincture . . . . 8.0 cc. (℥ ii)
      Apply as directed in ℞ 32.

34. ℞ Eugenol U.S.P. . . . . . . 30.0 cc. (℥ i)
      Use to saturate a 2 to 3 inch strip of ½ inch
      iodoform gauze and pack lightly into dry
      socket.

35. ℞ Guaiacol . . . . 15.0 cc. (℥ ss)
    Glycerin . . . . 15.0 cc. (℥ ss)
      Use in same manner as ℞ 34.

36. ℞ Phenobarbital. . . . . . . 30 mg. (gr. ss)
      1 tablet every 4 hours.

Hemostatic agents

37. ℞ Hydrogen peroxide, 3 to 10%
    solution. . . . . 120.0 cc. (℥ iv)
      Dilute with an equal part of water and hold
      a mouthful over bleeding socket; repeat as
      necessary.

38. ℞ Epinephrine hydrochloride,
    1:1,000 solution
      Saturate a 2 to 3 inch strip of ½ inch iodo-
      form gauze and pack well into socket, leaving
      it in for at least 72 hours.

39. ℞ Moccasin snake venom,
    1:3,000 solution   (vial)
      Use in same way as ℞ 38.

40. ℞ Thromboplastin, local   (vial)
    Use in same manner as ℞ 38.

41. ℞ Tannic Acid Glycerite U.S.P.   30.0   cc.   (ℨ i)
    Use in same manner as ℞ 38.

Miscellaneous

42. ℞ Sodium thiosulfate   (ampul)   1.0   Gm. (gr. xv)
    Contents of 1 ampul I.V., daily, for therapy
    of mercurial ptyalism.

43. ℞ BAL (2,3-dimercaptopropanol),
         10% solution in peanut oil
    3 mg./Kg. body wt., I.M., every 4 to 6 hours
    during the 1st 24 hours, less frequently (as
    indicated) thereafter.

44. ℞ Silver nitrate, 5% solution. .   30.0   cc.   (ℨ i)
    Apply to ulcer every 1 to 3 days.

45. ℞ Atropine sulfate . . . . . .   0.5   mg.   (gr. 1/120)
    1 tablet 2 to 4 times daily for ptyalism.

46. ℞ Pilocarpine hydrochloride. .   6   mg.   (gr. 1/10)
    1 tablet 3 times daily for aptyalism.

47. ℞ "Urecholine Chloride" . . .   5   mg.
    1 or 2 tablets for aptyalism.

48. ℞ Ascorbic acid . . . .   0.1   Gm.
    1 tablet 3 times daily.

EAR, NOSE AND THROAT

EXTERNAL EAR

FURUNCULOSIS

The auricle and canal frequently are sites of purulent skin infection. Predisposing factors are trauma, otomycosis, eczema, and accumulation of cerumen. The furuncle may be single, part of a general furunculosis or, occasionally, a complication of purulent otitis media (q.v.).

Onset of aural furunculosis may be acute. Patients commonly complain of a feeling of fullness in the ear, impaired hearing, and pain. Furuncles in the cartilaginous portion of the canal are the most painful. Those on the floor of the canal cause pain on mastication. The involved skin is reddened and may be so swollen as to narrow or entirely obliterate the canal and impair hearing temporarily. Adenopathy and postauricular swelling are often evident, but the latter is not so exquisitely tender as it is in mastoiditis (q.v.). Movements of the auricle and pressure on the tragus elicit pain.

Treatment

When the lesions are on the auricle, the treatment is the same as for furunculosis elsewhere (q.v.); when in the canal, furuncles usually respond well to continuous application of packs saturated with Burow's solution (R 8), or drops of metacresylacetate (R 4). Warm saline irrigations followed by gentle packing every 4 hours with cotton soaked in 70% alcohol may be beneficial (℞ 6). Other means of applying heat locally are usually effective in decreasing pain and hastening recovery. Incision should be postponed until fluctuation is well developed.

OTOMYCOSIS

Fungus infection of the external ear, causing either a sub-acute or chronic dermatitis. The most commonly incriminated fungi are *Aspergillus niger, flavus* and *fumigatus.* Poor local hygiene, swimming, or a warm, moist climate favors the infection.

Otomycosis frequently is asymptomatic but may cause itching, pain, or a stinging sensation in the canal. Pruritus may be extreme because this area is so richly endowed with cutaneous sense organs. Prolonged scratching causes thickening and lichenification of the skin, occasionally with exudation. The skin may be dirty gray or black in color. Smears made in potassium hydroxide mounts (*see* LAB. PROC.) will confirm the fungus etiology of the infection. Eczema (q.v.), which often is confused with otomycosis, frequently is secondary to purulent otitis media. Eczematous face and scalp eruptions also may spread to involve the ear.

Treatment

Many fungicidal preparations are available for treatment of this and other dermatomycoses (q.v.). Before treatment is begun the canal should be cleaned by irrigation, and swabbed with 70% alcohol. Good results have been obtained with a 2% thymol solution in metacresylacetate (℞ 1) applied in the form of packs or drops for at least 2 weeks. Other therapeutic agents recommended for similar use are 2% thymol in 70% alcohol (℞ 2) and insufflation of thymol iodide (℞ 3).

HERPES ZOSTER

A herpetic condition due to viral involvement of the facial nerve at its geniculate ganglion. Onset is acute and characterized by a feeling of fullness in the ear which often suggests acute eustachitis (q.v.). As the disease progresses pain, impaired hearing, or tinnitus is common. Nystagmus, vertigo, and vomiting due to vestibular involvement may be present. Slight pyrexia, up to 102° F., is common. Vesicles appear, the auricles become swollen and regional lymphadenopathy is evident. Temporary facial paralysis occasionally ensues.

Treatment

A regimen similar to that described under Herpes Zoster (q.v.) in the NERVOUS SYSTEM section should be instituted.

IMPETIGO CONTAGIOSA

A highly contagious disease, caused by staphylococci or streptococci, which may involve the external ear alone, occurs

*as an extension of the lesions from adjacent skin areas, or be
secondary to purulent otitis media.* (For further description
and treatment, *see* IMPETIGO CONTAGIOSA in the SKIN section.)

TUMORS AND MASSES

A variety of neoplasms may arise in the external canal,
among these being sebaceous cysts, osteomas, gummas, keloids,
keratoses, epitheliomas, and painful nodules. In patients with
gout (q.v.), tophi frequently occur in the external ear. Tumors
that occlude the external auditory canal may cause impaired
hearing and retention of cerumen. These often are the only
symptoms produced by sebaceous cysts (q.v.), or osteomas.
Keloids may appear following skin trauma (usually in dark-
complexioned individuals). Keratoses are scaly, flat lesions
with an inflammatory base that bleeds on removal of the
scales. Epitheliomas (q.v.) are identified by their characteristic
firm, elevated, rounded borders and waxy surface which later
breaks down and ulcerates. Painful nodule (chondrodermat-
itis nodularis) appears to be a low grade chronic inflammatory
disease involving the corium and cartilage: the lesion is tender,
immovable, and occasionally pinkish in color. Excision or
electrocoagulation is curative.

FOREIGN BODIES; CERUMEN

Foreign bodies, including insects, seeds, and stones, may become lodged in the external auditory canal. Impacted cerumen
occluding the canal often acts like a foreign body in impair-
ing the hearing and causing discomfort.

Treatment

Before removal is attempted the physician should determine
the nature of the foreign body and take measures to reduce
inflammation of the canal, if present (*see* Furunculosis). All
procedures should be undertaken with caution since injury
to the canal or tympanic membrane often results from poor
technic. Irrigation with warm water, although commonly used
for the removal of foreign material, is contraindicated for
hygroscopic and pointed bodies. Hygroscopic objects are best
washed out with 70% alcohol. Instrumentation is necessary for
removal of pointed bodies and those not washed out by irrigation. Because insects are attracted to light they often can be
encouraged to crawl out of the canal if a bright light is held
close to the ear. Floating out the insect with water, sometimes
after instilling alcohol or oil or a volatile anesthetic, is another
simple and often effective procedure.

Removal of impacted cerumen may be facilitated by preliminary softening with hydrogen peroxide or warm glycerin
and then dislodging the material with a stream of warm water.
Several repetitions of the procedure may be necessary.

TRAUMA

Because of its exposed position, the external ear often is subjected to such injuries as contusions, cuts, tears, burns, and frostbite. Contusion of the auricle frequently produces subcutaneous and subperichondrial bleeding. The resultant hematoma (othematoma) is a tense, round swelling which involves any portion of the auricle except the lobule.

Treatment

Cuts, tears, burns, and frostbite (q.v.) of the external ear are treated in the same manner as similar lesions in other parts of the body. For mild contusions, cold wet compresses may be applied. In severe injuries with massive hematoma, the blood should be aspirated before it coagulates. Pack folds of the auricle with wet pledgets of cotton and apply a pressure bandage. Change dressing at 48-hour intervals. Cauliflower ear (pugilist's ear) is the result of a neglected hematoma.

TYMPANIC MEMBRANE

MYRINGITIS

Inflammation of the tympanic membrane due to trauma or infection.

Traumatic Myringitis: This is commonly caused by irritant substances that gain access via the external auditory canal. Acute changes in pressure on either side of the tympanic membrane, such as occur in diving or in rapid ascent and descent in an airplane, may overstretch and thus cause inflammation of this delicate organ. The membrane is usually injected at the periphery or diffusely erythematous and may be perforated. Intense pain results.

Infectious Myringitis (Myringitis bullosa): Of probable viral origin, this usually is a complication or sequela of an upper respiratory infection. Onset usually is sudden, with excruciating pain, impaired hearing, and elevated temperature. The membrane and adjacent canal may be almost completely covered with blebs or vesicles, some of which are hemorrhagic in appearance. The condition may be mistaken for a full-blown otitis media, of which myringitis is one of the important manifestations. Such an error in diagnosis should be avoided, since simple myringitis ordinarily is self-limited, does not cause permanent damage to the tympanic membrane or hearing, and does not lead to complications.

Treatment

Pain in both traumatic and infectious myringitis may be controlled by any of the common analgesic preparations, such as acetylsalicylic acid and codeine (℞ 44). Warm instillations of a preparation such as Auralgan (℞ 7) are helpful in both conditions. Warm Burow's solution (℞ 8) often will quickly resolve the blebs of myringitis bullosa. Severe cases may require puncture of the blebs, and care must be exercised to avoid perforating the tympanic membrane.

MIDDLE EAR

EUSTACHITIS

(Acute eustachian salpingitis; Tubotympanic "catarrh")

Inflammation of the eustachian tube.

Because the eustachian tubes are outpouchings of the nasopharynx, they often are involved in upper respiratory infections. Violent blowing of the nose may force infected material into the tubal ostia, and thus initiate the disease process. Adenoid hypertrophy, enlarged inferior turbinates, prominent posterior septal deviation, or obstructing neoplasms may be predisposing factors. Extension of infection to the eustachian tubes occurs most commonly in children because in early life the tubes are almost straight so that both ends are at about the same level. Patients may complain of impaired hearing, pain, a feeling of fullness in the ears, and occasionally tinnitus or dizziness. Since this condition is so commonly synchronous with acute upper respiratory infection and leads to infection of the middle ear, these symptoms are only part of the entire symptom complex. Nasal examination usually reveals general congestion and profuse mucoid or mucopurulent discharge. The ear drum may be retracted and slightly injected (*see* Myringitis).

Treatment

Treatment depends upon control of the primary condition (*see* COMMON COLD). Relief often can be obtained by nasal instillation of a suitable vasoconstrictor such as 1% ephedrine sulfate (℞ 18) and aspiration of the secretions from the rhinopharynx. Steam inhalation, infrared radiation and diathermy are helpful measures. Chronic eustachian salpingitis may result from neglect of an acute attack or from repeated infections. Treatment includes eradication of predisposing factors (*see* above) and inflation of the eustachian tube when necessary.

OTITIS MEDIA; MASTOIDITIS

Inflammation of the middle ear (tympanum), which may be unilateral or bilateral; inflammation of the mastoid antrum and cells.

In the majority of cases the middle ear becomes infected by microorganisms from the nasopharynx, which enter via the eustachian tube (*see* Eustachitis). The infection rarely is traceable to trauma of the tympanic membrane (*see* Myringitis) or to metastatic involvement. The pathogens that may be encountered include viruses, hemolytic streptococci, pneumococci, staphylococci, *C. diphtheriae, Ps. pyocyanea, Myco. tuberculosis,* and *Esch. coli.* Middle ear infection frequently is a complication of hemolytic streptococcal infection (including scarlet fever), measles, mumps, pneumonia, or influenza.

ACUTE CONGESTIVE (CATARRHAL) OTITIS MEDIA

Earache (otalgia) of varying degree usually is present, often preceded or accompanied by a feeling of fullness, impaired hearing and, rarely, tinnitus. Mild constitutional symptoms may occur in children. Examination reveals injection of the tympanic membrane, diminution or distortion of the light reflex, partial obliteration of landmarks, and often retraction of Shrapnell's membrane. A fine hairline may mark the level of fluid in the tympanum. Air bubbles are seen occasionally, especially after the eustachian tube has been inflated. Bulging of the membrane seldom is present. The inflammation usually subsides within a few days, but may continue and become purulent or chronic.

Treatment

The primary disease must be controlled and the local condition treated in the same way as prescribed for eustachitis (q.v.). Pain may be relieved with analgesics (R 44 to 47). Instillation of warm preparations containing antipyrine and benzocaine, such as Auralgan (R 7), are soothing. Instillation of 70% alcohol (R 6) or metacresylacetate (R 4) also may be beneficial. Heat in the form of a hot water bag or copious irrigations with warm saline solution should be applied. In order to prevent spread of the infection, systemic administration of penicillin (R 36, 37, 38) or the sulfonamides (R 35) is recommended.

ACUTE PURULENT OTITIS MEDIA

The usual initial complaint is earache which is constant or intermittent and may radiate over the whole affected side of the head. There often is a feeling of fullness in the ear, with tinnitus or deafness, or both. Constitutional symptoms of pyrexia (up to 105° F. in children), chills, leukocytosis, and meningismus (q.v.) may be present. Tenderness frequently is elicited over the mastoid antrum. The tympanic membrane is red and bulging, landmarks are entirely absent and there is no light reflex. Differentiation from furuncle of the canal (q.v.) and bullous myringitis is made on the basis of otoscopic examination and absence of pain on firmly pressing the tragus or moving the auricle. Pain and pyrexia often subside spontaneously with drainage of the middle ear through a spontaneous rupture, or surgical incision of the membrane, or through the eustachian tube.

Complications

Observation of the patient for possible complications (q.v.) such as mastoiditis, petrositis, meningitis, lateral and sigmoid sinus thrombosis, brain abscess, labyrinthitis, and facial nerve paralysis (Bell's palsy), should be constantly maintained. These complications result from extension of the disease process to adjacent structures because of inadequate treatment, lowered resistance, or the presence of virulent organisms. Occasionally, they follow mastoidectomy.

Mastoiditis: A majority of middle ear infections are accompanied by some degree of mastoid involvement. Although there are cases in which acute mastoiditis occurs within a few days after the beginning of otitis media, in most instances obvious signs do not appear for 1 or 2 weeks. Pain behind the ear, fever, tenderness, increased aural discharge, deafness, post-auricular swelling and redness, and bulging or sagging of the external auditory canal are the more common symptoms encountered. Roentgen examination may be necessary for diagnosis of atypical cases. Rarely, a Bezold's abscess forms as a result of suppuration going through the medial aspect of the mastoid process into the neck. This will give symptoms of pain in the region of the sternocleidomastoid muscle, shoulder, and axillary region, impaired movement of the head, hyperemia, and fluctuation in the abscessed area.

Petrositis: Petrous involvement, although uncommon, is an extremely serious complication of otitis media, since extension of the infection to the meninges may occur. It is characterized by any combination of the following symptoms: retro-orbital pain, increased at night; profuse ear discharge (otorrhea); low grade fever, up to 102° F.; vertigo, and occasionally vomiting; irritability; paralysis of the 6th cranial nerve innervating the external rectus muscle; leukocytosis; X-ray evidence of petrous pyramid disease.

Sinus Thrombosis: Extension of the infectious process to the lateral and cranial sinuses or to the jugular bulb occasionally occurs as an early or late complication of acute otitis media. Findings in sinus phlebitis may include chills, a septic temperature, which is higher at night; headaches and vomiting; choked optic disks; metastatic abscesses and a positive blood culture. The condition of the patient is poor, as in any general sepsis.

Treatment

Since the early stages of suppurative otitis media are only a step beyond the acute congestive stage, similar treatment is applicable and may possibly abort the condition. The use of penicillin (℞ 36, 37, 38) and the sulfonamides (℞ 35) has reduced complications and the need for myringotomy and mastoidectomy. These drugs should be started early and continued until the symptoms completely disappear. Reliance upon them, however, should not replace careful observation and alertness, or performance of myringotomy in cases that do not satisfactorily respond to chemotherapy.

In performing myringotomy upon older children and adults a local anesthetic (℞ 17) may suffice, although a general anesthetic (e.g., ethyl chloride, Vinethene) is preferable. Infants should be wrapped in sheets, i.e., mummified, and a general anesthetic may or may not be necessary. Before myringotomy, cleanse and sterilize the canal by swabbing with hydrogen peroxide followed by the application of any mild antiseptic. Incision of the drum is best done in the posterior inferior quadrant. Immediately following incision or rupture of the membrane, the discharge is thin and pink; later it becomes thick and purulent. The canal should be loosely packed with sterile absorbent cotton, to be changed whenever saturated. The canal should be cleansed 3 times daily by instillation of warmed half-strength hydrogen peroxide (℞ 13), repeated each time until bubbling ceases. After this, the canal is washed out with a warm 1% solution of boric acid (℞ 16) or glycerite of hydrogen peroxide with urea (℞ 14) and mopped dry. Ear drops (℞ 4, 5) then are instilled. The external ear should be protected from irritating discharges by anointment with petrolatum. This form of therapy should be continued until the aural discharge has stopped.

Complications should be treated systemically with full dosage of penicillin (℞ 36, 37, 38), the sulfonamides (℞ 35) or streptomycin (℞ 40), according to the susceptibility of the causative organism (if it can be isolated for testing). A combination of 2 or all of these drugs may be indicated in cases of mixed infection. This medication is effective in most cases. Should it fail, myringotomy is indicated.

CHRONIC CONGESTIVE OTITIS MEDIA

This condition often follows repeated nasopharyngeal infections involving the eustachian tube, or attacks of acute otitis media. Onset is insidious; there is a gradual loss of hearing usually accompanied by tinnitus; otalgia is rare. Patients often experience vertigo and state that they hear well over the telephone, although to them their own voices sound unnatural. Examination reveals a thickened, lusterless, retracted tympanic membrane; absence or alteration of the light reflex; and sometimes the presence of a fluid level.

Treatment

Many regimens have been tried in this condition, usually with poor results. Inflation of the eustachian tube may produce improvement in cases with tubal obstruction (stenosis). When lymphoid pharyngeal hyperplasia is causing the deafness, radiotherapy or surgical removal of these tumors is effective. Some success has been reported from the use of Jacobson's solution (℞ 63), especially in the relief of tinnitus. Occasionally, X-radiation of the middle ear is beneficial. As a rule, however, the prognosis for relief of deafness is poor, and patients should be advised to employ a mechanical hearing aid or learn lip reading.

CHRONIC MASTOIDITIS
(Chronic purulent otitis media)

Acute mastoiditis usually precedes this disease. The outstanding symptom is a chronic purulent, fetid discharge from the ear (otorrhea). Pain, impaired hearing, and tinnitus may be present. Low grade fever often accompanies exacerbations. Examination of the drum reveals a perforation, through which pus exudes. Polyps and cholesteatomas may be found.

Treatment

Many physicians advocate daily scrupulous cleansing of the ear, either by the dry method, or by lavage with hot boric acid 1% solution (℞ 16) until the return flow is clear. Then the patient is made to lie on his sound side, and the ear is filled with an alcoholic solution of boric acid (℞ 9) or urea (℞ 10), which is allowed to remain for 5 minutes. Following this procedure the meatus should be protected with sterile cotton until the next treatment. Other ear drops that have been used with success are penicillin solution (℞ 12), metacresylacetate (℞ 4), mercuric oxycyanide (℞ 5), glycerite of hydrogen peroxide with urea (℞ 14), and sulfathiazole-urea (℞ 15). Some physicians prefer to insufflate a dry preparation such as urea powder (℞ 11) after the canals have been thoroughly cleansed and dried. Surgical intervention may be necessary in refractory cases, especially when intracranial complications are threatening.

INNER EAR
LABYRINTHINE DISEASE

Malfunction of the inner ear may be due to a variety of causes. One special, little understood, form of labyrinthine dysfunction is Ménière's syndrome (deafness, dizziness, nystagmus, and head noise). The following disorders may result in upset of the inner ear mechanism: (1) Suppurative labyrinthitis, which arises mainly from acute or chronic otitis media. Infrequently, it is the result of direct extension of infection from the meninges. (2) Cochlear otosclerosis (q.v.). (3) Trauma associated with brain concussion producing hemorrhage or fissuring in the labyrinth. (4) Cardiovascular diseases, including arteriosclerosis and vasomotor disturbances (angioneurotic octavus crises), which have been thought to be responsible for a form of Ménière's syndrome. (5) Congenital malformations of the labyrinth, usually associated with defects in the auditory or nervous system. (6) Allergy, which also has been suggested as the cause of Ménière's syndrome, through production of increased labyrinthine pressure and dilatation of the endolymphatic system (hydrops labyrinthi). (7) Endogenous or exogenous toxins, including drugs such as quinine, salicylates, and streptomycin, and bacterial products from foci of infection. (8) Blood dyscrasias such as leukemia.

Symptoms, Signs, and Diagnosis

The common symptoms of labyrinthine disease are deafness, vertigo (q.v.), nausea, and vomiting. There may be blurring of vision, nystagmus, and a tendency to fall in a certain direction. The symptoms of true labyrinthine disease are aggravated by head movements: the patient finds one special position of the head more comfortable than any other. Past-pointing is common (see Vertigo).

Suppurative labyrinthitis often is acute in onset and associated with fever of 100° to 101°F. Deafness may be sudden and complete. Facial nerve paralysis develops in the majority of cases.

Labyrinthine disturbance, characterized by recurring attacks of intense dizziness, nausea, and vomiting, a sensation of rotation of the body around its long axis, pronounced nystagmus, head noise, and partial to complete deafness is called Ménière's syndrome. This diagnosis should be made only after a complete examination has failed to reveal any other cause for the disturbance, since, as previously indicated, the cause of Ménière's syndrome still is in doubt.

Prognosis and Treatment

Diseases of the labyrinth have a guarded prognosis because the involved organ is delicate and easily damaged.

In suppurative labyrinthitis, control of the primary process is essential (see Otitis Media; see Meningitis). Correction of other conditions found to be etiologic is also indicated. Ménière's syndrome has been treated with a great variety of therapeutic agents, but owing to the variability in recurrence of attacks and the self-limiting character of the disturbance, it has been difficult to determine which one was effective. In the severe acute attack a quick-acting barbiturate such as pentobarbital I.V. (R 48) may give relief. Vasodilators such as Mecholyl (R 58) or nitroglycerin (R 59) may be beneficial. Scopolamine (hyoscine) hydrobromide (R 60) administered sublingually or subcut. often is effective. Many regimens have been recommended for prevention of recurrences, including removal of suspected foci of infection, inflation of the eustachian tubes, low salt diet plus ammonium chloride (℞ 61), quinine (℞ 62), Jacobson's solution (℞ 63), phenobarbital (℞ 50), pyridoxine (℞ 55), nicotinic acid (℞ 53), and an antihistaminic such as Neo-Antergan (℞ 52). If the condition recurs despite all medical therapy and becomes disabling, section of the vestibular portion of the auditory (8th) nerve may be indicated. Desensitization to histamine has been reported to prevent deafness frequently associated with Ménière's syndrome, or to result in restoration of hearing when auditory loss has occurred.

OTOSCLEROSIS

A chronic disease characterized by bony spongification of the labyrinth capsule and ossification of the annular ligament with resultant fixation of the stapes. Sound-conduction deafness results, except in instances where the cochlea is involved and a nerve type of deafness is produced, which is difficult to differentiate from other types of nerve deafness. The cause of otosclerosis is unknown, but a hereditary predisposition appears to exist. This disease occurs most commonly in females and is aggravated by pregnancy. Onset of otosclerosis usually occurs between the ages of 18 and 40 years.

Diagnosis

Progressive bilateral deafness and tinnitus are the prime manifestations of otosclerosis. Examination reveals a normal drum, a patent eustachian tube, loss of hearing for lower musical tones, and increased bone conduction. The Rinne (tuning fork) test will show impairment of air conduction but not of bone conduction.

Prognosis and Treatment

There is no known cure for otosclerosis. In slowly progressing cases, the disease process may cease before all hearing is lost. Prognosis is poor when onset occurs before the age of 20, or where there is a strong hereditary tendency to deafness. A mechanical hearing aid may be helpful. If not, the patient should be encouraged to learn lip reading. In selected cases the fenestration operation has proved beneficial.

TINNITUS

A wide variety of so-called "ear noises" are grouped under the general term "tinnitus." Usually, they are described as hissing, ringing, buzzing, thumping, whistling, or roaring. They may be constant or intermittent and often are accompanied by deafness (q.v.). Whatever their nature, they cause the sufferer great annoyance, especially in quiet surroundings. The causes of tinnitus are numerous, and may be classified as follows: Infectious processes such as myringitis, otitis media, labyrinthitis, petrositis, syphilis, meningitis; toxic disturbances due to large doses of quinine, streptomycin, or salicylates, or excessive smoking, or alcohol; cardiovascular diseases, including hypertension, aortic regurgitation, arteriosclerosis; tumors such as those in the cerebellopontine angle; otosclerosis; Ménière's syndrome; obstruction of the external auditory canal or the eustachian tube; endocrine disturbances; allergy; hysteria; dental disorders, especially malocclusion.

Treatment

Therapy is that of the primary disease (q.v.), although the many therapeutic regimens tried have resulted in variable degrees of success. When the cause cannot be determined, or control of the primary disease fails to bring relief, sedation with a bromide combined with chloral hydrate and chloroform (℞ 49) may be effective. Other medications of possible value are nitroglycerin (℞ 59) and quinine (℞ 62) in small doses. Nicotinic acid has been recommended in daily doses up to 300 mg. orally (℞ 53), or 25 to 50 mg. I.V. or I.M. (℞ 54).

DEAFNESS

Total or partial impairment of hearing which may result from a great variety of causes. Onset may be insidious or acute. Anomalies of the external auditory canal, eardrum, middle ear, or eustachian tube that interfere with the conduction of sound waves to the inner ear may be responsible. In this category are mechanical obstruction of the external auditory canal by foreign body, cerumen, furuncle, osteoma, or stenosis; perforation, scarring, or inflammation of the tympanic membrane; ankylosis of the ossicles; middle ear inflammation (acute or chronic), or tumor; otosclerotic involvement of the oval window margin which restricts the vibration of the stapes' footplate; obstruction of the eustachian tube by inflammation; stenosis, tumor, or lymphoid hypertrophy at the ostium.

Impaired hearing may be caused by disorders of the inner ear, 8th (auditory) nerve, cerebral pathways, or the auditory center. Included in this second group are infectious diseases involving these structures, such as meningitis, syphilis, typhoid, mumps, measles, and hemolytic streptococcal infection; tumors of the cerebellopontine angle, temporal lobe, 8th nerve or cochlea; trauma of these organs as from skull fracture; injury by such toxic substances as quinine, arsenic, alcohol, salicylates or mercury; psychogenic disturbances (malingering or hysteria); physiologic dysfunction such as occurs in senility and from excessive noise; otosclerotic involvement of the 8th nerve or cochlea; miscellaneous causes including congenital anomalies, leukemia, anemia, and myxedema.

Diagnosis

In determining the cause of deafness, a complete history should be taken including onset, duration, amount of impairment, previous diseases, and the patient's occupation. In many instances, a complete physical examination will be indicated. Gross testing of auditory acuity is done by estimating the distance at which whispering or the tick of an ordinary pocket watch can be heard. By using the audiometer a more exact determination of hearing at various intensities and frequencies can be obtained. With the aid of a tuning fork, air conduction deafness can be differentiated from nerve deafness. The Rinne test is a comparison of air and bone conduction. The stem of the vibrating tuning fork is placed on the mastoid process and when the patient indicates that he no longer hears the sound, the still-vibrating prongs are held opposite the auditory meatus; if then he hears it, the test is positive, and vice versa. In the normal individual sound is heard by air conduction (A.C.) about twice as long as by bone conduction (B.C.). The Weber test consists of placing the stem of the vibrating tuning fork on the patient's occipital prominence and asking him on which side he hears the sound more clearly. This is spoken of as the "lateralization test" because the bone-conducted sound is lateralized to the side where air conduction deafness is present, and to the healthy side in the presence of unilateral nerve deafness. Once the cause of deafness has been determined, treatment, if feasible, is directed to the underlying condition (q.v.).

EXTERNAL NOSE

Because of its particular structure and constant exposure, the nasal dermis is subject to a wide variety of skin diseases. Conditions commonly encountered (q.v.) are furunculosis (both of the skin and of the hair follicles within the nares), erysipelas, acne vulgaris, rhinophyma, burns, frostbite, eczema, and rhinoscleroma.

RHINOSCLEROMA

A chronic infectious granulomatous disease, causing sclerosis and hypertrophy of tissues in the nose and upper respiratory tract often responsible for ugly deformity. The etiologic agent is a gram-negative encapsulated bacillus (*Klebsiella rhinoscleromatis*). The lesions are nodular or diffuse enlargements of the areas involved. They are nontender, have a stony hardness, and may be dark purple or ivory in color. Biopsy of the hypertrophied tissue reveals the characteristic "Mikulicz" cells, which are large plasma cells containing clumps of the causative bacilli.

Onset of the disease is insidious, and the patient may have no complaints other than cosmetic throughout its course. Obstruction of the respiratory tract and paranasal sinusitis may occasionally occur as a result of the disease process.

Treatment

Good results have been obtained from X-radiation. Streptomycin (℞ 40) administered for 2 weeks also has been beneficial. In the more severe forms, surgery may be necessary to relieve obstruction and for plastic reconstruction of mutilated areas.

NASAL SEPTUM

DEVIATED SEPTUM

Septal deviation is the most common intranasal anomaly. It is readily seen on intranasal examination. Occasionally, it may be caused by trauma or a hypertrophied middle turbinate but usually it is of congenital origin. Great deviation of the septum may cause disturbances of breathing, interference with paranasal sinus drainage (see Sinusitis), or irritation due to pressure on adjacent structures. When symptoms arise that might be ascribed to the septal deviation, other possible primary causes for these symptoms should be considered, including a supervening sinusitis, degenerative changes of the turbinates (see Atrophic Rhinitis), allergy, lymphoid hyperplasia of Waldeyer's ring, and systemic disease such as leukemia (q.v.).

Treatment

Once all such factors have been eliminated and it is evident that the septal deviation must be corrected, submucous resection is indicated.

SEPTAL ULCER; PERFORATION

Ulcer and perforation of the septum occur occasionally in the course of systemic diseases such as syphilis, tuberculosis, diphtheria, and typhoid fever; as a result of exposure to chromic acid, tetryl, arsenic, and similar compounds; and commonly because of trauma from an intranasal foreign body or from picking the nose.

Treatment

Therapy consists of removing the primary cause. Locally, the single application of silver nitrate 5 or 10% solution may be beneficial (℞ 22, 23).

NASAL PASSAGES
ACUTE RHINITIS

The most frequent of the acute inflammatory nasal disorders, characterized by edema of the nasal mucosa, nasal discharge and obstruction (see COMMON COLD). Acute rhinitis is caused by a virus, to which no lasting immunity develops. Invasion of the nasal mucosa may occur in the course of bacterial infections elsewhere in the body by pneumococci, streptococci, staphylococci, *N. catarrhalis, C. diphtheriae,* or *H. influenzae.*

ALLERGIC RHINITIS
(Atopic rhinitis; Vasomotor rhinitis)

A nasal disturbance that often is confused with other forms of rhinitis, but is due either to hypersensitiveness of the nasal mucosa to an allergen (see ALLERGY *section), or in some individuals, to a type of vasomotor upset.* In the latter type (vasomotor rhinitis) the nasal mucous membrane suddenly becomes boggy, with itching, sneezing, and a serous discharge, in response to assuming the upright posture on arising; on exposure to cold, as in walking barefoot on a tile floor, to chilling drafts, or in the presence of emotional crises. Such attacks may be transitory, but are apt to recur with each repetition of the stimulus.

Treatment
Avoidance of the exciting factors provides the most benefit in vasomotor rhinitis. Symptomatic relief may be obtained by use of an ephedrine and barbiturate preparation (℞ 51) or an antihistaminic such as Neo-Antergan (℞ 52).

CHRONIC RHINITIS
(Hypertrophic rhinitis)

A chronic inflammatory process in which there is thickening of the nasal mucosa and submucosa, causing enlargement of the turbinates. Chronic irritation of any kind may be responsible for this disease. Among the many causes and contributory factors that have been incriminated are repeated upper respiratory infections, exposure to noxious materials, chronic sinusitis; nasal obstruction from septal deviation, bony spurs, and polyps; debility, poor nasal hygiene, and unfavorable climate.

Diagnosis
The chief complaints are obstructed nasal breathing and constant mucoid discharge. The obstruction may be responsible for mouth breathing which is associated with dry lips, coated tongue, and pharyngitis. Postnasal drip and an annoying throat tickle are frequent symptoms. Conjunctivitis, loss of the sense of smell associated with alteration in the sense of taste, or intermittent headache may be present. Rhinoscopic examination reveals a hypertrophic and congested mucous membrane

and enlargement of the inferior turbinates sometimes with polypoid degeneration. With thickening of the mucosa there may be an absence of contraction after application of a vasoconstrictor.

Treatment

All primary disorders should be eliminated, with particular attention paid to a possible allergic etiology. In milder cases, an alkaline spray (℞ 20) may be used to wash away mucoid discharge. Electrocautery or chemical caustic agents, such as 10% silver nitrate (℞ 23), or beads of trichloroacetic acid (℞ 27) or chromic acid (℞ 28) may be cautiously employed to reduce the hypertrophy of the inferior turbinates. The desired effect is contraction of the redundant tissues. Surgical removal of the hypertrophied posterior tips and lower borders of the inferior turbinates may be necessary in some cases.

ATROPHIC RHINITIS

Progressive atrophy of the internal nose associated with crust formation and nasal fetor in the later stages. The exact cause of this disorder is unknown. Among the many etiologic factors that have been suggested are chronic sinusitis, chronic rhinitis, endocrine dysfunction, blood dyscrasia, destruction of large areas of mucosa by infectious diseases such as syphilis or diphtheria, infection with a specific bacillus (Perez's bacillus), heredity, and dietary deficiency. In the course of intranasal atrophy, the lining epithelium loses its cilia and is transformed into a squamous form, the mucous and serous glands degenerate, venous plexuses are replaced by fibrotic tissue, and the bony structures may become smaller.

Diagnosis

Obstructed nasal breathing is a prominent complaint, often associated with excessive crust formation and nasal fetor (ozena). Dryness and irritation within the nose, and disturbance of the sense of smell (anosmia) which often is responsible for the patient's being unaware of his nasal fetor, are commonly encountered. Hawking, spitting, and blowing the nose are frequent, usually in unsuccessful attempts to remove secretions. On rhinoscopy, despite the complaint of nasal obstruction, the nares appear spacious, with scabs and pus adherent to a glazed, dry mucosa. Differentiation must be made from syphilitic ozena and chronic sinusitis.

Treatment

Measures should be taken to correct all primary or associated disorders. To control the ozena and remove the offensive crusts the patient should irrigate his nose twice daily (*see* Bedside Proc.) with warm alkalinized saline solution (℞ 19). In order to make sure that the fluid does not enter the eustachian tube, it should be permitted to flow gently, with no attempt by the patient to suck or blow it out violently. Another method for removal of crusts is by inserting a large tampon of absorbent cotton, either dry or soaked with Mandl's solution (℞ 24), into one nostril and letting it remain for 12 hours. The irritation thus produced causes increased secretion and the loosening of crusts, which come out on removal of the tampon. Next day, the other nostril is similarly treated. After the nose has been cleared of all crusts and pus, local medication may be begun. The following local applications have been advocated for office treatment once, twice, or thrice weekly: 3% zinc chloride in glycerin (℞ 26); 25% solution of glucose in glycerin (℞ 25); or Mandl's solution (℞ 24). Spraying the nose with estrone (1 mg. in oil) has been reported to give good results in some cases (℞ 32). Parenteral estrogen therapy also has been used beneficially. Good results have been reported from the use of neostigmine solution 1:2,000 sprayed into each nostril 4 times daily (℞ 34).

POLYPS

Semitranslucent, pedunculated myxomas which may cause nasal obstruction, headache, anosmia, or nasal discharge. They are a manifestation of hyperplastic rhinitis and are believed to result from repeated intranasal inflammation, such as occurs in chronic sinusitis and nasal allergy.

Treatment

Surgical removal is the treatment of choice. Underlying disorders should be corrected in order to prevent recurrence.

PARANASAL SINUSES
SINUSITIS, ACUTE AND CHRONIC

Inflammation of the accessory nasal sinuses.

Etiology

Sinusitis may be due to a great variety of microorganisms, including the coryza virus, streptococci, staphylococci and pneumococci. The following, alone or in combination, are predisposing causes frequently encountered; (1) inadequate drainage due to obstructive processes, e.g., deviated septum, enlarged turbinates, and polyps; (2) chronic rhinitis (q.v.); (3) general debility, such as follows a serious illness; (4) exposure to varying extremes in temperature or humidity, or both; (5) emotional upsets; (6) acute changes in intranasal pressure; (7) maxillary (dental) abscess; (8) allergy.

Symptoms and Signs

Acute Sinusitis: The onset may be sudden or gradual and often occurs in the course of other infections of the respiratory tract. Headache, nasal and postnasal discharge, pain and malaise are the manifestations commonly noted. Pyrexia, anorexia, vertigo, anosmia, photophobia, toothache, and generalized aches are frequent. Although commonly all of the sinuses are involved simultaneously (pansinusitis), the inflammatory process may be greater in some than in others. Likewise, it may begin in one sinus area and spread to others with varying degrees of rapidity. Tenderness is frequently elicited on pressure over those sinuses most affected. Periorbital edema also may be present. The amount of fever will vary with the severity of the attack, but usually does not exceed 102° or 103°F. High fever suggests a complication such as suppurative adenitis or bronchopneumonia. Leukocytosis also is moderate in degree.

Chronic Sinusitis: The findings are similar to those of acute sinusitis except that they usually are less in severity and number. Headache of a constant or recurrent type is not infrequently noted. The location of the headache is suggestive of the sinus or sinuses most involved. Complaints referable to the forehead and supraorbital region may signify frontal sinusitis. Maxillary sinusitis frequently is productive of pain in upper teeth, cheek, or frontal region. Sphenoid or ethmoid involvement commonly causes pain in occipital region, parietal region, root of nose, behind the eyes or in the neck, as well as psychic depression.

Frequent acute exacerbations characteristically occur and may be referred to by the patient as "recurrent colds." Unlike the common cold, the initial congestive phase, rhinorrhea and a definite prodromal period are absent or minimal.

Purulent maxillary sinusitis, fetid in character, usually is due to extension into the sinus of an alveolar abscess from an upper tooth. This condition may be either insidious or acute in its clinical manifestations.

Diagnosis

Examination often reveals either a serous mucoid or purulent discharge on the turbinates near the ostia of the involved sinuses. The nasal mucosa is boggy, red, and may be covered with exudate. Rarely, the nasal passages appear normal. In chronic sinusitis, hypertrophy or atrophy of the nasal mucosa, polyp formation and alterations in the turbinates may be noted.

X-ray of the sinuses is the most valuable single diagnostic aid, but is not infallible, since fluid, polyps, or thickened mucous membrane (especially that due to allergy) cannot be differentiated by this means. Changes may occasionally be noted on roentgenographic examination which appear suspicious but actually are not significant. Transillumination of the sinuses also may be helpful in diagnosis. Microscopic examination of nasal exudate stained with Wright's stain should be done to determine whether there is a predominance of eosinophils, which is indicative of an allergic etiology.

Complications

These include cervical adenitis, otitis media, acute bronchitis, bronchopneumonia, acute or chronic asthma, cavernous sinus thrombosis, osteomyelitis and, rarely, brain abscess from extension of an ethmoid or frontal sinusitis.

Treatment

In acute sinusitis and during exacerbations of chronic sinusitis, a vasoconstrictor drug in moderation (℞ 18), and steam inhalation may be used to advantage. These clear the airways and permit adequate drainage. Steam humidification of the inhaled air is especially valuable in soothing the respiratory passages (see BEDSIDE PROC.). In order to obtain optimum effect of nose drops, they should be administered with the patient in supine position, head tilted back so that the chin points toward ceiling and turned to the side being medicated. The excessive use of vasoconstrictors must be avoided since they may produce secondary vasodilatation with resultant nasal blockage and increased discomfort. Much benefit may be derived from cautious self-lavage of the nose with normal saline (see BEDSIDE PROC.). Such a procedure serves to wash out crusts and tenacious exudate. The use of mineral oil nose drops is generally inadvisable, due to their interference with normal ciliary action and the possibility of inducing oil aspiration pneumonia. Febrile patients should be put to bed and the fluid intake increased. Pain and headache may be controlled with anodynes (℞ 44 to 47). The systemic administration of sulfonamides (℞ 35), penicillin (℞ 36, 37, 38), or streptomycin (℞ 40), aureomycin (℞ 42), or Chloromycetin (℞ 43) has been recommended especially for those who appear toxic, have fever for more than 48 hours or who have complications. Choice of antibacterial agents depends on the causative organisms. Continue such therapy until the patient has been afebrile for 24 hours.

Aerosol inhalation of penicillin (℞ 39) or streptomycin (℞ 41), or a combination of both, at least 3 times daily, also has been found to be helpful. Once the airway has been cleared, physiotherapy with infrared, short-wave diathermy or ultraviolet rays may be efficacious.

Chronic sinusitis often poses a difficult problem. An allergic aspect of this disease may be prominent and necessitates measures to overcome such sensitivity (see ALLERGY section). Intranasal obstructive deformities may require surgical correction. Lavage of the involved sinuses often may provide relief to patients for short periods of time. Displacement-suction treatment often is helpful in relieving headache. About 5 to 8 cc. of warmed 1% ephedrine in isotonic saline is instilled in each nostril in the manner described above. The patient is instructed to rotate his head from side to side for about 2 minutes. Gentle suction then is applied to each nostril while the other nostril is kept closed and the patient repeats the consonant "K-K-K."

This process is repeated with isotonic saline solution until no more pus is present in the aspirated fluid.

A patient with chronic sinusitis should be instructed in the proper manner of blowing his nose and also cautioned against blowing it too often or too vigorously. The nose should be blown, with the mouth open, one nostril at a time. In order to avoid swallowing the profuse postnasal discharge often produced, warm saline nasal douches and frequent throat gargling should be performed. Such measures will relieve the uncomfortable feeling of nasal exudate adhering to the pharynx.

NASAL TRAUMA

Injury to the nose may result from laceration, contusion, fracture, burn, freezing, or intranasal foreign body. External lesions of the nose are treated in the same way as similar lesions elsewhere. Diagnosis of fracture frequently is made from the presence of deformity, crepitus, and radiographic evidence. When accompanied by bleeding (*see* EPISTAXIS) compound fracture should be suspected, and if it is found, the patient should receive penicillin (℞ 36, 37) prophylactically.

Children frequently insert foreign bodies into their noses, which may cause pain, sneezing, and foul discharge and result in serious irritation if not attended to promptly. Insects not infrequently gain entrance to the nose, with similar distressing symptoms.

Treatment

Fractures: These should be adequately cared for, since those occurring in childhood may result in obvious deformity or nasal obstruction which may cause the patient great distress in later life. Correction of a fracture shortly after it occurs, and before edema develops, may consist simply of manually molding the nose. Older and extensive fractures may necessitate elaborate surgical procedures. In all nasal corrections, care should be taken to produce an adequate airway and a good cosmetic effect.

Foreign bodies: In most instances, these can be dislodged by irrigation, suction, or forceps. Insects can best be dealt with by first killing them with a warm 20% chloroform solution spray before attempting extraction. In some instances, the topical application of a local anesthetic such as 2% cocaine (℞ 21) aids in removal.

EPISTAXIS

Hemorrhage from the nose is a common emergency that usually results from a local disturbance but may be associated

12

with a serious systemic disorder. Trauma (q.v.) from direct injury, nose-picking, fracture or intranasal foreign body is the most frequent cause. Other local causes are focal infections in the area, e.g., rhinitis, sinusitis and nasopharyngitis (especially when caused by *C. diphtheriae)*, nasal allergy, and intranasal tumors.

Nasal hemorrhage has been encountered in many systemic disorders such as measles, pertussis, rheumatic fever, scarlet fever, typhoid fever, bacteremia, hypertension, congestive heart failure, arteriosclerosis, and chronic glomerulonephritis. It may be the foremost symptom of hemorrhagic disorders such as telangiectasis (hereditary), scurvy, leukemia, thrombocytopenia, agranulocytosis, and hemophilia. Nasal hemorrhage also may occur as vicarious menstruation, associated with or replacing the sanguineous vaginal discharge, or as a complication of extensive liver disease with profound icterus.

Treatment

Since there are many diseases that may be responsible for this disorder, a thorough investigation should be made in any case of frequent epistaxis and the underlying disease corrected. Mild hemorrhage usually can be controlled by having the patient remain upright (with head bent forward) and apply pressure on the nasal alae. Cold applications to the neck and bridge of the nose may be effective. If the bleeding persists or is very profuse, cauterization with a bead of trichloroacetic or chromic acid (℞ 27, 28), or electric cauterization of the bleeding site may have to be resorted to.

Packing of the bleeding nostril with 1-inch gauze, oxidized cellulose or gelatin sponge soaked in epinephrine (℞ 29) or thrombin solution (℞ 30) may be necessary. Remove all packing after 24 hours in order to avoid middle ear infection. Postnasal hemorrhage may necessitate packing of the nasopharynx. A soft rubber urethral catheter (French 16) is threaded with heavy silk suture and passed through the nose to the posterior pharynx, where the suture is grasped and tied around a gauze sponge about 1 inch in diameter. Traction on the suture and catheter will draw the sponge firmly into the nasopharynx, after which the catheter is removed and the suture emerging from the nostril is anchored to the face with adhesive strapping. If danger of infection exists, institute penicillin (℞ 36, 37, 38) or sulfonamide (℞ 35) therapy.

TONSIL RING

The tonsils and adenoids, as part of Waldeyer's ring of lymphoid tissue which encircles the nasopharynx and oropharynx and serves as a protective organ at the ingress of the body, frequently are the sites of acute and chronic infection. Inflammation of these structures may be due to a variety of pathogenic agents including viruses, hemolytic streptococci, staphylococci, spirochetes, *D. pneumoniae,* and *C. diphtheriae.* Following a description of the more common conditions encountered in this area, their treatment is grouped at the end of the chapter.

ACUTE TONSILLITIS

Acute inflammation of the tonsil, most commonly due to group A hemolytic streptococci (see SCARLET FEVER*).* The onset usually is sudden, with chills and with fever up to 105° or 106°F. Malaise, headache, and varied bodily aches are frequently present. Severe pain in the tonsillar area, especially during swallowing, and swelling and tenderness of the lymph nodes at the ramus of the jaw are common complaints. Cough, and stiffness of the neck may cause additional discomfort.

Diagnosis

On examination, the tonsils appear enlarged, red, and spotted with a yellowish white purulent exudate oozing from the crypts. When the spots coalesce and cover the tonsil the resemblance to a diphtheric membrane (*see* DIPHTHERIA) is so pronounced that differentiation often is difficult. However, diphtheric membrane is gray, more adherent and has a tendency to bleeding on removal. Definite identification of the causative organism is best made by examination of smears and cultures.

Course and Prognosis

The course of acute tonsillitis usually is self-limited, but serious complications may occur. These (q.v.) include mechanical obstruction due to tonsillar enlargement; peritonsillar or retropharyngeal abscess; suppuration of the cervical lymph nodes; phlebitis of the internal jugular vein, bacteremia, endocarditis, acute rheumatic fever, and glomerulonephritis.

PERITONSILLAR ABSCESS
(Quinsy)

An acute suppuration, usually unilateral and located between the tonsil capsule and the constrictor muscle of the pharynx. Severe pain in the throat on the affected side, especially on opening the mouth, swelling and tenderness at the ramus of the jaw, cervical lymphadenopathy, edema of the uvula, nasal twang, and dysphagia are characteristic symptoms. The patient appears highly toxic and his temperature is between 101° and 105°F. Inspection shows the tonsil to be displaced mesially and downward. There may be pronounced edema of adjacent tissues, which masks the fluctuation of the abscess. Occasionally, the abscess ruptures spontaneously and drains.

ACUTE ADENOIDITIS

An acute involvement of adenoid tissue which usually occurs concomitantly with acute tonsillitis. It may, however, appear alone and be responsible for symptoms whose source may remain obscure because of the almost hidden position of the adenoids in the nasopharynx. Symptoms resemble those of acute tonsillitis (q.v.) but, in addition, nasal obstruction usually is prominent. Nuchal rigidity severe enough to warrant a spinal tap may be present. Involvement of the eustachian tube causes earache, and the physician should be on the alert for the development of otitis media.

CHRONIC TONSILLITIS

Chronic disease of the tonsils, usually accompanied by chronic adenoiditis, and both often resulting from repeated acute infections of Waldeyer's ring. In rare instances, the infection is tuberculous (*see* TUBERCULOSIS). Diseased tonsils or adenoids may cause local, constitutional, focal, or allergic disturbances. Local symptoms include recurrent sore throat, halitosis, chronic nasal discharge, and cervical lymphadenopathy. These patients have a tendency to develop colds frequently. Constitutional symptoms are asthenia, low grade fever, lassitude, and failure of growing children to gain weight. Infected tonsils and adenoids have been regarded as responsible for many systemic disorders on the ground that improvement of the disorders followed tonsillectomy or adenoidectomy. Bacterial allergy also has been attributed to these foci on a similar basis.

ADENOID HYPERTROPHY

Enlargement of adenoid tissue, most common in children and usually congenital, but which also may arise from repeated Waldeyer's ring infections. The enlarged nasopharyngeal structures obstruct the posterior nares and eustachian tubes and cause mouth breathing, oral fetor, nasal speech, postnasal discharge, cough, vomiting, and alteration of facial expression (adenoid facies). The occlusive process is conducive to repeated infection of the nose, paranasal sinuses, pharynx, tonsils, and middle ear. On examination of the oral cavity, dental malocclusion and a high arched palate may be noted. Digital palpation of the nasopharynx reveals the enlarged adenoid tissue.

Treatment

Abortive therapy may succeed in mild cases of acute tonsillitis or adenoiditis. It consists of painting the glands with a 10% solution of silver nitrate (℞ 23), Mandl's solution (℞ 24), or guaiacol in glycerin (℞ 31). In severe pyogenic infections, systemic administration of an antibiotic, such as penicillin (℞ 36, 37, 38), aureomycin (℞ 42), or Chloromycetin (℞ 43), or of a sulfonamide (℞ 35), or both, is helpful in preventing complications. In acute tonsillitis with tender painful cervical adenitis, an ice collar often will give considerable relief. The administration of penicillin or sulfonamide tablets as lozenges may help to reduce bacterial activity and ameliorate the local symptoms. Lozenges containing a local anesthetic, such as benzocaine (℞ 33), often will keep the patient quite comfortable; however, if it is necessary, analgesia may be obtained by use of Demerol (℞ 47), or codeine (℞ 46). Nutritious fluids should be given freely and the diet kept light. If tonsils or adenoids are the site of recurrent infection they should be removed, preferably during that period of the year when the incidence of respiratory infections is minimal and when poliomyelitis is not a known hazard. Peritonsillar abscess should be treated in the congestive phase with intensive systemic chemotherapy (℞ 35 to 38). Incision and drainage are indicated once fluctuation becomes evident. The oropharynx should be kept clean by frequent gargling (℞ 20).

Chronic tonsillitis, adenoiditis, and adenoid hypertrophy are best treated by surgical excision. Local applications of 5% silver nitrate (℞ 22) or Mandl's solution (℞ 24) weekly and periodic removal of caseous secretions by suction or irrigation may provide some relief of symptoms. Adenoid hypertrophy may be successfully resolved by exposure to radiation in the form of radon seeds. Such a procedure should be performed only by one experienced in this form of therapy.

PHARYNX

ACUTE PHARYNGITIS

Inflammation of the pharynx, most frequently viral in origin, but which may be due to streptococci, pneumococci, or C. diphtheriae. It often arises by extension of infection from the tonsils, adenoids, nose, or sinuses, or during the course of measles, streptococcicosis, diphtheria, Vincent's angina, or the common cold. A blood dyscrasia such as leukemia may, infrequently, be the cause. Occasionally, inhalation or swallowing of irritating substances is responsible.

Symptoms, Signs, and Diagnosis

Complaints of burning and dryness, or a lump in the throat are common. Chills and fever of varying degrees usually are present. Dysphagia, hoarseness, and cervical lymphadenopathy also are frequent symptoms. Stiffness of the neck may suggest meningitis. The pharyngeal mucosa is red and swollen. A membrane may be present with streptococcal pharyngitis, but is more common in diphtheria and Vincent's angina (q.v.).

Complications

Involvement of the retropharyngeal lymph nodes may cause abscess formation in this area. Retropharyngeal abscess also may follow tonsillitis, sinusitis, or perforation of the pharyngeal mucosa by a foreign body (e.g., fishbone). Dysphagia and dyspnea may be pronounced. Local pain and dysphonia are commonly present, plus constitutional symptoms of fever, chills, and malaise. The patient's head may be fixed because of interference with the action of the anterior vertebral muscles. A tender, fluctuant unilateral swelling usually is found in the retropharyngeal region. An X-ray of the vertebral region often helps in diagnosing doubtful cases.

Treatment

Medication is similar to that of acute tonsillitis (q.v.). If the abscess does not rupture spontaneously, it should be treated by proper surgical incision and drainage.

CHRONIC PHARYNGITIS

Chronic inflammation of the pharynx, most commonly due to prolonged irritation from disturbances in adjacent structures. Excessive or faulty use of the voice and the frequent ingestion or inhalation of irritating substances such as alcohol, smoke, and acid vapors also are frequent causes. In rare instances, chronic pharyngitis may accompany such constitutional diseases as syphilis and tuberculosis.

Symptoms and Signs

The entire pharynx may undergo either hypertrophic or atrophic changes. Hypertrophic changes consist of erythematous edema of the mucosa, frequently associated with follicular enlargement. The mucosa bleeds easily. It often is partially covered with a thick tenacious exudate which makes expectoration difficult and sometimes causes gagging, nausea, and vomiting. Atrophic pharyngitis is characterized by persistent crust formation on a glazed appearing mucous membrane. Chronic cough, tickling sensation, and dryness of the throat are the symptoms most commonly encountered in both forms.

Treatment

Determination of the primary cause and its eradication are essential. In the hypertrophic type, swabbing the throat with 5 or 10% silver nitrate (℞ 22, 23) or an iodine (Mandl's) solution (℞ 24) may be tried. A great variety of lozenges are commercially available, which may be used for their palliative effect.

LARYNX

ACUTE LARYNGITIS

Acute inflammation of the larynx.

Etiology

Acute upper respiratory infections such as the common cold, tonsillitis, pharyngitis, and sinusitis are the most frequent causes of acute inflammation of the larynx. Laryngitis also may occur in the course of pertussis, bronchitis, Vincent's angina, syphilis, pneumonia, influenza, measles, and diphtheria. Inclement weather, excessive use of the voice, inhalation of irritating materials, poor ventilation, and poor diet are possible predisposing factors.

Symptoms and Signs

The most prominent symptom usually is an unnatural change of voice. Patients may suffer from hoarseness and even aphonia, together with a sensation of tickling, rawness, and a constant urge to clear the throat. Symptoms will vary with the intensity of the process, which in turn depends on the etiology. Fever, malaise, dysphagia, and throat pain may occur in the more severe infections. Dyspnea may be apparent if there is edema of the larynx. Laryngoscopic examination reveals a mildly or highly engorged mucosa, which also may be edematous. Movement of the vocal cords frequently is impeded. If a membrane is present diphtheria (q.v.) must be suspected.

Treatment

When acute laryngitis occurs in the course of another disease it usually will resolve with cure of the primary disorder. The administration of penicillin either by inhalation (℞ 39), orally (℞ 38), or I.M. (℞ 36, 37), or by these methods combined, gives good results when the etiologic agent is penicillin-sensitive. Palliative therapy includes bed rest in a well humidified room, absolute rest of the voice, liberal ingestion of fluids, ice cream and ices and, if indicated for accompanying pharyngeal irritation, anesthetic lozenges containing benzocaine may be used (℞ 33). For the relief of cough and pain, cough syrups (℞ 56, 57) may be given. Steam inhalation, plain or medicated, is soothing and often hastens recovery (*see* BEDSIDE PROC.).

CHRONIC LARYNGITIS

Long-continued inflammation of the larynx usually resulting from repeated attacks of acute laryngitis. The condition also may be due to irritation from excessive drinking of alcohol, excessive smoking, abuse of the voice, exposure to irritating dusts or fumes, or the coexistence of long-standing inflammatory lesions of the nose, tonsils, or sinuses. Chronic laryngitis may be associated with a great number of disorders (*see* Hoarseness). The symptoms are similar to those of the acute form, but less pronounced. Treatment is based upon elimination, so far as possible, of the causative factors.

TUBERCULOUS LARYNGITIS

Primary tuberculosis of the larynx may occur but is infrequent. Most cases of tuberculous laryngitis are secondary to pulmonary tuberculosis (q.v.) and may appear relatively early in the disease.

Symptoms, Signs, and Diagnosis

Symptoms include hoarseness, irritation, dryness and, late in the disease, pain on swallowing. In the early stages, laryngoscopic examination may reveal only hyperemia and edema. In long-standing cases ulceration, tuberculoma or extensive deformity may be found. Diagnosis is made on the basis of a co-existing tuberculous process in the lungs, biopsy of the laryngeal lesion, or the finding of tubercle bacilli in the sputum, plus the clinical symptoms. Occasionally, a tuberculous patient may have inflammation of the larynx due to infection by bacteria other than *Myco. tuberculosis*.

Treatment

Pulmonary lesions should be treated concomitantly with the laryngeal lesions (*see* PULMONARY TUBERCULOSIS). Favorable results have been obtained from streptomycin administered by inhalation (℞ 41) and I.M. injection (℞ 40). In some instances, cauterization of the laryngeal lesions is indicated.

SYPHILITIC LARYNGITIS

Syphilitic involvement of the larynx usually is a manifestation of secondary syphilis. Primary laryngeal lesions occasionally occur as an extension of the disease from the pharynx. Gummas of the larynx may appear in tertiary syphilis. Hoarseness usually is the only clinical symptom of this infection. A painless luetic ulcer may be noted on laryngoscopic examination. (For treatment *see* SYPHILIS.)

HOARSENESS
(Dysphonia)

An unnaturally deep or harsh quality of the voice, usually the cardinal symptom of laryngeal disease, but often a manifestation of other disorders. Determination of the underlying cause is important since hoarseness often is the first symptom encountered in certain serious diseases. In a patient over 50, with hoarseness lasting one month or more, malignancy should be considered. A brief listing of the possible causes of dysphonia includes: (1) Infectious processes, both local and constitutional, such as acute laryngitis, chronic laryngitis, laryngeal abscess, laryngotracheobronchitis, tuberculosis, syphilis, diphtheria, Vincent's angina, influenza, measles, streptococcicosis, fungus infections, typhoid fever, smallpox, herpes, anthrax, leprosy, rhinoscleroma, trichinosis, glanders, rabies; (2) neurogenic disorders, including hysteria, C.N.S. tumors and injuries, laryngeal nerve disorders; (3) tumors, either benign or malignant, of the cords; (4) trauma; (5) allergy; (6) congenital anomalies such as double vocal cords, laryngocele, cervical fistula; (7) metabolic and endocrine disorders, including acromegaly, myxedema, and the laryngismus stridulus sometimes encountered in rickets; (8)

miscellaneous factors such as pressure from enlarged thyroid, myasthenia gravis, crico-arytenoid arthritis, or blood dyscrasias.

Treatment

Therapy of hoarseness consists of resting the voice, the use of mild sedatives, medicated steam inhalations, and other symptomatic measures while the cause of the condition is being determined and, where possible, eliminated.

PRESCRIPTIONS

(Wherever a prescribed "proprietary" is representative of a class of therapeutic agents, alternative proprietary preparations will be found listed in Part II.)

Ear Preparations

1. ℞ Thymol . . . .   0.6   Gm. (gr. x)
       Metacresylacetate . . . . .   30.0   cc. (ℨ i)

   > Warm and apply daily to affected ear as drops or as a moist pack.

2. ℞ Thymol . . . .   0.6   Gm. (gr. x)
       Ethyl alcohol 70% . . . . .   30.0   cc. (ℨ i)

   > Warm and apply daily to affected ear as drops or as a moist pack.

3. ℞ Thymol iodide

   > Insufflate powder daily into affected ear.

4. ℞ Metacresylacetate . . . . . .   30.0   cc. (ℨ i)

   > Warm and instill as drops into affected ear every 2 or 3 hours.

5. ℞ Mercuric oxycyanide . . . .   0.03   Gm. (gr. ss)
       Ethyl alcohol 70% . . . . .   30.0   cc. (ℨ i)

   > Instill as drops in affected ear 3 times daily.

6. ℞ Ethyl alcohol 70% . . . . .   30.0   cc. (ℨ i)

   > Warm and apply to affected ear 2 to 4 times daily as drops or as a moist pack.

7. ℞ "Auralgan"

   > Warm and instill in affected ear 3 times daily.

8. ℞ Aluminum Acetate Solution N.F.
       (Burow's Solution)

   > Dilute 1:5 with warm water and apply to affected ear 3 times daily as drops or as a continuous wet pack.

9. ℞ Boric acid . . . .   1.0   Gm. (gr. xv)
       Ethyl alcohol 70% . . . . .   30.0   cc. (ℨ i)

   > Keep affected ear filled with solution for 5 minutes.

10. ℞ Urea . . . . 3.0   Gm. (gr. xlv)
    Ethyl alcohol 70% . . . . 30.0   cc. (℥ i)

> Keep affected ear filled with solution for 5 minutes.

11. ℞ Urea (powder)

> Insufflate daily into cleansed affected ear.

12. ℞ Penicillin solution (500 u./cc.)

> Cleanse affected ear and instill as drops 3 times daily.

13. ℞ Hydrogen Peroxide Solution
    U.S.P.

> Use half-strength 3 times daily to cleanse affected ear.

14. ℞ Glycerite of hydrogen peroxide
    with carbamide (urea). . . 30.0   cc.   (℥ i)

> Instill as drops in cleansed affected ear, 3 times daily, mopping ear dry after each instillation.

15. ℞ Sulfathiazole . . . . 1.5   Gm. (gr. xxiiss)
    Urea . . . . 1.5   Gm. (gr. xxiiss)
    Anhydrous glycerin . . q.s. ad 15.0   cc.   (℥ ss)

> Instill as drops in cleansed affected ear twice daily.

16. ℞ Boric acid, 1% solution

> Warm and instill in affected ear 3 times daily, mopping the ear after each instillation; for irrigation, continue flow until return is clear.

17. ℞ Bonain's solution
    Phenol
    Menthol
    Cocaine hydrochloride. . āā 1.0   Gm. (gr. xv)

> Apply a moistened cotton wick firmly but cautiously against the tympanic membrane for 15 to 20 minutes; anesthesia is indicated by blanching of the drum.

Nose and Throat Preparations

18. ℞ Ephedrine sulfate, 1% solution   30.0   cc.   (℥ i)

> 5 drops in each nostril when necessary. (When indicated, the strength of solution used may be varied between 0.25 and 3%.)

19. ℞ Sodium bicarbonate. . . . . . 4.0   Gm. (℥ i)
    Sodium chloride. . . . . 4.0   Gm. (℥ i)
    Water. . . . . . . .q.s. ad 1,000.0   cc. (℥ xxxii)

> Warm and use twice daily as a nasal irrigation.

20. ℞ Alkaline Aromatic Solution N.F.

> Dilute with 2 parts of warm water and use as a nasal spray or a gargle.

21. ℞ Cocaine hydrochloride, 2% solu-
    tion . . . . 8.0   cc.   (ℨ ii)

> For topical anesthesia.

22. ℞ Silver nitrate, 5% solution . .   30.0   cc.   (ℨ i)

> For topical application.

23. ℞ Silver nitrate, 10% solution .   30.0   cc.   (ℨ i)

> For topical application.

24. ℞ Mandl's solution
    Iodine. . . . . 0.6   Gm. (gr. x)
    Potassium iodide . . . . . 1.2   Gm. (gr. xviii)
    Peppermint Oil U.S.P. . . 0.25 cc.   (ℳ iv)
    Glycerin . . . . . q.s. ad 30.0 cc.   (ℨ i)

> For atrophic rhinitis, apply to one naris at a time for 12 hours as a saturated cotton tampon, or as a spray 1 to 3 times weekly; for other conditions, use daily as a spray or gargle.

25. ℞ Dextrose. . . . . 15.0   Gm. (ℨ ss)
    Glycerin . . . . . . q.s. ad 60.0   cc. (ℨ ii)

> Spray affected nares 1 to 3 times weekly.

26. R Zinc chloride. . . . . 1.0   Gm. (gr. xv)
    Glycerin . . . . . . q.s. ad 30.0   cc. (ℨ i)

> Spray affected nares 1 to 3 times weekly.

27. ℞ Trichloroacetic acid (crystals)

> Place a few crystals on a wire loop and fuse into a bead by passing the loop repeatedly through an open flame. After cooling, apply bead cautiously to hypertrophied tissue or to bleeding nasal vessel.

28. ℞ Chromic acid (crystals)

> Prepare and apply in same manner as for trichloroacetic acid (℞ 27).

29. ℞ Epinephrine hydrochloride,
    1:1,000 solution

> Apply to bleeding nares as a saturated pack of gauze, oxidized cellulose, or gelatin sponge; remove after 24 hours.

30. R Thrombin, topical (ampul) 5,000   u.

> Dissolve contents of 1 ampul in 2.5 to 5 cc. isotonic saline and apply to bleeding nares as a saturated pack of gauze, oxidized cellulose, or gelatin foam; remove after 24 hours.

31. ℞ Guaiacol. . . . .   4.0   Gm. (ℨ i)
     Glycerin . . . . q.s. ad 30.0   cc. (ℨ i)

     Apply to throat every 4 hours by swab or spray.

32. ℞ Estrone in oil   (ampul) . . .   1   mg.

     Spray contents of 1 ampul into affected nares 1 to 3 times weekly or inject I.M. 3 times a week.

33. ℞ Benzocaine   (lozenges)

     Place 1 lozenge on tongue until dissolved, repeated as necessary for throat pain.

34. ℞ Neostigmine methylsulfate,
     1:2,000 solution

     Spray into each nostril 4 times daily.

Systemic Antimicrobial Agents

35. ℞ Sulfadiazine
     Sulfamerazine
     Sulfathiazole . . . . .āā   0.17   Gm. (gr. iiss)

     8 tablets initially, then 2 tablets every 4 hours.

36. ℞ Penicillin   (vial)

     250,000 u. I.M. every 12 hours.

37. ℞ Procaine penicillin   (vial)

     300,000 u. I.M. daily.

38. ℞ Penicillin   (oral tablets)

     100,000 to 200,000 u. orally every 3 hours, preferably on an empty stomach.

39. ℞ Penicillin 100,000   u.
     Physiologic salt solution . . .   4.0   cc.

     Inhale 1 or 2 cc. by aerosol every 3 hours.

40. ℞ Streptomycin   (vial)

     1 to 2 Gm. I.M. daily in divided doses.

41. ℞ Streptomycin . . . . 1.0   Gm.
     Physiologic salt solution . . . 20.0   cc.

     Inhale 1 cc. by aerosol every 2 hours.

42. ℞ Aureomycin   (capsules) . . .   0.25   Gm.

     25 to 100 mg./Kg. body wt./day divided into 4 to 8 equal doses.   Reduction of dosage is permissible following the acute phase of the disease.

43. ℞ "Chloromycetin"   (capsules) .   0.25   Gm.

     Administer as for ℞ 42, above.

Analgesics and Hypnotics

44. ℞ Acetylsalicylic acid . . . . . . 0.3   Gm. (gr. v)
      Codeine sulfate. . . . . 0.015 Gm. (gr. ¼)
        1 or 2 capsules every 3 hours.

45. ℞ Phenacetin . . . . 0.2   Gm. (gr. iii)
      Acetylsalicylic acid . . . . 0.2   Gm. (gr. iii)
      Caffeine . . . . 0.03   Gm. (gr. ss)
        1 or 2 tablets or capsules every 4 hours.

46. ℞ Codeine sulfate 30   mg. (gr. ss)
        1 tablet every 4 hours.

47. ℞ "Demerol Hydrochloride" . . 50   mg. (gr. ¾)
        1 tablet every 4 hours.

48. ℞ Pentobarbital sodium   (ampul)
      0.2 to 0.3 Gm. (gr. iii to v) I.V.

49. ℞ Chloral hydrate . . . . 2.0   Gm. (ℨ ss)
      Sodium bromide . . . . . 4.0   Gm. (ℨ i)
      Chloroform Water N.F. . . . 30.0   cc.   (ℨ i)
      Anise Water U.S.P. . . q.s. ad 60.0   cc.   (ℨ ii)
        1 teaspoon 3 or 4 times daily.

50. ℞ Phenobarbital 15   mg. (gr. ¼)
        1 or 2 tablets 3 times daily.

Antiallergic Preparations

51. ℞ Ephedrine sulfate 25   mg. (gr. ⅜)
      Phenobarbital 15   mg. (gr. ¼)
        1 capsule 3 times a day.

52. ℞ "Neo-Antergan Maleate" . . 50   mg.
        1 or 2 tablets 1 to 4 times daily.

Vitamins

53. ℞ Nicotinic acid 100   mg.
        1 tablet 3 times daily.

54. ℞ Nicotinic acid   (ampul)
      25 to 50 mg. daily I.V. or I.M.

55. ℞ Pyridoxine hydrochloride . . . 50   mg.
        1 or 2 tablets daily.

Cough Mixtures

56. ℞ Codeine phosphate . . . . . 0.25   Gm. (gr. iv)
      Ammonium chloride . . . . 10.0   Gm. (ℨ iiss)
      Tolu Balsam Syrup U.S.P. . . 30.0   cc.   (ℨ i)
      Terpin Hydrate Elixir N.F. . . .
              q.s. ad 120.0   cc.   (ℨ iv)
        1 teaspoon every 4 hours.

57. ℞ Methadone Hydrochloride
    N.N.R. . . . . 0.06 Gm. (gr. i)
    Papaverine hydrochloride . . 0.25 Gm. (gr. iv)
    Glycyrrhiza Syrup U.S.P. . . 30.0 cc. (℥ i)
    Terpin Hydrate Elixir N.F.
                q.s. ad 120.0 cc. (℥ iv)
    1 teaspoon every 4 hours.

Miscellaneous

58. ℞ "Mecholyl Bromide" . . . . 0.2 Gm. (gr. iii)
    1 or 2 tablets during an attack of Ménière's syndrome.

59. ℞ Nitroglycerin (hypodermic
    tablet) . . . . 0.3 mg. (gr. 1/200)
    1 or 2 tablets sublingually during an attack of Ménière's syndrome.

60. ℞ Scopolamine (hyoscine) hydro-
    bromide (hypodermic tablet) 0.6 mg. (gr. 1/100)
    1 tablet sublingually or subcut. for Ménière's syndrome.

61. ℞ Ammonium chloride (enteric
    coated) . . . . 0.5 Gm. (gr. viiss)
    2 tablets 3 times daily, taken in conjunction with a low salt diet.

62. ℞ Quinine sulfate . . . . 0.3 Gm. (gr. v)
    1 or 2 pills or capsules daily.

63. ℞ Jacobson's solution (ampul)
    Doses are given I.M. as follows: on days 1 and 2, 0.33 cc.; on days 3 to 8, 0.5 cc.; on days 9 to 12, 1 cc. Repeat for 3 series with 10 to 15 day rest periods between. If further courses are necessary, the rest period is lengthened to 30 days. In the presence of tinnitus, the maximum dosage must not exceed 0.5 cc.

ENDOCRINE

ENDOCRINE SYSTEM

The endocrine glands are structures which produce substances (hormones) that, when released into the blood stream, control a variety of body mechanisms. The more important hormones regulate growth, sexual development, the rate of body metabolism, and electrolyte balance. The various endocrine glands are interdependent. A disorder of one of the glands is often reflected in dysfunction of one or several of the others. The pituitary, commonly known as the master gland, produces hormones ("tropic" hormones) which influence the activity of adrenals, thyroid, parathyroids, and the gonads. These glands which respond to the tropic hormones of the pituitary are referred to as target glands. Certain disorders occurring because of hypo- or hyperpituitarism (q.v.) are recognizable as a result of deficient or excess stimulation of the target glands. For example, the major clinical features of panhypopituitarism (Simmonds' disease, q.v.) result from hypofunction of all the endocrines dependent on pituitary tropic hormones. Similarly, a disorder of one of the target glands may, in reverse, affect the pituitary. Overproduction of one of the hormones of a target gland may inhibit pituitary function.

As a result of the interaction among the endocrines it is often difficult to know which gland is responsible for a particular endocrinologic disorder. For example, Cushing's syndrome (q.v.) may occur either as a result of primary adrenal cortical disease or of adrenal cortical hypertrophy secondary to pituitary disease.

Because of the interdependence of the several endocrine glands, hormonal therapy is a complex matter. The administration of hormonal substances of a particular gland may, in addition to producing their primary replacement effect, secondarily stimulate or depress other endocrine glands. In some instances it may defeat the purpose of the original therapy.

At the present stage of development of endocrinologic therapy it is important to remember its limitations, and not expect dramatic clinical effects in all cases. For example, the great majority of individuals with hirsutism have no demonstrable endocrine disorder; the fat boy or girl usually is not an example of "glandular deficiency" and with proper dietary management develops normally by the time the age of 18 is reached; and testicular hypogonadism often is little benefited by replacement hormone therapy. There are, however, as will be seen in the ensuing chapters, certain well recognized endocrine disorders, many of which can be corrected by surgical or medical treatment. The designation of "glandular deficiency" or "polyglandular syndrome" should be applied with great caution and only where characteristic endocrinologic defects have been demonstrated.

THYROID

The thyroid gland is intimately concerned with the metabolism and storage of iodine. One of its most important functions is the production of an iodine-containing hormone, thyroxine, which has a controlling influence on the body's growth and metabolism. The production of thyroxine necessarily depends upon the presence and utilization of iodine in adequate amounts. Disorders of the thyroid are characterized chiefly by overproduction or underproduction of thyroxine, but other pathologic conditions may occur which have little effect on hormonal production. Thus, diseases of the thyroid may be divided into four general categories: (1) Those associated with a deficiency of hormone: hypothyroidism; (2) those associated with an excess of hormone: hyperthyroidism; (3) those without significant effect on hormone production: nodular, adenomatous goiters; (4) inflammatory conditions of the thyroid: acute and chronic thyroiditis.

HYPOTHYROIDISM
(Colloid goiter, Endemic goiter; Myxedema, Cretinism)

Hypothyroidism may arise from inadequate iodine consumption or from excessive intake of goitrogenic substances. Deficiency of iodine in water and food may induce simple enlargement of the thyroid (colloid goiter). Recently, the cyanate ion has been found to diminish the iodine content of the thyroid and thus cause compensatory hyperplasia. Excessive consumption of soybeans or cabbage or the use of drugs containing cyanate may produce goiter through this mechanism. Myxedema and cretinism are due to inadequate hormone production.

COLLOID (OR SIMPLE) GOITER

A diffuse, symmetrical enlargement of the gland, without hyperthyroidism. It is due solely to iodine deficiency and is endemic in geographic areas in which soil and water have a low iodine content. Although usually asymptomatic, the condition may show signs of thyroid hypofunction in a few cases (*see* Differential Diagnosis table). Pressure on the trachea is rare. The disorder usually becomes evident about puberty and tends to regress, with complete disappearance by the age of 20 to 25. Endemic goiter is of this type, and is so named because of its frequency in areas in which the soil and water lack iodine, such as the high mountainous regions of Europe and, in the United States, the Northwest, the Great Lakes Basin, and upper Mississippi Valley.

Pathology

Colloid goiter, early in the evolution of the disease, is characterized by thyroid hypertrophy and hyperplasia and a decrease in stainable colloid and in iodine content. Follicular epithelium changes from low cuboidal to high cuboidal, or even columnar, and infoldings and plications are present in the follicle walls. Sometimes new follicles seem to form and frequent mitotic figures are indicative of active growth. As the disease progresses involutionary changes occur which bring about colloid accumulation in the acini, and consequent acinar dilatation and flattening of the lining epithelium. A few islands of active hyperplasia usually remain. If the deficiency persists for years, cysts and adenomas may appear.

Symptoms, Signs, and Diagnosis

In the earlier stages, diagnosis depends upon the presence of a soft, symmetrical, smooth goiter, plus a history of low iodine intake or ingestion of goitrogens, with hyperthyroidism and pregnancy excluded. The basal metabolic rate usually is normal, or may be slightly low.

Treatment

Initially, the patient should be reassured that the tumor is not malignant. Seldom is the gland large enough to warrant surgical removal, although this may be desirable for cosmetic reasons or if there is pressure on adjacent structures. Iodine therapy (℞ 24, 25) begun in the early stages of simple goiter may produce excellent results, but when the colloid stage is reached it may be ineffective, though still worthy of trial. Iodine is most valuable as a prophylactic, and use of iodized salt should be urged, especially in endemic areas.

CRETINISM; INFANTILE MYXEDEMA

Cretinism: *A clinical syndrome encountered in infants and children, which results from a complete absence of thyroid hormone, the cause of which is unknown.* The condition is present at birth and is most common in areas where iodine-deficient goiters are prevalent. However, sporadic cases occasionally are found in infants with healthy parents, living in nongoitrous regions. **Infantile myxedema:** *A similar condition which develops in infants or children who apparently were previously normal.* Both conditions are due to a congenital or acquired lack of thyroid hormone.

Pathologic Physiology

In cretins the thyroid is greatly reduced in size, and its substance is replaced by fibrous tissue or by lymphocytes. Phagocytes appear to take up colloid. Follicles rarely are seen. The deficiency in the fetus produces profound metabolic changes, particularly diminished oxidation of fats, carbohydrates, and proteins. The entire physical and mental development of the child is retarded, as evidenced by delayed ossification of bones, delayed union of epiphyses, poor and late dentition, hypoplasia of the brain, and hypertrophy of the anterior pituitary.

Symptoms and Signs

Congenital cretinism is characterized by a thick skin, which later becomes dry, wrinkled, and sallow. The tongue is enlarged, the lips thickened, and the mouth open and drooling. The face is broad, the nose flat. The feet and hands are puffy, and the hands are spade-shaped. Umbilical hernia and potbelly develop in most cases. The infant is dull and apathetic, usually constipated, and has a subnormal temperature. Cretins are unusually large at birth, but due to defective development are small for their age as children, and as adults are dwarfs. The child's mental status varies from helpless imbecility to that of a dull but happy moron. In infantile myxedema, the clinical picture is more or less the same depending upon the age at onset and the amount of normal development that already has taken place.

Diagnosis

Cretinism may be suspected at birth, but diagnosis usually is made later. By the 3rd month the mother may report that the child shows symptoms of apathy, open mouth, large protruding tongue, and drooling. The characteristic facies, dry skin, subnormal temperature and lethargic behavior of the infant are contributory evidence. The diagnosis is established by findings of low basal metabolic rate, high serum cholesterol (see Differential Diagnosis table), and X-ray evidence of retarded skeletal development. Mongolism often is confused with cretinism, but can be distinguished by the slanting eyes, pink patches on the face, and normal shape of the hands. Differential diagnosis is confirmed by a therapeutic test with 0.5 gr. of desiccated thyroid twice a day. The subnormal temperature usually present in both conditions will become normal in the cretin within 48 hours.

Prognosis

Physical and mental dwarfism are inevitable in untreated cases of cretinism, but in cases discovered early and properly treated growth may become normal and great improvement in the mental status may be obtained, though it is questionable whether complete mental development will take place in the congenital cretin. The outlook is much better in acquired cases (infantile myxedema).

Treatment

Cretinism and infantile myxedema should be treated by administration of desiccated thyroid (℞ 1), begun promptly on diagnosis and continued throughout life. The use of this medication alone will affect the other systems by gradual metabolic restorations. The dietary intake of iodine should be adequate, and iodized salt is recommended.

Thyroid U.S.P.: Daily Dosage for Cretinism

		Metric	Grains
1–3	months	6 mg.	1/10
4–9	"	12 "	1/5
10–12	"	18 "	3/10
1–2	years	25–50 mg.	2/5–3/4
3–4	"	30–90 "	ss–iss
5–12	"	0.06–0.2 Gm.	i–iii

MYXEDEMA

The characteristic reaction to a lack of thyroid hormone in the adult, which may result from surgical excision or from primary atrophy or injury to the gland. It may, for example, follow toxic goiter. The condition is encountered predominantly in women and usually about the time of the menopause.

Symptoms and Signs

A history of a gradual change in the patient's personality is very important. This, coupled with the characteristic myxedematous facies, large tongue, slow and deep-toned speech, thickened edematous skin, and puffiness of the hands and face, especially about the eyelids, should suggest hypothyroidism. Mental apathy, drowsiness, and sensitivity to cold are common symptoms. In cases beginning before puberty amenorrhea may be present; after puberty, menorrhagia is a frequent symptom. Deafness is occasionally observed. Emaciation may be seen, especially in elderly apathetic patients, but overweight is more common.

Laboratory tests show a characteristic flattening of the complexes in all leads of the ECG, elevated total protein in blood and spinal fluid, and anemia. The anemia usually is of the iron-deficiency type—hypochromic and microcytic—but may be macrocytic in severe cases and simulate pernicious anemia. The basal metabolic rate is low, 35 to 40% below normal.

Diagnosis

The puffy facies of myxedema sometimes is mistaken for the facial edema of acute nephritis. The menorrhagia and anemia may lead to a false diagnosis of uterine tumor. Pituitary cachexia (Simmonds' disease) may simulate myxedema; differentiation can best be made by a therapeutic test with thyroid, to which myxedema responds quite promptly (usually inside 3 to 10 days). There also are states of hypothyroidism (i.e., low metabolic rate) without signs of true myxedema, the chief symptoms being undue fatigue, lack of energy, and sensitiveness to cold. Some individuals may have basal metabolic rates of around −15% to −20% without symptoms. These usually do not need any treatment.

Treatment

Under treatment with desiccated thyroid (℞ 1), which must be continued throughout life, the outlook for recovery is excellent, even in advanced cases of myxedema. The substance is given by mouth in tablet form and is safe and inexpensive. Parenteral administration of thyroid or thyroxin is unnecessary. The metabolic processes return gradually to normal, usually in about 30 days. During this time a daily dose of 30 mg. (gr. ss) thyroid should raise the basal metabolic rate of a completely myxedematous patient from approximately −40 to about −20; 60 mg. (gr. i) a day, to about −10; 0.1 Gm. (gr. iss), to about −5; and 0.2 Gm. (gr. iii) to variably higher levels. Overdosage may lead to rapid loss of weight, irritability, tachycardia, and even angina pectoris. It is therefore better to undertreat for the first few weeks by giving 30 mg. (gr. ss) daily, which can be administered in one dose at any time of the day. Some patients are relatively insensitive to thyroid and will require 0.3 Gm. (gr. v) or more a day as a maintenance dose.

SYMPTOMS AND BIOLOGIC EFFECTS OF THYROID HORMONE DISORDERS

Site of Hormone Action	Hyperthyroidism	Hypothyroidism
Cells and Tissues Generally 1. Calorigenic Mechanism	Sensation of warmth Increased sweating Warm, moist skin Increased appetite Weight loss	Chilliness Decreased sweating Dry, cold skin Decreased appetite Weight gain, or extreme thinness
2. Tissue Differentiation and Growth	Thyroid cell avid for iodine Increased uptake radioactive iodine Rapid growth of thyrotoxic children	Coarse, slow-growing skin, hair and nails Inflammatory eye lesions Diminished uptake radioactive iodine Dwarfism of the cretin
Circulatory System	Tachycardia; auricular fibrillation High pulse pressure Increased cardiac irritability Increased cardiac output Precordial pain (?)	Bradycardia Low pulse pressure Lowered cardiac tonus Decreased cardiac output Precordial pain
Muscular System	Myasthenia and muscular atrophy Creatinuria ECG: increased amplitude	Myxedematous muscle infiltration—weakness—hoarseness—macroglossia ECG: decreased amplitude Heart muscle edema
Nervous System	Tremor Palpitation Diarrhea, vomiting, nausea Overactivity Increased irritability Active cerebration Intoxication: psychosis	Complacency or nervousness Sleepiness or sleeplessness Constipation Underactivity (by EEG) Slow cerebration, poor memory Hearing loss
Blood and Other Body Fluids	Polyuria Increased blood volume Weight loss Increased excretion of sodium and potassium Increased drug tolerance High blood iodine Low sugar tolerance Hypocholesterolemia Increased excretion of calcium and phosphorus	Edema Decreased blood volume Weight gain (in part) Hyperproteinemia Increased deposit protein Increased spinal fluid protein Decreased drug tolerance Low blood iodine Albuminuria High sugar tolerance Hypercholesterolemia Decreased excretion of calcium and phosphorus

Site of Hormone Action	Hyperthyroidism	Hypothyroidism
Other Endocrine Glands	Increased sexual activity Oligomenorrhea or amen-orrhea Depressed adrenal (?)	Decreased sexual activity Menorrhagia or occasion-ally amenorrhea Sterility Failure to develop second-ary sex characteristics in cretins and juvenile myx-edemas
	Increased sensitivity to epinephrine	Decreased sensitivity to epinephrine

DIFFERENTIAL DIAGNOSIS IN THYROID AND OTHER DISORDERS

	Basal Metabolic Rate	Protein-bound Iodine, Blood	* Radio-active Iodine, Urinary Excretion	Blood Cholesterol
Normal	+ 15 − 15	3–7 gamma %	60–80%	140–240 mg./100 cc.
Hyperthyroidism, untreated	High	High	Low	Low
Hyperthyroidism, on iodine	High	High	Normal	
Hyperthyroidism Factitia	High	High	Normal	
Myxedema	Minus 30–40	Low	High	High
Hyperophthalmo-pathic Graves' Euthyroid	Normal	Normal	Normal	Normal
Hypometabolism (Non-myxedema)	Low	Normal		Normal
Pheochromocytoma	High	Normal	Normal	Normal
Polycythemia	High	Normal	Normal	Normal
Leukemia	High	Occasionally high	Normal	
Anorexia Nervosa or Starvation	Low	Occasionally high	Often in-creased	Occasionally high
Simmonds' Disease	Low			High
Hypertension	High	Occasionally high		Normal

* Measured after the oral administration of a fixed amount of radioactive iodine in the form of potassium iodide.

HYPERTHYROIDISM

(Thyrotoxicosis, Exophthalmic goiter; Parry's, Graves', or
Basedow's disease)

*A condition characterized by hyperplasia of the thyroid
glandular parenchyma, excessive secretion of its hormonal substance, increased rate of metabolism and often by exophthalmos.*
The cause of hyperthyroidism is unknown, but a strong familial
tendency to the disease has been observed. It often appears at
times of emotional or physical stress.

Pathology and Pathologic Physiology

Hypertrophy and hyperplasia are the principal findings. The
follicle cells increase in size and the wall of the follicle becomes
redundant and gives the appearance of papillary infoldings.
The lumen is thus smaller and contains less colloid. The swollen
follicle cells make a greater than normal amount of thyroid
hormone and release it into the circulation. Storage of hormone in the colloid is reduced. The protein-bound iodine is an
index of the excess hormone in the blood. The energy consumption of the body is increased. Oxygen consumption is
high, and hence the basal metabolic rate is elevated. Certain
individuals, however, may be in hyperthyroidism when their
basal metabolic rate does not exceed the upper limit of normal.
Blood cholesterol often is diminished. Glycosuria may appear
and existing diabetes may become worse. Creatinuria is a characteristic finding and is probably related to muscle wasting.

Symptoms and Signs (*see also* table)

In the classic form the disease is characterized by nervousness, weakness, sensitivity to heat, sweating, restless overactivity, weight loss usually with increased appetite, tremor, palpitation, and prominence of the eyes. Occasionally headaches,
nausea, abdominal pain or diarrhea are prominent features.
Older persons may be apathetic in hyperthyroidism, with either
heart failure or cachexia as the outstanding findings. The heart
is overactive with a high pulse pressure and systolic hypertension. The heart may be enlarged. Tachycardia or auricular
fibrillation is common. Hyperhidrosis often is prominent, and
the palms are warm and moist. The thyroid is diffusely enlarged, turgid with blood, and often a thrill or murmur (bruit)
is present over it.

Thyroid crisis, or storm, an acute exacerbation of all symptoms, accompanied by fever and extreme tachycardia, may occur, sometimes with fatal outcome. Such crises may be precipitated by infections, unusual emotional stress, or surgical operation, particularly on the gland.

Diagnosis

Hyperthyroidism is suggested by the history and physical
examination and confirmed by laboratory data. A history of

nervousness, a palpable thyroid and an elevated metabolic rate on a single observation frequently lead to a false impression of hyperthyroidism. The most important single test is the basal metabolic rate and this should be repeated to avoid errors. Normal rates range from +15 to —15. First tests frequently are without value because of the patient's excitement over this new experience. Likewise, care must be taken to make sure that conditions are truly basal. Coffee, cigarettes, food, exercise, lack of sleep, nervousness, and leak of oxygen through perforated eardrums are a few of the common sources of error. Tests done in the home or hospital when the patient first wakes give lower readings than those done in the laboratory. Sleep during the test may cause a lowered reading. In mild or moderate disease it is best to make a series of tests to establish the base line of metabolic rate.

The diagnostic table indicates other criteria that may be helpful. The blood cholesterol often is diminished in hyperthyroidism but this is by no means a reliable index. Certain persons with hyperthyroidism may have high blood cholesterol and others with myxedema have low values suggesting a separate disorder of cholesterol metabolism.

A blood picture of relative lymphocytosis and relative monocytosis with a normal total white count is characteristic of hyperthyroidism. Muscular changes in the patient with thyrotoxicosis lead to easy fatigue and even simulate myasthenia gravis, ocular palsies, or neurologic diseases. A test (quadriceps) for detection of muscular changes is to ask the patient, while seated close to the edge of a straight chair, to hold the leg extended horizontally. Normal persons usually maintain the position for more than 60 seconds, whereas the thyrotoxic patient lowers the limb in 20 to 30 seconds.

The clinical symptoms and laboratory tests make diagnosis fairly easy and it seldom is necessary to use a therapeutic test with iodine. Biopsy of the thyroid can be done safely but usually is reserved for the purpose of investigation.

Treatment

Despite recent advances in the treatment of hyperthyroidism, present methods do not reach the physiologic source of the disorder but rather tend to suppress the production of excess hormone in the thyroid gland or interrupt the cycle responsible for the hyperthyroid state. Currently, there are several methods by which this may be accomplished: Iodine (plain, by mouth); propylthiouracil, thiouracil, or other antithyroid agents; subtotal thyroidectomy; radiation therapy (external, radium collar, radioactive iodine).

Iodine: The mildly thyrotoxic person when first seen deserves a preliminary trial of iodine administered as 0.3 cc. (ℳ v) of saturated solution of potassium iodide/day (℞ 25), or Lugol's solution, 20 drops twice daily (℞ 24). There is no evidence to indicate that other forms of iodine are more effective. The element iodine is the essential ingredient. The course of the disease should be followed and the basal metabolism determined after 10 days of treatment. The response should be a diminution in symptoms and signs paralleling the fall in metabolic rate, and usually a rise in serum cholesterol over a period of 2 weeks. The goiter may enlarge further to a slight extent during the first few days, and then become smaller and firmer. Iodine by mouth causes an abrupt but only temporary remission in most cases of hyperthyroidism, and its continuation very rarely has a permanent effect; usually it allows the disease to follow its natural course of ups and downs, sometimes at a slightly lower level of metabolic activity, until the disorder either disappears entirely or becomes severe enough to warrant a change of treatment. Older patients, especially those with cardiac disturbances or nodular goiters, are less likely to respond to iodine.

If iodine is stopped, the signs and symptoms return in 1 to 2 weeks; if therapy is continued symptoms usually recur in 3 to 4 weeks (iodine escape). Continued observation of the patient and determination of the basal metabolic rate should continue every 2 to 3 weeks until his particular course has been estimated.

Thiouracil (℞ 26) is definitely effective in the treatment of hyperthyroidism, but it has two disadvantages: the gland remains large and vascular after its use, and toxic reactions are frequent. Drug fever or other allergic reactions occur in sensitive persons, and agranulocytosis may be a fatal complication. About 1 person in 10 reacts unfavorably to thiouracil.

Propylthiouracil (℞ 27) is relatively nontoxic and daily doses of 150 to 300 mg. ameliorate the disease, though improvement is slower than with iodine, ranging from 2 weeks to 3 months. A dosage of 100 mg. 3 times a day should be given until a normal or even slightly hypothyroid state is reached. This may take 3 to 6 weeks, or longer, and thereafter a maintenance dose of 50 mg. 3 times daily should be given for 6 months. The medication then may be stopped and the patient kept under observation. About 85% of cases thus treated remain in remission, while 15% relapse and require further treatment with the same drug or another form of therapy. Toxic reactions to propylthiouracil, which are rare, consist of drug fever, dermatitis, or slight depression of the white blood cell count.

Surgical treatment affords the patient a good chance of recovery without continuous medication. Postoperative recurrences are reported as 8 to 19%. In cases with one or more nodules and large cystic areas indicative of long-standing disease, surgical removal of the potentially malignant tissue is desirable. The higher incidence of carcinoma in the single nodule calls for surgical removal. In preparing the patient with moderate to severe hyperthyroidism for operation, a combination of iodine (℞ 24, 25) and propylthiouracil (℞ 27) has proved highly effective. Propylthiouracil renders the patient nontoxic in the first few weeks of treatment. The addition of iodine for 10 days before operation reduces the vascularity of the gland, which then bleeds less at operation and is more easily handled.

Contraindications to surgery at present are limited to those patients who are poor surgical risks, those who have previously undergone thyroidectomy, and those with a rare type of Graves' disease in which the eye signs exceed all other manifestations. These last mentioned patients are likely to be worse after operation and present a difficult problem in eye care, for which no satisfactory solution has yet been found. Administration of small amounts of thyroid (℞ 1), 15 to 60 mg. daily (gr. ¼ to i), has been suggested to suppress the production of thyrotropic hormone. Thyroid is given preoperatively along with iodine and propylthiouracil. Gradual reduction of the hyperthyroid state has been suggested as helpful in preventing the development of severe exophthalmos. When the latter is fully established, the administration of thyroid extract or thyroxin may alleviate it. Operations designed to decompress the orbit have been recommended. Special care of the eyes requires the assistance of an ophthalmologist, since bland protective ointment dressings often are required and suturing of the lids to prevent corneal ulceration may become necessary.

Radiation treatment of hyperthyroidism is of definite value but it must be done by skilled technicians. Roentgen radiation over the thyroid has been used successfully, but radioactive iodine is as effective and simpler to use. Although still in the experimental stage, this method holds great promise and should save the patient much time, money, and annoyance.

General measures: Successful treatment of hyperthyroidism depends chiefly on reducing the excess thyroid hormone in the circulation; when this is accomplished, the symptoms will disappear. Adequate nutrition should be maintained during this period, when the metabolic processes are greatly increased. A diet high in calories, especially carbohydrates, and vitamins is recommended.

The vocal cords should be examined before subtotal thyroidectomy and routine chest roentgenograms are desirable to exclude substernal thyroid, or a large thymus, and to measure the heart size.

Opinions differ on the use of sedatives in cases with severe nervous symptoms. Phenobarbital (℞ 34), 15 mg. (gr. ¼) at meals and 30 mg. (gr. ss) at bed time, is often sufficient to allay distress. Digitalis in therapeutic doses has no effect on the tachycardia in hyperthyroidism unless congestive heart failure or auricular fibrillation has developed (q.v.) Quinidine (℞ 37) is valuable in paroxysmal tachycardia or paroxysmal auricular fibrillation.

The use of many drugs or large doses should be avoided, as

the liver function often is diminished in hyperthyroidism.
Drugs definitely contraindicated are few, but one is atropine.
Its inhibitory effect on the vagus may increase the heart rate
and it may be a factor in producing thyroid crisis, or storm,
after operation. Thyroid storm is a medical emergency that
demands skillful management. Iodine (R 24, 25), propylthiouracil (R 27) and sedatives (R 34) should be given immediately.
I.V. glucose 10% solution in sterile distilled water, and the
added sparing action of adrenocortical hormone have been found
effective. Adrenocortical hormone (R 2), water extract, 1,000
dog u. subcut., followed by 250 dog u. every 2 to 4 hours, depending on the patient's reaction, is recommended.

NODULAR OR ADENOMATOUS GOITERS

*Goiters without significant changes in the circulating thyroid
hormone, including the nontoxic nodular goiters, cystic thyroids,
certain enlargements subsequent to pregnancy, and true tumors
of the thyroid.*

Etiology

The cause of each of these is unknown. The incidence of
thyroid nodules increases in each decade of life after 30 years.
Some observers believe that nodules are physiologically normal, representing areas of hyperplasia in response to the need
for hormonal balance. This view coincides with the fact that,
in regions of iodine-deficient goiter, the individual goiter of
long standing may gradually change from diffuse to nodular.
Likewise, in myxedematous persons with nodular goiters the
nodules may disappear under thyroid treatment.

Thyrotropin, the thyroid-stimulating hormone from the pituitary, also has been suspected as the stimulus causing the single
nodule. The single nodule becomes malignant more often than
multiple nodules, but the reason for this is unknown.

Pathology

Nodular goiters or adenomas are divided histologically into
colloid and fetal types. The colloid type shows large follicles
filled with colloid and low epithelium, while the fetal type has
small follicles, small lumens, and little colloid, although the individual cells may be large. The pathologic findings can be
confusing, as the changes may range from normal-appearing
thyroid tissue to undifferentiated cellular masses that may show
blood vessel invasion and appear malignant. The histologic
appearance and the biologic behavior of thyroid nodules may,
however, be quite at variance. The papillary cystadenomas
that show a disordered follicle formation with papillary infoldings are regarded as true tumors and potentially malignant.

Malignant tumors of the thyroid are difficult to classify. They
include adenocarcinoma, the extremely rare squamous cell carcinoma, carcinoma simplex or round cell tumors of rapid growth,
and the mixed cellular types. The highly differentiated type

that resembles normal thyroid, but yet metastasizes, may be an exception to the general classification in that it may produce thyroid hormone. Signs of rapid growth with the appearance of mitotic figures, lack of differentiation, and especially the characteristics of colonization seen in blood vessel invasion and distant metastases, usually are accepted as evidence of malignancy. Approximately 90% of malignant tumors of the thyroid take origin in a previously existing benign single nodule.

Symptoms and Signs

The patient with a goiter not producing hormonal change usually becomes suddenly aware of a mass in the neck, or someone else notices it. Pressure symptoms occur in about half the cases of nontoxic nodular goiter. Pain and tenderness are infrequent. Rarely, metastases from a small thyroid cancer may lead to the presenting complaints, which may be pulmonary symptoms, a skull nodule or the result of a destructive lesion somewhere in the skeleton, lymphatics or brain.

Diagnosis

The diagnosis of such goiters is made by seeing and feeling them. Transillumination occasionally helps to diagnose a cystic structure. Hardness, irregularity, and fixation to adjacent structures are presumptive signs of malignancy. Softness, mobility, multiplicity, and failure to grow suggest a benign lesion. A single nodule has 3 or 4 times the likelihood of being a true neoplasm as have multiple nodules. Hyperthyroidism should be excluded. Tracer doses of radioactive iodine are of value in determining the physiologic activity of thyroid tumors. Adenomas of the colloid or fetal type take up little of the tracer substance. Probably less than 3% of thyroid tumors have sufficient avidity for iodine to make treatment with radioactive iodine possible.

Surgical biopsy or exploration is the most important step in doubtful cases. Punch biopsy cannot be recommended as it is a blind and potentially hazardous procedure for such a vascular structure as the thyroid.

Treatment

Treatment depends upon whether surgery is indicated. Absolute indications for operative removal are pressure symptoms or a rapidly growing single nodule or other signs of malignancy. Some patients desire removal of their goiter from fear of cancer or because of the annoyance it causes. Both are valid reasons for operation.

If there are no absolute indications for surgery and the patient does not desire it, he should be observed every 3 to 6 months. Any change toward malignancy is an indication for immediate operation.

If the nodule appears after a physiologic upset (pregnancy, menopause, fear, fatigue, injury) conservative medical procedure is justified. Rest, avoidance of alcohol and nicotine, use of iodized salt, and even a trial of moderate doses of thyroid may be recommended while the patient continues under observation. Thyroid (℞ 1), 30 to 60 mg. daily by mouth, may be continued for weeks to months unless palpitation or weight loss ensues.

External radiation is of little value in these disorders. High hopes were held as to the value of radioactive iodine in the treatment of malignant tumors of the thyroid, but only in selected cases where an adequate uptake of the isotope is accomplished have the results been impressive.

THYROIDITIS
ACUTE THYROIDITIS

Acute inflammation of the thyroid gland. This is relatively uncommon, and in about half of the cases there has been antecedent infection of teeth, throat, or upper respiratory tract. Pathologically there are no distinctive features: the inflammation may progress to suppuration and abscess formation. Specific pathogenic organisms rarely are found. Onset usually is acute, with symptoms of swelling, heat, redness and tenderness over the gland, associated with fever and leukocytosis. There may be difficulty in swallowing and a tendency to keep the head flexed upon the chest. Hoarseness and stridor are uncommon. It sometimes is difficult to differentiate acute thyroiditis from acute cellulitis.

Treatment

Therapy should be similar to that commonly employed for acute laryngeal inflammation—bed rest and rest of the voice. The head should be kept flexed on the chest and moved as little as possible. An ice collar or warm, moist compresses may add considerably to the patient's comfort. Penicillin (℞ 31) in doses of 300,000 u. every 12 hours is advisable until fever and other signs of inflammation subside. If there is no response to penicillin, sulfadiazine (℞ 32) or streptomycin (℞ 33) may be substituted or added. Sedation (℞ 34) and an analgesic (℞ 35) every 4 hours may be advisable.

CHRONIC THYROIDITIS

A form of thyroiditis that develops gradually without previous trauma or infection and whose cause usually is unknown, although occasionally it has been shown to be due to syphilis or tuberculosis. There are two pathologic classes of idiopathic chronic thyroiditis: (1) A fibrous type described by Riedel (Riedel's struma), in which the gland is enlarged, hard, and adherent to adjacent structures but not to the skin; microscopically, fibrosis separates atrophic follicles; (2) a lymphoid type described by Hashimoto, characterized by extensive lymphoid infiltration with germinal centers in lymphoid follicles. Scattered cases of mixed types and even some containing amyloid have been described.

Diagnosis and Treatment

Differentiation of the fibrous or lymphoid type of chronic thyroiditis from neoplasm of the thyroid is practically impossible, except by histologic examination after biopsy or subtotal removal. Radiation treatment may be effective in the lymphoid type but should not be used unless diagnosis has been established. Both types of chronic thyroiditis often are associated with deficient hormone production. Basal metabolism determinations should be done frequently and thyroid administered if necessary (*see* Hypothyroidism).

PARATHYROID

HYPOPARATHYROIDISM
(Postoperative tetany; Parathyroid tetany)

A condition resulting from parathyroid hormone deficiency, characterized by a low serum calcium level, and manifested by a tendency to chronic tetany.

Etiology

Hypoparathyroidism usually follows accidental removal of or damage to several parathyroid glands during thyroidectomy. It also is seen after surgical correction for hyperparathyroidism (q.v.) when too much tissue has been removed. Idiopathic parathyroid deficiency has been reported but is extremely rare. The clinical manifestations begin about 24 hours postoperatively, and may be transient or permanent.

Symptoms and Signs

In the latent stages of tetany signs of increased neuromuscular excitability may be elicited. These consist of a neuromuscular response to a galvanic current weaker than is necessary to produce such a response in the normal—**Erb's sign;** hyperreflexia of the muscles innervated by the facial nerve following gentle tapping over the exit of the nerve from the stylomastoid foramen—**Chvostek's sign;** and the production of a tetanic contraction of the muscles of the forearm following temporary occlusion of its blood supply or pressure over a principal motor nerve of the arm—**Trousseau's sign.** When the condition is active, tonic contractions occur spontaneously, and may involve any muscle, especially those of the face, eyes, tongue and larynx. Breathing may be impaired, with the occurrence of laryngismus stridulus and marked cyanosis, so that tracheotomy may be necessary. Consciousness usually is unaffected. Cataracts may develop in inadequately treated patients with chronic hypoparathyroidism. The bones, by X-ray, usually show increased density. In severe cases generalized tonic convulsions may be prolonged and death result.

Low serum calcium and high phosphorus levels are the cardinal laboratory signs of hypoparathyroidism. Neuromuscular irritability is increased, dependent on the degree of hypocalcemia. Tetany usually appears when the serum calcium falls below 7.5 mg./100 cc.

Diagnosis

Tetany due to parathyroid deficiency is distinguished by a low serum calcium and high serum phosphorus level. However, tetany (q.v.) may result from other causes of hypocalcemia and from alkalosis. Such causes of hypocalcemia (rickets, osteomalacia, steatorrhea, and renal failure) can be distinguished by the absence of high serum phosphorus levels. Tetany resulting from alkalosis brought on by hyperventilation, usually follows some emotional disturbance. There may be a history of previous attacks. Respiratory neuroses of this type readily respond to holding the breath or rebreathing in a paper bag. Alkalosis resulting from excessive vomiting causes an alkaline urine, increased CO_2 combining power of the serum, and a low serum chloride level. Rarely, encephalitis, meningitis, and cerebral trauma may, by damaging the respiratory centers, cause hyperventilation and consequent alkalosis and tetany.

Treatment

Immediate specific therapy for tetany associated with a low calcium level is slow I.V. injection of 1 to 2 Gm. (gr. xv to xxx) of calcium gluconate (R 28). Relief is transient and the dose may be repeated every 6 hours if necessary. For maintenance, 15 to 30 Gm. of calcium chloride may be given orally in divided doses (R 29). Ammonium chloride (R 38) should be administered to keep the urine acid in reaction in order to avoid the formation of calculi.

For more permanent effects, parathyroid hormone (R 6) may be used, but the response is of short duration, because of the development of immunity to this substance. The administration of large amounts of vitamin D (R 41) is desirable to promote the absorption of calcium. The treatment of choice, however, is the oral administration of 2.5 to 12.5 mg. of dihydrotachysterol daily (R 30) until tetany is relieved; 1.25 to 5.5 mg. then is given once or twice a week to maintain the serum calcium at normal levels. Dihydrotachysterol should be supplemented with calcium salts (R 29). Because of the danger of hypercalcemia, maintenance dosage should be regulated by repeated determinations of the serum calcium. An aid in estimating blood calcium levels is provided by the Sulkowitch test (see LAB. PROC.) which measures urinary calcium content. Thyroid administration may help elevate the serum calcium, particularly when a thyroid deficiency (*see* Hypothyroidism) is present.

HYPERPARATHYROIDISM

(Parathyroid adenoma; Primary parathyroid hyperplasia; Osteitis fibrosa cystica)

A condition resulting from overactivity of the parathyroid glands, characterized by decalcification of the bones, nephrolithiasis and a relative elevation of the blood calcium. In the severe form, the type of decalcification is known as **osteitis fibrosa cystica.**

Etiology

The disease is due to an excess secretion of the parathyroid hormone caused by primary hyperplasia of all the parathyroid glands, or an adenoma of one or more of them resulting in a disturbance in the calcium and phosphorus metabolism.

Symptoms and Signs

The complaints are muscular weakness, hypotonia, anorexia, nausea, constipation, pain in the bones, polydipsia and polyuria. Skeletal involvement occurs in about two-thirds of the cases and is marked by rarefaction of the bones which may produce spontaneous fractures and collapse of vertebrae. In advanced stages the latter may result in marked decrease in body stature. The teeth are not affected. X-rays frequently reveal multiple bone cysts. Giant cell bone tumors and epulis are common. In prolonged cases, chronic nephritis develops, and the patients become bedridden. Death follows from renal insufficiency.

The serum calcium level usually is high (15 to 20 mg./100 cc.), but in the milder forms of the disease, it may be within normal limits. The level of serum protein should be determined, since a normal level of serum calcium in the presence of a low serum protein level is abnormal. The inorganic phosphorus level in the serum almost always is low (2 to 3 mg./100 cc.). Urinary excretion of calcium, deposition of calcium in the tubules (nephrocalcinosis), and renal stones are commonly found.

Diagnosis

Spontaneous fractures, or unexplained and recurrent nephrolithiasis, require investigation for the presence of a possible hyperparathyroid condition. Relatively high calcium and low phosphorus serum levels are essential to establish the diagnosis.

Osteitis deformans (Paget's disease) is differentiated by the presence of normal serum calcium and phosphorus levels in addition to the distinguishing clinical and roentgenographic features. In osteomalacia the serum phosphorus is low, but the serum calcium is normal or low and there is no increase in the calcium excreted in the urine.

Treatment

The treatment is surgical. Removal of the parathyroid adenoma offers an excellent chance for recovery, depending upon the extent of renal damage. The adenomas may be multiple and not infrequently are located in the mediastinum rather than in the neck. If diffuse parathyroid glandular hyperplasia is discovered, a subtotal parathyroidectomy should be performed. In severe cases, too much tissue may be removed with the result that hypoparathyroid tetany (q.v.) may appear postoperatively. To prevent postoperative tetany 6 to 12 mg. of dihydrotachysterol (℞ 30) should be given for several days postoperatively, and then sharply reduced to 1 mg. 2 or 3 times a week for several weeks. Blood calcium values should be checked for hypercalcemia and the urine should be kept acid in reaction to avoid the formation of calculi.

Following surgery, the symptoms often are rapidly alleviated. The giant cell bone tumors tend to disappear, and the bone cysts fill in slowly. A high calcium diet (*see* DIETS) supplemented with large amounts of vitamin D (℞ 41) and calcium (℞ 29) should be maintained for many months.

THYMUS

Normally, the thymus gland, present at birth, increases in size until puberty and then gradually atrophies and is replaced largely by fat. Its purpose and functions are not clear. The gland becomes hyperplastic in cases of hyperthyroidism, Addison's disease, acromegaly, myasthenia gravis, rickets, and status thymicolymphaticus, and also following gonadectomy. Malignant thymomas occur, which are highly invasive and respond poorly to radiation therapy. The association of thymoma with myasthenia gravis is sufficiently frequent to warrant investigation of the thymus in all cases of myasthenia. Occasionally, aberrant parathyroid tissue is found in the gland.

"Status thymicolymphaticus" and "thymic asthma" are terms that have been used to describe a syndrome in young infants manifested by cough, cyanosis, dyspnea, and suffocation. Convulsions and death may occur in severe cases. X-ray and autopsy findings reveal thymic enlargement, sometimes with tracheal compression. Prophylactic X-radiation of the gland may be advisable when enlargement is demonstrable in the roentgenogram.

It should be noted that some authorities are skeptical of the importance of the thymus in most of these cases, even when the gland is enlarged and, unless tracheal compression is definite, are inclined to ascribe the respiratory symptoms to other causes. Status thymicolymphaticus also is less commonly accepted than

13

it was formerly as an explanation for sudden death, such as
death under anesthesia.

PITUITARY

The endocrinopathies due to pituitary dysfunctions vary with
the portion of the gland involved. The clinical entities resulting from altered function of the anterior lobe of the pituitary are
caused by hyper- or hypofunction of its secretory cells, namely,
the acidophilic and basophilic cells. Diabetes insipidus is the
classic disturbance of the posterior lobe of the gland.

The following outline, although incomplete, may serve as a
practical classification:

> **Anterior Lobe**
>   **One cell type involved**
>   Acidophilic cells
>   Hyperfunction: Gigantism; Acromegaly
>   Hypofunction: Dwarfism
>   Basophilic cells
>   Hyperfunction: Cushing's Syndrome
>   Hypofunction: 1. Adiposogenitalism
>   (Secondary Hypogonadism)
>   2. Cryptorchism
>   **Both cell types involved**
>   Hypofunction: 1. Simmonds' Disease
>   2. Partial Hypofunction
> **Posterior Lobe**
>   Hyperfunction: Diabetes Tenuifluus
>   Hypofunction: Diabetes Insipidus

ANTERIOR LOBE DISORDERS

GIGANTISM; ACROMEGALY

*Growth disturbances caused by hyperfunction of the eosino-
philic cells of the pituitary.* **Gigantism** is characterized by
overgrowth of the long bones before epiphyseal closure, and
acromegaly by the overgrowth of the terminal parts of the
skeleton after epiphyseal closure.

Gigantism and acromegaly are caused by an overproduction
of the growth hormone elaborated by a simple hyperplasia,
adenoma, or carcinoma of the eosinophilic cells of the anterior
lobe of the pituitary.

Symptoms and Signs

Gigantism: Rapid and pronounced increase in skeletal
growth, muscular development and splanchnomegaly occurring
before epiphyseal closure are characteristic of hypophyseal gigantism. The height of these individuals varies from 6½ feet
to over 8 feet. The span is greater than the height. Somatic,
sexual and metabolic disturbances may occur. The B.M.R.
may be elevated and hyperglycemia may be present. Libido

is occasionally increased or prematurely lost. During the terminal phases of this disease, physical and mental deterioration, thoracic kyphosis and genital regression may ensue.

Acromegaly: Onset of symptoms usually is insidious. Gradual enlargement of the hands and feet and exaggeration of facial features are the earliest manifestations. The acromegalic appearance results from overgrowth of the frontal sinuses, protrusion of the jaw (prognathism) and accentuation of the orbital ridges, enlargement of the nose and lips and thickening and coarsening of the soft tissues of the face. Prognathism, ocular disturbances and muscular pains may be early complaints. Symptoms of hyperthyroidism and diabetes mellitus are not uncommon. Galactorrhea and hypertrichosis may occur in both sexes.

Diagnosis

Roentgenograms in acromegaloid gigantism and in acromegaly reveal enlargement of frontal sinuses, broadening of metacarpals, tufting of distal phalanges and occipital protuberances, and hypertrophy of soft tissues. The sella turcica usually is widened, markedly enlarged or eroded, but it may be normal in size. Coincident disturbances in the other glands of internal secretion help in differentiating this condition from simple gigantism.

Course and Prognosis

The disease may run a chronic course and in many instances it is self-limited. When a pituitary tumor is present, the prognosis depends on the nature and size of the growth.

Treatment

The treatment is not very satisfactory. X-radiation of the pituitary occasionally produces improvement. Surgical intervention is indicated for the relief of symptoms due to pressure on the optic chiasm. Attempts to inhibit the pituitary with estrogens and androgens have been unsuccessful.

PITUITARY DWARFISM

Arrest in statural growth due to deficiency of the growth hormone of the anterior lobe of the pituitary.

Etiology

The condition often is caused by a congenital or idiopathic hypofunction of the eosinophilic cells of the anterior lobe of the pituitary. Destruction of this portion of the gland may result from neoplasms, most commonly craniopharyngiomas, infectious processes, and infarction.

Symptoms and Signs

Retardation of normal growth, most severe when the condition occurs during infancy, is the outstanding feature of the disease. Sexual infantilism usually accompanies pituitary dwarfism. The development of normal intelligence usually is not impaired. A well proportioned body plus diminutive features in which many of the physical manifestations of childhood are retained throughout life is characteristic of the pituitary dwarf. Premature aging of the facies may occur and a wizened, owlish appearance may develop.

Diagnosis

The diagnosis is difficult. Roentgenographic studies of the sella turcica usually reveal it to be small or normal. In patients in whom suppression of function is due to a pituitary or parapituitary tumor, distortion of the sella may occur. The bone age is retarded. The sinuses are hypoplastic and the facial bones, in proportion to the cranium, are small. The calvarium is thin. The pituitary dwarf may show increased glucose tolerance and pronounced sensitivity to insulin.

Pituitary dwarfism is caused by hypopituitarism and must be differentiated from dwarfism due to cretinism and juvenile hypothyroidism, hypoovarian function, genetic or hereditary factors, achondroplasia, debilitating diseases, malnutrition, and renal rickets.

Treatment

Courses of polyvalent anterior pituitary extracts (R 7) may be tried, but the results obtained with growth-promoting extracts of the anterior pituitary gland have generally been unsatisfactory. If hypogonadism is present, skeletal growth may be stimulated with chorionic gonadotropin (R 8) or testosterone propionate (R 9) in the male, and with estrogens (R 12, 13) in the female. Such treatment should be started at the age at which puberty normally begins. Thyroid replacement therapy is indicated if hypothyroidism (q.v.) is present. A well balanced diet rich in proteins and minerals is of value.

PITUITARY BASOPHILISM
(Cushing's disease)

A condition characterized by obesity, atrophy of the skin, hypertension, plethora, osteoporosis, increase in androgen production, salt and water retention, disturbances in carbohydrate and protein metabolism and, in the female, by hypertrichosis.

Etiology and Incidence

The condition, though rare, is relatively more common among females. Hyperactivity of the adrenal cortex, either due to intrinsic adrenal disease such as hyperplasia, adenoma, or carcinoma (Cushing's syndrome), or secondary to anterior pituitary hyperfunction (Cushing's disease), is believed to be the mechanism causing the clinical manifestations. A pituitary basophile adenoma associated with hyperplasia of the adrenal cortex has been found in a high proportion of these cases. It is thought that this adenoma, or normal pituitary tissue under abnormal hypothalamic stimulation, results in an overproduction of pituitary adrenotropic hormone which then causes adrenal cortical hyperactivity. In some cases, pathologic changes cannot be found in the pituitary or adrenal. Further confusion arises from the fact that pituitary basophile adenomas and adrenocortical hyperplasia and neoplasms have been found in patients without Cushing's syndrome.

Symptoms and Signs

Obesity is usually encountered and is of the so-called buffalo type, i.e., confined to face and trunk, with the abdomen protruding, while sparing the extremities. Hypertrichosis of the face and chest and masculine distribution of pubic hair are conspicuous features in the female. Manifestations of atrophy of the skin are common findings. The plethoric appearance observed in these individuals is thought to be due to increased transparency of the skin. Purplish striae and purpuric spots result from poor skin matrix. The skin manifestations are thought to be part of a widespread tissue atrophy due to the protein deprivation. The blood pressure usually is very high, and may fluctuate. As the disease progresses, suppression of menstruation gradually sets in. Regressive ovarian function is reflected in an atrophic endometrium and in castrate vaginal smears. Diminished or absent libido is a prominent symptom, especially in the male. Osteoporosis, particularly of the vertebrae, is of frequent occurrence. Collapsed vertebrae, kyphosis and lumbar pain are common features. The decalcification is not primarily the result of a disturbance in calcium metabolism but is the result of a lack of bone matrix.

Hyperglycemia and glycosuria are frequently found. In many cases the fasting blood sugar is normal but when a glucose tolerance test is performed a decreased sugar tolerance curve is obtained. The diabetes is somewhat resistant to insulin. A negative nitrogen balance is present in Cushing's disease. The excessive protein loss is caused by hyperglyconeogenesis which results from the hyperadrenocorticism. The B.M.R. in many instances has been found to be elevated.

Diagnosis

Circulating eosinophiles are characteristically below 50/cu. mm. (normal: 75 to 150) in the presence of a high white count with relative lymphopenia. The sella turcica is not enlarged. Visualization of a shift of the kidney shadow on an I.V. pyelogram taken in the upright and recumbent positions, and perirenal air insufflation by one skilled in its technic may reveal the presence of an adrenal tumor. In the female, the syndrome must be differentiated from the truly masculinizing syndromes as found in adrenogenitalism, and arrhenoblastoma and other virilizing tumors of the ovary. Assay of urinary 17-ketosteroids usually reveals high values in the above conditions but is commonly not significantly elevated in Cushing's disease. Pituitary basophilism is characterized by muscular weakness, adrenogenitalism by muscular strength.

Treatment

The treatment is unsatisfactory and the prognosis poor unless an adrenal adenoma or a unilateral hyperplastic adrenal can be found and removed surgically with adequate substitution therapy (see ADDISON'S DISEASE). Operations on the pituitary are contraindicated. If bilateral adrenal hyperplasia is present deep X-ray therapy to the pituitary and both adrenals is indicated. Roentgen therapy, expertly administered, has been followed by a satisfactory response in some patients.

Endocrine therapy: Estrogen therapy (℞ 12, 13) designed to depress pituitary activity, is of limited value. Progesterone (℞ 16), 5 to 10 mg. I.M. daily, has been used with some success. Androgens (℞ 9) have given the most beneficial results but still leave much to be desired. It may seem paradoxical to administer androgens to a woman already hirsute, but the chief symptoms of the disease are due to protein lack, and testosterone has nitrogen-sparing properties. A high protein and high calcium diet (see DIETS) may improve the nitrogen balance.

ADIPOSOGENITALISM

(Adiposogenital dystrophy, Fröhlich's syndrome)

A condition characterized by a singular type of obesity and hypogenitalism.

Etiology

It is thought to be a hypothalamico-pituitary disorder. When the lesion is primarily hypothalamic, pituitary function is interfered with. Lesions in the hypothalamic-pituitary pathways also disturb the gonadotropic function of the pituitary. Occasionally, hypophyseal lesions are found (chromophobe adenoma), and not infrequently craniopharyngeal tumors and suprasellar lesions have been reported.

Symptoms and Signs

Adiposogenitalism most commonly is seen in adolescent boys and girls. The boys have a female type of fat distribution. The obesity usually is most marked around the trochanteric region and lower part of the torso. The skin usually is of delicate texture. The hands are pudgy with tapering fingers. Statural growth may be somewhat retarded or may be accelerated. The bones usually are small, and facies juvenile. These patients show hypotrichosis, hypogenitalism and frequently are socially maladjusted, although their intelligence is not impaired.

Diagnosis

Diagnosis is made on the basis of typical fat distribution and hypogenitalism. Girdle obesity without hypogonadism is purely dietary in origin. Delay in sexual maturation may occur in obese children from causes other than Fröhlich's syndrome. Hypofunction of the basophilic elements of the pituitary may result in various degrees of sexual infantilism and hypogenitalism.

Treatment

Dietary limitation is essential. Courses of gonadotropins, such as chorionic gonadotropin (℞ 8) beginning at the age of 11 to 12 and continuing until epiphyseal closure, have proved of value. Thyroid is advisable as adjunctive therapy if the B.M.R. is low (*see* Hypothyroidism).

CRYPTORCHISM

Delay or failure of descent of one or both testes.

Etiology

Cryptorchism may be due to anatomic barriers to testicular descent. Cases of cryptorchism which respond to gonadotropin therapy may have been caused by an insufficiency in the stimulus emanating from the pituitary. Cryptorchism is sometimes associated with infantilism or with adiposogenitalism.

Diagnosis

In some boys the cryptorchism may be false. The testes may be small and retract easily into the inguinal canal or the abdomen. Treatment is not indicated in this type of case because the testes will descend permanently into the scrotum at puberty.

Treatment

Descent occurs with glandular therapy in about 25% of the cases. Chorionic gonadotropin is the treatment of choice and should be started by the age of 3 years. Two or three courses of gonadotropins (℞ 8) should be tried at 2 to 3 month intervals. In some instances, better results are obtained when combinations of pregnant mare's serum (℞ 18) and chorionic gonadotropin (℞ 8) are administered. As soon as descent occurs, the therapy may be stopped or the dosage greatly reduced. Priming with small doses of testosterone propionate (℞ 9) for several weeks, followed by the gonadotropin therapy (℞ 8) has produced good results in what first appeared to be failures. If failure occurs after several courses of therapy, then such cases are gonadotropin-resistant or have anatomical barriers and surgical treatment is indicated. This is best undertaken before the 15th year.

SIMMONDS' DISEASE
(Panhypopituitarism)

A condition characterized by profound and progressive emacia-
tion due to a complete failure of anterior pituitary functions.

Etiology

Simmonds' disease may result from atrophy, hemorrhagic
necrosis, destructive tumor or chromophobe adenoma of the
pituitary. In the female the disease not infrequently follows a
difficult pregnancy or postpartum hemorrhage.

Symptoms and Signs

The clinical manifestations depend on the degree of loss of
function of the thyroid, adrenals, and gonads, all of which are
dependent on the pituitary. Genital and breast atrophy, loss
of pubic and axillary hair, loss of weight, premature aging,
lethargy, and weakness are prominent symptoms. Slow pulse,
hypotension, hypoglycemia, hypothermia, anorexia, and hypometabolism suggest polyglandular deficit. Terminally, somnolence, extreme emaciation, apathy, and cachexia occur.

Diagnosis

The B.M.R. is low. Carbohydrate metabolism is disturbed
and there is an increased tolerance for carbohydrate and hypersensitivity to insulin. Bouts of hypoglycemia may be frequent.
Excretion of 17-ketosteroids is minimal.

Anorexia nervosa (q.v.) may simulate Simmonds' disease.
Other diseases associated with marked emaciation are tuberculosis, gastric malignancy, and Addison's disease. These do not
exhibit the striking degree of hypometabolism and sexual regression of Simmonds' disease.

Treatment

Supportive therapy is of primary importance and usually
must be continued indefinitely. The administration of salt
(℞ 39), adrenal cortex extract (℞ 2), desoxycorticosterone
(℞ 5), and small doses of thyroid, 30 to 60 mg. (gr. ss to i) daily,
with multiple small feedings, has been recommended. Administration of androgens (℞ 9) to the male and estrogens (℞
12, 13) to the female may prove helpful. Therapy employing
cortisone or ACTH is currently giving encouraging results.

PARTIAL HYPOPITUITARISM

A term reserved for the milder forms of diminished function
of the target glands (thyroid, adrenal, and gonads) resulting
from partial pituitary failure.

Etiology

Partial or selective failure of the pituitary hormones which
stimulate all or some of the target glands, i.e., the thyroid,

adrenals, and gonads, may occur without evidence of an exciting cause. This condition may follow pregnancy, severe influenza, infectious processes or some locally destructive lesions.

Symptoms and Signs

There usually is evidence of decreased function of many of the target glands. Hypometabolism may be present due to lowered thyroid function. Lowered adrenal activity may be evidenced by hypotension and a tendency to asthenia and fatigue. Hypoglycemic reactions may be present. Poor gonadal function may manifest itself in sterility, loss of libido, amenorrhea in the female and impotence in the male. If the disease occurs early in adolescence, evidence of decreasd function of the growth and gonadotropic principles as manifested by diminished stature, retarded bone age and infantilism may be apparent.

Diagnosis

The B.M.R. usually is low, and increased carbohydrate tolerance and insulin sensitivity often are present. These patients may resemble in some respects a patient with mild Simmonds disease, and at times, a patient with severe hypothyroidism. The prognosis for life is good. Differentiation from mild forms of Addison's disease, myxedema, and functional nervous disturbances often is difficult.

Treatment

Polyvalent anterior pituitary extracts (℞ 7) are not too effective but may be of value in an occasional case. The courses of therapy should be relatively short (4 to 6 weeks) with long intervals (10 to 12 weeks) between courses. Substitutional therapy with the hormones of the target glands yields better results. Thyroid therapy (see Hypothyroidism) is indicated to compensate for deficiency of the thyrotropic hormone. Adrenal cortical hormones (℞ 2, 5) are rarely indicated but may be necessary where there is evidence of hypocorticalism. Cyclic estrogen and progesterone therapy (see Primary Ovarian Deficiency) encourages growth and stimulates the development of the breasts and genitals in the female. Courses of androgens (℞ 9) in the male result in increased stature, genital development, and increased muscular strength.

POSTERIOR LOBE DISORDERS
DIABETES TENUIFLUUS

A rare syndrome usually associated with pituitary and parapituitary tumors, accompanied by hypersecretion of the posterior pituitary antidiuretic hormone leading to water retention, and characterized by oliguria and an absence of undue thirst.

Posterior lobe hyperfunction must, for the present, be considered on a theoretical basis. Dystocia, hypertension, dysmenorrhea, and eclampsia have at times been regarded as due to excessive secretion of posterior lobe hormones.

DIABETES INSIPIDUS

A disorder of the pituitary gland, chronic in its manifestations and characterized by the excretion of enormous quantities of very dilute but otherwise normal urine, associated with a tremendous thirst.

Etiology

Diabetes insipidus results from the diuretic activity of the anterior lobe of the pituitary gland, unchecked by the antidiuretic hormone of the posterior lobe. Secretion of this antidiuretic principle is dependent on innervation through the supraopticohypophyseal tract. Injury anywhere along the tract may result in this symptom complex.

Cases may be separated into two main groups. The primary or idiopathic group, in which no organic disease is demonstrable, and the secondary or symptomatic group in which a variety of pathologic conditions are present. The lesions most frequently associated are cranial injury, especially fracture of the base of the skull, basilar meningitis, primary or metastatic brain tumors, especially those of the pituitary and neighboring structures, cerebral hemorrhage, encephalitis, syphilis, tuberculosis, and Hand-Schüller-Christian disease. A hereditary type has been described, and its association with congenital defects such as the Laurence-Moon-Biedl syndrome (obesity, hypogenitalism, retinitis pigmentosa, mental deficiency, polydactylism) is recognized.

Symptoms and Signs

The condition is uncommon and chiefly affects young adults, particularly males. The onset usually is insidious, with progressively increasing polydipsia and polyuria. However, the disease may be congenital, or the onset may be sudden, following an injury, emotional shock, or infectious disease. Enormous quantities of fluid are ingested and excreted (5 to 40 liters/day). The urine is pale, and of low specific gravity (1.001 to 1.006), but otherwise normal. Because of the tremendous polyuria, the skin is dry, sweating is markedly diminished and saliva decreased. Patients are usually constipated.

In patients with the idiopathic form, the only symptoms are those of the diabetes insipidus. In the secondary type, the symptoms of the associated lesion will be present, in addition to the polydipsia and polyuria.

Diagnosis

In a case in which diabetes insipidus is suspected, a urine concentration test should be performed (*see* LAB. PROC.). Inability of the patient to concentrate urine during the urine concentration test, is indicative of this condition. An injection of posterior pituitary extract (℞ 20) or pitressin (℞ 19) as a therapeutic test in doubtful cases will cause a temporary disappearance of the polyuria and polydipsia due to diabetes insipidus.

Diabetes mellitus is distinguished by glycosuria and the high specific gravity of the urine. Psychogenic polydipsia and polyuria can be differentiated from diabetes insipidus by giving the patient an infusion of 500 to 600 cc. of 2.5% saline solution over a period of 45 minutes. Hypertonic saline stimulates the release of antidiuretic hormone and a marked reduction in diuresis follows. This does not occur in patients with true diabetes insipidus. Chronic nephritis is recognized by the urinary findings of albumin and casts and the presence of hypertension.

Treatment

Definitive: When it is possible to discover the causative factor, measures directed toward its eradication should be instituted. Removal of intracranial tumors, or irradiation of inoperable tumors or the lesions of Hand-Schüller-Christian disease, has been followed by relief of diabetes insipidus. If the condition is syphilitic in origin, antiluetic therapy may be followed by a disappearance of the diabetic symptoms.

Symptomatic: Effective control of polyuria may be obtained in over 90% of the cases by administering preparations of the posterior pituitary gland. Of the injectable materials, Pitressin Tannate in oil (℞ 19) usually is the most satisfactory. Care must be taken to mix the material thoroughly before injection. Gentle warming may be needed if it is cold. A dose of 0.3 to 1 cc. should be given I.M., never I.V. The frequency of injection must be determined by trial. Control of the polyuria and thirst is variable, but usually it can be maintained 30 to 80 hours after an injection.

A less satisfactory method for prolonged treatment is injection of aqueous solutions. However, an acute antidiuretic effect of short duration may be obtained by using Posterior Pituitary Injection U.S.P., 0.1 to 1 cc. subcut. (℞ 20). Since this material is rapidly absorbed, the injection may be followed by unpleasant, and possibly dangerous, evidences of smooth muscle stimulation. Palpitation, facial pallor, faintness, nausea, intestinal cramps with desire to defecate, and uterine cramps may appear. Such side effects should be avoided by using smaller doses. In particular, pregnant or hypertensive individuals, as well as those with coronary insufficiency, should receive Pitressin Tannate in oil I.M. rather than the aqueous solution. The dose of Posterior Pituitary Injection U.S.P. is the minimal amount that will give an antidiuretic effect of several hours' duration without side effects; 0.1 to 1 cc. subcut. may be necessary. It also may be inserted into the nostril as a powder (inhaled like snuff) (℞ 23) or as a nasal spray (℞ 21) or jelly (℞ 22).

After the effectiveness of a posterior pituitary lobe preparation has been demonstrated with an injectable material, use of the drug as a snuff in powder form is the easiest, simplest, and least expensive method for long continued use. A large capsule containing 40 mg. (℞ 23) may be given daily for a few days as a trial dose to determine the efficacy of this amount. The capsule should be emptied on the back or palm of the hand and the material snuffed up the nose, or inserted into the nostrils with the tip of the finger. The patient soon learns to choose the proper amount of posterior pituitary powder and frequency of administration for the control of the polyuria.

Dietary measures may be tried if satisfactory symptomatic results are not obtained with posterior pituitary preparations. A diet low in salt, containing no more than 1 Gm. of protein/Kg. of ideal body weight, with sufficient calories to maintain normal body weight, usually results in some decrease in urine output.

PANCREAS

For a discussion of inflammatory disease of this gland, the reader is referred to the chapter on Pancreatitis. Diabetes Mellitus also is fully covered in a separate chapter (q.v.).

ADRENAL

ADDISON'S DISEASE

(Chronic adrenal cortical insufficiency,
Chronic hypoadrenocorticism)

An insidious and usually progressive disease due to adrenal cortical hypofunction, characterized by increasing weakness, abnormal pigmentation of the skin and mucous membranes, weight loss, hypotension, dehydration, gastrointestinal upsets, and occasional hypoglycemia.

Etiology and Incidence

Approximately one-half of the cases are due to adrenal cortical atrophy of unknown etiology. The remainder are a result of partial destruction of the gland by tuberculosis, rarely by neoplasm, amyloidosis, or inflammatory necrosis.

Addison's disease is found in approximately 0.4 per 100,000 of the population. It occurs in all age groups and about equally in both sexes. The incidence of partial adrenal cortical insufficiency ("hypoadrenia") probably is much higher. It tends to become manifest clinically under conditions of metabolic stress and trauma.

Pathologic Physiology

The adrenal cortex secretes a number of hormones which play important roles in the regulation of many metabolic functions.

In Addison's disease there is an increased elimination of sodium and chloride in the urine, and a decreased excretion of potassium, resulting in a low concentration of serum sodium and chloride and a high serum potassium. The changes in the electrolyte balance result in increased water excretion with severe dehydration, plasma concentration, hypotension, and eventual circulatory collapse subsequent to decreased circulatory volume. Desoxycorticosterone, a synthetic adrenal cortical hormone, is effective in maintaining normal electrolyte balance. Inadequate adrenal cortical function results also in disturbances of intermediate carbohydrate fat and protein metabolism. In the absence of certain other adrenal cortical hormones designated as Compounds A, E, and F, too little carbohydrate is formed from protein, too little fat and too much carbohydrate is broken down. This results in hypoglycemia (q.v.), and diminished liver glycogen. The lack of certain unidentified substances results in abnormal pigment metabolism and the deposition of melanin in the skin.

Symptoms and Signs

Weakness and easy fatigability are the first symptoms usually observed. Unlike the psychogenic type of fatigue, it becomes worse as the day progresses. Increased pigmentation is almost invariably present, but may be minimal or absent especially when there is an accompanying anterior pituitary insufficiency. Diffuse tanning of a somewhat ashen tint of both exposed and nonexposed portions of the body occurs, most characteristically at pressure points, skin folds, bony prominences, scars, and on extensor surfaces. Black freckles over the forehead, face, neck, and shoulders, areas of vitiligo often with small central pigmented patches, and bluish black discolorations of the areolas and of the mucous membranes of the lips, mouth, rectum, and vagina are common. Weight loss, dehydration, hypotension and small heart size are characteristic. Anorexia, nausea, vomiting, and diarrhea often occur. Decreased tolerance to cold, with hypometabolism (B.M.R. minus 15 to 20), usually is noted. Nervous and mental instability with dizziness and syncopal attacks may occur.

An adrenal crisis is characterized by a rapid intensification of symptomatology. It is associated with profound asthenia, severe pains in the abdomen, lower back, or legs, a fall in blood pressure to shock levels, and finally renal shutdown with azotemia. The body temperature usually is subnormal although severe hyperthermia occasionally is present. Crisis is most often precipitated by acute infection, trauma, operative procedures, and salt loss by diaphoresis during the summer months.

Laboratory Findings

The presence of a low serum sodium, below 130 milliequivalents/liter, together with the clinical picture, is suggestive of Addison's disease. The serum sodium may be calculated from the sum of CO_2 combining power and the serum chloride mEq. plus 10.

LABORATORY FINDINGS SUGGESTIVE OF ADDISON'S DISEASE

Blood Chemical (values given are per 100 cc.)	Low serum sodium (< 130 milliequivalents) High serum potassium (> 5 milliequivalents) Low fasting blood sugar (< 50 mg.) Decrease in CO_2 combining power (< 45 vols.) Elevated blood nonprotein nitrogen (> 30 mg.)
Hematologic	Elevated hematocrit Low leukocyte count (6,000 to 8,000) Relative lymphocytosis (35%) Mild eosinophilia (3 to 10%)
Basal Metabolic	B.M.R. of −15 to −20
Roentgenographic	Evidence of: Calcifications in the adrenal areas Renal tuberculosis Pulmonary tuberculosis Small heart size

Diagnostic Tests

1. Water test: Normal water diuresis is absent in adrenal cortical insufficiency. The patient is allowed no fluids after 7 P.M. His urine is collected from 10 P.M. to 7 A.M. inclusive. Water, 20 cc./Kg. is given by mouth at 7 A.M. followed by 4 hourly urine collections. If the volume of any of the hourly specimens exceeds that of the night collection, Addison's disease is unlikely. However, an inadequate diuresis following water ingestion is suggestive but not pathognomonic of Addison's disease alone.

2. 17-ketosteroid determination: The quantity of these androgenic breakdown products is determined chemically in a 24-hour urine specimen as a measure of general androgen production. If above 10 mg. in the female or 15 mg. in the male (where one-third is testicular), a diagnosis of Addison's disease is improbable.

3. ACTH test: Adrenal cortical response to pituitary adrenocorticotropin is measured by the eosinolytic action of certain cortical factors. Adrenocorticotropin, 25 mg., is injected I.M. and circulating eosinophils are determined just before the injection and 4 hours thereafter. A fall in circulating eosinophils of 50% or more effectively rules out Addison's disease.

4. Salt deprivation test: Salt preservation is impaired in Addison's disease. The patient is given a salt-poor diet containing less than 0.7 Gm. of sodium daily. After 2 to 4 days on such a diet, patients with Addison's disease will complain of the intensification of their symptoms and will show a definite fall in the serum sodium level and an increased excretion of urinary sodium and chloride over dietary intake. (CAUTION! There is the danger of precipitating an adrenal crisis when using this test. It should be performed in a hospital, and used only as an aid in the diagnosis of doubtful cases.)

Diagnosis

Various chronic infections may simulate Addison's disease. Exhausting chronic disease may be associated with secondary adrenal atrophy and a true Addison's disease picture. In tuberculosis there may be either adrenal tuberculosis, or secondary adrenal atrophy.

The chronic gastrointestinal diseases may be difficult to differentiate. Weakness of myasthenia gravis is specifically relieved by a therapeutic test with prostigmine. Chronic thyrotoxic myopathy shows an elevated B.M.R. and a good response to antithyroid treatment. In hyperparathyroidism there is an increased serum alkaline phosphatase and calcium, and a decrease in phosphorus, usually with a complicating diffuse osteofibrosis cystica. Spontaneous hypoglycemia shows weight gain rather than loss, and little response to insulin as opposed to marked sensitivity found in patients with Addison's disease. Salt depletion in terminal nephritis with severe renal tubular impairment, proves refractory to treatment with desoxycorticosterone. Simmonds' disease (q.v.) also should be differentiated.

Prognosis

Under constant care and appropriate therapy at times of crisis, infection, or surgery, a patient with relatively severe Addison's disease can enjoy a life that is only moderately restricted. The prognosis no longer is hopeless under continued substitution therapy. Active tuberculosis makes the prognosis worse.

Treatment

In addition to appropriate treatment of any complicating infection, such as tuberculosis, therapy should include:

Treatment of acute adrenal crisis (applicable also to the Waterhouse-Friderichsen syndrome, crisis occurring after adrenal surgery, and in the rare instances of postpartum adrenal hemorrhage): Acute adrenal crisis with shock requires adrenal cortical hormone replacement therapy, I.V. fluids and sodium chloride to combat dehydration, glucose to counteract hypoglycemia, and chemotherapy to limit spread of infection. The principles of treatment in adrenal crisis are similar to those in diabetic coma in that therapy should be adapted to the individual circumstances, with respect to size and weight of the patient, extent of dehydration and of shock, and presence or absence of a complicating infection. The following is a sample regimen:

To a patient in crisis, 250 cc. of human plasma or preferably 15 Gm. of concentrated human albumin is given I.V. with 30 cc. of aqueous adrenal cortical extract (℞ 2). This is immediately followed by 250 cc. of 10% glucose in saline, containing 100,000 u. of penicillin, at the rate of 100 drops/minute. This treatment may be repeated if shock persists. Once the blood pressure is stabilized, 1,500 cc. of 10% glucose in saline with 30 cc. of aqueous adrenal cortical extract (℞ 2) should be given I.V. and followed by a slow drip of 10% glucose in water, taking care not to exceed 3,500 cc. in a 24-hour period. Whole aqueous adrenal cortical hormone (℞ 2) also is given I.M. For the first 12 hours, 5 cc. is given hourly, then every other hour for 12 hours, then every 4 hours for 12 hours, and finally every 6 hours until the patient has eaten well for 2 days. Adrenal cortical extract in sesame oil (℞ 3) may be substituted for the aqueous extract and given in 1 cc. doses I.M. every 6 hours. Desoxycorticosterone acetate in oil (℞ 5) is given once during the first 24 hours in a 5 to 10 mg. dose I.M. in two or more sites, followed thereafter by 5 mg. or less daily. Penicillin (℞ 31) is given prophylactically during the entire period in doses of 300,000 u. I.M. every 12 hours. Fluids I.V. are discontinued as soon as the patient can take adequate amounts of fluids by mouth.

The appearance of edema, the loss of consciousness after temporary improvement, and the development of circulatory failure suggest overdosage of desoxycorticosterone acetate and parenteral fluids. Whole aqueous adrenal cortical extract will not give rise to toxic manifestations and should be used whenever a question of overhydration arises. Opiates, including paregoric, and barbiturates are contraindicated at all times in patients with Addison's disease. Antipyretics should be used only in small doses and with care. Glucose should not be given I.V. without concurrent plasma or albumin administration since it may lead to hyperpyrexia in the presence of adrenal cortical insufficiency. The addition of 2 Gm. of dibasic potassium phosphate to 1,000 cc. of the 10% glucose solution (resultant pH about 7.4) tends to prevent these episodes.

Interim treatment of chronic adrenal cortical insufficiency: Mild cases of adrenal insufficiency may be controlled by the oral administration of 3 to 6 Gm. of sodium chloride daily (℞ 39). In the more severe cases, the electrolyte disturbance may be controlled by the daily administration of desoxycorticosterone acetate in oil or by the subcut. implantation of desoxycorticosterone acetate pellets supplemented with 3 Gm. of sodium chloride by mouth. An initial I.M. dose of 0.5

mg. of desoxycorticosterone acetate in oil (℞ 5) is given, followed by daily increases of 0.5 mg. until the body weight, blood pressure or heart size shows a rapid and excessive increase. Thereupon, the dose is reduced by 10 to 20% and the patient is continued on this amount daily. The average daily dose of desoxycorticosterone acetate is 1 to 3 mg.

To dispense with the daily injections, one 0.125 Gm. or 0.075 Gm. pellet of desoxycorticosterone acetate (℞ 4) may be implanted subcut. in the subscapular region for every 0.5 mg. or 0.3 mg., respectively, of the material in oil used daily in a particular patient. One implantation usually is effective for 9 to 12 months.

Overdosage of desoxycorticosterone results in excessive salt and water retention and is accompanied by increase in heart size, hypertension, pitting edema, and stiffness of the joints and tendons leading to painful contractures. A flaccid paralysis of the extremities due to low serum potassium may occur. Desoxycorticosterone I.M. should be discontinued or the pellets surgically removed if signs of overdosage develop. Whole adrenal cortical extract is substituted since it does not cause dangerous salt retention yet does relieve weakness and hypoglycemia. Salt restriction and potassium citrate by mouth (℞ 40) also are used in the treatment of desoxycorticosterone overdosage.

A high carbohydrate and protein diet with 6 feedings a day is indicated, and at times of inadequate food intake, infections and other types of stress, whole adrenal extract (℞ 2) may be administered subcut. or I.M. in doses of 5 cc. 6 times a day, or adrenal cortical extract in oil (℞ 3) 1 cc. I.M. 3 times a day may be used.

Where evidence suggests that fat is not being properly absorbed by the intestine, absorption may be aided by the use of a wetting agent, such as the polyoxyethylene derivative of sorbitan monooleate, given as 1.5 Gm. doses with each meal (℞ 43).

Recent investigational use of the adrenocortical hormone, cortisone (Compound E), has proved so encouraging as to suggest that much of the foregoing therapy may soon need to be modified or replaced. Further observation, follow-up and evaluation will be necessary, however, before the efficacy of steroid treatment can be determined.

ADRENAL CORTICAL TUMORS
(Adrenogenital syndrome; Cushing's syndrome)

Secreting adrenal cortical tumors (adenomas, carcinomas) may give rise to relative overactivity of the androgenic factors (adrenogenital syndrome), the carbohydrate regulating factors

(Cushing's syndrome), or both, with varying degrees of increase in the activity of the salt and water retaining hormones. The adrenogenital syndrome is characterized by pubertas praecox in children, by overmasculinization in both sexes, with deepening of the voice, overgrowth of the beard, pubic hair, phallus or clitoris, and marked muscular development. A high 17-ketosteroid excretion usually is found. Cushing's syndrome (*see also* CUSHING'S DISEASE) is characterized by protein loss, obesity, weakness, often osteoporosis, diabetes mellitus, hypertension and marked capillary fragility. Excretion of 17-ketosteroids usually is normal. Tumors should be sought by pyelography, or, with due precautions, by perirenal air insufflation roentgenography, and removed surgically if located. Ample adrenocortical substitution therapy (*see* ADDISON'S DISEASE) must be provided during and after operation. It may prove helpful to administer pituitary adrenocorticotropin prior to operation to stimulate the contralateral atrophic adrenal gland.

PHEOCHROMOCYTOMA
(Chromaffinoma)

A chromaffin cell tumor, usually benign, causing hypertension through the production of excessive amounts of epinephrine. The tumor commonly arises in the adrenal medulla but often occurs in other chromaffin tissues (paraganglia, Zuckerkandl's body, thoracic sympathetic chain).

Symptoms and Signs

Hypertension, often precipitous in onset, with its usual associated manifestations is the cardinal symptom. Paroxysmal hypertension, in which the blood pressure reaches high levels for short periods of time (a few minutes to several hours), is characteristic of this disease. It is associated with pounding headache, a sense of impending death, a feeling of constriction in the extremities, and epigastric distress. Immediately after the attack the patient feels exhausted, sweats profusely, and may go into shock. This so-called typical syndrome of paroxysmal hypertension may not be present, however. Many cases cannot be differentiated clinically from essential or malignant hypertension.

Diagnosis

Pheochromocytomas are considered to be responsible for approximately 0.5% of all cases of hypertension. All hypertensive patients, especially children with hypertension, should be carefully studied for the presence of such a tumor. Removal of an epinephrine-producing pheochromocytoma generally results in cure of the hypertension.

The hypertension of hyperepinephrinemia may be abolished

temporarily by adrenolytic drugs. This is the basis for the test with Benodaine (benzodioxane) (℞ 42). A dose of 10 mg./sq. meter of body surface, as calculated from B.M.R. height and weight charts is administered I.V. over a 2-minute period. A hypotensive effect lasting 10 to 15 minutes is diagnostic of a pheochromocytoma. A pheochromocytoma of the adrenal medulla may be visualized by perirenal air insufflation roentgenography, or by exploration of the adrenal areas during sympathectomy. Tumors of the accessory chromaffin bodies cannot be detected by insufflation roentgenography.

Treatment

Surgical removal of the tumor is indicated.

OVARIAN DYSFUNCTION

PRIMARY OVARIAN DEFICIENCY

(Primary ovarian failure; Sexual infantilism; Turner's syndrome; Hypoovarianism)

A condition characterized by failure of ovarian function, hypoestrogenism, primary amenorrhea, sexual infantilism and sterility.

Etiology

Primary ovarian insufficiency is intrinsic and due to ovarian agenesis or arrest in development due to constitutional disease or severe malnutrition. The ovarian derangement is rarely organic. Usually, it is functional—an inherent or acquired inability of the ovarian follicles to grow, ovulate, and luteinize, despite adequate stimulation from the anterior hypophysis. The functional ovarian deficiency may be either congenital or acquired.

Symptoms and Signs

In the congenital type the facies remains childlike but later takes on a wizened appearance. The vaginal mucosa is atrophic and the uterus remains infantile. The breasts fail to mature. Pubic hair is absent or scanty. This type is characterized by an unusual length of the bones of the extremities, especially those of the lower limbs. This resultant disproportion in bony growth stigmatizes the congenital hypogonad as the eunuchoid female. Amenorrhea usually is primary or absolute.

The woman with the acquired type of primary ovarian deficiency is, on the contrary, normal in stature. The condition develops after closure of most of the epiphyses, when pelvic infections, overwork, and an improperly balanced or insufficient diet affect the ovaries adversely and it results in amenorrhea, hypoplastic generative organs, frigidity in some cases, dysmenorrhea, dyspareunia, and sterility.

Diagnosis

Urinary and blood gonadotropin determinations are diagnostic aids, for increased gonadotropins occur in primary ovarian insufficiency. X-ray of the bones may show the presence of osteoporosis. B.M.R. and cholesterol determinations are important to rule out cretinism and hypothyroidism. Glucose tolerance and insulin tolerance studies are of help. Increased carbohydrate tolerance and marked insulin sensitivity and hypoglycemia unresponsiveness may be expected in most cases of hypopituitarism. A careful physical and endocrine survey will help rule out nonendocrine and extraovarian diseases.

Sexual infantilism and amenorrhea may occur in many conditions other than primary ovarian insufficiency, selective hypopituitarism, or pituitary failure. In hypothyroidism, diabetes mellitus, severe nutritional disorders and severe constitutional illnesses, a similar syndrome may be present. In primary hypoovarianism a positive urinary or blood gonadotropin assay usually will be found. In hypopituitarism, pubic hair growth is absent, and therapeutic administration of estrogens does not result in hair growth. Congenital anomalies such as coarctation of the aorta, webbed neck and cubitus valgus sometimes coexist (Turner's syndrome).

Treatment

Primary ovarian failure can be treated best by substitutional therapy, i.e., cyclic courses of ethinyl estradiol (R 14), 0.02 mg. orally daily for 3 weeks every month or estrogens followed by progesterone, 10 mg. I.M. daily for 5 days (R 16), or anhydrohydroxyprogesterone (R 17). Sexual maturation, breast development, improvement in well-being and cosmetic appearance may be expected. Withdrawal bleeding will sometimes occur, usually after the 1st or 2nd month of therapy and thereafter, if sufficient estrogen or estrogen-progesterone therapy is administered. Psychotherapy sometimes is of value in the treatment of certain emotional states frequently seen to accompany primary ovarian insufficiency.

PUBERTAS PRAECOX

Precocious sexual maturity is "true" when all the events of the normal physiologic process are prematurely reproduced. In the female, it is "pseudo" or "false" when associated with granulosa cell tumor of the ovary or when due to hypothalamic or cerebral disease.

Etiology

Hyper-responsiveness of the ovaries to intrinsic gonadotropin activity is thought to be the etiologic factor in true pubertas praecox.

Symptoms and Signs

The syndrome is characterized by premature development of secondary sex characteristics such as breast and genital development, and the appearance of pubic and axillary hair. Body growth is temporarily accelerated in the direction of maturity. Cyclic menses occur, with ovulation and corpus luteum formation. Pregnancy, when it occurs in girls 6 to 12 years of age, belongs to this group. In pseudo pubertas praecox uterine bleeding is anovulatory.

Diagnosis and Treatment

Differentiation between true and pseudo pubertas praecox is important, since no treatment is necessary for the former. In pseudo pubertas praecox surgical removal, where possible, of the causal pathologic process (such as granulosa cell tumor of the ovary) will be followed by regression of the prematurely developed secondary sex characteristics, with cessation of uterine bleeding.

MENOPAUSE
(Change of life, Climacteric)

The transitional phase in a woman's life when menstrual function ceases. It may be natural, premature, or artificial, and often is attended by a complex imbalance of the glandular and autonomic nervous systems.

Etiology and Types

Natural menopause: This is a result of declining ovarian function due to aging of the ovaries and usually occurs between the 40th and 50th years. Most of the symptoms are due to a general endocrine imbalance resulting in autonomic nervous system instability. When ovarian regression is gradual the menopause may be asymptomatic but when decline of ovarian function is relatively rapid the symptomatology may be severe and last from a few months to many years.

Premature menopause: Cessation of ovarian function occasionally occurs between the 25th and 35th years. In some women spontaneous arrest of ovarian activity has occurred a few years after the menarche. Instances of its occurrence before the 20th year are recorded. It may be due simply to premature aging of the ovaries or may follow prolonged lactation, debilitating diseases or infectious processes. This syndrome usually is not as severe as the other forms of menopause.

Artificial menopause: This type occurs subsequent to surgical castration, X-radiation of the ovaries, or following radium implantation in the uterus. It usually is comparable to the more severe manifestations of the natural menopause.

Symptoms and Signs

Symptoms that may be encountered during the menopause are many and varied. In order of frequency, they include:

nervousness, menstrual disturbance, flushes and chills, excitability, fatigability and lassitude, depression and crying spells, irritability, insomnia, heart palpitation and precordial consciousness, vertigo, headaches, numbness and tingling, arthralgias and myalgias, sweating, formication, urinary frequency and incontinence and varied gastrointestinal disturbances. However, it is possible for many such symptoms to be due to organic disease rather than to the menopause itself.

Diagnosis

With menopausal patients it is important to evaluate possible psychogenic factors and to rule out organic disease, e.g., hypertension, pyelitis, cholecystitis, avitaminosis, or thyroid disturbance. The increased irritability and nervous manifestations during the stressful period of the climacteric are occasionally accompanied by thyroid enlargement, frequently with transient disturbances in thyroid activity. Clinical and experimental data suggest that such thyroid enlargement often is associated with hyperfunction. Usually, considerable improvement promptly follows rest, mild sedatives and estrogen therapy.

The frequent complaint of back pain during the climacteric should not be dismissed by the physician as something vague and due to advancing age. X-ray studies of the spine and pelvis commonly reveal osteoporosis. Osteoporosis is associated with hypoestrogenism; it may be seen either in primary ovarian insufficiency (q.v.) or in physiologic decline of ovarian activity (menopause). Postmenopausal osteoporosis is not evident until the climacteric is well developed or complete. At the climacteric, myalgias, arthralgias, and various forms of the arthritides are common complaints.

Treatment

Where psychic factors play a dominant role, psychotherapy and mild sedation (℞ 34) may be used to good advantage. Where depression is marked, amphetamine sulfate (℞ 36) frequently buoys the patient.

The menopausal patient with symptoms of major degree usually obtains gratifying relief from estrogen therapy. At the outset of treatment large doses of estradiol benzoate (℞ 15), administered parenterally at frequent intervals until the patient is stabilized, are recommended. Oral estrogens in the form of ethinyl estradiol, 0.02 to 0.04 mg. daily (℞ 14), or diethylstilbestrol (℞ 13), are then administered in descending amounts over a period of several months. Such a regular regimen is preferable to parenteral injections at irregular intervals based on symptomatology, since the latter method is apt to prolong the therapy unduly.

Estrogen therapy very occasionally may produce bleeding, sore breasts, nervous tension states, abdominal bloating and uterine cramps, and must be discontinued. In such cases testosterone propionate (℞ 9) may be tried alone, or preferably together with ethinyl estradiol, 0.02 mg. daily (℞ 14). Such combined therapy, as an empiric measure, has proved of utmost value in preventing some of the common complications in the treatment of the woman in menopause, such as uterine bleeding, sore breasts and pelvic discomfort. The ratio of androgen to estrogen therapy need not be high—merely that amount necessary to obviate the side effects or estrogens.

MALE HYPOGONADISM

A condition resulting from hypofunction of the endocrine or spermatogenic tissues of the testes. The following discussion is limited to the considerations of hypofunction of testicular endocrinous tissue; disorders of the spermatogenic tissues are discussed in the chapter on male sterility (q.v.).

Etiology

Hypofunction of the interstitial or secondary sex hormone producing cells (cells of Leydig) is of varied etiology. Hypofunction of the pituitary, the master endocrine gland, is a cause of hypogonadism. Panhypopituitarism is reflected by gonadal hypofunction as well as adrenal and thyroid hypofunction. "Idiopathic" eunuchoidism is thought to result from the lack of pituitary luteinizing hormone, one of the hormones of the pituitary which activate the gonadal interstitial cells. In these conditions there are no intrinsic defects in the cells of Leydig. Intrinsic defects of the interstitial cells are the most common causes of hypogonadism; these cells may be destroyed by X-radiation or infection; there may be a primary lack of gonadal tissue as a result of a congenital defect (primary eunuchoidism) or castration. When hypogonadism is due to intrinsic defects of the interstitial cells, assay of the blood or urine reveals the presence of pituitary follicle stimulating hormone (FSH).

Symptoms and Signs

Hypofunction of the interstitial cells of the testes occurring before the onset of puberty results in the eunuchoid state. The genitalia remain infantile and the voice is high pitched. There is female distribution of fat. The skin is soft, pale and sallow. Growth of facial and body hair is fine and scanty. Because of delayed epiphyseal union, overgrowth of the long bones is frequent. Muscular development is poor.

When this type of testicular failure occurs after the onset of puberty, few changes may result. The patient may complain of fatigue or hot flushes. Secondary sex characteristics show regression. Facial hair growth is diminished and less frequent shaving is required. Adipose tissue may be deposited in the

pectoral and trochanteric regions and over the mons pubis.
Sexual libido or ability usually is lessened. The voice and genitalia show little change.

When the reactions are severe, nervousness, psychosexual instability, depression, impaired mental acuity and ambition,
vasomotor disturbances and loss of libido may be prominent
complaints.

Treatment

The therapy must be selected appropriately so as to benefit
gonadotropin-responsive cases in which there is no intrinsic testicular disease, or the nonresponsive cases in which there is intrinsic disease. In the gonadotropin-nonresponsive cases (primary eunuchoidism) which constitute by far the larger group,
attempted stimulation of the interstitial tissue with gonadotropic hormones fails to produce male sex hormone and substitutional therapy with male sex hormone is therefore indicated.
Dosage should be individualized according to age in order to
avoid precocious puberty or premature closure of the epiphyses.
Before the onset of puberty, 5 to 10 mg. of testosterone propionate I.M. (℞ 9) may be given once or twice a week. In the
adolescent and in the adult 25 mg. I.M. 2 to 3 times weekly
usually gives optimal results. Methyltestosterone (℞ 10) may
be given by mouth or sublingually in doses of 10 to 30 mg. daily,
but is not as effective as parenteral therapy. Testosterone pellet
implantation (℞ 11) may be employed after the maximum development of secondary sex characteristics has been induced
with testosterone propionate. Therapy must then be continued
at a maintenance level indefinitely.

In the gonadotropin-responsive cases (secondary hypogonadism) administration of pituitary-like gonadotropic hormones
will stimulate the interstitial cells of the testes to produce the
androgenic hormone. Gonadotropin therapy should consist of
chorionic gonadotropin in doses of 200 to 1,000 u. I.M. 2 or 3
times/week (℞ 8). The addition of pregnant mare's serum
in doses of 100 to 300 u. (℞ 18) to the chorionic gonadotropin
may be effective in some cases. Adjunctive therapy with the
androgens is useful.

PRESCRIPTIONS

(Wherever a prescribed "proprietary" is representative of a
class of therapeutic agents, alternative proprietary preparations
will be found listed in Part II.)

Hormones

    1. ℞ Thyroid U.S.P. 15   mg. (gr. ¼)

        The dosage varies according to the patient's
        age, and severity of hypothyroid state. (For
        details, see text.)

2. ℞ Adrenal cortex extract, aqueous
    (vial)

> Administer subcut., I.M. or I.V. according to instructions given in the text (*see* ADDISON'S DISEASE).

3. ℞ Adrenal cortex extract in sesame
    oil   (vial)

> 1 cc. I.M. every 6 hours.

4. ℞ Desoxycorticosterone acetate
    (sterile pellets) . . . . .   0.12   Gm.

> Implant subcut. according to schedule given in text (*see* ADDISON'S DISEASE).

5. ℞ Desoxycorticosterone acetate
    in oil   (vial)

> 1 to 2 mg. I.M. daily; for Addison's disease, administer I.M. according to directions given in the text.

6. ℞ Parathyroid Injection U.S.P.
    (vial)

> 100 to 300 u. I.M., repeated in 12 hours if necessary; to be administered with calcium chloride (℞ 29) and vitamin D (℞ 41).

7. ℞ Anterior pituitary extract   (vial)

> 1 cc. I.M. daily for 4 to 6 weeks; subsequent courses may be given after a rest period of 1 to 3 months.

8. ℞ Chorionic gonadotropin   (vial)

> 200 to 1,000 u. I.M. 2 or 3 times a week for 6 to 8 weeks; subsequent courses may be given after a rest period of 1 to 2 months.

9. ℞ Testosterone propionate   (vial)

> 5 to 25 mg. I.M. every 2 or 3 days; when improvement occurs, the dosage should be gradually reduced to maintenance levels. For menopausal therapy, the dose is 25 mg. I.M. every 1 to 2 weeks.

10. ℞ Methyltestosterone 10   mg.

> 1 to 3 tablets daily, sublingually or orally.

11. ℞ Testosterone   (sterile pellets)

> Implant 0.1 to 0.3 Gm. subcut. for maintenance therapy after maximum response is obtained from I.M. administration of testosterone.

12. ℞ Estrone   (ampul)

> 0.2 to 0.4 mg. (2,000 to 4,000 I.U.) I.M. 1 or 2 times weekly.

13. ℞ Diethylstilbestrol. . . . . . . 0.25 mg.
    1 to 5 tablets daily.

14. ℞ Ethinyl estradiol . . . . . . 0.02 mg.
    Administer according to instructions given in
    the text (*see* PRIMARY OVARIAN DEFICIENCY;
    MENOPAUSE).

15. ℞ Estradiol benzoate (ampul)
    1.6 mg. I. M. once or twice a week.

16. ℞ Progesterone (ampul)
    Administer according to instructions given in
    various treatment sections in the text.

17. ℞ Anhydrohydroxyprogesterone . 10   mg.
    1 tablet 3 times daily for 5 days.

18. ℞ Pregnant mare's serum (ampul)
    100 to 300 u. I.M. 2 or 3 times weekly.

19. ℞ "Pitressin Tannate" in oil (ampul
    containing 5 pressor u./cc.)
    0.3 to 1.0 cc. (℔ v to xv) I.M. every 30 or
    more hours as required to control polyuria.

20. ℞ Posterior Pituitary Injection
    U.S.P. (ampul)
    0.1 to 1.0 cc. (℔ iss to xv) subcut., repeated
    every few hours if necessary.

21. ℞ Posterior Pituitary Injection
    U.S.P. . . . . 4.0   cc.   (℥ i)
    Sodium chloride, isotonic solu-
    tion . . . . q.s. ad 30.0   cc.   (℥ i)
    Use as a nasal spray as required to control
    polyuria.

22. ℞ Posterior Pituitary Injection
    U.S.P. . . . . 4.0   cc.   (℥ i)
    White Petrolatum U.S.P.
               q.s. ad 30.0   cc.   (℥ i)
    Apply ointment to nasal mucosa as required
    to control polyuria.

23. ℞ Posterior Pituitary U.S.P. . . 40   mg. (gr. ⅔)
    Apply contents of 1 capsule to nostrils like
    snuff, repeated as necessary to control poly-
    uria.

Iodides and Thyroid Depressants

24. ℞ Strong Iodine Solution U.S.P.
    (Lugol's solution) . . . . . 60.0   cc.   (℥ ii)
    20 drops in water twice daily.

25. ℞ Saturated Potassium Iodide Solution N.F. . . . . 15.0   cc.   (℥ ss)

    5 drops daily in water.

26. ℞ Thiouracil . . . . 0.1   Gm. (gr. iss)

    4 to 6 tablets daily until the B.M.R. becomes
    normal, after which the dosage is reduced to
    1 to 3 tablets per day.

27. ℞ Propylthiouracil 50   mg. (gr. ¾)

    1 or 2 tablets 3 times a day until the B.M.R.
    is normal; then, reduce dose to 1 tablet 3
    times daily for 6 months.

Antitetanic Agents

28. ℞ Calcium gluconate, 10% solution (ampul)

    10 to 20 cc. I.V., slowly, repeated every 6
    hours if necessary.

29. ℞ Calcium chloride

    1 to 2 teaspoons 3 or 4 times daily.

30. ℞ Dihydrotachysterol . . . . . 0.6   mg.

    2 to 5 capsules 2 to 4 times daily, followed by
    2 to 9 capsules once or twice a week depend-
    ing on the serum calcium levels.

Antimicrobial Agents

31. ℞ Penicillin   (vial)

    300,000 u. I.M. every 12 hours.

32. ℞ Sulfadiazine . . . . 0.5   Gm. (gr. viiss)

    4 to 8 tablets initially, then 2 tablets every 4
    hours.

33. ℞ Streptomycin   (vial)

    0.5 Gm. I.M. every 4 to 6 hours.

Miscellaneous

34. ℞ Phenobarbital 15   mg. (gr. ¼)

    1 or 2 tablets before each meal and at bed-
    time.

35. ℞ Acetylsalicylic acid . . . . . 0.3   Gm. (gr. v)

    2 tablets every 4 hours.

36. ℞ Amphetamine sulfate 5   mg.

    1 tablet in the morning and in the afternoon.

37. ℞ Quinidine sulfate . . . . . . 0.2   Gm. (gr. iii)

    1 or 2 capsules or tablets every 2, 3, or 4 hours
    until arrhythmia is controlled.

38. ℞ Ammonium chloride (enteric
        coated) . . . . 0.5   Gm. (gr. viiss)
        2 to 4 tablets 3 or 4 times daily.

39. ℞ Sodium chloride. . . . . 0.3   Gm. (gr. v)
        6 to 18 tablets daily.

40. ℞ Potassium citrate. . . . . . . 0.3   Gm. (gr. v)
        2 or 3 tablets or capsules every 6 hours.

41. ℞ Vitamin D
        10,000 u. daily.

42. ℞ "Benodaine" (Benzodioxane)
        (ampul)
        10 mg./sq. meter of body surface, adminis-
        tered I.V. over a 2-minute period (*see* Phe-
        ochromocytoma).

43. ℞ Sorbitan monooleate, polyoxy-
        ethylene derivative . . . . . 0.5   Gm.
        3 capsules with each meal. (Caution! The
        use of mineral oil during this treatment is
        contraindicated.)

EYE

CLINICAL EXAMINATION

The physician should follow a regular routine examination, so as not to overlook abnormalities involving any of the functions or structures of the eyes and their adnexa. Lacrimation, photophobia, and pain are nonspecific complaints. They may be caused by any of a variety of lesions in the lids, conjunctiva, cornea, or uveal tract, and by such conditions as glaucoma and errors of refraction. Therefore, the practitioner should be acquainted with the technic of performing a fairly complete eye examination, so that on all patients with symptoms referable to the eye, he may be able to locate and identify the lesion responsible.

Before an attempt is made to treat any eye complaint (except in emergency cases), the acuteness of vision of each eye separately and both together, with and without glasses, should be determined and recorded. The visual fields and function of the extraocular muscles may be roughly determined at this time. If the patient wears glasses, an approximation of the degree of ametropia (e.g., nearsightedness, farsightedness, astigmatism) may be estimated simply by looking through the lenses. Then, under a good light, a systematic objective examination of the eye should be begun. The eyelids should be examined for lesions of their margins and subcutaneous tissues. The regions of the lacrimal sacs should be palpated and an attempt made to express any contents up through the canaliculi and puncta. The lids then are everted, and the palpebral and bulbar conjunctiva and the fornices inspected for inflammatory exudate, follicular hypertrophy, injection, or other abnormalities. Next, the cornea should be closely examined. A drop of fluorescein (℞ 1) will make any corneal abrasion or ulcer present more apparent. The size and shape of the pupils and their reactions to light and accommodation are noted.

The interior of the eye should be examined with the ophthalmoscope. The pupil may be dilated with one drop of a 3% solution of ephedrine (℞ 2) or, for greater dilatation, a 1% solution of homatropine (℞ 4). Atropine should not be used because of its long-lasting action. The tension of the eyeball should always be estimated before dilatation, since the mydriatics may precipitate an attack of acute glaucoma in an eye with increased intraocular tension. After the ophthalmoscopic examination, 1 drop of 0.25% physostigmine (eserine) (℞ 8) should be instilled if homatropine or atropine has been used, or 1 drop of 1% pilocarpine (℞ 10) if ephedrine or a similar mydriatic has been used. Ophthalmoscopic examination will reveal lesions in the lens, opacities in the aqueous and vitreous humors, retinal lesions, and other defects that may be present. An approximation of the amount of ametropia may be obtained from noting the strength of concave or convex lenses necessary to bring the retina into clear focus. The retina, in addition to manifesting lesions peculiar to itself, such as primary optic atrophy, retinoblastoma, and retinal separation, may show changes related to systemic diseases. The retinal vessels, for example, reflect the general status of the systemic arteriolar bed. Many disease processes such as diabetes, nephritis, and hypertensive vascular disease may be evident on retinoscopy. In addition, changes in the dynamics of the cerebrospinal fluid secondary to increased intracranial pressure will be manifested by edema of the optic nerve disk.

The tonometer, slit lamp, corneal microscope, amblyoscope, and other instruments permit a more exact diagnosis, but their effective utilization requires special training and frequent use. The general practitioner can successfully care for many of the diseases of the eye, but he should be aware of his limitations and consult with one skilled in ophthalmologic diagnosis and therapy whenever in doubt.

INJURIES

Traumatic injuries to the eye or adjacent structures require meticulous examination to determine the extent of injury and the structures involved. For example, an apparently trivial wound may be the entrance point of a foreign body causing severe intraocular damage. Testing and recording the patient's vision is of particular importance, for the protection of the physician himself, the patient, and, in industrial cases, the employer. If the patient's condition contraindicates such examination, this fact should be recorded.

FOREIGN BODIES

1. Conjunctival and corneal: These are the most frequent eye injuries and, lacking proper treatment, the greatest cause of loss of vision, ranging from slight impairment correctable with lenses, to the total loss of an eye. A foreign body, in addition to possibly carrying bacteria into the cornea, causes corneal abrasions which may become secondarily infected and result in corneal ulcers and eventual panophthalmitis (q.v.).

Treatment

Adequate light, good anesthesia, and proper instruments are essential to ensure minimum trauma in removing embedded foreign bodies. An anesthetic, such as 2 or 3 drops of 0.5% Pontocaine (℞ 15), is instilled into the conjunctiva. Both lids are everted and the entire conjunctiva and cornea are inspected with a binocular lens (loupe). Conjunctival foreign bodies are flushed out with a stream of normal saline or wiped out with a sterile cotton applicator. A corneal foreign body, resistant to dislodgment by irrigation or to one wipe of the applicator, may be lifted out on the point of a sterile spud, scalpel blade, or myringotomy knife. Preceding and following removal of the object, the conjunctival sac should be thoroughly irrigated with normal saline. One drop of a 2% fluorescein solution (℞ 1) then is placed into the conjunctival sac and the excess washed out with normal saline or boric acid solution (℞ 21). Corneal abrasion due to foreign body trauma will stain green. If it is small, less than 1 mm. in diameter, no further treatment is needed; if larger, a mild anesthetic and antiseptic ointment such as butacaine sulfate with Metaphen (℞ 29) is placed in the sac and a firm patch fastened over the eye for 24 hours. A sulfonamide or penicillin ophthalmic ointment (℞ 53, 54, 57) may be used if the abrasion is large and potentially infected. The regenerative powers of the corneal epithelium are remarkable, and abrasions involving as much as half the cornea usually heal in 24 hours.

2. Global foreign bodies: The definitive treatment of intraocular foreign bodies must be referred to a specialist in major eye surgery, but certain emergency measures should be instituted immediately. The pupil is dilated with a 1% atropine solution (℞ 5) and a local anesthetic (℞ 15) instilled into the conjunctiva. Penicillin I.M. (℞ 50, 51) or a sulfonamide (℞ 52) by mouth, plus a sulfonamide or penicillin ointment (℞ 53, 54, 57) locally is indicated for preoperative treatment.

LACERATIONS; CONTUSIONS

Contusion of the lids ("black eye") if seen within the first few hours is best treated by cold compresses to stop further extravasation of blood into the subcutaneous tissues; this is followed by hot compresses, 12 to 24 hours later, to hasten absorption. Minor lacerations of the lids may be repaired with fine silk sutures. Major lacerations, especially those involving the lacrimal apparatus, should be repaired by a specialist in plastic surgery of the eye. Trauma to the globe itself may cause severe damage to any of the internal structures. Hemorrhage into the anterior chamber, laceration of the iris, cataract, dislocated lens, glaucoma, vitreous hemorrhage, retinal hemorrhage or detachment (q.v.), and rupture of the eyeball may result. Emergency treatment consists of alleviating pain (℞ 15, 16), keeping the pupil dilated with 1% atropine (℞ 5), and combating infection with penicillin or a sulfonamide given both locally and systemically (℞ 50 to 58). Definitive therapy should be instituted by a qualified eye surgeon.

BURNS

Burns of the eyelids are treated by closing the lids, cleansing them thoroughly with sterile saline or boric acid solution (℞ 21), and applying boric acid ointment (℞ 22) or vaseline gauze. Sterile cotton-waste pressure dressings then are put on and held in place by an elastic bandage or stockinet around the head. Débridement and frequent changing of the dressings should be avoided to prevent infection. Chemical burns of the conjunctiva and cornea are treated by copious washing of the conjunctival sac with suitable neutralizing agents for a minimum of 20 to 30 minutes. Sodium bicarbonate solution (℞ 19) is used for acid burns, and 2% acetic acid (℞ 20) for burns due to alkalies. Thermal burns of the cornea and conjunctiva should be immediately and thoroughly irrigated with normal saline. Pain is relieved and healing promoted by the use of ointment containing Holocaine and epinephrine (℞ 16), Metaphen (℞ 27), cod liver oil and Metaphen (℞ 28), butacaine sulfate and Metaphen (℞ 29), or Butesin (℞ 30), 3 to 4 times daily. Severe pain may require frequent instillations of 4% cocaine (℞ 18) or injections of Demerol (℞ 66) or morphine (℞ 67). The treatment of severe burns of the cornea and conjunctiva is in the specialist's province. Deep corneal ulcers, iridocyclitis, panophthalmitis (q.v.), and cicatricial deformities of the lids may occur as complications.

14

LACRIMAL APPARATUS
DACRYOSTENOSIS

Narrowing of the nasolacrimal duct, most often resulting from congenital stenosis. Obstruction usually becomes apparent at the age of 2 to 12 weeks as a persistent tearing (epiphora) of one eye or, rarely, both. It can be easily differentiated from the conjunctivitis following prophylactic silver nitrate installation at birth and from corneal abrasion or ophthalmia neonatorum (q.v.) by the severe lacrimation with relatively little conjunctival inflammation. Dacryostenosis with epiphora may occur in later life from chronic nasal infection with inflammatory obstruction of the duct. Fracture of the nose and facial bones may cause mechanical obstructon. Prolonged blockage from any cause usually leads to infection of the lacrimal sac (dacryocystitis [q.v.]).

Treatment

In infancy, most cases of congenital dacryostenosis can be cured by milking the contents of the lacrimal sac down through the nasolacrimal duct with fingertip pressure once or twice daily, and instilling 2 or 3 drops of an astringent collyrium (℞ 23) into the conjunctival sac at each feeding. If milking is unsuccessful, the punctum should be stretched with a dilator under local anesthesia (℞ 15) and normal saline gently forced through the nasolacrimal system with a fine blunt canaliculus needle. A drop of fluorescein (℞ 1) in the saline will make it easily detectable in the nose. When this fails, patency may be established by passing lacrimal sounds, under general anesthesia. In adults, when the obstruction is not complete, the use of probes of increasing sizes followed by irrigation with a mild astringent and antiseptic solution (℞ 23) sometimes is successful. When complete bony obstruction is present, or probing is unsuccessful, a new opening may have to be made surgically from the tear sac into the nasal passages.

DACRYOCYSTITIS

Inflammation of the lacrimal sac.

Etiology

Infection of the lacrimal sac usually is due to the common pyogenic organisms and is almost always secondary to obstruction of the nasolacrimal duct. In infants it occurs as a complication of congenital dacryostenosis (q.v.). In older persons it may result from obstructive lesions of the duct following nasal trauma, deviated septum, hypertrophic rhinitis, mucosal polyps, hypertrophy of the inferior turbinate, or residual congenital dacryostenosis.

Symptoms and Signs

In acute dacryocystitis, pain, redness, and edema about the

lacrimal sac, epiphora, conjunctivitis, blepharitis, corneal ulcer (q.v.), fever and leukocytosis may be present. In chronic dacryocystitis there often is only slight swelling of the sac. On pressure, pus may escape through the punctum. In some cases, the sac becomes distended by retained secretions to form a large mucocele. Repeated episodes of acute inflammation may result in a red, brawny indurated area over the sac. Occasionally, an abscess may rupture and form a draining fistula.

Treatment

Acute dacryocystitis is treated by frequent application of hot compresses; widening the canaliculus by surgical incision for evacuation of pus; incision and drainage if an abscess has formed; penicillin I.M. (℞ 50, 51), or a sulfonamide by mouth (℞ 52); and benzalkonium chloride or Metaphen drops (℞ 33, 34) into the conjunctival sac to prevent secondary infection of the lids, cornea, and conjunctiva. Sulfonamide drops (℞ 55, 56) should be avoided if possible because lid dermatitis often follows their use. Chronic dacryocystitis may occasionally be cured by dilating the nasolacrimal duct with probes, using local anesthesia (℞ 15, 16). This is followed by irrigation of the duct with antiseptic solutions such as Metaphen 1:3,000 (℞ 34), Phemerol (℞ 44), mild silver protein 10% (℞ 41), methylene blue (℞ 26), or zinc sulfate and boric acid solution (℞ 23). Contributory nasal or sinus abnormalities also should be treated. If conservative treatment is unavailing, open operation with removal of the lacrimal sac may be necessary to prevent development of a corneal serpent ulcer, which is likely in chronic dacryocystitis.

EYELIDS

BLEPHARITIS

Inflammation of the lid margins with redness, thickening, and usually the formation of scales and crusts or shallow marginal ulcers.

Etiology

Ulcerative blepharitis, the most common type, is caused by bacterial infection, usually staphylococcic, of the lash follicles and meibomian glands. The nonulcerative, squamous, or seborrheic type, the cause of which frequently is obscure, may be allergic in origin or associated with seborrhea of the face and scalp. Lowered resistance due to systemic infection and poor hygiene, inadequate diet, and refractive errors may be predisposing factors.

Symptoms and Signs

Itching, burning, and redness of the lid margins, edema of the lids, falling out of lashes, and conjunctival irritation with lacrimation and photophobia may be present in both types. The ulcerative type is associated with thick tenacious crusts adherent to the lid margins and lashes, which leave a bleeding surface when pulled away. Small pustules develop in the lash follicles and eventually break down to form shallow ulcers. Overnight, the lids become glued together by dried secretions. There often is a history of repeated sties and chalazions. The nonulcerative type is associated with greasy, easily removable scales on the lid margins, the so-called "granulated eyelids."

Both types are indolent, recurrent, and stubbornly resistant to treatment. Exacerbations of the nonulcerative type are merely inconvenient and unsightly. Repeated attacks of the ulcerative type result in loss of eyelashes, scarring of the lids, and occasionally corneal ulceration (q.v.). It is well to warn patients that recurrences are usual.

Treatment

Ulcerative Blepharitis: Treatment is both local and systemic. Locally, ointments of penicillin (℞ 57) or the sulfonamides (℞ 53, 54) used for a few days only, or Metaphen (℞ 27) will help clear the lid infection. Drops of penicillin (℞ 58) or the sulfonamides (℞ 55, 56), cautiously used or benzalkonium chloride (℞ 33) will combat the secondary infection of the conjunctiva and cornea. Drops may be used by day and ointment at night. Hot water compresses applied to the closed lids for 10 minutes 3 times/day help combat the acute phase. More severe cases require a sulfonamide orally (℞ 52) or penicillin parenterally (℞ 50, 51). Stubborn infections may be aided by a course of commercially prepared staphylococcus toxoid (℞ 62) or autogenous vaccine (℞ 64). Continued use of sulfonamides and penicillin, particularly when applied locally about the eyes, may sensitize some patients to these drugs; therefore, alternative treatment should be employed when possible. Never give these drugs to patients for self-use during recurrences.

Nonulcerative Seborrheic Blepharitis: Remission may be obtained by relieving an accompanying seborrhea of the scalp (q.v.). Massage of the lid margins with a salicylic acid and sulfur ointment (℞ 31) every other night for 2 weeks usually will remove crusts. Daily application of silver nitrate 0.5% (℞ 37), or 5% brilliant green (℞ 36) every other day, sometimes gives excellent results. Methylene blue with Holocaine and epinephrine drops (℞ 26), or zinc sulfate-epinephrine-boric acid collyrium (℞ 23) will relieve the secondary conjunctival irritation. Vitamin A (℞ 77), 25,000 I.U. daily for 2 weeks, is effective in cases due to a deficiency of this factor.

HORDEOLUM
(Sty)

An acute localized pyogenic infection of one or more of the glands of Zeiss or Moll (external hordeolum) *or meibomian glands* (internal hordeolum; meibomian sty).

Etiology

The staphylococcus usually is the responsible organism. Sties often are associated with and secondary to blepharitis (q.v.), uncorrected errors of refraction, poor general health, and infection elsewhere in the body. Recurrence is common.

Symptoms and Signs

External hordeolum begins with lacrimation and photophobia, a feeling of "something in the eye," and considerable pain and redness of the lid margin with a small, round, tender area of induration. Edema, though usually localized, may be diffuse. A small yellowish spot, indicative of suppuration, appears in the center of the area of induration in a day or so. The abscess soon ruptures with discharge of pus, relief of pain, and the formation of a central slough.

Internal hordeolum involving one of the meibomian glands (*see* Chalazion) is more severe. The pain, redness, and edema are more localized. Close inspection of the inner side of the lid margin in early cases shows a small elevation corresponding to the location of the affected meibomian gland. If seen at a later stage an abscess will be found, usually pointing on the conjunctival side of the lid following the long axis of the affected gland. Rarely, it points on the skin side. Following spontaneous rupture of the abscess, pain and swelling promptly subside. Recurrence is common.

Diagnosis

External sty usually is superficial, well localized, and appears to lie at the base of an eyelash. The internal sty is deeper and can be seen in the conjunctiva, through which it generally ruptures. Both types in their early stages may be difficult to distinguish from an exacerbation of blepharitis (q.v.). Blepharitis usually involves the entire margin of one or more lids. If the hordeolum lies near the inner canthus of the lower lid, it must be differentiated from acute dacryocystitis (q.v.), in which condition gentle pressure over the swelling generally causes pus to regurgitate through the inferior punctum.

Treatment

In the early stages, suppuration may be aborted by cold or hastened by hot compresses applied for 15 minutes 3 or 4 times a day. Penicillin (℞ 50, 51) or a sulfonamide (℞ 52) given systemically increase the chances of resolution without suppuration. As soon as suppuration is evident by the formation of a central yellow area, the sty should be incised with a sharp cataract knife. This is best done under a short-acting general anesthesia such as with Vinethene, nitrous oxide, or I.V. Pentothal. Benzalkonium chloride (℞ 33), Phemerol (℞ 44), or Metaphen (℞ 34) drops instilled into the conjunctiva every hour by day and an ointment such as yellow oxide of mercury (℞ 32) or Metaphen (℞ 27) at night are recommended to prevent the spread of infection to adjacent glands and the conjunctiva. In severe cases parenteral penicillin (℞ 50, 51) or an oral sulfonamide (℞ 52) may be necessary.

Attempt should be made to remove foci of infection elsewhere and to improve the general health of the patient. Adequate rest and nutrition are important. All cases should be refracted and have correcting lenses prescribed if necessary. When crop after crop of sties occurs despite the above measures, treatment with a commercial staphylococcus toxoid (℞ 62) or vaccine (℞ 63), or an autogenous vaccine (℞ 64) should be undertaken.

CHALAZION

Chronic granulomatous enlargement of a meibomian gland caused by occlusion of its duct, often following inflammation of the gland.

Symptoms and Signs

Symptoms are slight or absent except for a painless, slow-growing, round mass in the lid which is seen or felt by the patient. Conjunctival irritation is frequent with the larger chalazions. The skin can be moved loosely over the tumor, which may be seen in the tarsus of the lid, generally presenting subconjunctivally as a red or gray mass. There often is a recent history of sty or chronic blepharitis (q.v.). Occasionally, the tumor may suppurate to form an internal hordeolum (q.v.). When the mass is near the inner canthus in the lower lid, chronic dacryocystitis must be ruled out. Differentiation from chalazion can be made by pressure over a chronically inflamed lacrimal sac which, in dacryocystitis, will cause thick mucus to regurgitate through the puncta.

Treatment

In the early stages, absorption of the chalazion occasionally may be brought about by repeatedly massaging the lids with a yellow oxide of mercury ointment (℞ 32) in the conjunctival sac. Hot compresses for 10 to 15 minutes, 3 or 4 times daily, are useful. If this procedure fails, excision of the tumor under local anesthesia becomes necessary. After the chalazion is removed, methylene blue drops (℞ 26) 3 times a day and yellow oxide of mercury or Metaphen ointment (℞ 32, 27) nightly should be used until all postoperative reaction has subsided. Hot compresses also hasten absorption of the postoperative reaction. Occasional massage of the eyelids may aid in preventing recurrences.

ORBIT

ORBITAL CELLULITIS

An inflammation of the orbital tissues caused by extension of infection from the accessory nasal sinuses or teeth, trauma to the orbit, or metastatic spread from infections elsewhere. The usual symptoms are extreme pain in the orbit, exophthalmos, impaired mobility of the eye, swelling of the lid, chemosis, and fever with malaise. Possible complications are loss of vision due to optic neuritis, thrombophlebitis of the orbital veins resulting in cavernous sinus thrombosis, panophthalmitis (q.v.), and spread to the meninges and brain.

Treatment

Specific therapy in the form of penicillin (℞ 50, 51) or a sulfonamide (℞ 52) systemically, general supportive therapy including bed rest and ample fluids, with local hot applications to localize the infection are the principles of treatment. Demerol (℞ 66) or codeine and acetylsalicylic acid (℞ 68) should be given to relieve pain. Incision and drainage are indicated if suppuration is suspected.

CAVERNOUS SINUS THROMBOSIS

Thrombosis of the cavernous sinus usually resulting from direct spread of infection along the venous channels draining the orbit and face. It is most often secondary to orbital cellulitis or pyogenic infection of the skin in the central region of the face. Occasional cases are caused by metastatic spread from pyogenic foci elsewhere in the body. It is manifested by bilateral exophthalmos, papilledema, severe cerebral symptoms, and a septic temperature curve. The prognosis is grave.

Treatment

Systemic penicillin and sulfonamide therapy (℞ 50, 51, 52) and supportive care offer the best chance for cure. Prophylaxis by prompt and adequate treatment of pyogenic infections about the face is extremely important.

EXOPHTHALMOS

Protrusion of the eyeball that may occur as a result of inflammation, edema, tumors, and injuries of the orbit, or from cavernous sinus thrombosis, or because of enlargement of the eyeball, as in congenital glaucoma. In hyperthyroidism (q.v.), edema and lymphoid infiltration of the orbital tissues may cause a bilateral exophthalmos. Arteriovenous aneurysm involving the internal carotid artery and the cavernous sinus may produce a pulsating exophthalmos of one or both eyes.

Treatment

Ligation of the common carotid artery on the involved side is necessary in cases of arteriovenous aneurysm. The exophthalmos of hyperthyroidism may or may not subside upon controlling the thyroid hyperactivity. Severe cases may require surgical orbital decompression.

CONJUNCTIVA

ACUTE CATARRHAL CONJUNCTIVITIS

("Pink-eye," Koch-Weeks conjunctivitis)

A catarrhal form of acute conjunctival inflammation caused by various bacteria.

Etiology

The highly contagious epidemic form, usually occurring in the spring and fall and known as "pink-eye," is caused most often by the pneumococcus, occasionally by the Koch-Weeks bacillus. These organisms and *Neisseria catarrhalis, Hemophilus influenzae* and the meningococci, as well as the coliform bacilli, may be responsible for sporadic cases. Mixed infections are common. Frequently, no pathogens can be found. The disease often is associated with irritation from wind, dust, and smoke; intense light as from electric arcs, sun lamps, and reflection from snow; and with the common cold and the exanthems, especially measles.

Symptoms and Signs

Lacrimation followed by a discharge, at first watery and later mucoid or mucopurulent, with sensations of itching, smarting, and burning of the lids, and photophobia are common symptoms. Usually both eyes are involved. The products of inflammation may seal the lid margins together overnight and may transiently interfere with vision by adhering to the cornea. The conjunctiva of lids and fornices becomes bright red. Hyperemia and loss of transparency of the bulbar conjunctiva may occur. These symptoms are much more intense in the epidemic form. The discharge may become purulent, with considerable swelling of the lids, chemosis (edema) of the bulbar conjunctiva, and small subconjunctival petechial hemorrhages. In the milder, more common sporadic type, most patients get well in a few days to a week. The epidemic type, when due to the pneumococcus, may last 1 to 2 weeks, and when due to the Koch-Weeks bacillus, 2 to 4 weeks. The cornea is almost never involved in simple catarrhal conjunctivitis, but in the epidemic type, small corneal ulcers (q.v.), usually healing readily, are not uncommon.

Diagnosis

The bacterial forms of conjunctivitis may be identified by demonstrating the causative organisms in smears and cultures. Catarrhal conjunctivitis may be differentiated from inclusion blennorrhea and from vernal conjunctivitis (q.v.) by examining conjunctival scrapings. Inclusion bodies will be found in inclusion blennorrhea, and eosinophiles in vernal conjunctivitis. Retained corneal or conjunctival foreign bodies and corneal abrasion and ulcer (q.v.) may be ruled out as causes for conjunctival injection by examination with fluorescein (R 1) and a hand lens.

Conjunctival injection in conjunctivitis must be differentiated from the deep ciliary injection in iritis and acute glaucoma (q.v.). Ciliary injection is mainly circumcorneal, pink or lilac in color, and composed of fine straight deep vessels immovable when the conjunctiva is moved. Conjunctival injection in catarrhal conjunctivitis is present mainly in the fornices, is brick red in color, and composed of coarse tortuous superficial vessels movable with the conjunctiva.

Treatment

The disease usually is self-limiting, but treatment will shorten its duration and prevent complications. In mild cases, the use of dark glasses, application of cold compresses several times daily, boric acid or alkaline collyrium irrigations (R 21, 24, 25) 3 times daily, and instillation of a small amount of antiseptic ointment (R 32) in the conjunctival sac at bedtime usually is the only treatment necessary. If chronicity develops, zinc sulfate collyrium (R 23) or 0.5% silver nitrate (R 37) applied to previously anesthetized everted lids, followed by normal saline irrigations or mild silver protein drops (R 41), is indicated. Never put a patch over these eyes.

In severe cases, sulfonamide, penicillin, or aureomycin drops (R 55, 56, 58, 59), day and night, should be used, but with caution to avoid sensitization. Satisfactory results may be obtained in refractory cases due to the Koch-Weeks bacillus, *H. influenzae*, and *Ps. pyocyanea* by using streptomycin parenterally (R 60) and tyrothricin solution locally (R 61).

Recurrences may be prevented by avoiding exposure to excessive light, dust, smoke, and chemical irritants; correcting errors of refraction; and removing carefully and completely any conjunctival or corneal foreign bodies.

CHRONIC CATARRHAL CONJUNCTIVITIS

Inflammation of the conjunctiva characterized by chronicity with exacerbations and remissions over a period of months or years and symptoms similar to but less severe than those of acute conjunctivitis. The causal bacteria usually are similar.

Angular Conjunctivitis of Morax-Axenfeld: This is a special form of chronic catarrhal conjunctivitis, due to the Morax-Axenfeld bacillus, which affects chiefly the inner and outer angles of the conjunctival sac.

In all forms of chronic conjunctivitis, ectropion, overuse of the eyes, and continuous exposure to wind, smoke, dust, and other irritants are of considerable etiologic importance.

Symptoms and Signs

The symptoms, generally worse at night, consist of itching, smarting, and a feeling of "something in the eye." The palpebral conjunctiva is reddened and thickened, with a velvety appearance. The bulbar conjunctiva may be involved slightly or not at all. A scant mucoid secretion may be present. In the angular, Morax-Axenfeld type the redness is most intense near the inner and outer canthi. Scrapings from these regions usually reveal Morax-Axenfeld bacilli in large numbers.

Treatment

This consists of eliminating irritating factors, and the use of bland antiseptics such as methylene blue (℞ 26), Phemerol (℞ 44), or Metaphen drops (℞ 34). Scrubbing the everted anesthetized lids with 0.5% silver nitrate (℞ 37) weekly is useful. Frequent instillation of a 0.2% solution of zinc sulfate (℞ 23) is almost specific in Morax-Axenfeld conjunctivitis. Cortisone or ACTH, possibly with an antibiotic, may be helpful.

CONJUNCTIVITIS NEONATORUM
(Ophthalmia neonatorum)

A purulent conjunctivitis of the newborn, acquired from an infected birth canal during parturition. The majority of cases are due to the gonococcus, but staphylococcus, streptococcus, pneumococcus, and other bacteria sometimes are responsible.

Symptoms and Signs

Both eyes usually are affected. In gonorrheal cases, symptoms appear 12 to 48 hours after birth. Inflammation of the conjunctiva with serous discharge is rapidly followed by chemosis with bulbar injection and edema of the lids. In 1 or 2 days the discharge becomes purulent and extremely copious, and the other symptoms diminish. The acute condition may subside in 2 or 3 weeks, with conjunctival hypertrophy and chronic inflammation lasting for several months. Corneal ulceration (q.v.) is a frequent complication. Corneal perforation (q.v.) and panophthalmitis (q.v.) may occur. In nongonorrheal cases the incubation periods are longer, symptoms milder, and recovery is more rapid.

A prompt diagnosis of gonococcal conjunctivitis can be made by examining gram-stained scrapings from the retrotarsal fold in all newborn infants showing signs of conjunctivitis. With proper treatment, the prognosis is good.

Prophylaxis

Preventive measures are of first importance, and their routine use in hospitals has enormously reduced the incidence of blindness due to ophthalmia neonatorum. In all newborn babies, 2 drops of 1% silver nitrate solution ($\mathbb{R}$ 38) or, where legally permissible, a few drops of a penicillin solution ($\mathbb{R}$ 58) should be instilled into each eye immediately after birth. Expectant mothers known to have gonorrhea should be given appropriate therapy (*see* GONORRHEA) during pregnancy. If it is not possible to treat these women before delivery, the infant should be given penicillin both locally ($\mathbb{R}$ 58) and parenterally ($\mathbb{R}$ 50, 51) immediately after delivery.

Treatment

Parenteral and local penicillin or sulfonamide therapy is specific ($\mathbb{R}$ 50 to 58) and will immediately prevent spread of the infection to the unaffected eye. The conjunctival sac should be irrigated frequently with normal saline to prevent the purulent secretions from adhering to the cornea or conjunctiva. The pupils should be kept dilated with atropine ($\mathbb{R}$ 5) if corneal involvement threatens. Residual conjunctival hypertrophy may be reduced by periodic brushing of the everted and anesthetized palpebral conjunctiva with 0.5% silver nitrate ($\mathbb{R}$ 37). Irrigations of the conjunctival sac with mild silver protein solution ($\mathbb{R}$ 41) twice daily are indicated until all evidence of discharge has disappeared.

ADULT GONOCOCCAL CONJUNCTIVITIS

A severe form of purulent conjunctivitis in adults caused by the gonococcus, usually acquired by self-inoculation from a genital infection. Doctors and nurses may acquire the disease from gonorrheal patients. Usually, only one eye is involved. The clinical findings are similar to, but more severe than, those of ophthalmia neonatorum. Pain, blepharospasm, chemosis, and induration of the lids are more prominent. The disease begins after a 12- to 48-hour incubation period, reaches its peak about the 10th day, and subsides in 1 to 2 months. Complications, including corneal ulceration, abscess, perforation, panophthalmitis (q.v.), and blindness are more common than in ophthalmia neonatorum. Treatment is essentially the same as for the latter disease.

TRACHOMA
(Granular conjunctivitis, Egyptian ophthalmia)

A chronic contagious viral conjunctivitis, characterized by exacerbations and remissions, follicular hyperplasia of the pal-

*pebral subconjunctival tissue, corneal vascularization, and cica-
tricial shrinkage of the lids.*

Epidemiology

The disease is highly prevalent in Egypt, Palestine, Southern
and Central Europe, and the Far East. It is widespread among
American Indians and occurs endemically in the Southern
mountainous areas of the United States. It is most contagious
in its early stages and may be transmitted by direct contact
with trachomatous material or indirectly by handling contaminated articles (e.g., towels, handkerchiefs).

Symptoms and Signs

The incubation period averages about 1 week. There then is
a gradual onset of conjunctival congestion, edema of the eyelids, photophobia, and lacrimation, usually in both eyes, which
suggests catarrhal conjunctivitis. After 7 to 10 days small
follicles appear in the conjunctiva of the upper lids. These
gradually increase in size and number for 3 to 4 weeks and form
yellow-gray semitransparent "sago grain" granulations surrounded by inflammatory papillae. Pannus formation usually
begins at this time with invasion of the upper half of the cornea
by infiltration of loops of vessels from the limbus. In severe
cases, the entire cornea may become involved, reducing vision
to light perception only. Complete retrogression of the pannus
with restoration of corneal transparency then frequently occurs
spontaneously in uncomplicated cases. This stage of follicular
hypertrophy and pannus formation may last from several
months to one or more years, depending upon response to
therapy.

A cicatricial stage follows. The follicles and papillae gradually shrink and are replaced by scar tissue which often results
in entropion and obstruction of the ducts of the lacrimal gland.
Ulcers may form in ischemic areas of the pannus. Upon healing, the conjunctiva is smooth and grayish white. A varying
amount of corneal opacity with loss of vision is present resulting from pannus residuum, healed corneal ulceration with consequent scar formation, and xerophthalmia in which the corneal
epithelium becomes dull and thickened because of scarcity of
tears.

Diagnosis

In the early stage the presence of minute granular cytoplasmic inclusion bodies in Giemsa-stained epithelial conjunctival
scrapings helps to differentiate trachoma from acute catarrhal
conjunctivitis (q.v.). These inclusion bodies also are found
in the inclusion blennorrhea group of conjunctivitis (q.v.).
Observation of the development of the complete clinical picture will differentiate trachoma from this group. Vernal palpebral conjunctivitis (q.v.) has some similarity to trachoma

in its follicular hypertrophic stage: eosinophilia, absence of inclusion bodies in the scrapings, and milky flat tops of the papillae suggest vernal conjunctivitis.

Treatment

Excellent results may be obtained from oral and local sulfonamide therapy (℞ 52 to 56). Application of a copper sulfate stick (℞ 45) or a 1:500 solution of mercuric chloride (℞ 40) to the everted and anesthetized lids once daily, or instillation of 5% copper citrate ointment (℞ 46) into the conjunctiva twice daily, is valuable. Penicillin (℞ 50, 51, 57) also may be useful. Roller forceps expression of well developed granulations is indicated in the absence of severe inflammation. Occasionally, surgical removal of infected areas and plastic surgery of deformed lids may be necessary.

INCLUSION CONJUNCTIVITIS
(Inclusion blennorrhea, Swimming pool conjunctivitis)

An acute conjunctivitis caused by a virus of genital origin, known as inclusion blennorrhea in the newborn and swimming pool conjunctivitis in the adult.

Symptoms and Signs

In the newborn, after an incubation period of 5 to 7 days, an intense papillary conjunctivitis, swelling of the lids, chemosis, and a mucopurulent discharge develop. Epithelial cell inclusion bodies can be demonstrated in conjunctival scrapings. Both eyes are usually involved. Hypertrophied papillae lasting for several months may develop in both conjunctival folds. No corneal damage occurs. In adults the condition is less severe and more often unilateral. The secretion is less profuse, but the papillae are larger. Swelling of the preauricular glands on the side of the involved eye is not uncommon.

Treatment

In the newborn, local application of a sulfonamide ointment (℞ 53, 54) usually produces cure in a week. In adults, both oral and local sulfonamide therapy (℞ 52 to 56) often is necessary. In cases that have established chronicity prior to treatment, 5% copper citrate ointment twice daily (℞ 46) in addition to sulfonamide therapy is helpful. Protecting the uninvolved eye is important in preventing bilateral infection.

VERNAL CONJUNCTIVITIS
(Spring conjunctivitis)

A bilateral chronic conjunctivitis thought to be allergic in origin, with symptoms recurring in the spring and lasting through the summer. It is most often seen in males between the ages of 5 and 20.

Symptoms and Signs

Intense itching of the eyes, tearing, photophobia, conjunctival injection, and a tenacious mucoid discharge are characteristic. Smears of the discharge contain numerous eosinophiles. The palpebral or bulbar conjunctiva or both are affected. In the **palpebral form,** hard, flattened, square, pale pink to grayish granulations appear, packed together like cobblestones, chiefly in the upper lids. The uninvolved tarsal conjunctiva looks milky white. In the **bulbar** or **limbic** form, the conjunctiva in the region of the limbus becomes hypertrophied and grayish. Occasionally corneal ulcers develop.

Symptoms disappear during the cold months, and become milder with the passing of years. The lesions, however, persist throughout the year, and often throughout life.

Treatment

If a causal allergen can be found, desensitization and other appropriate therapy are indicated (*see* ALLERGY). The thick secretion should be washed out frequently with 3% sodium bicarbonate solution (Ŗ 19). Itching may be relieved by ice compresses and the cautious use of a Holocaine-epinephrine solution during the day (Ŗ 17), and an ointment of similar composition at night (Ŗ 16). In refractory cases, radium or solid carbon dioxide may be applied to the granulations.

PHLYCTENULAR CONJUNCTIVITIS
(Phlyctenular keratoconjunctivitis, Eczematous conjunctivitis)

A conjunctivitis, usually occurring in children, characterized by discrete nodular areas of inflammation known as phlyctenules, and resulting from the atopic reaction of a hypersensitive conjunctiva or cornea to an allergen. In most cases, the allergen is believed to be a product of the tubercle bacillus, staphylococcus, or other bacteria.

Symptoms and Signs

The phlyctenules appear, singly or in groups, as small yellowgray nodules most frequently at the limbus, but sometimes on the cornea and the bulbar conjunctiva. With conjunctival involvement there may be only mild itching and tearing. When the cornea is affected, blepharospasm, severe tearing, photophobia and pain may be prominent. The phlyctenules occur in crops lasting from several days to a week or two. They almost always ulcerate, but usually heal without scar formation. Frequent recurrence of corneal phlyctenules, especially when secondary infection occurs, may result in corneal opacity with loss of vision.

Treatment

In the uncomplicated conjunctival form, powdered calomel

dusted into the conjunctival sac once a day (℞ 48) or 1% yellow oxide of mercury ointment (℞ 32) applied to the lesions usually effects a cure. When corneal involvement occurs, atropine (℞ 5) and sulfonamide drops (℞ 55, 56) should be used to dilate the pupils and to prevent secondary infection. Holocaine and epinephrine ointment (℞ 16) can be used to relieve pain and blepharospasm. Dark glasses should be worn.

General treatment includes the removal of infective foci and correction of errors in diet and hygiene. A course of tuberculin or typhoid vaccine (℞ 65) may be tried in refractory cases. Recent results obtained with cortisone or ACTH in this and various other acute and chronic inflammatory eye conditions have been highly encouraging.

CORNEA

CORNEAL ULCER

A localized necrosis of corneal epithelium usually due to invasion by microorganisms following trauma or to spread of infection from adjacent infected areas.

Etiology

Pneumococcic, streptococcic, and staphylococcic infections complicating persistent or improperly removed foreign bodies of the cornea (q.v.) are the most common primary causes. Corneal ulcers also occur as complications of chronic blepharitis; conjunctivitis, especially catarrhal and gonorrheal; trachoma, dacryocystitis, and acute infectious diseases (q.v.). Disturbances in corneal nutrition secondary to keratomalacia and glaucoma (q.v.) and corneal exposure due to eyelid injuries and defective closure of the lids (lagophthalmus) occasionally are responsible. Ulceration may occur as a manifestation of corneal atopy as in phlyctenular conjunctivitis (q.v.). Dendritic keratitis (q.v.) due to the herpes virus often results in a refractory type of ulcer.

Symptoms and Signs

Pain, photophobia, blepharospasm, and lacrimation often are present. However, extensive corneal ulceration may occur with relatively few symptoms. The lesion appears at first as a dull grayish circumscribed superficial infiltration and subsequently undergoes necrosis and suppuration to form an ulcer. It can be stained green, and thus becomes more easily visualized, by placing 2 or 3 drops of fluorescein (℞ 1) into the conjunctival sac, after which the excess is washed out with normal saline. The ulcer may spread to involve the greater part of the cornea, or penetrate into its deeper structures. Corneal ulceration is usually associated with considerable ciliary injection, and blood vessels may be seen growing in from a point on the limbus nearest the ulcer. The serpiginous or serpent ulcer, which usually is due to the pneumococcus, occurs most often as a complication of chronic infections of the adnexa of the eye. It frequently develops in debilitated elderly persons, with or without such chronic infections. It often appears near the center of the cornea, grows rapidly in size and depth, and may destroy much of it.

Complications

The deeper the ulcer the more severe the symptoms and complications. Superficial ulcers usually have no sequelae. Ulcers deep enough to involve Bowman's membrane and the lamellas of the cornea heal with fibrous tissue replacement. This causes opaque scarring of the cornea, resulting in the formation of nebulas, maculas, and leukomas with consequent loss of vision. Iritis, iridocyclitis, corneal perforation with iris collapse, hypopyon (pus in the anterior chamber), panophthalmitis (q.v.), and destruction of the eye may occur in untreated cases, or in debilitated patients with or without treatment.

Treatment

Because of the seriousness of its complications, corneal ulceration should be treated only by a skilled ophthalmologist.

Small ulcers, 1 to 2 mm. in diameter, following aseptic removal of foreign bodies (q.v.), heal within 24 hours when treated with Metaphen ointment (℞ 27) and a firm patch. Larger ulcers occurring after corneal trauma, especially when infected, require a sulfonamide or penicillin ointment (℞ 53, 54, 57) in addition to an anesthetic ointment (℞ 16) and patching. The cornea should be examined with fluorescein (℞ 1) and retreated every 24 hours until healed.

In treating ulcers of several days' duration and increasing severity, atropine (℞ 5) should be instilled into the conjunctival sac until the pupil is widely dilated, in order to put the uveal tract at rest. The base of the ulcer should be cauterized with 3% silver nitrate (℞ 39) followed by immediate irrigation. A sulfonamide or penicillin ointment (℞ 53, 54, 57) then is placed inside the lower lid once daily for a few days only, and the eye patched. When pneumococci are found in scrapings from the ulcer bed, a few grains of Optochin (℞ 47) may be dusted onto the lesion and washed off with saline after 30 seconds. Parenteral penicillin (℞ 50, 51) or an oral sulfonamide (℞ 52) is beneficial when the ulcer is due to a susceptible organism. Tyrothricin drops (℞ 61) may sterilize an ulcer contaminated with sulfonamide-fast and penicillin-resistant staphylococci or streptococci. Streptomycin (℞ 60) is useful in ulceration complicating conjunctivitis due to the Koch-Weeks bacillus or other streptomycin-sensitive organisms.

Hot compresses to the eye several times daily often bring comfort and may aid in healing. Patching is necessary to prevent additional corneal irritation from lid movements. Ulcers secondary to blepharitis or conjunctivitis (q.v.) will clear up when these conditions are successfully treated. Paracentesis should be performed as soon as increasing severity of the ulcer becomes evident and corneal perforation threatens despite treatment.

Nonspecific therapy with 2 to 5 cc. of sterile boiled milk I.M. every other day for 5 days or typhoid organsims I.V. (℞ 65) often brings dramatic resolution of the lesion.

SUPERFICIAL PUNCTATE KERATITIS

A condition affecting one or both eyes and characterized by scattered fine punctate infiltrations in the superficial corneal layers. It often is associated with trachoma, staphylococcic dacryocystitis, blepharitis, and conjunctivitis (q.v.), or it may be due to a virus similar to the herpes virus. Occasionally, it complicates infections of the respiratory tract. The chief symptoms are photophobia, pain, lacrimation, and conjunctival injection, with diminution of vision when the pupillary area of the cornea is heavily involved. The lesions may last several months, after which there is almost complete absorption with little residual impairment of vision.

Treatment

The lesions may respond to treatment of the associated disease. Instillation of 2 or 3 drops of a 2% potassium iodide solution (℞ 42) 3 or 4 times daily is helpful. Atropine (℞ 5) is of value in relieving pain. A patch should be used to keep the eye at rest.

DENDRITIC KERATITIS

A chronic relapsing form of superficial corneal inflammation and ulceration caused by the herpes simplex virus, and characterized by an arborizing, many-branched lesion covering large areas of the cornea, and arranged like the veins in a leaf, with knoblike terminals. Early symptoms are a sensation of foreign body in the eye, lacrimation, photophobia, and mild conjunctival injection. Corneal anesthesia rapidly follows. Permanent nebulous scarring of the cornea frequently results.

Treatment

After anesthetizing the cornea with Pontocaine (℞ 15) or cocaine (℞ 18), the lesion is touched with a fine cotton point moistened with a saturated iodine solution (℞ 43). One treatment often is sufficient. Metaphen or yellow oxide of mercury ointment (℞ 27, 32) then is placed in the conjunctival sac and an eye patch is applied until healing is complete. Atropine (℞ 5) should be used to dilate the pupil in severe cases threatening uveal tract involvement. In treatment-resistant cases, grenz rays, ultraviolet radiation, or X-ray may be of use.

PHLYCTENULAR KERATITIS
(*see* PHLYCTENULAR CONJUNCTIVITIS)

INTERSTITIAL KERATITIS
(Parenchymatous keratitis)

A chronic infiltration, without ulceration, of the deep layers of the cornea, with uveal tract inflammation. Most cases occur in children between 5 and 15, as a complication of congenital syphilis. Both eyes are usually involved. Rarely, acquired syphilis or tuberculosis may cause a unilateral form of the disease in adults.

Symptoms and Signs

Photophobia, pain, lacrimation, and gradual loss of vision until only light perception remains are common symptoms. The lesion begins as a grayish infiltration in the deep corneal layers at the center or periphery, which soon spreads to involve the entire cornea. The cornea develops a characteristic groundglass appearance, obscuring the iris. Vascularization of the cornea then results from blood vessels growing in from the limbus and producing orange-red areas ("salmon patches"). Uveitis, in the form of iritis, iridocyclitis, and choroiditis (q.v.), is common. The inflammation and vascularization usually begin to subside after 1 to 2 months, with clearing of the cornea most noticeable at the periphery. The cornea may clear completely, or some opacity may remain. Vision may be impaired even when the cornea clears completely, if residual complications of iritis, iridocyclitis, or choroiditis remain.

Treatment

If syphilis (q.v.) is present, systemic treatment, together with fever therapy, is indicated. Recently, use of cortisone or ACTH has proved of value in shortening the course and limiting the complications of the corneal inflammation. Locally, atropine (℞ 5) is used to put the uveal tract at rest during the acute phase of the disease. Dionin (ethylmorphine) 1% (℞ 35) instilled into the conjunctival sac once daily and massage of the cornea through the closed lids 3 times daily with yellow oxide of mercury ointment (℞ 32) in the sac will hasten the healing process.

KERATOMALACIA
(Xerophthalmia)

A condition caused by systemic deficiency of vitamin A, and characterized by greasiness and dryness of the cornea, which becomes denuded of its epithelium. Corneal ulceration with secondary infection is common. The lacrimal glands and conjunctiva also are affected. Lack of tears causes extreme dryness of the eyes, and greasy spots appear on the bulbar conjunctiva. Night blindness (q.v.) often is associated. Specific therapy consists of vitamin A, 25,000 u. by mouth daily (Ŗ 77). Locally, atropine (Ŗ 5) and mild antiseptic ointments (Ŗ 27 to 30) are useful in combating secondary infection.

CORNEAL VASCULARIZATION
(Rosacea keratitis)

A condition that may occur as part of the symptom complex of riboflavin deficiency and is a common accompaniment of acne rosacea (q.v.). It arises from proliferation of small blood vessels growing from the limbus into the cornea. Dimness of vision, photophobia, and itching of the eyes are common complaints. It is frequently associated with cheilosis, glossitis, and angular stomatitis (q.v.). Excellent therapeutic results may be obtained by the oral administration of 10 mg. of riboflavin daily (Ŗ 80). Cortisone or ACTH may be helpful.

CATARACT

An opacity of the lens or its capsule, and which may be developmental or degenerative. **Developmental cataract** occurs congenitally or during early life as a result of heredity and nutritional or inflammatory disturbances. **Degenerative cataract** is characterized by gradual loss of transparency in a normally developed lens. This may be due to senile degenerative changes, the effects of heat, X-radiation, trauma, systemic disease (e.g., diabetes), uveal tract inflammation (cataracta complicata), and the ingestion of certain toxic substances (e.g., dinitrophenol).

Symptoms and Signs

The cardinal symptom is a gradual diminution of visual acuity. The degree of loss of vision depends upon the location and extent of the opacity. Well developed diffuse cataracts may reduce vision until only light perception remains. Myopia often develops in the early stages so that a presbyopic patient may discover that he can read without his glasses ("second sight"). Diplopia or polyopia occasionally is annoying. Pain is absent unless the cataract is secondary to intraocular inflammatory disease.

Diagnosis

Well advanced cataracts can be seen with the unaided eye as gray opacities in the lens. Ophthalmoscopic examination of the dilated pupil (*see* CLINICAL EXAMINATION OF THE EYE), with the instrument held approximately 2 feet away, usually will reveal less distinct opacities. Small ones will stand out as dark defects in the red reflex. A large cataract may obliterate the red reflex entirely. Slit lamp examination will give much more detailed information about the character, location, and extent of the lesion.

Gradual loss of vision in middle-aged or older patients is characteristic of both cataract and glaucoma (q.v.). Before dilation of the pupils for an ophthalmoscopic examination, an increase in intraocular tension should be ruled out. The vision lost through cataract is restored by operation, but the deterioration due to glaucoma mistakenly diagnosed as cataract may result in permanent blindness. Glaucoma must therefore be ruled out in every case.

Treatment

During the development of a cataract, frequent refractions and changing of eyeglass prescriptions will help maintain useful vision. Operative removal of the lens is necessary in cases with considerable impairment of vision. Age is no contraindication to surgery. Cataracts secondary to uveitis should not be operated upon for at least 6 months after all signs of inflammation have ceased.

UVEAL TRACT
IRITIS; IRIDOCYCLITIS

An acute or chronic inflammation of the iris. When the ciliary body is involved, as it almost always is, the condition is known as **iridocyclitis.**

Etiology

The causes are varied, and in many cases cannot be determined. Secondary syphilis is perhaps the most common of the known causes of iritis. Tuberculosis, sarcoidosis (uveoparotid fever), gonorrhea, diabetes, the "rheumatic state," and various acute infectious diseases are among the systemic causes. Tonsillitis, diseased teeth and gums, sinusitis, chronic genitourinary disease, and other foci of infection may be responsible. Iritis may complicate keratitis, corneal ulcer, and conjunctivitis (q.v.), trauma to the eye, and infections of or injury to the other eye (*see* Sympathetic Ophthalmia).

Symptoms and Signs

Severe throbbing pain in the eyeball, radiating to the forehead and temple and becoming worse at night, is the most distressing symptom. Photophobia and lacrimation may be present. Blurring of vision, transient myopia, and astigmatism occur. The eyeball is tender to palpation through the closed lids. The iris appears dull and swollen, brown irides become muddy, and blue and gray ones greenish. The pupil may be irregular, miotic, and react sluggishly or not at all to light and accommodation because of adhesions between the posterior surface of the iris and the capsule of the lens (posterior synechiae). Circumcorneal ciliary injection usually is seen. The aqueous appears turbid and a deposit of dustlike particles (keratitic precipitates) may be seen covering the posterior surface of the cornea. Pus may accumulate at the bottom of the anterior chamber (hypopyon).

With ciliary involvement, the symptoms are more intense. Swelling of the upper lid may occur; the circumcorneal injection is more severe; there is greater ciliary tenderness on palpation; and the aqueous is more cloudy with the formation of denser precipitates.

Diagnosis

Iritis and iridocyclitis must be differentiated (*see* accompanying table) from acute congestive glaucoma and the various forms of conjunctivitis (q.v.).

DIFFERENTIAL DIAGNOSIS

Acute Iritis	Acute Glaucoma	Acute Conjunctivitis
Small irregular pupil	Dilated pupil	Normal pupil
Severe circumcorneal injection	Circumcorneal and episcleral injection	Superficial conjunctival injection
Iris muddy and swollen	Iris congested and bulging	Iris normal
Lacrimation	Lacrimation	Mucous or mucopurulent discharge
Moderately severe pain	Very severe pain	Burning, but no severe pain
Considerable eyeball tenderness	Considerable eyeball tenderness	No eyeball tenderness
Eyeball tension usually normal	Tension increased	No change in tension
Cornea transparent, precipitates may be present on posterior surface	Cornea appears steamy	Cornea normal
Moderately decreased vision	Considerably decreased vision	Normal vision

Complications and Sequelae

Permanent posterior synechiae may occur, with seclusion of the pupil, in which the iris is bound down to the lens capsule throughout its entire pupillary margin. This results in a fixed

pupil, loss of communication between the anterior and posterior
chambers of the eye, and consequent bulging (iris bombée) and
atrophy of the iris from retained secretions in the posterior
chamber. Secondary glaucoma (q.v.), ending in blindness if
unrelieved, is an occasional complication. Vision may be obscured by corneal and anterior lens capsule deposits, exudate
filling the pupillary space (occlusion of the pupil), and inflammatory changes in the lens (cataracta complicata). Choroiditis
may occur.

Prognosis

Acute iritis usually lasts a number of weeks; chronic iritis
may last several months with a tendency to recur. Prognosis
is guarded because of the severity of certain complications.
Ciliary body involvement makes the outlook more serious.

Treatment

The treatment of iritis and iridocyclitis is essentially the
same. The patient should be put to bed in a room with subdued
light. Pain may be relieved with codeine and acetylsalicylic
acid (℞ 68). As soon as the diagnosis is established, vigorous
local treatment should be begun to prevent the formation of
posterior synechiae and to put the iris and ciliary body at rest.
Atropine (℞ 5) every 2 hours until the pupil is dilated and 3
or 4 times daily thereafter usually will maintain adequate dilatation. For children, an atropine ointment (℞ 6) is preferable
because the ointment base blocks the puncta and prevents absorption via the nasolacrimal duct, thus reducing the likelihood
of atropine toxicity. If adhesions have formed, the action of
atropine may be augmented by instilling drops of 1:1,000
epinephrine (℞ 3) or 4% cocaine (℞ 18). Subconjunctival
circumlimbal injection of atropine (℞ 5), epinephrine (℞ 3),
or both, frequently will free the most stubborn adhesion.

Dionin (ethylmorphine) (℞ 35) and the frequent application
of hot compresses several times daily aid in the absorption of
exudate and bring comfort. Pontocaine (℞ 15) will alleviate
pain.

Nonspecific therapy in the form of 2 to 5 cc. of sterile
boiled milk intragluteally every other day for 5 injections, or
typhoid vaccine I.V. every other day (℞ 65) is useful.

If the encouraging results now being reported following treatment of nonspecific iritis and iridocyclitis with cortisone or
ACTH are confirmed, the therapy of these and similar conditions will be drastically altered.

If syphilis or other disease or a focus of infection is responsible, vigorous specific therapy should be promptly instituted.

Surgical treatment may be required for hypopyon, persistent
posterior synechiae, secondary glaucoma, and the establishment of an artificial pupil.

CHOROIDITIS; CHORIORETINITIS

An inflammation, usually chronic, of the choroid. The overlying retina almost always is involved **(chorioretinitis).**

Etiology

Similar to that of iridocyclitis (q.v.) in that syphilis, tuberculosis, and focal infections are frequently causative. However, there is a large idiopathic group.

Symptoms, Signs, and Complications

Pain is absent unless the iris or ciliary body is involved. Various visual disturbances result from retinal displacement or involvement by inflammatory changes in the choroid. Retinal displacement may cause distortion of the size of objects (micropsia or macropsia). Peripheral retinal involvement will not result in easily noticeable visual defects, but careful visual field study reveals peripheral scotomas. Macular involvement causes reduction in or loss of central vision. Vitreous opacities may cause diffuse blurring of vision.

Complications include retinitis, retinal detachment, vitreous abscess (endophthalmitis), iridocyclitis, and cataract (cataracta complicata).

Diagnosis

The eye shows no external signs of inflammation in uncomplicated cases. The pupil is regular and reacts freely. Ophthalmoscopic examination reveals patches of exudation in the fundus varying in size, shape, and position according to the cause and extent of the choroiditis. Opacities and a general cloudiness of the vitreous may be evident. The exudates appear as yellow-gray areas with ill-defined margins. The retina overlying the choroid lesion becomes edematous and somewhat elevated; the retinal blood vessels are bent as they pass across these areas. In mild cases, the exudates may be absorbed, leaving little or no residual scarring. In the more advanced cases, white patches with rings of surrounding black pigment may be seen as a result of choroid and retinal atrophy, with patches of sclera showing through.

Treatment

Therapy directed against possibly causative infectious diseases or foci of infection is essential. Foreign protein injections of milk (2 to 5 cc. I.M.) or typhoid vaccine (℞ 65), or the use of cortisone or ACTH as recently tried with encouraging results, may hasten absorption of the exudates before permanent damage to the retina occurs. Atropine (℞ 5) may be used to immobilize the uveal tract and help prevent spread of the infection. Dark glasses and rest are indicated.

PANOPHTHALMITIS

A suppurative inflammation involving the entire eye, usually ending in its complete destruction. **Suppurative endophthalmitis** is a similar condition but is restricted to the uveal tract. It may be caused by pyogenic organisms gaining access to the interior of the eye through trauma, a perforating corneal ulcer, a septic embolus from an infectious process elsewhere, or extension from an orbital cellulitis or meningococcus meningitis.

Intense pain in the eye, rapid loss of vision, conjunctival and ciliary injection with chemosis, swelling of the lids, and rapid development of pus throughout the interior of the eye mark the course of the disease. Eventually, the sclera ruptures and the purulent contents of the eyeball drain out, leaving a blind shrunken globe. Severe constitutional symptoms of fever, malaise, and headache usually are present. Sympathetic ophthalmia does not occur.

Treatment

Systemic administration of a sulfonamide (R 52) or penicillin (R 50, 51) is indicated as for any pyogenic infection. Potent analgesics (R 66, 67) are necessary to relieve pain. Locally, hot compresses followed by incision and drainage of the sclera to allow the escape of pus are necessary. Enucleation is not advisable during the acute stage of the disease because of the danger of spreading the infection via the optic nerve to the meninges; it can be done for cosmetic purposes after the inflammation has subsided.

SYMPATHETIC OPHTHALMIA

An inflammation of the uveal tract in one eye ("sympathizing eye") *following a traumatic iridocyclitis of the other* ("exciting eye").

Etiology

The condition almost always occurs after a perforating injury involving the uveal tract, with a retained intraocular foreign body, or an operation on the exciting eye. The exact cause is unknown. An allergic reaction of the uveal tract of the sympathizing eye, or an infection via the optic chiasm are suspected causes.

Symptoms and Signs

Symptoms of uveal tract irritability such as photophobia, lacrimation, transient blurring of vision, neuralgic pain in the eye, and eyeball tenderness may develop in the sympathizing eye from several weeks to several years following injury to the exciting eye. During the period of irritability, proper treatment of the exciting eye—enucleation if necessary—will prevent further damage to the opposite eye. Otherwise, active inflammation develops, with ciliary injection, vitreal opacities, keratitic deposits, and other signs of acute iridocyclitis. A blind, atrophic eye often is the end result.

Treatment

Prompt, adequate treatment of an injured eye is of great importance in preventing a sympathetic ophthalmia. The eye should be enucleated when sightless or when the preservation of sight is unlikely, especially when the ciliary body is involved. During the stage of sympathetic irritability, enucleation of the exciting eye usually will have a beneficial result. When there is useful vision in the injured eye the question of enucleation is a difficult one because signs of irritability often subside without developing into an active sympathetic inflammation. However, once active inflammation has developed in the sympathizing eye, enucleation is of no value. In fact, the exciting eye may ultimately possess better vision than the sympathizing eye. Recently the use of cortisone or ACTH has proved encouraging as an aid in preventing the development of sympathetic ophthalmia.

In case sympathetic ophthalmia has developed, vigorous treatment may still salvage some useful vision. Treatment has consisted of atropine (℞ 5), Dionin (ethylmorphine) (℞ 35), hot wet compresses, and foreign protein injections as in iridocyclitis (q.v.). Sodium salicylate in large daily doses (℞ 69) may be tried. Cortisone or ACTH has been used effectively.

GLAUCOMA

A disease of the eye characterized by increased intraocular tension, and commonly causing impairment of vision ranging from slight abnormalities to absolute blindness. **Primary glaucoma** may be of an acute or chronic congestive (narrow angle) type or a chronic simple (wide angle) type. Congenital glaucoma (buphthalmos) also is a primary type. **Secondary glaucoma** results from preexisting diseases of the ocular structures.

PRIMARY GLAUCOMA

Etiology and Pathogenesis

The initial causes of primary glaucoma are not known. Advanced age, arteriosclerosis, vasomotor instability, hyperopia, and heredity are among the predisposing factors. The increase in intraocular tension is related to an imbalance between the production of aqueous and its escape through the normal channels of exit. Obstruction to the escape of intraocular fluid appears to be mainly responsible for this imbalance. In the narrow angle type (acute and chronic congestive glaucoma), the anterior chamber is shallow and the filtration angle is narrowed, making the canal of Schlemm inaccessible. A vasomotor disturbance resulting in an increase of intraocular fluid content may push the root of the iris forward against the angle and precipitate an acute attack. Disproportion between a small-sized globe and a relatively large ciliary body and lens, as in hyperopes, may result in a shallow anterior chamber, and cause the peripheral folds of the iris to crowd the angle. In the wide angle type (chronic simple glaucoma), the anterior chamber is of normal depth but there is an actual obstruction of the pores of the sclerocorneal trabeculae leading to the canal of Schlemm that makes drainage impossible.

CHRONIC SIMPLE (WIDE ANGLE) GLAUCOMA

This type occurs about 5 times as frequently as acute congestive glaucoma (q.v.). Progressive loss of sight, premature presbyopia, contraction of the visual fields, and scotomata may develop unnoticed by the patient over a considerable period of time. Central vision is not impaired until late in the disease. Occasionally, colored halos are seen about artificial lights. Foggy vision and impaired dark adaptations are complained of. Pain is not prominent.

Diagnosis

The eye shows few abnormal external signs. There may be minimal circumcorneal injection and moderate dilatation of the pupil. The tension is not increased so much as in acute glaucoma. The eyeball may not feel hardened on palpation, but examination with a tonometer usually reveals moderate elevation of tension. A provocative test may bring about a significant rise in intraocular tension in suspicious cases. A rise in tension after the patient has remained in absolute darkness for 1 hour, or has drunk 1 qt. of water or 2 cups of strong coffee, or has received eucatropine mydriasis (℞ 7), will help confirm the diagnosis. The earliest diagnostic changes found on examination are a contraction of the nasal side of the visual fields in the form of a right-angled defect, and a large scotoma in the region of the blind spot. Cupping or excavation of the disk may be visualized upon ophthalmoscopic examination in advanced cases. The disease usually begins in one eye and the second eye almost always becomes involved after a variable period of time, sometimes years later. Complete blindness due to optic atrophy (q.v.) eventually ensues in untreated cases.

Treatment

A good percentage of cases can be controlled (tension normalized) by a course of one of the miotics: pilocarpine (℞ 10), Floropryl (di-isopropyl fluorophosphate) (℞ 12), physostigmine (eserine) (℞ 9), Carcholin (℞ 13), or neostigmine (℞ 14). Since the response to these drugs varies in different patients, trial should be made to determine the most effective one for each case. Foci of infection should be eliminated. The patient should avoid fatigue and emotional upsets and the use of tobacco and coffee. If a satisfactory response to therapy is obtained, the visual fields and intraocular tension should be tested periodically to make sure the disease is being kept under control. When the tension cannot be normalized or the visual field shows increasing defects, operative treatment becomes imperative.

ACUTE CONGESTIVE (NARROW ANGLE) GLAUCOMA

Prodromal symptoms may occur, usually in the form of transitory attacks in which the patient complains of diminished visual acuity, seeing colored halos around lights, and some pain in the eye and head. If examination is made at such times, a somewhat dilated, poorly reacting pupil and rather shallow anterior chamber will be revealed. These attacks may last only a few hours and recur at intervals of weeks to years before a typical attack of acute glaucoma occurs. The acute attack is characterized by rapid loss of sight and sudden onset of severe throbbing pain in the eye, which radiates over the sensory distribution of the 5th nerve. Nausea and vomiting are frequent accompaniments. There is considerable swelling of the lids, lacrimation, circumcorneal conjunctival injection, chemosis, and a dilated fixed pupil. The cornea is steamy, the anterior chamber shallow, and the aqueous turbid. The eyeball tension is considerably increased. The fundus cannot be clearly visualized with the ophthalmoscope because of the turbidity of the media. After a few days of treatment the symptoms may subside, only to recur repeatedly. After each acute attack, vision becomes progressively poorer and the visual field more contracted. Examination of the fundus between acute episodes shows a gradual cupping of the disk increasing in severity with repeated attacks. The condition usually is unilateral, but occasionally may be bilateral.

The last stage of the disease when unrelieved by treatment is referred to as absolute glaucoma. The eye is blind due to progressive atrophy of the optic nerve head (*see* Optic Atrophy). The cornea is clear and often insensitive. The pupil is widely dilated and fixed, the iris atrophied, and the disk deeply excavated. Pain no longer is prominent but sometimes recurs at rare intervals. After a time, the eyeball may degenerate and become secondarily infected.

Treatment

An acute attack may be aborted in the prodromal period by the use of miotics as indicated in chronic simple glaucoma (q.v.) (℞ 9, 10, 12, 13, 14). If the patient is seen soon after onset of the acute attack more vigorous therapy with the miotics is indicated. Physostigmine (eserine) salicylate 1 or 2% (℞ 9) should be instilled every 10 to 15 minutes for 1 to

2 hours, and then every half hour for several hours until miosis occurs. Pilocarpine 2% (℞ 11) and the other miotics (℞ 12, 13, 14) may be used in the same manner. Morphine (℞ 67), in addition to relieving pain, also produces miosis. The opposite, normal eye should be kept in a miotic state during this period by instilling dilute solutions of physostigmine (℞ 8) or pilocarpine (℞ 10) as a precautionary measure. Injection of 100 cc. of 50% glucose I.V. (℞ 49) also may aid in decreasing intraocular tension. Ice packs to the eye help to reduce pain and congestion. If the tension has been brought down to normal by the strong miotics, a weaker one such as 0.25% physostigmine (℞ 8) or 1% pilocarpine (℞ 10) may be used 1 to 4 times daily for 4 to 5 weeks before discontinuing therapy. If there is no sign of relief within 6 to 8 hours, operative interference is necessary to avoid permanent loss of vision. Complete iridectomy is the operation of choice.

CHRONIC CONGESTIVE GLAUCOMA

The symptoms and signs are similar in character but less severe than in the acute form. Onset is more gradual and often occurs after a prodromal period as in the acute variety. The disease is more protracted but eventually ends in blindness if unrelieved.

Treatment

The use of miotics (℞ 9 to 14) as in the acute congestive form (q.v.) is indicated but treatment is less vigorous. If the disease is not controlled after several weeks of medical therapy, surgery becomes necessary to prevent optic atrophy. One of the filtering cicatrix operations is the procedure of choice.

CONGENITAL GLAUCOMA
(Buphthalmos, Hydrophthalmos)

In this condition, which is rare, the outflow of aqueous is obstructed by a congenital defect in the region of the angle of the eye or by a rudimentary or absent canal of Schlemm, with consequent increase of intraocular tension. The disorder usually is bilateral and is seen in infants and children. The eyeball becomes considerably enlarged, the cornea is thinned and bulging, the pupil large and fixed, and the anterior chamber very deep. As the disease progresses the disk is excavated and blindness often ensues.

Treatment

Miotics are of little value. Early operative interference offers the best chance of preserving useful vision.

SECONDARY GLAUCOMA
Etiology and Pathogenesis

This is caused by any abnormal condition that interferes with the flow of aqueous from the posterior chamber through the pupil into the anterior chamber to the canal of Schlemm. Inflammatory intraocular disease may prevent aqueous escape by causing complete posterior synechia, iris bombée, edema of the lens, iris, or ciliary body, and by forming exudates which alter the fluidity of the aqueous and plug the canal of Schlemm. Other common causes are trauma to the eye, operative procedures, intraocular tumors, thrombosis of the central retinal vein, and intraocular hemorrhage.

Treatment

Correction of the primary cause is necessary for cure. If the glaucoma is secondary to iridocyclitis, paracentesis of the anterior chamber in addition to the usual treatment is necessary (*see* Iridocyclitis). Miotics are not indicated. When due to blood in the anterior chamber, prompt operative interference is essential to prevent permanent blood staining of the cornea as well as optic atrophy. Inflammatory adhesions blocking aqueous escape require surgical correction in the form of iridectomy or cyclodialysis.

RETINA

RETINITIS

An inflammation of the retina, frequently bilateral, and commonly due to syphilis, tuberculosis, or spread from a focus of infection. It often occurs with, or secondary to, choroiditis (q.v.) or other uveal tract infection.

Symptoms and Signs

The most frequent symptoms are diminution of visual acuity, apparent distortion of the size and shape of objects, a variety of visual field defects, and a feeling of discomfort in the eyes, occasionally with photophobia. There seldom are any external signs and the diagnosis usually is made upon ophthalmoscopic examination. White or yellow exudates, varying in size, are seen in the vicinity of the retinal vessels and may partially obscure them. Flame-shaped superficial and rounded deeper retinal hemorrhages, with clouding of retinal details and congestion of the disk, may be observed. Opacities sometimes are seen in the vitreous. The lesions often heal with complete restoration of vision, but the involved portions of the retina may become atrophic, with impairment of vision corresponding to the size and location of the lesions.

Treatment

Retinitis complicating syphilis, tuberculosis, other infectious diseases or foci will respond to therapy of these primary causes. Local treatment is most unsatisfactory and consists of immobilizing the uveal tract with atropine (℞ 5), the use of smoked glasses, and absolute rest of the eyes.

CENTRAL ARTERY OBSTRUCTION

An uncommon vascular blockage causing sudden blindness, without pain, in one eye. It may be due to thrombosis in a sclerotic central retinal artery; embolism, often from an endocarditis or from crushing injuries to long bones (fat embolus); or, rarely, to spasm of the artery in an individual with a highly labile vasomotor apparatus. Ophthalmoscopic examination reveals characteristic findings. The fundus appears very pale except for the macular region, which is bright cherry red. The arteries are extremely thin and contain no blood. The veins also are thinner than normal and contain less than the normal amount of blood. If the obstruction is unrelieved, retinal degeneration takes place within a few days and sight is irretrievably lost.

Treatment

Therapy must be instituted within a few hours if restoration of vision is to be hoped for. Reduction of intraocular tension by vigorous massage of the eyeball and paracentesis of the anterior chamber may dislodge the embolus and allow it to pass into a smaller branch of the artery, thus limiting the amount of retinal ischemia. Inhalation of amyl nitrite (℞ 70), sublingual administration or subcut. injection of nitroglycerin (℞ 71), sodium nitrite by mouth (℞ 72), acetylcholine subcut. (℞ 73) or papaverine subcut. or I.V. (℞ 74) may relieve spasm of the artery. Deep heat by diathermy also may be useful.

CENTRAL VEIN THROMBOSIS

Complete obstruction of the central retinal vein by a thrombus, usually occurring in elderly patients with arteriosclerosis and cardiac disease. Idiopathic closure may occur in the younger age group. Vision is lost somewhat more slowly than in arterial obstruction. With complete closure of the vein, blindness develops in an hour or so. On ophthalmoscopic examination, the retinal veins are seen to be greatly distended. The fundus is congested and edematous, and numerous hemorrhages are present, often extending into the vitreous. If the thrombus is in a branch of the vein, these changes are limited to the area drained by the branch. Secondary glaucoma often develops as a result of increased intraocular venous pressure.

Treatment

The anticoagulants, heparin and dicumarol (℞ 75, 76), may prevent the further production of thrombi if only a branch is involved (*see* ANTICOAGULANT THERAPY). When complete thrombosis of the central vein has occurred, there is no effective treatment. Miotics (℞ 9 to 14) may help prevent glaucoma (q.v.).

RETINAL DETACHMENT

Partial or complete separation of the retina from the choroid. This is an uncommon condition and occurs most often in highly myopic eyes and as a result of shrinking of organized vitreal exudates following uveitis. Subretinal edema and tumor, choroidal hemorrhage, the use of potent miotics, and traumatic detachment are among other causes.

Loss of vision, ranging from a small field defect in minimal separation to complete blindness in total detachment, is the chief symptom. Ophthalmoscopic examination may reveal a flat detachment with irregularities in refraction of different parts of the retina and diminution of the light reflex or the characteristic, grossly irregularly folded, partially or completely detached retina.

Treatment

The prognosis after early treatment by an expert is excellent. If detachment is suspected, the patient should be put to bed immediately. It is necessary to bandage both eyes or prescribe pinhole glasses until expert help is available. Prompt operative reattachment by a skilled eye surgeon offers the only worth-while chance for cure.

RETINOPATHIES

Arteriosclerotic Retinopathy: This type usually is found in individuals with generalized arteriosclerosis and moderate hypertension. The walls of the retinal arterioles become thickened, thus narrowing the lumens and the contained columns of blood. This results in widened light reflexes, indentation of the veins at the arteriovenous crossings, and an increased ratio between the size of the venous and the arteriolar columns of blood. The arterioles are tortuous and the walls of the arteries may become visible as gray sheaths about the columns of blood. Hemorrhages may be seen in the vicinity of the vessels, and there may be areas of localized ischemia appearing as white plaques in the retina.

Hypertensive Retinopathy: This form is associated with essential hypertension, toxemia of pregnancy, and chronic glomerulonephritis with severe hypertension. Early in the course of such diseases, the fundi demonstrate generalized retinal arteriolar constriction (angiospasm) or resemble those seen in arteriosclerotic retinopathy (q..v.), with superimposed angiospasm. As the disease progresses numerous hemorrhages and white or gray exudates become prominent. The hemorrhages may be flame-shaped or round. Edema of the retina, especially in the macular region, appears as a white star-shaped figure. Signs of retinal ischemia are more evident than in arteriosclerotic retinopathy. In the most severe form of the disease the optic disk becomes edematous and resembles the choked disk (papilledema) caused by brain tumor. The absence of changes in the arterioles helps to differentiate the choked disk of brain tumor from the edematous disk of severe hypertension.

Diabetic Retinopathy: This usually occurs among elderly diabetics and often is associated with arteriosclerotic retinopathy. Numerous small, oval or round, white or yellow deposits in the retina grouped in and around the macular region are characteristic. They do not form the star-shaped figure seen in arteriosclerotic retinopathy, and there is no edema of the optic nerve or retina. Small, round hemorrhages are seen in the deeper retinal layers. In advanced cases, large fluffy deposits may fill the entire macular region.

Treatment

The general treatment is that of the underlying specific cause: hypertension, nephritis, toxemia of pregnancy, or diabetes (q.v.). In retinopathies with considerable angiospasm, smoking is contraindicated. Rutin (R 81), vitamin C (R 79) and vitamin K (R 82) may be of some value in diminishing the hemorrhagic tendencies.

OPTIC NERVE; VISUAL PATHWAYS
PAPILLEDEMA
(Choked disk)

A swelling of the nerve head caused by increased intracranial pressure or interference with venous return from the eye. It usually is bilateral, and occurs with brain tumor or abscess, cerebral trauma, cerebral hemorrhage, meningitis, and cavernous sinus thrombosis. Vision is not affected in the early stages. The blind spot gradually enlarges, and this is followed by progressive contraction of the visual fields. After a considerable time, if the intracranial pressure is not reduced, blindness ensues due to secondary optic atrophy (q.v.). Ophthalmoscopic examination reveals considerable elevation of the disk. The degree of elevation is determined by comparing the highest plus lens necessary to bring into sharp focus the most elevated portion of the disk with that used to see clearly an unaffected portion of the retina. A difference of as much as 8 diopters may be present. Engorgement and tortuosity of the retinal veins, as well as hemorrhages in the retina in the region of the disk, may be observed.

Treatment

This consists of correcting the factor causing increased intracranial pressure, if possible, or a palliative cerebral decompression operation. There is no local treatment.

OPTIC NEURITIS

An inflammation of the optic nerve restricted by definition to that portion of the nerve which is visible with the ophthalmoscope. Perhaps the most frequent cause is secondary syphilis. The neuritis also occurs with meningitis, encephalitis, acute febrile diseases, foci of infection, multiple sclerosis, and poisoning by methyl alcohol, carbon tetrachloride, lead, and thallium. It is almost always unilateral. The only symptom is a disturbance of vision varying from minimal contraction of the visual field with enlargement of the blind spot to complete blindness. The maximum reduction of vision frequently is reached within 1 or 2 days. In the early stages, ophthalmoscopic examination reveals hyperemia and minimal edema of the disk. In advanced cases the disk is more edematous, and appears whitish with a red center. The retina becomes edematous and its vessels engorged; exudates and hemorrhages may be present. The disease usually lasts for many months. Spontaneous remission or successful removal of etiologic factors early in its course usually results in more or less complete restoration of vision. The majority of cases, however, eventually go on to postneuritic optic atrophy (q.v.), with considerable to complete loss of vision.

Treatment

Removal of the underlying etiologic factor, if possible, is essential. Use of cortisone or ACTH has produced highly encouraging results. Typhoid vaccine I.V. (℞ 65) or other hyperthermic measures may be useful in cases due to multiple sclerosis or to undetermined causes. Large doses of thiamine (℞ 78) are worthy of trial.

RETROBULBAR NEURITIS

An inflammation of the orbital portion of the optic nerve, usually unilateral. Multiple sclerosis is responsible for a little more than half the cases. The remainder are due to the same factors that cause optic neuritis (q.v.). The clinical picture is marked by rapid loss of central vision often accompanied by pain in the orbit aggravated by movements of the globe. The fundus usually appears normal except for some hyperemia of the disk later in the course of the disease. Spontaneous remission often occurs in 2 to 8 weeks, with restoration of normal vision. In some cases a central scotoma may remain and pallor of the temporal portion of the disk may be evident. Frequent relapses are not uncommon, especially when the neuritis is due to multiple sclerosis. Each relapse leaves increased residual visual damage and temporal pallor. Optic atrophy (q.v.) and permanent total blindness may result.

Treatment

This is essentially the same as that of optic neuritis (q.v.).

15

OPTIC ATROPHY

Atrophy of the second cranial nerve, commonly divided into simple or primary atrophy and secondary or postneuritic atrophy. **Simple optic atrophy** results from a degeneration of the nerve fibers following retrobulbar neuritis (q.v.), most often due to syphilis, central retinal artery occlusion, glaucoma (q.v.), or any condition or drug (Tryparsamide) causing injury to the optic nerve along its intracanalicular or intracranial course. In **secondary optic atrophy,** degeneration of the nerve fibers is accompanied by scar formation upon the nerve head and follows optic neuritis and severe and prolonged papilledema (q.v.).

The amount of vision lost is directly proportional to the degree of nerve atrophy. Total blindness and a dilated and fixed pupil are the end results. Ophthalmoscopic examination of a simple optic atrophy reveals a white or grayish disk with sharp edges and a saucer-shaped excavation. The lamina cribrosa often is clearly visible. The retina usually is normal. The disk in secondary optic atrophy is dense white, its margins are irregular and indistinct, and it is covered by connective tissue which conceals the lamina cribrosa. Evidence of previous inflammation may be seen in the retina.

Treatment

Once the optic nerve has atrophied, nothing can be done to restore vision. Therapy, to be of any value, must be directed at the underlying factors causing damage to the nerve.

TOXIC AMBLYOPIA

A reduction in the acuteness of vision believed to be due to a toxic reaction in the orbital portion of the optic nerve. It usually is bilateral, and most often is caused by overindulgence in alcohol and tobacco. Prolonged exposure to carbon monoxide, carbon tetrachloride, arsenic, lead, and benzol are at times responsible. The condition begins as a small central scotoma which slowly enlarges and progressively interferes with vision. The visual disturbances are more pronounced in bright light. The peripheral fields usually are intact. In extreme cases, the scotoma may become absolute and result in complete blindness. Ophthalmoscopic examination commonly reveals no abnormalities. Pallor of the temporal side of the disk may develop late.

Treatment

Upon removal of the cause gradual improvement with restoration of normal vision usually takes place, although in extremely severe cases some residual impairment may remain. Thiamine (R 78) in high doses may hasten recovery.

HIGHER VISUAL PATHWAY LESIONS

Characteristic changes in the visual fields are noted, depending upon which portions of the optic pathways are damaged.

Lesions of the optic nerve will result in visual disturbances restricted to the eye innervated by the damaged nerve. Lesions in the region of the chiasm usually affect vision in both eyes. Pathologic changes in the central region of the chiasm, such as a pituitary tumor, will result in destruction of nerve fibers supplying the inner or nasal half of both retinas and consequently cause defects in the temporal visual fields. This is called a bitemporal hemianopsia. Lesions in the lateral portions of the chiasm, such as aneurysms of the internal carotid arteries, may destroy the nerve fibers supplying the outer or temporal side of the retina and cause defects in the nasal visual fields. This is called a binasal hemianopsia. A homonymous hemianopsia results from a lesion situated in the optic tract or cerebral cortex and is marked by loss of function of the right or left halves of both retinas corresponding to the optic tract affected. This, the most common type of hemianopsia, may be caused by brain tumor or cerebral hemorrhage (q.v.).

Treatment

The treatment is that of the primary lesion. There is no local treatment. When a diagnosis of hemianopsia is made, the above mentioned lesions should be looked for and corrected, if possible.

STRABISMUS

(Squint)

Inability of an eye to attain the normal convergence required for fixation of a near object; or the deviation of one eye from parallelism with its fellow. A **paralytic strabismus** results from paralysis of one or more of the ocular muscles and is characterized by limitation of the eye movements that are dependent upon the particular muscles involved. Diplopia becomes aggravated when the eye attempts a movement which it cannot perform because of paralysis of a particular muscle. In **nonparalytic** (concomitant) **strabismus** seen in childhood, the deviation from parallelism does not vary with ocular movements, and the power of individual muscles is intact. Usually no diplopia is encountered. A concomitant strabismus may be convergent, divergent, or vertical. Disuse of an eye, as in cases of severe refractive error or impaired vision due to disease, often results in a nonaccommodative strabismus in which the blind eye is rotated outward. **Latent strabismus** is a concomitant type in which the muscle imbalance is overcome by the fusion faculty, and is obvious only when fusion is suppressed artificially. Latent strabismus may result in blurring of vision, headache, and diplopia, especially after prolonged use of the eyes for close work.

Treatment

Strabismus should be treated only by a skilled oculist. Corrective glasses, orthoptic training, and surgical restoration of muscle balance are the methods used.

NYSTAGMUS

A rhythmic horizontal or vertical oscillation of the eyeballs, usually affecting both eyes, and generally becoming more pronounced when the eyes are turned in certain directions. Congenital nystagmus is the most common type and frequently is secondary to poor vision resulting from congenital abnormalities. Nystagmus developing in later life often is a sign of cerebellar, vestibular, or labyrinthine disease (q.v.). It is one of the cardinal signs of multiple sclerosis (q.v.). Prolonged use of the eyes with defective illumination and strained position, as in miners, and fatigue of the eye muscles, especially when due to errors of refraction, also may be causative. Vestibular stimulation, as in the Kobrak test (*see* VERTIGO), causes nystagmus.

Treatment

Correction of errors of refraction and other causes of eye strain will relieve the simple forms of nystagmus. Nystagmus due to labyrinthine, cerebellar, or vestibular disease usually ceases upon removal of these etiologic factors.

ERRORS OF REFRACTION

Emmetropia (normal refraction) exists when parallel light rays are focused clearly on the retina. **Ametropia** (abnormal refraction) may be of several varieties. **Hyperopia** (far-sightedness) is the most frequent form. The image is focused behind the retina, either because the eyeball axis is too short or because the refractive power of the eye is too weak. In **myopia** (nearsightedness), the image is focused in front of the retina because the axis of the eyeball is too long or the refractive power of the lens too strong. **Astigmatism** is a complex form of ametropia in which a difference in degree of refraction exists in several meridians of the eyeball. **Presbyopia** is the result of a physiologic change in the lens, which often develops with old age. This renders the lens less responsive to the process of accommodation. The presbyopic individual is unable to focus for near vision.

Treatment

Corrective therapy, by a skilled ophthalmologist, consists of the prescribing of suitable lenses to compensate for the refractive errors found.

PRESCRIPTIONS

(Wherever a prescribed "proprietary" is representative of a class of therapeutic agents, alternative proprietary preparations will be found listed in Part II.)

Staining Agent

1. ℞ Fluorescein sodium . . . . .   0.2   Gm. (gr. iii)
   Sodium bicarbonate . . . . .   0.3   Gm. (gr. v)
   Water . . . . .q.s. ad 10.0   cc. (℥ iiss)
   > Instill 1 drop in the eye and wash out the excess with normal saline.

Mydriatics

2. ℞ Ephedrine sulfate, 3% solution   8.0   cc. (℥ ii)
   > Instill 1 drop into eye for dilatation.

3. ℞ Epinephrine hydrochloride,
   1:1,000 solution . . . . . .   8.0   cc. (℥ ii)
   > 1 drop into eye 3 to 4 times daily as necessary.

4. ℞ Homatropine hydrobromide, 1%
   solution . . . .   8.0   cc. (℥ ii)
   > Instill 1 or 2 drops into the eye for dilatation.

5. ℞ Atropine sulfate, 1% solution .   8.0   cc. (℥ ii)
   > Instill 1 to 3 drops into conjunctival sac, depending on weight of patient, for dilatation of pupil.

6. ℞ Atropine sulfate, 1% ophthalmic
   ointment . . . .   4.0   Gm. (℥ i)
   > Apply inside lower lid 3 times daily as long as necessary for dilatation.

7. ℞ Eucatropine hydrochloride
   ("Euphthalmine"), 5% solution . . . .   8.0   cc. (℥ ii)
   > Instill 1 drop into eye for mydriatic effect.

Miotics

8. ℞ Physostigmine (Eserine) salicylate, 0.25% solution . . . .   8.0   cc. (℥ ii)
   > 1 drop in eye to facilitate recovery from mydriatic action of homatropine, or as often as necessary to maintain miosis.

9. ℞ Physostigmine (Eserine) salicylate, 1 to 2% solution . . . 8.0 cc. (ℨ ii)

Instill 1 drop into eye every 10 to 15 minutes
for 1 or 2 hours and then every half hour
until miosis occurs in acute glaucoma.

10. ℞ Pilocarpine nitrate, 1% solution 8.0 cc. (ℨ ii)

1 drop in eye to facilitate recovery from mydriatic action of ephedrine; or as often as necessary to maintain miosis.

11. ℞ Pilocarpine nitrate, 2% solution 8.0 cc. (ℨ ii)

Instill 1 drop into eye every 10 to 15 minutes
for 1 or 2 hours and then every half hour
until miosis occurs.

12. ℞ "Floropryl" (Di-isopropyl
fluorophosphate), 0.1% in pea-
nut oil . . . . 10.0 cc. (ℨ iiss)

1 or 2 drops daily in eye.

13. ℞ "Carcholin" (Carbamylcholine
chloride), 1.5% solution . . 8.0 cc. (ℨ ii)

Instill 1 drop into eye as often as necessary to
maintain miosis.

14. ℞ Neostigmine bromide, 5% solution . . . . 8.0 cc. (ℨ ii)

Instill into eye as often as necessary to maintain miosis.

Local Anesthetics

15. ℞ Tetracaine hydrochloride ("Pontocaine"), 0.5% solution . . 8.0 cc. (ℨ ii)

Instill 2 or 3 drops into conjunctival sac for
local anesthesia as often as necessary.

16. ℞ Phenacaine hydrochloride
("Holocaine") . . . . . 0.04 Gm. (gr. ⅔)
Epinephrine hydrochloride,
1:1,000 solution . . . 0.16 cc. (♏ iiss)
Ophthalmic ointment base . .
q.s. ad 4.0 Gm. (ℨ i)

Apply inside lower lid for local anesthesia.

17. ℞ Phenacaine hydrochloride
("Holocaine") . . . . . 0.1 Gm. (gr. iss)
Epinephrine hydrochloride,
1:1,000 solution . . . . 0.6 cc. (♏ x)
Boric acid . . . . 0.3 Gm. (gr. v)
Water . . . . q.s. ad 30.0 cc. (ℨ i)

1 drop into eye to relieve itching.

18. ℞ Cocaine hydrochloride, 4% solution . . . . 8.0   cc.   (℥ ii)

    1 drop in eye every 2 or 3 hours as necessary
    for pain.

Antiseptics, Caustics, and Collyria

19. ℞ Sodium bicarbonate, 3% solu-
tion . . . . .500.0   cc.   (℥ xvi)

    Irrigate conjunctival sac freely for burns due
    to acids.

20. ℞ Acetic acid, 2% solution . . 1,000.0   cc.   (℥ xxxii)

    Irrigate conjunctival sac freely for burns due
    to alkalies.

21. ℞ Boric acid, saturated solution 1,000.0   cc.   (℥ xxxii)

    Use freely as mild antiseptic eyewash.

22. ℞ Boric acid, 5% ointment . . . 30.0   Gm. (℥ i)

    Apply to burned areas of lids.

23. ℞ Zinc sulfate. . . . . 0.06   Gm. (gr. i)
Epinephrine hydrochloride,
   1:1,000 solution . . . . . 4.0   cc.   (℥ i)
Boric acid, 2% solution q.s. ad 30.0   cc.   (℥ i)

    Instill 2 or 3 drops in affected eye several
    times daily.

24. ℞ Boric acid . . . . 1.3   Gm. (gr. xx)
Sodium chloride . . . . . . 1.3   Gm. (gr. xx)
Camphor Water U.S.P.
Water . . . . . .āā q.s. ad 120.0   cc.   (℥ iv)

    Use warm in eyecup 3 times daily.

25. ℞ Sodium chloride . . . . . . 2.0   Gm. (℥ ss)
Sodium bicarbonate . . . . 1.8   Gm. (gr. xxvii)
Sodium borate . . . . . . 1.5   Gm. (gr. xxiii)
Camphor Water U.S.P. . . . 30.0   cc.   (℥ i)
Rose Water U.S.P. . q.s. ad 240.0   cc.   (℥ viii)

    Dilute with equal parts of water and use in
    eyecup 3 times daily.

26. ℞ Methylene blue . . . . . . 0.002 Gm. (gr. 1/30)
Epinephrine hydrochloride,
   1:1,000 solution . . . . . 1.0   cc.   (♏ xv)
Phenacaine hydrochloride
   ("Holocaine") . . . . . 0.02   Gm. (gr. 1/3)
Distilled water . . . .q.s. ad 8.0   cc.   (℥ ii)

    Instill 1 drop in affected eye 4 times daily.

27. ℞ "Metaphen" 1:3,000 ophthalmic
ointment . . . . 4.0   Gm. (℥ i)

    Apply inside lower lid of affected eye 3 or 4
    times daily as necessary.

28. ℞ Cod Liver Oil U.S.P. . . . . . 2.8   Gm. (gr. xlii)
    "Metaphen," 1:3,000 ophthalmic
    ointment . . . . . q.s. ad 4.0   Gm. (℥ i)
    Apply inside lower lid 3 or 4 times daily as
    necessary.

29. ℞ Butacaine sulfate . . . . 0.08 Gm. (gr. iss)
    "Metaphen," 1:3,000 ophthalmic
    ointment . . . . . . q.s. ad 4.0   Gm. (℥ i)
    Apply inside lower lid 3 or 4 times daily as
    necessary.

30. ℞ "Butesin Picrate" . . . . . . 0.04 Gm. (gr. ⅔)
    "Butesin" . . . . 0.04 Gm. (gr. ⅔)
    Ophthalmic ointment base q.s. ad 4.0 Gm. (℥ i)
    Apply inside lower lid 3 or 4 times daily as
    necessary.

31. ℞ Salicylic acid. . . . . 0.15 Gm. (gr. iiss)
    Sulfur, precipitated . . . . . 0.09 Gm. (gr. iss)
    Ophthalmic ointment base q.s. ad 30.0 Gm. (℥ i)
    Massage into eyelids every other night for
    two weeks.

32. ℞ Yellow mercuric oxide, 1 to 2%
    ophthalmic ointment . . . 4.0   Gm. (℥ i)
    Apply inside lower lid of affected eye.

33. ℞ Benzalkonium chloride 1:2,000
    solution . . . . 30.0 cc. (℥ i)
    1 drop in affected eye several times daily.

34. ℞ "Metaphen," 1:3,000 solution. 30.0 cc. (℥ i)
    1 drop in affected eye several times daily.

35. ℞ "Dionin" (Ethylmorphine hydro-
    chloride), 1% solution . . . 8.0   cc. (℥ ii)
    Instill 1 or 2 drops into conjunctival sac once
    daily.

36. ℞ Brilliant green . . . . . . 0.75 Gm. (gr. xii)
    Ethyl alcohol 70% . . q.s. ad 15.0 cc. (℥ ss)
    Apply to lid margins every other day until
    relieved of all crusting.

37. ℞ Silver nitrate, 0.5% solution . 30.0 cc. (℥ i)
    Gently swab on lid margins once daily.

38. ℞ Silver nitrate, 1% solution . . 30.0 cc. (℥ i)
    Instill 2 drops in each conjunctival sac of
    newborn and wash out the excess with normal
    saline solution.

39. ℞ Silver nitrate, 3% solution . . . 8.0 cc. (℥ ii)

   Touch base of corneal ulcer with small amount on cotton point. Irrigate eye immediately after application with normal saline.

40. ℞ Mercuric chloride, 1:500 solution . . . . 8.0 cc. (℥ ii)

   Apply with cotton applicator to everted lids once daily.

41. ℞ Mild silver protein, 10% solution . . . . 30.0 cc. (℥ i)

   1 to 3 drops in affected eye several times daily.

42. ℞ Strong Iodine Solution (Lugol's
          Solution) U.S.P. . . . . . 0.12 cc. (℥ ii)
       Potassium iodide . . . . . . 0.6 Gm. (gr. x)
       Water . . . . q.s. ad 30.0 cc. (℥ i)

   Instill 2 or 3 drops into eye 3 or 4 times daily as necessary.

43. ℞ Iodine Tincture U.S.P. . . . 0.3 cc. (℥ v)
       Glycerin . . . . 0.3 cc. (℥ v)
       Saturated Potassium Iodide
          Solution N.F. . . . . . . 0.6 cc. (℥ x)
       Iodine crystals . . . . . . 0.6 Gm. (gr. x)

   Apply on fine cotton point to ulcer.

44. ℞ "Phemerol Chloride," 1:5,000
          solution . . . . 8.0 cc. (℥ ii)

   2 or 3 drops in affected eye several times daily.

45. ℞ Copper sulfate (crystal)

   Rub crystal over inner surface of everted lid once daily.

46. ℞ Copper citrate, 5% ophthalmic
          ointment . . . . 4.0 Gm. (℥ i)

   Apply inside lower lid twice daily.

47. ℞ "Optochin Hydrochloride" . . 1.0 Gm. (gr. xv)

   Dust a small amount of the powder into the ulcer bed and wash off with normal saline after 30 seconds.

48. ℞ Calomel . . . . 30.0 Gm. (℥ i)

   Dust small amount into conjunctival sac once a day.

Hypertonic Solution

49. ℞ Glucose, 50% solution (ampul)

   Inject 100 cc. (℥ iiiss) I.V. over a 5-minute period.

Antimicrobial Agents

50. ℞ Procaine penicillin   (vial)

   300,000 u. I.M. every 12 to 24 hours for as
   long as necessary.

51. ℞ Penicillin   (vial)

   50,000 u. I.M. every 3 hours or 300,000 u.
   I.M. every 12 hours for as long as necessary.

52. ℞ Sulfadiazine . . . .   0.5   Gm. (gr. viiss)

   4 tablets as first dose, then 2 tablets every 4
   hours for as long as necessary.

53. ℞ Sodium sulfacetimide, 10%
   ophthalmic ointment . . .   4.0   Gm. (ℨ i)

   Apply inside lower lid of affected eye.

54. ℞ Sulfadiazine, 5% ophthalmic
   ointment . . . .   4.0   Gm. (ℨ i)

   Apply inside lower lid of affected eye.   (*Note:*
   if sulfadiazine is not available 5% sulfathiazole may be used.)

55. ℞ Sodium sulfacetimide, 30% solution . . . .   8.0   cc.   (ℨ ii)

   1 drop in conjunctival sac 4 times daily.

56. ℞ Sodium sulfadiazine, 5% solution . . . .   8.0   cc.   (ℨ ii)

   1 drop in conjunctival sac 4 times daily.

57. ℞ Penicillin, ophthalmic ointment
   (2,000 u./Gm.) . . . . .   4.0   Gm. (ℨ i)

   Apply inside lower lid of affected eye.

58. ℞ Penicillin solution (500 u./cc.).   8.0   cc.   (ℨ ii)

   2 drops in affected eye every 1 or 2 hours.

59. ℞ Aureomycin, ophthalmic solution
   (5 mg./cc.) . . . .   5.0   cc.

   2 drops in affected eye every 1 or 2 hours.

60. ℞ Streptomycin   (vial)

   0.25 Gm. I.M. every 6 hours.

61. ℞ Tyrothricin solution (300 micro-
   grams/cc.) . . . .   8.0   cc.   (ℨ ii)

   Instill 1 drop in eye every 1 to 3 hours as
   necessary.

Biologicals

62. ℞ Staphylococcus toxoid

   Administer according to instructions accompanying preparation.

63. ℞ Staphylococcus vaccine

    Administer according to instructions accompanying preparation.

64. ℞ Autogenous vaccine

    To be prepared from organisms present in infected area, and administered as required.

65. ℞ Typhoid vaccine (vial containing 100 million organisms/cc.)

    0.15 cc. as the initial dose I.V., followed by 1 dose every other day for a total of 5 injections increasing the dosage each time by 0.1 cc.

Analgesics

66. ℞ "Demerol Hydrochloride" (ampul)

    50 to 100 mg. I.M. every 6 hours as necessary.

67. ℞ Morphine sulfate

    8 to 15 mg. (gr. ⅛ to ¼) subcut. every 6 hours as necessary.

68. ℞ Codeine sulfate . . . . 0.03 Gm. (gr. ss)
    Acetylsalicylic acid . . . . . 0.6 Gm. (gr. x)

    1 capsule every 4 hours as necessary.

69. ℞ Sodium salicylate . . . . . 0.3 Gm. (gr. v)

    Give 1 grain/lb./day orally in divided doses.

Antispasmodics

70. ℞ Amyl nitrite (ampul) . . . . 0.3 cc. (♏ v)

    Crush ampul in handkerchief and inhale contents.

71. ℞ Nitroglycerin (hypodermic tablet) . . . . 0.3 mg. (gr. 1/200)

    1 or 2 tablets sublingually or subcut. Repeat in 30 minutes if necessary.

72. ℞ Sodium nitrite . . . . 60 mg. (gr. i)

    1 tablet 3 or 4 times daily.

73. ℞ Acetylcholine chloride (ampul) 0.1 Gm. (gr. iss)

    Contents of 1 ampul subcut. Repeat in 1 hour if necessary.

74. ℞ Papaverine hydrochloride (ampul) . . . . 60 mg. (gr. i)

    Contents of 1 ampul subcut. or I.V. Repeat in 1 hour if necessary.

Anticoagulants

75. ℞ Heparin (vial)

> 50 to 100 mg. I.V. twice daily. The total daily dosage should not exceed that required to raise the blood clotting time above 20 minutes (*see* ANTICOAGULANT THERAPY). To be given for 2 days only in conjunction with dicumarol (℞ 76).

76. ℞ Dicumarol 50   mg.

> Give 4 to 6 capsules the first day and then 2 to 4 capsules daily as long as prothrombin activity exceeds 25% of normal (*see* ANTICOAGULANT THERAPY).

Vitamins

77. ℞ Vitamin A 25,000   u.

> 1 capsule daily.

78. ℞ Thiamine hydrochloride . . . 10   mg.

> 2 tablets 3 times daily.

79. ℞ Ascorbic acid . . . . 0.1   Gm.

> 1 tablet 3 times daily.

80. ℞ Riboflavin 5   mg.

> 2 tablets daily.

81. ℞ Rutin 20   mg.

> 2 to 4 tablets 3 times daily.

82. ℞ Menadione 1   mg.

> 2 to 5 tablets or capsules daily.

GASTROINTESTINAL

DYSPHAGIA

Difficulty in swallowing, from any cause. Since the act of swallowing is a complex neuromuscular mechanism, the causes of this symptom are many. Dysphagia also includes those severe cases in which there is resultant regurgitation of food through the nose or mouth. Possible causes of dysphagia are listed below.

Congenital defects: These include cleft palate, atresia or narrowing of the esophagus, tracheoesophageal fistula, congenital esophageal diverticula.

Esophageal obstruction: This may result from fibrosis after swallowing corrosive chemicals, foreign bodies (bone, teeth), pressure from adjacent masses (tumor, thyroid enlargement, aortic aneurysm), dysphagia lusoria, acquired (traction) esophageal diverticula, esophageal varices, diaphragmatic (hiatus) hernia.

Neurogenic disturbances: In this group are poliomyelitis, postdiphtheritic paralysis, bulbar paralysis, pseudobulbar paralysis (bilateral paralysis of 9th to 11th cranial nerves), syphilis of the medullary area, lead or sodium fluoride poisoning, alcoholism, hysteria, encephalitis, cerebral vascular accidents.

Muscular dysfunction: This type of dysphagia may be caused by spasm (e.g., due to rabies, hysteria, tetanus, or cardiospasm), or myasthenia (e.g., myasthenia gravis).

Local irritation: The presence of esophagitis, pharyngitis, tonsillitis, laryngitis, glossitis, stomatitis, Ludwig's angina, mumps, regional abscesses, angioneurotic edema, or esophageal ulcer gives rise to dysphagia of varying degree.

Most of the above conditions are described elsewhere in the MANUAL and the reader is referred to appropriate chapters for details of diagnosis and treatment. When indicated, esophagoscopy and esophageal X-ray studies are especially useful in diagnosis.

ABDOMINAL PAIN

Pain in the abdomen is a symptom of many diseases, either intra-abdominal or extra-abdominal. It may be somatic or visceral in origin. Somatic abdominal pain is due to stimulation of the sensitive parietal peritoneum and therefore is well defined and well localized. Visceral pain is poorly localized and may be true pain (originating in the affected viscus) or referred (originating elsewhere in the body).

Etiology

Abdominal pain may arise from a multitude of disorders including the following:

I. Intra-abdominal Disorders

1. Gastrointestinal: Appendicitis, gastroenteritis, peptic ulcer, dysenteries, colitis, hernia (including internal hernias), constipation, intestinal obstruction (due to tumor, fecal impaction, hernia, volvulus, foreign body), intussusception, tumors, regional ileitis, diverticulitis, intestinal parasites, allergy, pylorospasm, perforation (by trauma, ulcer, or foreign body), congenital defects (e.g., bands, atresia, pyloric stenosis); and hunger, overfeeding, and accumulations of gas (particularly in infants).

2. Genitourinary: Renal colic (due to calculi, tumor, Dietl's crisis, aberrant renal vessel), urinary tract infection, tumors, renal carbuncle, foreign bodies, congenital anomalies (including patent urachus). Male: Prostatitis, epididymitis, torsion of undescended testicle. Female: Pregnancy and its complications (e.g., abortion, ectopic gestation, abruptio placenta; ruptured uterus; labor pains), pelvic inflammatory disease (including cervicitis and salpingitis), dysmenorrhea, ovulatory bleeding, torsion of a prolapsed ovary or of an ovarian cyst.

3. Hepatobiliary: Cholecystitis, biliary colic, hepatitis, liver abscess (secondary to amebiasis, pylephlebitis, or echinococciasis), cirrhosis, hepatomegaly, subdiaphragmatic abscess.

4. Pancreatic: Pancreatitis, islet cell tumor (hypoglycemia), carcinomas (particularly those obstructing the common bile duct).

5. Peritoneal: Peritonitis, either tuberculous or pneumococcal, or secondary to abdominal infections.

6. Vascular: Mesenteric thrombosis or embolism, splenic infarct, thrombophlebitis, abdominal or dissecting aneurysm.

7. Other: Mesenteric lymphadenitis, mesenteric cyst, torsion of omentum, lymphomas, splenomegaly.

II. Extra-abdominal Disorders

1. Cardiorespiratory: Pericarditis, coronary insufficiency, pneumonia, pleurisy, upper respiratory infections, esophageal disease (e.g., cardiospasm, ulcer, malignancy).

2. Neurologic and neuropsychiatric: Neuritis (including herpes zoster), radiculitis, tabetic (gastric) crisis, withdrawal symptoms of drug addiction, hysteria, decompression illness (caisson disease).

3. Hemic or metabolic: Hypoglycemia, acidosis, Schönlein's purpura, crises of hemolytic icterus or of sickle cell anemia.

4. Other: Acute systemic infections, spinal arthritis, metallic poisoning (e.g., due to lead, arsenic, gold, mercury).

Diagnosis

Differential diagnosis of abdominal pain depends upon a careful history, complete physical examination (preferably during an attack), and appropriate laboratory tests. The patient's description of the pain is most important. The physician should determine its duration and such characteristics as its onset, location, radiation, frequency, nature, and severity. Factors that aggravate or relieve the discomfort (e.g., effort, position, food, medication, menses) should be noted. Evidence of tenderness, spasm, distention, masses, or extra-abdominal disease must be sought. A rectal or pelvic examination is usually required. X-ray, blood and urinary studies are useful and, when indicated, additional laboratory tests should be performed.

A detailed or comprehensive discussion of the differential diagnosis of abdominal pain is not within the scope of this chapter. Further information on certain of the etiologic factors (see Etiology) and their treatment may be found elsewhere in the MANUAL; for others the reader is referred to standard textbooks. However, brief summarizations of some of the more common conditions that cause abdominal pain are given below.

Acute appendicitis: There usually is mild to severe abdominal pain and cramp, periumbilical or generalized at first, and then localizing in the right lower quadrant. Tenderness over the appendix is present. Later, the pain becomes more constant but less intense. A sudden cessation of pain may indicate perforation. Appendicitis may be simulated, especially by regional ileitis, colitis, Meckel's diverticulitis, salpingitis, and mesenteric lymphadenitis.

Peptic ulcer: Pain may be absent or present as a recurrent epigastric burning or pain to the right (duodenal ulcer) or to the left (gastric ulcer) of the midline, which ordinarily occurs 1 to 2 hours after eating. The pain may "bore" into the back if the ulcer is on the posterior wall and is penetrating. It is relieved by food and alkali. A complicating hemorrhage may produce intestinal cramps or be painless, whereas perforation causes acute, agonizing epigastric pain, muscle spasm, and often shock.

A change in the symptoms of a gastric ulcer should always suggest gastric malignancy. In the absence of an ulcer, gastric carcinoma usually is painless until the disease is far advanced.

Acute intestinal obstruction: Rapidly increasing, severe, colicky pain with complete relief between paroxysms is usual. Vomiting and distention are conspicuous. Obstipation is usual but small loose bowel evacuations may occasionally occur. The interval between paroxysms gradually decreases until the pain is constant but less severe. The pain is not relieved by vomiting and is usually aggravated by food or a laxative. If intestinal gangrene also is present, there is exquisite local tenderness and shock may rapidly ensue.

Mesenteric occlusion: Thrombosis or embolism of the mesenteric vessels causes sudden severe midabdominal or generalized abdominal pain which does not radiate. Vomiting is common but does not alleviate the pain. Blood in the stool is usual. The presence or history of auricular fibrillation, arteriosclerosis, or periarteritis nodosa assists in making the diagnosis.

Biliary disease: Gallbladder disease produces a sensation of epigastric fullness, which is most apt to occur after a heavy meal and is commonly relieved by belching or vomiting. If significant pain is present, it is maximal in the right upper quadrant, often radiating to the right scapula or shoulder. Obstruction of the cystic or common duct by a gallstone gives rise to sudden, severe, colicky pain which is felt most in the region of the gallbladder and persists for several hours, unless relieved by strong analgesics and antispasmodics. Tenderness and spasm usually are present in the gallbladder region.

Pancreatitis: Acute pancreatitis is characterized by sudden, agonizing, knifelike pain in the epigastrium which radiates into the back. Tenderness, muscle spasm, prostration, and shock are striking. A history of biliary tract disease is frequently elicited. Chronic pancreatitis has a history of one or more acute attacks or of cholecystitis. There is mild epigastric tenderness and pain.

Renal colic: Ureteral obstruction is ushered in by a sudden severe pain in the loin radiating along the involved ureter to the genitalia or inner thigh. Restlessness is prominent, the patient assuming bizarre positions in an effort to find relief. Nausea and vomiting, hematuria, frequency, lumbar tenderness and shock may be present. Symptoms and signs of urinary infection may occur concomitantly.

Tubal pregnancy: Pain is rare before rupture, at which time there is sharp, severe pain on the involved side. Shock and vaginal bleeding are common, and a history of a missed period is usual. Pelvic examination may reveal tender adnexa and a pelvic hematoma as a fluctuant mass in the cul-de-sac; manipulation of the cervix frequently is painful.

Acute salpingitis: There is pain in both lower quadrants, usually more severe on one side. A history of vaginal discharge or previous painful episodes is not unusual. Pelvic examination reveals tender adnexa, palpable tubes and a cervical discharge.

Twisted ovarian cyst: Torsion produces sudden severe pain in the lower abdomen and is frequently initiated by physical exertion. Pelvic examination reveals a definite, tender, cystic mass on the involved side.

Ovulation or mittelschmerz: The escape of blood into the peritoneal cavity as a result of ovulation may produce lower abdominal pain. The diagnosis is suggested by absence of pelvic findings and the expected onset of the next menses about 14 days later.

Heavy metal poisoning: Lead poisoning may produce intense abdominal colic which is relieved by pressure and usually is felt below the umbilicus. The colic is generally preceded by a long period of constipation. A history of exposure to lead, with facial pallor, the lead line, and basophilic stippling of the red cells should give the diagnosis.

Toxic reactions to therapy with arsenic, mercury, and gold salts also may be responsible for abdominal pain. The suicidal, homicidal and accidental use of arsenic and mercury compounds also must not be overlooked in obscure cases.

Thoracic disease: Coronary thrombosis, pericarditis, pneumonia, and pleurisy can cause epigastric pain and must always be considered in the differential diagnosis of abdominal pain. Failure to do so may lead to erroneous diagnoses and unnecessary surgery.

Neurologic disease: Neuritis, radiculitis, or herpes zoster of the lower thoracic nerves may produce pain over involved somatic segments. The severe abdominal pains (gastric crises) of tabes dorsalis or of decompression sickness (caisson disease, "the bends") may simulate an acute abdominal condition, and these disorders should be considered with cases of obscure etiology.

DYSPEPSIA

("Indigestion")

A symptom complex including nausea, heartburn, upper abdominal pain, flatulence and eructation, a sense of fullness and a feeling of abdominal distention, occurring during or after the ingestion of food.

Etiology

Indigestion may be caused by organic disease in the gastro-intestinal tract and by many diseases originating elsewhere in the body. Consideration will be given here mainly to the symptoms that occur in the absence of demonstrable organic disease.

Common causes of indigestion are eating too much or too rapidly, inadequate mastication (frequently due to poor dentition), eating during emotional upsets or severe mental strain, and swallowing large amounts of air. Other factors are excessive smoking, constipation, ingestion of poorly cooked foods, foods with high fat content, and certain kinds of food, such as cucumbers, radishes, and gas-forming vegetables (e.g., beans, cabbage, turnips, onions).

Most of the symptoms of indigestion result from altered gastric motor activity. Fats inhibit such activity, decrease the peristaltic waves, lower gastric tone, and prolong gastric emptying time. Moderate distention of the stomach stimulates motility, while marked distention, such as occurs from overeating, inhibits motility and may produce a sensation of epigastric distention and fullness, and nausea. Nervousness and anxiety tend to increase peristalsis, while fear, shock and depression tend to inhibit it and reduce gastric tone. Pain and physical fatigue also inhibit peristalsis. Drinking alcohol and coffee increases peristaltic activity, while smoking decreases it and tends to delay gastric emptying. Swallowed air in large amounts distends the fundus and gives rise to a feeling of epigastric fullness, distention, or pressure and the desire to obtain relief by belching. Spasm of the pylorus or antrum in a tense individual, when present prior to or during a meal, may be responsible for similar sensations. Constipation tends to produce symptoms by interfering with the normal passage of gas and feces toward the rectum.

Symptoms and Signs

Nausea may be produced by any condition that increases the tension upon the walls of the stomach, duodenum, or lower end of the esophagus. It may follow exposure to unpleasant odors, distention of the stomach or lower esophagus, or functional impairment of the normal forward propulsive movement of duodenal content. Nausea may be accompanied by a feeling of faintness, weakness, vertigo, headache, and sweating.

Heartburn is a popular term used to describe a sensation of burning in the epigastrium, a common complaint in chronic gastritis. It may result from the distention of any part of the esophagus, especially the lower, as by the sudden introduction of a large amount of fluid. It also can be caused by retention of regurgitated food and gastric content in the lower esophagus. It is not due, as was formerly believed, to excessive gastric acidity, as the same symptom often occurs in achlorhydria.

Flatulence is an excessive accumulation of gas in the stomach or intestine. There are two types of flatulence, gastric and intestinal. The accumulated gas in the stomach may be expelled by belching, while intestinal flatulence is relieved by the passage of flatus. In nervous individuals or those who gulp food and drink, an excessive amount of air is carried down into the stomach. In many neurotic patients "aerophagia," or the swallowing of air is quite common. Drinking large quantities of carbonated beverages is another way in which gas may enter the stomach. The accumulated gas produces a sensation of pressure, fullness, or distention in the epigastrium or precordial region. The patient tries to relieve the discomfort by belching, during which additional air may be swallowed, particularly if the mouth is kept closed. Successful expulsion of gas affords temporary relief. Extreme aerophagia may produce abdominal distention, a sensation of smothering, palpitation, dyspnea, cardiac pain, and even a fear of impending death. Similar complaints of gastric fullness and abdominal distention can arise from intestinal flatulence. The gas in this case is formed by fermentation or putrefaction of ingested material. It often is associated with abdominal cramps, and relief is afforded by the passage of flatus rather than by belching. Attempts at belching, however, are not uncommon in patients with intestinal flatulence and frequently the aerophagia so induced increases their discomfort.

A sensation of fullness or pressure in the epigastrium may be caused by overeating, swallowing of air, bolting of food, and eating when fatigued or emotionally upset.

Diagnosis

In all cases of indigestion, careful history, physical examination, and laboratory procedures are necessary to exclude organic disease before concluding that the indigestion is due only to functional disturbances. The clinical significance of nausea is closely linked to that of vomiting. In the absence of vomiting, nausea is a frequent symptom of nonhemolytic jaundice, chronic gastritis, gastric carcinoma and the early stages of cardiac failure, chronic renal disease, and pulmonary tuberculosis; nausea occurring after a headache may be due to migraine or a refractive error of the eyes. Nausea associated with pronounced vertigo suggests labyrinthine disease. Morning nausea is suggestive of pregnancy, gastritis, or chronic toxemias, especially chronic renal disease. When heartburn is present, lesions in the lower esophagus must be excluded. It is common with uncomplicated duodenal and pyloric ulcer and with chronic gastritis. Chronic cholecystitis or other intra-abdominal inflammatory conditions also may cause heartburn. Belching may occur in gastric atony or obstruction at the pyloric or cardiac orifices of the stomach, and is a frequent complaint of patients with gallbladder disease.

A sense of fullness or pressure in the epigastrium after meals may be experienced by patients with coronary sclerosis, scirrhous carcinoma of the stomach, linitis plastica, or fibrosis secondary to chronic gastritis or to syphilis. The feeling of distention or swelling in the abdomen may be associated with excessive gas formation such as occurs in achylia gastrica, chronic pancreatic insufficiency, chronic enteritis, deficiency states, affections of the liver and biliary passages, partial intestinal obstruction, ascites, large intra-abdominal or pelvic cysts or tumors, and diseases causing great enlargement of the liver or spleen. Food allergy (see GASTROINTESTINAL ALLERGY) must always be kept in mind when a patient complains of indigestion after eating some particular food.

Treatment

General: The patient should eat a balanced diet. At least an hour should be allowed for a meal. Food should be thoroughly chewed without haste and, when possible, meals should be taken in a pleasant, quiet, and relaxing environment. Smoking immediately before meals should be prohibited. The food should be properly cooked, appetizing, and eaten in moderate amounts. Following a meal, the patient should avoid excitement.

Specific: If a "to-and-fro" movement of barium in the duodenum has been demonstrated fluoroscopically, administration of Urecholine (R 55) may dispel nausea by propelling the duodenal contents in the proper direction. Striking results may also be obtained from the use of Urecholine in cases of intestinal flatulence. Nausea sometimes may be relieved by an injection of pyridoxine (R 104). For heartburn, despite evidence that it is not caused by excessive gastric acidity, prompt relief frequently is afforded by a dose of sodium bicarbonate (R 4). Eructation may be prevented by carefully instructing the patient how to avoid swallowing air. Nervousness and tenseness may be allayed by small doses of phenobarbital (R 66, 67). Sodium bicarbonate (R 4) or an effervescent drink may induce an eructation and afford relief from gastric flatulence. Repeated staccato-like eructations in cases of hysterical aerophagia can be interrupted only by inducing sleep with a sedative (R 68), or by constant suction applied with a Wangensteen or similar apparatus.

Constipation (q.v.) requires teaching the patient regular bowel habits and, if necessary, prescribing a mild laxative such as milk of magnesia (R 21), with or without cascara sagrada (R 22). For "spastic" or irritable colon, belladonna and phenobarbital (R 56) may be helpful.

ACHYLIA GASTRICA

Complete absence of gastric ferments and hydrochloric acid, even after stimulation with histamine. Achylia is present in 10 to 20% of all individuals. It is frequently associated with an atrophic gastritis.

Etiology

Primary achylia (achylia gastrica simplex) is probably congenital and usually persists throughout life. **Secondary achylia** frequently may occur in association with gastric cancer or polyposis, gastric syphilis, gastric resection, and gastric neurosis. It is always present in pernicious anemia, where a definite familial tendency also may exist. Less commonly, it may accompany any chronic debilitating disease, such as nephritis, diabetes mellitus, alcoholism, tuberculosis, cancer, hyperthyroidism, pellagra, sprue, cholecystitis, colitis, and parasitic infections. Achylia is not uncommon in otherwise normal individuals after 50 years of age.

Symptoms

Symptoms may be mild, severe, or absent, depending on gastric motility and intestinal digestion. Where gastric symptoms predominate, there may be anorexia, sour eructations, epigastric discomfort and, occasionally, vomiting of undigested food. Intestinal symptoms include diarrhea, borborygmi, and colic; constipation is frequent. When diarrhea is present, it tends to be persistent and severe.

Laboratory Findings

Diagnosis is made by demonstrating the absence of free HCl and ferments after the subcut. injection of 0.5 mg. of histamine. Histamine will induce gastric secretion in all cases except in true achylia gastrica. The total (combined) acidity is very low in primary achylia, but may be relatively high in the secondary form.

Prognosis

There is no cure for the primary disease, or for the secondary types when the gastric mucosa is atrophic or nonfunctioning, as in pernicious anemia. Persisting achylia gastrica is, however, entirely compatible with long life, especially when it causes few symptoms.

Treatment

The treatment of achylia gastrica is directed toward symptomatic relief and the correction of any underlying abnormality. Hydrochloric acid may be administered as such (℞ 15), or as glutamic acid hydrochloride (℞ 16). It allegedly alleviates symptoms by preventing rapid evacuation. The diet should be easily digestible, well balanced, and rich in vitamins (*see* DIETS). If hydrochloric acid therapy fails to alleviate the diarrhea, the diet is restricted to strained soups, broths, cocoa, rice, tea, boiled milk, hard-boiled eggs, cooked fish, and well cooked meats free of fat and fibrous parts. When indicated, bismuth subcarbonate (℞ 8) with or without paregoric (℞ 11) may be administered daily to combat the diarrhea. If constipation (q.v.) is pronounced, this should be treated appropriately. Coarse fruits and vegetables are to be avoided at all times; even when constipation persists. Gastric lavage frequently is effective in relieving nausea and vomiting.

GASTRITIS

Inflammation, acute or chronic, of the gastric membrane.

ACUTE GASTRITIS

An acute inflammation of the mucosa of the stomach, sudden and violent in onset and of brief duration. There are four types: **acute simple exogenous, acute corrosive, acute infectious, and acute suppurative gastritis.**

Etiology

(1) Acute simple exogenous gastritis may be caused by the ingestion of alcohol, sharp spices, salicylates, creosote, croton

oil, coal tar products, the sulfonamides, ammonium chloride, iodides, bromides, cubeb, quinine, Atabrine, very hot foods, allergenic foods by hypersensitive individuals (especially milk, eggs and fish), and by swallowed bacteria and their toxins. (2) Acute corrosive gastritis may be caused by swallowing strong acids or caustics, iodine, potassium permanganate, or salts of arsenic, mercury, zinc, or lead. (3) Acute infectious, or toxic, gastritis may occur in patients with influenza, measles, scarlet fever, diphtheria, bacteremia, pneumonia, or enteric fevers. (4) Acute suppurative, or purulent, gastritis is rare and may be caused by infection of the stomach with streptococcus, colon bacillus, pneumococcus, or *B. subtilis*.

Pathology

The following findings are characteristic: (1) Acute simple exogenous gastritis: Patches of intense hyperemia, excessive mucus, and occasional submucosal hemorrhage. (2) Acute corrosive gastritis: Necrosis, membrane formation, and a subsequent (frequently hemorrhagic) inflammatory reaction. (3) Acute infectious gastritis: Hyperemia, blood extravasations, and erosions of the mucosa. (4) Acute suppurative gastritis: Diffuse purulent inflammation of the submucosa with hyperemia of the serosa and hemorrhages, necrosis, erosions, and fibrin deposits in the mucosa. In some cases circumscribed abscesses of the submucosa may form and may even perforate through the serosa.

Symptoms and Signs

(1) Acute simple exogenous gastritis: Six to 24 hours after ingestion of the offending agent, there are symptoms of malaise, anorexia, epigastric pressure with a sensation of fullness, nausea, headache, vertigo, vomiting (affording temporary relief from gastric symptoms), prostration, and exhaustion. The tongue is coated, and there may be slight fever. The tendency is toward constipation unless the intestine also is involved. Symptoms subside within 24 to 48 hours. (2) Acute corrosive gastritis: Collapse with tachycardia, cyanosis, severe epigastric pain, and dysphagia, followed by excessive thirst, hematemesis, and melena. The abdomen is tender and rigid. (3) Acute infectious, or toxic, gastritis: This type is characterized by anorexia, a sensation of epigastric fullness, and vomiting. In the influenzal form, gross hemorrhages may occur. (4) Acute suppurative gastritis: A fulminating onset with severe epigastric pain, chills and fever soon is followed by severe prostration, dry tongue, weak and rapid pulse, cyanosis, rapid respiration, and vomiting. The abdomen is distended, tender and rigid.

Diagnosis

(1) Diagnosis of acute simple exogenous gastritis is based upon signs and symptoms, particularly if one of the causative factors is elicited in the history. (2) The history, plus evidence

of a corrosive agent on the lips or face, or in the mouth, provides the diagnosis of acute corrosive gastritis. (3) Anorexia with vomiting and epigastric fullness in a patient with a febrile illness should arouse the suspicion of acute infectious or toxic gastritis. (4) Diagnosis of acute suppurative gastritis usually is made at laparotomy or necropsy. This form may be extremely difficult to differentiate clinically from perforated peptic ulcer or acute pancreatic necrosis.

Treatment

1. Acute simple exogenous gastritis: During the acute illness the patient requires complete bed rest. On the 1st day, no solid or semisolid food should be given. If vomiting has not occurred, gastric lavage is indicated. For nausea, phenobarbital (R 66) often is beneficial. If pain is severe, Demerol (R 75) or methadone (R 72, 73) may be given. Morphine is contraindicated if the patient is nauseated or vomiting. Fluids in the form of water, bouillon with added salt, mineral water, hot tea with sugar, and thin soups may be given orally, if tolerated. If not, 5 or 10% glucose in saline should be administered I.V. From the 3rd day on, bland foods may be ingested. These include buttered toast, soft-boiled eggs, cooked cereals (e.g., farina, strained oatmeal), mashed potatoes, custards, junket, milk and cream, flavored gelatin desserts, and jellied consommé. Subsequently, broiled or boiled (but not fried) tender meats may be added; these should be well chewed. The bland diet (see DIETS) should be adhered to for at least 2 weeks to avoid transition of the acute attack into chronic gastritis or enteritis. A laxative may be advisable if there is no diarrhea from an associated enteritis.

2. Acute corrosive gastritis: Treatment must be prompt and energetic. It is directed toward relieving the initial collapse and removing or neutralizing the offending agent by gentle use of the stomach tube or by emetics and antidotes. The patient should be put to bed as soon as possible, preferably in a hospital. Blood, plasma, and sufficient parenteral fluids should be administered to maintain circulatory efficiency. For severe pain, Demerol (R 75) rather than morphine is recommended. The procedure for removing or neutralizing the poison—stomach tube, emetic, or antidote—will depend on the nature of the agent (see POISONING). An emetic should not be employed if the patient is vomiting profusely or is comatose, or if there is danger of further damaging the mouth and esophagus. Antidotes must be administered promptly and in sufficient amounts. The stomach tube, if used, should be a large one; it is contraindicated if there is danger of perforating the esophagus or stomach, especially when strong acids or caustics have been ingested. Gastric perforation requires emergency surgical repair. Food should be withheld during the first few days and then permitted only according to the regimen outlined above. A cathartic should not be given if there is danger of irritating the intestine by the corrosive agent. Late complications include esophageal stricture which may require dilatation, and pyloric obstruction which may require surgical correction.

3. Acute infectious gastritis: The primary disease is treated as indicated. For nausea, phenobarbital (℞ 66) may be prescribed. Starvation must not be permitted; the patient should be encouraged to eat a bland diet (*see* DIETS). During the period of decreased food intake, vitamin supplements in the form of multivitamin capsules are indicated.

4. Acute suppurative gastritis: Treatment is primarily surgical. Drainage of a localized abscess or gastrectomy for a diffuse phlegmon may lead to complete cure. Sulfonamides (℞ 107, 108), penicillin (℞ 109, 110), streptomycin (℞ 111), or dihydrostreptomycin (℞ 112) parenterally are indicated.

CHRONIC GASTRITIS

Chronic inflammation of the gastric mucosa, three types of which may be recognized gastroscopically: superficial, atrophic, and hypertrophic.

Etiology

The etiology of chronic gastritis is unknown. A wide variety of irritants have been suspected, but none has been established as specific.

Pathology

Chronic superficial gastritis is characterized by hyperemia of the mucous membrane, edema, and exudation. The mucosa is friable and small purpuric spots or ulcerations may be present. The chronic atrophic type is characterized by a gray or greenish gray discoloration and thinning of the mucosa, and by easily seen blood vessels in the thinned-out areas. Mucosal hemorrhages are frequent. Chronic hypertrophic gastritis is characterized by a dull, velvety, slightly swollen, loose and spongy appearance of the mucosa, usually with granular nodules which, if large, may be confused with true polyps. Erosions and small ulcerations frequently are present.

Anacidity, abnormal amounts of mucus, and prolonged gastric emptying time are more characteristic of the atrophic than of the hypertrophic type.

Symptoms and Signs

In chronic superficial or atrophic gastritis, the majority of patients have sensations of epigastric burning, fullness, or pressure. Anorexia, nausea, vomiting, and serious gross hemorrhages may occur. Loss of weight usually is more striking in the atrophic form.

In chronic hypertrophic gastritis, there is epigastric pain, frequently of the "ulcer type." It is more intense than in the superficial and atrophic forms, but is more readily relieved than ulcer pain. Nocturnal pain is frequent and tends to recur, especially after dietary indiscretions and emotional upsets. The clinical manifestations vary: some cases are symptomless despite the presence of ulceration, while others show severe symptoms. Serious gross hemorrhages and, less frequently, pyloric obstruction may occur. Physical examination rarely reveals anything except occasional epigastric tenderness, which is apt to be more diffuse than with peptic ulcer.

Diagnosis

Diagnosis of chronic gastritis usually is made by exclusion. Frequently, the presumptive diagnosis is peptic ulcer or malignant gastric neoplasm. These diseases, as well as reflex gastric symptoms of extragastric disease, must always be ruled out. Roentgen examination of the stomach is either noncontributory or, in the hypertrophic type, shows exaggeration of the mucosal folds. In the atrophic type, gastric analysis frequently reveals achlorhydria and excessive amounts of gastric mucus. Atrophic gastritis is a constant finding in pernicious anemia (q.v.). In the hypertrophic type, gastric acidity may be high or normal. High gastric acidity in a patient with ulcer-like symptoms but with a normal roentgenogram should suggest hypertrophic gastritis. The diagnosis of chronic gastritis is established by means of the gastroscope.

Treatment

All gastric irritants must be avoided, such as alcohol, nicotine, spices, condiments, salicylates, iodides, and harsh cathartics. The diet should be bland as for peptic ulcer (*see* Diets) and taken frequently in small amounts. Supplementary vitamins of the B complex and ascorbic acid must be given if meats and fresh fruits or juices are not tolerated. Foci of infection in the mouth and pharynx should be eliminated. The treatment of massive hemorrhage is similar to that of hemorrhagic peptic ulcer (q.v.).

Patients with atrophic or superficial gastritis, on getting up in the morning, should drink slowly a pint of warm water containing a teaspoon of salt. This may promote bowel movement and possibly wash away some of the overnight mucus that may be adherent to the gastric mucosa. For patients with achlorhydria, hydrochloric acid (℞ 15) or glutamic acid hydrochloride (℞ 16) may be helpful. Liver extract (℞ 93) I.M. may be useful. If such I.M. therapy is not feasible, desiccated hog's stomach (℞ 94) may be given by mouth. If the gastritis is associated with achlorhydria and a macrocytic anemia, intensive treatment for pernicious anemia is indicated (q.v.). Hypochromic anemia if present may respond to iron (℞ 95, 97).

For patients with intractable hypertrophic gastritis, the regimen should be identical with that used for active peptic ulcer (*see* DIETS). If acid is not successfully neutralized and pain is intractable, an antacid (℞ 2) 15 minutes before each hourly feeding is indicated. If this therapy does not afford relief, 200 to 400 cc. of a 15 to 20% solution of a protein hydrolysate-maltose mixture (in equal parts), calculated on a basis of 20 calories/lb. body wt. should be administered orally every 2 hours from 6 A.M. to 10 P.M. (℞ 99). After subsidence of acute symptoms, a bland diet supplemented with vitamins C and B complex, in frequent feedings, should be gradually resumed (*see* DIETS).

If there is any question of malignant change, radical subtotal resection of the stomach should be performed.

PEPTIC ULCER

A circumscribed erosion of the mucous membrane of the lower end of the esophagus, in the stomach or duodenum, or on the jejunal side of a gastrojejunostomy.

Etiology

The exact etiology of peptic ulcer is still obscure. Hypersecretion of acid gastric juice is an important factor in the production of a peptic ulcer and in the reactivation of healed ulcers. Peptic ulcers are not encountered in achlorhydric patients. Psychic disturbances such as increased emotional tension and psychologic conflicts play an exceedingly important though poorly defined role in the mechanism of ulcer formation.

Curling's ulcer, an acute gastroduodenal ulceration, is caused by severe burns of the body and may be related to hyperacidity caused by liberation of histamine.

Pathology

Peptic ulcers occasionally develop at the lower end of the esophagus and on the jejunal side of a gastrojejunostomy, but the majority occur on the lesser curvature of the stomach or in the first portion of the duodenum. They usually are single, although multiple ulcers of the duodenum or stomach or both have been described. Those occurring in the stomach tend to be larger than those in the duodenum, the former rarely exceeding 2 cm. and the latter, 1 cm. in diameter. The margins of the ulcer are sharp; the surrounding mucosa may be normal or inflamed; the floor of the crater usually is clean and consists of a thin layer of exudate overlying a deeper layer of granulation and fibrous tissue. In chronic ulcer the muscular layer may be replaced by fibrous tissue and the surrounding tissues distorted by scarring. The ulcer heals by scarring, the crater fills in and a smooth surface devoid of mucosa remains.

Whether carcinomatous change occurs at the base of a benign ulcer, or a peptic ulcer becomes superimposed on a carcinoma, thus giving a malignant lesion the appearance of benign ulcer, is more or less an academic question. Whatever the mechanism of its formation, a malignant lesion of the stomach may at times have all the characteristics of a benign lesion.

Symptoms and Signs

Pain, the outstanding symptom of peptic ulcer, has four distinctive characteristics: A uniform quality and location, a tendency to rhythmicity and to periodicity with periods of remission, and a proneness to become chronic. The pain varies in degree from a mild discomfort to a sharp, severe, sometimes penetrating sensation. It may be steady, aching or gnawing and is quite frequently described by the patient as a "steady hunger pain." When there is associated pylorospasm the pain may become sharp and cramplike. It is characteristically located in the epigastrium and usually is circumscribed so that the patient can indicate the spot with one finger point. In duodenal ulcer the pain is more likely to be located in the right epigastrium, in esophageal ulcer near the xyphoid or under the sternum, and in jejunal ulcer in the left midabdomen or even in the left lower quadrant.

The pain is related to the digestive cycle. It usually is absent before breakfast, appears during the day from 1 to 4 hours after meals and often is sufficiently severe at night to awaken the patient. It is relieved by foods and antacids and aggravated by alcohol and condiments.

The periodicity of the pain is a significant characteristic of the disease. Symptoms may last for a few days, a few weeks or several months and be followed by a variable period of spontaneous remission. It often is possible to relate the periods of exacerbation to episodes of psychic trauma or emotional tension. Other possible factors associated with exacerbations include fatigue, excessive use of tobacco or alcohol, dietary indiscretion and acute infections.

Besides pain, other common complaints are constipation, especially during periods of exacerbation, heartburn, acid eructations, and gastric distention. Symptoms occurring occasionally in uncomplicated peptic ulcer include nausea, vomiting, excessive salivation, anorexia and weight loss, diarrhea and anemia.

The tall asthenic individual is more likely to develop peptic ulcer than the stocky extroverted pyknic; however, there are exceptions to this tendency. Except for these constitutional characteristics, physical examination usually is entirely negative, although there may be slight to moderate tenderness in the epigastrium over the circumscribed area of pain, especially when elicited by deep pressure over the sensitive spot with a single thumb or finger. More acute or widespread tenderness suggests a penetrating ulcer with peritoneal irritation.

The chronicity of the disease is evidenced by the fact that the average duration of symptoms before initial discovery of the lesion is 6 to 7 years; occasionally symptoms have been present for 40 to 50 years before treatment is instituted.

Laboratory Findings

The hydrochloric acid content (both free and combined) of the stomach secretion is elevated, particularly after a test meal or an injection of histamine (*see* Lab. Proc.). X-ray examination of the gastrointestinal tract establishes the diagnosis in 95% of the cases. In gastric or duodenal ulcer the crater, when seen in profile, appears as a penetrating niche, but when viewed otherwise, appears as a circumscribed collection of barium surrounded by a clear zone. In certain acute cases of duodenal ulcer a crater sometimes cannot be demonstrated and one has to rely on secondary signs such as spasm, irritability, failure of the duodenal cap to fill, and spot tenderness. When such secondary signs are due to ulcer, re-examination soon after the acute symptoms have subsided frequently will reveal the crater. When there is scarring of the pylorus, or prolonged spasm, gastric retention is observed in the films taken 6 hours after the ingestion of barium.

As the ulcer in the duodenum heals, some contraction occurs, while in the stomach healing rarely gives rise to deformity except in those few cases where an hourglass deformity results. In ulcers of the stomach it usually is not possible to identify the ulcer site by X-ray after healing has taken place.

Gastroscopy, in the hands of the expert familiar with the appearance of lesions visualized in this way, may be of use in attempting to differentiate the benign from the malignant lesion of the stomach or in visualizing stomach or marginal ulcers not readily demonstrable by X-ray. It is, of course, of no use if the ulcer is in or distal to the pylorus. Esophagoscopy may be of assistance in visualizing an esophageal ulcer but the procedure should be performed with great caution to avoid the possibility of rupture.

Diagnosis

Diagnosis of peptic ulcer is based on clinical and laboratory findings as described, particularly the demonstration of the ulcer by X-ray. Since duodenal ulcers almost never undergo malignant change, the diagnosis is established as soon as the ulcer is demonstrated by X-ray. The differentiation, however, between benign and malignant ulcers of the stomach may be extremely difficult; indeed, at times microscopic examination will reveal evidences of malignancy despite all other evidence, clinical, roentgenologic and gastroscopic, to the contrary. The differentiation is, of course, exceedingly important since not only does it determine whether therapy shall be medical or surgical but also establishes the basis for subsequent management and prognosis.

The ulcer should be considered malignant and surgery advised if: (1) The ulcer is located on the greater curvature; (2) a histamine achlorhydria is present; (3) the crater is located on a subtraction defect *niche en plateau*; (4) the crater is surrounded by a translucent halo (Carman's meniscus sign); (5) the crater is greater than 2.5 cm. in diameter; (6) there is inability to demonstrate roentgenographically radiating mucosal folds emerging from the ulcer crater; (7) the contour of the ulcer niche is irregular; or (8) the crater is located distal to the incisura, especially when it is on the posterior wall.

In such cases it probably is advisable to apply a 3-week test period on a strict medical regimen in a hospital and if the lesion does not heal in that time and remain healed, surgery (gastrectomy, partial or complete) should be advised.

Treatment

The three basic principles important in healing a peptic ulcer are: (1) Rest—mental, physical, and gastric; (2) suppression of gastric motor and secretory activity; and (3) improvement of the nutritional status of the patient, particularly with regard to protein.

For gastric ulcer, 3 weeks of treatment on bed rest, preferably in a hospital, should be instituted in every case and the lesion examined by X-ray at the end of this time. If complete healing or at least striking improvement in the size of the lesion has not taken place, malignancy should be suspected and a competent gastric surgeon promptly consulted.

For duodenal ulcers much more latitude is permissible. In the acute phases when pain and apprehension are prominent, removal from home environment to the hospital is advisable. Hospitalization, however, need not extend beyond a week or two during which time the patient can be gradually educated to the factors important in precipitating ulcer symptoms and the basis sought for emotional conflicts, free from the presence of members of the family. Though possibly ideal, hospitalization is seldom essential in the treatment of uncomplicated duodenal ulcer. Rest at home for 7 to 10 days usually will control the acute symptoms and ambulation may begin as soon as the pain is under control and the dietary program well established.

In the acute phase, hourly feedings may be necessary and for this the first day Sippy regimen is satisfactory (*see* DIETS). In severe cases the progression of diet must be slow and it may be advisable to continue the progressive Sippy regimen through to the ambulatory ulcer diet reached on the 12th day. Where pylorospasm is severe and emptying of the stomach delayed, it may be necessary to prolong gruel feedings represented by the 7th day Sippy diet before incorporating ground meat into the diet. In most instances, however, one may begin with the 5th or 7th day diet and progress steadily to the ambulatory ulcer diet or remain on these gruel feedings until symptoms have subsided, then shift directly to the ambulatory ulcer diet with between-meal feedings of milk and crackers. Since ulcer diets are likely to be deficient in certain accessory food substances, it usually is advisable to prescribe multivitamin capsules once or twice a day. Furthermore, the possibility of hypercalciuria and the development of renal calculi during prolonged Sippy treatment must be kept in mind.

For patients depleted of proteins an intensive course of protein hydrolysate may be advisable. There are several useful oral preparations (*see* PROTEIN DEFICIENCY). The hydrolysate may be administered in addition to or as a substitute for the between-meal milk and cream feeding or it may be used as a mixture of equal parts of protein hydrolysate and maltose (℞ 99) in place of the hourly feedings of milk and cream in the 1st day Sippy regimen. When the hydrolysate is not tolerated orally or when protein depletion is particularly severe, amino acids may be administered parenterally as protein hydrolysates or as solution of amino acids (℞ 100) free of peptides. The latter usually is better tolerated and may be given I.V. at a rate of 1,000 cc. of solution in 1 to 2 hours. Each 1,000 cc. contains over 80 Gm. of amino acids so that the total daily requirement may be supplied in this manner.

Medication should be aimed at minimizing the hyperacidity and intestinal spasm. Hyperacidity usually can be controlled by frequent feedings; occasionally the additional use of alkali after meals and between feedings is required. The most useful antacid is a combination of aluminum hydroxide and magnesium trisilicate (℞ 1).

Sedatives should be given to allay anxiety and reduce nervous tension. Phenobarbital (℞ 66, 67) is the drug of choice and should be given 3 or 4 times daily. In addition, a bedtime hypnotic may be desirable (℞ 69, 70).

The control of intestinal spasm, particularly spasm of the pylorus, may be effected by the use of any one of several drugs with an atropine-like action (℞ 56, 59, 63).

The tendency to constipation, so frequently encountered with ulcer diets, may be effectively prevented by the use of liquid petrolatum nightly (℞ 23) and, if necessary, a small dose of milk of magnesia (℞ 21).

When the ulcer is associated with pylorospasm or with edematous and inflammatory narrowing of the pylorus, or with unusually high acidity, intractable persistent pain and vomiting may result. If these symptoms do not respond to dietary, antispasmodic, and neutralization therapy, special measures may be required.

Continuous Wangensteen or Levin tube aspiration of the excess acid gastric juice, and tube feeding of protein hydrolysate and maltose solution (℞ 99) or milk and cream at regular intervals, in small quantities sufficient to obtain sustained neutralization of the stomach and to restore protein balance and caloric requirement, often relieve this type of case. Since continuous aspiration of the hydrochloric acid from the stomach may lead to alkalosis, the pH of the blood should be closely followed by frequent serum chloride, CO_2 combining power, and total base determinations. Replacement of chlorides where necessary may be attained by the parenteral administration of physiologic saline. Transfusions of blood or plasma also may be desirable if protein depletion or anemia are prominent factors.

As soon as oral feedings are better tolerated, the tube feedings should be discontinued and the plan of treatment outlined for acute active ulcers instituted.

Continuous gastric aspiration with simultaneous jejunal feeding (℞ 99, 101) occasionally can be useful in the presence of intractable pain and in the absence of pyloric obstruction. This can be accomplished by the use of the Abbott-Rawson or similar tube arranged so that the open end of the aspirating tube rests in the stomach and the other opening in the jejunum. The blood chlorides and CO_2 combining power should be followed closely and any imbalance corrected promptly by the parenteral administration of the appropriate fluids and electrolytes.

In the absence of vomiting, intractable pain may be controlled by the continuous alkalinized drip method (℞ 102), or by a 24-hour aluminum hydroxide intragastric drip (℞ 3). Neither of these methods should be used in the presence of functional or organic pyloric obstruction. It should be emphasized that any form of gastric intubation is contraindicated in the presence of bleeding.

The value of vagotomy, surgically or medically induced, remains to be determined.

COMPLICATIONS OF PEPTIC ULCERS

PERFORATION

Acute perforations are 8 to 10 times more frequent in duodenal ulcers than in gastric ulcers, and both types occur but rarely in women. They constitute major surgical emergencies. Shortly after a perforation (a few minutes to 1 hour) the patient experiences agonizing abdominal pain (unless aged or moribund) and makes every effort to splint the abdomen and avoid undue movement. Respirations are costal and shallow, the leaves of the diaphragm are splinted, and beads of sweat appear on the forehead. There are no immediate evidences of peripheral vascular collapse, the pulse may be normal or slightly elevated, the blood pressure is not altered significantly, and the temperature remains normal or subnormal. The abdomen is boardlike and tender over the site of the ulcer. Peristaltic sounds are absent initially, but may return later. The initial state is followed by a reaction in which the classic signs of peritonitis with attendant shock predominate. The pulse and temperature become elevated, and the blood pressure falls. The abdomen distends and the rigidity abates somewhat. The tenderness may shift to the right lower quadrant or it may remain generalized depending on the dispersion of the gastric contents. Leukocytosis invariably accompanies the fever. X-rays of the abdomen often will demonstrate air in the abdominal cavity and if the patient is upright it may be seen under the diaphragm. However, inability to demonstrate pneumoperitoneum does not exclude the diagnosis of perforation.

Subacute or chronic perforations produce a less dramatic clinical picture and in fact may occur quite silently if the perforation is chronic and closure is effected by adherence of the ulcer site to pancreas or liver. Transient or intermittent seepage may result in the formation of a subphrenic abscess.

Diagnosis

The diagnosis usually is not difficult. In biliary or renal colic the frozen attitude of the patient and the boardlike rigidity of the abdomen are absent. In intestinal obstruction the pain is rhythmical and intermittent. In acute appendicitis the onset is more gradual and the pain less severe. In tabetic crisis and coronary occlusion there is no abdominal rigidity and the distribution of pain and other signs and symptoms of diagnostic value usually are present. Perforation of the gallbladder usually is indistinguishable from that of the stomach or duodenum; however, it usually occurs during or after an attack of acute cholecystitis. In acute pancreatitis, which is occasionally difficult to differentiate, the patient usually is in profound shock, abdominal rigidity is less widespread and less intense. The serum amylase and lipase are usually elevated but they also may be elevated when a peptic ulcer has penetrated posteriorly into the pancreas. At times, it may be impossible to differentiate between perforations of the duodenum and of the colon, particularly when they occur at the hepatic or splenic flexures of the transverse colon.

Treatment

Acute perforation of a peptic ulcer requires immediate operation; the earlier it is performed the better the prognosis. Eight to 10 hours after perforation the prognosis begins to become grave. Measures to prevent shock should be instituted immediately. A gastric tube should be passed into the stomach and the gastric contents aspirated continuously. Following operation, treatment to combat the expected peritonitis (q.v.) should be instituted. Clear fluids by mouth in small quantities usually may be given 24 hours after operation, with slow progression through gruels to an ambulatory ulcer diet within 10 to 14 days (see DIETS).

16

MASSIVE HEMORRHAGE

The early symptoms of massive hemorrhage consist of faintness, weakness, vertigo, and profuse perspiration. These soon may be followed by the passage of a large tarry stool or the vomiting of blood; the latter is a little more common in gastric than in duodenal ulcers. Syncope and collapse may occur if hemorrhage is sufficiently severe to produce a profound fall in blood pressure. The pulse in such cases becomes weak and rapid and thirst develops. The blood count and hemoglobin fall and the blood volume is restored by hemodilution. The BUN may be moderately elevated because of absorption of blood from the intestine and diminished blood flow through the kidneys secondary to the fall in systemic blood pressure.

Treatment

If the patient is not vomiting, a feeding program should be promptly instituted regardless of the severity of the hemorrhage or its continuance. The patient's blood should be promptly typed and adequate sources of suitable blood kept in readiness. If shock is present, suitable measures to combat it should be instituted immediately.

Bland liquid feedings, first of milk and cream or equal parts of cream and gelatin, or protein hydrolysate should be administered day and night every 2 hours, supplemented later by gruels and puréed vegetables. Administration of a full diet, in the form of purées (Meulengracht diet), from the 1st day of hemorrhage also has produced satisfactory results. The patient should be allowed as much food as he desires; the withholding of food is indicated if the patient is vomiting or the degree of shock does not permit alimentation. Restlessness may be controlled by the parenteral administration of a barbiturate (R 68) or, if accompanied by pain, by the use of morphine (R 74) or Demerol (R 75). (CAUTION! Discontinue morphine if nausea or vomiting results.)

Transfusions of whole blood or plasma or I.V. infusions of dextrose and saline may be given according to medical indications, i.e., if the pulse rate is markedly elevated (120 or more), the systolic blood pressure down to 90 or less, or when the red blood cell count is below 2,500,000. Iron (R 95, 97) should not be prescribed until the hemorrhage has ceased and the stools are free of blood.

OBSTRUCTION

Obstruction of the outlet of the stomach may be partial or complete and may be due to spasm, cicatricial stenosis, edema, or inflammatory swelling about a pyloric or duodenal ulcer. Symptoms and signs of obstruction include vomiting of food ingested during previous meals, foul gaseous eructation and, in individuals with thin abdominal walls, overactive and visible peristalsis which may be seen traveling from the left upper quadrant toward the umbilicus. If vomiting has been pronounced, there may be clinical and laboratory evidence of dehydration and alkalosis. Aspiration of the stomach in the morning after an evening meal containing identifiable food substances will show the food to be still present in undigested or partially digested forms. Roentgen examination of the stomach yields the most valuable evidence for it permits not only the determination of the site, nature, and extent of the obstructing lesion, but also the degree of retention. (The barium meal should be aspirated from the stomach as soon as the examination has been completed.)

Treatment

The stomach should be intubated and emptied night and morning, or constant suction applied in severe cases. Nourishment should be administered I.V. and should be aimed at correcting the dehydration, the acid-base imbalance and the hypoproteinemia (as described earlier in this chapter in the section on continuous gastric aspiration). If the stomach is aspirated night and morning, alkali and bland liquid nourishment should be given between aspirations, and total intake and output measured each 24 hours. After 48 to 72 hours, liquid feedings of milk and cream or protein hydrolysate-maltose solution (R 99) may be administered regularly, the suction being discontinued for about 2 hours after each feeding. If the feedings are returned to the suction bottle on resumption of suction, the obstruction has not been relieved. If obstruction has been due to spasm or edema, it usually will have been relieved at least partially at the end of 48 to 96 hours and entirely at the end of a week or 10 days. At the end of this period the stomach should be re-examined roentgenographically. If vomiting then occurs or if the stomach still is dilated, with little or no barium passing into the duodenum, or if aspiration in the evening reveals a quantity of 800 to 2,000 cc., surgical intervention is advisable.

HEMATEMESIS; MELENA

The vomiting of gross blood; the passage of tarry stools.

Etiology

Hematemesis almost always is followed by melena. Melena, however, frequently occurs without hematemesis, especially when bleeding takes place below the pyloric end of the stomach, as in a bleeding duodenal ulcer. Only occasionally will hemorrhage above the pylorus, such as caused by a ruptured esophageal varix, result in melena without hematemesis.

The most common causes of hematemesis and melena are peptic ulcer, gastric or duodenal (60%), bleeding esophageal varices in portal hypertension (8%), and gastric carcinoma (5%). A miscellaneous group responsible for about 3% of the cases consists of: (a) bleeding points in the nose, mouth, pharynx, or respiratory passages; (b) lesions of the esophagus, including benign or malignant tumors, esophagitis, peptic ulcer, diverticulum, foreign body, syphilis, tuberculosis and actinomycosis; (c) gastric lesions, including gastritis, benign tumors, syphilis, tuberculosis, hiatus hernia, traumatic injuries, and acute gastric dilatation; (d) lesions of the duodenum, including duodenitis, tumors, and erosion caused by gallstones or by neoplasm invading from nearby structures; (e) prothrombin deficiency as in hepatic and biliary tract disease, or following overdosage with dicumarol; (f) blood dyscrasias, including the purpuras, leukemia, polycythemia, hemophilia, and hemorrhagic disease of the newborn; (g) rupture of an aneurysm or abscess into the esophagus or stomach; and (h) blackwater fever, yellow fever, and scurvy.

A "cause undetermined" group comprises about 24% of the cases of hematemesis and melena. The bulk of the cases in this group undoubtedly are caused by many of the lesions mentioned above. However, these lesions may heal by the time it is considered safe to perform diagnostic procedures, and others may escape detection unless special technics of diagnosis are employed.

Symptoms and Signs

In hematemesis the appearance of the vomitus depends on the amount and character of the gastric content at the time the blood has been vomited as well as on the length of time the blood has been in contact with gastric secretion. Gastric acids convert the bright red hemoglobin into brown acid-hematin which is responsible for the "coffee ground" color of the vomitus. Bright red blood results from profuse hemorrhage and little contact with the gastric juices.

A tarry stool containing altered blood may be passed if 60 cc. or more of blood has entered the intestine and is eliminated by way of the large bowel. If there has been no spontaneous stool, the finding of tarry material on the gloved finger inserted into the rectum will aid in establishing the fact that bleeding into the gastrointestinal tract has occurred.

Concomitant symptoms depend largely on the severity of the hemorrhage and the efficiency with which the compensatory mechanisms are maintained. There may be no systemic symptoms of significance. In massive hemorrhage, however, the typical symptoms of shock occur (q.v.).

Azotemia is a frequent accompaniment of gastrointestinal bleeding. The degree of azotemia is proportional to the severity of the hemorrhage. The nitrogen retention is thought to be caused by the absorption of the decomposition products of the blood in the intestinal tract, and renal failure occurring secondary to shock.

Diagnosis

To determine the cause of gastrointestinal bleeding the conditions listed above must be considered. Ordinarily, X-ray, gastroscopy, and other procedures which might traumatize the bleeding site should not be undertaken until 1 or 2 weeks after bleeding has ceased, as indicated by the disappearance of blood from the stools.

Treatment

General: The patient should be placed at complete bed rest. The blood type and Rh grouping should be determined without delay and suitable blood made available and held in readiness. If the patient is apprehensive or restless, sodium phenobarbital (℞ 68) or Dilaudid (℞ 76) should be administered as frequently as necessary. Morphine should not be used because of its tendency to cause nausea. If pain is severe, Demerol (℞ 75) may be administered. If the systolic blood pressure is below 90 and the pulse rate above 140, then slow I.V. drip of 5% glucose in physiologic saline should be begun immediately and continued until plasma or whole blood can be substituted. Large quantities of blood or parenteral fluids should not be introduced into the circulation if the blood volume has not been diminished, otherwise the bleeding may be prolonged. In such cases fluids can be administered by hypodermoclysis (*see* SHOCK). The urinary output should be measured and recorded and sufficient fluid administered parenterally to maintain an output of at least 800 cc./24 hours. An ice bag may be placed on the abdomen for psychological reasons and to keep the patient from moving about unnecessarily. In patients who are in shock, oral alimentation is out of the question until recovery from the vascular collapse has occurred. In most cases of intragastric or duodenal bleeding, if nausea is absent, feeding can be promptly instituted (*see* treatment of hemorrhage from peptic ulcer). In bleeding from esophageal varices or, when solid or semisolid food is not deemed advisable, hourly feedings of albumin water, 5 to 10% sweetened gelatin, milk, protein hydrolysate solutions or strained fruit juices may be administered. After the 4th to 7th day, soft bland foods may be permitted.

Specific measures: These depend on the underlying disease causing the bleeding. Hemorrhage due to blood dyscrasias is best treated with transfusions of whole blood. In bleeding due to prothrombin deficiency the parenteral administration of vitamin K (℞ 105) will result in a restoration of a normal prothrombin blood concentration, provided the liver is not too badly damaged. Otherwise, transfusions of whole blood are indicated. If the patient is scorbutic, vitamin C (℞ 106) is indicated.

Laxatives and enemas are withheld until 3 or 4 days after all evidences of bleeding have disappeared. If anemia is present a soluble preparation of iron (℞ 96, 98) should be administered after stools have become normal in color. Specific therapy, if any, of the underlying disease process can be begun as soon as bleeding has ceased. The injection of sclerosing solutions into esophageal varices may be attempted if facilities and the services of a skilled esophagoscopist are available. Emergency surgery should be performed when bleeding continues despite a thorough trial of conservative therapy. Elective surgery, if indicated, can be performed subsequently when the patient is in good condition.

ACUTE GASTRIC DILATATION

Dilatation of the stomach characterized by the sudden loss of gastric tonus resulting in the intragastric accumulation of large quantities of fluid and gas.

Etiology

The exact cause of acute gastric dilatation is not definitely known. The majority of cases probably are due to a reflex inhibition of the gastric motor nerves via the autonomic pathways. Some are caused by obstruction of the terminal portion of the duodenum through compression by the superior mesenteric artery and vein.

From 60 to 70% of cases occur in the first 3 to 5 days following an operation. The incidence is greatest after abdominal operation, but any major operative procedure may be responsible. Severe trauma, immobilization in a body cast, prolonged labor, and a severe acute or chronic illness in which the patient is confined to bed also are occasionally causative.

Symptoms and Signs

A sensation of fullness in the abdomen, followed by epigastric pain and persistent vomiting or regurgitation of large quantities of bile-stained fluid are common initial symptoms. The upper abdomen becomes distended and tympanitic to percussion. Hematemesis may occur if the dilatation is not promptly relieved. The patient suffers severe thirst, dyspnea due to elevation of the diaphragm, and dehydration as manifested by loss of skin turgor, dry tongue, and oliguria. Alkalosis, tetany, and finally shock may develop as a result of fluid and electrolyte loss.

An anterior-posterior X-ray of the abdomen with the patient

in the supine position usually shows the typical shadow of a gas-filled stomach.

Diagnosis

The diagnosis usually is obvious when a bedridden patient suddenly becomes distended and begins to vomit profusely. The chief condition to be differentiated from acute dilatation of the stomach is a high mechanical obstruction of the small bowel. X-ray examination and auscultation of the abdomen usually suffice. In high obstructions the X-ray usually will reveal one or two dilated loops of small bowel, and increased borborygmi occurring concomitantly with abdominal cramps usually are present.

Treatment

The aim of treatment is threefold: to empty the stomach and keep it empty; to restore the blood electrolyte balance; and to relieve the dehydration.

The stomach can be emptied and kept empty most efficiently by constant mild suction through an indwelling Levin-type duodenal tube. This is the most important measure and is curative within 24 to 48 hours in the vast majority of cases. Urecholine (Ɽ 55) may be useful.

The blood electrolyte balance can quickly be restored by the adequate administration I.V. of isotonic saline solution. The amount required will vary with the individual case depending upon the level of the blood chlorides. It has been suggested that 0.5 Gm. of sodium chloride/Kg. body wt., in the form of isotonic saline solution, be given for each 100 mg./100 cc. that the plasma chlorides have dropped below the normal level. However, too much reliance should not be placed on such an arbitrary rule. Frequent blood chloride and CO_2 combining power determinations must be made to check adequately the amounts of saline solution needed.

Much of the dehydration will be corrected by the saline solution required for treatment of the hypochloremia, but additional amounts of 5 or 10% glucose in water should be given I.V. to ensure a urine output of about 1,000 cc. a day.

After 24 to 48 hours of this treatment, the duodenal tube can be clamped for a few hours and the patient allowed to take some fluid by mouth. If this does not stagnate in the stomach, the duodenal tube can be removed and oral feedings begun.

PANCREATITIS

Inflammation of the pancreas, which may occur as **acute pancreatitis,** *associated with a varying degree of inflammation and necrosis of the adjacent omentum and viscera, with or with-*

out hemorrhage; or **chronic interstitial pancreatitis,** *which is an inflammation, usually nonspecific, characterized by gradual replacement of the parenchyma by fibrosis.*

ACUTE PANCREATITIS

Etiology and Pathogenesis

The etiology of acute pancreatitis, a relatively infrequent condition, remains unproved although some cases may be a result of trauma, mumps, obstruction of the ampulla of Vater, or perforation or disease of adjacent viscera. Bacteriologic studies of the bile and pancreatic juices are inconsistent in their results and may be negative or reveal staphylococci, streptococci, or any of the intestinal bacilli. It is possible that such infection represents a secondary invasion. Owing to this uncertainty regarding etiology, any classification of the disease must rest upon clinical and pathologic bases. Thus, acute idiopathic pancreatitis may be considered in the following categories: (1) Nonhemorrhagic, showing (a) edema without fat necrosis (edematous or interstitial); or (b) edema with fat necrosis. (2) Hemorrhagic. It is impossible to know whether these forms are distinct entities or merely progressive stages of the same process. It is certain, however, that the mortality rate is vastly higher in the hemorrhagic form than in the nonhemorrhagic (*see* Prognosis).

The inflammatory changes have been attributed to the regurgitation of bile from the common bile duct into the major pancreatic duct. Bile salts will cause necrosis of the pancreatic cells, allowing release of pancreatic lipolytic and proteolytic enzymes which digest tissue, fat, and protein. The resulting fatty acids combine with calcium ions to form the insoluble "white soap" deposits which are the pathognomonic plaques of "fat necrosis." A rise in the concentration of serum lipase and amylase follows the local release and absorption of these pancreatic ferments. It is probable that digestion and necrosis of the vascular walls, with resultant hemorrhage, are similarly caused.

Symptoms and Signs

Onset usually is abrupt, with pain as the predominating symptom. Characteristically, it is constant, agonizing, centers in the epigastrium, and radiates to the back. Other typical symptoms in severe cases are nausea, vomiting, upper abdominal spasm and tenderness, decreased peristalsis, tachycardia, and vasomotor collapse. Since, theoretically, an obstruction of the ampulla of Vater by a common duct stone or by a spasm of the sphincter of Oddi may be an etiologic factor, especially in the hemorrhagic form, it is not surprising that many of the patients are jaundiced. In the average mild or moderate case, not requiring surgery, the patient's temperature ranges between

100° and 102° F., and the leukocyte count between 10,000 and 15,000. When necrosis and interstitial hemorrhage occur, the symptoms of shock are prominent, the pulse is rapid, blood pressure low, and the patient is pale and cyanotic with cold extremities and clammy skin. Death may ensue in a few hours.

Complications

Biliary tract disease complicates 75% of the cases. A common duct calculus occasionally is found. Acute cholecystitis is not uncommon and may prove to be the dominating complication and the determining factor in treatment.

Diagnosis

The symptoms of acute pancreatitis are nonspecific and therefore not diagnostic; many cases have been diagnosed only at operation. However, a definitive preoperative diagnosis can be made by enzyme studies, the most practical of which is the determination of the serum amylase by Somogyi's method. Pancreatitis is to be suspected when the amylase concentration reaches 300 Somogyi units or more (normal, 50 to 200 u.). The parotid glands also secrete amylase, however, and inflammation of these glands may produce a rise in the serum concentration. Nevertheless, a serum amylase of twice the normal value serves to differentiate acute pancreatitis from gastrointestinal diseases such as perforated ulcer, acute cholecystitis, appendicitis, and upper intestinal obstruction, and from coronary thrombosis and early pneumonia with pleurisy (q.v.).

Prognosis and Sequelae

The prognosis in acute hemorrhagic pancreatitis is exceedingly grave, the mortality rate being 60% as compared with only 5 to 20% in the nonhemorrhagic form. Where there is destruction of the islet cells, diabetes mellitus (usually mild) may result. Pancreatic abscess may be an early development when bacterial invasion is present, and in such cases the prognosis is less favorable. Following recovery there is a tendency to recurrence of the pancreatitis in the same or a different form. Repeated attacks, if not fatal, may ultimately produce fibrosis of the gland (chronic pancreatitis), with pancreatic insufficiency.

Treatment

Mild cases will respond to rest, sedation, adequate fluids, and maintenance of electrolyte balance, with recovery in 1 to 3 weeks. However, severe symptoms at onset, or progressive unfavorable developments that suggest advancing peritonitis (with or without biliary tract involvement) are indications for laparotomy, not to be performed, however, until the patient has been adequately treated for shock (q.v.). The administration of parenteral fluids is essential, and it may be necessary to give blood or plasma. Intubation of the stomach or small bowel (*see* BEDSIDE PROC.) usually is of value. Although the presence of infection cannot always be ascertained preoperatively, the prophylactic use of penicillin (℞ 109, 110), streptomycin (℞ 111), or dihydrostreptomycin (℞ 112), and sulfonamides (℞ 107, 108), is advisable. Morphine (℞ 74) should be given to relieve pain.

Because of the possibility of "regurgitation" or "common channel" as an etiologic factor, as well as the high incidence of biliary tract complication, surgical decompression of the biliary tract is frequently performed. Since the patient often is critically ill, a cholecystostomy, associated with drainage of the pancreas, usually is the operation of choice. In an attempt to relieve spasm of the sphincter of Oddi, procaine injection of the celiac ganglion or the administration of antispasmodics, such as atropine (℞ 57), may be tried.

CHRONIC INTERSTITIAL PANCREATITIS

Chronic inflammation of the pancreas, in which fibrosis is the prominent feature, of unknown etiology. It may be caused by repeated attacks of acute or subacute pancreatitis (q.v.). The acini and islet cells are damaged, resulting in pancreatic fibrosis. Rarely, tuberculosis, syphilis, or calculus in the gland may be responsible.

Symptoms, Signs, and Diagnosis

The symptoms are nonspecific. There often is a dull pain in the upper abdomen radiating to the back; postprandial discomfort and loss of weight usually occur. Stools are apt to be bulky, foul, and fatty owing to pancreatic deficiency. As the fibrosis proceeds, the pancreatic and common bile ducts may become partially or completely occluded. The resulting jaundice is likely to be fatal if not relieved, and it is this symptom which usually necessitates a definitive diagnosis. Although the jaundice usually is progressive, the bile seldom disappears completely from the stool. Glycosuria may appear, depending upon the extent of damage to islet tissue. The syndrome of jaundice, malnutrition, and weight loss suggests the possibility of pancreatic carcinoma. Since duodenal drainage may demonstrate only an obstruction of both the pancreatic and common bile ducts, laparotomy is necessary to determine the nature of the obstructing lesion. Undoubtedly, most cases of chronic pancreatitis go unrecognized, but once jaundice occurs and operation is required, the mortality rate is high.

Treatment

If jaundice is present, the patient should be prepared for operation on a regimen similar to that described for other biliary tract lesions complicated by obstructive jaundice (*see* CHOLECYSTITIS; CHOLELITHIASIS). The operative procedure must aim to establish the diagnosis and to restore the flow of

bile into the intestinal tract. Cholecystoenterostomy usually
has been resorted to, but resection of the obstructing pancreatic
tissue may prove more effective. Pancreatic extracts (R 17)
given after each meal may be helpful. Insulin may be necessary
if there is an associated diabetes (q.v.). The intestinal absorption of fat may be aided by the use of a wetting agent,
such as the polyoxyethylene derivative of sorbitan monooleate,
given as 1.5 Gm. doses with each meal (R 131).

GASTROENTERITIS; FOOD POISONING
ACUTE GASTROENTERITIS
(Acute gastroenterocolitis; Acute enteritis)

Acute inflammation of the lining of the stomach and intestine.

Etiology

Acute gastroenteritis may be caused by excessive indulgence
in alcohol, the virus of "intestinal grippe," allergy to certain
ingredients of food and drink, food poisoning (q.v.), drastic
cathartics, salicylates, Atabrine, cinchophen, colchicine, and
the heavy metals—arsenic, lead, mercury, and cadmium. It
may occur in many infectious diseases, especially typhoid fever,
bacillary dysentery, and cholera, or in uremic states and extensive burns.

Symptoms and Signs

The character and severity of the symptoms depend upon the
nature and the dose of the irritant, the duration of its action,
the resistance of the patient and the extent of involvement of
the gastrointestinal tract.

The onset is sudden, with anorexia and nausea followed by
vomiting, abdominal cramps, borborygmi, and diarrhea. If
the diarrhea is intense, burning and tenesmus in the rectum
develop. In very severe cases the discharges may contain blood
and mucus. Malaise and varying degrees of prostration usually
are present. Fever often occurs in acute gastroenteritis of infectious origin. With severe vomiting leukocytosis may reach
20,000 to 25,000. However, in most cases the leukocyte count
is normal. Persistent vomiting and diarrhea may result in
severe dehydration and shock. If the fluid lost by vomiting has
been excessive, alkalosis occurs; if the diarrhea has been more
prominent, acidosis is more likely to develop. In cases where
pronounced dehydration and acid-base imbalance have occurred,
headache and symptoms of muscle and nervous irritability may
be prominent.

The abdomen usually is somewhat distended, with areas of
tenderness more commonly in the lower abdomen than in the
upper quadrants. In severe cases there may be muscle guard-

ing. Intestinal gas often may be palpated. Borborygmi can be heard with the stethoscope, even when there is no diarrhea, an important differential from paralytic ileus.

Diagnosis

A history of the ingestion of a gastrointestinal irritant or of a previous food allergy may be obtained. Eosinophilia suggests allergy or parasitic infection. If the symptoms do not subside within 48 hours, stool examination and culture are indicated. Sigmoidoscopy is helpful in establishing the diagnosis in cases of ulcerative colitis and amebic dysentery. The acute "surgical abdomen" is usually excluded by the history of frequent stools, the low leukocyte count, and the absence of muscle spasm and localization of tenderness. However, diarrhea may occur at times in acute appendicitis and colonic malignancy.

Treatment

The patient should be placed at rest in a bed conveniently located to the bathroom. If this is not feasible, a bedpan or commode should be readily available. Nothing is permitted by mouth as long as nausea and vomiting persist. When they cease, light fluids such as warm tea, albumin, barley or rice water, strained broth, cereal gruel, or bouillon with added salt may be taken. If vomiting persists, I.V. infusions of 5% glucose in isotonic saline should be administered to ward off dehydration, anuria and acid-base imbalance. Blood plasma is indicated in severe cases when shock is impending. Laxatives should not be prescribed if the diarrhea is severe. Vomiting usually can be controlled by sedation with sodium phenobarbital (℞ 68) hypodermically, alone or with scopolamine (℞ 58). Demerol (℞ 75) or an antispasmodic (℞ 59) may be given for severe abdominal cramps. Morphine should be avoided because it increases intestinal muscle tone and also may cause vomiting. When warm liquids are well tolerated, the diet may be increased gradually to include cooked bland cereals, gelatin, jellied consommé, simple puddings, soft-cooked eggs, and other bland foods. If, after 12 or 24 hours, moderate diarrhea persists in the absence of severe systemic symptoms, paregoric (℞ 11, 12) or a prescription containing bismuth, belladonna, and kaolin (℞ 13) may be used.

CHRONIC ENTERITIS

Chronic inflammation of the mucous membrane of the small intestine.

Etiology

A residual inflammation of the small intestine of sufficient severity to produce symptoms occurs very rarely as a sequel to an attack of acute gastroenteritis, especially if the return to coarse foods has been too rapid. Alcoholic addiction, condiments, food roughage, salicylates, arsenic, antimony, lead, cadmium, and the constant use of cathartics may be responsible. Food allergy also may produce chronic enteritis especially when the allergen is a constituent of foods frequently ingested, such as milk, wheat, and egg protein. There are some individuals who have frequent loose stools for years without other evidence of disease and others who develop diarrhea readily whenever they are under emotional strain.

Symptoms and Signs

There usually is anorexia, postprandial nausea, fullness, some relief by belching, abdominal pain and a low grade diarrhea. The stools are free of mucus, pus, or blood. Tenesmus usually is absent. The abdominal pain is not severe and may be experienced in the periumbilical region, or in the upper hypogastrium.

Diagnosis

Diagnosis is made by exclusion. Achlorhydria is common. Roentgenologically, the barium meal arrives in the rectum ½ to 1 hour after its ingestion. Undigested food particles may be recognized in the stools and there may be large amounts of fat present. Regional ileitis, parasitic infection, tuberculosis, chronic amebic and bacillary dysentery, idiopathic ulcerative colitis, Addison's disease, hyperthyroidism, pernicious anemia, chronic pancreatitis, and sprue should be ruled out in all such cases. In a patient who has a chronic metal poisoning, abnormal amounts of a suspected metal may be found in the blood or excreta. The withdrawal of a suspected food allergen from the diet or the administration of an antihistaminic agent, when followed by improvement, is of diagnostic help.

Treatment

The patient should be placed on a low fat, bland diet with small meals, but with interval feedings, as in the 6-feeding bland diet regimen for peptic ulcer (q.v.). Food is to be eaten slowly. Vitamin supplements must be given. In achlorhydric patients, hydrochloric acid (℞ 15) may be tried but can be expected to have little effect except as an appetizer or tonic. In patients whose stools contain excessive amounts of fat and undigested meat fiber, pancreatin (℞ 17), bile salts (℞ 18), and calcium carbonate (℞ 6) to avert the danger of hypocalcemia, must be administered. In patients with chronic low grade diarrhea, folic acid (℞ 103) orally, or crude liver extract (℞ 93) I.M. is worthy of a trial. A preparation containing belladonna, bismuth, and kaolin (℞ 13) may be helpful for patients with small intestine hypermotility. Alcohol should be discontinued by patients who have been taking it regularly. For nervousness, small doses of phenobarbital (℞ 66, 67) are advisable. Suspected food allergens should be eliminated from the diet. If the allergenic substance is very widespread in the diet, an antihistaminic such as Neo-Antergan (℞ 123) should be prescribed.

FOOD INFECTION GASTROENTERITIS

An acute gastroenteritis following the ingestion of food contaminated with certain bacteria.

Etiology

Almost all of the cases are due to infection with the Salmonella group of organisms among which *S. enteritidis* of Gartner, *S. typhimurium*, and *S. paratyphi* A and B are the most common. Rarely, *Esch. coli*, alpha hemolytic streptococci, and *A. aerogenes* have been responsible for outbreaks.

Symptoms and Signs

The incubation period varies from 6 to 48 hours, with the majority of cases occurring about 12 hours after the contaminated food is ingested. The onset is abrupt with headache, chills and fever, muscle aches and prostration, and is accompanied by nausea and vomiting, abdominal cramps and severe diarrhea. In severe cases, the vomitus and rectal discharges may contain blood. Dehydration, acid-base imbalance, anuria, and shock may develop.

The attack usually lasts 24 to 48 hours; it may be so mild as to permit the patient to continue his usual activities. Rarely, it may be so severe as to result in death within 24 hours. The mortality varies from 0.4 to 1.5%.

Diagnosis

The diagnosis usually is easy when the patient is one of a group that became ill at about the same time after eating a certain food, and when the symptoms are typical. Gross examination of the food may reveal no evidence of contamination. Diagnosis is aided by demonstration of the bacteria in the food, or in vomitus, feces, blood, or urine of the patient. The organisms may persist in the stools for 7 to 10 days following infection. Agglutination tests seldom are positive until 6 or 8 days after the onset but are valuable diagnostic aids.

Treatment

Essentially the same as for acute gastroenteritis (q.v.). In severe cases of infectious diarrhea, streptomycin or dihydrostreptomycin may be of value. It should be given orally (℞ 117) or perhaps better by both oral and I.M. (℞ 111, 112) routes. Succinylsulfathiazole (℞ 118) also exerts an antibacterial action on the gram-negative coliform organisms and may be used as an alternative form of therapy.

STAPHYLOCOCCUS TOXIN GASTROENTERITIS

An abrupt and sometimes violent gastrointestinal upset caused by the ingestion of food contaminated with the staphylococcus enterotoxin.

Etiology

The ingestion of a preformed enterotoxin produced by staphylococci growing on a variety of foods, chiefly custards, cream-filled pastry, milk, processed meat, and fish, rather than an enteric infection with the staphylococcus organism, results in the disease. It probably is the most common type of food poisoning. Food handlers with staphylococcic skin infections are mainly responsible for its spread.

Symptoms and Signs

The incubation period usually is from 2 to 4 hours after the ingestion of food containing enterotoxin. The onset is abrupt with nausea, vomiting, abdominal cramps, diarrhea, and occasionally headache and fever. In severe cases, acid-base imbalance, prostration and shock may ensue. Very occasionally blood and mucus may be present in the stools. The attack is short in duration, most often lasting only 3 to 6 hours, with complete recovery. Fatalities are rare.

Diagnosis

The diagnosis is based on sudden onset after the eating of infected food, the patient's usually being one of a number of similarly affected individuals; the brevity of the symptoms; and the rapidity of recovery. Confirmatory evidence includes the isolation of staphylococci from suspected food, and the demonstration of the enterotoxin-producing ability of the organisms by the injection of culture filtrates into laboratory animals.

Treatment

The same as for gastroenteritis (q.v.).

BOTULISM

An acute intoxication manifested by neuromuscular disturbances, following the ingestion of food containing a toxin elaborated by Clostridium botulinum.

Etiology

The causative agent is one of several types of exotoxin elaborated by the sporulating, anaerobic bacillus, *Cl. botulinum*. This common soil bacillus may be present in the straw sometimes used as packing around the jars in which the housewife puts up vegetables and fruits. Poisoning in man is usually caused by toxin of type A or B, rarely by that of type E. The disease always is caused by the ingestion of improperly preserved food (today, usually a home-canned product), in which the toxin has been produced during the growth of the causative organism. The spores of *Cl. botulinum* are highly resistant to heat; in water, they require exposure for 5 hours at 212° F., or for 6 minutes at 248° F. to ensure their death. The toxins, however, are readily destroyed by heat; the cooking of fresh food at 176° F. for 30 minutes is a safeguard against botulism. In the United States, the preserved foods wherein the toxin is most commonly found are string beans, corn, spinach, olives, beets, asparagus, sea food, pork products, and beef. The disease occurs throughout the United States and has its highest incidence in California. In the West, type A intoxications predominate, whereas those due to type B toxin are more common in the Mississippi Valley and Atlantic Coast regions.

Symptoms and Signs

The onset of symptoms is abrupt, usually developing from 18 to 36 hours after ingestion of the toxin, though the incubation period may vary from 4 hours to 8 days. Following a short period of lassitude and fatigue, visual disturbances develop. These may include diplopia, diminution of visual acuity, blepharoptosis, loss of accommodation, and diminution or total loss of pupillary light reflex. In the typical case of botulism, vomiting and diarrhea are absent; these symptoms occur, however, in approximately one-third of the cases, and probably result from the ingestion of spoiled food rather than from botulinus toxin. After the onset of visual disorders, symptoms of bulbar paresis follow and include dysarthria, dysphagia, and nasal regurgitation. Difficulty in swallowing not uncommonly leads to aspiration pneumonia. The muscles of the extremities and trunk become weak. The disease is marked by the general absence of sensory disturbances, and the sensorium characteristically remains clear until shortly before death. Unless intercurrent infection develops, the temperature remains normal or subnormal. Routine studies of blood and urine reveal no pathognomonic changes. The spinal fluid usually is normal.

Diagnosis

The diagnosis of an isolated case of botulism is suggested only by the pattern of neuromuscular disturbances. The simultaneous occurrence of 2 or more cases following ingestion of the same meal makes the diagnosis less difficult. Confirmation of the diagnosis is obtained by the demonstration of botulinus toxin or of *Cl. botulinum* in suspected food, and occasionally by the demonstration of toxin in the circulating blood. Suggestive confirmatory evidence may be derived from the recovery of *Cl. botulinum* from vomitus and feces during life or from intestinal contents and, rarely, from viscera at autopsy. Further diagnostic aid may be gained from observing the development of botulism in pets that have eaten the same contaminated food.

Botulism may be confused at times with poliomyelitis, the several virus encephalitides, C.N.S. syphilis, myasthenia gravis, and poisoning due to curare or the belladonna alkaloids.

Prognosis

The mortality from botulism may be as high as 65%. Most of the fatal cases die between the 2nd and 9th days following the ingestion of the toxin, though deaths during the 1st and as late as the 16th day have been reported. Death usually results from respiratory paralysis or from secondary bronchopneumonia. In those who survive, the disease usually reaches its height in the first 10 days of illness. Recovery is characteristically very slow, and residual weakness of the ocular muscles may persist for many months. There are, however, no permanent sequelae.

Prophylaxis

Prophylaxis depends on proper home canning and adequate heating of food before serving. Food showing any evidence of spoilage should be discarded.

Treatment

If possible, the patient should be cared for in a hospital during the acute phase of botulism. Adequate facilities for care of so serious an illness are difficult to provide in the home.

Specific therapy: Although botulinus toxins are excellent antigens and give rise to potent antiserums, the use of such antiserums has been disappointing. Once symptoms have developed, it is doubtful if antiserum has any effect on toxin already "fixed" by the tissues. However, because of the possibility of the continued presence of circulating toxin, polyvalent antiserum should be administered. A dose of 10,000 to 20,000 units each of types A and B antiserum (℞ 127) should be given I.V. only after a negative history of allergy to horse serum has been elicited and the conjunctival and skin tests reveal no hypersensitivity. Epinephrine must be on hand at the time of injection for use in the event of an anaphylactic reaction.

The most important use of botulinus antiserum is in the protection of those exposed to contaminated food who have not yet developed symptoms of botulism. All persons exposed should immediately be treated with 10,000 u. each of types A and B antiserum following the appropriate tests for sensitivity to the antiserum. Such a measure may be lifesaving.

Supportive therapy: Supportive measures are most important in the treatment of botulism. The patient should be kept in a darkened room and denied all visitors save those immediately concerned with his care. To relieve anxiety and to provide sedation, chloral hydrate is a highly satisfactory drug and may be given orally (℞ 70) or rectally (℞ 71). Morphine should be avoided because of its depressant effect upon the already enfeebled respiration. One of the barbiturates (℞ 68, 69) may safely be employed. Oral medication and feeding must be carried out with caution because of the danger of aspiration, and the physician must be prepared to use rectal or parenteral routes of administration when dysphagia develops. It may be necessary to feed the patient I.V. for a number of days. The substances given in 24 hours should include water 2,500 to 3,500 cc., glucose 100 to 150 Gm., salt 8 to 16 Gm., and amino acids or protein hydrolysate 50 to 100 Gm. (℞ 99, 100). An attempt should be made to maintain a urinary output of at least 800 cc./day. If the patient has difficulty in swallowing his oropharyngeal secretions, they must be removed by suction at frequent intervals. The accumulation of such secretions may result in aspiration and be followed by pneumonia. If the patient is completely unable to swallow, tracheotomy may prove lifesaving by providing an adequate air passage and preventing further aspiration from the pharynx. If cyanosis develops from failing respiration or from pneumonia, oxygen can be administered readily by catheter through the tracheotomy tube. If respiratory paralysis seems impending, the patient should be placed in a respirator. To prevent atelectasis, the patient should be turned frequently and not allowed to lie on his back for extended periods. Penicillin (℞ 109, 110) in doses of 50,000 u. every 3 hours I.M. or 300,000 u. every 12 hours should be given prophylactically. Should aspiration pneumonia develop, it must be treated on the basis of the bacteriology of the sputum.

NONBACTERIAL FOOD POISONING

Poisoning due to ingestion of certain plants and animals containing a naturally occurring poison.

Etiology

Nonbacterial food poisoning can occur following the ingestion of (1) certain species of mushrooms such as *Amanita muscaria*, which contains the toxic alkaloid muscarine, and *Amanita phalloides*, which contains phalloidin or other toxins; (2) immature or sprouting potatoes, the active poison of which is solanin, though some of the reported outbreaks have undoubtedly been due to bacterial contamination; (3) mussels, at certain unpredictable times of the year; (4) grain, especially rye, which has become contaminated with the ergot fungus, *Claviceps purpurea*—ergot contains a number of active principles including ergotoxin, tyramine and ergamin (histamine); (5) fruits sprayed with salts of lead or arsenic and food stored in cadmium-lined containers. This type of food poisoning is referred to in the section on chronic gastroenteritis (q.v.).

Symptoms and Signs

(1) **Mushroom poisoning:** In muscarine poisoning due to *A. muscaria* the symptoms come on within a few minutes to 2 hours after ingestion. They consist of lacrimation, salivation, sweating, miosis, vomiting, abdominal cramps, diarrhea, thirst, vertigo, confusion, collapse, coma, and occasional convulsions. In poisoning due to ingestion of *A. phalloides*, the symptoms occur after 6 to 15 hours and are heralded by the sudden onset of abdominal pain, nausea, vomiting, and diarrhea. The stools and vomitus are often blood streaked. Dehydration and thirst

may become extreme. Jaundice due to liver damage follows in 2 or 3 days. Oliguria and anuria may develop. Symptoms resulting from C.N.S. damage usually are present. The physical signs include jaundice, palpably enlarged and tender liver, diminished tendon reflexes, hypotension, tachycardia, and a subnormal temperature. A remission of symptoms may occur but the eventual mortality is about 50%.

(2) Immature or sprouting potato poisoning: In poisoning due to the ingestion of immature or sprouting potatoes containing large amounts of solanin, there occur within a few hours, nausea, vomiting, abdominal cramps, diarrhea, mydriasis, vertigo, a sense of constriction in the throat, and prostration. The symptoms only rarely are severe, and practically all of the victims recover. Infrequently, jaundice and collapse may occur.

(3) Mussel poisoning: The first symptoms come on 5 to 30 minutes after ingestion of the mussel and consist of a numbness and prickling about the mouth. Nausea, vomiting, and abdominal cramps are followed by muscle weakness and peripheral paralysis. Death may occur as a result of respiratory failure.

(4) Ergot poisoning: Two types of symptoms may be seen, those referable to the circulatory system and those referable to the C.N.S. Circulatory symptoms usually are the first to become evident. Gangrene, due to vasoconstriction and thrombosis secondary to blood vessel intima damage, usually starts in the toes but also may appear in the fingers. Anginal pain, tachycardia, bradycardia, and elevation or lowering of the blood pressure may occur. Other symptoms which may appear include headache, nausea, vomiting, and diarrhea. In the convulsive form, the first symptoms are depression, weakness, drowsiness, often headache and vertigo, painful cramps in the extremities and pruritus. Muscle pains and cramps are followed by spasms which may continue for a few hours to several days. In severe cases, epileptiform convulsions and hemiplegia may occur. There may be tabetic manifestations and a fixed miosis.

(5) Metal contaminants: The symptoms due to ingestion of arsenic, lead, and cadmium are described in other sections. The gastrointestinal symptoms are referred to in the section on chronic gastroenteritis.

Diagnosis

The diagnosis is usually based on the clinical picture but especially on the history of ingestion of the offending agent. A careful scrutiny of the foods eaten should always be made as bacterial food poisoning may be confused with the poisoning due to foods containing natural poisons.

Treatment

General: The patient should be placed at absolute bed rest. If there has been violent vomiting or diarrhea or if the symptoms come on several hours after the food has been ingested, there is little to be gained by lavaging the stomach or administering an emetic as the offending agent has left the stomach. However, when indicated, the bulk of the poison should be removed from the digestive tract by gastric lavage. An emetic (℞ 19, 20) or saline cathartic (℞ 24) should be considered sufficient only in mild cases and never in mushroom or mussel poisoning. If nausea and vomiting persist, fluids containing salt and glucose should be administered parenterally to combat dehydration and changes in acid-base balance. Plasma or blood is indicated if shock threatens. Demerol (℞ 75) should be given for pain.

Specific: In poisoning due to the ingestion of muscarine, atropine (℞ 57) is a specific antagonist of the muscarine-like overstimulation of the parasympathetic nervous system. It should be given in doses of 1 mg. repeated every 1 to 2 hours subcut. or I.V. until the symptoms are controlled. In poisoning due to phalloidin a high protein diet supplemented by the I.V. administration of 10% glucose in saline and I.V. protein hydrolysate or amino acids mixture is indicated to help prevent severe liver damage. In the treatment of ergotism, arterial spasm may be combated by the use of amyl nitrite (℞ 60) by inhalation, nitroglycerin (℞ 61) or papaverine (℞ 62). An anticonvulsive agent (℞ 68) should be used when indicated. In poisoning due to arsenic, mercury, or cadmium (q.v.), BAL (2,3-dimercaptopropanol) (℞ 128) should be administered.

REGIONAL ENTERITIS

(Terminal ileitis; Granulomatous jejunoileitis; Crohn's disease)

A nonspecific granulomatous and inflammatory disease which usually affects the lower ileum but may involve other parts of the intestine. It is most frequent in young persons between 18 and 30, and more common in males than in females.

Etiology and Pathology

The etiology is unknown. The mucosa, all the structures of the intestinal wall, the adjacent mesentery, and the mesenteric glands are involved, first by edema, hyperemia and cellular infiltration, later by extensive fibrosis and localized abscesses. The mucosa bears shallow ulcerations and often develops a "cobblestone" appearance. Giant cells and epithelioid tubercles, such as are found in sarcoid, frequently appear in the intestinal mesenteric glands; but the tubercle bacillus cannot be isolated. The whole process renders the intestine thickened, indurated, stenosed, and inelastic.

The gross distribution of the lesions is variable: usually 8 to 12 inches of the terminal ileum is involved. The disease, however, may encompass almost all of the small bowel, sometimes extending up by direct continuity, at other times forming "skip areas" by leaving normal bowel between scattered patches of diseased tissue. Occasionally, skip areas appear in the large bowel.

Symptoms and Signs

The character of the symptoms depends on the extent and the chronicity of the process. An acute inflammatory process located in the ileocecal region mimics acute appendicitis and can hardly be differentiated before operation. In some cases, diarrhea may precede the acute attack, but this cannot be relied upon as pathognomonic of acute ileitis. In the chronic localized form of the disease, which is the one most commonly seen, there is diarrhea with cramping midabdominal pains and mild intermittent fever; often anorexia, loss of weight, and moderate malaise. As the enteric canal becomes more obliterated by the granulomatous process, symptoms of partial small-intestinal obstruction may supervene. In the chronic diffuse form, symptoms of obstruction are subordinate, but evidence of inflammation and malnutrition may be striking. Thus, some patients may exhibit constant low fever with recurrent exacerbations mounting up to 103° or 105° F. and accompanied by dull, diffuse abdominal pain. Others may show weight loss, hypoproteinemia, and vitamin deficiencies.

In early or inactive cases, the physical findings may be minimal. In active cases, abdominal tenderness, voluntary resistance, and masses are found, usually in the right lower quadrant. The mass consists of inflamed bowel with adherent mesentery and neighboring intestinal loops. It is large and firm, but not hard, and presents an ill-defined outline. It may later be added to by internal fistulous tracts and walled-off peritoneal abscesses. External fistulas from the inflamed ileum as well as localized anorectal fistulas sometimes occur.

Diagnosis

Diagnosis is established by means of X-ray. A barium enema that regurgitates through the ileocecal valve may suffice to demonstrate terminal ileitis, but usually an hourly study of the progress of a barium meal, or a "small-intestinal enema" given by duodenal tube, is necessary. Regional enteritis must be differentiated from the following (q.v.): functional gastrointestinal disorders, ulcerative colitis, tuberculous enterocolitis, sprue, Hodgkin's disease, and intestinal neoplasms. Functional disorders seldom manifest the symptoms which occur, singly or combined, in regional enteritis; i.e., weight loss, fever, hypochromic anemia, leukocytosis, elevated E.S.R., and occult blood in the stools. Ulcerative colitis is diagnosed by the proctoscopic and X-ray findings, and by the presence of gross pus and blood in the stools. Gastrointestinal tuberculosis (q.v.) is unusual in an adult with normal lungs.

Treatment

Early and acute cases may subside spontaneously. Chronic cases, however, progress slowly but steadily unless arrested by surgical means. Either resection of the involved bowel or an operation which by-passes the diseased areas is satisfactory. Unless all the involved intestine is resected or by-passed, however, the disease will be likely to recur. The rate of recurrence for all cases appears to be from 12 to 30%.

Medical management may be palliative, but it rarely cures the well established cases. Bed rest, a low residue diet (*see* Diets), supplemental vitamins, blood transfusions, liver injections (℞ 93), and antispasmodics (℞ 56, 57, 59) may produce temporary improvement, but relapses are almost invariable once the patient resumes his normal activities. The intestinal absorption of dietary fats and of oil-soluble vitamins may be aided by the use of a wetting agent, such as the polyoxyethylene derivative of sorbitan monooleate (℞ 131), given as 1.5 Gm. doses with each meal.

When inflammatory symptoms predominate, sulfadiazine (℞ 108) usually will reduce the fever. For the average case, succinylsulfathiazole (℞ 118) or phthalylsulfathiazole (℞ 119) is recommended, but the action of these drugs is confined to the intestinal lumen. Parenteral penicillin (℞ 109, 110) and streptomycin (℞ 111) or dihydrostreptomycin (℞ 112) are indicated if a generalized peritoneal infection is feared or a localized infection appears to be spreading. The efficacy of combined parenteral and oral streptomycin or dihydrostreptomycin (℞ 111, 112, 117) requires further evaluation as does the current investigation of the usefulness of cortisone or ACTH.

APPENDICITIS

Inflammation of the vermiform appendix.

Etiology and Pathology

Appendicitis usually is preceded by inadequate emptying of the appendix due to obstruction, stenosis, atonia, or kinking of the organ. Inflammation results from invasion of the appendiceal wall by any of the many bacteria present in the intestine. The appendix becomes edematous, and the blood supply is reduced. With extension of the infection to the peritoneal surface, the appendix is covered with a yellowish, fibrinous exudate.

Finally, gangrene may occur, followed by perforation. Rupture of the appendix permits dissemination of fecal matter into the peritoneal cavity and generalized peritonitis (q.v.) may result. If the surrounding loops of bowel or omentum, or both, become adherent to the inflamed appendix the purulent material is walled in as a localized abscess about the site of perforation.

Symptoms and Signs

Typically, appendicitis is heralded by pain in the umbilical or epigastric regions, commonly accompanied by anorexia, nausea and vomiting, but usually not by diarrhea (except, of course, when the patient has injudiciously been given a cathartic). After several hours this referred pain shifts to the right lower quadrant, and is continuous, dull or severe, accentuated by coughing, sneezing, or jarring.

The anterior abdominal wall may be splinted involuntarily and boardlike on palpation. More often there is a subtle increase in the resistance of the right rectus muscle as compared with the left. Localized tenderness in the right lower quadrant, usually at McBurney's point, is the most common and dependable physical sign. Direct rebound tenderness in the right lower quadrant, or referred from other areas to the right lower quadrant, is frequently elicited. On rectal or vaginal palpation, right lower quadrant tenderness may be noted. In thin individuals a local abdominal tumor occasionally can be palpated. Other possible physical findings are hyperesthesia of the overlying skin on light stroking and pain on abduction (obturator sign) or hyperextension (psoas sign) of the right thigh.

Acute appendicitis is usually associated with mild fever, 99° to 102° F., and a leukocytosis of 10,000 to 16,000, chiefly polynuclear; however, both temperature and white blood count may be normal. Further elevations in temperature and white count are often indicative of gangrene, rupture, spreading peritonitis, or some other clinical condition. The physician should not be deceived by an apparent diminution in local symptoms, since this often accompanies gangrene and diffuse peritonitis ("soft belly peritonitis").

Since the appendix may be located in almost any portion of the abdominal cavity, findings may vary greatly from those described above. A retrocecal or retroperitoneal appendix will cause minimal muscle guarding and tenderness. An appendix situated low in the pelvic cavity may cause tenderness only on rectal or vaginal examination. Because of congenital maldevelopment the appendix may be situated subjacent to the liver, or on the left side, and give symptoms referable to these areas.

Diagnosis

A disease frequently confused with appendicitis is mesenteric lymphadenitis (q.v.). Such an error is easily understood, because absolute differentiation often is impossible, as is the case with Meckel's diverticulitis (q.v.). Pelvic inflammatory disease (see GONORRHEA) also is commonly mistaken for acute appendicitis but may be ruled out by a careful review of the history and a pelvic examination. Occasionally, mittelschmerz (pain secondary to ovulation) or an ovarian cyst may have to be considered in diagnosis.

Gastroenteritis (q.v.) may be differentiated from appendicitis by the increased peristalsis productive of vomiting and diarrhea that is present; peristalsis in appendicitis is reduced.

Among the many other entities that may be confused with appendicitis are hemorrhagic pancreatitis, regional ileitis, strangulated hernia, volvulus, intussusception, nephrolithiasis, pyelitis, Dietl's crisis, typhoid fever, pneumonia, and diaphragmatic pleurisy (see ABDOMINAL PAIN). The administration of atropine sulfate (℞ 57) often is helpful in differential diagnosis, since conditions due to smooth muscle spasm are relieved by it, whereas the pain of appendicitis is not.

Prognosis

The over-all mortality rate for adequately supervised early appendicitis is very low, in some hospitals less than 1%. Once the disease process has progressed to rupture and diffuse peritonitis, the outlook is graver. Patients who have received an enema or a purgative are likely to develop peritonitis early.

Treatment

Early operation is imperative even when the diagnosis is in doubt, since it is safer to operate than to permit an atypical inflammatory process to progress on to gangrene, rupture, and peritonitis. Appendectomy should be preceded and followed by administration of penicillin (℞ 109, 110), with streptomycin (℞ 111), dihydrostreptomycin (℞ 112), aureomycin (℞ 113), or Chloromycetin (℞ 114). In instances of widespread peritonitis (q.v.) with evidence of peripheral vascular collapse, greatly elevated temperature, high pulse rate, and a very toxic appearance, operation should be postponed. Such a patient should receive massive antibiotic therapy to control both grampositive and gram-negative pathogens. Sulfonamide therapy (℞ 107) may be given in addition or as an alternative. Nothing should be given by mouth. Thirst may be quenched by rinsing the mouth with cold water. The patient should be kept at absolute bed rest. Demerol (℞ 75) may be used for sedation. Supportive therapy should include I.V. glucose, saline, and liberal blood transfusions. The administration of oxygen often is helpful, as is suction drainage by either a Levin or a Miller-Abbot tube (see CLIN. PROC.).

Continuation of fever for more than 7 days usually indicates a localization of the purulent process or an infectious process that will not respond to the combination of agents used. Any such localized abscess should be drained. Often, an abdominal abscess may drain spontaneously into the intestinal tract or vagina or may resolve completely. Occasionally, the abscess drains into the perinephric tissues, forming a perinephric abscess and causing intermittent fever, pain, and tenderness in the flank. Once conservative treatment has accomplished its purpose, appendectomy can be done at a later date as an elective operation.

It should be emphasized that conservative therapy may be

indicated for adults but usually not for children since they do poorly on such a regimen. Infants and children are best operated upon early.

At the time of operation, adequate drainage should be instituted if the peritoneal cavity is contaminated. It has been recommended by some that penicillin (℞ 115) and streptomycin (℞ 116) be instilled into the areas involved.

PERITONITIS

Inflammation, either acute or chronic, of the serous membrane that lines the abdominal cavity and covers its viscera.

Etiology

Infectious agents or foreign matter within the peritoneal cavity are responsible for the inflammatory process. Practically all pathogens that gain entrance multiply rapidly, since the peritoneum and the fluid elaborated by it for lubricative purposes are ideal culture media. The organisms most commonly encountered are the gram-negative coliform bacteria, which are normal inhabitants of the gastrointestinal tract.

The ways in which microorganisms may reach the peritoneum and cause infection include: (1) Gastrointestinal tract inflammation or perforation as a result of appendicitis, peptic ulcer, Meckel's diverticulitis, diverticulitis of the colon, bowel neoplasm, volvulus, intussusception, cholecystitis, typhoid fever, bacillary dysentery, and infection with intestinal parasites; (2) the female genital tract, as a means for allowing the entrance of gonococci, pneumococci, streptococci and tubercle bacilli; (3) abdominal wall penetration by bullet, knife, or similar object; (4) inflammation of contiguous organs, e.g., the kidney and pancreas; (5) the blood or lymphatic systems, especially as avenues for the spread of *Myco. tuberculosis*, *Str. hemolyticus*, and pneumococci.

Any of these routes also may give access to irritant foreign matter. The intestinal contents may soil the peritoneum as a result of a perforated ulcer or a ruptured viscus. The more common foreign materials which cause irritation of the peritoneum when in contact with it are bile from a ruptured gallbladder, bloody fluid from an ectopic pregnancy, and fluid from a ruptured cystic ovary.

Pathology

Initially, the peritoneal surface loses its transparent and glistening appearance, becomes dull, opaque and injected, and fibrin is laid down. An exudate is produced which is serofibrinous at first and later becomes purulent. Fluid accumulates in dependent pockets. With spread of the peritoneal reaction, coils of intestine and the omentum may be glued together by the exudate produced. Localization of the process often occurs, with abscess formation.

Symptoms and Signs

Clinical manifestations are highly variable since they depend on the type of etiologic agent, the pathologic process that develops, and the presence or absence of other disorders. With a localized peritonitis, such as may occur in appendicitis (q.v.), the patient complains of severe pain, usually at the site of the lesion. Local tenderness may be elicited. Progression of the inflammatory process is accompanied by rising temperature and pulse, chills, leukocytosis of 10,000 to 50,000, evidence of shock, vomiting, progressive constipation, and hiccups. Any or all of these symptoms may be encountered in the localized form but are more frequent in generalized peritoneal infections. In the early stages, hyperperistalsis due to irritation of the bowel may cause vomiting and diarrhea. Later, intestinal paresis supervenes and results in abdominal distention. When the peritonitis is due to perforation of a hollow viscus, signs of the presence of free fluid and gas may be elicited. Hiccups may indicate involvement of the diaphragmatic peritoneum.

To avoid movement and pressure, the abdominal musculature is involuntarily splinted, the patient draws up his thighs and hunches his shoulders, and his respiration becomes shallow. Abdominal wall rigidity is associated with direct and rebound tenderness. Rectal and vaginal examination may aid in confirming the localized tenderness and rigidity noted on abdominal palpation. In severe peritoneal inflammation the patient exhibits great anxiety, as evidenced by the characteristic "hippocratic facies."

As mentioned previously the clinical manifestations vary widely. In those cases in which large quantities of free fluid are produced, pain and other symptoms may shortly disappear, or be absent from the beginning. The latter often is the case in patients who are debilitated and in whom a deceptive "soft belly" peritonitis is present. The disappearance of pain often may be incorrectly interpreted as a sign of improvement, when it actually indicates further progression of the disease. Increased toxemia and tachycardia are usually noted at this time and confirm the gravity of the situation. Ascites often develops to such degree that mechanical distress is produced within the abdominal and thoracic cavities.

Chronic peritonitis may be responsible for any combination of the above symptoms, but the symptoms usually are milder and of longer duration than in the acute form. Fibrous adhesions caused by chronic peritonitis may result in intestinal obstruction (q.v.), with characteristic symptoms.

Diagnosis

Because peritonitis so often occurs as a complication, its presence usually is confirmed after determination of the primary disorder. Occasionally, differentiation must be made between peritonitis and renal colic, lead colic, pneumonia, rheumatic fever, twisted ovarian pedicle, and gastric tabes.

Procedures that may aid in evaluating peritoneal inflammation are determination of leukocyte count and E.S.R., abdominal paracentesis, roentgenography, peritoneoscopy, and exploratory laparotomy. The degree of elevation of white count and E.S.R. often is indicative of the severity of the inflammation, except in rapidly fulminating cases where very little elevation may have developed. Abdominal paracentesis may be used to reduce intra-abdominal pressure and also to obtain a specimen of the exudate for isolation of a causative organism. When the peritonitis is the result of intestinal perforation, radiographic examination usually will reveal the presence of gas free in the peritoneal cavity. Peritoneoscopy or laparotomy permits direct examination and evaluation of the peritoneal inflammation and also, in some cases, of the primary disorder.

Course and Prognosis

Recovery usually ensues when peritonitis remains localized. Once the disease process has progressed beyond the local area, the prognosis should be guarded and recovery depends on the adequacy of therapy, the resistance of the patient, and the virulence of the pathogen. If death occurs, it usually is due to toxemia and further complications such as pneumonia or intestinal obstruction. Residual abscesses frequently form following the acute phase of peritonitis. These pockets of suppuration usually are found in the iliac fossa, the pelvis, or the subphrenic region and either are slowly absorbed or, if no drainage is established, rupture into contiguous hollow organs. They may exist without producing symptoms or may be responsible for chills, fever and leukocytosis. The accumulation of pus may be identified by X-ray examination and confirmatory needling.

Prophylaxis and Treatment

Of great importance is the early and adequate treatment of lesions such as appendicitis, female pelvic infections, peptic ulcer, intestinal obstruction, cholecystitis, and carcinoma, which with unchecked progression are usually complicated by peritonitis. Preoperative and postoperative administration of antibacterial agents has done much to lower the incidence of peritonitis as a complication of abdominal surgery (see SULFONAMIDE THERAPY; ANTIBIOTIC THERAPY; PREOPERATIVE AND POSTOPERATIVE ROUTINE).

Removal of the focus of infection, drainage of the site, if necessary, and the administration of chemotherapeutic agents until the condition is well under control are the essential measures in treatment. Use of penicillin (℞ 109, 110) and sulfadiazine (℞ 107, 108) in combination is highly effective in controlling peritonitis arising from the gastrointestinal and female genital tracts, since the infection is nearly always a mixed one. Pneumococcic and streptococcic peritonitis also may be benefited by these drugs. Streptomycin (℞ 111), dihydrostreptomycin (℞ 112), aureomycin (℞ 113), or Chloromycetin (℞ 114) may be given in addition to the penicillin-sulfonamide combination until the causative organism has been isolated. Such a combination will adequately cover the bacterial spectrum, but it should not be continued injudiciously as "shotgun" therapy. Some physicians advocate the daily instillation of penicillin (℞ 115) and streptomycin (℞ 116) into a draining abscess cavity, claiming that a higher concentration of the drug is thus obtained in the area of the infection. Tuberculous peritonitis often may be adequately controlled by streptomycin therapy (*see* TUBERCULOSIS, GASTROINTESTINAL).

Bed rest and supportive measures are essential in the treatment of peritonitis. The intestinal tract should be taxed as little as possible, i.e., nothing should be given by mouth. Gaseous distention may be relieved by use of a rectal tube and Wangensteen suction (*see* CLIN. PROC.). Fluid and food requirements should be supplied by the parenteral administration of 5% dextrose solution, isotonic sodium chloride solution, or a solution of amino acids. Transfusions of blood or plasma may be helpful. Pain may be controlled by hypodermic injection of an analgesic such as codeine (℞ 77), Demerol (℞ 75), morphine (℞ 74) or methadone (℞ 73) once the diagnosis has been established, but analgesics should not be given beforehand since they may mask important signs and symptoms.

COLITIS

Two widely differing forms of colitis will be discussed: **chronic ulcerative colitis,** a serious and often fatal disease; and **mucous colitis,** or "irritable colon," a relatively innocuous functional disorder.

CHRONIC ULCERATIVE COLITIS

A chronic, nonspecific, inflammatory and ulcerative disease of the colon, accompanied by systemic symptoms and characterized by remissions and relapses.

Etiology

Although the etiology is unknown, the disease has been attributed variously to infection with streptococcus (the diplostreptococcus of Bargen), dysentery bacilli, or *Bacterium necrophorum*; to psychogenic disorders, in which nervous stimuli induce spasms which damage the colonic tissue and thus permit bacterial invasion; and to an allergic reaction of the bowel to ingested allergens.

Pathology

Ulcerative colitis begins with hyperemia, edema, thrombi, and intramural hemorrhages in the submucosa and mucosa of the colon. The mucosa appears red and shiny; even slight trauma may cause bleeding into the bowel. Subsequently, cellular infiltration with polymorphonuclear leukocytes takes place, and minute abscesses form directly under the mucosa. Proctoscopic examination shows a finely granular mucosa and the tiny abscesses appear as yellowish spots. Soon the mucosa overlying the abscesses and hemorrhages breaks down to form a red, spongy surface dotted with myriads of tiny ulcerations oozing blood and pus. As the mucosa becomes progressively involved, the inflammatory and hemorrhagic processes also extend into and destroy the muscular coats of the bowel.

Arrest or healing may occur at any stage, but even in mild cases, mucosal structure does not return to normal; residual scar tissue gives it a granular, "pockmarked" appearance and renders it so friable that it bleeds readily. After severe attacks, the destroyed mucosa and musculature are extensively replaced by fibrous tissue, which, as it contracts, forms crevices and pseudopolyps giving a rough cobblestone appearance to the bowel lining. At the same time, fibrosis of the musculature causes thickening of the bowel wall with loss of elasticity and contractility, and narrowing of the lumen. A reactivation of the colitis in such an altered bowel may lead to the formation of large, irregular mucosal ulcerations.

The usual case of chronic ulcerative colitis begins in the rectosigmoid area and, if not controlled, extends upward, eventually to involve the whole colon and sometimes even the terminal ileum. Two other varieties of ulcerative colitis are recognized: (1) a diffuse form which appears to attack most of the large bowel simultaneously and is characterized by watery and purulent rather than by bloody discharges; and (2) a regional or segmental form, where a granulomatous, stenosing inflammation is sharply confined to one, or occasionally several, local areas of the colon.

Symptoms and Signs

Ulcerative colitis may occur at any age, but most frequently it attacks young adults of either sex during the 2nd to 4th decades of life. Onset may be acute and fulminant, but more often is insidious and slow, beginning with an increased urgency to move the bowels, mild lower abdominal cramps, or the appearance of bloody mucus in the stools. If the process extends upward, the stools become looser, and eventually the patient may have 10 to 20 bowel movements daily, often associated with severe cramps and distressing rectal tenesmus, from which there is no respite at night. The stools may contain watery feces mixed with pus, blood, and mucus, but characteristically consist almost entirely of blood and pus. Systemic symptoms at onset are anorexia, moderate malaise, and mild evening temperature. Extension of the inflammatory process is marked by a fluctuating, often high, fever, some leukocytosis, severe anorexia with nausea and vomiting, anemia, and rapid inanition.

When the ulcerative process is confined to the rectosigmoid, the feces may be normal, or even hard and dry. Between bowel movements, however, there are rectal discharges of mucus, grossly loaded with red and white blood cells. Systemic symptoms are mild or absent.

In the fulminant type, the patient is suddenly seized by violent diarrhea, severe cramps, high fever, and profound toxemia. The stools are watery and contain foul fecal matter mixed with pus. Gross blood often is present.

Physical signs are relatively few. In addition to the systemic evidences of infection, abdominal tenderness may be present, particularly in both lower quadrants. In severe cases, the abdomen is distended and tympanitic. On rectal examination, the mucosa feels soft and velvety.

Complications

Local complications include hemorrhoids, anal fissures and fistulas, perirectal abscess, perforation with peritonitis, thickening and shortening of the colon with stenotic areas leading to obstruction, or general rigidity preventing normal bowel function even when the colitis is quiescent, and pseudopolyp formation with malignant degeneration. Systemic complications in addition to weakness, anorexia, and weight loss include hypochromic anemia, hypoproteinemia, nutritional deficiencies, pyoderma, arthritis, stomatitis, erythema nodosum, endocarditis, hepatitis, splenomegaly, and clubbing of fingers. Children are retarded in growth and manifest sexual immaturity.

Diagnosis

Diagnosis of chronic ulcerative colitis can be established and confirmed by proctosigmoidoscopy and, except in early cases, by barium enema. Radiography reveals a shortened, spastic colon with absent haustral markings. In most instances, however, the history and an adequate stool examination suffice. The finding, by gross and microscopic examination, of large numbers of red and white blood cells in the rectal discharges rules out functional disorders such as "irritable colon" (mucous colitis). Large amounts of pus are uncommon in amebic colitis; nevertheless, this disease should be excluded by careful examination of fresh and warm stool specimens for motile *E. histolytica*. If amebiasis cannot be excluded, a course of antiamebic therapy (q.v.) may be tried as a therapeutic test. Bacillary dysentery is usually a self-limited disease which is identified by stool culture and examination of the blood for specific antibodies. Cancer of the bowel usually occurs in older age groups, does not cause much fever, and rarely leads to purulent rectal discharges, but proctoscopic and radiologic examinations are needed to rule out this disease. Tuberculous enterocolitis (q.v.) producing rectal discharges of blood and pus is extremely unlikely except in a few patients with advanced pulmonary tuberculosis.

Prognosis

The patient may succumb to a rapidly progressive initial attack, the immediate cause of death being an exsanguinating hemorrhage from a colonic ulcer or from perforation of the colon with peritonitis, or general debility and toxemia with a terminal complication such as bronchopneumonia.

More often ulcerative colitis is a disease of remissions and exacerbations. Such repeated attacks incapacitate the patient and render him a partial or complete invalid.

Treatment

Prime objectives in treating ulcerative colitis are to support the patient's strength and nutrition so that his own defense mechanisms may combat the disease, and to rest the bowel as much as possible.

Supportive: Strict bed rest, liberal fluid intake, and a low residue diet, with all substances that might irritate or stimulate the bowel eliminated (see DIETS) are indicated. Efforts should be made to maintain a high caloric intake, and to this end medications should be given after meals. In general, 3 or 4 daily feedings permit the highest caloric intake. Appetizing natural food is better than highly concentrated food mixtures fortified with powdered milk, protein digests, or yeast preparations. Protein digests to be given by mouth are used only if adequate nitrogen balance cannot be maintained otherwise (see PROTEIN DEFICIENCY). In general, however, such concentrated nutrients may stimulate intestinal activity and induce nausea and anorexia. If the patient cannot eat or drink fluids, nutriments and vitamins should be given parenterally.

Vitamin B complex should be provided by I.M. injections of crude liver extract (℞ 93), with additional vitamins, particularly vitamin K (℞ 105), by mouth. Iron (℞ 95 to 98) to combat anemia can be used in quiescent or mild cases, but it may be poorly tolerated.

In all patients seriously ill with ulcerative colitis, repeated transfusions of 500 cc. of whole blood are of utmost importance. They are indicated as general supportive measures even if not necessary to correct anemia and hypoproteinemia. Liberal use should be made of analgesics (℞ 74, 75, 76) and antispasmodics (℞ 57, 58, 59) to depress the activity of the bowel; a combination of tincture of belladonna and deodorized tincture of opium (℞ 10) every 4 to 6 hours is recommended. Opiates (℞ 9) should be given by the clock, not according to the number of stools. General sedation (℞ 66 to 70) as well often is necessary. Medications that thicken bowel discharges (℞ 5, 7, 8, 14), alone or in combination, can be tried but they rarely allay the inflammation of the colon and may stimulate colonic motility by increasing the fecal bulk. Similarly, rectal or colonic instillations, irrigations, or enemas of any type have little place in the treatment of a disease which, above all, requires rest for the bowel.

Antibacterial agents: Although it is unproved that ulcerative colitis is an infectious disease, various antibacterial agents often are used with success, possibly because secondary infection is thereby controlled. Sulfonamide preparations that primarily affect the intestinal flora and are poorly absorbed (℞ 118, 119) are used extensively. However, they act chiefly on the mucosal surface, and probably exert little effect on severe active processes in the intestinal wall. A systemically-acting sulfonamide like sulfadiazine (℞ 107, 108) may control the inflammation more effectively in such cases. Sulfonamides, particularly those easily absorbed, must be used with extraordinary care in ulcerative colitis, since the patient may be drinking little liquid, may be vomiting, and is losing fluid in sweat and bowel movements. Thus, urinary complications are likely to ensue unless a urinary output of at least 1,500 cc. a day can be ensured (*see* SULFONAMIDE THERAPY).

Penicillin (℞ 109, 110), or streptomycin (or dihydrostreptomycin) (℞ 111, 112), or both, are useful, particularly in desperately sick patients with high fever and toxemia, or those with impending perforation. In addition, oral administration of streptomycin (℞ 117) may decrease the intestinal flora. However, it is doubtful whether the antibiotic penetrates diseased tissue; and a theoretic hazard from this therapy is the proliferation of resistant bacterial strains and the development of vitamin B complex and K deficiencies.

Antistreptococcus horse serum, prepared with Bargen's vaccine, for severe cases has been recommended. In chronic cases, dysentery bacilli or autogenous vaccines have been used, but such vaccines and bacteriophage are of questionable benefit and are not readily available. Sometimes, however, ulcerative colitis improves following a vaccine-induced hyperpyrexia. Consequently, nonspecific treatment with I.V. typhoid vaccine (℞ 129) may be used in young, afebrile patients with chronic ulcerative colitis, who otherwise are free from disease. The initial course of serum or vaccine injections should always be given in a hospital, with due precautions against allergic reactions.

Psychotherapy: The patient with ulcerative colitis is discouraged and apprehensive. Furthermore, he is most likely to be an abnormally dependent and introspective type of person, a condition which probably plays an important role in the pathogenesis of his disease. Therefore, the physician must give him encouragement and be tolerant toward his many complaints. Sedation (℞ 66) is indicated. After the patient has recovered from the acute illness, psychotherapy may help to prevent recurrences. In any case, the lot of the colitis patient must be improved. As far as possible, emotional problems must be solved and difficult environmental factors eliminated.

Other treatment: Elimination diets (*see* Diets), if tried, should exclude notorious allergens (e.g., milk, wheat, eggs, oranges, chocolate). Severely ill patients may be fed a non-allergenic mixture of predigested amino acids and glucose. Treatment employing cortisone has recently been tried, with some reported success.

Surgery: If medical treatment fails, surgical measures are indicated. These consist of ileostomy, followed in many cases by colectomy. The ileostomy is permanent; there is no hope of eventual ileocolonic anastomosis. Operative intervention is imperative if colonic obstruction or neoplasm develops. A debilitated patient who has steadily gone downhill, or one with perforation or severe hemorrhage, is admittedly one in whom medical therapy has failed, but such a patient has little chance of surviving a "last-ditch" operation. In general, surgical intervention should be considered in the following circumstances: (1) When there is an acute process, high fever, over 10 rectal discharges daily uncontrolled by opiates, and a steadily downhill course despite medical treatment for 2 weeks. (2) When there is a chronic process involving the whole colon (as shown by barium enema), which produces progressive malnutrition and remains unimproved after 2 months of medication. (3) When the disease is in remission in a patient who has had repeated previous attacks and can be expected to have more, and whose colon is seen by X-ray to be extensively and diffusely damaged by fibrosis and pseudopolyps.

MUCOUS COLITIS
("Irritable Colon")

A common functional disorder of the large bowel, in which motor, dehydrating, and mucus-secreting activities are variably deranged, with constipation as the characteristic manifestation.

Etiology

Numerous irritating factors, singly or combined, probably produce irritable colon: psychogenic stimuli in patients who are tense, anxious and hurried; long-standing faulty habits, such as rapid and irregular eating, or repeated failure to heed the urge to move the bowels; abuse of laxatives and enemas; allergy to foods.

Pathologic Physiology

Instead of orderly storage and evacuation of fecal material, the irritable colon exhibits irregular, uncoordinated, and non-propulsive contractions, particularly in the sigmoid. These retard the evacuation of feces, which become excessively dehydrated and hard. Gas is not absorbed or expelled normally, but is trapped or compressed, causing sensations of bloating and fullness. There is excessive formation of the mucus normally produced in the bowel. In some patients, the unintegrated contractions and spasms are sporadically replaced by a period of hyperactive propulsive waves causing frequent and loose bowel movements.

These disorders produce an injected mucosa which may even manifest slight pinpoint bleeding on trauma, but there is no cellular infiltration or other evidence of inflammation in mucous colitis.

Symptoms and Signs

The chief symptom is chronic constipation with the passage of hard, dry stools covered with mucus. In some cases, pure mucus is passed when the patient strains at stool. Bowel movements are incomplete and unsatisfactory. Bouts of diarrhea may interrupt the constipation. Colic is unusual, but an aching distress over the sigmoid or cecum, occasionally radiating to the back, epigastrium or left upper quadrant, is a frequent complaint. Moderate manual pressure may relieve this distress but, conversely, tight clothing often aggravates it. There are no systemic symptoms, although the patient may have accompanying headache, insomnia, morning anorexia, tiredness, and symptoms of indigestion from the same cause that produced the colitis. Physical examination often, but not always, reveals lower abdominal tenderness. In many cases a tender, contracted, ropelike sigmoid may be palpated.

Diagnosis

A history of chronic bowel disorders, often associated with other functional symptoms, is typical. Stool examination may be negative or reveal considerable mucus. Hemorrhoids may complicate the constipation and cause streaks of blood to show in the feces. When blood is found, however, and in all cases that present diagnostic problems, proctoscopic and barium enema X-ray examinations are indicated to rule out cancer and other organic local diseases.

Treatment

Therapy of the irritable colon will hardly be successful unless both psychologic and physical aspects are treated.

Psychologic: The patient who has been told he has mucous colitis must be freed from fear and made to realize that it is a functional, not inflammatory, disorder; that it is not fatal, and is vastly different from serious forms of colitis which he may have heard about. Breaking the patient of a laxative or enema habit is principally a matter of fortifying his will power. He should be warned that the omission of these measures may, for a time, aggravate his symptoms, but will bring ultimate improvement. He also must be disabused of the idea that his constipation is the cause of other complaints, such as headache, lassitude, and indigestion, and informed that there is no evidence to support the theory of "intestinal intoxication."

Rest and relaxation may be achieved by sedation (℞ 66). Curtailment of excessive physical or mental activity and, if possible, bed rest for a period of 1 or 2 weeks may be advisable. Certain cases doubtless require expert psychotherapy.

Intestinal: There are two basic principles: The colon must again be conditioned to expel feces in response to normal stimuli, and no foods or medicines are to be taken which might irritate the bowel. The patient is instructed as follows: (1) Eat regularly, following a soft or low residue diet (*see* DIETS). (2) Try to move the bowels at the same time every day, at least 10 minutes in the attempt. Do not strain. Since the ingestion of food on an empty stomach activates intestinal peristalsis, the best time for establishing a regular bowel habit is 15 to 45 minutes after breakfast. The daily bowel routine must faithfully be adhered to. (3) Use no laxatives or enemas except as instructed. If there is no bowel movement for 3 days, a saline or oil enema may be taken (*see* BEDSIDE PROC.).

For the patient habituated to laxatives, it may be necessary to keep the stools soft temporarily with a hydrophilic colloid (℞ 28) or mineral oil (℞ 23). If more than 1 oz. of mineral oil is given daily, a deficiency of fat-soluble vitamins may be induced. Once reasonable bowel regularity has been reestablished, the dose of mineral oil or hydrophilic colloid is slowly reduced over a period of weeks until the patient is taking no laxatives whatever.

Spasm and deranged bowel function are treated by liberal application of heat to the abdomen. Antispasmodics yield variable results but should always be tried. While atropine and related substances (℞ 57, 63) usually are satisfactory, other preparations (℞ 59) may be substituted if atropine causes uncomfortable side effects, has been used for a long time, or has proved ineffectual. Combinations of these antispasmodics with a sedative (℞ 56) are extensively employed. In general, antispasmodics should not be given continuously for more than 2 months.

Diarrheal episodes are treated with demulcent substances that thicken the feces (℞ 5, 7, 8, 14). When diarrhea is alternating with constipation, however, control of the constipation by a bowel-training regimen usually eliminates the diarrhea as well.

DIVERTICULOSIS; DIVERTICULITIS

Diverticula: *mucosal sacculations which protrude from the intestinal lumen through the bowel wall, occurring most commonly in the colon, particularly the sigmoid.* When uncomplicated, the disorder is described as **diverticulosis;** when inflammation is present, as **diverticulitis.**

DIVERTICULOSIS

Etiology and Pathology

The nature of the mural defects permitting these herniations is unknown, but the intestinal wall is said to be weakened where penetrated by blood vessels. Diverticula, when fully developed, are spherical pouches connected with the intestinal lumen by narrow necks. The spherical portion is composed almost entirely of serosa and mucosa, with few muscular elements. The incidence of diverticula increases with age and probably with obesity. Almost 10% of persons over 45 have diverticulosis.

Symptoms and Signs

Diverticulosis of the colon causes no symptoms, and abdominal complaints should not be ascribed to it. Some patients may complain of symptoms suggesting an irritable colon, but the irritable colon syndrome probably is coincidental with diverticulosis rather than causal.

Diagnosis and Treatment

Diverticulosis of the colon is diagnosed by 24-hour examination after a barium meal, by barium enema, or by air-contrast enemas. Occasionally, an experienced observer can make the diagnosis by sigmoidoscopy. If the patient has had no symptoms referable to his colon, no treatment is indicated. If he suffers from a coincidental irritable colon (mucous colitis, spastic constipation [q.v.]), therapy for this condition should be instituted. If he has had attacks of diverticulitis in the past, a low residue diet is recommended (*see* DIETS). The stools should be kept soft, but not liquid, by nonirritating laxatives (R 23, 28) as needed (*see also* CONSTIPATION). Stronger laxatives and enemas are best avoided.

DIVERTICULITIS

Etiology and Pathology

Diverticulitis occurs when the diverticular neck becomes obstructed, as by edema or a fecalith. The ensuing stasis favors the multiplication of bacteria and infection of surrounding tissues, as a result of which the walls of the involved diverticulum, the nearby musculature of the colon, and the adjoining serosal fat participate in an inflammatory reaction. This may follow one of several courses: the process remains localized and subsides spontaneously within a few days, or spreads and culminates in local abscess formation; edema or spasm resulting from the inflammatory reaction may obstruct the intestinal lumen; the involved diverticulum may perforate, leading to localized or generalized peritonitis; if the affected diverticulum lies next to the urinary bladder, a sigmoidovesical fistula may be formed; incomplete healing or repeated recurrences of acute diverticulitis may eventuate in a chronic process which thickens the bowel and its fatty appendages. Chronic diverticulitis also may lead to intestinal obstruction or the formation of sigmoidovesical fistulas.

Symptoms and Signs

Acute diverticulitis produces fairly constant pain, usually in the left lower quadrant. Because of associated intestinal spasm and reflex disorders of gastrointestinal motility, the patient may have nausea, vomiting, abdominal distention, and inability to pass gas or feces. Malaise, chills and fever occur in proportion to the degree and extent of the inflammatory process. If abscess formation, large bowel obstruction, or peritonitis develops, symptoms characteristic of these disorders (q.v.) supervene. In chronic diverticulitis, the patient feels dull, nagging pain. Constipation, occasionally diarrhea, and moderate gaseous distention often are prominent. Recurrent lower abdominal cramps may signify partial obstruction of the colon. Urinary frequency and urgency suggest that the inflammatory reaction is contiguous to the bladder. The occurrence of gas in the urine signifies a patent fistula. In either acute or chronic diverticulitis tenderness and resistance occur almost invariably over the affected bowel, usually accompanied by some abdominal spasm. If abscess formation or chronic induration of the sigmoid has taken place, a mass may be palpable in the left lower quadrant.

Diagnosis

In acute diverticulitis, the leukocyte count is over 10,000; in chronic diverticulitis, it often is normal. Occasionally, gross blood appears in the stools. The diagnosis is best achieved by barium and air-contrast enemas which demonstrate diverticula, spasms, obstruction, and deformity of the intestinal lumen. The principal condition to be differentiated is carcinoma, which, if concurrent with diverticulosis, may be impossible to distinguish. Proctosigmoidoscopy is always indicated.

Treatment

Acute diverticulitis without complications is treated conservatively with bed rest and application of heat to the lower abdomen by hot water bottle, heating pad, or flaxseed poultice (*see* BEDSIDE PROC.). An antispasmodic (℞ 57, 59, 63) should be given in doses larger than those used in chronic conditions. Opiates (℞ 74, 76) are given for only two purposes: to relieve severe pain and, in case of perforation or near-perforation, to rest the bowel in an attempt to prevent generalized peritonitis.

Antibiotics and sulfonamides are indicated both to combat the infection and to hinder its extension. Streptomycin or dihydrostreptomycin (℞ 111, 112), penicillin (℞ 109, 110), or sulfadiazine (℞ 107, 108) can be given, singly or in appropriate combinations. Sulfonamides that act principally within the intestinal lumen (℞ 118, 119) probably do not reach the inflamed diverticulum (*see also* SULFONAMIDE THERAPY, and ACID-BASE AND ALLIED DISORDERS). Laxatives are contraindicated, but the patient may benefit from a daily bland, saline or oil enema (*see* BEDSIDE PROC.). This should be given slowly and not forced past any partially obstructing point.

In chronic diverticulitis, treatment consists of local application of heat, a liquid or low residue diet (*see* DIETS), moderate doses of antispasmodics (℞ 57, 59, 63) and nonirritating laxatives (℞ 23, 28) to keep bowel movements soft. Cleansing enemas with saline or oil only (*see* BEDSIDE PROC.) also may be beneficial.

Surgical intervention is indicated for the following complications of acute or chronic diverticulitis: abscess formation without resolution, perforation, fistula formation, intestinal obstruction, or repeated attacks of acute diverticulitis. It is likewise necessary where the possibility of cancer of the colon cannot be excluded by other means.

MECKEL'S DIVERTICULUM

A congenital sacculation resulting from incomplete obliteration of the vitello-intestinal duct. It may be found 1 to 5 feet proximal to the ileocecal valve and occurs in 1 to 2% of the population. It is subject to ulceration with hemorrhage and to inflammation. Ulceration or intussusception usually is a disease of childhood, but inflammation may occur at any age. When Meckel's diverticulitis is acute, it simulates acute appendicitis. A chronic process may lead to obstruction of the small intestine. Treatment is invariably surgical.

INTESTINAL OBSTRUCTION

A condition in which the passage of intestinal contents is arrested or seriously impaired.

Etiology

The causes of intestinal obstruction may be classified as mechanical, vascular, or neurogenic. Mechanical causes include extrinsic factors such as bands and adhesions, pressure on the gut from tumors in surrounding structures, and incarceration of a loop of bowel in a hernial ring; intrinsic factors such as impacted foreign body or feces, enteroliths, parasites (Ascaris), and gallstones; and lesions in the bowel wall such as neoplasms and strictures of the bowel, intussusception and volvulus. Vascular causes include embolism or thrombosis of a large blood vessel resulting in infarction of a bowel segment. The neurogenic group consists of the adynamic or paralytic ileus seen in pneumonia and peritonitis, and following abdominal surgery or injuries to the spinal cord.

Symptoms and Signs

The clinical features of this condition vary, depending upon whether the obstruction is complete or incomplete, high or low in the intestinal tract, and simple or strangulated.

Complete mechanical obstruction of the small intestine results in severe intermittent cramplike periumbilical pain. Vomiting soon follows; the higher the obstruction the sooner the vomiting. At first, vomiting is synchronous with the pain, but later it occurs at irregular intervals and becomes fecal in character. Abdominal distention is minimal if the obstruction is high but is conspicuous if obstruction is low in the small bowel. Rigidity of the abdominal wall is absent. Occasionally, peristaltic waves are seen coincident with the colicky pains. Peristaltic sounds are present.

Partial obstruction of the small intestine is characterized by recurrent attacks of cramplike abdominal pain, occasionally associated with vomiting. The amount of distention varies with the degree of obstruction.

The symptoms of complete obstruction of the colon are insidious in onset. Abdominal distention and vomiting develop later or not at all and pain is less severe than in small bowel obstruction. Partial obstruction of the colon often is characterized by diarrhea alternating with constipation and mild intermittent cramplike pains in the lower abdomen. If the obstructing lesion is in the distal portion there may be a decrease in the caliber of the stools.

Adynamic or paralytic ileus is marked by severe abdominal distention and absence of peristaltic sounds or colicky pains.

Strangulation as a complication of incarcerated hernia, volvulus, intussusception, or infarction usually gives symptoms of complete bowel obstruction and in addition shock and peritonitis which increase in severity with time and in proportion to the length of bowel involved. Blood is occasionally passed per rectum in a strangulated obstruction.

Diagnosis

A thorough history and careful evaluation of the development of the symptoms and signs usually is sufficient for diagnosis. X-ray is the most valuable diagnostic tool. A flat film of the abdomen may show extremely dilated loops of bowel. The site of obstruction may be evident if the dilatation is confined to a portion of the abdomen. An upright abdominal X-ray may show fluid levels in stepladder fashion in dilated loops of bowel. A barium enema will reveal colonic obstruction, but it should be employed with caution lest a partial obstruction be made complete by impaction of the barium proximal to the point of obstruction. A gastrointestinal series should not be done if intestinal obstruction is suspected.

Treatment

The aim of treatment is to restore the continuity of the bowel lumen quickly and with as little risk to the patient as possible. Operative procedures upon a distended bowel are dangerous; therefore every attempt should be made to relieve distention preoperatively. This can be done by applying mild constant negative pressure to an indwelling tube inserted through the nose into the stomach, duodenum, or intestine. The Wangensteen modification of the Levin tube and the double-lumen Miller-Abbott tube are most commonly used (*see* BEDSIDE PROC.). Simple obstructions of the small intestine may be relieved by suction alone, but continuation of such conservative treatment for longer than 48 hours may be dangerous unless repeated X-ray examinations show a decrease in the amount of distention or the passage of gas into the lower bowel. Operation should not be delayed by attempts at conservative treatment in cases of strangulation obstruction or of acute obstruction of the colon. Patients treated by suction usually do not require narcotics. Sedation (℞ 66) is of value for the relief of restlessness.

Inhalation of oxygen in high concentration (80%) tends to decrease the gaseous component in intestinal distentions. However, if this is carried on continuously for long periods of time there is danger of oxygen poisoning. Therefore, the treatment should be interrupted for 20 to 30 minutes 3 times a day.

Fluids should be administered parenterally in order to relieve dehydration, to furnish sufficient sodium chloride to restore the plasma chloride level to normal, and to cover the metabolic needs of the patient until he can safely ingest and absorb liquids. Enough fluid should be given to replace that lost by suction and also to ensure the production of 1,000 cc. of urine daily. This may be accomplished by alternating the administration of 1,000 cc. of isotonic saline, 5% glucose in saline, and 5% of an amino acids preparation in 5% glucose and saline until the desired total is reached. For patients with chronic or partial obstruction, low residue diets (*see* DIETS) and 1 or 2 oz. of mineral oil daily are recommended.

Neostigmine methylsulfate (℞ 64), or Urecholine Chloride (℞ 55) is of value in the treatment of adynamic ileus. Blood transfusions and other measures indicated in the treatment of shock should be given to patients with a strangulated segment of bowel.

The operative treatment of intestinal obstruction is divided into two phases. One phase includes enterostomy and colostomy as a preliminary measure to obtain decompression of a distended bowel. The other includes a number of procedures directed against the obstructing mechanism. These should not, however, be employed in the presence of severe distention except in cases of strangulation, where the additional risk must be accepted.

CONSTIPATION

(Colon stasis)

Difficult or infrequent passage of feces, with stasis in part or all of the large bowel. It is not generally realized that healthy persons may have normal bowel movements as often as 2 or 3 times a day, or as seldom as once every 3 or 4 days. Many people become intensely worried and frightened if they do not have at least one movement a day; they expect dire consequences and ascribe numerous unrelated symptoms to their "constipation." Actually, the feces may be withheld for a considerable period of time before undesirable symptoms occur. Ideally, however, the bowels should move regularly, daily or every other day. The infrequency of movements is not so serious as the difficult passage of hard dry stools, or fecal impaction. When this becomes habitual or when an individual is unable at any time to evacuate his bowels without a laxative, medical attention is required. Chronic constipation predisposes to secondary infectious colitis, diverticulitis, fissures, and hemorrhoids.

Etiology

Atony of the bowel is the usual cause of constipation characterized by hard dry stools without abdominal pain. Constipation with abdominal pain more often is due to a spastic or hypertonic condition, the so-called "irritable colon." Loss of power to function normally may result from the abuse of self-administered cathartics, which is widely prevalent; from lack of exercise, habitual failure to respond to the urge to defecate, improper diet, and inadequate fluid intake. Anorectal disease (q.v.) and spasm of the rectal sphincter may be responsible; also any condition that produces loss of general muscle tone, such as fatigue, infectious disease, chronic debilitating disease, and malnutrition. Psychologic disturbances are an important cause of constipation. Additional causes are systemic diseases producing venous stasis; endocrine upsets; gastric disorders such as achylia, hyperchlorhydria, cancer, ulcer, or atony; a preceding diarrhea; fissures of the rectum and hemorrhoids; intestinal obstruction by such conditions as strangulated hernia, tumors, or foreign bodies; malposition of the uterus; and peritonitis. Congenital anomalies of the large bowel, such as stenosis, hypertrophy, and dilatation (megacolon), or atony due to inadequate parasympathetic innervation, are less frequent causes.

Stasis may develop in any part of the colon. Rectal stasis

(dyschesia) may be due to relaxation or laceration of the pelvic floor or to loss of sensitivity in the rectal mucosa owing to habitual repression of the desire to defecate. Stasis in other sections may result from redundancy of the pelvic colon or splenic flexure, from adhesions of the cecum or hepatic flexure, from ptosis of the transverse colon, or from colonic spasm. The large bowel may be affected throughout its entire length from similar causes or from megacolon (Hirschsprung's disease). It may become dilated by gas following operation, or in cases of peritonitis and other severe infectious diseases such as lobar pneumonia—often to the point of paralytic ileus (q.v.). Obstruction of the sigmoid or rectum may result in complete colon stasis. Megacolon is a congenital condition characterized by extreme dilatation and hypertrophy of the colon.

Symptoms, Signs, and Diagnosis

In any patient complaining of constipation, digital examination of the rectum is the first step in diagnosis. This often will reveal a large hard mass of feces presenting at the anus. Persons who have not previously been constipated and who develop increasing difficulty in defecation should be suspected of having some organic disease that may be interfering with bowel function. A complete examination must be made to determine the underlying cause. Proctoscopy may reveal anorectal disease (q.v.) or some form of local obstruction. Individuals with constipation due to faulty habits may complain of nothing more than anorexia and difficulty or infrequency of evacuation. In such cases and in cases secondary to systemic disease, X-ray examination of the colon will reveal no abnormality. When obstruction causes the symptom complex of ileus (q.v.), the bowel movements and even the passage of gas cease entirely. The patient has symptoms of vomiting, severe abdominal pain, and collapse. The passage of blood, frank or occult, in the stools sometimes indicates a malignant growth or hemorrhoids. Rectal stasis is marked by the more or less constant presence of a fecal mass in the rectum while the patient feels no desire to defecate. Diagnosis can be made by digital examination. Stasis occurring beyond the rectum can be demonstrated when X-ray examination shows retention of the contrast medium for 48 hours or longer. In the spastic state, it is seen chiefly in the transverse colon and usually is accompanied by pain and tenderness in the left iliac region or over the entire length of the colon, due to descending-colon spasm. Spastic tender segments of the bowel can be rolled under the fingers. The X-ray film may reveal dilatation atony in the descending colon from decompensation of intestinal musculature in the presence of obstruction. The patient may show the symptom complex of "biliousness," i.e., anorexia, coated tongue, bad taste in the mouth, flatulence, pyrosis, nausea, abdominal distention, pressure sensations; subicteric tint; palpitation, extrasystoles; headache, vertigo; moderate rise of temperature, leukocytosis; abnormal color and consistency of stools. When spasm is present, pain and regional tenderness are added clinical manifestations. Stasis of the entire colon is revealed by X-ray. Megacolon occurs most frequently in children, who usually exhibit retarded growth and a large protruding abdomen. In this condition, evacuation of the bowels may not occur for weeks or months unless artificially induced.

Treatment

Any existing local or systemic disease or abnormality that may cause the constipation should receive appropriate treatment. Faulty hygiene should be corrected. Any laxatives the patient may be using habitually must be abandoned. The diet should contain sufficient cellulose, or "residue," to give bulk to the feces (see DIETS). Intake of vitamins, especially thiamine and B complex, and of fluids, should be increased. Adequate exercise (e.g., walking) is beneficial, particularly if the patient normally leads a sedentary life. He should at all times, if possible, go to the toilet immediately he feels the urge to defecate.

Psychotherapy plays an important part. The patient should be made to understand that it is not necessary to have a bowel movement every day and that no serious consequences are to be expected from moderately infrequent evacuations. The constipating after-effects of most cathartics should be explained. He should be encouraged to eliminate unnecessary nervous tension and worry of all kinds as far as possible. Autosuggestion frequently is of great value in establishing a regular bowel habit. The patient should accustom himself to go to the toilet at a regular time each day—preferably after a meal, when he is free to relax—and to remain at the stool without impatience long enough to give the bowels ample opportunity to move.

Bed patients often suffer from rectal stasis, and it is a good rule in such cases to order an enema of warm physiologic saline solution or 2% sodium bicarbonate whenever the bowels have not moved for 48 hours (see BEDSIDE PROC.). In ambulatory patients, an oil retention enema at bedtime followed by a small warm water enema in the morning has proved effective. A glycerin suppository often produces satisfactory results. In cases of obstruction, enemas may be employed if peritonitis or perforation has not occurred.

When, for any reason, "roughage" cannot be ingested in the diet, bulk can be given the feces by administration of such nonabsorbable agents as agar (R 26), emulsion of agar and mineral oil (R 27), mucilaginous extracts of psyllium seed (R 28), or methylated cellulose (R 25).

Irritating cathartics generally are to be condemned. Not only do they tend to cause spasm of the bowel after their temporary effect is over, but they are distinctly dangerous in the presence of an undiagnosed appendicitis (q.v.). It is a safe rule to avoid any drug likely to stimulate intense peristalsis (e.g., castor oil) when the patient complains of abdominal pain or where evidence of exaggerated intestinal muscular activity is found. In cases of obstruction, cathartics definitely are contraindicated. For certain bed patients, however, or for those persons in whom it is necessary to break the laxative habit, the following drugs may be used, with caution: Milk of magnesia (℞ 21), or cascara sagrada tablets (℞ 29). When prompt relief is required, the quick-acting saline cathartics such as magnesium sulfate (Epsom salt) may be given (℞ 30).

In cases of rectally impacted feces with rectal tenesmus that prove refractory to enemas and cathartics, manual breaking up and removal of the fecal mass must be resorted to. In chronic rectal stasis, the rectum must be kept empty. The patient should regularly attempt to evacuate his bowels by the method of autosuggestion described above. If this fails, he should, while still at the stool, take a small cool enema of 1 pint of water containing 1 teaspoonful of salt. This routine should be carried out every day, preferably at the same hour.

For spastic colon, oil enemas are recommended. About 200 cc. of oil, such as olive oil, should be injected every night at bedtime until the feces are freed from hard lumps. The feces may be kept soft also by the oral use of liquid petrolatum (℞ 23) or emulsion of agar and liquid petrolatum (℞ 27). If leakage of oil from the rectum occurs, dosage should be reduced or psyllium seed (℞ 28) substituted. Antispasmodic drugs of the atropine group (℞ 57, 63) combined with an analgesic (℞ 65), plus heat to the abdomen, are indicated for relief of painful spasm, and a temporary diet free from roughage should be prescribed. As soon as the colic has subsided, a coarse diet must be given and increased as tolerated.

In chronic cases of upper-colon stasis, the bowel should be put at rest by a restricted diet, such as sweet milk or buttermilk every 2 hours, for a few days. The bowel contents may be kept liquid by administration of salines, e.g., effervescing sodium phosphate or sodium sulfate combined with alkali when a stronger effect is needed. If nervous irritability is excessive, a sedative may be given (℞ 66). When the symptom complex of "biliousness" is present, an effective cathartic should be administered. If a high residue diet can be tolerated, this may enable the patient to get along without a cathartic; otherwise, a smooth diet with an occasional saline laxative must be employed.

Gaseous distention of the colon following operation or infectious disease, if mild, can be treated by local heat applications and moderate ingestion of nonirritating foods. If there is localized spasm, atropine (℞ 57) and barbiturates (℞ 56, 66) may be given.

Congenital anomalies, such as stenosis of the bowel, must be treated surgically. Constipation due to megacolon may be temporarily relieved by administration of laxatives or enemas, or both. However, surgery with excision of the bowel and lumbar sympathectomy offers the best hope of recovery in such cases.

TUBERCULOSIS

OROPHARYNGEAL TUBERCULOSIS

A form of tuberculosis which, when it occurs, usually is secondary to pulmonary tuberculosis. In the mouth, painful ulcers with undermined edges and yellowish gray bases may appear on any of the mucous membranes. Similar ulcers may be present on the margin or dorsum of the tongue. Painful ulcers in the nasopharynx and pharynx proper also are seen occasionally. Tuberculous tonsillitis usually is not diagnosed clinically until ulceration has occurred. However, routine histopathologic examination of specimens obtained by tonsillectomy reveals an incidence of tuberculous tonsillitis of about 1%.

Treatment

Streptomycin (R 111) or dihydrostreptomycin (R 112) given I.M. is of distinct value in the treatment of oropharyngeal lesions. Cauterizing the ulcers with 5% trichloroacetic acid (R 130) every 7 to 21 days as necessary may be of value. Resistant lesions may be electrodesiccated with high frequency current, or irradiated with ultraviolet.

ESOPHAGEAL TUBERCULOSIS

A rare condition, characterized by ulceration and cicatrization of the esophagus, most often occurring as a result of direct extension from tuberculous mediastinal lymph nodes, with traction diverticula sometimes ensuing.

TUBERCULOSIS OF THE STOMACH

A rare disease of the stomach, always secondary to tuberculous infection elsewhere, usually by extension from contiguous regional lymph nodes. The acid gastric juice and the absence of lymph follicles in the gastric mucosa possibly discourage the formation of primary gastric tuberculous lesions following the ingestion of tubercle bacilli. The tuberculous lesion may exist as single or multiple ragged ulcers with undermined edges or it may appear as a hypertrophic lesion resembling a tumor. It usually occurs in the prepyloric region on the lesser curvature. Diagnosis is difficult because the symptoms and X-ray findings as a rule do not differ from those present in peptic ulcer (q.v.) or gastric carcinoma (q.v.).

Treatment

Active measures should be taken for the control of the primary lesion, usually located in the lungs (q.v.). A smooth, low residue, high protein diet (*see* DIETS) may be of value. Resection becomes necessary in about 60% of the cases.

TUBERCULOUS ENTEROCOLITIS

*A form of tuberculosis involving the intestine, and which is
the most common complication of pulmonary tuberculosis.* In
50 to 90% of patients dying of pulmonary tuberculosis, tuberculous lesions are found in the intestinal tract.

Pathogenesis

Most cases undoubtedly are due to enterogenous infection.
Tubercle bacilli swallowed in the sputum of patients with cavities in the lungs are largely responsible. Hematogenous dissemination to the intestinal wall may account for a few of the
cases. The primary form of intestinal and mesenteric lymph
node tuberculosis probably is due to the ingestion of milk or
meat containing the bovine strain of tubercle bacillus. It most
often is seen in infants and children in countries where bovine
tuberculosis is not well controlled.

The lesions of intestinal tuberculosis may occur in ulcerative
or hypertrophic forms. The **ulcerative** form usually first involves the ileocecal region, the portion of the intestinal tract
richest in lymphoid tissue. From there the lesions spread up
and down the gut. The ulcers are shallow with undermined
edges and necrotic floors and occasionally encircle the bowel.
The entire large bowel and a considerable portion of the small
intestine may be involved. Lymphatic spread to the mesenteric
lymph nodes may occur, healing with cicatricial contraction of
the bowel leading to intestinal obstructions is less frequent, and
perforations resulting in peritonitis are rare. The **hypertrophic**
form of the disease is characterized by the formation of tuberculous granulation tissue. The bowel wall becomes thickened
and indurated. The granulation tissue may form a tumor-like
mass usually in the right lower quadrant, which may gradually
encroach upon the lumen of the bowel and eventually result in
obstruction. This form of the disease may be very difficult to
differentiate from a neoplasm of the bowel.

Rectal involvement commonly occurs via the enterogenous
route. It is characterized by ulceration, ischiorectal abscesses
and fistulas.

Symptoms and Signs

The clinical manifestations depend upon whether a predominantly ulcerative or hyperplastic intestinal tuberculosis is present. Symptoms of well advanced pulmonary tuberculosis also
are often evident. An increase in the general symptoms of
tuberculosis without a parallel increase in the severity of the
pulmonary disease is highly suggestive of the presence of intestinal tuberculosis.

The **ulcerative** form of the disease is characterized by increasing fever, wasting and anemia. Abdominal pain is colicky,
paraumbilical, usually confined to the lower half, and generally
greater upon defecation. Tenderness is slight or absent unless

definite peritonitis develops. Diarrhea occurs in most patients, occasionally with gross or occult blood and pus or mucus.

The clinical picture in the **hypertrophic** form of intestinal tuberculosis results largely from mechanical factors. The induration of the bowel wall and the tumor mass cause chronic constipation, occasionally alternating with attacks of diarrhea, visible peristalsis, and colicky pains. Localized areas of tenderness and a tumor mass, most often in the ileocecal region, may be palpated. Partial or complete intestinal obstruction may develop and necessitate surgical intervention. Almost always signs and symptoms of ulceration eventually develop, as manifested by the appearance of fever, diarrhea, and possibly blood and pus in the stool.

Diagnosis

The occurrence of the symptoms and signs outlined above in a patient known to have pulmonary tuberculosis is highly suggestive of tuberculous enteritis. The identification of tubercle bacilli in the stool is significant only if there are no open tuberculous lesions in the lungs. Proctoscopic and sigmoidoscopic examinations should be made, although the tuberculous lesions usually are not far enough down the tract to be visualized. X-ray studies of the small and large bowel demonstrating the presence of filling defects, spasm, narrowing of the lumen of the bowel, and hypermotility with rapid emptying of involved segments of gut are indicative of tuberculous enteritis, especially if the patient has pulmonary tuberculosis.

Tuberculosis of the bowel must be differentiated from regional ileitis, neoplasms (especially those of the cecum), chronic ulcerative colitis, syphilis, lymphogranuloma venereum and other chronic stenosing infections of the rectosigmoid and rectum.

Treatment

Streptomycin (℞ 111) or dihydrostreptomycin (℞ 112) I.M. has proved to be of definite usefulness in treating these lesions. Oral antibiotic (℞ 117) supplementation may be of value. In addition, the same principles employed in the treatment of other forms of tuberculosis are necessary. Rest, fresh air; smooth, low residue, high protein diet; vitamin supplements, and heliotherapy are recommended. If the diarrhea is troublesome, bismuth subcarbonate (℞ 8) may give relief. Where evidence suggests that fat is not being properly absorbed by the intestine, absorption may be aided by the use of a wetting agent, such as the polyoxyethylene derivative of sorbitan monooleate (℞ 131) given as 1.5 Gm. doses with each meal.

Localized hyperplastic tuberculous lesions, especially in the ileocecal region, may be excised with good results by a one-stage resection with intestinal anastomosis. Persistent partial intestinal obstruction, complete intestinal obstruction, and perforation of the bowel require surgical intervention.

INTESTINAL PARASITIC INFECTIONS

Common Name	Synonyms and Varieties	Distribution	Portal of Entry	Form Present in Stool
ROUNDWORMS Giant intestinal roundworm	Roundworm *Ascaris lumbricoides*	Cosmopolitan. More common in warm, moist climates.	Mouth	Eggs
Hookworm	*Ancylostoma duodenale* (Old World hookworm) *Necator americanus* (Tropical hookworm)	Common in warm, moist climates.	Skin (usually of feet)	Eggs
Strongyloides stercoralis	*Anguillula stercoralis*	Southern states.	Skin (usually of feet)	Larvae
Pinworm	Seatworm *Oxyuris vermicularis* *Enterobius vermicularis*	Cosmopolitan. More common in warm, moist climates.	Mouth	Eggs Adults (may be found peri-anally)
Threadworm	Whipworm *Trichuris trichiura* *Trichocephalus trichiurus*	Cosmopolitan. More common in warm, moist climates.	Mouth	Eggs
TAPEWORMS Dwarf	*Hymenolepsis nana**	Common in children in S. E. states.	Mouth	Eggs* Segments of the adult worm**
Beef	*Taenia saginata***	Cosmopolitan.		
Pork	*Taenia solium***	Rare in U.S.; freq., Mexico.		
Fish	*Diphyllobothrium latum**	North'n Minn. and Mich.		
FLUKES	*Fasciolopsis buski*† *Heterophyes heterophyes*† *Metagonimus yokogawai*† *Echinostoma ilocanum*† *Fasciola hepatica*†† *Paragonimus westermani*†††	Rare in U.S. and only as infections imported from Orient or tropics.	Mouth	Eggs
PROTOZOA *Giardia lamblia* *Endameba histolytica* (see AMEBIASIS)	*Lamblia intestinalis* *Giardia intestinalis* *Cercomonas intestinalis* *Megastoma entericum*	Cosmopolitan. More common in warm, moist climates, especially in small children.	Mouth	Cysts

ENCOUNTERED IN NORTH AMERICA

Source of Infection	Most Common Symptoms	Therapeutic Agents (Listed in Order of Efficacy) Prescriptions, pp. 541 to 543	Remarks
Fecal contamination of soil (eggs)	Colicky pains Diarrhea "Acute abdomen"	1. Hexylresorcinol (℞ 81) 2. Tetrachloroethylene with oil of chenopodium (℞ 82) 3. Santonin (℞ 83)	May cause intestinal, bile or pancreatic duct obstruction or bronchial symptoms.
Fecal contamination of soil (larvae)	Anemia Diarrhea Retarded growth	1. Tetrachloroethylene with oil of chenopodium (℞ 82) 2. Carbon tetrachloride (℞ 84) 3. Tetrachloroethylene (℞ 85)	Prophylaxis based on use of sanitary privy and wearing of shoes.
Fecal contamination of soil (larvae)	Intermittent diarrhea	1. Gentian violet (℞ 86)	Prophylaxis based on use of sanitary privy and wearing of shoes.
Fecal contamination (eggs); autoreinfection common	Itching around anus Convulsions in children	1. Gentian violet (℞ 86) 2. Hexylresorcinol (℞ 81)	Entire family frequently infected and should be treated. May cause acute appendicitis.
Fecal contamination of soil (eggs)	Diarrhea Nausea and vomiting Anemia Retarded growth	1. Tetrachloroethylene with oil of chenopodium (℞ 82) 2. Carbon tetrachloride (℞ 84) 3. Hexylresorcinol (℞ 81)	Entire family frequently infected and should be treated. May cause acute appendicitis.
Poorly cooked meat and fish (except dwarf tapeworm, fecal contamination)	Abdominal discomfort Diarrhea or constipation	1. Oleoresin of aspidium (℞ 87, 88) 2. Carbon tetrachloride (℞ 84) 3. Hexylresorcinol (℞ 81) · 4. Tetrachloroethylene (℞ 85)	Frequently no symptoms. May cause intestinal obstruction. Potential systemic cysticercosis from *T. solium*.
Contamination of water and food by infected snails	Diarrhea† Cholecystitis†† Hemoptysis††† Abdominal pain Anasarca Retarded growth	1. Carbon tetrachloride (℞ 84) 2. Tetrachloroethylene (℞ 85) 3. Hexylresorcinol (℞ 81) 4. Emetine hydrochloride (℞ 90)†† †††	Frequently no symptoms.† Liver parenchyma necrosis.†† Possible intestinal obstruction.
Fecal contamination (human)	Diarrhea Abdominal pain	1. Atabrine (℞ 78) 2. Chloroquine (℞ 89) 3. Carbarsone (℞ 79) 4. Stovarsol (℞ 80)	Frequently no symptoms. (Eosinophilia may accompany intestinal parasitic infections.)

* ** † †† †††

Symbols indicate related items

NEOPLASMS

Benign or malignant tumors may occur in any part of the alimentary tract; their cause is unknown. Benign growths are relatively rare, whereas the malignant neoplasms are responsible for more than one-third of all cancer deaths.

The clinical manifestations of such tumors depend on their size, location, and pathologic characteristics (ulcerating, benign or malignant). Diagnosis requires a careful history, complete physical examination, and demonstration of the tumor by X-ray (barium or air contrast studies), or appropriate endoscopic examination of the esophagus, stomach, sigmoid, or rectum. Needle or punch biopsy is indicated when the growth is accessible by endoscopy. Other diagnostic aids include gastric analysis, blood count, and testing for occult blood in the stool (*see* LAB. PROC.).

The treatment is surgical. Essential to good therapeutic results are an early and accurate diagnosis, particularly with malignant growths, and proper preoperative preparation of the patient. Once metastases are evident (clinically or at operation), the prognosis is hopeless and therapy is palliative and supportive.

BENIGN TUMORS

Benign growths include fibroma, neurofibroma, myoma, adenoma, lipoma, hemangioma, papilloma, and single or multiple polyposis. Some of these tumors may bleed easily and cause hematemesis or melena, particularly the hemangiomas, adenomas, papillomas and polyps, but they usually are asymptomatic unless and until sufficiently large to cause symptoms of obstruction. Cancer must be ruled out in all cases of a suspected benign condition, particularly in patients over 35 years of age. Intussusception may complicate an intestinal neoplasm. Multiple polyposis of the colon may produce symptoms resembling those of ulcerative colitis (q.v.). The diagnosis is made by X-ray or endoscopy, and the benign status confirmed by biopsy before or at operation. Malignant degeneration of adenomas, papillomas, and polyps is common. Surgical excision of the tumor area is indicated for those benign tumors which are symptomatic or are liable to malignant degeneration.

MALIGNANT TUMORS

Malignant growths are common in individuals over 40. Males are affected more frequently, particularly by cancer of the stomach.

Symptoms and Signs

Small growths may produce no complaints, or there may be the usual symptoms common to cancer: weakness, anorexia, weight loss. As the tumor grows larger, symptoms of obstruction ensue, often with evidence of bleeding (hematemesis or melena) due to ulceration and anemia. After a variable period of time, untreated and poorly treated cases develop metastases to local and distant points, death occurring due to cachexia, hemorrhage, perforation, or infection.

The symptoms produced by the enlarging tumor depend on its location within the alimentary canal.

Esophagus: Increasing dysphagia and cachexia; rarely pain or bleeding.

Stomach: Cancer may be present for 2 or 3 years before it produces symptoms such as dyspepsia, epigastric pain, nausea, vomiting. There may be a history suggestive of peptic ulcer (q.v.), from which it must often be differentiated. Although early carcinoma of the stomach may be relatively silent, anorexia, epigastric discomfort (sometimes leading to pain), nausea and vomiting are frequently experienced. Dysphagia or pylorospasm may be present if the lesion involves the cardia or pylorus respectively. Bleeding, as evidenced by fresh or old (coffee ground vomitus) blood or tarry stools, may occur at any time during the course of the disease. A macrocytic hyperchromic anemia, often indistinguishable from pernicious anemia, is not infrequently associated with gastric cancer. Chronic gastritis often precedes or accompanies gastric cancer. Gastric analysis usually reveals hypochlorhydria or achlorhydria, lactic acid, Boas-Oppler bacilli, and often occult blood.

Small Intestine: Malignant growths are rare. Partial obstruction is manifested by dyspepsia, constipation and, rarely, melena.

Colon: Sigmoidal growths cause obstruction early, with symptoms of increasing constipation (often alternating with diarrhea), streaking of stools with red blood (rarely massive hemorrhage), cramps, and cachexia. In cancer of the ascending colon, obstruction is unusual until late in the disease. However, ulceration of the growth occurs early, the resultant bleeding causing a severe microcytic hypochromic anemia even before intestinal function is disturbed.

Rectum: There may be a sense of rectal discomfort, with a change of bowel habit. Painless bleeding is common. In advanced cases, rectal obstruction supervenes.

Anus: A painful malignant ulcer usually is evident.

Diagnosis

The diagnosis depends on X-ray or endoscopic demonstration of the growth. Most rectal cancers can be palpated with the finger. Cancer should be suspected and searched for in any individual over 35 who complains of weakness or anorexia, weight loss, recently acquired gastric symptoms, alteration in bowel habit, hematemesis or melena, or has an unexplained macrocytic hyperchromic, or a severe microcytic hypochromic anemia. The presence of a palpable abdominal mass usually indicates the case is hopeless; this is certain when there are metastases, including the Virchow node in gastric cancer.

Prognosis

If the neoplasm is discovered early and treated properly, permanent eradication or a 5-year "cure" is possible. Usually, however, the course is progressively downward, death eventually occurring in 1 to 3 years due to cachexia, hemorrhage, or a terminal infection.

Treatment

In the absence of evident metastases, radical excision of the growth is indicated. Roentgen therapy preoperatively sometimes is useful in anal ulcers. If metastases are demonstrable, therapy is merely palliative and symptomatic, since the outlook will not be significantly improved by removal of the primary growth.

ANORECTAL DISORDERS

A number of conditions of related anatomical origin are here discussed. In many instances there is an overlapping of symptomatology, while several methods of examination and modes of treatment are similar. Neoplasms of this region are discussed in a separate chapter (q.v.).

ANAL FISSURE

An interruption of the continuity of the lining surface of the anal canal, frequently accompanied by inflammation.

Etiology

Any object that lacerates the anal skin may produce a fissure. The most common causes are passage of a hard constipated stool, anal stenosis, hypertonicity of sphincter muscle, fish bones, careless instrumentation, overenthusiastic divulsion, childbirth, cryptitis, or other inflammatory condition rendering anal tissues more susceptible to injury. A simple tear of the epithelium appears first, usually in the posterior midline. If this does not heal in a few days, inflammation occurs, with attendant swelling of the surrounding tissues, and a sentinel pile of Brodie appears at the outer end of the fissure.

Symptoms, Signs, and Diagnosis

The principal symptom is pain on defecation, that subsides but recurs in the next half hour. There may be slight bleeding. Fissures must be differentiated from syphilitic chancre, which is not painful and usually is laterally located; from chancroid with very painful multiple ulcers; and from tuberculous ulcers, which frequently are lateral, may be painless, and usually are associated with tuberculosis elsewhere in the body.

Treatment

Maintain soft stools by means of liquid petrolatum (℞ 23) or sulfur with or without reinforcement by other laxatives (℞ 31). Following each stool, a cupful of cool water should be injected into the rectum to keep the latter clean.

The superficial fissure is the only one on which topical applications can be used successfully. For this purpose liquified phenol (℞ 51), ichthammol (℞ 32), silver nitrate 5% (℞ 50), or balsam of Peru 20% (℞ 33) is recommended. This local treatment, with the insertion of an analgesic suppository (℞ 34) after defecation, may produce healing. Cure often is obtained by gentle dilation of the anal sphincter either with anal dilators or the gloved finger. Dilation should be performed twice daily, with rectal instillation of cod liver oil (℞ 35) at bedtime. In the presence of excessive sphincter spasm, application of a local anesthetic (℞ 36) may help to induce relaxation.

The deeper fissure cannot be improved by topical applications. Infiltration with a local anesthetic solution (℞ 126), plus dilation with the lubricated finger can be tried before resorting to surgical excision and drainage. If a good result is to be obtained from excision, it is important that part of the external sphincter be severed.

CRYPTITIS

An inflammation of the crypts of Morgagni, the saclike cavities of rectal mucosa just above the anorectal line, which readily catch small foreign bodies or particles of feces. Pressure and necrosis of this material may produce infection in the crypt wall, which spreads rapidly in the submucosal plane. The usual symptom is pain, dull or sharp, which is increased by bowel movements. It often is accompanied by sphincter spasm, which may result in constipation. Digital examination reveals tenderness of the inflamed crypt, and when infection is present, pus can easily be expressed.

Treatment

The pain may be alleviated by instillations of warm olive oil (℞ 37) or of an ichthammol 25% solution (℞ 38) twice a day. A sitz bath or hot boric acid compresses (℞ 39) frequently give relief. Maintenance of soft stools is desirable during the acute phase of the inflammation. If symptoms do not subside under the treatment described, the affected crypt may be excised under local anesthesia, a blunt hook in the crypt outlining the area for excision. Bleeding usually is slight and controllable by pressure. Sitz baths or hot compresses are used in the healing stage. Gentian violet, 1% solution (℞ 40), may be painted on the wound every other day. Insert the finger into the rectum every 3rd day to prevent bridging during healing.

ABSCESS

Anorectal abscesses are divided arbitrarily into those situated above the levator ani muscles, and those below. The supralevator abscesses are either in the rectal wall or in the supralevator space, in which case they are called pelvirectal and in some cases retrorectal abscesses. The infralevator group includes ischiorectal abscesses and those involving the skin only.

Etiology

With the exception of the cutaneous variety of anorectal abscess the infection usually is secondary to inflammation of one or more of the crypts of Morgagni. The infection spreads, often without causing symptoms of cryptitis, and an abscess develops in one of the many rectal or perirectal sites. The supralevator abscesses also may originate from infection in the broad ligament or in the male pelvic organs, from traumatism, and from inflammatory processes in the rectal mucosa. Organisms frequently found are *Esch. coli*, staphylococci and streptococci.

Symptoms and Signs

The usual symptoms of inflammation and abscess formation are found in the anorectal region. A painful swelling with redness and induration readily suggests the cutaneous or ischiorectal abscess. Fever may be present with the latter. Insertion of the finger into the anal canal usually is painful. Supralevator abscesses are more difficult to detect. An abscess above the levator muscles may cause fever and a boggy tender mass anterolaterally in the midrectal region. There may be peritoneal irritation resulting in tenderness and muscle guarding in the lower quadrants of the abdomen. Except for the retrorectal type, supralevator abscesses cause no tenderness near the anus. Abscesses within the wall of the rectum produce a heavy, dull ache. Tuberculous abscesses are characteristically without pain and tenderness.

Treatment

Abscess in the anorectal area requires incision and drainage. Failure to give proper treatment may result in spread of the infection. A frequent complication of perirectal abscess is fistula formation (q.v.).

FISTULA IN ANO

Anorectal fistulas are deep sinuous passages leading from the anorectal canal and usually opening through the skin near the anus. They may be single or multiple. Complete fistulas have openings at both ends; incomplete fistulas, an internal opening only. Those with one or more outlets in the perianal skin are called external; those that communicate with the rectum but do not necessarily penetrate the skin, internal.

Fistulas occur as a sequel to abscess formation, and usually are of the complete external type. These are identified by a chronic or recurrent purulent discharge in the skin near the anus. A small, blunt metal probe passed through the external opening will follow the tract and emerge into the anal or rectal canal. The origin of the inflammation usually is at the anorectal line, often in a crypt of Morgagni. Multiple skin openings in the perianal region may lead to tracts that practically surround the anterior or posterior halves of the anus, and these are known as horseshoe fistulas. Incomplete internal fistulas can be discovered only by proctoscopy.

Treatment

This is invariably by surgical excision of the infected tract. It must be done with great skill to avoid injury to the external sphincter muscle, which might result in fecal incontinence.

PROCTITIS

An inflammatory disease of the rectum with manifestations varying in accordance with the agent causing the inflammation.

Etiology

Acute catarrhal proctitis may be due to food allergy, over-indulgence in alcohol, localized drug reactions (e.g., to tribromoethanol solution or paraldehyde administered per rectum), reaction to cathartics, heavy infestation with intestinal worms, neurogenic disorders, trauma, fecal impaction, foreign bodies, rectal irrigations with hot solutions, prolapse and procidentia. **Chronic hypertrophic proctitis** usually is a sequel to acute proctitis and involves the pelvic colon as well as the rectum. **Chronic atrophic proctitis** is associated with prolonged constipation in debilitated elderly individuals, and is frequently restricted to the rectum. Specific types of proctitis are due to infection with the organisms that cause amebic and bacillary dysentery, chronic ulcerative colitis, venereal infections including lymphopathia venereum, and tuberculosis; also to radium emanations. Diverticulitis and cancer of the sigmoid colon with irritating discharges can cause a secondary proctitis.

Symptoms and Signs

Clinical symptoms vary in type and degree with the etiologic agent. In general, they consist of diarrhea, with or without blood and pus; rectal discomfort, tenesmus (painful, long-continued, ineffectual straining at stool), fever, and pain. **Chronic atrophic proctitis** is accompanied by constipation, but there may be recurrent episodes of diarrhea. **Acute catarrhal proctitis** is characterized by a hyperemic mucosa with a granular appearance and ulcer formation, and blood and pus in varying amounts. **Chronic hypertrophic proctitis** results in thickening of the mucosa, narrowing of the rectal lumen, and a glairy mucous exudate. Atrophic proctitis is characterized by a thin, dry mucosa.

In the specific types, generalized inflammation of the mucosa, with pus and blood, and ulcer formation in the acute stages, are present. Amebic ulcers are fairly deep and often located on the valves of Houston as well as higher up in the rectum. In bacillary dysentery, the ulcers are not characteristic; they usually are superficial with a brown base. Those of ulcerative colitis are numerous, small, and scattered diffusely throughout the sigmoid colon and rectum. Lymphopathia venereum produces ulcerative or papular lesions with a reddened and edematous mucosa in the acute stages. Radiation proctitis in the early stages exhibits a hyperemic mucosa with a granular appearance.

All the specific and acute types may progress to chronic proctitis, not necessarily resembling the acute condition. Radiation proctitis and that of lymphopathia venereum are particularly likely to develop rectal stricture. Chronic ulcerative colitis and proctitis frequently produce inflammatory polyps which tend to undergo malignant change.

Diagnosis

Proctoscopic examination, bacteriologic and microscopic investigation of the feces, and a careful evaluation of the history are essential to a diagnosis. Other aids are the examination of scrapings of the base of ulcers, agglutination tests of the blood serum for bacillary dysentery, and barium enema X-ray studies.

Treatment

Acute catarrhal proctitis: The underlying cause must be determined and eliminated. General measures to allay irritation and promote recovery are rest in bed, high vitamin nonirritating diet, including white meat and fish and excluding roughage; mineral oil (R̸ 23), rectal irrigations with physiologic saline (R̸ 41) or soda bicarbonate 2% solution (R̸ 42), and instillation of 2 oz. of warm cod liver oil (R̸ 35) or ichthammol 25% solution (R̸ 38) into the rectum daily.

Chronic hypertrophic proctitis: The determination and elimination of the causative factor is fundamental. A diet similar to that for acute catarrhal proctitis is indicated. Rectal irrigation with one of the following solutions is soothing: physiologic saline (R̸ 41), potassium permanganate 1:8,000 (R̸ 43), tannic acid 1% (R̸ 44). Ulcers may be treated by local application of 5% silver nitrate solution (R̸ 50). Warm olive oil, 2 oz. (R̸ 37), instilled into the rectum twice daily allays irritation. Bismuth salts (R̸ 8) help prevent putrefaction.

Chronic atrophic proctitis: A nutritious nonirritating diet is in order. To counteract the constipation often present, liquid cascara, 4 cc. (R̸ 22), is given at bedtime. This should not be continued indefinitely. Enemas may be necessary to aid in emptying the bowel. Rectal instillation of mineral oil, 3 oz. (R̸ 23), at bedtime is useful for lubrication.

Infectious proctitis due to intestinal parasites *(Endamoeba histolytica, Ascaris lumbricoides, Oxyuris vermicularis, Taenia saginata* and *solium)*, to lymphopathia venereum, or to gonococcal infection, or **proctitis with chronic ulcerative colitis,** should be treated as outlined under the respective diseases (q.v.). For **irradiation proctitis** treatment includes bland diet, water or saline enema after each defecation, rectal instillation of cod liver oil (℞ 35), anesthetic preparations in oil (℞ 45) to relieve pain, and colostomy for intractable bleeding or stricture formation.

HEMORRHOIDS
(Piles)

Dilatations of the veins of the hemorrhoidal plexus, with low grade inflammation and thrombi usually developing. The lesions may be **internal** (above the pectinate line) or **external** (below the pectinate), or may extend over both areas.

Etiology

Hemorrhoids may result from any condition that produces rectal venestasis, such as constipation, pregnancy, enlarged prostate, rectal disease, diverticulitis of the sigmoid, uterine tumors, urethral stricture, obesity, and sedentary occupations. There is a definite herditary predisposition to the development of hemorrhoids.

Symptoms and Signs

External hemorrhoids: These appear as small, rounded, purplish tumors covered with skin, which become more prominent when the patient strains at stool. Unless the veins are thrombosed, the lesions are soft and seldom painful, although they may produce a sense of fullness at the anus. Thrombotic hemorrhoids usually are multiple, nodule-like on palpation, and painful. They appear suddenly and enlarge rapidly. Defecation is accompanied by tenesmus and an increase of pain. These lesions may become highly inflamed, break down, and bleed profusely as a result of local trauma. External hemorrhoids tend to undergo spontaneous remissions and exacerbations; during remissions they appear at the mucocutaneous junction as tabs of hypertrophied tissue which may be asymptomatic or may itch severely.

Internal hemorrhoids: These develop above the sphincter and generally are multiple. They are soft, purple, irregular in shape, and covered by a thin layer of mucous membrane. Minor injuries cause bleeding and ulceration. Bleeding usually is the objective symptom, but a dull backache and sense of incomplete evacuation often are experienced first. There is a tendency to prolapse, which is precipitated by straining at stool and is accompanied by painful and disabling thrombosis. Constipation, leakage of mucus from the anus, and itching are frequent complications. Severe prolapse often is associated with strangulation.

Diagnosis

External hemorrhoids are readily diagnosed by direct examination; internal ones, from the symptoms and by digital and proctoscopic examination.

Hemorrhoids are the most common cause of rectal bleeding. The blood is bright red in color and usually is seen coating the surface of a formed stool. Other conditions causing bright red blood in the stool which must be differentiated include neoplasms of the lower bowel and rectum (q.v.), bleeding polyps, diverticulitis, and colitis. As a rule, bleeding from lesions high in the gastrointestinal tract causes tarry stools (see HEMATEMESIS; MELENA). However, bright red blood may be passed if the hemorrhage is massive and intestinal hypermotility is present.

Prophylaxis

During quiescence, recurrences may be prevented by keeping the stools soft with bulk diets (see DIETS) and if necessary by nonirritating laxatives such as mineral oil (R 23). The anus at all times must be kept scrupulously clean, which is difficult to accomplish when the hemorrhoids are external. After each stool the area should be washed with cold water and a soft sponge, then thoroughly dried and sprinkled with talcum powder. When the hemorrhoid is internal, about 60 cc. of cold water should be injected after each bowel movement and immediately ejected with gentle pressure. Thus, the folds of the anus can be kept clean. The crypts can be cleansed with the finger wrapped in moist cotton.

Treatment

Constipation must be corrected by mild measures, as outlined above. Drastic catharsis is contraindicated. Warm olive oil, 2 to 3 oz. (R 37), injected rectally through a small rubber catheter is soothing. Thrombosed external hemorrhoids respond well to hot sitz baths or the application of hot compresses of boric acid solution (R 39). The clots may be removed by incision and evacuation under local anesthesia to obtain relief more quickly. Protruding internal hemorrhoids should be reduced digitally if edema and strangulation do not prohibit this maneuver. Recumbency in the prone position and cold applications make it easier subsequently to squeeze out the edema (gently) and get the mass through the sphincter. Application of a local anesthetic (R 45) astringent antispasmodic ointment (R 46) or an iodoform tannic acid salve (R 47) also may be helpful; after reduction, the ointment may be injected into the rectum, or a suppository (R 34) inserted. Opium may be added to each suppository to relieve pain.

Hemorrhage usually clears up spontaneously; if it does not, epinephrine solution 1:1,000 applied with cotton is helpful.

Injection therapy: Simple uncomplicated internal hemorrhoids without severe prolapse, ulceration, infection, or strangulation are suitable for injection. (External hemorrhoids should never be so treated.) A safe average amount of the sclerosing solution to inject into the submucosa in any one hemorrhoid is 1 cc. Moderate distention of the pile is the proper result. If the injection is made into the mucosa, blanching appears and a slough will follow. A week later, if the patient has shown no sign of sensitivity to the solution, more than one injection can be made. The following preparations are recommended: 5% solution of quinine and urea hydrochloride (R 52); 5% solution of sodium morrhuate (R 53); or 5% solution of phenol in oil (R 54). Surgical excision is indicated when conservative measures are not successful.

PROLAPSE OF THE RECTUM

Partial prolapse: *simple eversion of the rectal mucosa through the anus.* Complete prolapse: *eversion of the entire rectal wall.* Partial prolapse, the more common form, usually is seen in infancy, early childhood, and old age. A predisposing condition in children is the absence of a sacral curve; this causes the rectum to become a straight tube when the patient sits. Abnormal motility of the rectal mucosa upon the submucosa also is contributory. In elderly persons, decreased muscle tone plays an important role. In all age groups, straining at stool is the chief precipitating factor; it may be associated with diarrhea or constipation. In early cases the tissue returns spontaneously into the rectum. As the condition progresses, protrusion occurs not only after a stool but also on coughing or any strong muscular exertion, and the tissue must be replaced manually. Later developments are mucoid discharge with slight bleeding and congestion and ulceration of the exposed mucosa. Rarely, gangrene may occur due to constriction by the sphincter muscle.

Treatment

The first step is manual replacement of prolapsed tissue. If this cannot be accomplished by ordinary manipulation, the insertion of a soft paper cone occasionally is helpful. Anesthesia may be necessary at the time for muscular relaxation. Bowel movements must be controlled by appropriate means to reduce straining. Diet should be low in residue. Hemorrhoids or polyps, if present, should be removed, as they predispose to prolapse. In small children, especially, regular bowel movements at the same time each day should be induced. Mineral oil (R 23), or olive oil (R 37) by rectum, will produce a soft stool. A small cold water enema before each movement is helpful. If feasible, the child should be placed in a recumbent or semirecumbent position for defecation. In any case, prolonged sitting at stool is to be avoided. The buttocks are best strapped together after defecation to prevent prolapse.

Older patients should be instructed to contract the sphincter muscle repeatedly through the day to improve its tone. Faradic current stimulation in the elderly or debilitated may increase the tone considerably.

Injection of a sclerosing solution into the submucosa of the lower rectum through a proctoscope is advantageous in mild prolapse. Preliminary sedation may suffice to keep the patient quiet. The solutions recommended are the same as those for hemorrhoids (℞ 52, 53, 54). The injections are made at several points, 0.5 to 1 cc. at a time, the highest injection being made first. A total of 3 to 5 cc. may be injected into a child at one treatment, and repeated in a week if necessary. Surgical treatment is indicated for severe prolapse.

INJURIES

Traumatic injuries of the rectum may be caused by operation, instrumentation, foreign bodies (q.v.), fracture of pelvic bones, or penetrating wounds from without; trauma from an enema nozzle has been reported. Pain is always present, and this together with the history and digital and proctoscopic examination readily affords the diagnosis of minor injuries. Hemorrhage may appear, and even a small amount of blood in the bowel lumen usually indicates penetration of the bowel wall. Inability to distend the rectum or sigmoid with air confirms the presence of perforation. If the peritoneal cavity has been entered, shock and peritonitis rapidly ensue.

Small lower rectal wounds may be sutured. If the injuries are extensive and involve the sphincter or the urethra, a colostomy is indicated. Wounds in this region are particularly subject to infection, and antibiotics and gas gangrene antiserum should be administered in all serious cases.

FOREIGN BODIES

Foreign bodies in the rectum usually have passed down through the gastrointestinal tract or have been inserted through the anus. Almost any kind of article may be found, ranging from screws and bone splinters to metal rods and whole drinking glasses and bottles. The patients usually are infants, children, or psychopathic or drunken individuals. The foreign body may cause rectal discomfort, pain, bleeding, or other symptoms depending upon its size, nature, and location. An exact history, if obtainable, is of great aid in diagnosis, particularly when insertion has been made through the anus. Usually, the object can be palpated or visualized through the proctosigmoidoscope; if it is too high up for this, radiographic examination is of value. Examination should be made with great care to avoid further damage to the tissues.

Removal of the object often presents a problem. In the

case of large, hollow glass articles, such as drinking glasses, bottles, or test tubes, with the open end toward the anal orifice, the following procedure is recommended: Fill the foreign object with plaster of Paris and remove after the plaster has hardened. Incorporation of a string or rubber catheter in the plaster provides the means of traction. Broken edges of glass should be covered with gauze, if possible, or the tissues otherwise protected against laceration during withdrawal of the object. The suction from above which holds a large, round object in place may be overcome by boring a hole through the foreign body, if its nature permits. Rubber-shod clamps help in grasping smooth objects. Local anesthetization of the sphincter muscle is necessary when large articles are to be removed. Very small particles—of glass, for example—can best be eliminated by having the patient ingest bulky food, such as coarse cereals or whole-grain bread.

PRURITUS ANI

A chronic constant or intermittent perianal itching of varying etiology. The perianal region is especially susceptible to development of the vicious scratch-itch cycle because its skin folds encourage retention of fecal matter, it provides an ideal environment for the growth of parasitic organisms, and the skin is highly sensitive.

Etiology

The possible causes of this ailment include (1) mechanical factors: poor anal hygiene, minor trauma secondary to defecation, instrumentation, irritating soaps, and tight clothing; (2) allergic conditions: atopic eczema, contact dermatitis, and food sensitivity; (3) local rectal disease: hemorrhoids, proctitis, cryptitis, anorectal papillitis, fissures, fistulas, and skin tags; (4) infectious and parasitic agents: fungi (Monilia), Trichomonas, pediculi, and intestinal parasites; (5) psychogenic: sexual maladjustment, psychoneurosis, habit; and (6) systemic disease: genitourinary or gynecologic disorders, and the various conditions that cause jaundice.

Symptoms and Signs

The pruritus may extend from the anus to the labia or scrotum, but occasionally the process is reversed, with vulvar or scrotal pruritus coming first. The paroxysms of itching often are worse at night. They are aggravated by heat and improper cleansing following defecation.

In early cases, the lesion may be one-sided or confined to a patch, but usually it is circumanal extending for variable distances over the perineum. The skin around the anus is erythematous, with excoriations, and may be dry or moist. The radiating skin folds are accentuated by edema. In chronic cases, the skin has a whitish gray, sodden appearance, is less erythematous but shows evidence of lichenification, fissuring, excoriation, and accentuation of the skin folds.

Treatment

The possibility of cure is good, provided the single or multiple causative factors have been determined and a specific therapeutic regimen instituted. Not infrequently, however, even when all such factors have been eliminated, the pruritus continues because of skin changes that have taken place. Therefore, the following treatment should be instituted regardless of etiology. (Hospitalization is necessary in severe cases.)

1. Anal hygiene: This includes a bland, low residue diet (*see* DIETS), with toilet training, to ensure a soft bowel movement once daily, at the same hour, preferably on arising in the morning. Anal manipulations as by enemas or prostatic massage, should not be allowed because of their tendency to stimulate itching. The patient is instructed to carry out the following routine after each bowel movement: (*a*) cleanse the anus with a water-moistened cotton pad; (*b*) use a sitz bath, already prepared with tepid water containing a soapless detergent in a large basin, for 5 minutes. Assume a squatting position so that the buttocks are spread apart and the anus can be adequately cleansed. The solution then should be washed off the anus and genitalia in a sitz bath of clean warm water. Dry the parts with a soft towel, using patting movements.

2. Sedation: Barbiturates (℞ 66) are desirable for sedation. The optimum dosage varies and must be determined by the response of the individual patient.

3. Local therapy: Tepid sitz baths with potassium permanganate (℞ 48) or local compresses with silver nitrate solution (℞ 49) are recommended during the acute phase. In cases with pyogenic or fungus elements, Castellani's paint (℞ 120) diluted with an equal amount of water, or full strength, is applied locally 1 to 3 times a day; Desenex (℞ 121) or Pragmatar (℞ 122) can be used in the same way. A mild, cooling antipruritic shake lotion (℞ 125) frequently is useful when there is considerable lichenification; this lotion leaves a thick, heavy coating after the water evaporates. Thephorin, a relatively new antipruritic agent (℞ 124), is effective in a significant percentage of patients. However, it should be emphasized that the use of antipruritic agents is not a substitute for an etiologic approach to therapy in each patient.

4. X-ray: Among the local measures, superficial X-radiation given by a qualified physician affords a modality that frequently produces dramatic relief by decreasing the pruritic hyperexcitability.

5. Surgical methods: Many surgical means have been devised for the relief of pruritus ani, ranging from tattooing to Ball's undercutting operation. This purely symptomatic approach is frequently unsuccessful and surgery should be limited to the correction of specific pathologic conditions.

No attempt has been made to discuss treatment of the diseases causing pruritus ani, which can be found in the appropriate chapters. Resistant cases should be referred to the dermatologist or the proctologist for study and therapy.

PRESCRIPTIONS

(Wherever a prescribed "proprietary" is representative of a class of therapeutic agents, alternative proprietary preparations will be found listed in Part II.)

Antacids

1. ℞ Magnesium trisilicate. . . . 0.45 Gm. (gr. vii)
   Aluminum hydroxide. . . . 0.24 Gm. (gr. iv)
   1 powder after each meal.

2. ℞ Magnesium trisilicate. . . . 0.5 Gm. (gr. viiss)
   1 or 2 tablets or powders in water 15 minutes before each feeding.

3. ℞ Dried Aluminum Hydroxide
   Gel U.S.P., 7% solution . 200.0 cc. (℥ viss)
   Distilled water. . . . . . . 600.0 cc. (℥ xx)
   Allow mixture to drip into stomach through small nasal tube at rate of 30 drops/minute, day and night, for as long as is necessary to control symptoms. (CAUTION! Aluminum hydroxide is contraindicated when there is pyloric obstruction or bleeding into the gastrointestinal tract.)

4. ℞ Sodium bicarbonate . . . . 0.3 Gm. (gr. v)
   Crush 2 tablets in a glass of water and drink slowly.

5. ℞ Aluminum Hydroxide Gel
   U.S.P.
   2 tablespoons 3 or 4 times a day.

6. ℞ Precipitated calcium carbonate. . . . . 1.0 Gm. (gr. xv)
   1 powder in water 1½ hours after each meal.

Antidiarrheal Agents

7. ℞ Bismuth subcarbonate . . . 15.0 Gm. (℥ ss)
   Kaolin . . . . 15.0 Gm. (℥ ss)
   Water . . . . .q.s. ad 200.0 cc. (℥ viss)
   1 teaspoon every 4 hours as necessary.

8. ℞ Bismuth subcarbonate . . . 1.0 Gm. (gr. xv)
   1 or 2 powders, with water, at bedtime.

9. ℞ Deodorized Opium Tincture
   U.S.P. . . . . 30.0 cc. (℥ i)
   5 to 10 drops in water every 4 to 6 hours.

10. ℞ Belladonna Tincture U.S.P. . 6.0 cc. (℥ iss)
    Deodorized Opium Tincture
    U.S.P. . . . . . .q.s. ad 30.0 cc. (℥ i)
    5 to 10 drops in water every 4 to 6 hours.

11. ℞ Camphorated Opium Tincture
    U.S.P. (Paregoric) . . . 60.0 cc. (℥ ii)
    1 or 2 teaspoons every 4 hours.

12. ℞ Camphorated Opium Tincture
    U.S.P. (Paregoric) . . . 30.0 cc. (℥ i)
    Bismuth subnitrate. . . . 15.0 Gm. (℥ ss)
    Cinnamon Water U.S.P.
    q.s. ad 60.0 cc. (℥ ii)
    1 teaspoon every 2 hours.

13. ℞ Belladonna Extract U.S.P. . 0.5 Gm. (gr. viiss)
    Phenobarbital. . . . . . 0.4 Gm. (gr. vi)
    Bismuth subnitrate. . . . 24.0 Gm. (℥ vi)
    Kaolin . . . . 45.0 Gm. (℥ iss)
    Peppermint Oil U.S.P. . . 0.12 cc. (♏ ii)
    1 teaspoon before each meal until diarrhea
    has subsided.

14. ℞ Kaolin
    1 to 2 tablespoons in water 3 or 4 times daily.

Digestants

15. ℞ Diluted Hydrochloric Acid
    U.S.P. . . . . 120.0 cc. (℥ iv)
    1 teaspoon in at least ½ glass of water, to
    be sipped through a straw during each meal.

16. ℞ Glutamic acid hydrochloride. 0.3 Gm. (gr. v)
    2 or 3 capsules with each meal (each capsule
    is equivalent to 10 drops of Diluted Hydro-
    chloric Acid U.S.P.).

17. ℞ Pancreatin U.S.P. . . . . . 0.3 Gm. (gr. v)
    2 to 6 tablets after each meal.

18. ℞ Oxbile Extract U.S.P. . . . 0.3 Gm. (gr. v)
    1 tablet 1½ hours after each meal.

Emetics

19. ℞ Apomorphine hydrochloride
    6 mg. (gr. 1/10) subcut.

20. ℞ Ipecac Syrup U.S.P. . . . . 30.0 cc. (℥ i)

    1 to 3 teaspoons every 15 minutes until vomiting is induced.

Cathartics

21. ℞ Milk of Magnesia U.S.P.

    1 to 3 tablespoons at bedtime.

22. ℞ Cascara Sagrada Fluidextract U.S.P.

    1 teaspoon at bedtime.

23. ℞ Liquid Petrolatum U.S.P.

    1 or 2 tablespoons at bedtime; for rectal instillation, instill 3 ounces at bedtime.

24. ℞ Sodium sulfate

    2 tablespoons in ½ glass water.

25. ℞ Methylated cellulose . . . . . 0.5 Gm. (gr. viiss)

    3 to 6 tablets daily with at least 1 glass of water.

26. ℞ Agar U.S.P. . . . . 15.0 Gm. (℥ ss)

    2 to 4 teaspoons dissolved in water and followed with a full glass of water, daily.

27. ℞ Emulsion of agar and mineral oil

    1 to 2 tablespoons daily, taken with water.

28. ℞ Psyllium Hydrophilic Mucilloid with Dextrose N.N.R.

    1 to 4 teaspoons in a full glass or two of water.

29. ℞ Cascara Sagrada Extract U.S.P. . . . . 0.3 Gm. (gr. v)

    1 or 2 tablets at night.

30. ℞ Magnesium sulfate

    1 teaspoon in water.

31. ℞ Sulfur . . . . 0.6 Gm. (gr. x)
    Potassium bitartrate . . . . 0.2 Gm. (gr. iii)
    Senna U.S.P. . . . . 0.1 Gm. (gr. iss)

    1 or 2 capsules at bedtime.

Emollients and Antiseptics

32. ℞ Ichthammol N.F. . . . . . . 30.0 Gm. (℥ i)

    Apply undiluted once daily to lesion.

33. ℞ Peruvian Balsam. . . . . . . 6.0 Gm. (℥ iss)
    Castor oil. . . . . . .q.s. ad 30.0 cc. (℥ i)

    Apply locally once daily.

34. ℞ Iodoform . . . .   0.15 Gm. (gr. iiss)
     Opium Extract N.F. . . . . .   0.02 Gm. (gr. ⅓)
     Belladonna Extract U.S.P. .   0.01 Gm. (gr. ⅙)
     Cocoa Butter U.S.P. . .q.s. ad   2.0   Gm. (℥ ss)
     1 suppository in rectum night and morning.

35. ℞ Cod Liver Oil U.S.P.
     Instill 2 ounces into the rectum at bedtime.

36. ℞ Benzocaine . . . .   0.03 Gm. (gr. ss)
     Phenol . . . .   0.05 Gm. (gr. ¾)
     Benzyl alcohol . . . . . .   0.50 cc. (♏ viiss)
     Expressed Almond Oil U.S.P.
                         q.s. ad   5.0   cc. (♏ lxxv)
     For local anesthesia of anal fissure.

37. ℞ Olive oil
     Warm and instill 2 to 3 ounces into rectum
     morning and night.

38. ℞ Ichthammol N.F. . . . . .   30.0   Gm. (℥ i)
     Glycerin . . . . . .q.s. ad 120.0   cc. (℥ iv)
     Instill 2 ounces into rectum twice daily.

39. ℞ Boric acid, 5% solution
     Apply locally as a warm compress.

40. ℞ Gentian violet, 1% solution .   30.0   cc. (℥ i)
     Apply to area of excised crypt every 2 days.

41. ℞ Sodium chloride, 0.85% solu-
         tion
     For irrigating rectum; use 1 pint at 110° F.
     twice a day.

42. ℞ Sodium bicarbonate, 2% solu-
         tion
     For irrigating rectum; use 1 pint at 110° F.
     twice a day.

43. ℞ Potassium permanganate,
         1:8,000 solution
     Use 1 pint as a rectal irrigation.

44. ℞ Tannic acid, 1% solution
     Use 1 pint as a warm rectal irrigation.

45. ℞ Benzocaine . . . .   4.0   Gm. (℥ i)
     Olive oil . . . . . .q.s. ad 120.0   cc. (℥ iv)
     Instill 2 ounces into rectum daily.

46. ℞ Belladonna Ointment U.S.P.
     Tannic Acid Ointment U.S.P.
                         āā   30.0   Gm. (℥ i)
     Apply freely within the rectum and ex-
     ternally.

47. ℞ Iodoform . . . . 4.0 Gm. (ʒ i)
   Tannic acid . . . . 2.0 Gm. (ʒ ss)
   White Petrolatum U.S.P.
   q.s. ad 30.0 Gm. (ʒ i)

   Apply freely within the rectum.

48. ℞ Potassium permanganate . . 0.12 Gm. (gr. ii)

   Dissolve 2 tablets per gallon of water and
   use as sitz bath for 20 minutes twice daily.

49. ℞ Silver nitrate, 0.1% solution

   Apply locally as compresses.

Caustic and Sclerosing Agents

50. ℞ Silver nitrate, 5% solution . . 30.0 cc. (ʒ i)

   Apply topically once daily.

51. ℞ Liquified Phenol U.S.P. . . 30.0 cc. (ʒ i)

   Apply once daily to lesions, undiluted.

52. ℞ Quinine and Urea Hydrochloride, N.F., 5% solution
   (vial)

   For injection treatment of internal hemorrhoids.

53. ℞ Sodium morrhuate, 5% solution (ampul)

   For injection treatment of internal hemorrhoids.

54. ℞ Phenol . . . . 1.5 Gm. (gr. xxiiss)
   Olive oil . . . . . q.s. ad 30.0 cc. (ʒ i)

   For injection treatment of internal hemorrhoids.

Agents Affecting the Autonomic Nervous System or Smooth Musculature

55. ℞ "Urecholine Chloride" . . . 5 mg.

   2 to 5 tablets orally or sublingually immediately after each meal.

56. ℞ Belladonna Tincture U.S.P. 30.0 cc. (ʒ i)
   Phenobarbital Elixir U.S.P.
   q.s. ad 180.0 cc. (ʒ vi)

   1 teaspoon ½ hour before each meal and at
   bedtime.

57. ℞ Atropine sulfate (hypodermic tablet)

   0.6 mg. (gr. 1/100) orally or subcut. every
   6 hours if necessary.

   For muscarine poisoning: 1 mg. (gr. 1/60)
   subcut. or I.V. every 1 to 2 hours until
   symptoms are relieved.

58. ℞ Scopolamine (Hyoscine) hydrobromide
   0.4 mg. (gr. 1/150) subcut.

59. ℞ A synthetic antispasmodic
   (For available products *see* dose
   table of ALTERNATIVE PROPRIE-
   TARY PREPARATIONS.)

60. ℞ Amyl nitrite (ampul) . . . 0.2 cc. (♏ iii)
   Crush 1 ampul in handkerchief and inhale
   fumes.

61. ℞ Nitroglycerin (hypodermic
   tablet) . . . . 0.3 mg. (gr. 1/200)
   Dissolve 1 or 2 tablets under tongue as necessary.

62. ℞ Papaverine hydrochloride
   (ampul)
   15 to 60 mg. (gr. ¼ to i) I.V. repeated as
   necessary.

63. ℞ Belladonna Tincture U.S.P. . 30.0 cc. (℥ i)
   10 to 15 drops in water before meals and at
   bedtime.

64. ℞ Neostigmine methylsulfate,
   1:2,000 solution (ampul)
   0.5 to 1 cc. (♏ viii to xv) subcut. 2 or 3
   times daily.

65. ℞ Atropine sulfate . . . . . . 0.0003 Gm. (gr. 1/200)
   Acetylsalicylic acid . . . . 0.3 Gm. (gr. v)
   Acetophenetidin . . . . . 0.2 Gm. (gr. iii)
   1 capsule 3 times daily.

Sedatives and Analgesics

66. ℞ Phenobarbital . . . . 15 mg. (gr. ¼)
   1 or 2 tablets every 4 hours.

67. ℞ Phenobarbital Elixir U.S.P. 240.0 cc. (℥ viii)
   1 teaspoon after each meal and at bedtime.

68. ℞ Phenobarbital sodium (ampul)
   0.1 to 0.3 Gm. (gr. iss to v) subcut. or I.M.

69. ℞ Pentobarbital sodium . . . 0.1 Gm. (gr. iss)
   1 capsule at bedtime.

70. ℞ Chloral hydrate . . . . . . 0.3 Gm. (gr. v)
   1 to 3 capsules at bedtime.

71. ℞ Chloral hydrate . . . . 1.0   Gm. (gr. xv)
Cottonseed oil . . . q.s. ad 60.0   cc. (℥ ii)

> Emulsify and instill rectally every 6 hours
> if necessary.

72. ℞ Methadone Hydrochloride
N.N.R. 5   mg.

> 1 or 2 tablets every 4 hours for pain.

73. ℞ Methadone Hydrochloride
N.N.R.   (ampul)

> 2.5 to 10 mg. I.M. every 4 hours for pain.

74. ℞ Morphine sulfate

> 10 to 15 mg. (gr. ⅙ to ¼) subcut. every 4
> hours.

75. ℞ "Demerol Hydrochloride"
(ampul)

> 50 to 100 mg. I.M. every 4 hours for pain.

76. ℞ "Dilaudid Hydrochloride"
(ampul)

> 2 mg. (gr. 1/30) subcut.

77. ℞ Codeine phosphate 30   mg. (gr. ss)

> Subcut. every 4 hours for pain.

Anthelminthics

In prescribing the anthelminthics, the recommended dosage regimen must not be exceeded. If the drug is one that is administered as a single dose, or in fractionated doses within a matter of hours, it is given in the morning and with the stomach empty. A saline purgative, such as sodium sulfate (℞ 91) or magnesium sulfate (℞ 92), is administered both the night before and 2 to 5 hours following the specific medication. Symptoms of intestinal obstruction, perforation, or appendicitis contraindicate anthelminthic medication or purgation until such crisis is past.

It is frequently necessary to treat the anemia resulting from the helminthic infection before administering an anthelminthic. If the anemia is severe, repeated blood transfusions may be indicated. For an anemia of moderate degree, ferrous sulfate (℞ 97) 0.2 Gm. 3 times daily for 10 to 12 days usually suffices.

78. ℞ "Atabrine" . . . . 0.1   Gm. (gr. iss)

> 1 tablet 3 times a day for 5 days.

79. ℞ Carbarsone . . . . 0.25   Gm. (gr. iv)

> *Adults:* 1 tablet daily for 7 to 10 days;
> course may be repeated, if necessary, after
> a rest period of 10 days.
> *Children:* Total dose of 75 mg./Kg. body
> wt. is given over a 10-day period.

80. ℞ "Stovarsol" (Acetarsone) . .   0.25 Gm. (gr. iv)

> *Adults:* 2 tablets daily for 7 to 10 days.
> *Children:* 0.05 to 0.2 Gm. (gr. ¾ to iii)
> daily, according to age, for 7 to 10 days.

81. ℞ Hexylresorcinol . . . . . .   0.1 Gm. (gr. iss)

> Orally, required number of tablets swal-
> lowed whole with water as a single dose.
> *Adults and children over 12 yrs. of age:*
> 1.0 Gm. (gr. xv)
> *Children:* 8 to 12 yrs., 0.8 Gm. (gr. xii)
>   6 to 8 yrs., 0.6 Gm. (gr. x)
>   Under 6 yrs., 0.1 Gm. (gr. iss)/yr.
>   of age.

82. ℞ Tetrachloroethylene . . . .   2.7 cc. (♏ xl)
    Chenopodium Oil N.F. . . .   0.3 cc. (♏ v)

> Dispense in 0.5 or 1 cc. amounts in soft
> gelatin capsules.
> *Adults:* 3 capsules (3 cc.), repeated after
> 5 days if necessary.
> *Children:* 0.2 cc. (♏ iii)/yr. of age.
> (CAUTION! The patient should remain in
> bed and take no food until a copious bowel
> evacuation results from saline catharsis
> given 2 hours after medication.)

83. ℞ Santonin . . . .   30 mg. (gr. ss)

> *Adults:* 0.1 to 0.2 Gm. (gr. iss to iii), orally
> as a single dose.
> *Children:* 10 mg. (gr. ⅙)/yr. of age, orally
> as a single dose.
> (CAUTION! Visual disturbances, vomiting,
> convulsion. Do not repeat.)

84. ℞ Carbon tetrachloride

> Administer orally as a single dose dispensed
> in gelatin capsules.
> *Adults:* 2 to 3 cc.
> *Children:* 0.1 cc. to 0.2 cc. (♏ iss to iii)/yr.
> of age.
> (CAUTION! Contraindicated in the presence
> of renal or hepatic diseases, or concurrent
> ascaris infection. No alcohol should be
> taken on the day of treatment and the drug
> should not be repeated until after 3 weeks.)

85. ℞ Tetrachloroethylene

> Dispense in gelatin capsules containing 0.5
> or 1 cc. and administer as a single dose.
> *Adults:* 3 cc. (♏ xlv)
> *Children:* 0.2 cc. (♏ iii)/yr. of age.

86. ℞ Gentian violet (enteric
    coated) . . . .   30 mg. (gr. ss)

> *Adults:* 2 tablets 3 times a day for 16 to 18
> days.
> *Children:* 1 to 3 tablets daily, according to
> age, for 10 days.

87. ℞ Aspidium Oleoresin U.S.P.

> To be administered after a 24- to 48-hour
> period of starvation. During that time,
> only liquids and broths are permitted; a
> saline cathartic is indicated daily for 2 days
> before treatment.
> Dispense in capsules, each containing 0.6 cc.
> (♏ x).
> *Adults:* 2 capsules every 30 minutes for 3
> doses (total, 3.6 cc.).
> *Children:* 0.06 cc. (♏ i)/yr. of age, every 30
> minutes for 3 doses.
> All bowel movements for 48 hours should be
> carefully examined to discover if the head of
> the tapeworm has been passed. In any
> case, therapy should not be repeated unless
> and until segments of the tapeworm again
> appear in the stools. Contraindications:
> Nephritis, pregnancy.

88. ℞ Aspidium Oleoresin U.S.P. .   4.0   cc.   (℥ i)
    Acacia Mucilage U.S.P. . . 30.0   cc.   (℥ i)
    Sodium sulfate, saturated
    solution. . . . . 30.0   cc.   (℥ i)

> Prepare patient as for ℞ 87. Administer by
> transduodenal intubation. Following ad-
> ministration, examine bowel movement as
> in ℞ 87.

89. ℞ Chloroquine diphosphate
    ("Aralen Diphosphate") .   0.25   Gm. (gr. iv)

> 2 tablets every 12 hours for 3 to 5 doses.

90. ℞ Emetine hydrochloride
    (ampul)

> 40 to 60 mg. (gr. ⅔ to i) I.M. daily for 6 to
> 10 days. (CAUTION! Therapy should be
> promptly terminated if signs of toxicity,
> such as generalized myositis and particu-
> larly, myocarditis, appear.)

91. ℞ Sodium sulfate (Glauber's
    salts), saturated solution

> 1 to 2 ounces the night before and 2 to 5
> hours after the administration of a vermi-
> fuge.

92. ℞ Magnesium sulfate

> 3 to 6 teaspoons in water taken the night
> before and 2 to 5 hours after a vermifuge.

Hematinics and Nutritional Supplements

93. ℞ Liver Injection (Crude) U.S.P.
    (vial)

> 2 to 6 cc. I.M. 2 or 3 times a week for 2
> weeks, then once or twice weekly thereafter.

94. ℞ Powdered Stomach U.S.P.

> 1 tablespoon in water or fruit juice 3 times
> daily.

95. ℞ Ferrous gluconate . . . . 0.3 Gm. (gr. v)
    1 tablet 3 times daily, after meals.

96. ℞ Ferrous gluconate, 5% elixir . 240.0 cc. (℥ viii)
    2 teaspoons 3 times a day.

97. ℞ Ferrous sulfate . . . . . . 0.2 Gm. (gr. iii)
    1 or 2 tablets 3 times daily.

98. ℞ Ferrous Sulfate Syrup N.F. . 240.0 cc. (℥ viii)
    2 teaspoons 3 times a day.

99. ℞ Protein hydrolysate powder
    Maltose. . . . . . . āā q.s.

    Dissolve required amount (20 calories/lb.
    body wt.; 1 Gm. of mixture yields 3.8 cal-
    ories) in sufficient boiling water to make a
    15 to 25% solution. Allow to cool and
    store in refrigerator. Administer 200 to 400
    cc. every 2 hours by mouth or by the drip
    intragastric method (5 cc./minute). Vita-
    mins should be added in the form of as-
    corbic acid, brewers' yeast, thiamine hydro-
    chloride, riboflavin, nicotinic acid, vitamin
    K, and vitamins A and D. Iron may be
    administered in liquid form as elixir of fer-
    rous gluconate or ferrous sulfate.

100. ℞ Amino acids, 10% solution
    (sterile bottle)

    Administer I.V. as needed at the rate of 120
    to 160 drops/minute.

101. ℞ Protein hydrolysate . . . . 225.0 Gm. (℥ viiss)
    Milk. . . . . 1,440.0 cc. (℥ xlvii)
    Eggs, 3
    Maltose . . . . 240.0 Gm. (℥ viii)
    Vegetable purée . . . . . . 120.0 Gm. (℥ iv)
    Ascorbic acid . . . . 0.3 Gm. (gr. v)
    Dried Yeast U.S.P. . . . . . 90.0 Gm. (℥ iii)
    Percomorph Liver Oil N.N.R. 0.6 cc. (♏ x)
    Sodium chloride . . . . . . 5.0 Gm. (gr. lxxv)
    Ferrous gluconate . . . . . 1.0 Gm. (gr. xv)
    Liver Extract U.S.P. . . . . 30.0 Gm. (℥ i)
    Water . . . . q.s. ad total fluid requirements.

    Warm the milk, mix the protein hydrol-
    ysate, maltose, yeast powder, salt, and liver
    extract powder. Add to the warm milk and
    mix thoroughly. Dissolve the ascorbic acid
    tablets in a small amount of cold water and
    add to the milk mixture. Beat the eggs and
    add to the milk mixture. Add the per-
    comorph oil to the formula and refrigerate
    until ready to use. Warm each feeding to
    body temperature just before intragastric or
    intrajejunal administration.

102. ℞ Milk. . . . . 1,000.0 cc. (℥ xxxii)
       Sodium bicarbonate . . . .   5.0 Gm. (gr. lxxv)

> Allow mixture to drip into stomach through
> small nasal tube at rate of 30 drops/minute,
> day and night, as long as is necessary for
> control of acute symptoms. (CAUTION!
> Alkalosis.)

103. ℞ Pteroylglutamic (folic) acid   5   mg.

> 1 or 2 tablets 3 times daily.

Vitamins

104. ℞ Pyridoxine hydrochloride
       (Vitamin B₆)   (ampul)

> 100 mg. subcut.

105. ℞ Menadione in oil   (ampul)

> 5 mg. I.M. every 8 hours for hypoprothrom-
> binemia.

106. ℞ Ascorbic acid . . . .   0.1   Gm.

> 4 to 8 tablets daily initially, then 1 tablet
> daily.

Antimicrobial Agents

107. ℞ Sodium sulfadiazine   (ampul)

> 5 Gm. I.V. initially followed by 2.5 Gm.
> I.V. every 8 to 12 hours.

108. ℞ Sulfadiazine. . . . .   0.5   Gm. (gr. viiss)

> 2 tablets every 4 hours.

109. ℞ Penicillin   (vial)

> 30,000 to 50,000 u. I.M. every 3 hours or
> 300,000 u. I.M. every 12 hours.

110. ℞ Procaine penicillin   (vial)

> 300,000 u. I.M. every 12 to 24 hours.

111. ℞ Streptomycin   (vial)

> For nontuberculous conditions:
> 0.5 Gm. I.M. every 4 to 6 hours.
>
> For oropharyngeal or gastrointestinal tuber-
> culosis: 1 Gm. I.M. daily for 42 to 90 days,
> or until healing if this occurs sooner.

112. ℞ Dihydrostreptomycin   (vial)

> For nontuberculous conditions:
> 1 to 2 Gm. I.M. daily.
>
> For oropharyngeal or gastrointestinal tuber-
> culosis: 1 to 2 Gm. I.M. daily for 42 to 90
> days, or until healing if this occurs sooner.

113. ℞ Aureomycin (capsules) . . 0.25 Gm.

    25 to 100 mg./Kg. body wt./day divided into 4 to 8 equal doses. Reduction of dosage is permissible following the acute phase.

114. ℞ "Chloromycetin" (capsules) 0.25 Gm.

    Administer as for ℞ 113.

115. ℞ Penicillin (vial)

    Dissolve 500,000 to 1,000,000 u. in 20 to 40 cc. Water for Injection U.S.P. and instill into the peritoneal cavity at operation, or daily into a peritoneal abscess.

116. ℞ Streptomycin (vial)

    Dissolve 1 Gm. in 20 cc. Water for Injection U.S.P.; instill into peritoneal cavity at operation, or daily into a peritoneal abscess.

117. ℞ Streptomycin (vial)

    0.25 to 1 Gm. dissolved in fruit juice, taken orally every 6 hours.

118. ℞ Succinylsulfathiazole. . . . 0.5 Gm. (gr. viiss)

    15 to 30 tablets (0.25 Gm./Kg. body wt.) as the initial dose, then ⅙ of initial dose every 4 hours as long as required.

119. ℞ Phthalylsulfathiazole. . . . 0.5 Gm. (gr. viiss)

    6 to 10 tablets daily in divided doses.

Fungicides

120. ℞ Castellani's paint

Basic fuchsin, saturated alcoholic solution	10.0 cc.	(ʒ iiss)
Phenol, 5% solution . . .	100.0 cc.	(ʒ iiiss)

    Filter and add:
    Boric acid. . . . . 1.0 Gm. (gr. xv)

    After 2 hours, add:
    Acetone . . . . 5.0 cc. (♏ lxxv)

    After 2 more hours, add:
    Resorcin . . . . 10.0 Gm. (ʒ iiss)

    Use half or full strength and apply twice daily. (CAUTION! Sensitization! Keep in dark, stoppered bottle and discard after 1 month.)

121. ℞ "Desenex" (ointment) . . . 60.0 Gm. (ʒ ii)

    Apply to affected parts 2 times daily.

122. ℞ "Pragmatar" . . . . 60.0 Gm. (ʒ ii)

    Apply to perianal area 1 to 3 times a day.

Antihistaminics

123. ℞ "Neo-Antergan Maleate". .   50   mg.
     1 or 2 tablets 4 times daily.

124. ℞ "Thephorin," 5% ointment .   60.0   Gm. (℥ ii)
     Apply to perianal area.

Miscellaneous

125. ℞ Coal Tar Solution N.F. . .   10.0   cc.   (℥ iiss)
       Calamine. . . . .   23.0   Gm. (℥ vi)
       Talc . . . .   23.0   Gm. (℥ vi)
       Glycerin . . . .   10.0   cc.   (℥ iiss)
       Distilled water. . . .q.s. ad 100.0   cc.   (℥ iiiss)
     Apply to affected area daily.

126. ℞ Quinine and urea hydrochlo-
     ride, 1% solution   (ampul)
     Inject 1 or 2 cc. into sphincter below an anal
     fissure to induce relaxation.

127. ℞ Botulism Antitoxin N.N.R.
     (vial)
     10,000 u. or more I.V. after testing for sen-
     sitivity.

128. ℞ BAL (2,3-dimercaptopropanol),
     10% solution in peanut oil
     (ampul)
     To be given deeply I.M. in accordance with
     procedure outlined in text under toxic mani-
     festations of gold; *see* RHEUMATOID ARTHRI-
     TIS.   *See also* ARSENIC POISONING; CAD-
     MIUM POISONING; MERCURY POISONING.

129. ℞ Typhoid vaccine   (vial)
     Dilute and administer I.V. 5 to 15 million
     organisms initially; each subsequent I.V. in-
     jection is given every other day for 10 in-
     jections, each dose being 50% larger than
     the preceding one.   Thereafter, ⅓ of the
     largest dose given is administered once or
     twice a month.   (CAUTION! If the result-
     ant fever ever exceeds 105° F., or if there is
     marked prostration or aggravation of the
     colitis, discontinue fever therapy.)

130. ℞ Trichloroacetic acid, 50%
     solution. . . . .   15.0   cc.   (℥ ss)
     Touch ulcer with small amount of acid on
     cotton applicator; repeat every 7 to 14 days
     if necessary.

131. ℞ Sorbitan monooleate, polyoxy-
     ethylene derivative. . . .   0.5   Gm.
     3 capsules with each meal.   (CAUTION!
     The use of mineral oil during this treatment
     is contraindicated.)

GENITOURINARY

GENITOURINARY SYSTEM

The genitourinary tract with its multiple component parts, its varied functions and extensive anatomical distribution, may be a most important site of disease at any age. Possible disorders include congenital anomalies, infections of many types, neoplasms, calculi formation, vascular diseases, and traumatic injuries. Frequently, these conditions do not produce clear-cut symptoms, so that the genitourinary system must be carefully considered in all patients who present an indefinite symptomatology, as well as in those whose complaints directly involve the tract.

CONGENITAL ANOMALIES

Congenital anomalies involve the genitourinary system more frequently than any other system. The kidneys and ureters especially may be the site of congenital defects. Such anomalies may produce mechanical difficulties and cause urinary stasis, infection, calculi, hypertension, and renal insufficiency. Congenital defects always must be considered in the presence of obscure abdominal or genitourinary symptomatology. Diagnosis depends on radiography and cystoscopy. The treatment is usually surgical, but no renal surgery must be undertaken until the functional capacity of the other kidney has been tested and found adequate.

KIDNEY

In its formation from the urogenital ridge together with its rotation and ascent to its permanent position, the kidney is subject to many anomalies. These include unilateral or bilateral agenesis, supernumerary organs, fused or horseshoe kidneys, and malposition. **Aberrant renal arteries** from the aorta to the lower pole of the kidney may cross and obstruct the ureter, giving rise to symptoms resembling renal colic. Treatment should be confined to the relief of obstructions or infection.

Polycystic disease is a rare familial condition in which the parenchyma of both kidneys is replaced largely by cysts. The diagnosis is established by pyelograms. The extensive involvement required to produce palpably large kidneys often is associated with hypertension, albuminuria, cylindruria, and hematuria. The cysts gradually increase in size, producing progressive renal insufficiency, so that a fatal uremia is frequent before the age of 55. Operative incision of the cysts may relieve the pressure on adjacent tissue temporarily, but should never be attempted in a patient who already is uremic. Medical treatment is similar to that for chronic nephrosclerosis (q.v.).

URETER

The ureters may have ectopic openings (into the urethra, prostate, vagina, uterus, urachus, or bowel), duplication, strictures, valves, and diverticula. Occasionally, the ureter passes behind the vena cava with resultant ureteral obstruction. Diagnosis is made by radiography and the therapy is operative.

BLADDER

Anomalies include agenesis, double bladder, diverticula, persistent urachus, exstrophy of the bladder, and obstruction of the bladder neck by valves or strictures. Therapy when necessary is surgical.

URETHRA

The urethra may be absent, imperforate, or open on the dorsal (epispadias) or ventral (hypospadias) surface. Congenital obstruction may be due to stenosis, valves, or hypertrophy of the verumontanum. Treatment is surgical.

UNDESCENDED TESTICLE

In true cryptorchism the testes fail to descend along the gubernaculum and remain within the abdominal cavity. This condition usually is bilateral and may be due to a hormonal deficiency. Partial descent of the testis is more common and is due to an ectopic attachment of the gubernaculum which leads the testis down to an ectopic site in the inguinal canal, in the subcutaneous tissues of the groin, in the perineum or in Scarpa's triangle. This condition usually is unilateral. Undescended testes are more subject to trauma, torsion, tumor formation, and developmental failure. A congenital hernia usually is present concurrently with cryptorchism. The diagnosis is made by palpation and inspection in a warm room with the patient quiet. Pressure over the internal inguinal ring with the flat of the hand will keep the testis from retreating into the abdominal cavity while the inguinal canal is palpated. The presence of secondary sex characteristics or any response to chorionic gonadotropin treatment implies the presence of at least one testis.

Treatment consists of a trial of 500 u. of chorionic gonadotropin subcut. 3 times a week for 6 weeks, any time between the ages of 6 and 13 years (R 30). If effective, descent will be evident within 2 to 3 months. If partial descent is noted, an additional course of about 3,000 u. (total) may be given unless secondary sex characteristics develop too rapidly. If there is no response, an orchiopexy and hernioplasty should be done. Large accompanying hernias may demand very early operation. Psychiatric complications are fewer if the operation is done at the age of 6 years but some testes will descend spontaneously up until the age of 13. Treatment can be initiated any time between these limits, but preferably between 6 and 9 years of

age. Cryptorchid patients often are sterile, even after orchiopexy.

TRAUMATIC LESIONS

Injury to the genitourinary tract usually is due to penetrating wounds, crushing injuries, blows over a hollow viscus,
the accidental inclusion of ureters in sutures, and torsion of
the testis due to an elongated mesorchium.

The primary symptom of injury to the urinary tract is hematuria. In general, all cases with genitourinary injuries should
be treated prophylactically with large doses of penicillin and
sulfadiazine or streptomycin (R 17 to 25). Diversion of the
urinary stream should be done freely and retrograde X-ray
studies should be preferred to other methods of diagnosis.

KIDNEY

Penetrating missiles, crushing automobile injuries or direct
blows over the kidney may injure it. Other viscera often are
injured concurrently. Contusions, hematomas, splits in the
parenchyma, ruptures of the pedicle or fragmentation of the
kidney can occur. These are usually, but not always, accompanied by hematuria. A local mass may occur due to a hematoma or urinary extravasation. Infection of this mass may
occur despite chemotherapy. Shock usually is brief but severe
shock due to a torn pedicle or concurrent massive intraperitoneal hemorrhage may require immediate operation. Both
I.V. and retrograde pyelograms may be necessary for accurate
localization of the point of injury. Pedicle injury will not be
revealed by retrograde pyelograms and shock may interfere
with the I.V. type. The psoas line often is obscured by the
perinephric hematoma just as it is obscured in perinephric
abscess. In general, kidney injuries should be treated conservatively. Operation is required only for exsanguinating hemorrhage or infection of the retroperitoneal hematoma and at
operation every effort should be made to repair the kidney.
Nephrectomy, when indicated, should be done only if the
contralateral kidney has been demonstrated to be functionally
adequate.

URETER

Ureteral injuries occur with only the most severe penetrating
wounds, with accompanying injury to the bowel, abdominal viscera or spine usually outweighing the injury to the ureter. The
ureters are occasionally included inadvertently in surgical sutures, causing hydronephrosis followed by urinary fistulas. The
diagnosis of ureteral wounds is difficult. Urine may leak through
the wound intraperitoneally or form a large subcutaneous mass.

Methylene blue can be given by mouth to identify any drainage as urine and the diagnosis can be confirmed by I.V. pyelogram or retrograde ureterogram. The severed ends must be approximated over a splinting catheter with urinary diversion by simultaneous nephrostomy. Small wounds of the ureter may heal spontaneously even without drainage of the extravasated urine.

BLADDER

A very light blow can rupture the distended bladder, either into the peritoneum or extraperitoneally. Intraperitoneal rupture may not show signs of peritonitis at first, since the urine often is sterile. However, it will quickly become evident that there is free fluid in the peritoneal cavity. Extraperitoneal rupture with perivesical infiltration of urine produces pain, increasing abdominal spasm, and a mass in the space of Retzius which can be felt suprapubically. A diagnosis of ruptured bladder is best made by catheterizing the patient, injecting about 200 cc. of radiopaque dye and taking AP and oblique roentgenograms of the entire abdomen. The extravasated dye can be seen easily. X-rays taken with the patient lying on one side may reveal the intestines floating on top of the urine in the peritoneal cavity. Intravenous pyelograms and cystograms should not be depended upon to reveal a ruptured bladder, nor is the introduction and extraction of measured amounts of fluid a dependable method. Treatment consists of suprapubic cystotomy with suture of the tear in the bladder, aspiration of the free urine from the peritoneal cavity, and suprapubic drainage for a period of about 2 weeks.

URETHRA

Straddle injuries, tears due to misguided or forceful introduction of instruments, or tears due to trauma to the pelvis are the common causes of urethral injury. Any fracture of the pubic bones must always be suspected of having an accompanying urethral rupture. There is pain at the point of injury, bleeding from the penis independent of urination, and extravasation and hematoma in the perineum. The patient tries to void but usually can express only a drop or two of blood. The diagnosis is made by attempting to pass a catheter for a cystourethrogram. If the torn ends of the urethra are separated a catheter will not pass. Oblique urethrograms will reveal the site of the tear. Tears in the bulb are repaired in the lithotomy position. Tears of the prostatic or membranous urethra are approached suprapubically and repair should be preceded by a suprapubic cystostomy.

PENIS AND SCROTUM

Gunshot wounds, avulsions of the skin when clothing is caught in industrial machinery, and lacerations due to foreign bodies applied to the penis are the most common lesions. Conservative débridement, the suturing of defects and the use of sliding or burrowing skin grafts from the adjacent loose skin are the principles to be followed in treatment.

TESTIS

Penetrating wounds of the testis should be débrided of only the most grossly damaged fragments since, with careful closure of the defects, some regeneration may occur. Traumatic epididymitis, orchitis, and hydrocele are rare and hematocele may be differentiated by the accompanying ecchymosis. Torsion of the testis often is due to a long mesorchium which allows the testis to rotate within the tunica vaginalis. (For a description of this condition, see SCROTAL MASSES.)

NEOPLASMS

KIDNEY

Renal neoplasms may arise in the kidney parenchyma, pelvis or capsule. Of such tumors, 70% are "clear cell" carcinomas (hypernephromas) which tend to be encapsulated and slow growing; 10% are highly invasive "granular cell" carcinomas; 10% are tumors (papillary or squamous) arising from the epithelium of the renal pelvis; and 5% are rare tumors such as sarcomas or the adenosarcomas of Wilms, which usually are found in children.

Symptoms and Signs

Hematuria is the cardinal symptom, occurring in well over half the cases. Dull pain, mass in the flank, anemia, and cachexia may occur singly or in combination. Blood clots may obstruct the ureter, causing colic. Wilms' tumors in children usually do not bleed and are first discovered as large, far advanced masses in the abdomen.

Diagnosis

Diagnosis is made by means of retrograde pyelogram, which should be done in all cases with hematuria. The I.V. pyelogram may give additional information but usually is not diagnostically adequate alone. Pyelograms will show enlargement or irregularity of the renal outline, elongation of the calyces, which appear to be drawn out into the tumor, or compression of the pelvis or calyces. Aortography and the finding of tumor cells in the urine may assist in marginal diagnoses.

Simple cysts of the kidney can be safely differentiated from tumors only by operation. Hydronephrosis can be differentiated by retrograde pyelograms. Splenic, pancreatic, adrenal and bowel masses can be differentiated by roentgenographic studies, including perirenal air insufflation.

Prognosis

The prognosis for a 5-year arrest is poor since the first symptoms usually occur only after the tumor has grown large. A sign of poor prognosis is failure of the involved kidney to excrete dye injected I.V., which implies invasion of the renal vessels.

Treatment

Immediate surgical excision, before metastasis, is the only effective treatment. Radiotherapy to inoperable tumors and their metastases may be palliative. Wilms' tumors should be removed at once and radiotherapy then given to the entire abdomen. Very large Wilms' tumors may be reduced in size by a short preoperative course of radiotherapy.

BLADDER

Neoplasms of the epithelium lining the bladder, which may be "benign" initially, have a tendency to become invasive or to recur following removal, so that the ultimate prognosis is poor. Their cause is unknown, although industrial exposure to certain aniline dyes can cause bladder papillomas. There are two general types: (1) Papillary epitheliomas, benign or malignant, with fronds growing out into the bladder lumen. (2) Invasive squamous cell epitheliomas, resembling large indurated, necrotic bladder ulcers. These tumors tend to extend rapidly toward the cavity or outside the bladder.

Symptoms

Painless hematuria is the cardinal symptom, and every patient with hematuria should be examined for bladder tumor. Obstruction of the ureteral orifices or the bladder neck may cause uremia. Infection of the surface of the tumor may bring on dysuria, pyuria, burning, and frequency. Debilitating and even fatal hemorrhages occur, and metastases may develop, first locally, and later at distant sites, especially the bones. Suprapubic mass and severe pain in the pelvis and legs are terminal manifestations.

Diagnosis

Cystograms and cystoscopic biopsy are essential for diagnosis. I.V. pyelograms will show whether or not the tumor is obstructing the ureteral orifices. Bimanual examination under anesthesia may give further indication of whether or not the tumor has invaded and penetrated the bladder wall.

Prognosis

If the tumor is confined to the epithelium, the prognosis is good. If it has invaded but not penetrated the muscular bladder wall, treatment may effect a cure in about 50% of cases. If extension has progressed beyond the bladder wall, the prognosis is extremely poor.

Treatment

Treatment depends on the size of the tumor and the degree of invasion of the bladder wall. Very small benign papillomas may be safely fulgurated through the cystoscope. Tumors under 2 cm. in diameter, located on the bladder dome may be resected surgically or treated by fulguration and the insertion of radium needles or radon seeds, preferably at open cystostomy. Tumors which are multiple, very large, recurrent, or are around the ureteral orifices or bladder neck and which have not yet penetrated the bladder wall, require total cystectomy. This is preceded by transplantation of the ureters so that they open into the sigmoid or through the skin.

Tumors which have penetrated the bladder only locally, can sometimes be treated successfully with interstitial radium needles which radiate the adjacent tissues as well. Million-volt roentgen therapy gives temporary palliation but less intense roentgen therapy is of little value.

MISCELLANEOUS GENITOURINARY TUMORS

For prostatic neoplasms the reader is referred to the chapter on Prostatism. Urethral tumors are similar to bladder tumors except that obstruction is the prime symptom. Radium therapy is the preferred form of treatment. Local metastases are common even when the patients are first seen. Epitheliomas of the glans penis occur only in uncircumcised males. Any chronic penile ulcer in a man over 40 should be biopsied for carcinoma. Very small lesions are treated with radium. Larger lesions are treated by partial or total amputation of the penis and radical dissection of the inguinal lymph channels. Testicular tumors are slightly more common in patients with cryptorchidism. Histologically, they are either teratomas or seminomas, and are first noted by the patient as a hard, heavy enlargement of the testis which is easily traumatized. This mass is solid and opaque, with a normal vas deferens. Only about 25% of the tumors (teratomas) give a positive Ascheim-Zondek. An I.V. pyelogram should be done before operation to detect displacement of the ureter by lymph node metastases. Treatment is radical removal, with postoperative X-radiation of the preaortic lymph nodes up to the level of the kidneys.

ADRENAL

Tumors of the adrenal gland can arise from either the cortex or the medulla. Both types may cause metabolic symptoms long before they metastasize, due to their excessive hormone secretion.

Adrenal medullary tumors (see PHEOCHROMOCYTOMA) cause episodes of violent hypertension with lesser bouts of prolonged hypertension due to the liberation of free epinephrine, which they produce in large quantities. Trauma or pressure over the tumor may precipitate an attack, with pounding of the heart, headache, sweating, and syncope, and often a feeling of impending death. In patients with this tumor, therapeutic test with Benodaine (benzodioxan) will relieve the symptoms by neutralizing the hypertensive effects of circulating epinephrine.

Adrenal cortical tumors (q.v.) may appear simply as inert masses in the flank, but more commonly they cause changes in the body due to the liberation of steroid hormones. Overmasculinization of both sexes (adrenogenitalism), with deepening of the voice and overgrowth of the beard, pubic hair, and phallus or clitoris is seen. More rarely the changes resemble those observed in Cushing's syndrome (q.v.); i.e., obesity of the body, moon face, thick "buffalo" neck, and changes in the hormone excretion. Adrenal cortical tumors which cause these changes should be located by I.V. pyelograms and perirenal aerograms and removed surgically.

FISTULA

Chronic urinary fistulas (e.g., vesicovaginal, perineo-urethral, and those leading from the suprapubic bladder, ureters, or kidney pelvis) may result from trauma or abscesses which open these structures to the outside. Obstruction to the flow of urine through the normal channels will perpetuate a fistula, and chronic infection or the presence of foreign bodies also may keep it open.

Treatment includes diversion of the urinary stream above the fistula, elimination of any existing infection by appropriate means, and removal of all obstructions or foreign bodies in the normal passages. If these measures are not followed by healing, the walls of the sinus must be dissected out and a meticulous layer closure done.

STRICTURE
URETER

Stricture or narrowing of the ureter may be due to congenital narrowing, abnormal pressure from adjacent vessels or tumors, renal ptosis, metastasizing neoplasms; trauma following penetrating wounds, passage of a renal calculus, or accidental injury during operative procedures; or inflammatory changes due to infections, particularly tuberculosis. The symptoms and signs are those of recurrent urinary tract infection with or without hydronephrosis (q.v.). Diagnosis is by means of history, laboratory examination, and I.V. and retrograde ureterograms. Renal ptosis may be associated with attacks of renal colic (Dietl's crisis).

Treatment of ureteral stricture usually is disappointing, but should be attempted as soon as feasible after the earliest possible diagnosis. Dilatation, plastic repair, or nephrectomy should be tried in that order.

URETHRA

Etiology

Stricture of the urethra is sometimes congenital, but usually acquired. In congenital cases there may be simple narrowing of the canal, or the canal may be obstructed by folds of redundant mucosa in the posterior wall, forming valvelike flaps. Acquired strictures are caused by infection (particularly gonococcal), by trauma, and by chemical irritation with resultant fibrosis. A nonorganic, temporary spasm of the membranous portion of the urethra may be produced by a posterior urethritis or urethrocystitis, or by rough instrumentation, strongly acid urine, calculi, organic stricture, psychic disturbances, or dietary, alcoholic, or sexual excesses.

Symptoms and Signs

There may be a history of recurrent urethral discharge and of abnormalities in the urinary flow, such as decreased caliber and force of the stream, hesitancy, frequency, intermittency, terminal dribbling, and occasional bleeding. Continued obstruction to the urinary stream may lead to symptoms of back pressure and ascending involvement of the urinary tract (infection, hydronephrosis). The diagnosis is suspected from the history and is confirmed by obstruction to attempted careful passage of a bougie, sound, or endoscope.

Treatment

Many strictures can be avoided by the proper management of acute urethritis (q.v.) and of traumatic injuries to the urethra. Therapy of existing stricture consists of gradual dilation over prolonged periods with appropriate filiforms, bougies, and sounds. Any etiologic factor still present (e.g., chronic infection) should be eliminated. Surgical intervention is indicated when (1) strictures are impenetrable, or are not amenable to dilation because of length or density; (2) uremia or urosepsis makes relief of the obstruction imperative; (3) the stricture is complicated by extravasation, periurethral abscess, suppuration, or fistula, or (4) protracted programs of dilation are not feasible. Surgical measures include dilation under anesthesia, meatotomy, internal and external urethrotomy, resection of congenital valves or strictured areas, and suprapubic cystostomy. Subsequent adequate dilation is an important feature of the after-care of all strictures.

CALCULI

Urinary calculi may be found in the kidney, ureter, bladder, or urethra, and usually are composed of crystalline concretions of calcium oxalate, calcium phosphate, uric acid, or cystine.

Etiology and Incidence

The cause is unknown. Calculi probably begin on the renal papillae as small plaques which break free and act as nuclei, around which the urinary salts are precipitated. Precipitation is more probable in the presence of infection, stasis, high urinary concentration, xanthinuria, during therapy with sulfonamides and in conditions associated with the hyperexcretion of phosphorus, calcium (hyperparathyroidism, excess calcium ingestion, hypervitaminosis D, long periods of immobilization) and uric acid (myeloid leukemia, polycythemia vera, gout). Cystinuria is responsible for some calculi and often is familial and sex-linked to the female. Hardness of drinking water is not a factor. Alkaline urine favors the development of phosphate stones whereas acid urine precipitates cystine, uric acid, urates, and oxalates. Calculi occur more frequently during middle life and in males (3:1). Negroes are less frequently affected.

Pathology

The size of a calculus varies from very small gravel to a large stag-horn stone which may fill the renal pelvis. Calcium oxalate stones usually are small, dark, rough, and hard, while calcium phosphate stones tend to be soft, white, chalky, and frequently stag-horn in shape. Uric acid stones are commonly small and yellow but they may be of any color. Cystine calculi often are stag-horn shaped and have a waxy, almost translucent appearance. Calculi may be multiple and bilateral. Migration of a stone may cause obstruction with resultant stasis, infection, and clinical manifestations. Persistent or repeated obstruction leads to pyonephrosis or hydronephrosis.

Symptoms and Signs

The clinical manifestations will vary with the size and location of the calculus. Small, smooth stones may be passed without any difficulty. Large stones may remain stationary within the renal pelvis for years without symptoms (silent calculi) or there may be only intermittent lumbar discomfort and albuminuria. When a stone enters and obstructs the ureter, renal colic occurs. There is excruciating pain which originates in the back or flank and radiates across the abdomen and into the groin, genitalia, and inner aspect of the thigh. The agony and writhing of the patient are extreme. There may be nausea, vomiting, sweating, frequency, urgency, chills, and shock. Examination reveals slight soreness over the involved kidney and ureter, spasm of the abdominal muscles, albuminuria, and microscopic (rarely gross) hematuria. The attack may last up to several hours, and there may be residual lumbar soreness and microscopic hematuria for several days.

Intermittent or persistent obstruction to the flow of urine leads to stasis, infection, hydronephrosis, and renal destruction. If the obstruction is bilateral, anuria and uremia ensue.

Vesical calculi may be quiescent or they may produce bladder irritation, with resultant pain, frequency, dysuria, hematuria, pyuria, and albuminuria. Passage of such stones through the urethra usually is uncomplicated. Rarely, there may be sudden obstruction of the urethral orifice or impaction of an irregular stone within the proximal urethra.

Roentgenograms may reveal a characteristic shadow, but the X-ray frequently is inconclusive, in which case I.V. or retrograde pyelography is indicated.

Diagnosis

Diagnosis is based on the above symptoms and signs plus the findings on roentgenographic and cystoscopic examination. The constant agonized movements of a patient with renal colic is an important diagnostic point, since a patient with intraperitoneal inflammation usually lies quietly. The symptoms of urinary calculi must be differentiated from appendicitis, gallbladder disease, peptic ulcer, pancreatitis, coronary occlusion, tabetic crisis, and lesions of the spine. Renal colic also may occur in Dietl's crisis (intermittent hydronephrosis) and ureteral obstruction due to spasm, stricture, tumor, or aberrant vessels.

Prophylaxis

Etiologic factors predisposing to the development of urinary calculi should be avoided or corrected. Chronic urinary stasis and infection must be relieved as promptly as possible. Hyperexcretion of calcium should be guarded against as occurs, for example, in hyperparathyroidism, or overlong therapy with the Sippy regimen in the treatment of peptic ulcer. Long periods of immobilization are undesirable; patients who are in casts or bedridden should have their position changed frequently, fluids should be forced, and the urine kept acid. Fluid intake should exceed 3,000 cc. daily if circumstances favorable to renal calculus formation are present. The reaction of the urine may be regulated in the hope of preventing precipitation. If phosphate stones are forming, the urine should be kept acid; if oxalates or urates are being precipitated, the urine should be kept alkaline.

Treatment

If the stone is small, and there are no complications, expectant treatment is indicated. The patient should receive adequate amounts of fluid (3,000 cc. daily), morphine (℞ 44, 47) and an antispasmodic (℞ 28, 29). In the presence of a large stone, or one which remains impacted, or with any complication (infection, severe hematuria, hydronephrosis, renal insufficiency), special urologic or surgical procedures are immediately indicated to relieve the obstruction, remove the calculus, or both. Existing complications should receive appropriate therapy.

HYDRONEPHROSIS

Dilatation of the kidney pelvis and calyces beyond their normal capacity of 3 to 10 cc.

Etiology

Hydronephrosis occasionally is present at birth. Most commonly, however, it is a result of obstruction or atony of the urinary tract which, if allowed to progress, will result in anoxia and pressure atrophy of the functioning kidney tissue.

Mechanical obstruction: (1) Strictures of the ureter may occur, usually at the ureteropelvic junction, due to aberrant vessels, congenital narrowing, renal ptosis, tumors, calculi, metastasizing neoplasms of the cervix or bowel, ureterocele or ligatures accidentally applied during operation. (2) Obstructions to the bladder neck or urethra may be due to abnormalities such as stricture; benign prostatic adenoma; carcinoma of the prostate, bladder, urethra, or glans penis; or congenital valves of the prostatic urethra.

Inflammatory obstruction: Urinary tract infection, both tuberculous and nontuberculous may produce narrowing and obstruction.

Atony: In pregnancy, atony of all the musculature of the urinary tract may occur. Rarely, in children, where it probably is due to a congenital defect in the innervation, most likely peripheral, atony also may be seen. These children usually die from resultant infection and uremia.

Pathologic Anatomy

The renal parenchyma undergoes pressure atrophy in a retrograde manner starting with the collecting tubules, which dilate and atrophy. The muscular walls of the pelvis and calyces dilate and are replaced by fibrous tissue. A functionless sac results.

Symptoms and Signs

These are variable and may include an asymptomatic abdominal tumor; recurrent attacks of pain, either dull and nagging or colicky with a permanent or transitory tumor (Dietl's crisis); pyuria, fever, and tenderness, where renal infection predominates; hematuria which is not persistent and occurs in approximately 10% of all hydronephrosis as a result of congestion; associated gastrointestinal symptoms, such as dyspepsia and epigastric pain; uremia, in the terminal stages.

Diagnosis

The history includes episodes of pain in the flank, chills and fever, a mass and, rarely, hematuria. The character of the pain varies but tends to be colicky; a recurrent mass may be transitory or permanent. Pyuria, especially in children and young adults, may be the only sign. Urologic examination includes detailed I.V. and retrograde pyelograms. A rapid clear drip from the ureteral catheter usually indicates a hydronephrosis. After the opaque medium has been injected and the catheter removed, a determination of the amount of retention is imperative. The normal kidney empties in about 8 minutes.

Prognosis

The outlook is good if the obstruction is unilateral, amenable to repair and the kidney not too badly damaged. If the infection has not seriously impaired the parenchyma, a large percentage of function will return when adequate drainage is provided. If bilateral, the prognosis should be guarded. Generally speaking, in cases with atonic ureters, pelves and bladder, the outlook is grave despite chemotherapy to combat infection.

Treatment

All obstructions should be removed surgically, or if slight, by urethral or ureteral dilatation. If kidney function does not then return, a nephrectomy should be done.

Nephropexy, pyeloplasty, lysis of obstructing bands and aberrant vessels at the ureteropelvic junction, elimination of valves or kinks in ureters or urethra, the opening of ureteroceles, prostatectomy, and the dilation of strictures are employed when indicated. After obstructions are removed, any residual infection is eradicated (see Chronic Pyelonephritis).

Temporary drainage for acute obstruction may be obtained by ureteral catheter or nephrostomy if necessary. Cutaneous ureterostomy, for tuberculous ureteral obstruction, will often prolong life.

TUBERCULOSIS

Infection of the genitourinary tract caused by the Myco. tuberculosis, which usually is blood-borne from a distant focus such as a pulmonary lesion, or one in the gastrointestinal tract, lymph nodes, or bone.

Pathology

Small lesions in the renal parenchyma may caseate, liquefy, and break down, leaving large ragged cavities in the medulla, lined by sloughing tuberculous granulations. This process gradually destroys the infected kidney and, if unchecked, hastens the breakdown of the opposite kidney. Infection may spread to the ureters, seminal vesicles, vasa, and epididymides. The prostate or epididymides are occasionally infected by blood-borne tubercle bacilli without renal infection. These dangerous foci often are unrecognized as tuberculous until a miliary dissemination occurs from them.

Symptoms and Signs

The cardinal symptom of urinary tuberculosis is frequency of urination. Burning, terminal dysuria, spasm and hematuria may occur as the condition grows worse. (Every case of long-standing cystitis should be investigated for tuberculosis.) Fatigue and weight loss result from the urinary pain and frequency, which disturb the patient's sleep. Dull pain often occurs over tuberculous kidneys.

Genital tuberculosis is evidenced by nodules in the prostate, seminal vesicles, vasa, or epididymides. The tuberculous prostate is sometimes soft, however, and cannot be distinguished from other forms of prostatitis. All tuberculous nodules are acutely tender and swollen at first but subside gradually into smaller, very firm nodules or ridges. Draining scrotal sinuses always should be investigated for tuberculosis.

Diagnosis

Surgical renal tuberculosis is diagnosed by means of X-ray and repeated urine cultures. Ragged, moth-eaten pockets are seen replacing or extending from the calyces. The ureters are irregularly narrowed and dilated, in different segments. Guinea-pig inoculation and cultures are preferable to direct smear. In late cases, secondary infection often is prominent.

Suspected tuberculous prostates should not be massaged. Suspicious, large, nodular epididymides should be removed carefully, especially if they show advancement of the disease or draining sinuses. A complete examination of the good kidney must be carried out to make sure there is adequate function and no tuberculosis. All other foci of tuberculosis in the body must be evaluated and stabilized. A reaction to the tuberculin test is obtainable in cases of genitourinary tuberculosis.

Prognosis

The disease usually is progressive and the prognosis for spontaneous arrest is poor.

Treatment

The original tuberculous focus of infection and other foci should be appropriately treated prior to or concomitantly with treatment of the genitourinary infection. If only one kidney is tuberculous it should be removed surgically. If the corresponding ureter is narrowed by strictures, it too should be removed completely. Following nephrectomy, the cystitis and prostatitis may subside. Any chronic epididymal nodule that shows signs of progressive disease or has a draining sinus should be removed surgically and the stump of the vas exteriorized.

Bilateral renal tuberculosis or tuberculosis in solitary kidneys should be treated with streptomycin or dihydrostreptomycin (R 25). Even if the lesion is too large or refractory to heal, the diminution in symptoms usually is gratifying.

NONSPECIFIC INFECTIONS

Specific infections of the genitourinary tract (e.g., tuberculosis, gonorrhea) are discussed elsewhere (q.v.). Here are described the more common nonspecific infections attacking the kidney, perirenal tissues, ureters, bladder, urethra, and other urogenital structures. Each is presented as a clinical entity, but a discussion of over-all chemotherapy appears at the conclusion of the chapter.

ACUTE PYELONEPHRITIS

An acute diffuse pyogenic infection of the kidney pelvis and underlying parenchyma. Since there always is some parenchymal involvement in infections of the renal pelvis, both pyelitis and pyelonephritis will be considered as a single entity—acute pyelonephritis being the most common kidney infection and often bilateral.

Etiology

Infection occurs by way of the blood stream or lymphatics from foci elsewhere, by direct spread from adjacent structures, or by ascending infection due to urinary back pressure. Anatomic or pathologic factors, such as strictures, calculi, tumors, prostatic hypertrophy, or extrinsic pressure of the gravid uterus, cause obstruction to the urine and predispose to infection. Females are especially liable to this infection, particularly during childhood and pregnancy. Any pyogenic bacterium may be the causative organism, but the colon bacilli, staphylococci, streptococci, *Proteus vulgaris,* and *Bacillus pyocyaneus* are the ones most frequently found. Mixed infections are common.

Pathology

The kidney is enlarged, soft, and dark in color due to venous stasis. Throughout the cortex are scattered areas of hemorrhage and leukocytic infiltration, which may go on to local suppuration and abscess formation. The renal pelvis shows similar evidence of inflammation with increased vascularity and areas of petechial hemorrhage.

Symptoms and Signs

Onset is rapid and characterized by chills, fever, abdominal pain, backache, and evidence of toxemia, often with an associated gastrointestinal upset, nausea and vomiting. The temperature is septic in type. Total urinary output may be decreased; frequency and urgency may become prominent symptoms due to irritation of the bladder by infected urine. On physical examination the abdomen will sometimes present some degree of rigidity which requires careful differentiation from that produced by intra-abdominal disease. If the rigidity is absent or slight, a tender enlarged kidney may sometimes be palpable. Costovertebral tenderness generally is present on the affected side. In severe cases the disease may go on to urinary suppression and death from uremia. With removal of obstructive factors and the proper use of chemotherapy to control intrinsic and extrinsic infection, the condition may subside completely. More commonly, in the absence of such treatment, the infection goes on to the chronic form (q.v.) with acute exacerbations at varying intervals.

Diagnosis

Diagnosis of acute pyelonephritis usually is not difficult, particularly when urinary symptoms (frequency and dysuria) and laboratory confirmation are present. Microscopically, the urine contains pus, red blood cells, and cellular casts; in the female only catheterized specimens are reliable. Leukocytosis and an elevated E.S.R. are associated with acute pyelonephritis. Urine culture should be made to determine the infecting organism before the institution of treatment. Radiographic studies may be invaluable in determining the cause and extent of the disease. A scout film of the entire abdomen in conjunction with I.V. pyelograms, taken in the erect and supine positions, usually will demonstrate any calculi or obstruction in the upper tract. Any ptosis of the kidney with angulation and blocking of the ureter will be seen on the upright film. During the initial acute attack no characteristic X-ray changes due to infection are seen in the kidneys. Urethral catheterization after voiding is essential to determine whether residual urine is present from bladder neck or urethral obstruction, or bladder dysfunction of a neurogenic type. Rectal examination and the passage of urethral sounds in the male patient help to determine the presence or absence of prostatic hypertrophy or urethral stricture. All patients not responding promptly to treatment, in whom a demonstrable and easily remediable cause cannot be found, require a complete urologic investigation.

Treatment

Antibacterial therapy (*see* below) should be instituted as soon as the diagnosis has been established and urine culture obtained. In the acute phase, bed rest and an adequate urinary output (to 1,500 cc. daily) are essential. Sedation (B 54, 55, 56) and analgesia (B 46) may be required. If nausea and vomiting are prominent symptoms, parenteral fluids are indicated to maintain a proper fluid balance. If residual urine is present in the bladder, continuous catheter drainage should be instituted. Ureteral catheterization may be needed to drain urine from above a ureteral obstruction. After the acute symptoms have subsided, every effort must be made to eliminate any obstructions or foci of infection that might prevent complete cure.

CHRONIC PYELONEPHRITIS

A slowly progressing infection in the renal pelvis and parenchyma, frequently bilateral.

Etiology

The condition may have its origin in an acute pyelonephritis (q.v.) in childhoood, especially in females, or during pregnancy. In males it usually is associated with some obstructive lesion, such as large "stag-horn" renal calculi or prostatic hypertrophy. The common etiologic agent is the colon bacillus, *P. vulgaris*, or a related organism. Infrequently, one of the gram-positive cocci may be responsible.

Pathology

The kidney is smaller than normal and the capsule strips with difficulty. The ureters and pelves have varying degrees of chronic infection and scarring. The renal parenchyma may show cloudy swelling, scarring, or suppuration with destruction of kidney tissue. Not infrequently there is an associated glomerulonephritis or arteriolar change.

Symptoms, Signs, and Course

Chronic pyelonephritis runs a protracted course, often extending over many years. There may be recurring acute episodes of fever, pain in the back or flank, and pyuria, with or without dysuria. When bilateral it is usually associated with moderate hypertension, albuminuria, and sometimes with mild symptoms of renal insufficiency such as headache, fatigue, and anemia. In the advanced stages of the disease, the kidney loses its ability to concentrate urine and the BUN rises to uremic levels. In this phase the disease often is indistinguishable from chronic glomerulonephritis.

Diagnosis

Diagnosis is made by the history, and the evidence of chronic infection: pyuria, episodes of fever, and positive urine culture. X-ray studies may reveal progressive dilatation of the calyces and ureter.

Treatment

Treatment of the infection in its acute phases is the same as that of acute pyelonephritis (q.v.). In the chronic stage, careful search should be made for renal calculi, polycystic kidney, congenital anomalies, or prostatic hypertrophy, and the appropriate therapeutic measures instituted.

Chronic unilateral pyelonephritis, with hypertension and progressive renal insufficiency, has been described, with cure following surgical removal of the affected kidney. However, proved instances of such surgical cures are extremely rare.

PERINEPHRITIC ABSCESS

(Perirenal abscess,
Perinephric abscess, Perinephritis)

Inflammation or suppuration in the fatty tissue surrounding the kidney and lying within the perirenal fascia (Gerota's capsule).

Etiology

This second most frequent of the nonspecific infections in or around the kidney most commonly arises by hematogenous or lymphogenous spread from foci other than the kidney. The focus usually is some pyogenic skin infection of staphylococcal or streptococcal origin. Occasionally, it may develop by direct spread from a perinephric hematoma secondary to trauma, a renal carbuncle, pyelonephritis, migration of an appendiceal abscess or other retroperitoneal infection. When this occurs, the infecting organisms are the same as in the primary site.

Symptoms and Signs

Onset may be sudden with fever, chills, nausea, vomiting, and prostration, or it may be more gradual with weakness, malaise and low grade fever. Tenderness and pain in the costovertebral region invariably occur during the course of the disease. A tender mass may be palpable in the flank, partially obscured by involuntary muscle spasm.

Diagnosis

This depends on the history, physical examination, particularly the presence of costovertebral tenderness, and radiologic findings. Routine laboratory procedures are of little diagnostic value. Urinary changes do not occur without concomitant renal involvement or approximation of the infection to the kidney, pelvis, and ureter. Anterior abdominal tenderness with voluntary muscle spasm requires differentiation from similar signs due to an acute abdominal disease. A flat film of the abdomen, plus pyelograms taken in both the supine and erect positions, is indicated. Diagnostic X-ray signs to be looked for are obliteration of the kidney shadow and psoas muscle outline, diminished kidney mobility, diminished diaphragmatic motility, and occasionally distortion of the kidney pelvis, ureter, or both. Scoliosis of the lumbar spine may be evident, with the concavity toward the involved side. Retroperitoneal lymphosarcoma sometimes resembles a perinephritic abscess.

Treatment

Therapy consists of supportive measures, such as parenteral fluids, transfusions, bed rest, sedatives (℞ 54, 55, 56), and analgesics (46), and prompt institution of antibacterial therapy (*see* below) to combat systemic as well as local infection. Rarely, the infection is aborted before suppuration occurs, by prompt antibacterial therapy. Surgical drainage under general anesthesia is required when localization occurs.

RENAL CARBUNCLE

(Cortical abscess, Focal suppurative
nephritis, Septic infarct of the kidney)

An area of suppuration in the renal cortex.

Etiology

The causes are similar to those of perinephritic abscess (q.v.), which it sometimes precedes. It usually is a hematogenous infection, secondary to a suppurative process of the skin, and therefore usually coccal in origin, *Staph. aureus* predominantly.

Pathology

The lesion is a true carbuncle in that it consists of coalescing centers of suppuration. Multiple carbuncles may occur.

Symptoms and Signs

These are essentially the same as with perinephritic abscess (q.v.).

Diagnosis

The condition is difficult to differentiate from perinephritic abscess. Urinalysis may show varying amounts of cellular elements, but the well circumscribed lesions usually do not produce urinary changes. Pyelograms showing distortion of one or more of the calyces indicate the possibility of a small expanding lesion of the renal cortex.

Treatment

(*See* Perinephritic Abscess.) In the fulminating case, in conjunction with chemotherapy, prompt surgical drainage is indicated as soon as the patient's general condition permits.

URETERITIS

An acute or chronic inflammation of the ureter, associated with, and secondary to, pyelonephritis (q.v.). The diagnosis and management are those appropriate to combat the primary kidney infection.

CYSTITIS

An acute or chronic inflammation of the urinary bladder.

Etiology

Cystitis rarely is a primary condition. It usually is secondary to an infection of the kidney, prostate or urethra. The bladder epithelium normally is highly resistant to infection, but continued drainage of infected urine from a pyelonephritis, infected drainage from an epididymovesiculitis or prostatitis, prolonged irritation from foreign bodies or calculi, ascending infection from a diseased urethra, or prevention of normal bladder emptying by a hypertrophied prostate, urethral stricture or neurogenic disturbance, may so wear down the tissue resistance that disease is established. Following major surgical procedures, childbirth and prolonged bed rest, lowered resistance, plus inadequate bladder emptying, predisposes to the development of cystitis. The incidence is high in cases of poorly controlled diabetes mellitus.

Pathology

This may vary from slight increase in vascularity of the trigonal region to generalized edema and ulceration. Bullous edema or cyst formation occurs in many chronic infections. Cystitis of long duration may produce a thick-walled, contracted bladder of small capacity. Calcareous incrustations of the epithelium result from chronic infections due to the urea-splitting bacteria.

Symptoms and Signs

Acute Cystitis: Frequency and burning during urination are the most frequent complaints and, in severe cases, they may lead to a continual urge to void. Pain is present in the perineal and suprapubic regions. Terminal hematuria is frequent. Chills, fever and systemic manifestations, when present, may be due to bacteremia.

Chronic Cystitis: The symptoms and signs are the same as above but present to a lesser degree.

Diagnosis

The history, physical examination and presence of pus in all portions of the voided urine (shown by the 2-glass test) suggest the diagnosis. Examination of the external genitalia, rectal examination in the male and pelvic examination in the female, passage of sounds to locate urethral strictures and catheterization for residual urine, may be necessary to rule out diseases of the lower genitourinary tract as possible causes. The upper tract, including the kidneys, ureters and bladder, should be investigated by X-ray, and by I.V. pyelograms taken in both the erect and supine positions. If the cause still is not apparent, further check should be made for foci of infection elsewhere in the body, with particular attention to any existing rectal or pelvic disease. Urologic consultation is needed in doubtful cases and cystoscopy should be done when the acute symptoms have subsided.

Treatment

As with the other nonspecific urinary infections, antibacterial therapy (*see* below) should be started as soon as the urine culture has been obtained and workup begun. Fluid intake should be kept above 2,500 cc. daily unless specifically contraindicated by other existing diseases or by type of medication being given. Analgesics (℞ 46) and sedatives (℞ 54, 55, 56) are administered to control severe symptoms. Bladder sedatives such as Pyridium (℞ 9) or mixtures containing tincture of hyoscyamus (℞ 51) are of value. Severe tenesmus will require an opiate (℞ 47) which may be given in conjunction with belladonna in a rectal suppository (℞ 45, 49). Alkalinization (℞ 68) of a strongly acid urine, aside from having a bacteriostatic effect, relieves the symptoms of burning and urgency. Bladder irrigations (*see* BEDSIDE PROC.) are indicated in chronic cystitis; potassium permanganate (1:5,000) or silver nitrate (1:5,000) are most commonly used, daily at first, then 2 or 3 times/week. The long-standing case with bladder contraction responds best to irrigations and gradual dilation of the bladder, using increasing amounts of an oily mixture (R 10). The patient should be advised against the use of alcoholic beverages and highly seasoned foods, which would tend to increase bladder irritability. In all cases, the search for, and elimination of, the predisposing cause should be undertaken at the same time that local treatment is begun. Adequate drainage of urine from the bladder must be assured. Diabetes mellitus (q.v.), if present, should be controlled immediately.

URETHRITIS, PROSTATITIS, SEMINAL VESICULITIS

Acute or chronic infections of the respective organs concerned. In the male, posterior urethritis and some degree of prostatitis generally coexist. The latter may be either primary or secondary to the urethritis. Prostatitis may occur without seminal vesiculitis, but rarely is the reverse true. Anterior urethritis in the male and urethritis in the female may occur independent of other conditions, but are usually associated with infection and even abscess formation of the periurethral glands. The incidence of urethritis and prostatitis is high in young males (20 to 35 years). Seminal vesiculitis is a relatively uncommon disease.

Etiology

Any or all of these conditions frequently but not invariably follow gonorrheal infection, and the presence of the latter must be excluded by repeated examinations of smears and by cultures. Seminal vesiculitis and prostatitis may be due to hematogenous spread of infection from other foci. They also may follow benign prostatic hypertrophy, if the normal drainage of these organs is obstructed and infected urine is present.

Pathology

Urethral infection by pyogenic organisms is generally limited to the epithelial and subepithelial layers where increased vascularity, accumulations of leukocytes and desquamation of the surface epithelium are noted. Prolonged infection results in squamous cell metaplasia and stricture formation by fibrosis. Somewhat similar inflammatory changes occur in the prostate gland and seminal vesicles and here the picture is further complicated by the presence of glandular structures which become filled with purulent exudate and which are converted to abscess cavities if drainage is prevented.

Symptoms, Signs, and Diagnosis

With nonspecific urethritis a discharge is present which may

19

vary from mucopurulent to purulent, but which usually is small in amount and is most commonly observed on arising in the morning. A frequent complaint is of itching about the urethral meatus, with some burning on urination. Systemic symptoms are unusual. If the disease has gone on to stricture formation, diminution in the size of the urinary stream is noted (*see* STRICTURE, Urethra). With associated chronic prostatitis and seminal vesiculitis, the findings are the same, plus some pain in the sacral or perineal region and, frequently, diminution of libido. Rectal examination discloses a normal-sized or slightly enlarged prostate gland which is tender to touch, soft in consistency and with pus cells present in the wet smear of the expressate. The chronically infected seminal vesicle, however, may be either small and fibrotic or large and distended. Normally, the vesicles are somewhat tender, and this sensitiveness may be lessened by chronic infection. Disease of the urethra is differentiated from cystitis by examination of the voided urine collected in several glass receptacles. In urethritis, only the first urine voided contains the pus and mucous shreds, but in cystitis these findings are distributed throughout the specimens. In acute prostatitis and seminal vesiculitis all signs and symptoms are exaggerated. Fever and malaise occur and the pain of acute seminal vesiculitis may radiate to the groin, testicle or flank region, simulating renal colic. In either condition, rectal examination discloses an exquisitely tender, distended organ, which is fluctuant when abscess formation occurs.

Treatment

Bed rest, sedation (℞ 54, 55, 56) and intensive antibacterial therapy (*see* below) are indicated during the acute phase. Opiates may be administered as rectal suppositories (℞ 45, 49), as required for pain, which often is severe. Hot sitz baths 2 or 3 times/day give considerable relief (*see* BEDSIDE PROC.). Instrumentation and rectal massages are contraindicated until the acute symptoms have subsided. Even then, the gentlest massage of the infected prostate or seminal vesicle may cause an acute and dangerous exacerbation with dissemination of the infection. Antibacterial therapy during the chronic stage is wasted unless local treatment is undertaken at the same time. Urethral dilatation with metal sounds promotes proper drainage of the infected urethra and neighboring glands. Massage of the prostate, seminal vesicles, or both, following the passage of sounds empties them of retained infected secretions and tends to increase the local circulation. Massage is carried out after the bladder has been filled with an antiseptic solution (silver nitrate 1:5,000 or potassium permanganate 1:5,000). The solution is retained for 10 to 15 minutes longer and the patient then is asked to void. Diathermy may be given to the infected prostate gland by inserting a special electrode into the rectum. Long-standing chronic urethritis and prostatitis frequently will respond to instillations of an antiseptic and astringent solution, such as 5% argyrol or 0.5% silver nitrate, directly into the posterior urethra by means of a posterior urethral instillator. This should be done in conjunction with prostatic massage. Chronic seminal vesiculitis refractory to treatment may respond to dilatation of the ejaculatory ducts. This is carried out through a urethroscope and requires the knowledge and skill of a trained urologist. The treatment of chronic urethritis in the female consists of dilatations and local applications of antiseptic and astringent solutions (*see* above). Cystitis (q.v.) must be eliminated as a complicating infection. Surgical drainage of infected periurethral glands (Skene's) or lacunae may be necessary. Elimination of possible foci in the cervix or vagina is essential.

ANTIBACTERIAL THERAPY OF NONSPECIFIC URINARY TRACT INFECTIONS

All obstructions, foreign bodies, and calculi must first be removed. Distant foci of infection must be eradicated. If these measures cannot be carried out, complete cure cannot be expected, although chemotherapy still may minimize the infection. The proper chemotherapeutic or antibiotic agents must be selected on the basis of urine and blood cultures.

Pyridium (R 9): This relatively nontoxic drug has an analgesic effect on the mucosa of the urinary tract and a mild bacteriostatic action. It may be given with safety for long periods of time, as in chronic pyelonephritis, cystitis, urethritis, and prostatitis, to control the symptoms and to lessen the danger of acute exacerbations. It has almost no bactericidal action, and cure of urinary infections is not anticipated by its use. It is contraindicated when kidney function is markedly impaired and in severe hepatitis. The patient should be informed that it will give a reddish color to the urine.

Methenamine (R 11): This relatively nontoxic drug liberates formaldehyde in an acid urine. To ensure adequate concentration, urinary output must be restricted to approximately 1,200 cc./24 hours, and maintained at pH 5.5 or less. Urinary acidity is obtained by the use of ammonium chloride (R 7), or sodium acid phosphate (R 12) administered midway between doses of methenamine. Because of its low bactericidal action the use of methenamine is limited. It is indicated in infections due to *Esch. coli* which have become resistant to streptomycin and the sulfonamides, or where sensitivity to these drugs exists. It may be given for long periods of time without ill effects and is nontoxic in the presence of renal insufficiency. It is contraindicated in acidosis.

Mandelic acid (R 13, 14, 15): One of the older urinary antiseptics, this has been largely replaced by the sulfonamides. A better bactericidal agent than methenamine, the indications for its use are the same, plus the fact that it often is the drug of choice in combating *Str. fecalis* infections. Its action depends on an acid urine (*p*H 5.5 or lower) and adequate concentration (as above). It may cause transient nausea, vomiting, or diarrhea. Rarely, microscopic hematuria is observed during its use. Mandelic acid is contraindicated where there is impaired renal function, since severe acidosis and renal damage may result. The sodium, ammonium, and calcium salts are used in therapy. Sodium mandelate (℞ 14) requires an additional acidifying agent (℞ 7, 12). The course of treatment is 10 to 14 days and may be repeated after 1 or 2 weeks' rest.

Neoarsphenamine (℞ 16): Its use is limited to resistant coccal infections, especially those due to *Micro. catarrhalis*, *Staph. aureus* and *Str. fecalis*. If no improvement is obtained after 3 doses, further treatment with this drug is not indicated.

Sulfonamides (℞ 17 to 21): These have largely replaced the older urinary antiseptics. They are used both in small doses over long periods of time to combat the low grade or chronic urinary infections and in large doses, in combination with penicillin, for the treatment of acute infections with toxemia and systemic symptoms, as seen in acute pyelonephritis, prostatitis, seminal vesiculitis, and perirenal or renal abscess formation. Sulfadiazine (℞ 17, 18) is the drug of choice in urinary tract infections; it may be given alone or in combination with the other sulfonamides (℞ 19, 20, 21). Sulfathiazole is of almost equal worth, and sulfacetamide and sulfamerazine also are used effectively. They are bacteriostatic in infections due to certain of the gram-negative bacilli, to hemolytic streptococci and the staphylococci. The enterococci, especially *Str. fecalis*, are resistant to this group of drugs and streptomycin or mandelic acid is required.

Combinations of sulfonamides (℞ 19, 20, 21) may be given in small doses with relative safety for prolonged periods of time without alkalinization of the urine. The combination offers the additive therapeutic effects of the separate agents, but the individual solubilities are not influenced by the presence of other sulfonamides, hence crystalluria is not a problem (*see* SULFONAMIDE THERAPY).

Penicillin (℞ 22, 23, 24): This is the drug of choice in all coccal urinary infections, being superior to the sulfonamides in such cases. In mixed bacillary and coccal infections penicillin is given in conjunction with sulfadiazine or streptomycin. It is ineffective against the gram-negative bacilli and only moderately effective against *Str. fecalis*, *Str. nonhemolyticus* and *Str. viridans*. Other organisms may become resistant after prolonged administration. Parenterally administered penicillin leaves the body almost exclusively through the kidneys and thus high urinary concentrations are obtained. Only 10 to 25% of orally administered penicillin reaches the kidneys and, therefore, 4 to 10 times the parenteral dose must be given for equivalent effect.

Streptomycin or dihydrostreptomycin (℞ 25): In addition to being useful in genitourinary tuberculosis (q.v.), these antibiotics are indicated in urinary infections due to the gram-negative bacilli and some of the gram-positive bacteria (*B. subtilis, Staph. albus, Staph. aureus, Str. fecalis, Str. alpha hemolyticus, Str. nonhemolyticus, Str. pyogenes,* and *Str. viridans*), but only if *in vitro* tests have shown the particular strain of organism to be streptomycin-sensitive. Since resistance, once developed, lasts 6 months or more, therapy should await removal of all foci, foreign bodies, and calculi which might prevent complete eradication of infection. Streptomycin and dihydrostreptomycin are largely excreted in the urine and have their optimum effect in an alkaline medium, hence alkalinization by giving adequate amounts of sodium bicarbonate (10 to 20 Gm./day) is indicated except with infections due to *P. vulgaris,* where alkalinity favors bacterial growth. A total daily dosage of either drug of 2.0 Gm. is sufficient for most urinary infections, with 3.0 Gm./day required if bacteremia is present. With this dosage and by limiting the course of treatment to 3 to 10 days, the danger of toxic symptoms is avoided. Furthermore, restriction of fluids to 2,500 cc. daily will tend to give higher concentration of the antibiotics in the urine.

Both **aureomycin** (℞ 26) and **Chloromycetin** (℞ 27) have been used successfully in treating infections caused by susceptible organisms.

NEPHRITIS

Classification

Nephritis properly indicates an inflammatory disease of the kidneys, but as commonly understood often includes changes due to degenerative and vascular disease and pyogenic infection. Diffuse bilateral nonsuppurative diseases of the kidneys often are grouped as varieties of Bright's disease. These include glomerulonephritis ("inflammatory Bright's disease"), nephroses ("degenerative Bright's disease"), and nephrosclerosis ("arteriosclerotic Bright's disease").

Glomerulonephritis is characterized by inflammatory changes in the glomeruli, presumably the result of an allergic response to infection, usually streptococcic, elsewhere in the body. Glomerulonephritis starts as an acute generalized disease, affecting the capillaries throughout the body, in which the chief lesions are in the kidneys. Chronic glomerulonephritis develops in 10 to 20% of cases of acute nephritis.

The various forms of the **nephroses** are characterized by degeneration of the epithelial cells of the renal tubules, usually caused by exogenous poisons (e.g., mercury, arsenic), interference with the blood supply (shock), or severe toxemia. Nephrosis must be distinguished from the **nephrotic syndrome** (q.v.) which primarily is associated with long continued massive albuminuria.

Of the **nephroscleroses,** renal arteriolosclerosis associated with essential hypertension is the more serious. Renal arteriosclerosis occurring with the generalized arteriosclerosis of the aged very seldom results in renal insufficiency of great degree.

In all types of chronic kidney disease (glomerulonephritis, nephrosclerosis, and chronic pyelonephritis [q.v.]) there is progressive destruction of nephrons with subsequent reduction in kidney function. In the late stages, the symptoms of each type are very similar and are due to renal insufficiency. An accurate diagnosis may be impossible at this time without a complete history of the onset and course of the disease.

ACUTE DIFFUSE GLOMERULONEPHRITIS

A disease characterized pathologically by diffuse inflammatory changes in the glomeruli of the kidneys, lesser lesions in other small arteries throughout the body, and an increase in the permeability of the systemic capillary bed; and clinically by edema, albuminuria, hematuria and hypertension. Renal insufficiency frequently is present.

Etiology

Acute glomerulonephritis usually follows some form of infection. In about 85% of cases this is a streptococcic infection of the upper respiratory tract. Scarlet fever, streptococcic skin infections, pneumonia, and bacterial endocarditis are less frequent causes. The disease is much more common in childhood and adolescence than in adult life.

Symptoms and Signs

Onset usually is abrupt, although sometimes insidious, and occurs 1 to 3 weeks after the subsidence of the infectious process. Headache, fever up to 101° F., anorexia, nausea and vomiting are common initial nonspecific symptoms. Hematuria and a decrease in the urinary output are frequent findings and complete suppression of urine may occur. Edema develops in about two-thirds of the cases. It may be noticed first as puffiness of the face and eyelids and later may appear in dependent parts or become generalized. Convulsions as a result of cerebral edema may occur, particularly in children. Hypertension, usually moderate and transient, is present in about 35% of the cases. The eyegrounds are normal as a rule, but may show hemorrhages and papilledema. Not uncommonly some degree of congestive heart failure develops. Renal insufficiency produces uremia in 2 or 3% of the patients.

Laboratory Findings

The urine may be scanty, highly colored, smoky, or frankly bloody. Specific gravity is usually maintained at normal limits. Microscopic hematuria is the most characteristic finding. Between 2 to 4 Gm. of albumin is excreted daily in the average case, and casts, white blood cells, and epithelial cells are of common occurrence. Anemia is unusual during the acute stage of the disease, unless hematuria is severe. In most instances there is a sharp rise of the antistreptolysin titer in the blood. Tests of renal function reveal no insufficiency in about 50% of the patients with acute glomerulonephritis. In the severe cases, especially those with considerable oliguria and hypertension, nitrogen retention may occur, along with reductions in the rate of excretion of phenolsulfonphthalein and urea clearance, and a fall of plasma protein.

Diagnosis

Acute diffuse glomerulonephritis must be differentiated from the following conditions (q.v.): acute pyelonephritis which is accompanied by high fever, pain in flank, pus and bacteria in urine; renal tumor, stone, or tuberculosis which causes albuminuria and hematuria, but does not cause edema or red cell casts; febrile and orthostatic albuminuria, in which there is no edema, hypertension, or hematuria, and casts, if present, are only hyaline; passive congestion of heart disease which may cause albuminuria, casts, and occasionally a few red blood cells in the urine, but other signs of heart failure usually are obvious.

Prognosis

The fatality rate in acute nephritis is said to be between 5 and 10%; however, since many mild cases go unrecognized and recover without treatment, these figures are undoubtedly too high. Congestive heart failure is the most common cause of death in acute nephritis. Death not uncommonly occurs following recurrent convulsive seizures of hypertensive encephalopathy. Uremia accounts for about 2% of the fatalities. Most patients with severe acute nephritis recover completely.

The time required for recovery is exceedingly variable, ranging from a few days to one year, but once recovery has been established an immunity results which prevents future attacks or recurrences in most instances. Patients whose illness starts with definite signs and symptoms of acute glomerulonephritis following a recognized infection usually do better than those whose illness begins insidiously with only albumin and red cells in the urine. These latter patients are most likely to develop chronic glomerulonephritis.

Prophylaxis

The proper treatment of the causative infection is the best method of preventing nephritis. The use of penicillin and the sulfonamides, with the resultant rapid control of infectious diseases, has reduced the incidence of acute nephritis. A specimen of urine should be examined 2 weeks after any upper respiratory infection due to a streptococcus, so that a mild nephritis, if present, can be detected.

Treatment

Bed rest is the most important therapeutic measure and is indicated until all symptoms have subsided and the urine is normal. This usually occurs in 2 to 6 weeks, but occasionally may require several months. After the urine has returned to normal, there usually is no recurrence of albuminuria when the patient is up and about. He may be returned to full activity as quickly as his strength permits.

During the first few days of illness, because of anorexia and nausea, the diet is best restricted to fruit juices, tea, or milk. When nausea no longer is present, a more liberal diet—cereals, gruels, ice cream, fruits, bread, milk—may be allowed. Albuminuria is no indication for restricting protein. Only in the severest cases of acute nephritis, where there is pronounced nitrogen retention, is there any need to restrict protein for more than a few days. In most cases, the patient should be back on a normal diet in 10 to 14 days. However, as long as edema is present, sodium chloride should be restricted. No added salt should be used in or after cooking. Since it is the sodium ion that increases the tendency to water retention, other sodium salts, such as sodium bicarbonate or sodium citrate, also must be avoided.

The fluid intake should be adjusted according to the volume of urine. Severe oliguria requires reduction of intake since excessive fluid only increases the edema and may precipitate heart failure. A workable rule is to allow 1,000 cc. more fluid daily than the volume of the previous day's urine. Diuretic drugs or hypertonic solutions are ineffective and may be harmful in acute nephritis.

If signs of congestive heart failure (q.v.) appear, a digitalis preparation should be given in adequate doses. Caffeine citrate (℞ 58) or caffeine sodium benzoate (℞ 59) may be used as an adjuvant to digitalis in extreme cases. Venesection may be helpful if the venous pressure becomes unusually elevated.

If a severe hypertensive encephalopathy develops, convulsive seizures may be prevented by the administration of magnesium sulfate by mouth (℞ 36) to help reduce cerebral edema by dehydration, and by vein (℞ 37) for its C.N.S. depressant action. I.V. hypertonic glucose solution (℞ 39), venesection, and lumbar puncture also may be of use.

When there is any evidence that a streptococcic infection still persists, penicillin (℞ 22, 23) should be given, although there is little evidence that the course of the glomerulonephritis will be modified by the drug. Penicillin is preferable to the sulfonamides since in the presence of oliguria these may increase the renal damage.

Anuria complicating acute nephritis should be treated by

attempting to improve the circulation and raise the blood pressure (when this is below 100 systolic) by whole blood transfusion, plasma, isotonic solution of sodium chloride, or glucose infusions; ephedrine sulfate (℞ 60); Neo-Synephrine (℞ 61); or if indicated, digitalis (*see* CONGESTIVE HEART FAILURE).

When suppurative sinusitis, otitis or mastoiditis, does not yield promptly to chemotherapy it should be treated surgically; diseased tonsils should not be removed until the nephritis has subsided. Diathermy to the kidney region, X-ray treatment, and surgical decapsulation of the kidneys have not proved of value.

CHRONIC DIFFUSE GLOMERULONEPHRITIS

A chronic inflammatory disease of the kidney, characterized pathologically by fibrosis and hyalinization of the glomeruli, degeneration of the tubules, and vascular sclerosis, and clinically by progressive renal insufficiency.

Etiology

The role of infection in chronic nephritis is obscure. It not infrequently develops after an acute nephritis. The disease often is aggravated by streptococcic infections. The antistreptolysin titer, however, usually is low.

Symptoms and Signs

These vary with the stage of the disease. During the latent or asymptomatic period the only evidence of disease may be albuminuria and microscopic hematuria. Massive edema characteristic of the nephrotic syndrome (q.v.) may develop when albuminuria is severe and prolonged, reducing the plasma protein. Almost always the latent and nephrotic phases develop into the typical clinical picture of chronic glomerulonephritis. The majority of patients so afflicted seek attention because of edema, headache associated with hypertension, exertional or paroxysmal dyspnea, or because albuminuria was found on a routine examination. Such patients may appear in good health for a number of years, evincing disease only when cardiac or renal failure develops. Hypertension is a constant finding, and the heart often becomes enlarged as a consequence. As the disease progresses the edema may become less noticeable, but nocturia and polyuria may develop. Retinitis, characterized by retinal exudates and hemorrhages and impaired vision may be noted. Most of these patients eventually die in uremia (q.v.), but death from cardiac failure as a result of hypertensive heart disease or cerebral hemorrhage is not uncommon.

Laboratory Findings

The blood may remain normal for years, but anemia usually develops in the later stages of the disease. The urine varies in character with the stage of the disease. Early in the course of chronic nephritis, albuminuria and hematuria are conspicuous. As the disease advances these findings become less striking, except during periods of acute exacerbation. With increasing renal insufficiency the specific gravity of the urine becomes fixed between 1.008 and 1.012, the BUN and creatinine become greatly elevated, and progressive diminution of renal function as measured by the PSP excretion test and the urea clearance test becomes evident.

Diagnosis

In the presence of a clear-cut history of a preceding attack of acute nephritis following an acute respiratory infection, chronic glomerulonephritis is not difficult to recognize. However, if the patient is first seen when the disease is in a late stage, and the past history is unknown, it may be impossible to differentiate it from nephrosclerosis or bilateral pyelonephritis. The presence of severe hypertension, cardiac enlargement, changes in the eyegrounds, and anemia will help to distinguish an exacerbation of the chronic form from acute glomerulonephritis. Arteriolar nephrosclerosis, bilateral pyelonephritis with or without stones, renal tuberculosis, and polycystic disease may give similar urinary findings, and also may terminate in uremia; hence they are difficult to differentiate.

Treatment

Although the prognosis of chronic glomerulonephritis is ultimately bad, there are variations in the disease's rate of progress, which at times may be modified by therapy.

In the **latent stage** of the disease, avoidance of fatigue, and periodic examinations to detect the development of other symptoms are the only measures indicated. Reassurance, encouragement, and the avoidance of unnecessary limitations in the diet and activity are important in the care of the patient and will prevent unnecessary invalidism. If activity of the kidney lesions develops, as manifest by increased hematuria or edema, the patient should be urged to remain in bed until it subsides. Dietary restriction is not indicated merely on the basis of albuminuria. The amount of protein in a normal diet does not injure the kidneys, and the protein lost as albumin in the urine must be replaced. Restriction of protein intake tends to reduce further the plasma proteins and also leads to the development of anemia.

In the **nephrotic stage**, bed rest is indicated. Salt intake should be restricted to less than 1 Gm./day. Sufficient protein, about 100 Gm./day, should be given to maintain nitrogen equilibrium. (For details of diuretic and other therapy, *see* The Nephrotic Syndrome.)

Headaches, sleeplessness, and irritability associated with hypertension may be relieved by mild sedatives: bromides (℞

50, 52), chloral hydrate (℞ 53, 56), or phenobarbital (℞ 54, 55). These are best used intermittently or alternately. Daily rest periods of 1 or 2 hours are of great importance. A warm bath at night, or a small dose of a barbiturate at bedtime (℞ 54, 55) will often promote sleep. Unnecessary physical exertion should be avoided. The bowels should be regulated with a saline or other laxative. Free catharsis may be resorted to for the relief of hypertensive headache (℞ 36).

Cardiac insufficiency requires bed rest and should be treated as congestive heart failure (q.v.). However, the problem of fluid regulation is difficult. Salt must be rigidly restricted. Water should be allowed liberally since with the loss of concentrating power by the kidney, urine volume must be maintained at 2,000 cc. or more per day to prevent nitrogen retention. Diuretic drugs should be used with extreme caution if renal insufficiency is advanced since mercurial diuretics may increase albuminuria and hematuria, and ammonium chloride may increase an already existing acidosis resulting from retention of sulfates and phosphates. Of the diuretic drugs, caffeine (℞ 58, 59) and those of the xanthine group, such as aminophylline (℞ 1, 2) and theobromine (℞ 3), are the safest. They should be given intermittently, on alternate days, or for only 2 or 3 days at a time, since they lose their effect when given continuously. The daily dose may be increased gradually until diuresis is obtained or evidence of toxicity (nausea or vomiting) appears.

The anemia which occurs in chronic nephritis is extremely resistant to treatment. Iron, preferably in the form of ferrous sulfate (℞ 65) may be given. If the anemia is macrocytic, liver extract (℞ 66) by injection or folic acid by mouth (℞ 67) may be tried. Transfusions provide temporary relief.

In the stage of early nitrogen retention without edema or symptoms of congestive heart failure, strenuous physical exertion should be avoided, although walking on the level is permissible. The diet should be well balanced, containing 50 to 60 Gm. of protein and enough carbohydrate to meet the caloric requirements (*see* DIETS). Vitamin supplementation may be desirable. Salt should not be rigidly restricted at this stage, since the kidney is unable to conserve salt, and a gradual depletion of the body salt may take place. Fluid intake should be between 2,500 and 3,500 cc./day. There should be frequent rest periods and at least 9 hours in bed at night. When nitrogen retention becomes severe and undue drowsiness develops, the treatment is that indicated for uremia (q.v.).

ARTERIOLAR NEPHROSCLEROSIS

A kidney lesion present in most cases of essential hypertension which in its benign form consists of sclerosis of the smaller renal arterioles, especially the afferent glomerular arterioles, with subsequent fibrosis, ischemic necrosis, and destruction of glomeruli.

Symptoms and Signs

The disease runs a benign course in the great majority of patients, and in its early stages is marked only by symptoms of hypertension (q.v.). Abnormalities in the urine or decrease in kidney function do not appear for many years. During the later stage albuminuria, and occasionally hematuria, develop; the latter, however, usually is intermittent, rather than continuous as in glomerulonephritis. Death usually results from cardiac failure or cerebral hemorrhage before there has been enough destruction of kidney tissue to produce uremia.

In a small number of patients with severe hypertension, particularly those in the younger age group, the disease runs a much more rapid course; renal insufficiency develops quickly and death occurs due to uremia. This is called **malignant hypertension**, or **malignant nephrosclerosis**. Pathologically, the characteristic findings, in addition to the arteriolosclerosis, are areas of necrosis in the walls of the arterioles.

Diagnosis

Benign nephrosclerosis occurs in adults, generally beginning after the age of 35 with hypertension antedating any change in the urine. This is of great help in differentiating arteriolar nephrosclerosis from glomerulonephritis, in which the urinary changes antedate the hypertension. Malignant nephrosclerosis is differentiated from glomerulonephritis by the rapidity of onset of severe hypertension, quickly followed by renal involvement.

Treatment

The treatment of benign nephrosclerosis is that of essential hypertension (q.v.). The treatment of malignant nephrosclerosis is that of chronic glomerulonephritis (q.v.) and of uremia (q.v.).

DEGENERATIVE NEPHROSES

A group of kidney lesions due to a wide variety of causes, including poisons and trauma, characterized by degeneration of the tubules and producing renal insufficiency.

Etiology

Crushing injuries, burns, transfusions of incompatible blood, shock, and sulfonamide poisoning produce degenerative lesions in the distal tubules (lower nephron nephrosis). Mercury and arsenic affect chiefly the proximal tubules (upper nephron nephrosis). Tubular degenerative lesions also are caused by infectious disease (diphtheria, pneumonia, typhoid, syphilis) and severe acid-base imbalance.

Symptoms and Signs

A decrease in urine output is a constant finding. Complete "renal shutdown" (anuria) is not uncommon. The small amount of urine produced is of low specific gravity and contains widely varying amounts of albumin and red blood cells. Edema is rare, except when due to excessive infusions. At first the blood pressure is low or normal, but a slight elevation frequently develops after 4 or 5 days. Because of the loss of renal concentrating power and the small volume of urine, urea, and other waste products accumulate rapidly in the blood. Regeneration of tubular epithelium with resumption of renal function often occurs in 5 to 10 days in the mild or moderately severe case. Uremia is the cause of death in the severe cases.

Treatment

Since the tubular epithelium has great powers of regeneration, the problem is to keep the patient alive until this can take place. In cases of poisoning from mercury or other heavy metals, BAL (R 69) is the most effective therapeutic agent. If anuria has developed, no diuretic will be effective until some regeneration of tubular epithelium has taken place. During this time care must be taken not to drown the patient by excessive infusions. To replace fluid loss resulting from evaporation from the skin and lungs, 750 cc. of 15% glucose in water I.V. should be given daily until spontaneous diuresis occurs. Resumption of urine secretion may be masked by bladder retention; if there is any doubt, the bladder should be catheterized. When the flow of urine is reestablished, the volume can often be increased by I.V. infusions of isotonic solution of sodium chloride or 5% glucose solution.

When renal damage is due to sulfonamides it is important to be sure that the ureters are not mechanically blocked by precipitated drug. Prompt treatment of shock in injury, burns, and at operation is more effective in preventing development of renal lesions than are efforts to cure them. Some patients with less severe involvement, who maintain a urine volume of 500 to 1,000 cc./day but who have increasing nitrogen retention, can be saved by administering sufficient fluid to maintain a minimum urine output of 3,000 cc., until concentrating power is restored.

Recently, measures have been devised to keep the patient alive until regeneration of the tubular epithelium can occur. Peritoneal irrigation, "artificial kidney," and renal decapsulation have been tried with varying degrees of success.

THE NEPHROTIC SYNDROME

A term applied to those cases of renal disease, from whatever cause, characterized by massive edema and albuminuria.

Etiology

The nephrotic syndrome may occur during a stage of glomerulonephritis, in lipoid nephrosis, amyloidosis of the kidneys, and in syphilitic nephritis.

Symptoms and Signs

Edema, usually developing insidiously, at first gravitational and later generalized, is the only abnormal finding on physical examination. Albuminuria and decreased serum albumin are characteristic of the syndrome. An elevated serum cholesterol and a low basal metabolic rate usually are present. There is no hypertension, nitrogen retention, or appreciable decrease in kidney function. The specific gravity of the urine is not restricted.

Diagnosis

In the nephrotic stage of glomerulonephritis there usually is a history of acute nephritis, and red cells as well as albumin generally are present in the urine. There may be elevation of blood pressure and moderate nitrogen retention. The nephrotic stage of glomerulonephritis tends to disappear after a few months or several years, to be followed by the clinical manifestations of chronic glomerulonephritis.

True lipoid nephrosis may be impossible to differentiate without a long period of observation. It is a rare disease of childhood. The onset is insidious, without previous recognized infection, and the prognosis is relatively good. Death may result from secondary infection, especially pneumococci. However, over 50% of these young patients recover and remain well.

Syphilitic nephrosis may develop during the secondary stage of syphilis. The Wassermann test is positive, and the response to antisyphilitic therapy is dramatic.

Amyloid nephrosis usually is due to a chronic suppurative focus, e.g., tuberculosis or osteomyelitis. The Congo red test sometimes is of value in supporting a diagnosis of amyloidosis (q.v.), but only if 90% or more of the dye is retained.

Treatment

Treatment must be directed toward eradication of the primary infection. Complete bed rest is mandatory with anasarca, and advisable for most of the day if the edema is more than minimal. Adequate protein intake and salt restriction are the main therapeutic measures. The diet should contain about 100 Gm. of protein/day, which usually is sufficient to maintain a positive nitrogen balance. The attempt to stimulate regeneration of plasma proteins by feeding diets higher in protein content has generally been unsuccessful. The restoration of plasma protein by plasma transfusions or injections of salt-poor human serum albumin may be followed by diuresis, but since a large portion of the injected protein is lost in the urine, the benefit usually is only temporary. Occasionally, however, a remission of several months' duration follows. Large amounts of protein must be given: at least 500 cc. of whole plasma or serum, or 50 Gm. of salt-free serum albumin, daily for 10 days.

Sodium restriction is imperative. Salt intake should be below 1 Gm., preferably below 0.5 Gm./day. Most so-called salt substitutes are sodium salts, therefore unacceptable. A fair substitute contains 2 parts potassium chloride, 2 parts potassium citrate, 1 part ammonium chloride. With salt rigidly restricted, thirst is diminished, and a fluid intake of 1,000 to 1,500 cc./day safe.

Diuretic drugs often help to reduce edema, the most generally effective having been the mercurials, Mercuzanthin (R 4), Salyrgan-Theophylline (R 5), or Mercuhydrin (R 6). Mercurial diuretics are most effective when combined with an "acid-producing" salt, such as ammonium chloride (R 7), or the latter alone may be sufficient. Since mercurials lose their diuretic effect after about 3 days, they should be given intermittently. The effect of their I.M. injection may be increased at times by 0.5 Gm. of aminophylline (R 2) given I.V. 1 hour previously. With no nitrogen retention, urea (R 8) often is effective. At times the xanthine diuretics, especially aminophylline (R 1, 2), or theobromine (R 3) are helpful, given intermittently in courses of 2 or 3 days. Occasionally, thyroid extract (R 31) in large doses up to 0.3 Gm. or more/day may be useful.

Recently, investigational use of cortisone or ACTH has produced prompt diuresis in patients in the nephrotic phase of glomerulonephritis, together with reversion of blood chemistry findings toward normal. Further study is necessary before such results can be fully evaluated.

KIDNEY FUNCTION TESTS

The kidney function tests, when properly correlated with the clinical findings and the microscopic and chemical examination of the urine, aid in determining on a quantitative basis the degree of impairment of renal function. These tests measure renal function, but not necessarily the extent of kidney damage. Kidney function may be severely impaired because of extrarenal factors such as cardiac failure and dehydration without there being significant renal damage.

Since the functions of the kidneys are multiple, a disease may interfere with one function while leaving others intact. Ideally, kidney function tests should give specific information as to the rate of glomerular filtration and tubular reabsorption and secretion. While the inulin and diodrast clearance tests do give this sort of quantitative information, many laboratories are not equipped to do them. In general use are the more practical tests described below which do not measure specific functions but rather determine the kidney efficiency as a whole.

The tests of renal function may be classified as follows: (1) tests for the accumulation of metabolic products in the blood as a result of the inability of the kidneys to excrete them (blood nonprotein nitrogen, blood urea nitrogen, blood creatinine); (2) those tests which determine quantitatively the efficiency of renal function by comparing the amount of an excretable substance in the urine to its concentration in the blood (urea clearance test); (3) tests of the ability of the kidney to form a concentrated or dilute urine (concentration and dilution tests, see LAB. PROC.); and (4) tests dependent upon the ability of the kidney to excrete certain dyes and other substances (phenolsulfonphthalein, urea concentration test).

The **blood urea nitrogen** (BUN), **blood nonprotein nitrogen** (NPN), and the **blood creatinine tests** are measures of the amount of the products of protein catabolism. Azotemia or abnormally increased nitrogen retention in the blood (BUN>18 mg./100 cc., NPN>35 mg./100 cc., creatinine>1.8 mg./100 cc.), may occur because of an inability of the kidneys to excrete these substances at such a rate as to keep their blood concentrations within normal limits. In renal insufficiency from whatever cause, the blood concentration of these substances may far exceed the normal values. The discovery of azotemia should alert one to the possibility of renal disease, but the chief value of these tests is that severe nitrogen retention in kidney disease points to a bad prognosis. Minimal or moderate renal damage usually does not result in abnormal nitrogen retention, and at times even severe renal damage may be present without abnormalities of the blood chemistry. These tests should be interpreted only in the light of the complete clinical picture, since azotemia may occur as a result of extrarenal factors such as dehydration, digestive tract bleeding or shock. An increase in the blood creatinine, however, usually occurs most strikingly in renal azotemia (uremia) and is therefore more specific for renal disease.

The **urea clearance test** is used to determine the equivalent amount of blood from which urea has been completely removed (cleared) by the kidney per minute. This is accomplished by comparing the amount of urea excreted in the urine over a given period to the blood urea concentration during the same period. In renal insufficiency the equivalent amount of blood completely cleared of urea falls drastically. This test is more sensitive than the tests of nitrogen retention and in addition is somewhat more specific for renal disease.

The **concentration and dilution tests** are of great value and simple to perform. With advancing renal disease the kidney loses the ability to produce a highly concentrated or very dilute urine. In performing these tests, water is first restricted in an attempt to produce a concentrated urine, and then forced in an effort to create a diuresis of urine of low concentration. The normal kidney concentrates urine to a specific gravity over 1.025 and dilutes down to as low as 1.002. In severe renal disease the specific gravity of the urine becomes fixed between 1.008 and 1.012 and fluctuates very little in response to changes in the fluid intake.

The **phenolsulfonphthalein test** depends on the ability of the kidney to excrete certain dyes. It is one of the most frequently used tests for a quantitative estimate of gross kidney damage. The test is based upon an increasing impairment of dye excretion more or less paralleling the severity of renal damage. Extrarenal factors also may depress dye excretion. In suspected unilateral renal disease, this test can be modified so that it can be applied to obtain urine from kidneys individually by means of catheterizing each ureter.

Some authorities advocate testing the excretory concentration power of the kidney by means of the **urea concentration test.** They feel this is a valid criterion, in that urea, easily administered by the oral route, is a product that the kidney is called on to excrete constantly as one of its normal functions.

While these tests give an approximation of renal function they are not particularly informative as to the type of pathologic involvement. The microscopic and chemical examinations of the urine remain the most important laboratory criteria for the identification of renal disease.

UREMIA

The toxic clinical condition associated with renal insufficiency and the retention in the blood of nitrogenous urinary waste products (azotemia).

Etiology and Types

Kidney insufficiency may be due to (1) nephritis, bilateral pyelonephritis, polycystic kidney disease, complete ureteral obstruction, bilateral cortical necrosis (generally associated with some debilitating disease such as tuberculosis or with the puerperium); (2) congestive heart failure; (3) crush syndrome, extensive burns or transfusion reaction; (4) poisons (in particular mercury and carbon tetrachloride); or (5) other agents producing diffuse renal lesions, such as sulfonamide crystals or hemoglobinuria. Azotemia may be extrarenal in origin when the cause is a condition in which reduced renal blood flow has led to the nitrogen retention, as in dehydration or shock. Some of the manifestations of uremia are the result of acid-base and allied disorders (q.v.), while others are thought to be due to retained but as yet unidentified waste products.

Convulsions are rare in true uremia. When convulsions occur in kidney disease, they are presumed to be mainly due to cerebral edema, and occur chiefly in acute glomerular nephritis and severe hypertension (hypertensive encephalopathy). In these, nitrogen retention usually is minimal. The convulsions are best spoken of as pseudo-uremic, and the condition described as acute convulsive uremia.

Symptoms, Signs, and Chemistry

The symptoms of uremia are headache, restlessness, muscular twitchings, mental disturbances, nausea, vomiting, and sometimes diarrhea. Anorexia, which continues, may have preceded the acute symptoms. Generalized pruritus may likewise continue, being usually associated with a dirty yellowish discoloration of the skin, but it occurs only when the blood nonprotein nitrogen is elevated. Pain from a polyneuritis may increase the patient's discomfort. The signs and symptoms of dehydration or acidosis are usually present. There is retention of urea, creatinine and other waste products. Anemia is common. Terminally, if the nitrogen retention is great, gingival and buccal mucous membrane ulcers may occur, and an erroneous diagnosis of scurvy may be made. These lesions are representative of those which may at this stage involve the entire gastrointestinal tract. Vomitus may be copious, and consist of foul, salty, brownish or greenish brown material which leaves a marked fetor oris. Also terminally, fibrinous pericarditis may occur.

The acidosis results chiefly from two factors: retention of phosphates and sulfates, and failure of the diseased kidney to form ammonia by which the base substances in the body are conserved. Because of the failure to excrete phosphates, a compensatory reduction in ionized calcium occurs, and hyperexcitability of the neuromuscular mechanism follows. In some instances, sodium bicarbonate given to combat the acidosis, even in relatively small doses, may precipitate tetany.

Prognosis

The prognosis is poor, unless the uremia is due to a remediable cause, such as a lower nephron nephrosis (see Degenerative Nephroses), or ureteral obstruction. However, remissions of weeks' or months' duration are occasionally encountered. Convulsions occurring in hypertensive encephalopathy usually portend early death, while those occurring in acute nephritis may not have a similar implication.

Treatment

If anuria with gradually developing uremia is present, fluid intake should be restricted to replace the amount of fluid lost through the skin, in respiration, and from vomiting or diarrhea. This may be accomplished by the daily I.V. administration of 750 to 1,500 cc. of 15% glucose in water until diuresis begins.

Saline is contraindicated during this period unless large amounts of electrolytes are being lost because of vomiting or diarrhea. The glucose serves to reduce protein breakdown and hence retards the development of azotemia.

If, as in a chronic nephritis, large amounts of salt and water are excreted, I.V. or subcut. injection of as much as 80 cc. of normal saline/Kg. body wt. is indicated. Care must be taken not to overburden the right side of the heart. Convulsions or other evidence of cerebral edema are contraindications. If in the presence of congestive heart failure it is deemed necessary to administer fluids, the subcut. route is obligatory. The injections should be repeated until the urine is of satisfactory volume, or until developing edema, excessive weight gain, or the intake-output chart proves that the fluid intake has exceeded the kidneys' remaining excretory capacity. Distressing hyperpnea (from acidosis) may be relieved by the cautious administration of sodium bicarbonate (R 40) by mouth. If nausea prevents use of the oral route, alkali may be given by injection as 5% sodium bicarbonate solution (R 41), or ⅙ molar sodium lactate (R 42).

If tetany (q.v.) develops, calcium gluconate (R 43) I.V., is indicated. The same therapy may be used to relieve the muscular twitching of uremia. Because of the marked anorexia, the patient is permitted any foods he will take. Salt restriction is not indicated except when convulsions or edema are present. When congestive heart failure is present, all other therapy must be secondary to its treatment (q.v.). Purgation, colonic irrigation, and sweating not only are theoretically incorrect, but also usually are deleterious in practice. Blood transfusion is the only effective treatment for anemia. Sedatives (R 56, 57) should be used for the headache and restlessness, but drug intoxications must be guarded against when renal insufficiency is present. Vomiting may be difficult to control. Gastric lavage with warm water or the I.M. injection of magnesium sulfate (R 38) may be helpful. Magnesium sulfate also is effective for the control of convulsions. The dose may be repeated in 3 to 4 hours. However, should severe respiratory depression occur following such therapy, it can be relieved by an I.V. injection of calcium gluconate (R 43).

Cerebral edema may be reduced by I.V. injection of 100 to 150 cc. of a 50% solution of glucose (R 39), repeated if necessary in 6 to 8 hours. Lumbar puncture for the relief of pressure may be indicated. Until the convulsions and the headache have ceased, salt should be rigidly excluded and the fluid intake restricted. Chloral hydrate (R 56), or paraldehyde (R 57) are the most effective sedatives. Venesection rarely is beneficial. Excessively high blood pressure can be combated by inhalations of amyl nitrite (R 62), repeated doses of nitroglycerin (R 63) or, more effectively, with erythrol tetranitrate (R 64). When the patient has been free of convulsions for 24 hours, treatment should become that of the underlying condition.

In uremia due to reversible processes, such as transfusion or sulfonamide reactions, the use of the artificial kidney, or peritoneal lavage may be indicated. Surgical decapsulation is recommended by some authorities.

ANURIA

Complete suppression of urinary secretion.

Etiology and Types

Prerenal anuria results from inadequate blood flow through the kidneys, either because of low blood pressure, decrease in blood volume, or both. It occurs in hemorrhagic and traumatic shock, in Addison's disease, postoperatively, and may be encountered whenever the systolic pressure falls below about 70 mm. for any cause.

Renal anuria (i.e., due to lesions in the kidney itself) occurs in acute glomerulonephritis, eclampsia, cortical infarction, tubular necrosis, transfusion reactions, or blocking of the renal tubules with crystals of certain sulfonamide drugs.

Postrenal anuria is due to mechanical obstruction in the renal pelvis or ureter by stone, blood, sulfonamides, or tumor. Accidental ligation of the ureters during surgical procedures may occur. Very occasionally, obstruction of one ureter may produce a reflex vasoconstriction in the other kidney, and anuria. Reflex anuria also may follow simple catheterization.

Diagnosis

There may be remarkably few associated symptoms; headache, vomiting, and lumbar pain frequently are present. Urea, nonprotein nitrogen, and creatinine rise rapidly in the blood, but convulsions are rare and the mind remains clear almost to the end. Anuria must be sharply differentiated from failure to void urine accumulated in the bladder. The differentiation is made by passing a catheter. Failure to empty the bladder may be due to prostatic obstruction, vesical calculus, urethral stricture, a lesion of the spinal cord, or from "toxic" causes, as occasionally in severe febrile diseases.

Prognosis

The severity of symptoms and prognosis varies with the duration of the anuria. Recovery is rare after prerenal anuria lasting more than a few hours, but may occur after a period of several days in the other types.

Treatment

The treatment of anuria depends upon its cause. When due to shock (q.v.), all efforts must be directed to raising the blood pressure above critical levels. Plasma and blood transfusions, plus the treatment of the condition causing shock, are necessary. Infusions of dextrose and saline are of little value except to restore depleted body fluids. Diuretics are ineffective. Peripheral vasoconstrictors, such as ephedrine (℞ 60) or Neo-Synephrine (℞ 61), may be helpful. In Addison's disease (q.v.), and possibly in the hypotension seen in severe infections, appropriate therapy with adrenal cortical extract or desoxycorticosterone should be given in addition to saline infusions.

In the anuria of acute nephritis (q.v.) no treatment will be effective until the swelling of the glomerular capillary endothelium diminishes. Hot applications to the loins and high, hot colonic irrigations may be of some value. Diuretics, hypertonic solutions of sodium chloride or of dextrose are ineffective. Sweating and free purgation cannot replace urine secretion. Hemolytic transfusion reactions should be treated appropriately (see INFUSION REACTIONS). In anuria from poisoning, with destruction of the renal tubules, little can be done until the epithelial cells have begun to recover, which may require 4 to 10 days. During this period, overzealous infusions lead to such complications as edema or pleural effusion. The fluid intake should not exceed the output (including any loss by the bowels) by more than 1,000 cc., preferably given in the form of 10 or 15% glucose in water I.V. daily. Once some urine flow has been reestablished, fluid intake should be augmented by I.V. infusions of physiologic saline. The plasma chloride level should be followed, for if only dextrose solutions are given, it may fall to dangerous levels. When plasma levels cannot be obtained, it is well to give 1 liter of physiologic saline for every 2 liters of 5% glucose. If blockage of ureters or renal pelves with sulfonamide crystals is not relieved by forcing fluids and alkalization of urine (see SULFONAMIDE THERAPY), cystoscopy and ureteral catheterization may be required. At times, I.V. administration of 2 or 3 liters of saline may reestablish urine flow. In cases caused by stone in the ureter, accidental ligation, or obstruction due to new growths, surgical treatment is imperative.

PROSTATISM

Obstruction of the bladder outlet by the prostate.

Etiology and Incidence

As a result of the lengthened life span, more men are living beyond the age of 60. Enlargement of the prostate is found in 40% of such men, half of whom have symptoms, which may be due to benign hypertrophy, carcinoma, or fibrosis of the prostate. The cause of benign hypertrophy or of carcinoma is unknown. Fibrosis may follow inflammation of the prostate but this is most common at an earlier age (30 to 50 years).

Pathology

Benign prostatic hypertrophy begins as multiple fibroadenomatous nodules which appear simultaneously under the epithelium of the posterior urethra. These enlarge concentrically, compressing the normal prostatic tissue laterally against the anatomic capsule of the prostate. This shell of normal prostatic tissue is the so-called surgical capsule. Rarely, the hypertrophic mass may push out into the bladder lumen as well, forming a pedunculated ball-valve type of "middle lobe."

Prostatic carcinoma arises in the posterior lobe adjacent to the rectum. It is unrelated to benign prostatic hypertrophy and sometimes occurs simultaneously with it. It most often is a slow-growing adenocarcinoma which penetrates the capsule of the gland and metastasizes to adjacent tissues and the bones.

Bladder infection, dilatation, trabeculation, diverticulum formation, calculus formation, hydronephrosis, uremia, hypertension, and sepsis may result from prostatic obstruction.

Symptoms and Signs

Large congested prostatic lobes cause bladder irritability even before they begin to obstruct the urinary passage. Urgency, frequency, and smarting may occur although the stream still is normal in size. Partial urinary obstruction follows, with nocturia, increased frequency, incomplete emptying of the bladder, a small feeble stream and straining on urination. Bleeding may occur due to congestion of the prostatic lobes. An insidious onset over the course of several years may result in chronic retention with overflow dribbling and a developing uremia. Elevation of the blood pressure, cardiac decompensation and the mental confusion of early uremia must be watched for in the prostatic patient. Acute obstruction may ensue when the enlarged lobes become congested and completely block the narrowed outlet. This may be precipitated by ingestion of spicy foods or alcohol, attempting to hold the urine too long, exposure to cold, or immobilization in bed. Anuria (q.v.) and uremia (q.v.) are the consequences of continued back pressure and obstruction. Prostatic cancer produces urinary obstruction only after the entire gland is invaded.

The stagnant residual urine behind an obstructing prostate easily becomes infected and increased frequency and dysuria then occur, together with chills, fever, nausea and vomiting.

Suprapubic dullness or bulging of the distended bladder and enlargement of the prostate as detected by rectal examination (although intravesical middle lobe enlargements are missed this way) are the usual findings.

Diagnosis

Any male over 40 years of age with the above urinary symptoms should be suspected of prostatism. Patients in whom onset of the condition has been prolonged may fail to complain of obstruction, since they have forgotten what it is to urinate freely. Digital rectal examination usually will reveal an enlarged gland, but fibrosis of the bladder neck, median bars across the lower edge of the neck, or pedunculated intravesical middle lobes cannot be detected by rectal examination. Most prostatic cancers are readily detected by their enlargement, hardness and fixation. If the urine is sterile and has little or no pus in it, catheterization should be deferred until urinary antiseptics can be given prophylactically or until the patient can be prepared for operation should this prove necessary. A single catheterization then is permitted. Catheterization after the patient has tried to empty the bladder will reveal the amount of residual urine and also will reveal urethral obstructions. Catheterization also will indicate lengthening of the prostatic urethra in benign prostatic hypertrophy, since enlarged middle lobes make it necessary to insert the catheter almost to the hilt before it draws urine. Cystoscopy, best deferred until the patient is ready for operation, will demonstrate bars, fibrosis, enlarged intruding lobes, intravesical middle lobes, calculi, and bladder tumors. An I.V. pyelogram, NPN determination, ECG and chest X-ray are useful in evaluating the patient preoperatively. Urine concentration tests are the most accurate kidney function tests which are practical. Urethrograms taken in the oblique projection demonstrate the type of enlargement and may help to differentiate carcinoma from benign prostatic hypertrophy. The serum acid phosphatase rises only after a prostatic carcinoma has penetrated its capsule. X-ray of the pelvis and spine for osteoblastic metastases and biopsy of the prostate gland are other methods of differential diagnosis. All doubtful nodules which are confined to the prostate should be biopsied perineally with the patient prepared for total perineal prostatectomy, should examination of a frozen section indicate carcinoma.

Complications

These include cystitis, vesical diverticula, calculi, prostatitis, pyelonephritis, hydronephrosis and hydroureter, renal insufficiency, or uremia.

Treatment

If symptoms are mild, if residual urine is under 3 ounces (90 cc.), if kidney function is good, and if there are no diverticula or calculi, palliative treatment is permissible. Congestion of the enlarged prostrate may be relieved by the use of a hard seat on chairs and by avoiding cold, dampness, long rides in automobiles and trains, alcohol, pepper, and sexual excesses. The urge to urinate must be obeyed at once and the bladder must never be permitted to be overdistended. Transitory difficulty in urination may be relieved by sitting down in a tub of hot water to urinate. Intensive therapy (*see* NONSPECIFIC INFECTIONS) must be used to combat any infection which occurs. Inoperable carcinomas may be benefited by castration or hormone treatment. Estrogens (℞ 32, 33) may result in slight shrinkage of the gland, but must be given in large doses for a period of 3 months or more. Testosterone propionate may increase the bladder tone slightly but it is definitely contraindicated in any case where the possibility of prostatic carcinoma exists. Prostatic massage with the evacuation of large amounts of prostatic fluid is of only the most transitory help.

Surgical: Acute retention, acute infection, calculi in the bladder, large bladder diverticula, or an increase in symptoms or of residual urine are indications for operation. An indwelling urethral catheter can almost always be inserted if a stylet is used. This will permit the BUN to drop and the infection to subside under chemotherapy. A preliminary cystostomy or bladder puncture is only rarely necessary, as in the presence of severe cardiac disease, uremia, or bleeding. Prostatectomy is performed as soon as the patient's condition has improved sufficiently. Ordinarily, suprapubic prostatectomy is a quick, easy, effective operation. Transurethral resection is especially useful when the gland is relatively small, in cases with fibrosis or a bar at the bladder neck, and in cases where carcinoma does not recede quickly on estrogen therapy. Poor-risk patients can be handled best by this method, with or without preliminary cystostomy. Total perineal prostatectomy is indicated for small carcinomas, or badly infected prostates containing calculi. Retropubic prostatectomy without opening the bladder provides the best hemostasis and the most comfort for the patient. It is best suited to large glands in patients who can stand the longer operation.

NEUROGENIC BLADDER

A condition in which the urinary bladder becomes hypotonic or hypertonic due to lesions of the central nervous system or disturbances of peripheral innervation, resulting in difficulty of micturition, inability to empty the bladder completely, or incontinence.

Etiology

Neurosyphilis, trauma, tumors, and degenerative diseases involving the brain, spinal cord, cauda equina, and sacral nerve roots are the most common causes. The type of bladder dysfunction depends on the site and severity of the damage to the nervous mechanism controlling bladder action. Lesions above the nuclear centers in the sacral cord abolish voluntary control, leaving the reflex arc to function uninhibited. Lesions of, or peripheral to, the sacral nuclei abolish both voluntary and reflex control, the bladder emptying only by overflow dribbling or through the application of direct pressure over the distended bladder.

Symptoms, Signs, and Types

The paralytic bladder occurs immediately following an acute injury or disease of the spinal cord. The bladder is toneless, and overflow dribbling is constant. Depending on the extent of the cord lesion, this phase may persist for a few days to several months. Usually, within 6 weeks, the patient either recovers normal bladder function or develops one of the following permanent patterns of neurogenic bladder: (1) The **atonic (flaccid) bladder:** This results from lesions involving the sensory roots of S_2, S_3, or S_4. The capacity of the bladder is great and it can be palpated suprapubically. Overflow dribbling is continuous and cystometrograms show no pressure within the bladder. Sensation is absent, rendering catheterization or instrumentation painless. (2) The **automatic (reflex) bladder:** This condition usually develops in patients with complete supranuclear transection of the cord or severe brain damage. Sensation is lost. The bladder capacity is variable and, as soon as its maximum is reached, it empties itself reflexly with little or no warning "aura." Residual urine is minimal in these cases. The interval between voidings depends on the bladder capacity; if this is small, the patient is said to have a spastic bladder. (3) The **autonomous bladder:** This is due to interruption of both the afferent and efferent components of the reflex arcs of the bladder. Sensation is absent except for a feeling of overdistension. Overflow dribbling is almost constant and the quantity of residual urine is large.

Diagnosis

Cystometrograms should be done weekly during the phase of spinal shock following acute neurologic lesions. Increases in intravesical pressure will herald the return of ability to void. Also, the development of one of the 3 patterns of neurogenic bladder behavior can be observed. Cystoscopic examination or cystogram will show the contour of the bladder outlet and will reveal any obstructing prostatic tissue or hypertrophy of the internal sphincter at the bladder neck. X-rays of the urinary tract and an I.V. pyelogram should be done every 3 to 6 months to detect possible calculus formation or excessive dilatation of the kidneys from back pressure. Urinary output, urinalysis, and urine cultures should be followed carefully to guard against alkalizing infections which cause stones to form. Estimations of residual urine should be frequent.

Treatment

In patients in spinal shock urinary overflow should be permitted until an indwelling urethral catheter (No. 18 Foley) can, with rigid asepsis, be safely inserted. Either gravity or tidal drainage then should be instituted (*see* BEDSIDE PROC.). Intermittent catheterization should never be done. Suprapubic cystostomy should be carried out only when an indwelling urethral catheter proves unsatisfactory. The possibility of epididymitis resulting from the catheter is no contraindication as it can be treated with appropriate chemotherapy or surgery. Any infection must be prevented or treated energetically. Calculus formation can be prevented by a fluid intake of 3,000 cc. or more of water daily and by measures to keep the urine from remaining alkaline. Diseases such as syphilis, diabetes, and pernicious anemia involving the C.N.S. should be treated specifically. Large residual urines should be reduced by pressing upon the bladder to make emptying more complete, by having the patient void while standing or lying face down, and by transurethral resection of any bladder neck obstruction such as prostatic tissue or rims of hypertrophic muscle around the internal vesical orifice. Automatic (reflex) spastic bladders are best treated by tidal drainage until a capacity of 250 to 300 cc. is achieved. Thereafter, clamping of the catheter for increasing periods of time (up to 3 hours) will "train" the detrusor reflex. Spastic bladders also may be helped by partial or complete pudendal nerve block or by anterior rhizotomy. Patients with atonic bladder must develop a system of periodic voiding with complete continence between times.

For overflow dribbling, a rubber funnel to hold the penis can be strapped to the body, or a watertight sleeve for the penis can be fashioned from a condom and attached to a rubber tube and reservoir which is strapped to the patient's leg. Cunningham incontinence clamps can be used to compress the penis and keep the patient dry for short periods. Some patients cannot be made to void a satisfactory amount and are continually wet. These must have a permanent urethral catheter or (less desirably) a suprapubic tube. If these measures do not suffice to prevent uremia, bilateral cutaneous ureterostomies should be done.

ENURESIS

Involuntary bed-wetting during sleep by a child over 3 years of age. Enuresis must be differentiated from true **incontinence**, which may occur when the patient is awake, and from **neurogenic bladder** (q.v.)—conditions that are seen in any age group.

Etiology

Enuresis may be due to functional, urologic, or general causes. **(1) Functional causes** include persistence of, or return to, the automatic reflex voiding of infancy owing to lack of training, emotional instability, neuroses, or environmental maladjustments. **(2) Urologic:** There may be local irritation from meatal or urethral strictures, phimosis, redundant prepuce, adherent clitoris, balanitis, urethritis, trigonitis, cystitis, highly acid or alkaline urine, infections of the upper urinary tract, or pinworms. Increased urine volume secondary to diabetes, excessive fluid intake, or the consumption of diuretic beverages, may be responsible. **(3) General:** Various contributing factors include systemic diseases (e.g., tuberculosis), spicy foods, fatigue, hypothyroidism, epilepsy, mental deficiency, and local defects (e.g., spina bifida).

Diagnosis

This requires the consideration and search for all possible etiologic factors by physical examination and complete urologic work-up. Psychiatric study may be required to identify cases due to emotional instability or maladjustment.

Prognosis

The outlook is favorable in children who have no mental deficiency or severe organic disease. Proper training and habit formation and the correction of local abnormalities usually are effective. If enuresis persists beyond puberty, despite conscientious and thorough therapy, the prognosis must be guarded in all cases, regardless of the cause.

Prophylaxis

A habit of voiding regularly about every 4 hours should be established in all children by the 3rd year. Training should start at about 15 months, as this usually is the age at which the normal baby begins to stay dry for approximately 2 hours. It should not be started too early or done too forcefully lest the child come to hate going to the bathroom. A prerequisite should be a child's special toilet seat, preferably one that rests on the floor (as a potty-chair). This tends to overcome the feeling of insecurity produced by sitting on a high bowl and the fears often engendered by flushing the toilet. The child should be placed on the toilet seat every 2 hours, kept there for a few minutes, and not urged to pass urine. He will soon learn to urinate only when placed on the toilet and, by the age of 2, will begin to express his need to go there. Parents should not punish the child for accidents brought on by preoccupation or excitement. Finally, he should learn to use bathrooms other than his own when away from home.

Treatment

Local and systemic abnormalities (*see* Etiology) must receive appropriate therapy. Regular bladder habits should be established. The enuretic child should be required to empty his bladder at bedtime and should be completely awakened just before the usual time of bed-wetting (generally about 2 hours after going to sleep) and required to urinate again, in the proper receptacle. The time interval for awakening can be gradually increased, and the routine may be abandoned after 6 months if enuresis ceases. Heavy bed clothing should be avoided. The patient should never be reproached or punished for bed-wetting, but always praised and rewarded for any improvement. It is better to call his attention to a dry bed, than to a wet one. Excitement and fatigue are to be avoided; a quiet outdoor life, an afternoon nap, and curtailment of activity toward bedtime should be instituted. If excessive nervous irritability persists despite this regimen, mild sedation is indicated (℞ 54, 55). Coffee, tea, cocoa, spices, salt, and sweets should be avoided, especially at the evening meal, which should be light and dry (e.g., bread, cereal, custard, fruit, or jello). Fluids should be moderately restricted after 4 P.M., only one glassful taken with supper and none permitted before retiring. However, restriction of fluid must not be overdone, lest the urine become overconcentrated.

Emotional instability or maladjustment should be investigated and treated. It may require the help of a psychiatrist to identify the faults of both the parents and the child.

Methyltestosterone (℞ 34) by mouth, 10 to 30 mg. daily in divided doses for a period of 1 to 3 months, may be tried in patients of either sex. If there is no response within 2 weeks, the oral therapy should be supplemented by weekly I.M. injections of 10 to 25 mg. each (℞ 35). With improvement in bladder control, the dosage is gradually decreased. If all other forms of therapy fail, treatment aimed at increasing irritability of the detrusor mechanism can be tried. Local application or instillation of silver nitrate solution 1:5,000, the passage of catheters or sounds, or ingestion of tincture of cantharides (℞ 70) will occasionally produce this effect. This may cause the patient to wake before bed-wetting occurs, through the stimulus produced by a small accumulation of urine.

INTERSTITIAL CYSTITIS

(Hunner's ulcer)

Middle-aged women are susceptible to a type of infiltration of the bladder wall which makes it shrink and decrease in capacity with resultant pain, splitting of the epithelium, and bleeding if the bladder is filled to any useful capacity. The etiology is unknown. Typical symptoms are frequency both day and night, with pain so severe as to cause sphincter spasm and intermittent urination, followed by abrupt relief on voiding. Cystoscopy often reveals a cherry red spot in the center of a stellate scar. As the bladder is distended, the lesion can be seen to crack open and bleed. Treatment is difficult. The lesions may be fulgurated with the cystoscopic electrocoagulating needle, or the bladder may be dilated under analgesia with silver nitrate solution, starting at a strength of 1:10,000 and increasing it to 1:1,000 over a period of 3 weeks as rapidly as the patient can tolerate the higher concentrations. Often, the two methods of treatment can be combined.

SCROTAL MASSES

Scrotal masses may be due to epididymitis, hernia, varicocele, hydrocele, spermatocele, testicular tumor, orchitis, torsion of the testis, lymphedema, hematocele, lipoma, gumma, metastatic tumor, and rare fatty or connective tissue tumors of the scrotum.

Epididymitis may occur as a complication of urethritis or prostatitis (particularly gonorrheal), prostatectomy, or following the use of indwelling catheters. The onset usually is acute with pain, fever, and the appearance of a hard, tender nodule in the tail of the epididymis. The infection rapidly subsides with bed rest, scrotal support, ice bags, and the use of appropriate antibiotic or chemotherapeutic agents. However, the epididymis usually remains blocked to the passage of sperm. Tuberculous epididymitis may have a more insidious onset and often is complicated by the development of chronically draining sinuses; epididymectomy, with prophylactic streptomycin or dihydrostreptomycin 2 days before and 19 days following the operation, is the treatment of choice.

Hernia usually is reducible and transmits an impulse upon coughing; therapy is surgical. A **varicocele** resembles a bag of worms in the scrotum. A suspensory should suffice since many varicoceles recede after marriage. Persistent symptomatic varicoceles require operation. **Hydrocele** may be congenital or secondary to trauma or infection of the scrotal contents. It transilluminates and does not reduce or give an impulse when the patient coughs. It may be complicated by **hematocele** or **pyocele.** An acute hydrocele should be treated by bed rest, scrotal support, and the application of either heat or cold. Hematocele or pyocele requires incision to permit evacuation or drainage. Congenital hydroceles should be observed for several years, since many will disappear by early childhood. Injection treatment (using sclerosing solutions) should be used very cautiously because of the danger of confusion with hernia. Aspiration of fluid is only palliative and makes subsequent operation difficult. Operative treatment is safe and satisfactory. **Spermatocele** resembles hydrocele but lies above the testis and contains sperm. It is best removed surgically.

Testicular tumors: Any painless, hard mass in the scrotum

which does not recede markedly within a few days should be
explored as a possible testicular tumor. Such growths are more
common in undescended testes. Adrenal rests and metastases
from distant tumors also may become evident as scrotal masses.
Gynecomastia and a positive urine pregnancy test indicate a
chorionepithelioma. Therapy consists of a radical orchidec-
tomy followed by radiation therapy. Patients with chorionepithelioma should receive pregnancy tests at 3 to 6 month
intervals to detect metastases. Individuals with metastases at
the time of diagnosis should be treated only with radiation.

Orchitis: Acute orchitis occurs usually in an adolescent as a
complication of mumps, but may accompany syphilis or any
acute infection. Fever, pain, and swelling of the involved
testicle are evident, plus the clinical manifestations of the
primary disease. Atrophy of the involved gonad commonly
follows. Therapy consists of bed rest, scrotal support, ice
bag, and the treatment of the primary disease. (For the treatment of mumps orchitis, *see* MUMPS.) Torsion of the testis
usually is found in an undescended testicle or one with a long
mesorchium. It may occur when the patient turns in bed or
as a result of strenuous work or exercise. The testis is acutely
tender, swollen and is held high in the scrotum. Rarely the
twisted cord can be felt above it. As the testis becomes
gangrenous because of occluded circulation, there is nausea and
vomiting, scrotal edema, fever, and leukocytosis. Immediate
operation is indicated to untwist the cord, followed by the use
of a suspensory and an ice bag. If the testis already is gangrenous, it must be removed.

Miscellaneous: Urinary extravasations from the anterior
urethra will cause abscesses which may point in the scrotum.
These should be treated surgically, as should lipoma of the
cord, elephantiasis, and rare tumors of the supportive tissues.

PRIAPISM

*Painful abnormal erection of the penis, which may be quite
persistent.* It results either from neurologic diseases, or painful stimuli, such as bladder calculus, urethritis or prostatitis;
or from obstruction of the blood vessels that drain the penis,
as from thromboses due to neoplasms, hematomas, cellulitis,
leukemia, or other blood dyscrasias.

Treatment

Appropriate measures should be taken to eliminate the underlying disorder. Locally, protective cotton padding should be
placed around the penis, and cradles over the body to hold
away the bedclothes. The skin is kept soft with lotions or ointments. Priapism due to neurologic disturbances may respond

to spinal or caudal anesthesia and sedation, if treatment is given early. If the condition is allowed to persist, the vessels will thrombose, causing permanent engorgement and edema. The thrombotic type of priapism is difficult to control. Large-caliber needles (No. 12) can be inserted into each end of both corpora cavernosa and the thrombi washed out by through-and-through irrigation with normal saline.

IMPOTENCE

The inability of the male to perform the sexual act. This is in contradistinction to **sterility** (q.v.), which implies inability to fertilize the ovum.

Etiology and Incidence

Impotence is physiologic in childhood and old age. Furthermore, there is a wide variation among normal individuals as to the frequency of coitus and the duration of active sex life. Pathologic impotence is a symptom which may result from any of the following conditions: **(1) Diseases of the genitalia:** These include structural defects, such as phimosis, micropenis, hypospadias and epispadias, balanitis, penile ulcers, urethritis, scrotal masses, orchitis, and prostatitis (truck and taxi drivers are particularly subject to traumatic prostatitis). **(2) Endocrinopathies,** such as hypogonadism, hypopituitarism, hypothyroidism. **(3) Systemic disorders:** Diabetes mellitus, all debilitating diseases, and infectious lesions of the spinal cord, excessive fatigue, chronic poisoning, as in alcoholism or drug addiction, and excessive exposure to X-radiation. **(4) Psychic factors,** such as a feeling of inferiority caused by premature ejaculation, fear of impregnating the partner or of contracting a venereal disease; or revulsion from the partner or her surroundings. Psychic impotence frequently is specific (e.g., for the wife, the virgin, or the prostitute) rather than absolute.

Diagnosis

Since impotence may accompany many diseases, a careful clinical study is necessary in all cases to discover any underlying cause. The history and a complete physical examination will suggest the diagnosis and indicate required laboratory procedures. Of particular importance is a history of penile lesions, urethritis, systemic diseases, alcoholism, or exposure to X-radiation. The patient's body type should be noted, the presence of secondary sex characteristics confirmed, and the testes palpated for size and location.

Psychic factors are responsible for most cases of male impotence. A diagnosis of psychoneurosis demands that organic causes have been ruled out and requires a thorough investigation into the psychologic makeup, marital relationship, and sex habits of both marital partners.

Treatment

Therapy is aimed at the correction of the underlying disease. Structural defects of the genitalia require surgical repair. Local or systemic disorders should receive appropriate therapy. Gonadotropins (R 30) are indicated for hypogonadotropic states, being given in doses of 1,000 u. twice weekly for 10 weeks. Testosterone, 25 mg. I.M. for 2 or 3 doses, followed by oral methyltestosterone, is useful in cases of primary testicular failure and in the "male climacteric" (R 34, 35). Thyroid (R 31) is indicated for hypothyroidism. Testosterone should not be used in patients with normally functioning testes, since the drug depresses spermatogenesis and may be a prostatic carcinogen. Aphrodisiacs (R 70) are of little worth except for their psychologic value. However, in cases of functional impotence, the moderate ingestion of alcoholic beverages (by those not opposed to their use) prior to attempted coitus is frequently successful in lessening the interfering inhibitions. Premature ejaculation, which produces impotence through discouragement and a sense of inferiority, may often be corrected by more frequent coitus or by the precoital application of an anesthetic ointment containing 5% benzocaine to the glans penis (R 71).

When impotence persists in the absence of any evident organic condition, a thorough and judicious psychiatric study is indicated. Detailed sex education is advisable in all cases.

MALE STERILITY

Relative or absolute inability of the male to fertilize the ovum.
It may or may not be associated with **impotence** (q.v.).

Etiology

Inability of the male to impregnate the female results from absence of any of the requisite physiologic factors; i.e., production of a sufficient number of normal spermatozoa by the germinal tissue of the testes, their unobstructed passage through the seminal tract, and their deposition well within the vaginal vault during coitus. This sequential process may be interfered with by any of the following conditions. (1) Failure of spermatogenesis due to congenital absence of the testes, cryptorchidism, testicular atrophy (following orchitis or trauma), hypogonadism, thyroid or pituitary deficiency, chronic diseases and nutritional deficiency states, overtreatment with testosterone, overexposure to X-radiation, and senility. (2) Obstruction of the seminal tract following infections of, or surgical procedures on, the epididymis, vas, seminal vesicles, prostate, or urethra. (3)

Defective deposition of ejaculate, due to impotence, penile abnormalities (e.g., hypospadias), or premature ejaculation.

Symptoms and Signs

Aspermia (absence of seminal fluid) is associated with urethral stricture and structural defects in the prostate such as may follow prostatic surgery. Azoospermia (absence of sperm in the semen) is due to obstruction of the seminal tract, to germinal aplasia, or to the end stages of tubular atrophy or fibrosis. Oligospermia (lowered semen sperm count) is caused by partial duct blockage or by retarded or suppressed spermatogenesis. The finding of necrospermia (high percentage of nonmotile sperm) in a specimen of semen usually denotes faulty collecting or handling, but may be due to prostatic or seminal vesicle infections.

Diagnosis

Two careful semen analyses should be done, each after 3 or more days of continence. The entire ejaculate must be collected (see Lab. Proc.). The time of collection is noted on the stoppered bottle, which should be kept at body temperature until it can be brought (as promptly as possible) to the laboratory.

Normal counts are 80 to 200 million spermatozoa/cc. Counts below 60 million indicate relative infertility. Low counts usually are associated with an increased number of abnormal sperms. Abnormal forms should not exceed 15% in a normal specimen. Motility should be above 15% after 2 hours at room temperature and should persist to some degree for 24 hours. If both analyses are normal the fault lies either in the wife or in improper sex technic.

When the semen analysis reveals a deficiency, a careful workup is in order. Of particular importance is a history of exposure to X-rays, or of severe febrile disease, mumps, venereal disease, cryptorchidism, nutritional deficiency, and endocrine imbalance. Evidence of physical exhaustion, overwork, nervous strain, drug addiction, or alcoholism must be sought. On physical examination the body type should be noted carefully, the presence of secondary sex characteristics confirmed, the testes palpated for size, location, firmness, and sensitivity to pressure. Careful palpation of each vas and epididymis may reveal nodules or thickening which would obstruct the ducts. Rectal examination may reveal obstructing nodules in the prostate or seminal vesicles, and a wet smear of the prostatic expressate will reveal prostatitis if present. Urethritis is demonstrated by cloudiness in the first glass of a 2-glass urine test. Penile abnormalities such as hypospadias should be noted. A sound should be passed to exclude urethral stricture.

Testicular biopsy in cases of diminished sperm count is the only accurate method for diagnosing an underlying disease process. This can be done under either local or pentothal anesthesia. If the testis is found to be hopelessly damaged the patient should be told that treatment is useless. If the biopsy findings are normal in the presence of azoospermia, obstruction of the epididymis, vas, or ejaculatory duct is to be suspected. X-ray studies of the vas may locate the site of obstruction.

Treatment

Adequate therapy requires the correction of any underlying disease. Deficiency states should be corrected by the use of appropriate foods and vitamin supplements. The routine use of vitamin E is recommended by some (R 72). Chorionic gonadotropin (R 30) may be tried for retarded spermatogenesis, but it generally has given disappointing results. Testosterone is contraindicated since it depresses spermatogenesis. Undue exposure to X-radiation should be avoided. When indicated, thyroid (R 31) often gives excellent results.

The treatment of seminal tract obstruction requires the use of appropriate chemotherapeutic agents to combat any existing infection, together with surgical correction of any obstruction amenable to surgery. Anastomosis of a previously divided vas sometimes produces successful results.

Improper sex technic should be eliminated. The physician should stress the need for regular coitus 2 or more times weekly, particularly at the probable time of ovulation. The wife must be advised not to douche following coitus and to remain in a reclining position for 2 to 4 hours after intercourse. If the semen drains out, she should elevate her hips on pillows. Premature ejaculation and impotence (q.v.) should receive appropriate therapy. If normal coitus is impossible, artificial insemination with the husband's semen should be tried several times, particularly in cases with oligospermia.

PRESCRIPTIONS

(Wherever a prescribed "proprietary" is representative of a class of therapeutic agents, alternative proprietary preparations will be found listed in Part II.)

Diuretics

1. R Aminophylline . . . . 0.1 Gm. (gr. iss)
   1 or 2 tablets daily.

2. R Aminophylline (ampul)
   0.25 to 0.5 Gm. (gr. iv to viiss) I.V., slowly,
   1 hour before a mercurial diuretic.

3. R Theobromine calcium salicylate . . . . 0.5 Gm. (gr. viiss)
   1 or 2 tablets 3 times daily after meals.

4. ℞ "Mercuzanthin"   (ampul)

> 0.5 cc. I.M. initially as a test dose followed by
> 1 to 2 cc. I.M. every 5 to 7 days as necessary.

5. ℞ "Salyrgan-Theophylline"
   (ampul)

> 0.5 cc. I.M. initially as a test dose followed by
> 1 to 2 cc. I.M. every 5 to 7 days as necessary.

6. ℞ "Mercuhydrin"   (ampul)

> 0.5 cc. I.M. initially as a test dose followed by
> 1 to 2 cc. I.M. every 5 to 7 days as necessary.

7. ℞ Ammonium chloride   (enteric
   coated) . . . .   0.5   Gm. (gr. viiss)

> 2 to 4 tablets 4 times daily.

8. ℞ Urea . . . .   45.0   Gm. (℥ iss)
   Syrup U.S.P. . . . . q.s. ad   90.0   cc.   (℥ iii)

> 2 to 4 teaspoons 4 times daily after meals.

Urinary Antiseptics and Antimicrobial Agents

9. ℞ "Pyridium" . . . .   0.1   Gm. (gr. iss)

> 2 tablets 3 times daily.

10. ℞ Phenol . . . .   0.6   Gm. (gr. x)
    Guaiacol . . . .   9.0   cc.   (♏ cxxxv)
    Chlorobutanol . . . . . .   1.2   Gm. (gr. xviii)
    Olive oil. . . . . . .q.s. ad   180.0   cc.   (℥ vi)

> Use for bladder irrigations.

11. ℞ Methenamine . . . .   0.3   Gm. (gr. v)

> 3 tablets every 6 hours, administered with a
> urinary acidifier (℞ 7, 12).

12. ℞ Sodium biphosphate. . . .   30.0   Gm. (℥ i)
    Water. . . . . . . .q.s. ad   120.0   cc.   (℥ iv)

> 1 teaspoon 4 times daily.

13. ℞ Calcium mandelate . . . .   0.5   Gm. (gr. viiss)

> 6 tablets 4 times daily, after meals and at
> bedtime for 10 to 14 days.

14. ℞ Sodium mandelate . . . . .   0.5   Gm. (gr. viiss)

> 6 tablets 4 times daily, after meals and at
> bedtime for 10 to 14 days, given in combina-
> tion with an acidifying agent (℞ 7, 12).

15. ℞ Ammonium mandelate. . . .   0.5   Gm. (gr. viiss)

> 6 tablets 4 times daily, after meals and at
> bedtime for 10 to 14 days.

16. ℞ Neoarsphenamine   (ampul)

    0.2 Gm. (gr. iii) I.V. followed by 1 or 2 injections of 0.3 Gm. each at 5-day intervals; continue therapy only if improvement is noted.

17. ℞ Sulfadiazine . . . .   0.5   Gm. (gr. viiss)

    8 tablets initially, then 1 or 2 tablets every 4 hours.

18. ℞ Sodium sulfadiazine   (ampul)

    2.5 Gm. I.V. every 6 to 12 hours.

19. ℞ Sulfadiazine
    Sulfathiazole. . . . . . .āā   0.25 Gm. (gr. iv)

    4 tablets (or capsules) initially, followed by 1 or 2 tablets 4 times daily.

20. ℞ Sulfadiazine
    Sulfacetamide . . . . . .āā   0.25 Gm. (gr. iv)

    4 capsules initially, followed by 1 or 2 capsules 4 times daily.

21. ℞ Sulfadiazine
    Sulfathiazole
    Sulfamerazine . . . . . .āā   0.17 Gm. (gr. iiss)

    8 tablets (or capsules) initially, followed by 1 or 2 tablets 4 times daily.

22. ℞ Penicillin   (vial)

    30,000 to 100,000 u. I.M. every 3 hours.

23. ℞ Procaine penicillin   (vial)

    300,000 u. I.M., every 12 to 24 hours.

24. ℞ Penicillin   (oral tablets)

    100,000 to 300,000 u. orally every 3 hours.

25. ℞ Streptomycin or dihydrostreptomycin   (vial)

    For nontuberculous infections: 2 to 3 Gm. daily, I.M., in divided doses. For genitourinary tuberculosis the average dose of streptomycin or dihydrostreptomycin is 1.8 Gm. I.M. daily for 90 to 120 days.

26. ℞ Aureomycin   (capsules). . .   0.25 Gm.

    25 to 100 mg./Kg. body wt./day divided into 4 to 8 equal doses. Reduction of dosage is permissible following the acute phase of the disease.

27. ℞ "Chloromycetin"   (capsules).   0.25 Gm.

    Administer as for ℞ 26.

Antispasmodics

28. ℞ Papaverine hydrochloride
(ampul)

30 mg. (gr. ss) subcut. every 3 hours if necessary.

29. ℞ A synthetic antispasmodic
(For available products *see*
dose table of ALTERNATIVE
PROPRIETARY PREPARATIONS.)

Hormonal Substances

30. ℞ Chorionic gonadotropin   (vial)

500 to 1,000 u. I.M. 2 or 3 times a week.

31. ℞ Thyroid U.S.P.   15   mg. (gr. ¼)

1 to 6 tablets daily.

32. ℞ Diethylstilbestrol   1   mg.

10 tablets daily for 10 days; then 5 tablets
daily for 10 days; then 3 tablets daily for life.

33. ℞ Ethinyl estradiol . . . . .   0.05   mg.

10 tablets daily for life.

34. ℞ Methyltestosterone   10   mg.

1 to 3 tablets daily.

35. ℞ Testosterone propionate   (vial)

For enuresis: 10 mg. I.M. once a week.   For
impotence: 25 mg. I.M. 2 or 3 times a week
for 4 to 6 weeks.

Fluids and Electrolytes

36. ℞ Magnesium sulfate

Dissolve 2 to 4 teaspoons in ½ glass of water
and drink daily as necessary.

37. ℞ Magnesium sulfate, 10% solution   (ampul)

10 cc. I.V. daily as necessary.

38. ℞ Magnesium sulfate, 25% solution   (ampul)

5 to 10 cc. I.M.

39. ℞ Glucose, 50% solution
(ampul)

25 to 150 cc. I.V. to combat cerebral edema.

40. ℞ Sodium bicarbonate

1 to 5 teaspoons hourly with copious quantities of water until acidosis is controlled.

41. ℞ Sodium bicarbonate, 5% solution   (ampul)
   6 cc./Kg. body wt. I.V. or subcut.

42. ℞ Sodium lactate, 1/6 molar solution   (sterile bottle)
   25 cc./Kg. body wt. I.V. or subcut.

43. ℞ Calcium gluconate, 10% solution   (ampul) . . . . .   1.0   Gm. (gr. xv)
   Contents of 1 ampul slowly I.V. to control convulsions.

Analgesics and Sedatives

44. ℞ Morphine sulfate . . . . . .   20.0   mg. (gr. 1/3)
   Atropine sulfate . . . . . .   0.6   mg. (gr. 1/100)
   Subcut.; half this dose may be repeated if necessary.

45. ℞ Morphine sulfate . . . . . .   0.015 Gm. (gr. 1/4)
   Belladonna Extract U.S.P. .   0.03 Gm. (gr. ss)
   Cocoa Butter U.S.P. . q.s. ad   2.0   Gm. (℥ ss)
   Insert one suppository rectally every 2 hours if necessary.

46. ℞ Codeine sulfate. . . . . . .   0.03 Gm. (gr. ss)
   Acetylsalicylic acid . . . . .   0.6   Gm. (gr. x)
   1 capsule as needed for pain.

47. ℞ Morphine sulfate
   8 to 15 mg. (gr. 1/8 to 1/4) subcut.

48. ℞ "Demerol Hydrochloride"   (ampul)
   50 to 100 mg. subcut.

49. ℞ Powdered Opium U.S.P. . .   0.06 Gm. (gr. i)
   Belladonna Extract U.S.P. . .   0.015 Gm. (gr. 1/4)
   Cocoa Butter U.S.P. . q.s. ad   2.0   Gm. (℥ ss)
   Rectal suppository as necessary for tenesmus.

50. ℞ Sodium bromide . . . . . .   0.3   Gm. (gr. v)
   2 or 3 tablets 3 or 4 times daily.

51. ℞ Potassium citrate. . . . . .   30.0   Gm. (℥ i)
   Hyoscyamus Tincture U.S.P.   30.0   cc. (℥ i)
   Water. . . . . .q.s. ad 120.0   cc. (℥ iv)
   1 or 2 teaspoons 3 or 4 times daily.

52. ℞ Potassium bromide . . . . .   10.0   Gm. (℥ iiss)
   Peppermint Water U.S.P.
   q.s. ad 90.0   cc. (℥ iii)
   1 teaspoon 3 times daily.

53. ℞ Chloral hydrate. . . . . 6.0 Gm. (ʒ iss)
    Acacia Mucilage U.S.P. . . . 30.0 cc. (ʒ i)
    Cinnamon Water U.S.P.
                  q.s. ad 90.0 cc. (ʒ iii)
> 1 teaspoon 3 times daily.

54. ℞ Phenobarbital Elixir U.S.P. . 120.0 cc. (ʒ iv)
> 1 teaspoon as needed.

55. ℞ Phenobarbital . . . . 30 mg. (gr. ss)
> 1 tablet 3 times daily.

56. ℞ Chloral hydrate. . . . . . . 0.3 Gm. (gr. v)
> 2 to 6 capsules; the smaller dose may be repeated in 1 to 3 hours, the larger in 6 hours.

57. ℞ Paraldehyde . . . . 60 cc. (ʒ ii)
> 1 teaspoon hourly until effective; rectally the dose is 0.25 cc./Kg. body wt., administered as a 10% solution in isotonic sodium chloride, and repeated in 10 to 12 hours if necessary.

Cardiovascular Agents

58. ℞ Citrated Caffeine U.S.P. . . 0.3 Gm. (gr. v)
> 1 tablet or capsule every 3 hours as necessary.

59. ℞ Caffeine and Sodium Benzoate
    Injection U.S.P. (ampul) . 0.5 Gm. (gr. viiss)
> Contents of 1 ampul subcut. every 3 hours as necessary.

60. ℞ Ephedrine sulfate (ampul)
> 25 to 50 mg. (gr. ⅜ to ¾) subcut.

61. ℞ "Neo-Synephrine Hydrochloride" (ampul)
> 5 to 10 mg. subcut. or I.V.

62. ℞ Amyl nitrite (ampul). . . . 0.3 cc. (♏ v)
> Crush in handkerchief and inhale fumes from 1 ampul every 30 minutes when awake.

63. ℞ Nitroglycerin (hypodermic
    tablet) . . . . 0.3 mg. (gr. 1/200)
> 1 or 2 tablets sublingually or subcut., repeated as necessary.

64. ℞ Erythrol tetranitrate . . . . 30 mg. (gr. ss)
> 1 or 2 tablets 3 times a day.

Hematinics

65. ℞ Ferrous sulfate . . . . 0.3 Gm. (gr. v)
> 1 or 2 tablets 3 times daily after meals.

66. ℞ Liver Injection U.S.P. (vial)
   4 to 8 u. I.M. once or twice weekly.

67. ℞ Pteroylglutamic (folic) acid .   5   mg.
   1 tablet 2 or 3 times daily.

Miscellaneous

68. ℞ Potassium citrate. . . . . .   0.3   Gm. (gr. v)
   3 to 6 tablets or capsules 4 times daily.

69. ℞ BAL (2,3-dimercaptopropanol),
   10% solution in peanut oil
   (ampul)
   0.3 Gm. I.M. followed by 0.15 Gm. every 4
   hours to a total of 0.6 to 0.7 Gm. Then 0.15
   Gm. twice daily for 4 to 7 days.

70. ℞ Cantharides Tincture N.F. . .   8.0   cc.   (℥ ii)
   1 drop in water 3 or 4 times daily.

71. ℞ Benzocaine. . . . .   1.5   Gm. (gr. xxii)
   White Petrolatum U.S.P.
                    q.s. ad   30.0   Gm. (℥ i)
   Apply to glans penis just prior to coitus.

72. ℞ Alpha tocopherol (Vitamin E)   25   mg.
   1 to 2 tablets or capsules 3 times daily.

GYNECOLOGIC AND OBSTETRIC

AMENORRHEA

Absence of menstruation, which may be primary or secondary, and either functional or physiologic.

Etiology

Amenorrhea may be pituitary in origin, e.g., lack of primary follicle-stimulating hormone (FSH), or normal FSH with deficient luteinizing hormone (LH). It may be due to primary or secondary ovarian failure or, occasionally, to an unresponsive end organ, such as an undeveloped uterus. Amenorrhea may occur in hypohormonal conditions such as Simmonds' disease, normal or premature menopause, hypothyroidism, and anorexia nervosa; in such hyperhormonal conditions as pregnancy, lactation, persistent corpus luteum, granulosa cell tumor, arrheno-

blastoma, and in certain pituitary and adrenal cortical hyperplasias or tumors. Menstruation frequently is suppressed in
metabolic disturbances associated with thyroid disease, diabetes
mellitus, obesity, malnutrition (low protein consumption) and
starvation, as well as in C.N.S. and psychopathic disturbances or
following systemic illnesses such as influenza, mumps, or tuberculosis. In many cases no explanation can be found.

Diagnosis

A carefully taken history and a complete physical examination are essential. The general physical examination should
include an X-ray of the chest as well as complete laboratory
studies. Pelvic examination will reveal existent congenital abnormalities and disease of the pelvic organs.

The evaluation of endocrine function should include the thyroid, the hypophysis, adrenals, and ovaries. X-ray of the sella
turcica should be considered as a means of establishing the
presence of pituitary adenomas. Ovarian function can be
studied indirectly by obtaining a series of endometrial biopsies,
since the endometrium reflects the changes that take place in
the ovary.

Types and Treatment

General principles: Before hormonal therapy for amenorrhea is instituted, an attempt should be made to correct any
existing dietary deficiencies or excesses, as well as unfavorable
environmental and psychologic situations. This alone is frequently followed by cyclic menstruation. In delayed menses
not due to conception, neostigmine methylsulfate (℞ 8) may
be successful in bringing on menstruation within a week.

Primary amenorrhea: The adult female who has never
menstruated is said to have primary amenorrhea. Examination may reveal hypoplastic uterus and genitalia. A course of
estrogen (℞ 1, 4) followed by a course of progesterone (℞ 6, 7)
to imitate cyclic production of gonadal hormones will sometimes bring on a menstrual flow if administered for at least 2
months. Thereafter, simultaneous administration of both estrogen (℞ 2) and progesterone (℞ 6), or these combined (℞ 12),
in high dosage for 2 or 3 consecutive days in each month may
be beneficial. The administration of gonadotropins usually
proves futile. Estrogens should be given over a long period of
time, not only to induce menses but also to promote the development of secondary sex characteristics.

Secondary amenorrhea: Amenorrhea is secondary when a
woman of childbearing age gives a history of having menstruated more or less regularly in the past but has had no signs
of catamenia for some time. Short courses of gonadotropin
(℞ 11) or combined estrogen-progesterone therapy (℞ 12) are
recommended. In certain of the metabolic disturbances (hyperthyroidism or diabetes mellitus), pituitary extracts are contra-

indicated, while the steroids (estrogen and progesterone) will do no harm and possibly some good. It should be emphasized, however, that secondary amenorrhea is but the expression of some disturbance elsewhere, and therapy should be directed to the underlying endocrinopathies, infections, and organic or metabolic disorders rather than the amenorrhea itself. Hormones should be employed with caution in those cases demonstrating or giving a history of neoplastic disease.

Functional amenorrhea: Bleeding at irregular intervals varying from 2 to 12 or more months is called functional amenorrhea. It in itself does not necessarily require therapy. When a patient is in good health otherwise, but is fearful or apprehensive because of her menstrual irregularities, she should be given reassurance that it has no organic basis and encouraged not to worry about her condition. Not infrequently a trial of thyroid medication (R 14) proves beneficial in the amenorrheic patient with a normal or subnormal B.M.R. Endometrial biopsy is highly desirable for those patients in whom endocrine imbalance is suspected, since in general the endometrium mirrors ovarian function and provides clues to therapy. For instance, if repeated endometrial biopsies show the presence of atrophy, ovarian deficiency may be assumed; this may be primary or secondary to hypofunction of the anterior pituitary gland. Many patients in this latter group respond well to cyclic courses of gonadotropins (R 11). Best results follow priming by an estrogen (R 1, 4). If the endometrial biopsy persistently reveals a hyperplastic endometrium, the administration of gonadotropins does not seem to be indicated. The prime purpose of therapy in this group is to put both ovary and certain components of the anterior pituitary "at rest." This is best accomplished by substitutional therapy of cyclic courses of estrogen (R 1, 4) and progesterone (R 6, 7) in moderately large doses.

Complete salvage and satisfactory regulation of the cyclicity may be expected in many patients in this group if properly timed estrogen-progesterone therapy (R 1, 7, 12) is carried on for a period of 4 to 8 cycles. In this group, the ultimate success achieved by substitutional therapy probably is due to various contributing factors, of which priming of the uterus, physiologic resting of the ovaries, and mediation of anterior pituitary function are the most important. The I.M. administration of progesterone (R 6) alone in 10 mg. doses parenterally for 3 days or the use of anhydrohydroxyprogesterone (R 7) orally in doses of 30 mg./day for 5 days will suffice in most instances to induce "progesterone withdrawal bleeding," but ultimate reestablishment of cyclic function has been observed to follow more frequently from the combined estrogen-progesterone (R 12) method of therapy.

Physiologic amenorrhea: During pregnancy and lactation, amenorrhea is physiologic. The endometrium during lactation usually is atrophic, indicating that the lactogenic hormone has prevented the release of gonadotropic hormones primarily, or has inhibited the ovaries secondarily. Occasionally, the inhibition is not complete and ovulation may take place—which accounts for the occasional occurrence of conception during lactation.

DYSMENORRHEA

Painful menstruation, a symptom which may occur without any evident organic cause (**primary** or **essential dysmenorrhea**) *or as a symptom of pelvic pathology* (**secondary dysmenorrhea**). Dysmenorrhea must be distinguished from the so-called physiologic menstrual distress in which there may be headache, lassitude, nausea, vomiting, pelvic fullness, and nervousness, but no pain.

Etiology

Primary (essential) dysmenorrhea may be associated with overwork, hysteria, or an endocrine imbalance. Secondary dysmenorrhea may be due to uterine hypoplasia or malposition, pelvic inflammatory disease, pelvic tumors (particularly submucous uterine fibroids), endometriosis, mechanical obstruction to the menstrual flow (e.g., small external os), systemic disease (e.g., anemia, tuberculosis, syphilis), masturbation, and nasal congestion (engorgement of the "genital spots"). Secondary dysmenorrhea may be aggravated by psychic and emotional factors.

The basic cause which produces the pain is unknown, and probably varies in different individuals. Uterine spasm, contractions, or ischemia each has been considered responsible. It is established that dysmenorrhea will occur only in ovulatory cycles, i.e., in a uterus that has been acted upon by progesterone. Anovulatory cycles are painless.

Symptoms and Signs

Typically, primary dysmenorrhea begins shortly after the menarche and ends with the first pregnancy, whereas secondary dysmenorrhea may occur at any time during the reproductive life of the patient. The pain is cramplike, mild to severe, and usually located in the lower abdomen. It is sometimes associated with the expulsion of endometrial casts (membranous dysmenorrhea) or clots. In some patients, the pain is felt mostly in the thighs and back. It may occur just before or during menstruation and persist for a few hours or throughout the menstrual period. A complete physical and pelvic examination may be negative (primary dysmenorrhea) or indicative of the underlying pathologic condition (secondary dysmenorrhea).

Treatment

General: Postural exercises intended to improve pelvic circulation and to stretch the pelvic ligaments are sometimes beneficial. Fatigue, nervous tension, and exhaustion must be avoided at all times by regulated exercise, adequate rest and sleep, and the use of a mild sedative (℞ 38). The patient must be encouraged to accept and ignore the condition by continuing her daily routine. Mild analgesics (℞ 32, 33, 34) and antispasmodics (℞ 18 to 21), administered separately or in combination, to the degree necessary, are indicated to make the pain endurable. Codeine (℞ 34) may be permitted, but other habit-forming opiates are to be avoided. Heat often gives relief and may be applied with a hot water bottle or electric pad. Psychotherapy is essential for all patients in whom the condition is incapacitating. Childbirth often is followed by the disappearance of dysmenorrhea.

Specific: Any pelvic or systemic disorder must be corrected by appropriate measures. Dilatation of a narrow cervical canal may give relief for 3 to 6 months. Uterine malposition may require a pessary or a uterine suspension. Cauterization of the "genital spots" in the nose is sometimes beneficial. Pelvic inflammatory disease may necessitate the use of chemotherapy or pelvic diathermy. Occasionally, surgical measures are indicated for patients with fibroids, endometriosis, infection, or for those who are approaching the menopause.

Hormones have been widely used in the treatment of dysmenorrhea, with variable results. It is impossible to evaluate just how much psychotherapy has to do with the results obtained by hormonal therapy. Estrogens (℞ 1, 4) promote vascularization and growth of hypoplastic reproductive organs. Given in sufficient dosage, estrogens also will suppress ovulation and their discontinuance will be followed by painless withdrawal bleeding.

Progesterone (℞ 6, 7) decreases uterine motility and may relieve the spasmodic type of dysmenorrhea when given for 7 days prior to and during menstruation. After such treatment with progesterone for 3 or 4 successive cycles, dysmenorrhea may not occur again for variable periods of time.

Testosterone (℞ 9, 10) in moderate doses is harmless and often effective. Its mode of action is uncertain but may be that it produces neutralization of estrogens, the suppression of ovulation, or a direct action on the hypophysis or the uterus. Chorionic gonadotropin (℞ 13) and thyroid extract (℞ 14) also have been effective in some cases.

Presacral neurectomy may be of benefit in certain selected cases in which the dysmenorrhea is primary, spasmodic, midline, not relieved by other measures, and which occurs in a psychologically stable person.

LEUKORRHEA

("Whites")

A common gynecologic disorder characterized by an abnormal, usually whitish and nonbloody, discharge from the genital tract.

Etiology

Leukorrhea is not in itself a disease but a symptom of some disorder in the genital tract or elsewhere in the body. Infection of the vagina or cervix with bacteria, protozoa, or fungi is the direct cause. Predisposing causes are parasitic infection; foreign body; pelvic congestion; retained placenta; chemical, thermal, or X-radiation injury; endocrine disturbances; allergy; avitaminosis; trophic disturbances; senility; tuberculosis or other debilitating disease requiring prolonged bed rest; hypersecretion; uncleanliness. While the possible primary and predisposing causes are almost innumerable, *Trichomonas vaginalis* infection probably is the most frequent direct cause of the discharge. Many cases are due to infection with Monilia organisms. Gonococcal, spirochetal, staphylococcal, streptococcal, pneumococcal, and tuberculous infections are less common causes.

Types

Leukorrhea in infancy and childhood: The vulva alone usually is involved, rarely the vagina. The vulva becomes irritated from soiled undergarments, dirt, intestinal worms, or masturbation. Foreign bodies are sometimes responsible. Gonococcus or Monilia must be sought as the probable etiologic factor. Other microorganisms, such as staphylococcus, colon bacillus, and *M. catarrhalis*, frequently are found. The discharge usually is white and the vulva is swollen, red, tender, and covered with a slimy secretion.

Leukorrhea in young virgins: A transient vulvitis or vulvovaginitis is sometimes noted in this group. Persistent leukorrhea in young girls often is ascribed to the same causes as are found in infants and young children. However, at puberty there frequently is a clear viscid uninfected discharge for which no cause can be discovered and which is probably due to overactivity of the cervical glands; it is of no clinical importance.

Leukorrhea in sexual maturity: The secretions may come from the vulva, vagina, cervix, or fundus. *T. vaginalis*, fungus, gonorrheal, postabortive, and puerperal infections are the usual contributing factors. When the discharge is profuse, yellowish in color, and associated with burning on urination, gonorrhea must be considered in the differential diagnosis. The irritating, profuse discharge which causes itching usually is due to *T. vaginalis* or some form of fungi. Brownish spotting with localized pelvic discomfort suggests extrauterine pregnancy.

Leukorrhea in senile women: A clear, watery, or bloody and foul discharge suggests the possibility of cancer. A creamy discharge, often bloodstained, suggests *T. vaginalis* vaginitis. Mycotic vaginitis is sometimes encountered in the senile woman.

Pathologic Physiology

Cervix: Much the most frequent cause of leukorrhea is infection of the cervix, commonly due to cervical damage during delivery. Infection and actual maceration of the squamous epithelium of the portio lead to the downgrowth of the columnar epithelium from the endocervix onto the visible portio. This produces the characteristic shining mucopurulent-covered cervical erosion. The excessive alkaline mucus and the persistent infection give rise to disturbances in the pH of the vaginal secretion which favor the growth of mixed bacteria and other vaginal pathogens. This sequence of events is the common background of leukorrhea and its treatment involves recognition of the cervical factor in its production. Further healing of the cervical lesion occurs by invasion beneath the columnar epithelium of the vaginal epithelium of the portio (epidermization); this epithelium matures to normal vaginal epithelium.

Vaginal tissue: The normal vagina is remarkably resistant to infection except in childhood and after the menopause when the mucosa is thin and lacks normal resistance. Vaginitis may occur in the adult when the pH is abnormal, commonly as a result of primary disturbances and excess secretion from the infected or damaged cervix. Other causes of vaginal leukorrhea include tumors, foreign bodies, and trauma of various kinds.

Vulva: Strictly defined, the discharge associated with vulvitis is not leukorrhea. Inflammation of the vulva may be associated with external lesions or with discharges from the generative tract. In general, it tends to occur in the absence of endocrine support as before puberty and after menopause.

Symptoms and Signs

An annoying discharge may be the only symptom of leukorrhea. However, as in the case of some mycotic infections, the discharge may be scanty or absent, and an intense itching the main symptom. Depending upon the extent of involvement of the vagina and vulva, vaginismus or dyspareunia may be the chief complaint.

Laboratory Findings

The offending organisms may be discovered by microscopic examination of the secretion. The secretion is diluted with normal saline and examined under the microscope for *T. vaginalis* or fungi. Parasites and fungi are recognized without staining if the secretion is fresh. Identification of the gonococcus may be made by smear and culture from the urethra and cervix.

Diagnosis

A study of the leukorrheal discharge often will give valuable clues as to the factors concerned in the production of the leukorrhea.

White discharge: A creamy white or viscid and clear discharge is associated with pelvic inflammation and congestion, and endocervicitis.

Yellow discharge: This type often is due to gonorrhea. It also may result from cancer of the cervix, a pelvic abscess draining into the vagina, or a purulent nongonorrheal infection of the vagina or cervix, and commonly with *T. vaginitis* or mycotic infection.

Watery discharge: A discharge of this type is of special significance late in life, when it may be caused by cancer of the cervix or body of the uterus. Congestion of the uterus, submucous uterine myomas and intermittent hydrosalpinx are other possible causes.

Bloody discharge: A blood-tinged discharge, occurring late in life, suggests the presence of cancer. Submucous myomas and cervical polyps also may be responsible.

Foul discharge: The presence of a foreign body or necrotic tissue is suggested by a malodorous discharge. Decomposed placental remains, sloughing submucous fibroid, or cancer of the cervix may be suspected.

Treatment

An intensive effort should be made to remove any causal or incidental factors before chronicity of the leukorrhea becomes established and thus more difficult to relieve. Systemic diseases such as tuberculosis, syphilis, and cardiac or hepatic disorders, if present, should receive appropriate treatment (q.v.). Polyps and neoplasms must be removed, and any other pathologic condition in the genital tract suitably treated. In intractable chronic cases the patient's husband also should be examined for infection and, if necessary, placed under treatment. Therapy of any existing uterine and cervical lesions must be undertaken as soon as leukorrhea is diagnosed.

General: Patients seen for the first time are examined for Trichomonads and Monilia, for evidence of residual gonorrheal infection and for lesions of the cervix. Palpation and stripping of Skene's ducts should be done. The endocervix is carefully inspected, not only for evidence of obstruction but also for mucous discharge, poorly draining pockets, and localized areas of unhealthy tissue. Treatment of any residual gonococcal infection (q.v.) should be undertaken. In the absence of localized infection of Skene's ducts, and provided there are no gross deformities or extensive lesions of the cervix, and no trichomonad or mycotic infection, relief may be obtained from the use of an iodine douche (2 cc. tincture of iodine to 1 qt. of hot tap water) once or twice weekly, or more often if necessary; or a daily douche with hypertonic saline (2 tbsp. of table salt in 1 qt. of tap water) or alum (1 heaping tsp. of powdered alum in 1 qt. of tap water). The office treatment of annoying nonspecific leukorrhea includes cleansing the vagina and cervix with cotton pledgets, maintenance of an open cervical canal, topical application to the endocervix of 5% trichloroacetic acid or a silver nitrate stick, electric cautery of raw or redundant areas, and painting the vaginal walls and vulva with 1% acriviolet solution.

T. vaginalis vaginitis: Vioform suppositories (℞ 29) may be used nightly, followed by a saline or alum douche in the morning. This treatment continued for a week or two usually results in temporary arrest of the infection. Intensive treatment, employing silver picrate, has given good results. The vagina is insufflated once a week with 5 Gm. of 1% silver picrate powder, and a silver picrate vaginal suppository (℞ 30) is inserted nightly by the patient. Silver picrate produces sensitization in some patients. Douches and coitus are to be avoided. A good response is sometimes achieved by the use of lactose tablets (℞ 31) as a means of restoring the normal vaginal flora.

Postmenopausal (senile) vaginitis: Estrogenic therapy is of great value in many of these cases. Vaginal suppositories of stilbestrol (℞ 5) are sometimes efficacious. Estrogens given orally (℞ 1) may be used if menopausal symptoms are present.

Most mycotic infections of the vagina (q.v.) are amenable to simple treatment with gentian violet solution.

Skene's duct infection: Penicillin therapy (℞ 22) is effective in these infections, when the causative organism is penicillin-sensitive. If relief is not obtained from such medication, excision of the infected ducts is indicated.

The diseased cervix: A 5% solution of trichloroacetic acid produces good results in some cases of chronically diseased endocervix. Treatment may be repeated at intervals of 10 days if necessary. Surgical treatment in the form of electric cautery or cervical conization is never to be employed during the active infection or during pregnancy. Such procedures should be carried out only immediately after a normal menstrual period.

VAGINAL MYCOSIS

(Vulvovaginal mycosis, Diabetic vulvitis, Diabetic vulvovaginitis)

Infection of the vagina (and usually the vulva) with a fungus.

Etiology

Monilia albicans (Candida albicans) is the most common pathogenic fungus causing this condition. Sugar fosters the growth of Monilia, hence increased amounts of glycogen in the vaginal mucosa furnish a good nutritive medium for the organism. In association with diabetes, mycotic vulvar infection occasionally occurs, the so-called "diabetic vulvovaginitis." Vaginal mycotic infection may sometimes result from lowered local resistance to these organisms. Pregnancy predisposes to infection by *M. albicans,* due to increased glycogen content of the mucous membranes of the vulva and vagina.

Symptoms and Signs

The predominant symptom is vulvovaginal pruritus which may vary from a mild to a distressing, unrelenting itch. In the pregnant woman, this condition develops after the 3rd month and reaches its greatest intensity around the 6th or 8th lunar month. Upon delivery or soon after, it subsides. Usually there is excessive secretion and, on speculum examination, fairly numerous white plaques or considerable quantities of caseous material are seen in the vagina. Varying degrees of vaginitis usually result from vaginal mycosis. At times there may be little or no leukorrhea, pruritus being the only symptom.

Laboratory Findings

Material obtained from the discharge or scrapings of the vulva and vagina will reveal, on a moist slide preparation, the typical mycelia and conidia. The buds of fungi are seen to be about the size of white blood cells and can be readily demonstrated by the Gram stain. The mycelia are revealed as long filaments with bamboo-like junctions.

Diagnosis

The diagnosis of vaginal mycosis is generally based upon the history of vulvar itching with or without leukorrhea. Examination of moist slide preparations of material obtained from the vagina will demonstrate the offending organisms.

Severe monilial infections sometimes resemble leukoplakia with kraurosis, especially in diabetics. Monilia must be carefully searched for, since mycosis, unlike kraurosis vulvae, is curable without surgery.

Treatment

There is no specific, but a few local applications of a 1% gentian violet solution (℞ 26) or of a 10% ointment of sodium propionate (℞ 28) will suffice to eradicate the infection in most cases. Stubborn infections often respond to the application of Lugol's solution (℞ 27) diluted 4 or 5 times. Grenz ray or other radiation therapy may produce excellent results in cases with intractable vulvar pruritus, but must be administered by a physician experienced in these procedures. Sedatives (℞ 38) may be of value in relieving local pruritus.

DYSPAREUNIA; VAGINISMUS

Dyspareunia, *painful or difficult coitus,* is frequently due to **vaginismus,** *spasm of the vagina,* but other factors such as lesions or anomalies of the female genitalia sometimes are responsible.

Primary dyspareunia and vaginismus: The honeymoon type of dyspareunia is the most striking example of primary vaginismus. It begins with the first attempts at sexual intercourse, and usually is introital. The spasm may be psychogenic or may result from local trauma, such as hymenal tears, lacerations of the fourchette, or bruises of the urethral meatus. Subsequent to the injury, superficial ulcerations may develop, which prove painful to the touch. Forceful pressure against a sensitive urethra during coitus may be a factor. Many of the patients show introital lesions due to inflammatory conditions, such as skeneitis, bartholinian abscess or cyst, inflammation of the labial sweat glands, or nonspecific infection. Irritation may result from the use of improperly fitted or inadequately moistened prophylactics; other cases may be due to the mechanical trauma caused by pubic hairs introduced into the vagina during coitus. Congenital septum also may cause dyspareunia.

Secondary dyspareunia and vaginismus may be quite unrelated to the honeymoon, in some cases developing many years later. Menopausal involution, dryness and thinning of the mucosa may be at fault. Sometimes an acute onset may follow roentgen sterilization. In a few women these conditions may result from tight perineorrhaphies following plastic repair. Overtightness of an episiotomy repair and kraurosis have been known to result in dyspareunia. Retroflexion of the uterus with prolapsed ovaries is at times responsible for both conditions. Endometriosis, vaginitis and pelvic inflammatory disease may cause painful coitus.

Psychogenic factors: When the dyspareunia with or without vaginismus is not due to local causes, or when local symptoms are overshadowed by nervous symptoms, it indicates a psychologic defense mechanism developed by the patient. The defense may be directed against sex and intercourse in general (e.g., due to excessive egotism, faulty upbringing, ignorance of the anatomy and physiology of the reproductive organs, old-maidishness, fear of pregnancy, aversion to the partner possibly due to a previous love affair, or some physical defect discovered in him after marriage). Even such offenses by the partner as lack of consideration in preliminaries, bromhidrosis, or halitosis may form the basis of aversion and subconsciously the beginning of sexual resistance and defense.

Diagnosis

Invariably, pain during or following coitus is the chief complaint. Additional reasons for consulting the physician may include failure of intromission, dysmenorrhea, amenorrhea, sterility, menorrhagia, and metrorrhagia, or symptoms due to cystocele or rectocele. Local introital lesions and uterine displacements are readily detected, although anesthesia may be required to overcome the spasm induced by even a gentle vaginal examination. In the absence of such obvious conditions, the dyspareunia must be attributed to psychologic causes. Great tact and understanding are necessary in order to draw from a patient the origin, or even the existence, of her fears and aversions. In many cases, the original psychic lesion is deeply buried in the subconscious and is not recognized or even remembered by the patient herself.

Prophylaxis

Ignorance, misinformation, and fear, as well as the presence of disease and of anatomic defects, congenital or postoperative, are primarily responsible for dyspareunia and vaginismus. Premarital examinations for both partners, with a frank explanation of the reproductive organs and their functions, including the physiologic and psychologic factors involved in sexual intercourse, and wise guidance in its technics, may go far in preventing dyspareunia and vaginismus. Any existing lesions or defects should be corrected if possible. If indicated, a gradual stretching of the hymen before marriage helps to minimize the initial pain, which often sets up an aversion to subsequent coitus, with resultant vaginismus and dyspareunia. Occasionally, a perineotomy may be necessary to correct an unusually tight introitus.

Treatment

The treatment of uncomplicated primary or "honeymoon" injuries is not difficult. Temporary avoidance of intercourse is important, and separate beds should be advised. Hot sitz baths may be helpful.

In mild secondary cases, lubrication of the vagina usually affords relief. For the pronounced changes seen in older patients (senile vaginitis) local estrogenic preparations (℞ 3) may be used. In some cases pain can be prevented by freely using a lubricant just before coitus, and by a more posterior intromission which avoids pressure on a sensitive urethra.

The treatment of demonstrable lesions should be along orthodox lines. Cysts or abscesses should be excised; inflamed labia are to be kept clean and dry; leukorrhea is treated in the usual manner (q.v.). If the vulva is swollen and painful, a wet dressing of aluminum acetate may be applied locally (℞ 46). At times, codeine (℞ 34) and sedation (℞ 38) may be indicated. Retroflexion and prolapsed ovaries can often be corrected by a pessary. Pelvic inflammation may require bed rest, heat (diathermy), and penicillin (℞ 22). Stretching the vagina by mercury colpeurysis may be of value in some chronic conditions of secondary contracture of the pelvic connective tissues. Trauma to sacrouterine ligaments may result from ill-fitting diaphragms, and in such cases proper adjustment or elimination of the diaphragm is indicated.

Patients without evidence of introital or deep lesions, whose vaginismus is due to psychogenic factors, and those who exhibit healed local lesions may be treated by the insertion of a well lubricated test tube. During the first week a tube about ⅝ inch in diameter is used. The patient should be in the position for gynecologic examination. The tube should be introduced deeply and allowed to remain in place for 10 minutes. This procedure should be carried out by the physician at each visit, at least 3 times a week. Self-insertion also is practiced by the patient twice daily, under the physician's supervision. During the 2nd week a larger test tube, 1 inch in diameter, should be used in the same manner. A 3rd week of this treatment may be indicated for some patients. This procedure has both mechanical and psychologic advantages. It helps to stretch the vagina and accustom its nerve endings to the presence of a foreign body, and at the same time the physician may impress upon the patient that, after diligent insertion of the tube for 3 weeks, she will find coitus not only painless but also pleasurable.

Psychotherapy may be applied, when indicated, by the methods outlined under Prophylaxis (q.v.). If some fault in the husband is responsible for a patient's aversion to coitus, he should be interviewed and instructed in better methods of personal hygiene and technic. Unreasonable fears on the part of the patient should be allayed, if possible, by information and explanation of natural processes. However, great caution must be exercised by the physician in employing psychotherapy for long-standing cases of dyspareunia and vaginismus, or for those in which the causative psychic trauma cannot be brought to light. Such cases should be referred to a competent psychiatrist.

FRIGIDITY

Incapacity of the female for normal pleasure in sexual intercourse.

Etiology and Incidence

Frigidity in women is much more common than its counterpart, impotence, in men. More than 50% of married women are so affected, either partially or completely. Many never achieve orgasm at any time in their lives. Often frigidity may persist for a certain period after marriage and then, under favorable conditions, normal response will develop.

The cause of frigidity is predominantly psychologic. It may be due to faulty sex instruction during girlhood, in which all matters pertaining to sex often are presented as shameful or wicked. Such connotations cannot immediately be purged from the consciousness upon marriage. The condition may result also from too brief preliminary love-making on the part of the husband. The sex reactions of most women are aroused more slowly than those of most men and, even when they have been aroused, a woman usually does not attain the orgasm so rapidly as her partner and often is left unsatisfied and disappointed. Impotence (q.v.) in the husband which prevents him from maintaining a sufficiently prolonged erection has the same effect, and a pattern of failure is initiated in the wife that tends to become permanent. In other instances, the husband may be at fault by physical offensiveness so that intimate contact with him becomes repugnant. All such conditions inhibit the wife's orgasm. Fear of pregnancy, when children are not desired, may be responsible, while in some other instances, an unconscious homosexuality may contribute to the frigidity.

All cases of frigidity are not, however, of psychogenic origin. A large number of women may become excited under the preliminary steps of love-making and welcome the consummation of the act, but actually suffer from vaginal anesthesia, which prevents them from having any local pleasurable sensation. In rare instances, certain organic diseases of the nervous system, such as multiple sclerosis, transverse myelitis, tabes dorsalis, and anterior poliomyelitis, may cause frigidity. Failure of orgasm under such conditions is readily understandable, and its relief depends upon recovery from the disease.

The ill effects of frigidity are insidious and far-reaching. Marriages in which sexual intercourse gives mutual satisfaction are not easily broken, and the converse is true. The attitude of many women, who accept it as a duty but feel neither pleasure nor displeasure in it, is discouraging to the husband and often leads him to seek a more satisfactory union outside of marriage. Moreover, many wives who have missed the normal enjoyment of sexual intercourse are prone to become neurotic and to suffer from premenstrual tension because their psychosexual needs have never had conscious expression. This also may be a factor in producing more troublesome menopausal symptoms in later life. Some women, frigid for psychologic reasons, are likely to develop vaginismus and dyspareunia (q.v.).

Any interference with a free flow of psychic energy into the sex act may reduce the secretions of the mucous glands of the vagina, whose function it is to make coitus easier. In other words, the woman may consciously submit to coitus while unconsciously trying to deny entrance of the penis by withholding these secretions.

Prophylaxis and Treatment

Nothing so promotes sexual success as an unworried state of mind, pleasure in the partner's personality, and a proper attitude toward the act itself. Many women can enjoy sexual intercourse during a vacation, when they are free from household responsibilities and worries, but cannot do so when they return home and resume the burdens of everyday life.

In the vast majority of cases, frigidity can be prevented by wise sex education, which should be given equally to boys and girls as soon as they are able to understand it and before sex has taken on an emotional color. In the treatment of frigid married women, the psychologic factors must be carefully elicited and evaluated. Many cases call for intensive psychotherapy which, if properly directed by a well trained physician or a psychiatrist, often will produce good results. If the husband is at fault, he should be interviewed and advised. A small amount of an alcoholic beverage (if there is no personal objection to such substances), taken by the wife a short time prior to coitus, is relaxing and often conducive to successful intercourse. Although various drugs and hormones have been tried in the treatment of frigidity, they have shown only limited usefulness. In some women the male hormone, methyltestosterone (℞ 10), taken orally, has yielded good results, but the estrogenic hormones generally have proved unsatisfactory. The so-called aphrodisiac drugs, such as cantharides, yohimbine, and damiana, are of no value.

UTERINE BLEEDING

Physiologic bleeding from the uterus, via the vagina, occurring in normal menstruation and, in some women to a lesser degree, at the time of ovulation. Abnormal forms of uterine bleeding, include menstruation of excessive duration or amount, or both **(hypermenorrhea, menorrhagia),** too frequent menstruation **(polymenorrhea),** and nonmenstrual bleeding **(metrorrhagia).**

Etiology and Diagnosis

Complications of pregnancy: These include abortion, ectopic pregnancy, bleeding from the placental site, retention of gestational products, hydatiform mole or chorionepithelioma. A history or signs of pregnancy or abortion will be present in these conditions. The cervix may be patulous. Expulsion of grapelike material (in hydatiform mole), or persistence of a positive Aschheim-Zondek or Friedman test (in chorionepithelioma) may occur. Pain usually is present and cramplike in character. A parametrial mass may be palpated in tubal pregnancy, with or without evidence of intraperitoneal hemorrhage; the leukocyte count usually is under 12,000.

Malignant tumors of the uterus: Abnormal bleeding at, or any bleeding after, the menopause must always be taken as evidence of uterine cancer until proved otherwise. The bleeding may be scanty or profuse, often is associated with leukorrhea, and frequently follows strain, douche, or coitus. Pain is unusual until extension of the tumor has occurred. Diagnosis is based on pelvic examination, inspection through a speculum, biopsy or curettage, and microscopic examination (Papanicolaou technic) of the cellular flora in the vagina and cervix. Schiller's test may be used if lesions of the cervix are suspected of being malignant.

Uterine polyp (cervical or intrauterine): This may cause sudden menorrhagia or irregular and recurrent "spotting," particularly after exertion or coitus; it may be accompanied by leukorrhea. Cervical polyps are most common in women over 40 years old with a history of chronic cervicitis. Cervical polyps usually can be seen on inspection, whereas intrauterine polyps can be diagnosed only by curettage. All polyps should be examined microscopically for evidence of malignancy.

Uterine myomas occur in about 40% of women over 40 years of age. Hypermenorrhea, polymenorrhea, dysmenorrhea, leukorrhea and pressure symptoms on adjacent structures may all be evident. A history of repeated spontaneous abortions is common. Bimanual examination reveals smooth, hard, single or multiple tumors, inseparable from the uterus.

Uterine abnormalities: Bleeding may be caused by such conditions as uterine malposition or subinvolution, lacerations of the cervix, and the vascular congestion which accompanies cervicitis, endometritis, and pelvic inflammatory disease. Diagnosis is established by the history, bimanual pelvic examination, and inspection of the cervix. Cervical biopsy or endometrial curettage is indicated in all doubtful cases to rule out uterine malignancy.

Malignant tumors of the ovary or fallopian tube occasionally are responsible for uterine bleeding. Diagnosis may be made by pelvic examination.

Endometriosis: This may be associated with pelvic pain, dysmenorrhea, hypermenorrhea, or polymenorrhea in a young woman. There also may be sterility, dyspareunia, and pressure symptoms. Bimanual examination may reveal an adherent fundus, shotty nodules, or ovarian cysts.

Constitutional (systemic) **disorders:** In this group are blood dyscrasias, hypertension (uterine apoplexy), cardiac decompensation, poisoning (e.g., by lead or phosphorus, or due to alcoholism), cirrhosis of the liver, hypoprothrombinemia and vitamin B deficiency. Diagnosis will depend on the history, a thorough physical examination, appropriate laboratory tests, and the ruling out of local causes within the pelvis by repeated examinations. A diagnostic curettage is indicated in all doubtful cases.

Vaginitis, particularly senile vaginitis, is sometimes responsible for abnormal vaginal bleeding which must be differentiated from uterine bleeding. Senile vaginitis is characterized by a thin, glistening mucosa with small petechial hemorrhages, in a patient who has passed the menopause.

In infants and children, bleeding may be due to true pubertas praecox (q.v.), adrenal tumor, granulosa cell tumor of the ovary, or sarcoma of the cervix or ovary. The history and physical examination will suggest the diagnosis.

Endocrinopathic (so-called "functional") **bleeding** may be suspected when abnormal uterine bleeding occurs at puberty or adolescence, or in an otherwise healthy woman approaching the menopause. A rational approach to this group of etiologic factors requires an understanding of the probable endocrine mechanism controlling normal menstruation. Briefly, menstruation is thought to occur as follows: Sufficient stimulation of the ovaries by the follicle-stimulating hormone of the pituitary leads to the formation of a mature graafian follicle, which elaborates increasing amounts of estrogenic hormone during its maturation. Under the influence of this hormone, the uterine endometrium grows (proliferative phase). Rupture of the follicle (ovulation) is followed by the formation of a corpus luteum under the influence of the luteinizing hormone of the anterior pituitary gland. Continued stimulation of the endometrium by both estrogen and progesterone from the corpus luteum produces a secretory type of endometrium. In the absence of conception, regression of the corpus luteum occurs within 10 to 12 days, resulting in a fall in the estrogen and progesterone levels, spasm of the endometrial spiral arterioles, and shedding of the secretory endometrium resulting in a normal bleeding (menstruation). It is this periodic fall in the estrogen-progesterone level that is directly responsible for menstruation. (The thyroid and adrenal glands also are important factors, but their part in normal menstruation is not fully understood.) Aberration from this normal process may produce abnormal bleeding of the following types:

1. Anovulatory bleeding: Failure of rupture of the graafian follicle and resulting absence of corpus luteum formation occasionally may produce alarming bleeding. Such cycles are, of course, infertile. They are most frequently seen near puberty and menopause but do occur at other times. Endometrial biopsy (not curettage!) just before the expected bleeding will show a proliferative endometrium and if bleeding follows at the expected time, the cycle is proven to be anovulatory. Anovulatory bleeding has its major significance in the sterile patient. When a series of such follicles develop but do not rupture or when continuous estrogen stimulation from any other source is present, an exaggeration of proliferative changes in the endometrium, known as endometrial hyperplasia, occurs.

2. Bleeding due to endometrial hyperplasia: Elaboration of estrogen over a prolonged period without cyclic falls in estrogen level (and therefore no shedding of the endometrium) leads to continued proliferation of the endometrium, often with cystic dilatation of the glands. Such an endometrium tends to bleed, and profusely, with any fall in the estrogen level. Excessive estrogenic stimulation of the endometrium also may result from granulosa cell tumors of the ovaries, overtreatment with estrogenic hormones and perhaps from vitamin B complex deficiency (which impairs the ability of the liver to destroy circulating estrogen).

3. The remaining causes of so-called "functional" bleeding are of obscure origin and probably are due to endocrine imbalance involving the thyroid, pituitary, or adrenal glands. "Functional" bleeding (a bad but frequently used term) may arise in a normal or even an atrophic endometrium. The sudden discontinuance of estrogenic therapy is usually followed by withdrawal bleeding within 7 to 9 days. Diagnosis of endocrinopathic bleeding requires curettage and repeated physical examinations to rule out organic disease. As a rule, bleeding associated with pain or leukorrhea is due to some local organic cause.

Treatment

Supportive: Prolonged or excessive bleeding may produce a severe anemia and may exhaust the patient. General supportive measures are bed rest, sedation, a high protein, high caloric diet with supplementary multivitamin capsules (*see* DIETS), and hematinics (*see* ANEMIA). Rarely, blood transfusions are indicated. Uterine oxytocics, such as ergonovine (R 15) may be effective as a purely temporary measure, in that they produce uterine contraction and thereby lessen the bleeding.

Specific: The treatment of uterine bleeding is that of its underlying cause, as outlined below:

The management of hemorrhage due to abortion is covered in the chapter on Abortion (q.v.). A diagnosis of ectopic pregnancy is an indication for immediate laparotomy. Hydatiform mole should be removed by curettage, and the specimen examined for malignant changes (chorionepithelioma). Chorionepithelioma necessitates a hysterectomy, with frequent Aschheim-Zondek or Friedman tests postoperatively to check on possible recurrence. Other causes of pre- and postpartum hemorrhage require specific measures as indicated by their character.

Cervical cancer should be treated with intensive radium and deep X-ray therapy by a qualified radiologist. Cancer of the fundus usually requires a total hysterectomy with bilateral salpingo-oophorectomy, with or without preoperative radium and postoperative X-radiation. Metastases should be treated with radiation; the value of large doses of testosterone propionate, 25 mg. I.M. daily (℞ 9), remains to be determined. Cervical polyps may be removed by torsion or by cautery, whereas intrauterine polyps can be removed only by curettage; all specimens should be examined microscopically for evidence of malignancy.

Fibromyomas which are large (10 cm. or more in diameter) or which are causing much bleeding should be removed by hysterectomy. Where needed surgery is contraindicated or refused, radiation (in castrating doses) may be employed, but only after a diagnostic curettage has ruled out uterine malignancy. Uterine malposition should be corrected by pessary or surgery, and lacerations repaired.

Pelvic infections should be treated with appropriate antibiotic or sulfonamide therapy (q.v.), or both. Cervical cauterization or conization, pelvic diathermy, and surgery may be indicated in selected cases of cervicitis and pelvic inflammatory disease.

Malignant tumors of the ovary or fallopian tube and granulosa cell tumors require prompt surgical removal. The therapy of endometriosis usually is surgical, although radiation of the ovaries (in castrating doses) will hasten the menopause and thereby result in involution of the endometrial implants.

Systemic disorders (q.v.), such as anemia, leukemia, hemophilia, purpura, scurvy, hypertensive vascular disease, congestive heart failure, hypoprothrombinemia, avitaminosis B, poisoning by lead or phosphorus, alcoholism, and cirrhosis of the liver, require appropriate therapy.

True pubertas praecox (q.v.) requires no treatment. Senile vaginitis is treated with estrogens (℞ 5), but only after cancer of the fundus or cervix has been ruled out. Other forms of vaginitis require acidification of the vaginal secretion, plus other appropriate therapy.

Endocrinopathic ("functional") bleeding will respond, in variable degree, to many different measures. It must be reemphasized that all organic pathologic conditions must be ruled out, particularly during the cancer ages, before a case can be diagnosed as one of so-called "functional" bleeding. Curettage, by removing a sizable portion of the bleeding endometrium, is not only of diagnostic value but often proves sufficient in itself to control the bleeding, at least temporarily. Numerous hormones have been employed, each with some measure of success, but selection of the proper hormone requires knowledge of the responsible hormonal imbalance.

1. Anovulatory bleeding: This usually is self-limited and requires only supportive care, particularly when it occurs at puberty or during the menopause. Should the amount of bleeding become alarming, it may be controlled by large doses of diethylstilbestrol, 10 mg. daily (℞ 4), which will promptly elevate the estrogen level above the point at which bleeding occurs. This dose level may be maintained for a sufficient time to permit the patient to recover her general health and to correct the blood loss. Discontinuance of estrogenic therapy should then be gradual, so as to avoid production of withdrawal bleeding. Anovulatory bleeding which gives rise to sterility may be treated best through procedures designed to improve general constitutional well-being. Nongynecologic diseases must be recognized and treated. Disturbances of thyroid function should be looked for; even in the presence of normal thyroid function, ovulatory cycles sometimes follow administration of thyroid (℞ 14). Experiences with pituitary substance administration have been disappointing. Chorionic gonadotropin (℞ 13) is sometimes effective in causing regression of the estrogen-producing follicles.

2. Endometrial hyperplasia: Therapy will depend on the underlying cause. Endometrial hyperplasia due to administration of estrogens will cease following withdrawal of the drug. Granulosa cell and theca cell tumors should be surgically removed. Immediate control of the bleeding itself usually may be accomplished by complete curettage, which also permits a histologic diagnosis. As with anovulatory bleeding, administration of estrogens (℞ 4) will promptly elevate the blood estrogen level above the point at which bleeding can occur, thus controlling the hemorrhage; however, this is of only transient value and may even cause further growth of the already overproliferated endometrium. Anemia (q.v.) should be corrected by the use of transfusions and blood-building measures.

Endometrial hyperplasia occurring at the menopause requires curettage to rule out uterine malignancy and to control excessive bleeding. About 50% of such patients are cured by curettage alone. Should bleeding recur, sterilization by X-ray is indicated.

3. Obscure types of "functional" bleeding: These may respond to therapy with thyroid (℞ 14), testosterone (℞ 9), estrogen (℞ 4), or progesterone (℞ 6). In these cases, treatment is necessarily empiric, since the single or complex underlying cause usually is obscure or not understood. After the childbearing period, severe "functional" bleeding is best treated by hysterectomy or castrating doses of X-ray.

PRENATAL AND POSTNATAL CARE

The desirability of medical supervision for all women throughout pregnancy and following delivery is well recognized. As a guide to the physician, the accepted minimum standards of procedure are outlined here.

Prenatal Routine

When pregnancy is first suspected, the patient should go to her physician for examination. If a diagnosis of pregnancy is established, a careful history should be elicited, including all past illnesses, such as scarlet fever, diphtheria, tonsillitis, rheumatism, syphilis, tuberculosis (or exposure to it), rickets, heart disease, and urinary tract infections; also operations, accidents, and abnormal discharges from the genital tract, together with treatment received. A careful scrutiny of the patient's menstrual history is essential. This includes the patient's age at menarche; frequency, amount, and duration of the flow; any changes occurring after marriage; and the presence or absence of dysmenorrhea or other menstrual disturbances.

A complete history of previous pregnancies and labors also is important. The following information should be sought: number of pregnancies, length of gestation, termination of labor; complications of any pregnancy, such as convulsions, headaches, swelling of extremities, visual disturbances, infections, hemorrhages, and length of time confined to bed. The results of previous laboratory tests, e.g., urinalyses, blood counts, and hemoglobin determinations, should be ascertained, if possible.

The status of living children should be inquired about: their number; their physical and mental condition; weight at birth, whether they were premature or full term; if breast fed, for how long. If born dead and macerated, how long before birth did fetal movements cease; what was the cause of death?

The family history should include any history of hypertension, diabetes, tuberculosis, multiple pregnancies, mental disease, or congenital anomalies.

Information concerning the present pregnancy should include the date and character of the last menstruation. If quickening already has occurred, at what date; are there any symptoms such as nausea and vomiting, bleeding, headache, shortness of breath, edema, or visual disturbances? Has albuminuria or elevation of blood pressure been discovered?

Next, a careful physical examination is made—if possible, at the first visit. Pulse and respiration rates, temperature, blood pressure, and body weight are determined. The patient's nutritional status and the condition of the skin, tonsils, teeth, breasts, abdominal wall, and extremities are noted. Auscultation of heart and lungs (as well as of the fetal heart if the pregnancy is advanced) should be done at this time.

If a vaginal examination is made early in pregnancy, it must be done gently to avoid risk of abortion. In the presence of vaginal bleeding at any time during gestation, examination should be rectal rather than vaginal, unless the strictest aseptic technic is observed. During the last month of pregnancy vaginal examination should not be attempted without rigid aseptic precautions. Provided internal pelvic measurements have been taken, a rectal examination at this time usually is sufficient. The examiner should note the following: signs of pregnancy, condition of the cervix, neoplasms, if any, and presenting parts.

Pelvimetry is an important prenatal consideration. Mensuration should include intercristal, interspinous, external conjugate and transverse diameters of the outlet. Measurement of the diagonal conjugate is best accomplished 6 weeks before term. At the time the diagonal conjugate is measured the examiner should palpate the sacrum and ischial spines to rule out any possible midpelvic contraction. Deformity of the sacrum may suggest a rachitic pelvis.

A complete urinalysis should be made as well as blood serologic tests for syphilis, Rh factor studies, blood typing, and hemoglobin estimation. If venereal disease other than syphilis (q.v.) is suspected, cultures and smears should be taken, and appropriate treatment instituted as necessary. A chest X-ray and Mantoux tuberculin test should be provided, to rule out tuberculosis or other pulmonary disease.

Following the physical examination, the patient should be instructed about diet, exercise, rest, sleep, and recreation, clothing (including shoes), baths, and general care of the skin and breasts, and bowel and kidney function. Advice concerning coitus during pregnancy also may be given. If a home delivery is contemplated, instructions regarding hygiene of the home and preparations for the delivery are given.

The patient should be warned to report promptly to the physician if any of the following symptoms appear: constipation, shortness of breath, colds or other respiratory infection, sore throat, cough, headaches, persistent nausea and vomiting, dizziness, visual disturbances, pain in the lower abdomen, bleeding, swelling of hands and feet, fever, dysuria, or diminished urinary output.

During the 1st and 2nd trimesters, the patient should be seen monthly, then every 2 weeks or oftener as required, then every week in the final month. At each visit, the patient's general condition, blood pressure, pulse, and weight should be checked, and urinalysis done. The physician should make a thorough abdominal examination, including auscultation of the fetal heart, especially in the later months, in order that the growth of the child may be followed. Abnormal presentation, if it exists, should be noted, for possible correction prior to labor.

The diet should contain a sufficient number of calories and an adequate amount of protein and minerals (see DIETS). If these requirements are not met by diet alone, nutritional supplements are mandatory.

In primiparas, lightening should take place within 2 weeks of the estimated date of confinement. If the fetal head is not fixed in the pelvis as term approaches, disproportion should be ruled out by careful pelvimetry, X-ray, and by manual efforts to determine the cephalopelvic relationship. Consultation should be sought if necessary. X-ray studies also may reveal a multiple pregnancy. Vaginal examinations, when the patient enters labor, should be made only when definitely indicated, and then only under strictest aseptic conditions. Whenever possible, primiparas and women who have experienced serious difficulty during previous labors should be delivered in a hospital. Multiparas with a satisfactory history may be confined at home if absolutely necessary.

Formula for Predicting Date of Delivery

A convenient method is to count back 3 months from, and add 7 days to, the 1st day of the last menstrual period. For example, if the patient last began to menstruate on March 1, then December 8 will be the presumable date of confinement.

Postnatal Routine

Postnatal care should begin before the patient leaves the delivery room. A thorough search for lacerations should be undertaken, and any necessary repairs made at this time. The patient should be observed by the physician for at least 1 hour following delivery, particularly for evidence of uterine hemorrhage. When bleeding occurs, the fundus, if relaxed, should be gently massaged to induce contraction and to control the hemorrhage. Ergonovine (℞ 15), 0.2 mg. (gr. 1/320), is indicated to maintain uterine contraction and lessen the danger of postpartum bleeding.

Subsequent postnatal follow-up includes care of the vulva, to which sterile perineal pads are applied routinely at least 3 or 4 times daily. Urination should be encouraged within 10 to 12 hours following delivery. Catheterization is employed only if absolutely necessary (see BEDSIDE PROC.). Early ambulation is desirable whenever possible; some physicians allow their patients up within 24 to 36 hours after delivery. This has resulted in fewer postpartum infections and complications. Temperature, pulse, and respiration are to be recorded daily. Cleansing enemas may be given after the 4th day.

Severe after-pains may be relieved by an analgesic combination such as acetylsalicylic acid 0.6 Gm. (gr. x) with codeine 30 mg. (gr. ss), given 3 or 4 times daily (℞ 35).

Painfully congested breasts should receive early attention. An ice bag, elevation by means of a snug binder, artificial emptying of the breasts after nursing, and proper nursing care will give considerable relief. If suckling is contraindicated for any reason (see LACTATION DISTURBANCES), diethylstilbestrol, 5 mg. once or twice daily (℞ 4) begun before lactation and continued for 5 to 7 days, will suppress milk formation. (CAUTION! Subinvolution of the uterus.)

The patient's diet should be nutritious and simple for the 1st day postpartum, following which a regular diet may be prescribed. A liberal fluid intake and a high protein diet are advisable once milk secretion is established (*see* DIETS).

The patient may be examined and discharged on or after the 8th day. Should subinvolution of the uterus be present, it is treated by douches using 4 liters of warm saline daily (*see* BEDSIDE PROC.) and ergonovine, 0.2 mg. (gr. 1/320) every 4 hours for 4 to 6 doses (℞ 15). Coitus is to be avoided for 6 weeks postpartum.

The normal puerperal patient should report to her physician at the end of the 6th week, at which time a complete recheck of her general physical condition and a thorough pelvic examination should be made. Any erosions of the cervix may be cauterized. Information and advice concerning future pregnancies should be given before the patient is dismissed. Reexamination at the end of 6 and 12 months is suggested as a further precaution against late postpartum complications.

CARE OF THE PREMATURE INFANT

The term "premature" is generally considered to refer to an infant weighing less than 2,500 Gm. (5.5 lb.) at birth, regardless of the period of gestation.

Prematurity increases the hazards of the neonatal period because of the functional and anatomic immaturity of various organs. Thus: (1) Respiratory difficulties (asphyxia, anoxia, aspiration pneumonia) may appear due to undeveloped alveoli, weak respiratory musculature, weak gag and cough reflexes, and anemia. (2) The body temperature fluctuates erratically, fever or subnormal temperatures resulting from moderate exposures to heat or cold, respectively. (3) Disturbance of water and electrolyte balance occurs because of a decreased rate of glomerular filtration. (4) Rickets is frequent, due to faulty absorption of fat and (fat soluble) vitamin D. (5) Hemorrhagic diathesis may complicate the increased capillary fragility already present; this condition may be further aggravated by anoxia and by inadequate body reserves of vitamins C and K. (6) Inability of the immature liver to manufacture prothrombin results in prothrombin deficiency. (7) A paucity in the volume of bone marrow and decreased storage of iron (which is stored largely during the last trimester) are principally responsible for the severe anemia which often is present. (8) Infections are frequent, due to poor placental transmission of maternal antibodies and to the relative inability of the premature infant to manufacture his own.

Environment

Hospital care of the premature infant, whenever possible, is preferable since expert nursing care is of utmost importance. However, the following outline of therapy can be adapted to be carried out in the home, should home care be necessary. Vitamin K preparations 2 to 5 mg. should be given orally or I.M. to the mother during labor, and I.M. to the infant at birth. The child should be isolated in an incubator or bassinette, maintained between 80° and 85°F., which temperature is adjusted as necessary to stabilize the infant's rectal temperature between 97° and 99°F. External clothing, other than a clean dry diaper, is to be avoided. Inhalation of an atmosphere containing 30 to 50% O_2 is necessary during at least the first few hours after birth and before and after meals thereafter; CO_2, 5 to 10%, may be added to promote deep breathing. All feedings should be carried out in this environment. Baths (oil) are best avoided during the first week; in fact, the incidence of skin infections may be lowered by allowing the vernix to remain on the infant's body and removing it only from the face. Unnecessary handling or overtreatment may unfavorably influence the prognosis.

Feeding

The first feeding is given 12 hours after birth and consists of a formula containing 5% glucose (or lactose) and 0.25% sodium chloride. By using a rubber-tipped medicine dropper for feeding, the formula may be deposited on the back of the tongue. One dropperful is given initially; subsequent feedings are given every 2 hours, being increased by increments of up to 4 cc. (3 i) if accepted and tolerated by the infant. After 24 hours, a weak milk formula (10 calories/oz.), preferably breast milk if available, is given every 2 hours in amounts slightly less than the largest previously accepted volume of glucose formula. Some of the latter may be administered if tolerated after each milk feeding. The volume of each subsequent milk feeding may be increased by 1 to 2 cc. as required.

During the first few days, maintaining the fluid intake is more important than meeting the caloric requirements. If oral intake is inadequate, fluids (preferably Ringer's Lactate Solution U.S.P.) are given parenterally in amounts not exceeding 10 to 15 cc./lb. at any one time. Gavage feeding may sometimes be necessary. After 24 to 72 hours, further increases in the amount, concentration, and interval between feedings may be made as indicated. The milk formula may be fortified with protein concentrates and carbohydrates, but fats are to be avoided as much as possible. Ascorbic acid, 25 mg. daily, is given on the 5th day and increased to 100 mg. daily by the 10th day. Vitamin D therapy, 1,000 I.U. daily, preferably in a water-soluble form, is instituted on the 10th day, the daily intake being gradually increased to 1,500 to 2,000 I.U. by the end of the 1st month. Other vitamin supplements may be given, although their need is not urgent. The regimen outlined above should be continued until the infant's weight is approximately 6 pounds.

21

The prognosis is more favorable with each passing day of survival. However, the birth weight and the degree of prematurity also influence the final outcome; thus, although most deaths due to prematurity will occur during the first few hours of life, it is not uncommon for very small infants (less than 3 pounds) to succumb after 3 to 5 days, due to exhaustion. Surviving prematures may be expected physically to lag behind other children of the same age during the first 2 years of life; however, by their 3rd birthday, any developmental deficits usually will have been fully overcome by the premature infant and average development can be expected thereafter.

ABORTION

The interruption of pregnancy prior to the period of fetal viability. The term as here used includes those cases commonly referred to as miscarriages.

Etiology

Abortion may be spontaneous or induced. When induced for other than therapeutic reasons, it is known as a criminal abortion.

Spontaneous abortions may be caused by: (1) acute infectious diseases; (2) systemic diseases, such as nephritis, diabetes, anemia, and cardiac failure; (3) poisons, especially lead; (4) uterine disease, including tumors, displacement, infection, adhesions; (5) dietary deficiencies; (6) trauma, due to instrumentation, abdominal blows, convulsions, strenuous exercise; (7) hormonal imbalance involving the thyroid, ovary, pituitary (premature involution or removal of the corpus luteum may occasionally be responsible for abortion); (8) diseases of the fetus or fetal membranes, and germ plasm deficiencies. Rarely, abortion may be due to syphilis, eclampsia, or pernicious vomiting. In a large number of patients, abortion may occur without evident cause.

Induced abortions may follow instrumentation, administration of oxytocics, or exposure to radiation.

Pathology

Up to the beginning of the 8th week of pregnancy, the ovum is relatively poorly protected and nourished. As a result, abortion (which may go unrecognized) is frequent during this period, with the entire ovum usually being expelled. From the 8th to the 12th weeks inclusive, fetal attachment and nutrition improve, so that the incidence of abortion decreases. However, should abortion occur, the tendency at this period is for chorionic elements to be retained. After the 12th week, the placenta is firmly attached and abortion is less likely. Further, the danger period during which the function of progesterone production is taken over by the placenta from the corpus luteum has passed. Abortion now simulates labor, but the placenta may be partially or completely retained after expulsion of the fetus. If all the products of conception are retained for several months, a "fleshy mole" may develop.

Types

Depending on time of occurrence and other factors, abortion may be classified as threatened, imminent, inevitable, incomplete, complete, missed, septic, habitual, or therapeutic.

THREATENED ABORTION

The ovisac has not yet been detached. Vaginal bleeding occurs, and may be slight or profuse. Slight intermittent pain may or may not be present and it may precede or follow bleeding. The cervix is closed and there is no shortening of the cervical canal.

Treatment

Unless an ectopic pregnancy is suspected, vaginal examination is contraindicated lest it aggravate the condition. Absolute bed rest is essential. Coitus, douches, and drastic catharsis must be avoided. Constipation may be relieved with glycerin suppositories, mineral oil, or milk of magnesia. If bleeding continues, morphine (℞ 36) is given and repeated every 6 hours if necessary. Expectant therapy may be continued as long as bleeding is not profuse and there is reason to believe the fetus is alive. Decidual biopsy has been recommended as a means of determining fetal viability; if a normal decidua is obtained from the lower anterior uterine wall, every attempt should be made to avoid an abortion. Neither the Aschheim-Zondek nor Friedman test is a reliable guide in determining the advisability of interference. The value of progesterone (℞ 6), with or without an estrogenic substance (℞ 4), is debatable but has many advocates.

IMMINENT ABORTION

Bleeding and colicky pain progressively increase. Signs of profound blood loss may be evident. The cervix is effaced or patulous.

Treatment

Therapy varies with the symptoms. If hemorrhage is not great, expectant treatment as for threatened abortion may be carried out, but only in a hospital. If hemorrhage is alarming, the uterus must be emptied by means of a curet or ovum forceps. Supportive therapy with fluids or whole blood should be carried out as indicated. After the uterus is emptied, ergonovine (℞ 15) may be prescribed. When evacuation of the uterus is not immediately possible, a vaginal pack may be inserted to control excessive bleeding, but it introduces an added hazard of infection.

INEVITABLE ABORTION

In addition to the symptoms of an imminent abortion, the membranes are ruptured or the ovum protrudes through a dilated cervix.

Treatment

When bleeding is not excessive, spontaneous complete abortion should be awaited. Such observation can be carried out safely only in a hospital. If hemorrhage is profuse, the uterus should be emptied. Prior to the 8th week, a curet or ovum forceps may be used to remove the ovisac. After the 8th week, the finger is used to separate the fetal tissues from the uterus. When immediate intervention is not possible, a vaginal pack may be tried as a temporary expedient.

INCOMPLETE ABORTION

Bleeding is due to retained products of conception and continues until such secundines are expelled or removed.

Treatment

Expelled material should be carefully examined under water but this method does not always demonstrate retained material. If examination shows retention of fetal membranes, or if an incomplete abortion is suspected, the curet (before the 8th week) or the finger should be used to empty the uterus. After the 16th week, vaginal hysterotomy may be necessary to evacuate the uterus.

COMPLETE ABORTION

All the products of conception are expelled. Pain and hemorrhage cease, although blood-stained discharge may last for several days.

Treatment

Therapy is supportive. Blood-building measures (*see* ANEMIA) with bed rest for a week, and observation until involution is complete, are indicated.

MISSED ABORTION

In these cases the ovisac is retained for some time after the death of the fetus. Following the symptoms of a threatened or imminent abortion, the breasts become smaller (occasionally, lactation may occur) and a brownish vaginal discharge persists. The uterus ceases to grow and the laboratory tests for pregnancy become negative.

Treatment

Whenever possible, spontaneous expulsion of the fetus should be awaited. If intervention is required, the uterus is emptied with a curet, before the 8th week, and with the finger and ovum forceps after that time. In advanced pregnancy, vaginal hysterotomy may be necessary.

SEPTIC ABORTION

Treatment

In the presence of active infection, local treatment of any type of abortion is to be avoided. Sulfonamides (℞ 24) and antibiotics (℞ 22) should be used freely. In addition, frequent blood transfusions may be useful.

Pitocin (℞ 16) or quinine (℞ 17) often hastens the expulsion of the ovisac and assists in controlling hemorrhage. When the temperature has been normal for 4 or 5 days and after the cervix is dilated, necessary instrumentation may be performed. If severe hemorrhage requires earlier intervention, any instrumentation must be done most gently and intensive antibacterial therapy continued.

HABITUAL ABORTION

Prophylaxis

The patient who habitually aborts is difficult to treat. She should have the benefit of a complete physical examination. Any pathologic condition present that can be corrected without major surgery should be cared for. As soon as the patient conceives, she should be placed on the following regimen: She should refrain from coitus, douches, and drastic catharsis. She should avoid strenuous physical activities and long-distance or jolting travel. She should be given sufficient thyroid (℞ 14) to make up for any deficiency. The patient's B.M.R. and her symptoms are safe guides as to dosage; 1 grain daily can be prescribed if the basal rate is 0 to –10, 2 grains daily when it is –10 to –20, and 3 grains when the rate is from –20 to –30.

Progesterone (℞ 6) has been used extensively, but its effectiveness is questionable. A daily dose of 5 to 10 mg. can be given for an indefinite period, at least until the patient feels life. If anhydrohydroxyprogesterone (℞ 7) is used orally, the dose is 50 mg. daily.

Estrogens are being tried in women who habitually abort, with the idea that these may stimulate placental formation of progesterone. The physician can prescribe diethylstilbestrol 50 mg. daily until fetal viability is reached (℞ 4). The value of this medication still is to be proved.

THERAPEUTIC ABORTION

This can be carried out if the patient's life or health is seriously jeopardized by the continuation of the pregnancy. Such a decision is often difficult to make and must never be reached without consulting with at least one other physician. In many cases of therapeutic abortion, some procedure to render further pregnancies impossible will need to be considered.

NAUSEA, VOMITING OF PREGNANCY

("Morning sickness," Pernicious vomiting of pregnancy, Hyperemesis gravidarum)

Nausea and vomiting occurring in pregnancy, usually in the early months, and of varying severity.

Etiology and Incidence

Many theories have been advanced to account for the nausea and vomiting which still occur in almost 50% of all pregnancies, although the incidence and severity of pernicious vomiting have decreased greatly in recent years. In the production of the abnormality, hunger has been thought to be a contributing factor and a neurogenic element undoubtedly plays an important part. Current postulations concerning etiology include (1) a sharp rise in the titer of chorionic gonadotropin, which parallels the period of maximal nausea and vomiting, and (2) the rapid increase in estrogen level, since exogenous estrogens in large dosage can produce identical symptoms.

From a consideration of these and other theories, it seems most likely that a metabolic dysfunction probably results in an upset in carbohydrate metabolism with incomplete oxidation of fatty acids. Psychogenic factors are important in the production of such disturbances and may consist of an unconscious or conscious desire to get rid of an unwanted pregnancy, a fear of pain or death, or upsets attendant upon changing from an active to a more sedentary life. Any circumstance that causes mental disturbance is apt to exacerbate the vomiting. Nausea and vomiting also may be precipitated by excessive swallowing of saliva in the abnormal condition known as salivation (ptyalism) of pregnancy (*see* SALIVARY DISORDERS).

Pathology

Severe vomiting of pregnancy is sometimes associated with serious liver damage. Necropsies in such cases usually have shown severe necrosis in the central portion of the lobules or a widespread fatty degeneration similar to that seen in starvation. Hemorrhagic retinitis, which develops in some cases, is a serious complication and indicates a grave prognosis: the mortality rate in patients with toxic retinitis is over 50%.

Symptoms and Signs

The nausea and vomiting appear at about the 5th or 6th week of pregnancy and last for a few weeks to 2 or 3 months, sometimes longer. The symptoms vary in severity from simple "morning sickness" to the pernicious vomiting which may end fatally. Morning sickness begins with a feeling of nausea when the patient gets up; she is unable to retain her breakfast, but by noon the symptoms have disappeared and she feels well until the following morning, unless the symptoms are restimulated by some idiosyncrasy of taste or smell. Occasionally, this cyclic nausea of pregnancy may appear as "afternoon" or "evening" sickness instead of the usual morning form. The condition usually clears up without treatment in 1 to 3 weeks, during which time a few pounds of weight may be lost. In some cases, morning sickness undergoes transition into the pernicious type of nausea and vomiting. A small percentage of pregnant women develop severe, persistent vomiting lasting from 4 to 8 weeks or longer, and lose 10 to 20 pounds in weight. Some patients show an even greater loss of weight, accompanied by drying of the skin and even jaundice. The term "pernicious vomiting" should be limited, however, to a small group of cases in which severe symptoms of starvation are superimposed on the vomiting syndrome. In rare instances, toxic retinitis occurs, which may lead to impairment of vision. Examination of the eyegrounds often reveals subhyaloid hemorrhages.

Laboratory Findings

The outstanding chemical changes accompanying severe vomiting are a slightly increased nonprotein nitrogen and uric acid, decreased blood chlorides and blood CO_2 combining power, and diminished urinary output with concentration of urine, increased specific gravity and the presence of acetone bodies. Hypoglycemia sometimes is present.

Diagnosis

Diagnosis generally is based upon the evidence of pregnancy plus the symptomatology and laboratory findings. However, concurrent diseases that may be responsible for the vomiting must be ruled out by thorough examination.

Treatment

The degree of vomiting, and the extent of starvation or dehydration, if present, should be determined first. Psychotherapy is helpful in most of the mild cases. Lack of a sense of security predisposes to unrest. The patient should be given a careful explanation of her condition, so that she will know what to expect. Unwarranted fears should be dispelled, and assurance given that she and her baby will receive proper care. A diet should be outlined, although if the patient can safely be allowed to cater to her own desires during the first 2 or 3 months, eating when and what she pleases, this will help to relieve her immediate discomfort. Frequent small feedings are helpful. Frequently, eating a cracker before getting out of bed, and avoiding excessive amounts of fluid intake will prevent the nausea. Phenobarbital (℞ 38) often is extremely helpful. Anorexia often may be combated successfully by the administration of 10 to 15 u. of insulin (always with a protective quantity of carbohydrate amounting to 2 Gm./u.), 20 minutes before mealtime. A high vitamin intake is desirable, particularly the B complex and vitamin C.

If the nausea, and especially the vomiting, become severe, hospitalization is necessary. It is advisable to isolate all these patients admitted to the hospital even when no psychiatric element is involved. During the first 24 hours, food and water by mouth should be withheld and 2,500 to 3,000 cc. of fluid given I.V. in the form of 5 to 10% glucose solution in saline or distilled water. (A 5% solution may be given subcutaneously, but this route of administration now is seldom employed, unless for reasons of psychic persuasion in appropriate cases.) After the 24-hour period, small quantities of light solid food are given every hour from 9 A.M. to 9 P.M. with fluids such as orange juice, ginger ale, milk, or broth between times. From the 3rd day on, 6 small meals are given daily, with ample fluids. In the average case, vomiting ceases after the first few days on this regimen, but sometimes it is necessary to repeat the routine of starvation, fluids, and small meals once or twice.

When there is extremely severe vomiting and dehydration, especially with signs of liver damage, it is essential to administer glucose and saline solutions at fairly frequent intervals; no time must be lost in restoring as far as possible the water balance of the body. Pyridoxine hydrochloride I.V. ($\mathbb{R}$ 45) has proved of great value in some cases. Sometimes the patient with severe vomiting develops a true acidosis, as shown by an appreciable drop in the CO_2 combining power of the blood to about 30 volumes/100 cc. The acidosis must be corrected by appropriate measures (see ACID-BASE AND ALLIED DISORDERS).

It is imperative that routine and repeated ophthalmoscopic examinations be carried out for every patient admitted to the hospital with nausea and vomiting of pregnancy. At the first appearance of hemorrhagic retinitis the pregnancy should be interrupted. Even in the absence of a developing retinitis, should the patient not respond (which rarely happens) to the therapy outlined above, as evidenced by a continual loss of weight, jaundice, and increasing pulse rate, termination of the pregnancy should be considered. If a therapeutic abortion is decided upon, it must be performed before evidence of liver destruction appears, otherwise the outcome may be fatal either immediately or within a day or two.

TOXEMIC AND OTHER DISORDERS OF PREGNANCY

PREECLAMPSIA AND ECLAMPSIA

Preeclampsia: *A dangerous toxic disturbance, usually developing late in pregnancy and characterized by hypertension, albuminuria, excessive weight gain and edema, generally considered to be the precursor of eclampsia.* **Eclampsia:** *In addi-*

tion to the symptoms and signs of preeclampsia, a condition, one of the most dreaded complications of pregnancy, characterized by convulsions and coma, which may progress to a fatal termination.

Etiology and Incidence

The cause of preeclampsia and eclampsia remains unknown. Theories, none of which is yet completely accepted, include endocrine imbalance, metabolic disorder, fluid and electrolyte imbalance, and absorption of toxins from the placenta or fetus.

Eclampsia is unknown in animals and rare in primitive human races. It is estimated that 5% of women delivered in hospitals in the U.S.A. show evidence of preeclampsia or eclampsia. From 90 to 95% of cases occur after the 30th week of pregnancy, 80 to 90% before the 30th year of age, and more than 75% in primiparas. The incidence is 6 to 10 times higher in cases of multiple pregnancy (e.g., twins), 3 to 4 times higher in the presence of hydatiform mole, and considerably increased in patients with polyhydramnios. The incidence also is increased in diabetic individuals.

Pathogenesis and Pathology

Extensive, severe changes are found in the tissues when death results from eclampsia. These are toxic in nature and indicate the violence of the disorder rather than specific effects which might point to the causal mechanism.

The basic pathologic mechanism of eclamptogenic toxemia is generalized arteriolar spasm, which in extreme degree may result in tissue anoxia. Arteriolar constriction can be demonstrated during life by means of ophthalmoscopic examination. The lesion long considered pathognomonic of eclampsia is hemorrhagic portal necrosis of the liver. This is not present in all cases, however. Thrombosis of the portal vein may occur. Edema of the brain and kidneys is common, and the placenta often contains anemic infarcts and increased deposits of intervillous fibrin.

A prominent factor in the pathologic physiology of the disorder is the increased retention of sodium and water by the tissues.

Symptoms and Signs

Symptoms usually are completely lacking in the early stages. Occasionally, however, complaints may include vague malaise, anorexia, headache, or weakness. Definite signs are increased blood pressure, excessive weight gain, edema greater than the usual slight swelling of the feet, and albuminuria. Dangerous symptoms are severe persistent headache, drowsiness, amnesia, vertigo, visual disturbances (spots or flashes, blurred or double vision, blindness), and precordial or epigastric discomfort. Signs of severe or increasing involvement are nausea and vomiting, edema of the disks, hematemesis, jaundice, steadily increasing blood pressure, tachycardia, respiratory changes, water retention, increasing widespread edema, lessened urinary output, and severe albuminuria. Twitching of the extremities is ominous and may herald the onset of convulsions. Eclampsia may appear suddenly, a convulsion being the first manifestation; infrequently, severe eclamptic coma has been known to develop without convulsions. In most cases, however, one or more of the premonitory symptoms or signs are present for some time and can be recognized by the careful observer.

The convulsions of eclampsia are dramatic; the patient stiffens, the pulse becomes rapid and hardly perceptible; respirations are irregular and hissing; breath-holding causes deep cyanosis. The eyes bulge and stare or roll from side to side. Teeth are clenched and frothy saliva appears about the mouth and nostrils. The body becomes rigid, with arms and legs stiffly extended. This tonic state persists a few moments and then gives place to and alternates with the wild, violent, thrashing movements of the clonic phase. The violence is so great that bones have been broken. The patient may fall from bed and sustain serious injury. During the convulsion, death can occur, as a result of cardiac arrest or cerebral hemorrhage, but this is rare except in extremely severe cases. Labor often is brought on by eclamptic convulsions, and occasionally delivery is precipitated by the strain. The course varies greatly: there may be a single convulsion followed by a brief partial coma, or multiple convulsions (as many as 200 have been recorded) growing progressively worse. Usually, the entire attack lasts only a few minutes; the spasms subside and are succeeded by coma. Death may seem imminent at this time, but almost always the patient begins to improve. A pulse rate continuing above 120, respirations above 40, or temperature above 102° F. are unfavorable signs.

Laboratory Findings

Proteinuria is the most consistent finding, varying from 0.5 Gm./day to as high as 40 Gm./day (in severe cases). A relatively high globulin fraction of the proteinuria and a decrease in the urinary urea nitrogen and urinary chlorides are usual. The blood uric acid content is increased, while the CO_2 combining power and the pH may be decreased. The NPN and BUN usually are not elevated except in actual eclampsia when, as a result of oliguria or anuria, the levels may be high. Blood sugar is reported to be low during a convulsion. In severe cases the hematocrit often reveals elevated blood concentration.

Diagnosis

Excessive weight gain (over 100 Gm./day), increased blood pressure, or albuminuria (over 0.5 Gm./day) establishes a tentative diagnosis of preeclampsia. Rapid increase in these manifestations and the development of gastrointestinal disturbances, eye signs, or cerebral signs indicate severe preeclampsia or impending eclampsia. Convulsions or coma during late pregnancy without evidence of other disease are considered to be due to eclampsia.

Differentiation from renal diseases is difficult, and often a positive diagnosis cannot be established until revealed by the course of events. Renal disease is frequently found before the last trimester. Cellular elements in the urine and fixed specific gravity, with albuminuric retinitis, and history of preexisting renal disease (q.v.) or infections likely to cause renal damage, help in differentiating renal involvement from preeclampsia. Kidney function tests are of value only in certain cases, since findings may be normal until damage is severe. Diagnosis may have to await evidence of increasing kidney involvement long after delivery, the clue being the persistence of symptoms.

Hypertensive vascular disease (q.v.) also is difficult to distinguish in certain cases. Hypertension appearing early in pregnancy, eyeground changes suggestive of hypertension in the absence of albuminuria or excessive weight gain, or a history of previous hypertension should suggest hypertensive disease rather than preeclampsia. Severe hypertension developing after the 30th week of pregnancy is practically always indicative of preeclampsia.

Preeclampsia and eclampsia can coexist with either hypertensive or renal disease. In a doubtful case it probably is wise to consider and treat the patient as suffering from preeclampsia and eclampsia primarily, when complete diagnostic studies have failed to distinguish the cause of symptoms.

Convulsions and coma of eclampsia are generally similar in appearance to convulsions and coma from other causes (q.v.). Therefore, patients seen for the first time in the convulsive state or in coma should be given a complete study, although symptomatic emergency treatment must be established at once.

Course and Prognosis

Mild preeclampsia usually is benign and in most cases responds readily to simple therapeutic measures. Severe preeclampsia treated immediately and vigorously usually does not progress and is often ameliorated. If actual eclampsia develops, it may be mild or severe. In the severe type, convulsions continue, urinary output remains below 700 cc./day and circulatory failure or deep coma develops. With the mild form, manifestations are less dramatic and eclamptic patients with pronounced edema (wet eclampsia) usually fare better than those with little edema.

Usually, evidence of eclampsia disappears within a week, except for such occasional residual complications as separation of the retina, pneumonia, puerperal psychosis, or injuries incurred during convulsions. Continued hypertension, edema, or positive urinary findings indicate hypertensive or renal disease, and suggest that they contributed to the eclampsia, were coincident with it, or were residuals of it.

While preeclampsia and eclampsia do not commonly recur in subsequent pregnancies, women who have experienced these disorders are more likely to be afflicted than are women who have thus far escaped. The maternal death rate in eclampsia averages 13%. Fetal mortality is approximately 50%.

Treatment

Mild preeclampsia usually responds to adjustment of diet, rest, and sedation. The office visits, with blood pressure determinations and urinalysis, should be more frequent (see PRENATAL AND POSTNATAL CARE). Daily weight records are mandatory, and measurements of fluid intake and urinary output are of value when made accurately. Patients are given a diet adequate in protein and liberal in carbohydrate but low in sodium, and are cautioned against adding salt during cooking or at the table. They also should avoid sodium-containing remedies such as bicarbonate of soda. The diet should be supplemented with vitamins. If serum proteins are low, additional protein is indicated; administration of amino acids mixtures may be necessary. Fluid restriction to 500 or 1,000 cc./day, with rigid salt reduction, is called for only if the patient shows excessive weight gain due to fluid retention, or edema and reduced urinary output. Ammonium chloride (R 44) may be given for 6 days and the course repeated, after a rest period of 6 days, to enhance urinary output. Mercurial diuretics apparently are of little value. Bed rest, 10 hours at night and 1 hour twice a day, in addition to sedation with barbiturates (R 38, 39) may be required.

Hospitalization or absolute bed rest is indicated if the patient's condition becomes progressively worse, weight gain exceeds 100 Gm./day, blood pressure remains above 150/90 or increases, or proteinuria reaches 3 Gm./day.

One or more of the following developments indicates severe preeclampsia, and termination of the pregnancy must be considered: a diastolic blood pressure persistently over 110 or one that rises to 120, or a systolic pressure staying above 170; albuminuria in excess of 5 Gm. protein each 24 hours (0.5 to 3 Gm./day is serious—over 3 Gm., ominous); daily weight gain in excess of 100 Gm. under sodium and fluid regulation; sudden appearance of extensive edema, oliguria, hematuria, or anuria; cerebral, visual, or gastrointestinal disturbances; jaundice; pulse rate of 120 or more, pulmonary edema, cyanosis; increase of NPN or BUN; high or increasing hemoglobin, hematocrit, serum protein concentration, uric acid, or specific gravity of the blood.

At this stage, all efforts should be directed at preventing the convulsions of eclampsia. Medical treatment affords the lowest mortality; surgery, except in highly skilled hands, significantly increases it. Fulminating preeclampsia which does not respond to medical treatment may require termination of the pregnancy. This should be done by the most conservative means feasible. If the patient is near term, induction of labor usually is successful, but if she is much more than a month from term, cesarean section often is necessary. From the standpoint of the fetus, premature termination of pregnancy entails the balancing of risks: the hazards of prematurity as compared with the danger of succumbing *in utero* because of the maternal toxemia.

General measures include placing the patient in a separate room, preferably darkened, with an experienced attendant constantly present to prevent disturbance and to record regularly pulse, respiration, and blood pressure readings.

Fluid intake is charted and urinary output measured. An indwelling catheter is advisable. An antieclamptic diet of water, fruits and juices may be given unless the patient becomes unconscious. Elimination may be aided by soapsuds enemas (*see* BEDSIDE PROC.), but if convulsions have occurred, this procedure should await effective sedation. Urinary retention is combated by administering hypertonic dextrose, 1,000 cc. of a 20% solution in distilled water being given over 30 to 50 minutes. If this is ineffective, or if pulmonary edema is feared, higher concentrations, 800 cc. of 30% or 400 cc. of 50% glucose, may be used. Approximately 200 Gm. glucose in a 20 to 25% solution, injected over 40 to 60 minutes 2 or 3 times a day, gives best results. A urinary excretion of at least 30 cc./hour is the objective. Normal saline, Ringer's bicarbonate, or glucose in saline solutions are contraindicated because of their sodium content.

Dangerous hypertension is treated by sedation with sodium phenobarbital (℞ 39), Sodium Amytal (℞ 40), or magnesium sulfate injections (℞ 43). Pulmonary edema or other evidence of congestive heart failure should be appropriately treated (q.v.).

If convulsions occur, at least 2 and preferably the first 3 of the following drugs are used: magnesium sulfate (℞ 42) 50% solution, 12 cc. I.M. (gluteus) and 4 cc. after each convulsion until paroxysms are controlled; or 20 cc. of a 10% solution (℞ 43) may be injected I.V. and repeated hourly for 5 doses. No more than 25 Gm. magnesium sulfate should be injected in 24 hours, and less if anuria persists. Sodium Amytal (℞ 40) subcut. every 8 or 12 hours or chloral hydrate (℞ 41) by rectum every 6 to 12 hours often is effective, and other sedatives, such as paraldehyde (℞ 37), have been used with good results, but I.V. injection of the Sodium Amytal (℞ 40) may be necessary to control the convulsions. Morphine sulfate (℞ 36) may be given I.V., but is less desirable, especially just before delivery.

[A modified Stroganoff regimen, using morphine hypodermically and chloral hydrate per rectum, may be employed to induce narcosis: Initially, morphine 15 mg. (gr. ¼) is administered; 1 hour later, chloral hydrate 1.3 to 2.6 Gm. (gr. xx to x1); 2 hours later, morphine 15 mg. (gr. ¼); 4 hours later, chloral hydrate 2 Gm. (gr. xxx); 6 hours later, chloral hydrate 1 to 2 Gm. (gr. xv to xxx); 7 hours later, chloral hydrate 1.3 Gm. (gr. xx). This routine may have to be altered to some extent, according to the condition of the patient.]

Once convulsions have occurred, examinations and manipulations should be infrequent. Tongue depressors wrapped with gauze, a clothespin, or a special mouth-gag should be available to prevent biting of the tongue during the convulsion. The patient should not be restrained or held, but extra care must be taken to prevent injury from thrashing about or falling.

The ensuing coma is treated in the usual way (q.v.), with oxygen and cardiac supportive measures. If the blood CO_2 combining power is lowered, acidosis (q.v.) should be corrected, but no solutions containing the sodium ion should be administered.

If the patient is in active labor, with evidence pointing to easy delivery, rupture of the membranes may hasten delivery. If not, and convulsions are not controlled by medical treatment after 8 to 12 hours' trial, labor should be induced, provided the cervix is effaced and delivery can be completed within 18 to 24 hours. Cesarean section is not indicated as a treatment for eclampsia. It may very occasionally be necessary in eclampsia because of the usual obstetrical indications for such a proceeding, such as cephalopelvic disproportion, and then only when the baby is alive and probably undamaged. The choice of anesthesia is important because of the likelihood of liver damage. Local anesthesia is successful and popular.

Although termination of pregnancy usually results in almost immediate amelioration of symptoms, it must be remembered that postpartum eclampsia can occur, and the patient should be carefully watched for at least a week thereafter.

HYPERTENSIVE DISEASE DURING PREGNANCY

The patient with underlying hypertensive vascular disease which remains uncomplicated may go through pregnancy with little additional risk to herself, but with a higher than average expectancy of miscarriage or fetal death. In about half of such hypertensive patients, however, preeclampsia does become superimposed; when this occurs, there is a significant increase in risk both to the mother and to the fetus. Furthermore, when renal impairment accompanies hypertension and pregnancy, the prognosis always is serious. Hypertension may be distinguished from preeclampsia by its existence prior to pregnancy or by failure of the blood pressure to return to normal following termination of pregnancy. Hypertensive vascular disease and preeclampsia (q.v.) can occur together. It also must be remembered that severe, persistent preeclampsia may result in a permanent hypertension.

RENAL DISEASE IN RELATION TO PREGNANCY

Nephrosis and nephritis (q.v.) are almost invariably aggravated by pregnancy. Serious disturbance of renal function, often terminating in uremia, is common. The first pregnancy may cause only mild exacerbation, but serious disturbances are likely to occur in subsequent pregnancies. Women with severe renal disease are advised to avoid conception, since termination of pregnancy does not always bring relief of symptoms.

OTHER DISORDERS DURING PREGNANCY

Excessive salivation (ptyalism) may occur in pregnancy and give rise to severe gastrointestinal disturbances with resulting malnutrition (*see* SALIVARY DISORDERS). Herpes gestationis is a condition in which herpetic lesions, beginning in early pregnancy, show a predilection for the umbilical area. The lesions may rarely progress to cover the whole skin surface, including mucous membranes and conjunctiva. Severe cases may result in miscarriage, and secondary infections sometimes lead to death (*see* HERPES SIMPLEX). Acute yellow atrophy of the liver (q.v.) now is considered a separate disorder, although, approximately 60% of all cases occur during pregnancy.

PUERPERAL SEPSIS

(Childbed fever)

Any infection within the female genital tract occurring during the puerperium, or as a complication of abortion. (Puerperal infection may be presumed to exist in the presence of a temperature elevation to 100.4° F. on any two successive days, exclusive of the first 24 hours following delivery, and during which other causes of fever are not apparent.)

Etiology

Normal labor produces multiple small bruises, abrasions and lacerations which increase susceptibility to infection. Prolonged labor, premature rupture of the membranes, retention of pieces of placenta, membranes or blood clots, and the existence of a relaxed rather than a firmly contracted uterus following delivery all encourage infection. Intercurrent infection (pneumonia, grippe), heart disease, hemorrhage, or any condition which lessens the vitality of the patient predisposes to infection. Multiple examinations, instrumentation, or operative procedures also increase the hazard.

For about 75% of cases the source of infection is endogenous, i.e., originated by organisms ordinarily present in the genital tract or by organisms carried by the blood from some preexisting focus elsewhere (e.g., tonsillitis, bronchitis). For the remainder the source is exogenous; the organisms may be inoculated by the physician or attendant through faulty aseptic technic; droplet contamination from the nose or throat of attendants or visitors may occur; the patient's hands may transmit organisms from her throat or a skin abscess; and sexual intercourse just prior to labor has been responsible. Illegal abortions commonly produce puerperal infections.

Anaerobic streptococci are responsible for most cases of puerperal infection, but such infections usually are relatively benign. On the other hand, the beta hemolytic streptococcus is one of the most virulent organisms, but fortunately infections due to this organism are infrequent, constituting only about 1% of all cases of puerperal infection. Certain strains of *Staph. aureus* or *Staph. albus* exhibit hemolytic properties and can produce serious infections. *Cl. tetani,* the gas-forming *Cl. welchii,* and *C. diphtheriae* also may be responsible for severe puerperal infection. Bacteria associated with decomposition and putrefaction, ordinarily nonpathogenic, can on occasion cause severe or fatal puerperal infection (sapremia). Mixed infections are the rule, however.

Pathology

The effects vary according to the site and extent of the infection, the virulence and characteristics of the invading organisms, and the state of local and general resistance of the patient. Infection within the genital tract may be superficial, confined to clots and bits of placenta or membranes, and producing its effects through absorption of toxic by-products; cellulitis leading to abscess formation may occur; infection may extend to adjacent tissues or to the peritoneum; or the organisms may be rapidly invasive, spreading through lymph channels to the blood, producing a serious or fatal bacteremia.

Symptoms and Signs

Clinical manifestations vary. The onset may be insidious or sudden. Early symptoms frequently are indistinguishable from normal complaints during the puerperium. Restlessness, irritability, anorexia, general malaise, or localized discomfort are suggestive. Change in the character of the lochia is significant, sudden and complete cessation especially so. Pain is present only when there is involvement of the pelvic cellular tissues or if distention of the uterus occurs. The leukocyte count is of little value early since a count of about 9,000 with variation from 6,000 to 12,000 is considered normal through the 4th day postpartum. Definite symptoms are essentially similar to those of any other acute infection. Malaise, prostration, nausea, and vomiting may occur; pain varies according to the site and nature of the infection; temperature, pulse and respiration are increased, and the leukocyte count and sedimentation rate are elevated.

Diagnosis

Chills, fever, tachycardia, vomiting, abdominal pain or rigidity occurring in a pregnant or puerperal woman must always suggest puerperal infection until proved otherwise. Pyelitis, mastitis, phlegmasia alba dolens (milk leg), respiratory infection, malaria, or appendicitis must be excluded. Blood cultures (aerobic and anaerobic) should be taken at least once a day for 3 days. Examination of the perineum is indicated and may reveal infection of a laceration or episiotomy. If the local findings are negative and the infection is severe, a bimanual examination must be made. This must be performed gently, carefully, with the strictest aseptic precautions, and by only one examiner (to avoid unnecessary manipulation). At this time, cultures (aerobic and anaerobic) can be obtained from the uterus. If the infection fails to subside, the bimanual examination must be repeated once a week to determine whether masses are forming about the uterus, or whether, if such masses already are present, they are pointing or softening.

Puerperal infection may be vulvar, vaginal, cervical, endometrial, or parametrial. Uterine or pelvic abscesses, pelvic thrombophlebitis, or peritonitis may develop. Degenerated myomas are especially prone to abscess formation during the puerperium. The diagnosis of local perineal or vulvar involvement is simple, and vaginitis is easily discerned. With endometritis, the temperature may vary from 100.4° to 104° F. Tachycardia and lower abdominal pain usually are present. The severity and duration depend upon the virulence of the organism and the drainage from the uterus. If the fever persists more than 3 or 4 days, the infection has probably extended beyond the endometrium. Parametritis (pelvic cellulitis) is distinguished by persistence of fever for days or weeks, with evidence of local peritoneal reaction and the development of induration about the uterus. Abscess of the uterine wall or pelvic abscess is evidenced by increasing but remittent temperatures, chills, a high leukocyte count, and the development of a softened area in the pelvic mass. With thrombophlebitis of the pelvic veins, proof of its presence usually is impossible until femoral thrombosis or embolism develops (*see* THROMBOPHLEBITIS).

Embolism may occur any time, from a few days to 3 months following delivery. Daily chills usually accompany thrombophlebitis, especially when due to one of the types of anaerobic streptococci. Peritonitis during pregnancy or puerperium may be completely atypical. Rigidity and constipation are rare, while distention is the most common sign. Tenderness and tympanites are present over the lower abdomen, but there is no actual rigidity. There may be vomiting; fever usually is present and is high terminally, while the pulse rate is much higher than the fever justifies. Frequently there are rales at the lung bases, with impairment of the percussion note due to splinting of the diaphragm. This may be confused with pneumonia. There may be a leukocytosis, which, if present, is rarely high. Occasionally there is a leukopenia. Vomiting, dehydration, oliguria, or anuria may follow.

Prognosis

Before the days of asepsis, epidemics of childbed fever with mortality rates of 90% were not uncommon. Even with the sulfonamides, puerperal infection was the greatest cause of maternal death (about 38% of maternal deaths). The antibiotics have reduced the death rate further but puerperal infection still is a serious threat. Tetanus, gas gangrene, streptococcal infections of epidemic nature, and infections characterized by the formation of cellulitis and abscesses are generally more treatment-resistant, and morbidity and mortality rates remain somewhat higher with any of these types.

Extensive endometritis, salpingitis, salpingo-oophoritis, and parametritis often result in sterility and varying degrees of chronic debility. Infectious emboli from pelvic thrombophlebitis often produce pulmonary complications. Mild gonococcal infections have occasionally caused bacteremia and fatal endocarditis. On the other hand, early recognition of puerperal infection and prompt treatment can in the great majority of cases effect a complete cure without sequelae.

Treatment

Every effort should be made to prevent puerperal sepsis by the use of approved obstetrical technics and the rigid maintenance of asepsis. Isolation: Any pregnant or puerperal patient with a fever, or with other evidence of severe infection, must be isolated, preferably in a single room separate from the obstetrical and delivery floors. Attendant personnel for these patients should not work on the obstetrical or delivery floors, and strict isolation technic must be maintained.

If puerperal infection is suspected, culture should be taken initially and specific treatment begun at once. Treatment can be modified later, if necessary, according to the bacteriologic report. Penicillin (℞ 22) may be administered in doses of 50,000 to 100,000 u. every 3 hours. Combined therapy with both streptomycin or dihydrostreptomycin (℞ 23) and penicillin (℞ 22) is preferred by many. Streptomycin or dihydrostreptomycin is given in 0.5 Gm. doses I.M. every 4 to 6 hours according to the severity of the infection. Sulfadiazine (℞ 24, 25), alone or in combination with the above, may be administered in amounts sufficient to maintain the blood concentration between 10 and 15 mg./100 cc.

General measures include absolute bed rest; light or liquid diet, or nothing by mouth, depending upon the nature of the infection; maintenance of fluid balance and nutrition by parenteral injections when necessary; restoration of the hemoglobin to 12 Gm./100 cc. by blood transfusions if the patient is anemic; and sedatives for the relief of pain (℞ 34, 36). Ascorbic acid and adequate amounts of any suitable vitamin B complex, administered daily, are of value (*see* NUTRITIONAL DEFICIENCIES).

Management of complications: (1) Where there is an infected episiotomy or laceration, sutures are removed, permitting adequate drainage. (2) In acute endometritis, having the patient move about frequently in bed and raising the head of the bed may be tried (early ambulation probably is a preventive), but insurance of adequate uterine drainage probably is the best treatment. A blunt packing forceps may be introduced into the uterine cavity, opened and gently withdrawn, to make certain that there is proper drainage through the cervix. Oxytocics are of questionable value and may be potentially dangerous. (3) For parametritis or pelvic cellulitis, purely symptomatic treatment includes codeine (℞ 34) or morphine (℞ 36) for pain, ice bag to lower abdomen (1 hour on, 1 hour off), or external heat. Pelvic examination is necessary every 5 to 7 days to determine the status of the infection. (4) In pelvic abscess, as soon as suppuration can be detected, it is to be drained through the cul de sac. A large, soft, perforated rubber tube is inserted and left in place for 2 to 3 weeks. The patient is allowed out of bed 24 to 48 hours after drainage has been established. (5) In uterine abscess, if the infection persists and it can be determined that it is localized in the uterine wall, hysterectomy may be indicated. (6) For pelvic thrombophlebitis treatment is symptomatic. For pain, codeine (℞ 34) or morphine (℞ 36) may be given. Ligation of ovarian or uterine veins, or removal of the uterus is rarely indicated. If there is evidence of or reason to suspect embolism, the use of anticoagulants is indicated (*see* ANTICOAGULANT THERAPY). (7) If generalized peritonitis occurs, specific therapy with the sulfonamides and antibiotics is to be intensified. The patient is given nothing by mouth, continuous drainage of the gastrointestinal tract is instituted by means of Wangensteen drainage or Miller-Abbott tube (*see* CLIN. PROC.), and nutrition and fluids are supplied by parenteral methods. Encouragement and reassurance are especially valuable in these serious cases. Anemia must be combated by the use of blood transfusions, and daily vitamin supplements are indicated. Oxygen administration (*see* CLIN. PROC.) is valuable in the profoundly toxic case, especially when abdominal distention interferes with respiratory movements. (8) For the treatment of patients who develop bacteremia, *see* the chapter on Sepsis.

LACTATION DISTURBANCES

Many conditions may interfere with normal milk secretion in the nursing mother, including anatomical anomalies, injuries to the breast, psychic, and metabolic disturbances, and infections such as mastitis. Such disturbances are frequently encountered at economic levels where adequate postpartum care is difficult to obtain.

Etiology

Anomalies of the duct structure and nipple may be responsible for the seldom encountered complete inability to produce milk, as would the congenital lack of one or both breasts; such conditions are extremely rare. Abnormally enlarged breasts also may be due to developmental anomalies, and as a rule, function poorly. Complete absence of milk, from any cause, is called agalactia.

The more common disturbances of nursing are due to deficient secretion, mammary congestion, or mastitis. Deficient milk secretion may result from many causes. It sometimes follows postpartum pituitary necrosis, in which there is almost immediate involution of the breast without evidence of lactation. Other conditions favoring scanty secretion include obesity of the breasts; inadequate suckling stimulus; exhausting diseases incidental to or resulting from pregnancy; pituitary hormone insufficiency; resumption of nursing after breast inflammation has necessitated its interruption; malnutrition; emotional disturbances; conception during lactation; and childbearing at an early or advanced age.

Excessive milk secretion (polygalactia), sometimes with spontaneous flow (galactorrhea), is occasionally observed but the flow usually subsides in a few days. Little is known of the causes of this condition. It has been reported to continue in some cases for months or even years after breast feeding has been discontinued.

Diagnosis

In agalactia, the infant is usually distressed, unsatisfied, cries, and often refuses the breast. There is no milk, and pain occurs in the breasts and at times radiates to the back. Polygalactia and galactorrhea are readily diagnosed by the excessive secretion of milk, which often continues to flow from the breasts even when they are tightly bound. Fissured nipples, which usually appear between the 3rd and 5th day of puerperium, are easily recognized on inspection. Pain, which usually is present, prevents nursing, milk is retained, and the mother often has insomnia and even fever. Mastitis may be readily diagnosed from the local findings and history of bruises or fissures, which give access to bacteria present on the skin, usually staphylococci. Pain in the breast is increased while nursing. There may be slight fever for a day or two preceding the attack.

Onset sometimes is marked by a chill, and fever usually is about 103° F. but sometimes as high as 105° F. The affected breast is red, tender, and painful. Several lumps may be palpated. Suppuration is indicated by remittent fever, chills, swelling, and formation of a large, hard lump. Fluctuation is generally not elicited until much later. When submammary abscess develops, the symptoms become aggravated, the breast is edematous and the skin assumes a dusky red appearance with a bluish tinge. Cervical and axillary lymph nodes may become enlarged. In very severe cases a fatal bacteremia may ensue.

Prophylaxis

In general, scrupulous cleanliness of the breasts, and especially the nipples, provides protection against infections that might result from fissures and bruises. The area should be gently washed with warm water before and after each nursing, and carefully dried to prevent chapping of the skin.

If the infant does not suck vigorously enough, the breasts often become hard, swollen, and tender (generally about the 3rd day after delivery) due to excess of retained milk, and there is a slight rise in the patient's temperature. In such cases, the breasts should be emptied by an electric or water breast pump and then gently massaged from the periphery toward the nipple, after which a firm binder is applied. If the nipple is painful, it is essential to remove the infant from the breast and to keep the breast empty by means of a breast pump. Usually, after a day or two, suckling can safely be resumed. If, for any reason, breast feeding is considered undesirable, lactation can safely be suppressed by the judicious administration of diethylstilbestrol (℞ 4). Acetylsalicylic acid and codeine (℞ 35) are useful for relief of pain during engorgement.

Treatment

Either agalactia or inadequate secretion of milk can be treated primarily by improving the mother's nutrition with a high caloric diet (*see* DIETS) supplemented by vitamins. An abundance of milk and other fluids should be prescribed. Moderate outdoor exercise such as walking is to be encouraged.

Complete evacuation of the breast is the best stimulant to milk secretion, hence breast pumps frequently are of benefit. Extending the intervals between feedings may stimulate the infant to more vigorous sucking. All local lesions of the nipple should receive prompt attention. Supplemental feeding of the infant may be required, especially if the agalactia results from conception during the period of lactation. Psychotherapy may be indicated in cases due to emotional disturbances.

Galactorrhea often is a stubborn affection. Breast binders may be of some value. Diethylstilbestrol (℞ 4) frequently gives relief. Attention should be given to any needed improvement of the patient's general health, nervous condition, and environment. Atropine (℞ 18) given internally inhibits the formation of milk. Extremely stubborn cases sometimes require X-radiation, in moderate dosage, administered by a physician experienced in its use. Fluid, fat and carbohydrate intake should be reduced and proteins and vitamins increased.

Cracked, ulcerated, or fissured nipples require discontinuance of breast feeding until healing has occurred. The nipples should be kept dry and exposed to the air for more rapid healing. The breasts may be emptied by breast pump unless lactation is being permanently discontinued. If a blister develops, this should not be opened and the child should be withheld from the breast for 36 hours, or longer if necessary.

If mastitis develops, breast feeding should be discontinued immediately. A snug supporting binder and an ice bag may relieve pain. Penicillin (℞ 22) is of great value in most cases. Irrespective of temperature and leukocytosis, if the lesion does not subside in a few days, the presence of an abscess must be considered, for which surgical treatment is indicated.

PRESCRIPTIONS

(Wherever a prescribed "proprietary" is representative of a class of therapeutic agents, alternative proprietary preparations will be found listed in Part II.)

Hormonal Substances

1. ℞ Ethinyl estradiol. . . . . . . 0.02 mg.

   Amenorrhea: 1 tablet daily for 24 days followed by ℞ 6 or 7.
   Dysmenorrhea: 2 or 3 tablets daily for 14 to 21 days after onset of menstruation.
   Menopause: 1 to 3 tablets daily.

2. ℞ Estradiol benzoate   (ampul)

   1.66 mg. I.M. daily for 2 or 3 days each month.

3. ℞ Estrone (suppositories) 2,000 I.U.

   Insert 1 suppository into the vagina nightly for 12 nights.

4. ℞ Diethylstilbestrol   (tablets)

   Amenorrhea: 0.5 to 1.0 mg. daily for 24 days.
   Dysmenorrhea: 2 to 3 mg. daily for 14 to 21 days after onset of menstruation.
   Menorrhagia: 10 mg. daily until excessive hemorrhage is controlled.
   Suppression of lactation: 5 or 10 mg. daily for 5 to 7 days following delivery.
   Threatened or habitual abortion: 50 mg. daily until period of fetal viability is reached.

5. ℞ Diethylstilbestrol (suppositories) . . . . 0.5 mg.

> 1 suppository inserted into the vagina once or
> twice daily for 4 to 8 weeks.

6. ℞ Progesterone (ampul)

> *Amenorrhea:* 10 mg. I.M. daily for 2 or 3
> days, preceded by ℞ 1, or with ℞ 2.
> *Dysmenorrhea:* 2 to 5 mg. I.M. daily for 7
> days before expected menses and continu-
> ing until flow ceases.
> *Menorrhagia:* 10 mg. I.M. daily for 6 days.
> *Threatened or habitual abortion:* 5 to 25 mg.
> I.M. daily.

7. ℞ Anhydrohydroxyprogesterone . 5 mg.

> *Amenorrhea:* 6 tablets daily for 5 days, pre-
> ceded by ℞ 1.
> *Dysmenorrhea:* 10 to 12 tablets daily for 7
> days before expected menses and continu-
> ing until flow ceases.
> *Habitual abortion:* 50 mg. daily.

8. ℞ Neostigmine methylsulfate,
1:2,000 (ampul)

> 1 cc. (0.5 mg.) daily subcut. for 2 to 4 doses.

9. ℞ Testosterone propionate (vial)

> *Dysmenorrhea:* 10 mg. I.M. every 1 or 2 days
> for 4 to 8 injections, either immediately
> following a menstrual period or during the
> 8 to 10 days preceding an expected period.
> *Metastatic carcinoma:* 25 mg. I.M. every 1 or
> 2 days.
> *Functional bleeding:* 10 to 25 mg. I.M. 3
> times a week.

10. ℞ Methyltestosterone . . . . . 10 mg.

> *Dysmenorrhea:* 3 tablets daily by mouth for
> 8 days immediately preceding or following
> a menstrual period.
> *Frigidity:* 1 or 2 tablets daily.

11. ℞ Pregnant mare's serum (vial)

> *Amenorrhea:* 500 u. I.M., 3 times weekly for
> 2 or 3 months.

12. ℞ Estradiol benzoate⎱ampul · · 2.5 mg.
Progesterone ⎰ 12.5 mg.

> *Amenorrhea:* Contents of 1 ampul I.M. daily
> for 2 or 3 consecutive days each month.

13. ℞ Chorionic gonadotropin (vial)

> *Dysmenorrhea:* 200 to 500 u. I.M. every other
> day during the 7 to 19 days preceding an
> expected menstrual period.
> *Anovulatory bleeding:* 200 to 500 u. I.M. daily
> until hemorrhage is controlled.

14. ℞ Thyroid U.S.P. . . . . 15 mg. (gr. ¼)

> 1 to 8 tablets daily as required. (*See* dosage regimen under HABITUAL ABORTION.)

Uterine Stimulants

15. ℞ Ergonovine maleate . . . . . 0.2 mg. (gr. 1/320)

> 1 tablet every 4 hours for 6 doses.

16. ℞ "Pitocin" (ampul)

> 0.1 to 0.5 cc. subcut., as often as every ½ hour for 4 to 6 doses if necessary.

17. ℞ Quinine sulfate . . . . 0.2 Gm. (gr. iii)

> 1 tablet or capsule every hour for 5 doses.

Antispasmodics

18. ℞ Atropine sulfate . . . . 0.5 mg. (gr. 1/120)

> 1 tablet every 4 to 6 hours.

19. ℞ Papaverine hydrochloride . . . 0.1 Gm. (gr. iss)

> 1 tablet or capsule every 4 to 6 hours.

20. ℞ Whisky

> 1 ounce every 6 hours.

21. ℞ A synthetic antispasmodic

> (For available products *see* dose table of ALTERNATIVE PROPRIETARY PREPARATIONS.)

Antimicrobial Agents

22. ℞ Penicillin (vial)

> 50,000 to 100,000 u. I.M. every 3 hours or 300,000 u. I.M. every 12 to 24 hours.

23. ℞ Streptomycin or dihydrostreptomycin (vial)

> 0.5 Gm. I.M. every 4 to 6 hours.

24. ℞ Sulfadiazine . . . . 0.5 Gm. (gr. viiss)

> 4 to 6 tablets initially, then 2 tablets every 4 hours.

25. ℞ Sodium sulfadiazine (ampul)

> 2.5 Gm. (gr. xxxviiss) I.V. every 8 to 12 hours.

26. ℞ Gentian violet, 1% solution

> Apply to vaginal mucosa every 1 or 2 days for 4 or 5 applications.

27. ℞ Strong Iodine Solution U.S.P. (Lugol's Solution)

> Dilute 1:4 or 1:5 with water and apply to vaginal mucosa every 1 or 2 days for 4 or 5 applications.

28. ℞ Sodium propionate . . . . . 12.0   Gm. (ℨ iii)
    Hydrophyllic Ointment U.S.P.
                q.s. ad 120.0   Gm. (ℨ iv)

    Apply to vaginal walls daily for 4 or 5 applications.

29. ℞ "Vioform" (suppositories) . . 0.25   Gm. (gr. iv)

    Insert 1 vaginal suppository into the vagina (posterior fornix) nightly.

30. ℞ Silver picrate

    Insufflate 5 Gm. into the vagina once a week and insert 0.13 Gm. (gr. ii) as a suppository into the vagina nightly.

31. ℞ Boric acid . . . . 0.3   Gm. (gr. v)
    Glucose . . . . 0.3   Gm. (gr. v)
    Lactose . . . . 0.3   Gm. (gr. v)

    Insert 1 or 2 tablets or capsules into the vagina at night.

Analgesics and Sedatives

32. ℞ Acetylsalicylic acid. . . . . 0.3   Gm. (gr. v)

    2 or 3 tablets every 4 to 6 hours.

33. ℞ Acetylsalicylic acid . . . . 0.22   Gm. (gr. iiiss)
    Acetophenetidin . . . . . 0.16   Gm. (gr. iiss)
    Caffeine . . . . 0.03   Gm. (gr. ss)

    2 capsules or tablets every 4 hours.

34. ℞ Codeine phosphate   (hypodermic
    tablets) 15   mg. (gr. ¼)

    1 to 4 tablets depending upon severity of pain, orally or subcut. every 4 hours.

35. ℞ Acetylsalicylic acid . . . . 0.6   Gm. (gr. x)
    Codeine sulfate . . . . . 0.03   Gm. (gr. ss)

    1 tablet or capsule 3 or 4 times daily.

36. ℞ Morphine sulfate

    10 to 15 mg. (gr. ⅙ to ¼) subcut. every 6 hours if necessary.

37. ℞ Paraldehyde

    0.5 cc./Kg. body wt. rectally as a 10% solution in olive oil.

38. ℞ Phenobarbital 30   mg. (gr. ss)

    1 to 3 tablets 3 times a day.

39. ℞ Phenobarbital sodium   (ampul)

    0.3 Gm. (gr. v) subcut. or I.V. every 8 to 12 hours.

40. ℞ "Amytal Sodium"   (ampul)
    0.25 to 0.5 Gm. (gr. iv to viiss) I.V. or subcut.
    every 8 to 12 hours.

41. ℞ Chloral hydrate . . . .   3.0   Gm. (gr. xlv)
    Starch U.S.P. . . . .   4.0   Gm. (℥ i)
    Warm water   . . . . .q.s. ad 90.0   cc.   (℥ iii)
    Instill 1 to 3 ounces in rectum every 6 to 12
    hours for relief of eclamptic convulsions.

42. ℞ Magnesium sulfate, 50% solution
    (ampul)
    12 cc. I.V. or I.M. followed by 4 cc. after each
    eclamptic convulsion.

43. ℞ Magnesium sulfate, 10% solution
    (ampul)
    20 cc. I.V. or I.M. repeated hourly for 5 doses
    if eclamptic convulsions have occurred.

Miscellaneous

44. ℞ Ammonium chloride   (enteric
    coated)   . . . .   0.5   Gm. (gr. viiss)
    20 tablets daily in divided doses for 6 days;
    course may be repeated after a rest period of
    6 days.

45. ℞ Pyridoxine hydrochloride (Vita-
    min B_6)   (ampul)
    50 to 100 mg. I.V.

46. ℞ Aluminum Acetate Solution N.F.
    (Burow's Solution)
    Dilute 1:10 or 1:20 and apply as cold com-
    presses to the affected parts 4 times daily.

INFECTIOUS AND PARASITIC

FEVER AND CHILLS

Fever: *An elevation of body temperature above the normal range.* In persons confined to bed, temperatures exceeding 98.6° F., and in persons recently moderately active, temperatures above 99.0° F., constitute fever. Rectal temperatures usually are 0.5° to 1.0° F. higher than oral. Fever may be:

1. Hyperthermic: Marked by high temperatures, usually reaching 105° F. or above.

2. Sustained: Average daily temperature exceeds normal.

3. Intermittent: Temperature falls daily to normal or below, then rises again.

4. Remittent: With daily rise and fall of temperature, but without return to normal.

5. Hectic (septic): With daily temperature swings of major degree, and frequently chills and sweats.

6. Relapsing: Febrile episodes alternating with a day or days of normal temperature.

Chill: *An attack of involuntary shivering, with a sense of coldness, and pallor of the skin.* Chills usually are followed by fever.

Etiology

Fever results when the heat production of the body exceeds its heat loss. A chill ushers in a great increase in heat production with relatively slight change in heat loss. Cerebral lesions that damage the thermal centers, located in the hypothalamus, affect the body temperature. The most common cause of fever, however, is a disease process altering the control of heat dissipation. Tumors, infections, vascular accidents, or trauma may directly affect the hypothalamus or the descending nerve tracts leading from it, and thus disturb the mechanism of heat regulation.

Low grade fever may accompany thyrotoxicosis, leukemia, and Hodgkin's disease, probably due to increased heat production associated with increased metabolic rate. Medication with dinitrophenol or the sulfonamides also may cause fever by the same mechanism. Conditions that give rise to hyperpyrexia through restriction of heat loss are high environmental temperatures with humidity and stagnant air, dehydration in infants, ichthyosis and other generalized skin diseases when the patient is in a warm atmosphere, and congenital absence of sweat glands. Elevation of temperature, probably by effect upon the thermoregulatory centers, may be caused by extensive tissue injury. Such injury may be due to bacterial, rickettsial, and viral infections; to parasitic infestations; to severe trauma; or to myocardial infarction, cerebral hemorrhage and thrombosis, and peripheral arterial occlusions. Malignant neoplasms commonly are accompanied by a febrile course. The hectic fever and daily chills sometimes seen with hypernephroma may simulate an infectious disease. Conditions causing massive intravascular hemolysis, such as hemolytic transfusion reactions, drug sensitivity reactions, and crises in sickle cell anemia, usually cause a rise of temperature.

Such conditions as serum sickness, periarteritis nodosa, rheumatic fever, rheumatoid arthritis, and erythema nodosum, as well as inflammatory diseases of unknown origin, cause fever, probably as a result of tissue destruction.

Chills usually follow, in about an hour, the introduction into the blood stream of a foreign substance, such as bacteria, bacterial vaccines, bacterial products (pyrogens), or parasites. There is good evidence that a hypothalamic center exists which, when stimulated, results in a chill. Foreign materials introduced into the circulation injure tissue and probably liberate substances capable of stimulating this "chill center." Malaria, pneumococcal pneumonia, and bacteremia secondary to localized pyogenic infections are common conditions characterized by chills. Many other infections, as well as transfusion reaction, and reaction to I.V. typhoid vaccine, pulmonary infarction, and hypernephroma, may be accompanied by chills.

Diagnosis

Fever is usually encountered in conjunction with other symptoms and signs, and consideration of all the data frequently suggests the diagnosis. The type of temperature curve also will often give a clue to the underlying disease. A "staircase rise" for a few days, followed by remittent fever for 1 to 3 weeks, with a staircase descent to normal, indicates the possibility of typhoid or paratyphoid fever. Typhus typically produces a sudden rise with sustained high fever for 7 to 10 days and a gradual fall reaching normal about 2 weeks after onset. A fever curve showing high daily spikes with descent to normal in between (hectic type) often is seen in pyogenic infections such as acute osteomyelitis, empyema, or intra-abdominal abscess. Short febrile periods alternating with one or more days of normal temperature (relapsing fever) are seen chiefly in only 4 conditions that occur in the United States: malaria, rat-bite fever, relapsing fever (due to *Spirillum recurrentis*), and chronic meningococcal septicemia.

Extremely high temperatures, above 106.5°F., are rare and almost all are neurogenic, from head injury, massive cerebral hemorrhage, or brain surgery. Dehydration may result in hyperpyrexia in infants. Rarely, in the course of rheumatic fever, very high fever may occur secondary to cerebral involvement. Ingestion of extracts of poison ivy (*Rhus toxicodendron*) has induced cerebral edema and hyperpyrexia. Fever of staphylococcal septicemia may reach high levels.

In fevers of undetermined origin, a careful history often gives important clues; for example, a history of drinking well water should suggest typhoid; proximity to rats, typhus; working in meat-packing plant, brucellosis; being bitten by a rat, rat-bite fever; drinking unpasteurized milk, typhoid, or brucellosis; contact with rat-infested water, Weil's disease; contact with wild rabbits, tularemia; contact with hides or skins, anthrax; tick bite, Rocky Mountain spotted fever; contact with parrots, psittacosis. Frequently repeated physical examination may yield a new sign which leads to the diagnosis. Physical signs of hilar pneumonia, lung abscess, empyema, peritonitis, or of hepatic, subdiaphragmatic or perinephric abscess should be repeatedly sought. The skin should be examined daily for evidence of rash or petechiae. Enlargement of spleen or lymph nodes may be a diagnostic sign. Any patient with prolonged fever and a heart murmur should be studied for subacute bacterial endocarditis.

In any undiagnosed febrile illness, blood cultures should be taken in groups of 3 to 6 daily for several days. Skin and agglutination tests should be repeated if typhoid, brucellosis, or a rickettsial disease is suspected, since a rise in titer as disease progresses is more significant than a single titer. Malaria must be considered, and a search made for parasites. Under therapeutic trial of antibiotics or the sulfonamides, the persistence of fever does not necessarily exclude the presence of infection, since many strains of staphylococci, for example, will resist enormous doses of penicillin, as will undrained pyogenic abscesses containing penicillin-susceptible organisms. X-ray studies may reveal a neoplastic process. Biopsy of enlarged lymph nodes, subcutaneous nodules, chronic skin lesions, or tender muscle tissue may yield a definite diagnosis of, respectively: lymphoma or metastatic carcinoma; disseminated lupus erythematosus or periarteritis nodosa; tuberculosis, Boeck's sarcoid, pemphigus, or other febrile skin disease; trichinosis or dermatomyositis.

Treatment

General principles: Basic treatment of fever must be directed to its cause, but in some cases it is necessary to treat the fever itself together with its complications and sequelae. It first must be decided, however, whether the pyrexia is harmful or beneficial. High body temperature is thought to enhance antibody production and perhaps to help mobilize other defense mechanisms during infections. Certain microorganisms are inhibited by febrile temperatures, e.g., gonococcus and *T. pallidum*. On the other hand, fever often is useless as a defense mechanism (as in neoplastic disease) and may be harmful. Prolonged fever is debilitating, since the associated increased metabolism is not matched by necessary intake of food (particularly protein), fluid, and electrolytes. Fever following vascular occlusion increases demands of tissues for oxygen and nourishment and is therefore harmful. Extremely high fever may in itself be fatal.

Alteration of the temperature curve by antipyretic measures disturbs a valuable indicator of the disease course. This must be weighed against the desirability of temperature reduction. Antipyresis is indicated when fever makes the patient restless and uncomfortable. It usually is justified in acute illness when the temperature exceeds 105° F., but in prolonged illness a temperature above 103° F. may deserve therapy, even if the patient is not complaining. Other symptoms often overshadow the patient's awareness of fever.

Hydrotherapy with cold head compresses or an ice cap, a sheet bath, an ice water enema, or by general sponging, is the method of choice in reduction of fever (see BEDSIDE PROC.). No effort should be made to reduce the temperature below 101° F. When heroic measures are indicated, as in heat stroke (q.v.), immersion of the patient's trunk and extremities in ice water is necessary. The ice water should be stirred and the patient steadily massaged. The tubbing should be discontinued when rectal temperature falls to 103° F.; otherwise hypothermia and shock may result. A good response can be expected in 10 to 40 minutes. Less vigorous methods are apt to be ineffective in heat stroke.

Drugs may be given, but are less safe than hydrotherapy. The common antipyretics are the salicylates (e.g., acetylsalicylic acid, sodium salicylate); aniline derivatives (acetanilid, acetophenetidin, phenetidin); pyrazolone compounds (aminopyrine and antipyrine); and cinchoninic acid derivatives (cinchophen and neocinchophen). These drugs all act on the thermoregulatory centers to increase heat loss by inducing cutaneous vasodilatation and increasing perspiration. The salicylates are the safest. Aniline derivatives are somewhat more toxic but reasonably safe. Since pyrazolone compounds occasionally cause agranulocytosis, and cinchoninic acid derivatives have produced acute yellow atrophy of the liver, they should not be used as antipyretics. Any of the drugs given to a patient with high fever may result in a sudden fall of temperature and general circulatory collapse. When used as antipyretics, the average oral adult doses are: acetylsalicylic acid and sodium salicylate (R 1, 2), 0.3 to 1 Gm. (gr. v to xv) every 3 or 4 hours; acetanilid (R 7), 0.2 Gm. (gr. iii) and acetophenetidin (R 8), 0.3 Gm. (gr. v). These drugs do not alter the course of febrile illnesses, but simply reduce fever. In acute rheumatic fever (q.v.), the dosage is entirely different, as the salicylates are not solely antipyretic or analgesic but also have a "specific" effect on the joint inflammation.

In neurogenic hyperpyrexia, as seen in cerebral vascular accident, head trauma, and following brain surgery, hydrotherapy and antipyretic drugs are seldom effective. These patients usually die with extremely high temperature. Barbiturates may be tried. In neurogenic fever it seems that the heat-conserving mechanisms overact for a number of hours following destruction or injury to the heat-dissipating center in the anterior hypothalamus. Sodium pentobarbital (℞ 25) and sodium phenobarbital (℞ 23, 24) are thought to paralyze the overacting heat-conserving center. These drugs may be given in repeated doses of 0.3 Gm. (gr. v) at intervals indicated by the response. The patient may thus be tided over the period of hyperpyrexia (48 hours in some cases). He may be left with an impaired temperature-regulating mechanism but spared death from excessive fever.

Special care: Maintenance of fluid and electrolyte balance usually is more important than reducing the temperature. Since fluid loss is increased in fever, the patient should be induced to drink water every hour, or fluids should be administered parenterally (*see* CLIN. PROC.). If fluid loss is excessive and salt intake low, supplementary sodium chloride, 1 to 2 Gm. three times daily, should be given. Nutrition should be maintained by a high protein, high vitamin diet (*see* DIETS) given in frequent small feedings. Multivitamin preparations containing thiamine (vitamin B_1) 10 to 25 mg.; riboflavin (vitamin B_2) 2 to 6 mg.; nicotinic acid 5 to 20 mg.; ascorbic acid (vitamin C) 50 to 100 mg.; vitamin A 3,000 to 8,000 u.; and vitamin D 400 to 800 u., may be administered daily in prolonged febrile diseases.

Nursing care: Persons with prolonged fevers require scrupulous attention to oral hygiene (*see* BEDSIDE PROC.) to prevent stomatitis and parotitis. Herpes simplex (q.v.) often accompanies febrile illnesses. Daily soap-and-water bed baths, followed by an alcohol back rub, contribute materially to the patient's comfort and morale as well as providing ordinary cleanliness. A clean dry skin and frequent turning in bed (together with adequate protein intake) provide the best prophylaxis against decubitus ulcers (q.v.).

Care of patients during fever therapy (Malarial): Syphilitic patients being treated with induced malaria require careful supervision. High caloric diet and liberal fluid intake are essential. Ephedrine sulfate (℞ 119), 25 mg. (gr. ⅜), should be given to combat the hypotensive effect, and sodium chloride 2 Gm. three times daily on the day of a paroxysm will balance the extra sodium chloride loss in the sweat. The urine should be examined microscopically and for albumin after each chill. Temperature should be determined every 4 hours during the afebrile period and every 15 minutes during a paroxysm. Blood pressure should be recorded twice daily. Weight, hemoglobin level, icteric index, and blood nonprotein nitrogen level should be determined once a week. Appropriate antimalarial therapy (*see* MALARIA) should be given to conclude the paroxysms after approximately 50 hours of temperature over 103°F. Chills usually can be alleviated by I.V. injection of calcium gluconate (℞ 150), 1 Gm., administered slowly. If it is given rapidly, the chill is apt to return after a few minutes.

22

DIFFERENTIAL DIAGNOSIS OF

Condition	Incubation (days)	Period of Communicability	Symptoms and Signs
Chickenpox (Varicella)	14–21	From 1 day prior to onset of symptoms until all lesions have crusted over (usually about 6 days after appearance of rash).	Chills, moderate fever, headache and malaise.
Smallpox (Variola)	10–14	Usually from 24 to 48 hours before onset of symptoms and until all crusts have disappeared.	Abrupt onset with chills, fever, rapid pulse and respiration, and frequently nausea and vomiting. Also severe headache, backache, and muscular pains.
Scarlet Fever (Scarlatina)	3–5	Usually from 24 hours before onset of symptoms until 2 to 3 weeks thereafter, or even longer if complications occur, e.g., sinusitis or otitis media.	Chills, fever, sore throat, vomiting; strawberry tongue; cervical lymphadenopathy; circumoral pallor.
Measles (Rubeola)	7–14	From 2 to 4 days before appearance of rash until 2 to 5 days thereafter.	Fever, coryza, cough, conjunctivitis, photophobia, Koplik's spots; frequently pruritus.
German Measles (Rubella)	14–21	From 1 day before onset of symptoms until perhaps 1 day after disappearance of rash.	Malaise, fever, headache, rhinitis; postauricular and postoccipital lymphadenopathy, with tender nodes.
Exanthem Subitum (Roseola infantum)	Not known	Unknown	Infants affected. High fever, splenomegaly.
Infectious Mononucleosis	5–15	Undetermined	Malaise, headache, fever, sore throat, splenomegaly and generalized lymphadenopathy.
Drug Rash	History of use of drug	None	Variable, including fever, malaise, arthralgia, nausea, photophobia, pruritus.

THE COMMONER EXANTHEMS

| Eruption | | | Laboratory Findings |
Site	Character	Onset; Duration	
Usually first on trunk, later spreading to face, neck and extremities; infrequently on palms and soles.	Lesions discrete; progress from macule to papule to vesicle; appear in crops, hence the various forms are present simultaneously. Crusts develop after vesicle rupture.	1 day after onset of symptoms; persists for 1 to 2 weeks.	None of significance.
First on face, neck, upper chest and hands. Most numerous on exposed body surfaces; palms, soles, pharynx may be involved.	Shot-like papules changing to vesicles and finally to umbilicated pustules, which become confluent as they enlarge. Usually only one crop of lesions, in contradistinction to chickenpox.	On 3rd or 4th day; persists for 2 to 5 weeks.	Initially, leukopenia; later, during pustular phase, leukocytosis.
Face, neck, chest, abdomen, spreading to the extremities. Entire body surface may be involved.	Diffuse pinkish red flush of skin, with punctate "goose flesh" feel. Positive Rumpel-Leede sign and Schultz-Charlton blanching reaction.	On 2nd day; lasts 4 to 10 days.	Granulocytosis; throat culture positive for *Str. hemolyticus.*
Forehead, face, neck, and then spreading over trunk and limbs.	Maculopapular; brownish pink in color and irregularly confluent.	3 to 5 days after onset of symptoms; lasts 4 to 7 days.	Granulocytic leukopenia.
Face, neck and spreading to trunk and limbs.	Fine pinkish macules which become confluent.	1 or 2 days after onset of symptoms; lasts for 1 to 3 days.	Leukocyte count usually normal or low.
Chest and abdomen, with moderate involvement of face and extremities.	Either diffuse macular or maculopapular.	On 4th day; simultaneously the temperature returns to normal and remains so; rash lasts 1 to 2 days.	Granulocytic leukopenia.
Most prominent over trunk.	Occurs in 15% of cases, as a morbilliform, scarlatiniform, or vesiculate rash.	Appears 5 to 14 days after onset of illness; lasts 3 to 7 days.	Heterophile antibody test of Paul-Bunnell is positive; leukocytosis with atypical enlarged lymphocytes ("mononucleosis").
Generalized, or, in some instances, restricted to exposed surfaces.	May be morbilliform, scarlatiniform, erythematous, acneform, vesicular, bullous, purpuric, or exfoliating.	Variable	Agranulocytosis may be present; drug may be detected in urine.

MEASLES

(Rubeola, Morbilli)

A highly contagious acute disease characterized by fever, cough, coryza, conjunctivitis, eruption (Koplik's spots) on the labial or buccal mucous membrane, and a spreading maculo-papular cutaneous rash.

Etiology and Epidemiology

Measles is caused by a filtrable virus which attacks man and may be transmitted experimentally to certain monkeys. It has been grown on the chorioallantoic membrane of chicken embryos.

The disease occurs in epidemics, almost always in the spring months. In urban areas of relatively stable population, epidemics appear at intervals of 3 to 4 years, with small localized outbreaks during the spring of intervening years. The virus is spread largely by droplet spray from the nose, throat, and mouth of persons in the prodromal or early eruptive stage of the disease. Indirect spread by persons or objects seems to be rare. The intermediate host of the virus, between epidemics, is not known, nor is the virus known to be perpetuated by healthy carriers. In urban areas, measles is largely a disease of pre-school and young school children. Mothers who have had measles give their infants a relative immunity for most of the first year of life. Thereafter, susceptibility is very high, as evidenced by the fact that approximately 98% of the population has frank measles at some time, usually during childhood. In isolated rural areas, epidemics of measles occur at irregular intervals, and some individuals may escape until late childhood or adulthood. Severity of symptoms varies from epidemic to epidemic, probably due to a difference in strains of the causative virus. The period of infectivity begins 2 to 4 days before the rash appears and lasts for 2 to 5 days thereafter. The slight desquamation that follows the rash is not infective, and the virus disappears from nose and throat secretions by the time the rash clears up.

Symptoms and Signs

After an incubation period of 7 to 14 days, prodromal symptoms of fever, coryza, hacking cough, and conjunctivitis appear. Within 24 to 48 hours, Koplik's spots may be seen, usually situated on the buccal mucosa opposite the 1st and 2nd upper molars. These spots (tiny white papules surrounded by an inflammatory areola) are pathognomonic of measles. When they are numerous, the entire background may be erythematous. There is a definite pharyngitis and inflammation of the laryngeal and tracheobronchial mucous membranes. The patient's temperature rises rapidly. The characteristic rash appears 3 to 5 days after onset of symptoms, beginning at the hairline on the face and neck. The first lesions are irregular macules, which soon become maculopapular and spread rapidly (within 24 to 48 hours) to the trunk and extremities, at the same time beginning to fade on the face. When the disease is at its height, the temperature may reach 104° F. or more, there is swelling of the face, particularly about the eyes, with conjunctivitis, photophobia, a hacking cough, extensive rash, and a bothersome pruritus. The leukocyte count is low. Constitutional signs and symptoms parallel the severity of the eruption and vary considerably with the epidemic. About the 4th day, the fever falls by lysis, the patient feels much more comfortable, and the rash fades rapidly leaving a coppery brown discoloration which is followed by a branny desquamation beginning on the face. With particularly severe rashes, there may be hemorrhage into the maculopapular lesions, which may become confluent in various areas.

Complications

Measles renders its victims highly susceptible to other infections, especially those due to streptococci, staphylococci, pneumococci, and *H. influenzae*. It also seems to nullify the patient's resistance to tuberculosis and is thus particularly dangerous in tuberculous individuals. Bronchopneumonia and otitis media are common complications, but both respond to treatment with sulfonamides or penicillin. Most of the complications develop as the rash begins to fade. The continuance or recurrence of fever, change in blood count from leukopenia to leukocytosis, and the development of malaise, pain or prostration signify the development of some complication. The most dreaded is encephalitis (q.v.). This usually occurs 3 to 6 days after the onset of the exanthem. Encephalitis occasionally may be noted when the rash has disappeared and only a slight cutaneous pigmentation remains. It is ushered in by high fever, convulsions, and coma. The spinal fluid shows an increase of lymphocytes, usually more than 50 and less than 500/cu. mm. (*see* table, SPINAL FLUID FINDINGS IN HEALTH AND DISEASE, page 986). The encephalitis may be of short duration with recovery in a week or so, or may be prolonged and terminate in serious C.N.S. impairment or death.

Diagnosis

Measles may be suspected in a child who has coryza, photophobia, and evidence of bronchitis, although before the rash appears diagnosis can be made with certainty only by identifying Koplik's spots. These, followed by high fever, malaise, low leukocyte count, and skin eruption with its characteristic cephalocaudal progression, make confirmation of the early diagnosis fairly easy. In measles, the leukocyte count usually is 5,000 or less. If septic complications occur, a polymorphonuclear leukocytosis is seen.

The diagnosis of measles in adults may be missed at first because of its unexpectedness. When suggestive symptoms appear in grownups with no past history of the disease, the possibility of measles should be kept in mind.

Differential diagnosis includes consideration of rubella, scarlet fever, drug rashes, serum sickness, and exanthem subitum. The distinguishing features of rubella are its mild course with few or no constitutional symptoms, low fever, normal blood count, usual absence of a recognizable prodrome, and short duration. Scarlet fever may at first be suggested by the pharyngitis and fever of measles, but the leukocytosis of scarlet fever is missing: the appearance of Koplik's spots and the skin rash of measles clarifies what might temporarily be a difficult diagnosis. While the diagnosis is pending, the patient should be isolated from those with rubella or scarlet fever as well as from healthy children. It is extremely dangerous to expose patients with measles to infection by streptococci, to which they are highly susceptible. Drug rashes, such as those caused by phenobarbital and the sulfonamides, may closely resemble the eruption of measles. Absence of the typical prodrome and failure of the rash to progress from head to trunk are helpful in distinguishing drug rashes. Here, as in all cases, the history is of great importance. Exanthem subitum (q.v.) produces a skin rash similar to that of measles, but usually can be differentiated by its high initial temperature, the absence of Koplik's spots and malaise, and the fact that the rash appears after the fever has subsided. Moreover, exanthem subitum seldom is seen in children over 3 years of age.

Prognosis

Measles usually is a benign infection with a low mortality rate and one attack apparently confers lifelong immunity. However, the disease may be followed, particularly in infants, by bronchopneumonia and other bacterial infections which may be fatal. Postmeasles encephalitis, which also may be fatal, occurs only about once in 1,200 to 1,500 cases.

Prophylaxis

Measles may be prevented or modified by passive protection with convalescent serum administered after exposure. The value of convalescent serum or placental globulin, and more recently of the gamma globulin fraction of pooled adult plasma, is well established. Following an attack of measles, specific antibodies can be demonstrated and these persist throughout life. Like all antibodies, they are most abundant in the gamma fraction (fraction II of Cohn) of the blood. The gamma fraction of pooled serum globulin (immune serum globulin, human) is so high in measles antibodies that amounts ranging from 0.3 cc. to 5 cc. are enough to modify or prevent the disease when administered at the proper time. It may be considered desirable for an exposed child to have a mild attack of measles, at a favorable time (as in warm weather, when the risk of complicating infections is lowest), in order to secure immunity. This can be accomplished by giving smaller doses, but the dosage has not yet been standardized. Inasmuch as complete passive protection following one exposure to measles lasts for only 3 to 6 weeks and then leaves the patient as susceptible as before, it should be reserved for individuals to whom measles would be unusually dangerous. These include children under 2 years of age, and prevention or modification should be tried for all under 4 years. Even more necessary is complete protection of children who have scarlet fever or debilitating diseases of any kind, most especially tuberculosis. Mere modification of measles should never be attempted in tuberculous patients: complete protection from every exposure until the disease has been healed for many years is the ideal management. Gamma globulin (℞ 94), currently available in most communities through local health departments, is the most reliable and safest of the several agents that may be used. It should be given as soon as possible after exposure. If treatment is postponed for 6 or 7 days, complete prevention of an attack is unlikely, but some modification can be expected when given up to the 10th or 12th day. Gamma globulin should always be given I.M., according to the dosage schedule accompanying each vial.

With the doses recommended, relative passive immunity lasts for at least 3 weeks, but probably disappears entirely after 6 weeks. Reexposure then calls for treatment as before.

Convalescent serum or plasma from a person recently recovered from measles may be used in doses of 5 cc. to 20 cc. I.M., according to the age of the treated subject. The time factor is the same as for gamma globulin.

Treatment

After the rash appears, treatment of measles is symptomatic and aimed at preventing complications. Strict confinement to bed is advisable until the rash clears up. Thereafter, the patient should be protected from cold and dampness for about 10 days or 2 weeks. Since strong light and glare cause discomfort, the patient should be turned away from the principal source of light. There is no proof that light is injurious to the vision or that darkness will protect the eyes from the blindness that so rarely occurs. If cough is troublesome, give a suitable cough syrup (℞ 144). Increasing the humidity in the room may soothe the mucous membranes and allay the cough. During illness, the patient's appetite is poor; the diet should be fluid or soft, with fluid intake carefully maintained while fever persists. Pruritus may be relieved by phenolated calamine lotion (℞ 124). Whether to give antibacterial agents such as sulfadiazine or penicillin for 4 or 5 days to prevent complications must be decided for each case. If the illness is mild these drugs are not indicated. When the sulfonamides are given, the patient's urine should be kept reasonably dilute. The patient with measles should not be exposed to other infections, including the common cold. If essential attendants have "colds" at any stage, they should wear masks and keep their hands scrupulously clean.

If encephalitis occurs as a complication, its treatment is principally symptomatic. Spinal fluid máy be carefully withdrawn to relieve excess pressure. Glucose, 50 cc. of a 50% solution (℞ 149), also may be given I.V. to lower the spinal fluid pressure temporarily. Convalescent serum in large amounts, 50 to 200 cc. I.V., has been suggested, but its value has not been proved. The temperature, which is likely to range between 105° and 107° F., must be held to safe levels by administration of acetylsalicylic acid (℞ 1) and by sponging the skin with tepid water or alcohol. Ice packs and cold enemas may be used if necessary.

GERMAN MEASLES

(Rubella, Three-day measles)

An exanthematous, contagious disease with mild constitutional symptoms.

Etiology and Epidemiology

German measles is caused by a filtrable virus. The virus is spread by droplet spray from nose and throat and, like measles, the disease may be air-borne for short distances. Rubella is less contagious than measles, which probably accounts for the fact that children often do not contract the disease and cases in young adults are frequent. The incubation period is 14 to 21 days.

Epidemics may occur at irregular intervals during the spring months. One attack protects for life. Newborn infants seem particularly immune to rubella, but lose their immunity before 1 year of age.

Symptoms and Signs

Adults may experience fever and malaise with German measles, but characteristically they complain of few or no constitutional symptoms. Headache, stiffness of the joints, and a slight feeling of lassitude are symptoms often noted. Mild catarrhal pharyngeal symptoms at the very onset are frequent. The prodrome is short. The older child or adult often becomes aware of the disease by noting the morbilliform rash on chest, arms or forehead. Sometimes it is the characteristic postauricular lymphadenopathy, discovered while washing, or on combing the hair, that calls attention to the disease. Tender adenopathy of postcervical and postoccipital glands are characteristic signs and, in the presence of the typical rash, they aid in diagnosis.

The skin eruption of rubella is at times very similar to that of measles (rubeola) but is usually more evanescent. At the onset of the eruption there may be a flush, particularly on the face, which suggests scarlet fever. The rash of rubella begins on the face and neck and quickly spreads to trunk and extremities. It usually lasts 3 days and the very slight skin discoloration remaining as the rash fades may disappear in a day. A mild enanthem on the palate is present. There is a definite reddening of the pharynx at the onset of rubella, but no complaint of sore throat. The skin eruption is rarely pruritic.

Diagnosis

This includes a consideration of measles, scarlet fever, secondary syphilis, drug rashes, and infectious mononucleosis. Rubella is differentiated from measles by the absence of Koplik's spots, definite coryza, or photophobia. The measles patient is sicker, and his illness lasts longer. It is only during or on the first day of rubella that the eruption may resemble that of scarlet fever. Mild scarlet fever has more constitutional symptoms. The leukocyte count is elevated in scarlet fever—normal in rubella. A day's observation usually leaves no doubt as to which disease is present. The eruption and adenopathy of rubella can, of course, be closely simulated by the manifestations of secondary syphilis. However, the adenopathy of lues is nontender, the skin eruption is more bronze in color and the mucous membrane lesions of the two diseases are entirely different. A quantitative serologic test should be done if there is doubt, and repeated observations made. Infectious mononucleosis also may cause an adenopathy and skin rash which might be confused with those of German measles. In the former disease, the initial leukopenia, followed by leukocytosis and the presence in the blood smear of many typical mononuclear cells, is characteristic. As a rule, the angina of infectious mononucleosis is a prominent part of the patient's complaints, and the malaise is almost always distinctly greater and of much longer duration than that encountered in rubella.

Prophylaxis

Few, if any, states require quarantine for rubella, but a warning sign and reporting are generally required. Isolation need not be prolonged beyond 1 week and it is the consensus that the patient will no longer pass the disease when his rash has faded and he is afebrile.

Until recently, there seemed to be no reason to attempt prevention of rubella. It is associated with a low fatality rate, and has only one possible severe complication—encephalitis—which is exceedingly rare. The linking of the disease with congenital anomalies now makes it imperative to protect women who are in the first trimester of pregnancy. In such cases, exposure should be followed at once by administration of human gamma globulin (℞ 94). This should be repeated in 10 days. If convalescent serum is available, fairly large doses, 10 to 30 cc. I.M. are suggested at the same intervals. So real is the danger of rubella to the fetus during the first 2 to 3 months of gestation that it has been suggested that young girls be exposed to the disease so as to have it before their reproductive period.

Treatment

Uncomplicated German measles requires little or no treatment. If itching is present, antipruritic lotion or powder may be applied (R 124, 127). Rarely, otitis media (q.v.) complicates rubella, and requires appropriate treatment.

EXANTHEM SUBITUM

(Roseola infantum, Pseudorubella)

An acute disease of infants characterized by fever, absence of localizing signs or symptoms and the appearance of a rubelliform eruption which follows the critical fall of temperature.

Etiology and Epidemiology

The cause and mode of spread of exanthem subitum are unknown, although it is believed to be communicable. The disease occurs most often in the spring and the fall. Minor local epidemics have been reported.

Symptoms and Signs

In exanthem subitum, high fever (103° to 105°F.) begins abruptly and persists for 3 or 4 days without any evidence of the cause. Convulsions are common during this period. There is leukopenia with relative lymphocytosis. In many instances the spleen is slightly enlarged.

Usually, on the 4th day the fever falls by crisis, and the macular or maculopapular eruption appears. It is profuse on the chest and abdomen and mild on face and extremities. At this stage the temperature is normal and the child feels and acts well. The evanescent rash, in mild cases, may escape notice.

Diagnosis

If the disease is known to be in the community, exanthem subitum should be suspected when a child between the ages of 1 and 3 develops a persistent elevation of temperature, and all the usual examinations fail to reveal its cause. In many instances, a presumptive diagnosis can be made with considerable confidence.

Treatment

Therapy is exclusively symptomatic. The use of acetylsalicylic acid (R 1), in a dosage appropriate for the age of the child, and tepid water or alcohol sponges to keep the fever below 103° F. are indicated. The treatment of convulsions (q.v.), is covered elsewhere. When the temperature falls to normal and the eruption appears, the patient is so nearly well that further treatment is unnecessary.

CHICKENPOX

(Varicella)

An acute infectious disease, usually ushered in by mild consti-tutional symptoms, followed shortly by an eruption appearing in crops, and characterized by macules, papules, vesicles, and crusting.

Etiology and Epidemiology

In almost all respects the infecting organism of chickenpox behaves as a virus and the host response to it also suggests its viral nature; however, no virus has yet been cultured from lesions or from nose and throat secretions of patients. A pos-sible relationship between chickenpox and herpes zoster is sug-gested by the occasional occurrence simultaneously of the two conditions in the same family.

This disease shares with measles the highest rate of com-municability. Most adults are fortunate enough to have had the disease in childhood. Chickenpox occurs in epidemics every 3 to 4 years—the period required to develop a new group of susceptibles. These epidemics occur in winter and early spring. Susceptibility to chickenpox remains high from birth until the disease is contracted. Although some infants under 6 months seem to have a partial immunity, most of them do not.

Chickenpox is believed to be spread by infected droplet spray from the nose and throat. Apparently the agent floats in the air for at least a short time. The period of greatest communi-cability is during the short prodrome and the early stages of eruption. When the final lesions have crusted over, the pa-tient probably is no longer able to transmit the disease. Most health departments require isolation of the patient until all these crusts have come off.

It is not believed that there are carriers of chickenpox in the sense that diphtheria or typhoid may be carried by persons long recovered. Also, indirect contact, as through third persons or objects, is thought to play no part in spreading the disease.

Symptoms and Signs

During the 3rd week after exposure and about 24 to 36 hours before the first series of lesions appears, the child coming down with chickenpox may have a mild headache, low grade fever and some malaise. Patients over 10 years of age are more likely to have some or all of these prodromal symptoms and signs. In small children, the prodrome is usually unrecognized;

in adults it, like the disease, is a time of fever and severe malaise.

The initial rash may be accompanied by an evanescent flush or morbilliform eruption. Following the appearance of the characteristic "tear drop" vesicle surrounded by a red areola, the diagnosis usually can be made. In severe cases, the eruption may be generalized; otherwise the face and extremities are partially spared. When but a few lesions are present, the upper trunk is the frequent site. Lesions may occur on the mucous membranes.

The typical lesion of chickenpox progresses from macule to papule to vesicle within 24 to 48 hours. The latter stage is diagnostic, as the monolocular vesicles containing clear fluid stand out from their dime-sized areolas like drops of water on wax paper.

Complications

Secondary infection of the chickenpox vesicle by streptococci may lead to erysipelar sepsis, scarlet fever, or rarely gangrene of the skin. Acute hemorrhagic nephritis is an occasional sequel to chickenpox complicated by streptococcic infection. Staphylococci also may infect the vesicles with resultant impetiginous lesions. Vesicles on the mucous membrane of the larynx or trachea may cause severe dyspnea. Pneumonia may complicate severe cases of chickenpox. Post-chickenpox encephalitis is rare and, like that following measles, is likely to occur toward the end of the disease or within a week or so following its termination. Transverse myelitis, cranial nerve palsies and multiple sclerosis-like clinical manifestations have occurred apparently as complications of chickenpox. While death may occur from encephalitis, the prognosis for complete recovery from C.N.S. complications is generally good.

Diagnosis

Differentiation between chickenpox and smallpox is less often necessary nowadays because of the rarity of the latter disease. While individual lesions of the two diseases might be confused, several characteristics differentiate them. Chickenpox has 3 or 4 distinct series of lesions with approximately one day separating each series. Thus after a day or so the patient clearly has lesions in various stages of development, a condition not found in smallpox where all lesions are of approximately the same developmental age. The lesions of smallpox are deeper seated than those of chickenpox and have a "shotty" feel when palpated with some pressure. Perhaps the most outstanding difference between smallpox and chickenpox is that fever and malaise are most severe preceding the eruption in smallpox, but are at peak when the eruption is at peak in chickenpox. In chickenpox, pustulation does not characteristically follow vesiculation, which fact further differentiates it from smallpox. Diseases other than smallpox which must be included in the differential diagnosis include secondary syphilis, impetigo, infected eczema, insect bites and stings, drug rashes, dermatitis venenata, hydroa estivale, and herpes zoster.

Prophylaxis

There is no vaccine for protection against chickenpox. Gamma globulin (℞ 94), in doses several times those effective against measles, may have some preventive or modifying action against chickenpox but proof is not yet conclusive. Convalescent serum can be used, if available, to protect selected patients, but as a rule there seems no need for such measures.

Treatment

The mild case of chickenpox requires only simple symptomatic treatment, chiefly the application of antipruritic lotion (℞ 124) or powder (℞ 127) to control the bothersome itching. Because of the frequency of staphylococcic or streptococcic infection in the vesicular lesions, the child should be carefully bathed with soap and water and clothed in clean underclothing. His hands should be kept clean and the nails clipped. It is not advisable to apply antiseptics to the individual lesions unless they become secondarily infected. A single infected vesicle may be treated with penicillin ointment (℞ 31); widespread involvement is treated most effectively by I.M. administration of penicillin (℞ 28, 29).

SMALLPOX

(Variola)

An acute, highly contagious disease, initiated by sudden severe constitutional symptoms, characterized by a progressive cutaneous eruption that often results in permanent pits and scars on healing.

Etiology and Incidence

Smallpox is caused by a filtrable virus, closely related to vaccinia virus that causes cowpox. It is present through all stages of the disease, in the vesicle, pustule, crust, nasopharyngeal secretion, excreta, and in the blood. The virus resists drying and may be transmitted in the dried scales of the lesions, or it may be air-borne in the droplets of nasopharyngeal secretions. This disease may be transmitted directly from person to person or by contact with contaminated clothing or household articles.

The disease is endemic in the tropics, but occurs throughout the world in areas where vaccination is not practiced. All ages, sexes, and races are susceptible.

Symptoms, Signs, and Course

Incubation period: Usually 10 to 12 days, but extremes from 5 to 31 days have been observed.

Pre-eruptive stage: Onset is abrupt with distressing chills, fever to 103° or 104° F., rapid pulse and respirations, prostration, severe headache and muscular pains. Persistent vomiting may be an early symptom especially in children, among whom delirium, convulsions and coma may be the outstanding manifestations. A prodromal, transient (24 to 48 hours), morbilliform, scarlatiniform, or hemorrhagic (petechial) rash may appear on the thighs and abdomen. During this period, the patient is acutely ill, diarrhea or constipation may occur and the temperature may increase to 106° or 107° F.; however, the severity of these symptoms gives no indication of the type of eruption to follow.

Stage of eruption (3rd day): The severe symptoms usually lessen considerably with the appearance of the eruption. The lesions are pink-red macules of varied dimensions which appear first on the forehead, temples, perioral region, and anterior surface of the wrists. Rapid spread throughout the scalp, face, ears, neck, forearms, and hands, follows. Extension to the trunk, abdomen, lower extremities, palms, and soles may be complete within 24 hours. These macules disappear on pressure. By the 2nd day of the eruption, the lesions become papules by the increased induration of their base and give a shotty feeling under the skin. By the 3rd day of the eruption, the papules are converted into hemispherical (2 to 3 mm.), multilocular, umbilicated, hard vesicles with a glistening surface, containing clear serum and a pinkish areola at the base. These may become confluent as their number increases. Unlike the vesicles of chickenpox, these are in the skin rather than on the surface.

Stage of suppuration (5th or 6th day of eruption): A secondary rise of the temperature and return of general symptoms, the "suppurative" fever of smallpox, which usually is less intense than that of the initial stage, makes its appearance at this time and persists until the involution of the eruptive process. The vesicles mature, a pearly appearance develops, the contents gradually increase in turbidity and become frankly purulent. These pustules assume a yellowish or grayish white appearance as the areola broadens and deepens in color to a purplish red. The lesions on the trunk and extremities usually are less confluent than those on the face, and lag somewhat in development, while those on the hands and feet may be quite confluent and produce severe pain, especially in the palms and soles. Edema of the loose areolar tissue about the face distorts the features and may cause almost complete closure of the eyes. Mucous membranes near external surfaces exhibit denudation of the epithelial surface, erosions or superficial ulcerations. Involvement of the nasal mucosa, mouth, pharynx, larynx, vagina, urethral meatus, or rectum may occur and is severe and painful. During the pustular stage, soreness of the skin is the patient's chief complaint. There may be a leuko-penia earlier, but a leukocytosis develops with the onset of suppuration.

Period of involution: By the 8th or 9th day of the eruption in uncomplicated cases, general improvement begins; the pus-tules on the face have reached their greatest development and begin to regress by shrinking and rupturing. The exuding pu-rulent material dries on the skin in the form of dirty, yellowish, malodorous crusts. The inflammatory edema and redness around the pustules slowly subside, exudates dry, and the crusts begin to fall off in about one week. This drying stage is com-monly accompanied by intense itching. Reddish brown stains at the site of the pustules may persist for months. Hair of the head, beard, or eyebrows may be lost and the nails of the fingers and toes may be shed. After the decrustation, which requires 1 to 2 weeks, the extent of permanent injury ("pock-marks") is evident. The amount of scarring depends on the depth of the destructive inflammatory process; involvement of the epiderm alone produces no scars, but involvement of the true skin results in the characteristic pits.

Other Forms, Complications and Sequelae

A confluent form of smallpox may occur. The lesions on the face, head, palms, and soles may coalesce with maturation of the pustules, and the entire skin of the head and extremities may become a massive superficial abscess. Great facial disfig-urement may ensue and skin of the hands and feet may be shed entirely.

Two severe, usually fatal, hemorrhagic varieties of the dis-ease may occur: (1) Purpura variolosa develops in the first few days of the disease, usually before the formation of the papules, and is characterized by extensive hemorrhages into the corium. Death may follow in 2 to 6 days. (2) Variola pustulosa hemor-rhagica is characterized by hemorrhage into the areola of the pock itself. The earlier the hemorrhage, the graver the prog-nosis. Recovery from this form of smallpox is very rare.

A mild form of smallpox (varioloid), with a scattered, super-ficial rash that rarely produces scars, may be seen, especially in those who may have partial immunity from previous vac-cination. In this form, there is no secondary rise of fever and the whole course may be considerably shortened.

Complications and various sequelae may ensue: impetiginous lesions, furuncles and subcutaneous abscesses are the most com-mon. Erysipelar gangrene of the skin, ocular and aural compli-cations occur occasionally, but lesions of the myocardium and central nervous system are rare.

Diagnosis

The diagnosis of smallpox cannot be based on any one char-acteristic symptom. It must depend upon history of exposure, prevalence of an epidemic, history of vaccination, careful consideration of the symptoms, and appearance and distribution of the eruption.

During the initial stage, smallpox must be differentiated from severe cases of influenza, typhus, meningitis, and typhoid fever. The prodromal rash of smallpox may easily be confused with measles or scarlet fever. In the papular and vesicular stage, especially in the modified or "varioloid" form, it may be confused with chickenpox, generalized vaccinia, and at times with syphilis and drug eruptions.

While the diagnosis of typical florid smallpox is not difficult, when it appears in the modified form it may present great difficulties. It is only by vigilance and the most meticulous observation of the suspected case that error can be avoided. Serologic and virus identification tests are valuable but not generally available.

Prognosis

Where vaccination has been strictly enforced the mortality of the disease has been minimal. The mortality of unmodified smallpox in unvaccinated individuals is 20 to 50% or more. There is great variation in different epidemics. In modified smallpox (varioloid) the mortality is less than 2%.

Prophylaxis (Vaccination)

The efficacy of smallpox vaccination is unquestioned. It imparts practically complete immunity against the disease. Immunity develops within 8 days of a successful vaccination and lasts for 2 to 5 years or longer. However, exposure to smallpox requires vaccination or revaccination within 24 to 48 hours to assure full protection. Partial protection, however, with modification of the subsequent attack of smallpox may often be gained even if vaccination is delayed several days.

The usual and preferred site for vaccination is the posterolateral aspect of the upper third of either arm over the deltoid muscle. For cosmetic reasons, females frequently ask to be vaccinated on the lateral aspect of the upper thigh, the buttock, or on the inner surface of the lower third of the leg. Because of the greater sensitivity of these parts and because the frequent involvement of the femoral and inguinal nodes causes much more discomfort and pain and may incapacitate the individual, such sites are better avoided.

The site chosen should be cleansed with soap and water if necessary, followed by the application of a quickly evaporating skin antiseptic such as alcohol, ether or acetone. The prepared area must be completely dry before vaccination. A small drop of vaccine is placed on the skin, which then is gently stretched taut. A sterile needle, held like a pencil, as nearly horizontal to the skin surface as possible, is pressed gently through the drop of vaccine into the outer layer of the skin 10 to 15 times. (The point of the needle is not pushed into the skin, rather the whole pointed end is pressed downward against the skin.) When done properly this procedure is rapid, painless, and does not draw blood. The multiple punctures can readily be confined to an area ⅛ inch in diameter. Other methods include acupuncture, wherein the needle is held perpendicular to the skin and the point pushed directly into the superficial layers 8 to 10 times, or the scratch method, by which 2 to 4 small ¼-inch scratches are made through the drop of vaccine. With this latter method control is somewhat more difficult, blood frequently appears, and the resulting vaccination is more likely to become secondarily infected and form a larger, more unsightly scar.

Following vaccination, it is best to permit the drop of vaccine to dry completely before allowing replacement of the clothing. However, the drop may be blotted with a pledget of sterile dry cotton or gauze to shorten the period of drying. No dressing, cover, or "protective hood" of any sort should be used. With infants, clothing usually covers the site, but older children and adults must be warned not to touch or scratch the area, not only to prevent secondary infection but also to avoid autoinoculation of other sites. Should the vesicle of the primary or accelerated reaction break and discharge the fluid exudate, exposure to air for 10 to 30 minutes permits drying and the formation of a fibrinous crust, thereby avoiding the necessity of a cover. However, for marked reactions secondarily infected with purulent discharge, the standard surgical treatment of any purulent skin inflammation is indicated, including wet dressings if necessary.

Results or "takes" are classified according to size, nature and time of appearance: (1) **Primary vaccination** (vaccinia, "take") indicates absence of immunity. A small pink-red papule appears in 3 to 5 days, vesicles form and the lesion attains its greatest diameter in 8 to 14 days following the vaccination. At first the vesicle is filled with a clear serous fluid and surrounded by a red areola; later, the contents become turbid and a pustule forms. The dome of the pustule gradually flattens out and fuses with the base, forming a crust which, if unmolested, is ready to fall off in about 3 weeks. A glistening red scar remains for a considerable time, but within 1 or 2 years becomes white and pitted (vaccination mark). (2) **Accelerated vaccination** (vaccinoid, "mild take") indicates existence of partial immunity. The stages here are similar in appearance to those of primary vaccination, but the size of the reaction is less, and the whole course is shortened or accelerated. The papule appears within 24 to 48 hours and the maximum reaction is reached in 5 to 7 days. A small scar (vaccination mark) may result. (3) An **"immune" reaction** (early or sensitivity reaction) consists of a very small papule developing within 8 to 24 hours, often with marked itching, which disappears in 3 to 5 days. This is commonly considered an indication of immunity, but may represent sensitivity only. Many authorities insist upon the formation of a tiny vesicle before considering this to represent immunity or a "take." However, when a potent vaccine and proper technic have been used, this reaction generally is accepted as the equivalent of a "take" and representative of immunity.

The patient should always be warned that headache, malaise, fever, and regional lymphadenopathy usually accompany the primary vaccination and more severe forms of the accelerated type. Occasionally, bed rest and elevation of the arm or leg are necessary. In most cases, however, the symptoms subside in 1 or 2 days without requiring treatment. A generalized vaccinia may occur with development of constitutional symptoms and a red papular rash over the body which usually subsides in several days. Occasionally, multiple vesicular lesions appear in the vicinity of the vaccination site. Secondary infection of the vaccination is rather common, but other complications such as postvaccinal encephalitis or tetanus are rare. Autoinoculation or vaccination of the face, lips, conjunctiva, and other areas is possible from transmission of the infectious exudate; also, other individuals may be inoculated from contact with the serum or crust of an active vaccination.

Following vaccination, the site should be examined in 2 or 3 days, again on the 5th or 7th day, and finally on the 7th or 9th day to ensure proper evaluation of the reaction. If such a schedule is impractical, the patient may be recalled on the 7th day only, since by this time the "immune" reaction will have disappeared, the accelerated reaction will be at its height or subsiding, and the primary reaction will be in the early vesicular stage and still developing; however, misinterpretation is possible because of normal variations in reactions. Causes of failure include use of impotent vaccine (outdated; not properly refrigerated), improper cleansing of skin prior to vaccination (not cleansed, not dried, or vaccine inactivated by the presence of antiseptic), or the use of an ineffective method of vaccination. In this event, the vaccination should be repeated in 1 month, or sooner if necessary—provided that the necessity outweighs the possibility of a severe "double vaccination." If unsuccessful then, an attempt should be made each 3 months until a successful "take" has been obtained. Failure to react is no guarantee of immunity.

Infants from the age of 1 week on may be vaccinated. In any event vaccination is preferable prior to the 6th month and should always be performed before the 1st year (see ROUT. IMMUN. PROC.). A repeat vaccination is indicated before a child enters school, and at any time in adult life that an epidemic threatens, or travel to an endemic area is contemplated. Ideally, vaccination of all persons should be repeated about every 5 years.

Infantile eczema, impetigo, tuberculosis, diabetes, and debilitating disease are, in general, contraindications to vaccination. For these cases, the urgency of vaccination must be weighed against the physical status of the patient. Following successful smallpox vaccination, the blood serum of many individuals will cause false positive Wassermann or Kahn reactions for several months, and this fact must be borne in mind when evaluating such reactions.

Treatment

There is no specific treatment for smallpox. Therapy is directed toward making the patient comfortable, maintenance of nutrition and local treatment of the lesions.

Isolation: The treatment of the patient with smallpox should be undertaken only in a hospital for contagious disease. The most meticulous, rigid isolation technic and the help of specially trained personnel are required (*see* BEDSIDE PROC.).

General treatment: The use of an air mattress, to reduce injuries to lesions on the back, and cradles to lessen contact with bed covers will contribute to the patient's comfort. Every effort should be made to maintain nutrition. Patients with painful pharyngeal or laryngeal lesions, for whom swallowing is difficult, may require a liquid diet. When these lesions subside, or to patients who do not develop such lesions, a bland nutritious diet may be given (*see* DIETS). Adequate daily intake of liquids is important. To attain this, parenteral administration of fluids may occasionally be necessary.

Local heat to the back and legs may relieve the severe muscular pains; ice bags may allay the intense headache; tepid sponge baths are sedative and help reduce the high fever.

Sedatives: Sedation is indicated in the invasive stage and later in the eruptive period when distress is acute. Bromides, (R 17) or a barbiturate (R 15) may be used in small doses for short periods and, in exceptional instances, codeine (R 10) or morphine (R 11) may be used in small amounts; paraldehyde (R 18) or chloral hydrate (R 19) may be of benefit in delirium.

Penicillin: Recent reports indicate that favorable results may be obtained from the use of penicillin (R 28, 29) parenterally for reduction of the effects of secondary bacterial invaders in the vesicular and pustular stages. The indications for penicillin therapy are even more clearly defined in the secondary bacterial complications of smallpox.

Local treatment: There is a variation of opinion concerning topical applications at the height of the eruptive stage. Some authorities advise frequent or continuous warm baths: others forbid bathing.

During the periods of pustulation and desiccation, baths in very weak antiseptic solutions are recommended for removing the purulent exudate and possibly reducing skin infection (R 145, 146).

Local impetiginous areas respond to application of 2% ammoniated mercury (℞ 89). Simple ointments such as vaseline containing 1% phenol (℞ 90) help to soften and remove crusts and to soothe the skin. Itching may be lessened by the use of lotions containing 1% phenol or mercuric chloride 1:1,000 solution (℞ 124, 125).

The mouth should be cleansed frequently with a mildly antiseptic mouthwash (℞ 108). Gargles and hot irrigations benefit the pharyngeal lesions (℞ 109). The eyes require cleansing with weak saline solution, and the lid margins should be kept moist with 5% boric acid ointment (℞ 87), 1% yellow oxide of mercury ointment (℞ 88), or 5% sulfadiazine ophthalmic ointment (℞ 47). Swabbing of the lid margins daily with a 2% silver nitrate solution (℞ 92) also is recommended as a protective measure. Lesions about the rectum and genitals may require similar special care.

MUMPS
(Epidemic parotitis)

An acute, contagious, viral disease, usually causing painful enlargement of the salivary glands, most commonly the parotids; after puberty, involvement of the testes or ovaries, C.N.S., pancreas, or breasts may occur.

Etiology and Incidence

The causative agent of mumps is a filtrable virus. It is found in the saliva of patients, where it may be present for at least 24 hours before swelling of the salivary glands develops, and throughout the entire period of glandular enlargement. It is probable that the virus enters through the mouth. It has been isolated from the blood; and, in patients with signs of C.N.S. involvement, from the spinal fluid.

Spread is by droplet infection or direct contact with materials contaminated with infected saliva. Mumps is endemic in heavily populated areas but may occur in epidemics when large numbers of susceptible individuals are brought together under crowded conditions such as occur in Army camps during a period of mobilization. The peak incidence is in late winter and early spring. Most of the cases occur in children between 5 and 15 years of age but the disease is unusual in children under 2 years. Infants up to 10 months are ordinarily immune. However, the disease may occur at any age, and cases in the older age groups are most often seen in young men and women from rural areas. One attack of mumps usually produces immunity, though second attacks may occur in from 7 to 10% of cases.

Symptoms and Signs

During the incubation period of from 14 to 21 days following exposure, the patient feels entirely well. Chilly sensations, headache, anorexia, and generalized malaise mark the onset. This is accompanied by a low to moderate fever which may last from 12 to 24 hours before any involvement of the salivary glands is noted. In mild cases, these prodromal symptoms may be absent. Pain on chewing or swallowing is the earliest symptom of parotitis. It becomes aggravated by swallowing acid liquids such as vinegar or lemon juice, only when the parotid duct is obstructed by edema. The patient exhibits marked sensitivity to pressure over the angle of the jaw. With the development of parotitis, the temperature frequently rises to 103°–104° F. Swelling of the gland reaches its maximum about the 2nd day and is associated with swelling involving the cheek and area below the ear. In most cases, both parotid glands are involved. Occasionally the submaxillary and sublingual glands may also be swollen, or more rarely may be the only glands affected. In such cases, there is swelling of the neck beneath the jaw. The oral openings of ducts of the involved glands are "pouting" and slightly inflamed. The skin over the glands may become tense and shiny. Involved glands are acutely tender during the febrile period which lasts from 24 to 72 hours.

Complications

The disease may involve organs other than the salivary glands, more commonly in patients past puberty. These other organs may be involved without primary disease in the salivary glands. This has become apparent through the use of the recently developed specific serologic methods of diagnosis.

Orchitis: Inflammation of the testicles develops in about 25% of postpuberal male patients. Swelling of the testes usually begins about 5 to 7 days after the appearance of the enlargement of the salivary glands and may rarely occur without involvement of the salivary tissue. Testicular involvement is preceded by a rise in temperature, increased malaise, headache, and sometimes nausea and vomiting. The swollen testis may become 2 to 3 times normal size and extremely painful and sensitive to touch. In about 15% of cases, both testes may be involved. The swelling disappears in from 7 to 10 days. The gland may show a decrease in size, indicating atrophy, in about 50% of untreated cases. Sterility results only if the atrophy is bilateral; it is not accompanied by loss of hormonal function.

Meningoencephalitis: Involvement of the central nervous system may develop in any age group and in either sex. About 10% of all cases show some clinical evidence of nervous tissue irritation such as severe headache, drowsiness, and nausea and vomiting. This complication customarily appears at the end of the 1st week of the disease and may be associated with stiffness of the neck and a positive Kernig's sign. These symptoms vary greatly in severity and usually disappear in less than a week. Almost always the prognosis is good, although deafness, facial paralysis, or death may occur rarely. The spinal fluid of most patients with mumps meningoencephalitis is under increased pressure and shows more than 10 cells/cu. mm., mostly lymphocytes, and protein levels greater than 30 mg./100 cc. On the other hand, when lumbar punctures are done routinely on patients with mumps, these abnormal spinal fluid findings may be discovered in individuals with no C.N.S. symptoms. This suggests that the virus often is present in nervous tissue.

Pancreatitis: Toward the end of the 1st week, a few patients may have a sudden onset of severe nausea, vomiting, and abdominal pain most severe in the epigastrium, suggesting pancreatitis. Such symptoms disappear in about one week and the patient recovers completely.

Miscellaneous: Oophoritis, prostatitis, nephritis, mastitis and involvement of the lacrimal glands are occasionally seen. Edema of the tissue over the sternum may be seen with involvement of the submaxillary glands.

Laboratory Findings

The leukocyte count usually is within normal limits averaging from 5,000 to 7,000 cells/cu. mm., with some relative increase in the number of lymphocytes. In certain cases in which the inflammation of the glands is severe, there may be an increase in the number of polymorphonuclear leukocytes.

Diagnosis

The diagnosis of typical cases of mumps during an epidemic is simple, but sporadic cases present a more difficult problem. The swelling of the parotid or other salivary glands due to the virus of mumps must be distinguished from: (1) bacterial parotid involvement occurring in streptococcal throat infections, diphtheria, or debilitated patients with poor oral hygiene, typhoid or typhus fevers; (2) Mikulicz's syndrome, a chronic, usually afebrile condition; (3) malignant tumors of the salivary glands; (4) postoperative parotitis; and (5) obstruction produced by a calculus in Stenson's duct. Enlarged lymph nodes along the mandible may be mistaken for swollen salivary glands.

Meningoencephalitis due to mumps virus must be differentiated from lymphocytic choriomeningitis and nonparalytic poliomyelitis.

The development of a specific complement fixation test for the presence of antibody for the virus of mumps in the blood serum has made it possible to make a definite diagnosis of infection with this virus even when the clinical syndrome is not characteristic. Two serial serum specimens are essential, one taken early in the disease and the second 10 days or more after onset. The demonstration of an increase in antibody titer for mumps is diagnostic. This test makes it possible to determine that a patient has been infected with mumps virus in the absence of parotid swelling, for example, in such cases as only show symptoms and signs of a meningoencephalitis. At the present time, only certain laboratories are prepared to carry out the test, but others should soon be able to do so.

Prognosis

In uncomplicated mumps, the prognosis is excellent. However, relapses may occur occasionally after about 2 weeks. In complicated cases, testicular atrophy may follow orchitis, and deafness or facial paralysis has been known to occur following involvement of the nervous system.

Prophylaxis

Patients should be isolated as soon as they become ill, since the saliva is known to be infectious for at least 24 hours before symptoms appear. The patient should remain in isolation until the glandular swelling subsides. Regulations vary in different localities but quarantine usually is not required. Contacts giving a previous history of mumps may be allowed full freedom. Susceptible individuals should be examined daily from the 14th to 21st days after exposure, to detect cases early and prevent spread of infection. This is especially important in school children. The I.M. administration, to susceptible individuals, of 20 cc. of gamma globulin specially prepared from mumps convalescent serum, during the first few days of exposure will probably protect a large percentage of those exposed. However, this material is not generally available. The use of pooled convalescent serum is not advisable due to the danger of infecting the patient with the virus of homologous serum jaundice. Pooled serum from normal adults, or the gamma globulin prepared from such serum pools, appears of little value due to a low content of mumps antibodies. Vaccines prepared from egg tissues infected with mumps virus have been shown to produce immunity in man. Their general use awaits further trial and preparation of a standard vaccine.

Treatment

Treatment is purely symptomatic. Patients should remain in bed until they are afebrile. However, strict bed rest does not appear to reduce the incidence of complications. Most patients obtain relief from the local application of heat over the affected glands, though an occasional patient may prefer an icebag. Scrupulous attention must be paid to mouth hygiene to prevent secondary bacterial infections. Mild cleansing mouthwashes (R 107, 108) are useful. Ingestion of ample fluids should be encouraged and constipation prevented with the use of a laxative (R 140) when necessary. A soft diet (q.v.) eliminates some of the pain caused by chewing. Analgesics (R 1, 9) may be used for general malaise, and a barbiturate, such as phenobarbital (R 15), for sedation as necessary.

When available, the administration to adult males of 20 ml. of gamma globulin prepared from mumps convalescent serum as soon as the diagnosis of mumps is made causes a reduction in the incidence of orchitis.

The treatment of the complications also is essentially symptomatic. Patients with orchitis should be placed on absolute bed rest, the scrotum supported in cotton on an adhesive tape bridge between the legs to avoid any tension. Cold applications often afford relief from pain. Codeine and acetylsalicylic acid (B 9) may be used to relieve discomfort. If the scrotal swelling is severe and the pain excruciating, surgical treatment by incision of the tunica vaginalis may be necessary to relieve the pain and shorten the period of disability. This may prevent or minimize subsequent atrophy of the involved testicle.

In pancreatitis, if nausea and vomiting are severe, oral feedings should be withheld, and fluid balance restored by I.V. administration of glucose and saline solutions. Fluids such as fruit juices and thin, fat-free soups may be given by mouth as soon as vomiting ceases.

Meningoencephalitis, in severe cases, may require lumbar puncture with removal of some spinal fluid in an attempt to reduce intracranial pressure and relieve the headache. Analgesics (B 1, 9) may be used further to relieve pain. Sedation (B 15) is needed to treat the associated restlessness. Except for its use in diagnosis, lumbar puncture usually is not necessary in mild cases.

WHOOPING COUGH

(Pertussis, Kink-cough)

An acute, highly communicable, infectious disease, characterized by a paroxysmal or spasmodic cough which usually ends with a prolonged, high-pitched crowing inspiration, commonly known as the whoop, and occasionally accompanied by vomiting.

Etiology and Epidemiology

Hemophilus pertussis, a small nonmotile gram-negative coccobacillus, is the causative agent. *B. bronchisepticus* closely resembles this organism, as does *B. parapertussis.* The latter causes a disease, parapertussis, which at times is indistinguishable from pertussis, although usually it is milder and less frequently fatal.

Whooping cough is endemic throughout the world and reaches epidemic proportions every 2 to 4 years in a given locality, variations according to seasons being insignificant. The disease occurs at all ages, usually following the first exposure. Customarily, infants possess no protective antibodies against *H. pertussis,* and 50% of all cases occur before 2 years of age. One attack usually confers lifelong immunity, but second attacks occasionally are reported.

Transmission generally is by aspiration of *H. pertussis* disseminated into the air by a patient, particularly in the catarrhal and early paroxysmal stages of the disease. Transmission by contact with contaminated articles is probably rare. Carriers may be implicated, but patients usually are not infectious after the 8th week. It is thought that dogs and cats can contract and spread the disease.

Symptoms and Signs

The incubation period is on the average from 7 to 14 days and probably never extends beyond 3 weeks. *H. pertussis* invades the mucosa of the nasopharynx, trachea, bronchi, and bronchioles, causing an increased secretion of mucus, which at first is not thick. Later, it becomes viscid and tenacious. Typically, the disease lasts about 6 weeks, and is divided into 3 stages, catarrhal, paroxysmal, and convalescent. The onset of the **catarrhal stage** is insidious, generally with sneezing, lacrimation, or other signs of coryza; poor appetite; listlessness; rarely fever; and a hacking cough at night, which gradually becomes diurnal.

After 10 to 14 days the cough becomes **paroxysmal;** rapidly consecutive coughs (as many as 5 to 15 or more) occur. These are followed by a hurried, deep inspiration, which produces the whoop. After a few normal breaths another paroxysm may begin, the whoop being repeated from 1 to 20 times with each attack. In severe cases, these attacks may recur as often as 50 times in 24 hours. Crying, sneezing, chilling the skin, violent muscular effort, inhaling irritating substances, or overfilling the stomach with food or liquid may increase paroxysms, as may psychic disturbances, such as fright and anger, and mimicry. They may be particularly troublesome at night. During or following the paroxysms copious amounts of viscid mucus may be expelled. However, in infants and young children, this usually is swallowed. Vomiting subsequent to paroxysms, or due to gagging because of the tenacious mucus, also is characteristic.

The **convalescent stage** usually begins within 4 weeks; paroxysms are not as frequent or severe, the patient appears less ill, and vomiting decreases. The child often retains an ability voluntarily to initiate paroxysms and vomiting, which he may use to gain his own ends. Aside from this, the development of bronchitis or a cold within a year may cause a prompt recurrence of these manifestations.

Fever and objective physical findings in uncomplicated pertussis often are minimal. Cases may be so mild that whooping and vomiting are absent. On the other hand, infants or the aged, without exhibiting the characteristic whoop, may be critically ill with a bronchopneumonia or other complication of the disease.

While the blood changes in pertussis are typical, absence of a leukocytosis does not rule out the disease. Leukocyte counts usually vary between 15,000 and 20,000, rarely reaching 50,000. Differential counts usually reveal 60 to 80% of small lymphocytes. During convalescence moderate eosinophilia frequently is present. The urine may contain albumin and casts, and uric acid output may be doubled or trebled.

Complications and Sequelae

The most frequent complications are those associated with the respiratory tract, including, in infants, asphyxia. Convulsions are not uncommon. Pneumonia, in particular bronchopneumonia, is responsible for the majority of the fatalities, and is a frequent complication in old people and in children under 3 years of age. Secondary to the increased intrathoracic pressure during paroxysms, interstitial emphysema, subcutaneous emphysema, and pneumothorax may occur, but are infrequent. Bronchiectasis, particularly in debilitated children, is a fairly common sequela, as is residual emphysema. Atelectasis may result from occlusion of a bronchiole by a mucous plug. An ulcer of the frenum of the tongue may develop, because of wounding by the lower incisors during paroxysms. Increased intracranial pressure may hemorrhage into the brain, the eyes, the skin, and mucous membranes. Umbilical hernia occasionally occurs; also prolapse of the rectum. Brain damage from cerebral hemorrhage, cerebral edema, or encephalitis may result in spastic paralysis, mental retardation, or other neurologic disorder. Otitis media is frequent.

Diagnosis

Distinguishing pertussis in its catarrhal stage from bronchitis or influenza is occasionally difficult. A lymphocytosis of 50% or more in an afebrile or slightly febrile child over 3 years of age with a suspicious cough usually indicates pertussis. In the catarrhal and early paroxysmal stages, 80 to 90% of the cases yield positive cultures of *H. pertussis*. More consistent results are obtained by the nasal swab method. Small sterile cotton swabs on 28-gauge, zinc-coated wire which may be passed into the region of the middle turbinates or through the nostril to the nasopharynx are desirable for this purpose. Standard Bordet-Gengou media should be used, and the plates smeared with one loopful of aqueous solution of penicillin (1,000 u./cc.) at time of inoculation. Or the cough-plate method may be used, in which the plate is held 4 inches from the patient's mouth during a paroxysm of coughing. A patient may develop parapertussis with symptoms clinically indistinguishable from those of pertussis, and even though immune to the latter. Antibodies, as demonstrated by the agglutinin titer and by complement fixation and mouse protective tests, appear during convalescence from pertussis, and after successful immunization.

The results of skin tests for immunity have in the past not always been reliable. However, a new intradermal test that employs purified agglutinogen and gives a tuberculin-like reaction in immune individuals, has yielded consistently accurate results in those tested, with the possible exception of young infants. Usually, the test becomes positive about 3 weeks after onset of the disease.

Prognosis

In children below 4 years of age, pertussis is dangerous, and of the acute infectious diseases it perhaps ranks first as a cause of mortality in infancy. Before 6 months of age, the death rate may be as high as 25%, but with good medical care this should not exceed 2 to 4%. In older children and adults, except the aged, the disease is troublesome but rarely serious.

Prophylaxis

Persons ill with pertussis should be quarantined from susceptible family members, also from cats and dogs; further, exposed individuals should be isolated from susceptible unexposed persons for at least 2 or 3 weeks.

Active Immunization: This may be started as early as 2 to 3 months of age (*see* Rout. Immun. Proc.). A triple antigen, combining pertussis vaccine and the toxoids of tetanus and diphtheria, is recommended by some, for two reasons: First, the antigenic response to the pertussis vaccine is greater when the vaccine is mixed with toxoid; second, the number of injections necessary for the various immunization procedures is materially reduced. At approximately 4-year intervals thereafter booster doses of saline pertussis vaccine should be given to ensure retention of immunity. After 4 or 5 years of age, the triple antigen is contraindicated, since constitutional reactions are too frequent. As dosages of these antigens and those of other preparations subsequently to be mentioned vary, the manufacturer's directions contained in the package should be followed.

Passive Immunization: Success with this procedure depends upon early administration of hyperimmune serum following exposure to pertussis. Unfortunately, the susceptible infant or child often is well along in the incubation period when the disease is recognized in the individual to whom he was exposed. Either hyperimmune human or rabbit serum is used. (Caution! *see* serum, *under* Treatment.) When exposure is continuous, these injections should be repeated every 7 to 10 days until danger of infection has passed.

Dosage: Human serum: (1) Vacuum-dried, 1 dose, equivalent to 20 cc. of whole serum, I.M. (℞ 104). (2) Gamma globulin fraction (℞ 94), 1 dose of 2.5 cc. I.M., never I.V. Refined rabbit serum: 1 dose of 4 cc. I.M. (℞ 104). Before using a rabbit serum preparation, test patient for sensitivity.

Treatment

General: If the disease is not severe, bed rest usually will be unnecessary for older children, who may be permitted quiet outdoor play on warm, clear days. Activity and extreme changes of temperature stimulate attacks of coughing. The patient's room should be maintained constantly at 65° to 70° F., at the same time admitting fresh air. Frequent small meals are preferable, and it is helpful, particularly with younger children, to give solid foods and liquids separately. Refeeding 15 to 30 minutes after a meal is vomited is essential in maintaining good nutrition, as is providing an adequate fluid intake. Parenteral fluids are administered if necessary, particularly in critically ill infants. The use of an abdominal binder may be helpful in infants or other weak children, especially those with rickets. In young infants the use of suction to remove excess mucus from the throat may be lifesaving. When possible an electric suction apparatus should be kept at hand. Otherwise, a mouth-suction apparatus or, less preferably, a large ear syringe or enema bulb may be used. In the presence of cyanosis which is not immediately relieved by removing the mucus, oxygen therapy should be used. Vinethene or chloroform inhalations, preferably the former, may be needed to ward off suffocation or convulsions when the paroxysms are frequent or severe. In such instances intubation, as used in diphtheria, may be instituted with benefit. An infant's nose, mouth and throat should be cleaned at least once daily with warm water, physiologic saline, or 2% sodium bicarbonate solution. Mineral oil should not be instilled in the nose to soften nasal crusts.

Local applications: Steam inhalations with, but probably as effective without, compound tincture of benzoin (℞ 141), may allay the bronchitis and cause the viscid exudates to be expelled with more ease.

Drugs: Expectorant cough mixtures are of little value and may increase nausea and vomiting. Mild sedatives such as phenobarbital (℞ 15) are useful for promoting rest and sleep. Codeine (℞ 10) and paregoric (℞ 128) also are used but opiates should be avoided if possible, as should indiscriminate use of any drug. In the more severe cases, instilling rectally 2 to 8 cc. of ether as a 25% solution in olive oil may be helpful. Streptomycin has been administered in pertussis by nasal instillation, aerosol, and parenterally with beneficial effects, especially when given early in the course of the disease (*see* ANTIBIOTIC THERAPY). Aureomycin (℞ 35) and Chloromycetin (℞ 36) have been used with some success but require further evaluation. Although *H. pertussis* is not sensitive to penicillin, often a complicating condition such as bronchopneumonia or otitis media will be due to other organisms which are sensitive to the drug. Penicillin (℞ 28, 29) therefore should be given in full therapeutic doses to individuals exhibiting such complications. Since sulfadiazine (℞ 37) and sulfamerazine (℞ 38) appear to be somewhat effective against *H. pertussis,* one of these also should be given, possibly in all severe cases and particularly when a complication is present. Of the calculated daily dose of sulfadiazine, ¼ (or perhaps ½ in the case of a critically ill infant) may be given initially and ⅛ of the total daily dose administered thereafter at 4-hour intervals. Dose for children is 30 to 60 mg. (gr. ss to i)/lb. body wt./24 hours, the larger dose being advised in most instances, with not more than 8 Gm. (ℨ ii) in 24 hours. Sulfamerazine, more slowly absorbed and excreted, is given in doses of 30 to 50 mg. (gr. ss to ¾)/lb. body wt./24 hours, the larger dose usually being advisable in the case of this compound also, with ¼ the calculated dose (or ½; *see under* sulfadiazine above) being given initially and thereafter the proportionate fractions of the daily dose at 8- to 12-hour intervals. An alkali such as sodium citrate or sodium bicarbonate should be given with the sulfonamide (*see* SULFONAMIDE THERAPY). The urine should be observed for crystalluria or other evidence of renal irritation, the white cell count repeated at least once every 3 days, and the patient examined daily for rashes, pallor, or jaundice.

Serum: In treating pertussis, hyperimmune human or rabbit serum (℞ 104) is of definite value as conjunctive therapy, especially in younger children and infants. With critically ill infants in particular, there appears to be a better therapeutic response following I.V. injection of the serum. For this purpose vacuum-dried human serum has definite advantage, although a refined rabbit serum may be administered I.V. with caution. In every instance, lack of sensitivity to a rabbit serum preparation must be ruled out before it is used. The dose of vacuum-dried human serum is calculated in terms of original volume. By adding 8 cc. of Water for Injection U.S.P., the residue from 20 cc. of serum may be restored to the liquid state. (This serum may be obtained from the Philadelphia Serum Exchange when unavailable elsewhere.) **Dosage:** (1) Vacuum-dried human hyperimmune serum; (*a*) critically ill infants, 40 to 60 cc. I.V., repeated 1 or 2 times at 24-hour intervals; (*b*) average cases, 20 cc., I.M. or I.V., repeated 3 or 4 times at 24- to 48-hour intervals. (2) Refined rabbit serum: Depending both on the severity of the illness and the product being used, the dose varies from 4 to 8 cc., preferably I.M., repeated 3 or 4 times at 24- to 48-hour intervals.

Neither the gamma globulin fraction of human nor that of rabbit hyperimmune serum is safe for I.V. use, as at present prepared. Of the two forms available for I.M. administration, the human serum is preferable. Approximately 2.5 cc. of either type is equivalent to 20 cc. of whole serum. **Dosage:** Gamma globulin fraction (℞ 94) of either human or rabbit serum, according to the severity of the illness, 2.5 to 5 cc. I.M., repeated 3 or 4 times at 24- to 48-hour intervals. Given in this way, serum seldom causes unfavorable reactions.

INFLUENZA
(La Grippe, "Flu")

A highly contagious acute disease caused by a filtrable virus and characterized by fever, prostration, aches and pains, and inflammation of the respiratory mucous membranes.

Etiology and Epidemiology

Acute uncomplicated influenza with recovery is the most frequently encountered variety of this disease. It is generally believed that these cases are of virus origin. The known viruses causing influenza are designated as types A and B. The disease can be reproduced in both man and animals with viruses isolated from patients with influenza. There is an increase in the virus antibody titer in the serum of patients with the clinical syndrome. Rarely, as in the pandemic of 1918, a fatal outcome is frequent due to unusual virulence of the virus or secondary bacterial invasion, or both.

Secondary bacterial pneumonia following influenza is most often due to hemolytic streptococcus, staphylococcus, pneumococcus, *Klebsiella pneumoniae, Hemophilus influenzae.* Fatal cases have been reported in which an influenza virus and one of these bacteria have been isolated from the same lung.

The disease may be sporadic or epidemic. Epidemics occur every 1 to 4 years, and develop rapidly, since most persons are susceptible to the virus and its incubation period is brief (1 to 3 days). Influenza also may become pandemic, spreading to all parts of the world. The last pandemic was in 1918–19, during which more than 10 million people died of the disease. Following an attack, a partial or complete immunity persists for up to 1 year.

Symptoms, Signs, and Complications

The onset of influenza usually is sudden and often marked by chills or chilly sensations and fever. Constitutional symptoms are prominent and consist chiefly of prostration, generalized aches and pains most pronounced in the back and legs, headache, weakness, and anorexia. There is a subjective sense of anxiety. Symptoms in the respiratory tract usually are moderate, with sore throat, unproductive cough, mild substernal distress, and sometimes coryza. The soft palate, posterior part of the hard palate, tonsillar pillars, and posterior pharyngeal wall may be reddened, but exudate is not seen unless there also is a secondary bacterial infection.

In mild cases, the temperature rises to 101° or 102° F. and lasts for 2 or 3 days; in severe cases it reaches 103° to 104° and continues, with a corresponding degree of prostration, for 4 or 5 days. The acute symptoms usually subside rapidly with the cessation of fever, although weakness, sweating, and fatigue may continue for several days and occasionally for weeks.

Persistence of fever, cough, and other respiratory symptoms beyond 5 days suggests secondary bacterial invasion. When this occurs, crepitant or subcrepitant rales may be detected, usually at both pulmonary bases posteriorly. The cough increases and sputum is produced.

The most important and dangerous complication is secondary bacterial pneumonia. Other possible complications are bronchitis, sinusitis, otitis media, and cervical lymphadenitis.

Diagnosis

In uncomplicated cases, examination of the chest usually reveals no abnormality. In distinguishing influenza from other infections of the respiratory tract, consideration should be given to the mode of onset, whether an influenza epidemic is in progress, the severity of constitutional symptoms, the presence or absence of exudate or a membrane on the tonsils. The leukocyte count is low in uncomplicated influenza, sometimes reaching a definite leukopenia with a relative lymphocytosis. The diagnosis of influenza may be confirmed by the isolation and identification of one of the influenza viruses, A or B. With the common cold, severe constitutional symptoms are absent. With tonsillitis due to hemolytic streptococcus, although severe systemic symptoms often are present, there usually is an exudate or a membrane over the tonsils which is absent in influenza. Especially during epidemics, the clinical manifestations of influenza may include pulmonary symptoms simulating those of atypical pneumonia.

The prodromal symptoms of a number of other infectious diseases, such as the common exanthems, virus pneumonia, infectious mononucleosis, infectious hepatitis, lymphocytic choriomeningitis, yellow fever, smallpox, and rickettsial diseases, may simulate those of influenza in their systemic manifestations. Exacerbations of incipient pulmonary tuberculosis often resemble influenza by the presence of fever, constitutional symptoms, and cough. The frequent recurrence of influenza-like syndromes may lead the physician to suspect tuberculosis.

A complicating pneumonia may be suspected when the patient's temperature fails to subside after 4 or 5 days or if a secondary rise occurs. It is probable that the "relapses" frequently seen in influenza are really due to bacterial infection of the lung. In addition to signs of bronchopneumonia on physical examination, leukocytosis, with young granulocytes in the blood smear, is a particularly valuable diagnostic sign in bacterial pneumonia. The cough becomes productive, and other symptoms of pneumonia develop if bacterial infection of the lungs is present and remains unchecked.

Prognosis

In uncomplicated influenza, recovery is the rule. Even in cases complicated by severe bacterial pneumonia, the sulfonamide drugs and the newer antibiotics may be expected to decrease the fatality rates. One attack of influenza frequently renders the patient temporarily immune to that same causative virus, but apparently not to others.

Prophylaxis

Patients with influenza should be isolated if possible. Although the spread of the viral disease is not appreciably curbed by this means, it probably will protect the patient from pathogenic bacteria in the respiratory tracts of persons with whom he comes in contact, whether they be carriers or patients with active infection.

Vaccines prepared from representative strains of influenza virus are available commercially and have proved effective in preventing influenza. Evidence of their prophylactic value has been obtained in experimental animals and also in human volunteers exposed to the virus. Careful studies of a number of epidemics also have shown a low incidence of influenza among vaccinated persons as compared with control groups. The vaccinated individual develops immunity within 2 weeks. However, it must be emphasized that influenza due to strains of virus not represented in the vaccine may occur sporadically or in epidemic form in vaccinated persons. The vaccine should be given subcut. in a dose of 1 cc. to adults and 0.5 cc. to children. One inoculation a year, preferably in the fall, is necessary for protection. In addition, if serologic study indicates a sporadic or early case due to the specific viruses, prompt inoculation of contacts may be effective in preventing the development of influenza and subsequent epidemic spread.

Local reactions to the vaccines, such as redness, swelling, tenderness, and heat, or general reactions with fever and constitutional symptoms are not uncommon. They may be minimized by giving the total amount of vaccine in divided doses at 1 or 2 day intervals. Intradermal inoculation with 0.1 cc. doses is under trial in an attempt to minimize reactions and conserve material, and preliminary reports indicate an excellent antibody response.

Severe immediate reactions are very rare, but may occur with fatal results. Their incidence can be reduced by taking a careful history concerning sensitivity to eggs, since the vaccines are made from virus grown in chick embryos and contain egg protein. Some authorities recommend a preliminary intradermal test dose of 0.01 cc. of the vaccine. In any case, epinephrine should be kept at hand ready for immediate use when vaccine is administered, and the patient should be closely watched for half an hour or more after the injection.

Treatment

Since there is no specific chemotherapy available and vaccines are useless once the disease has become established, treatment is symptomatic. Patients should remain in bed during the acute stage of the disease and for 24 to 48 hours after the temperature has become normal and medications have been withdrawn. The diet should be light, with fluids up to 3,000 or 3,500 cc. daily, and laxatives if necessary.

The constitutional symptoms of acute uncomplicated influenza are severe, but fortunately the antipyretic and analgesic drugs are helpful (℞ 1, 4, 9, 10). Care should be taken not to allow the reduction of temperature caused by antipyretic drugs to confuse the original diagnosis or to give a false sense of security regarding the clinical course and development of complications. The clinical syndrome in individual cases often is atypical enough to make it impossible to be sure that it actually represents influenza. In such cases, it may be desirable to give antipyretic drugs for the relief of constitutional symptoms, but it should be realized that they lower the temperature artificially and nonspecifically in other diseases as well as influenza. For the same reason, it is usually wise to discontinue antipyretics or diminish the dose as soon as the temperature becomes normal, so that a secondary rise will not be obscured.

Treatment of respiratory symptoms may not be necessary in the less severe cases, but often it is desirable to administer mild remedies. One or 2 drops of 0.25% Neo-Synephrine (℞ 116) in isotonic salt solution may be instilled into the nose every 3 hours to relieve nasal obstruction. Gargles of warm isotonic salt solution are valuable for sore throat. The inhalation of steam may alleviate respiratory symptoms to some extent and also prevent the drying of secretions. A codeine cough mixture often is indicated (℞ 144).

The onset of secondary bacterial pneumonia usually is gradual and for a considerable time it may be difficult to predict whether bacterial pneumonia will develop. During this period of uncertainty, the prophylactic administration of antibacterial agents such as the sulfonamides or penicillin is justified, especially as early use enhances their effectiveness. In severe epidemics with a high incidence of secondary bacterial infection, it may become desirable to administer these drugs routinely even though no signs of pneumonia are detected when the patient is first seen. The dosage and methods of administration are discussed in the chapter on pneumonia (q.v.), and these need not be altered when the drugs are given prophylactically or for suspected early infection. Other less serious complications (q.v.), such as sinusitis, otitis media, or lymphadenitis, also may require chemotherapy with the sulfonamides or penicillin, or with streptomycin if the infection is due to *H. influenzae*.

Ambulation following an atack of influenza should be undertaken gradually and full activity postponed until weakness, dizziness, and easy fatigue have practically disappeared. Premature activity is likely to precipitate a relapse.

23

INFECTIOUS MONONUCLEOSIS
(Infectious lymphadenosis, Glandular fever)

An acute infectious disease, characterized clinically by the constitutional symptoms of an infection and generalized lymphadenopathy; pathologically by hyperplasia of lymphatic tissue throughout the body; hematologically by the appearance of abnormal lymphocytes in the circulating blood; and serologically by the presence of a heterophile agglutinin.

Etiology and Incidence

Although no etiologic agent has been found, the disorder probably is due to a virus. It occurs in epidemic form (especially in children, and in young people, such as in colleges or other institutions), as well as in sporadic form. In epidemic form, it behaves like an easily transmitted infection, which probably is air-borne.

Symptoms and Signs

The term "glandular fever" denominates the two main features of the typical case: lymphadenopathy and fever. Following an incubation period of 5 to 15 days, there are vague, grippe-like symptoms, such as malaise, fatigue, headache, and chilliness. In addition, symptoms reflecting involvement of the lymphatic tissue in various systems may occur. When the central nervous system is affected, the patient has severe headache, signs of meningeal irritation (photophobia, eyeball tenderness, stiffness of the neck), and neuritic pains. When the lungs are involved, chest pain, dyspnea, and cough result. When the heart is infiltrated, tachycardia, cardiac arrhythmias, and electrocardiographic changes may occur. When the mesentery or the gastrointestinal tract itself is involved, abdominal pain, nausea, and jaundice may occur. Transitory erythematous eruptions of the skin are occasionally seen. Common clinical types of the disorder are: **glandular,** in which lymphadenopathy is prominent; **febrile,** marked by fever; and **anginose,** in which pharyngeal symptoms and signs are outstanding. Because of the diffuseness of the pathologic infiltration, the symptomatology may be so varied as to be extremely confusing. However, the typical case of infectious mononucleosis is characterized by a grippelike syndrome, sore throat, headache, and findings of lymphoid hyperplasia on examination. Splenomegaly occurs in about 50% of the cases, cervical or generalized lymphadenopathy in almost every case, and hepatomegaly in about 10%.

Complications

Infectious mononucleosis usually is benign, but in rare cases such serious complications as the following may occur: (1) **Secondary infection** of the throat with Vincent's organisms or streptococci. **(2) Liver:** The liver, like other organs, becomes infiltrated with lymphocytes. Rarely, however, true hepatitis may simulate the disease. The two diseases probably are related since it sometimes is virtually impossible to distinguish between them except by the heterophile agglutination studies, for even frank infective hepatitis may show "atypical lymphocytes" in the blood. **(3) Spleen:** Rupture of the spleen sometimes occurs, either spontaneously or following excessive diagnostic palpation. Hypersplenism (q.v.), the physiologic counterpart of the anatomic enlargement of the spleen, may occur and give rise to a reduction in various blood cells. It may be in the white cells (leukopenia), red cells (anemia), or platelets (thrombocytopenia), or in all three (pancytopenia). Occasionally, the anemia is hemolytic in nature.

Diagnosis

Two measures are of prime importance: examination of the blood smear, and immunologic study of the blood serum. Most clinical laboratories are adequately equipped to supply both these types of information.

Hemogram: The characteristic finding is a great number of atypical lymphocytes, which are larger than adult lymphocytes, stain more darkly, and frequently show vacuolization of nucleus and cytoplasm. There is extreme variability in size and staining characteristics from cell to cell. The total leukocyte count usually is elevated to about 15,000 (although it may range from 1,000 to 30,000), and of these the atypical lymphocytes form 10 to 90%. Neither anemia nor thrombocytopenia is ordinarily present. These characteristic atypical lymphocytes are virtually pathognomonic of infectious mononucleosis, although a few may be found in infectious hepatitis and (rarely) in malaria. Other changes in the blood smear are extremely rare (see Complications).

Heterophile Agglutination Test (Paul-Bunnell): The blood serum of patients with infectious mononucleosis contains peculiar immune bodies, "heterophile agglutinins," or "heterophile antibodies," which are capable of agglutinating the red cells of other species, particularly sheep. A high titer of these substances—over 1:40 dilution of the serum itself— in the serum of a patient with clinical indications of infectious mononucleosis, establishes the diagnosis beyond doubt. The antibodies, however, may appear at varying times after onset of the illness (a few days to 4 weeks), and several determinations may therefore be necessary. Similar heterophile antibodies, which sometimes occur in serum sickness and in normal individuals, can be differentiated by special treatment of the serum.

The abnormality in the serum may give rise to changes in other tests whose positivity also depends upon abnormalities in the serum. Thus, some cases of infectious mononucleosis (about 10%) show a false positive Wassermann reaction and most cases also show a positive cephalin flocculation reaction (cephalin-cholesterol flocculation test of Hanger). Under these circumstances, the latter may not signify liver disease, but merely an abnormality in the blood serum. However, hepatitis and infectious mononucleosis are occasionally found together.

In cases in which the C.N.S. symptoms are prominent, examination of spinal fluid will frequently disclose findings similar to those of lymphocytic choriomeningitis, i.e., increase in pressures, in lymphocytes and in protein (*see* table, SPINAL FLUID FINDINGS).

The disease must be differentiated from the various acute infections (both bacterial and viral), the lymphomatous disorders (leukemia, lymphosarcoma, Hodgkin's disease), German measles, and infectious hepatitis (q.v.).

Prognosis

The disease usually spends itself in 1 to 3 weeks, although it may linger for 2 or 3 months. It leaves no sequelae. In rare cases, death may occur from splenic rupture, severe hemolytic anemia, or thrombocytopenia with purpura. With careful observation and treatment, the prognosis is almost uniformly excellent.

Treatment

Therapy is almost entirely symptomatic, although aureomycin (℞ 35) has been tried with some reported success. Bed rest should be enforced during the acute phase of fever and malaise and should be prolonged in cases simulating hepatitis. Fluids must be administered liberally, both by mouth and, in cases of severe illness and high fever, I.V. as glucose in saline or water. Antipyretic measures are indicated when the temperature becomes high (about 103°F. in adults, 104°F. in children). These include medication (℞ 1, 4), sponging with tepid water or alcohol, a cold wet draping sheet in high fevers, and (rarely) packing in ice if the fever rises to 106° or 107°F. Sore throat may be alleviated by the use of a gargle (℞ 112) and anesthetic lozenges (℞ 13). Secondary infection by pyogenic organisms responds to treatment with a sulfonamide (℞ 37) or penicillin (℞ 28, 29).

The value of convalescent plasma (30 to 300 cc.), obtained from patients who have recently recovered from the disease, remains to be determined. Because of the possibility of splenic rupture, palpation of the greatly softened spleen should be avoided once the diagnosis is fairly definite. In the rare cases in which rupture occurs, emergency splenectomy is indicated. Rupture may be suspected in the presence of constant, severe, unexplained abdominal pain; signs of peritoneal irritation due to free blood in the peritoneal cavity; and signs of blood loss (anemia, leukocytosis, pallor, tachycardia, shock). In cases complicated by hemolytic anemia or severe thrombocytopenia, splenectomy should be done if the complication does not clear up spontaneously within a few days or after 2 or 3 transfusions.

DIPHTHERIA

An acute contagious bacterial disease characterized by the formation of a fibrinous pseudomembrane upon the mucosa, usually that of the respiratory tract. Occasionally, other mucous membranes are involved, and sometimes the skin or open wounds. An accompanying toxemia may produce, among other changes, degeneration of peripheral nerves and of muscles, particularly those of the heart.

Etiology and Epidemiology

Diphtheria is caused by *Corynebacterium diphtheriae* (Klebs-Löffler bacillus). Ordinarily, the organisms find lodgement on the mucous membranes of the tonsil and, as they multiply, produce lethal exotoxins which lead to death of the host cells in the vicinity.

Diphtheria is spread chiefly by infected secretions of the nose and throat expelled by persons who have the disease in a preclinical or postclinical phase, or by apparently well carriers. Sporadic cases of diphtheria usually result from exposure to carriers who may never have had the disease in recognized form; cases occurring during an epidemic usually are traceable to other clinical cases. Milk or other food may serve as a carrier of diphtheria organisms. Before active immunization was widely employed, diphtheria epidemics occurred in most communities every 3 or 4 years, with peak case incidence in children of preschool age. Enlarged tonsils and adenoids increase susceptibility to diphtheria and also increase the severity of symptoms.

Diphtheria carriers: Routine throat cultures of school and pre-school children taken during late winter months usually reveal a few apparently healthy carriers of diphtheria organisms. The number varies widely—it may be as low as 2 or 3 or as high as 40 to 50/1,000. Many of these children will be found on further test (virulence test) to harbor avirulent or harmless bacteria of the diphtheria or diphtheroid groups. Any campaign to seek carriers, by throat cultures obtained from healthy persons, also must provide for virulence tests before subjecting suspects to isolation and treatment.

Pathology

Significant pathologic lesions are found in the respiratory

passages and oropharynx, and in the heart, central nervous system, and kidneys. Local lesions are characteristic: the diphtheria bacillus first destroys a layer of superficial epithelium, usually in patches, and the resulting exudate coagulates to form a grayish pseudomembrane containing leukocytes and dead epithelial cells which have undergone coagulation necrosis (diphtheritic necrosis). The membrane is formed in the wake of the spreading infection and does not indicate the extent of involvement. The actual zone of bacterial multiplication and area of toxin absorption is wider and deeper than the size of the membrane. This explains the increase in size of the membrane often observed after adequate antitoxin has been given.

The diphtheria organism elaborates an extremely powerful soluble exotoxin, which damages not only the host cells at the site of infection but also distant organs to which it is carried by the blood stream. The heart muscle fibers lose their characteristic appearance and staining qualities, and if many are affected, heart failure results. This often is sudden and fatal, but may be preceded for several days by changes in pulse, blood pressure, and ECG. Even in mild cases of diphtheria, the kidneys may be damaged by the toxin, with consequent cloudy swelling and an interstitial nephritis with extensive cellular infiltrations between the tubules, resulting in albuminuria. If the patient recovers from diphtheria, the kidneys return to normal.

Degenerative C.N.S. changes occur in most of the severe cases and their extent is directly proportional to the duration of infection before antitoxin is given. In missed cases, when patients survive without antitoxin, the incidence of nerve damage is particularly high.

Symptoms and Signs

Diphtheria is typically an angina and a toxemia. The incubation period of 2 to 4 days and the prodromal period of 12 to 24 hours are among the shortest in diseases caused by bacteria. Initially, the patient with tonsillar or faucial diphtheria has only a slightly sore throat, an elevation of temperature (100° to 104°F.), and a rising polymorphonuclear leukocytosis. In small children, who are not likely to show any signs of illness until the disease is well established, a membrane often is present at the first examination. In older children and adults, complaints of sore throat and fatigue may antedate the appearance of membrane by several hours. As the disease progresses, difficult swallowing and signs of toxemia become prominent, and severe prostration may occur. Edema of the pharynx and more particularly the larynx obstructs breathing. If the pseudomembrane involves the larynx (and the trachea and bronchi) it may cause partial obstruction by encroachment on the lumen of the air passage, or, becoming detached, may suddenly produce complete obstruction. The lymph glands of the neck enlarge and in severe cases the whole neck may become so swollen as to present the appearance of "bull neck." If the nose is affected, a serosanguineous discharge, often unilateral, may appear.

Complications and Sequelae

The milder forms of diphtheria may be accompanied by otitis media, or peritonsillar abscess. Such severe complications as bronchopneumonia, myocarditis, and nerve palsies occur in a high percentage of cases, especially in patients receiving antitoxin late in the course of the disease. Bronchopneumonia is a frequent complication of diphtheria of the larynx and tracheobronchial tree, and of septic faucial forms of the disease. Intubation and tracheotomy often may be followed by pneumonia, due to the unavoidable introduction of various bacteria, especially in infants and young children.

Myocarditis (q.v.) is the most dangerous complication and is particularly common in patients with pronounced nasopharyngeal involvement. Death from toxic myocarditis may occur suddenly during an early stage of the illness or even during convalescence. Frequently, the presence of myocarditis is unsuspected and is discovered only by the most careful examination. A rapid, thready pulse, labored cardiac action, soft and blurred heart sounds, and a loud systolic murmur are the usual indications. With less extensive involvement of the myocardium the only abnormality may be a prolongation of the P-R interval or inversion of the T waves in Leads 1 and 2. In later stages, bradycardia and partial or complete heart block may be noted. Blood pressure may remain almost normal even in fatal cases; but as toxemia progresses it may fall, coincident with the onset of decompensation, cardiac arrhythmia, and a diastolic gallop rhythm. As circulation fails, the liver becomes large and painful, and nausea and vomiting may occur. In all instances, albuminuria is a consistent finding, not as evidence of renal stasis secondary to circulatory failure, but as a signal of the widespread toxic insult to the parenchyma of all viscera.

Toxic neuritis occurs in 5 to 20% of all hospitalized diphtheria cases and the resulting paralysis is one of the most serious sequelae. The muscles of the soft palate are generally affected first, and a nasal "hot potato" speech, and regurgitation of liquids through the nose on attempts at swallowing, indicate glossopharyngeal and vagus nerve involvement. Diplopia or strabismus may reveal 3rd, 4th, or 6th nerve involvement. In severe cases where antitoxin was not administered before the 5th or 6th day, death is likely and may be preceded by such severe nervous system damage as paralysis of intercostal muscles or of the extremities. The paralyses sometimes require 2 to 5 weeks to reach their greatest intensity and several weeks more to disappear. Residual neuropathy occasionally results.

Diagnosis

The diagnosis of diphtheria is seldom missed on thorough examination. In very early cases, it may have to await confirmation by culture of the organism from a throat swab. If there is any doubt about the nature of a membrane observed on the tonsils, fauces, or pharynx it should be regarded as diphtheritic and treated as such. Any suspicious patch of membrane or exudate should be observed at least twice daily until its nature is determined. A rapidly spreading membrane, particularly one that grows from the tonsil onto the pillars and pharyngeal wall, is likely to be diphtheritic. Typically, the membrane is of a dirty gray color, but this alone is not a reliable diagnostic sign. A serosanguineous nasal discharge is strongly suggestive of nasal diphtheria and when found should be cultured, and the patient should be isolated. If membrane is not found elsewhere, antitoxin may be withheld until results of the culture are reported. Increasing dyspnea with aphonia strongly suggests laryngeal diphtheria, and direct laryngoscopic examination should be made, during which material for culture also can be obtained. The Schick test (q.v.) is of no value in the diagnosis of clinical diphtheria, as too much time is required to determine its results.

Diagnosis of diphtheria in a wound or an area of burned skin may be made by culture of membrane or serosanguineous discharge from the lesion. Chronic otitis media may be caused by diphtheria organisms, as can be revealed by culture.

(NOTE: Most city and state health departments furnish culture media and will supply a bacteriologic report on throat cultures in less than 24 hours.)

Prognosis

The case fatality rate of diphtheria varies with the type of treatment and site of infection. Nasopharyngeal, laryngeal and the hemorrhagic forms are the most fatal. The over-all fatality rate is approximately 10%. (For other details of prognosis, *see* Complications and Sequelae.)

Prophylaxis

Immunity to diphtheria depends on antibodies, which can be demonstrated by the Schick test, or by toxin-neutralizing studies using experimental animals. Antibodies are formed by the individual under one of the following conditions: active immunization by toxoid injections, recovery from clinical diphtheria, or sufficient (repeated) subclinical infections with the diphtheria organism. The last named method, formerly important, becomes less so as the incidence of diphtheria progressively decreases. A fourth way of acquiring immunity to diphtheria is passively, through injection of preformed antibodies. The immunity thus produced lasts only 2 to 3 weeks, and the method should be used only to afford temporary protection to susceptible individuals exposed to infection, where constant supervision is impossible. (Diphtheria nowadays does not have a high attack rate even among exposed susceptibles; therefore, such persons should not receive antitoxin routinely, but should be examined and have throat cultures daily for at least a week after exposure.)

Active immunization against diphtheria should be afforded all children—beginning, ideally, between the 3rd and 9th months of life. At 2 years, a "booster" injection of toxoid should be given, and another just before the child enters school. Many excellent preparations of diphtheria toxoid are available from state health laboratories and private manufacturers. Toxoids precipitated or stabilized with such metallic salts as those of aluminum, or other substances that prolong absorption, are recommended. At least 2 injections are needed. Many physicians use diphtheria toxoids combined with pertussis vaccine or tetanus toxoid, or both; 3 injections of these combinations at intervals of 3 to 6 weeks is thought best.

Schick test: Dilute diphtheria toxin (1/50 MLD toxin/0.1 cc. of testing solution) is injected intradermally to determine susceptibility or immunity. (At the same time, a control test with heated, and therefore inactivated, test material is made to rule out sensitivity to culture proteins.) The results are read 72 to 96 hours later. If the subject has an antibody level sufficient to neutralize the toxin, there will be no local reaction **(negative test)** and the individual usually does not contract diphtheria when exposed. Susceptibility is indicated by an area, 1 cm. or more in diameter, of inflammation and induration at the site of injection **(positive test).**

Management of an outbreak: (1) Quarantine all patients until they have recovered clinically and at least 2 throat cultures are negative for *C. diphtheriae*. If positive cultures persist after clinical recovery, do a virulence test and continue isolation if organisms are virulent. Tonsillectomy sometimes is necessary to clear up such a carrier. (2) Examine throats, make cultures, and do a Schick test on all contacts. (3) Persons with positive throat cultures and Schick tests are potential cases of diphtheria and should be isolated and treated. (4) Those with negative cultures but positive Schick tests are susceptibles and need daily examination, with repeated cultures. (5) Those with negative cultures and Schick tests are presumably safe, from personal and public health standpoints. (6) Persons with positive cultures and negative Schick tests are carriers and must be isolated until a virulence test is performed. If the organisms carried are avirulent, specific treatment is unnecessary and these individuals may be released from further observation.

Treatment

Antitoxin (℞ 93) should be administered as early as possible in clinical diphtheria. The dose ranges from 5,000 to 20,000 or 40,000 u. according to the severity of symptoms and the patient's age. Children under 2 years should be given 5,000 or 6,000 u.; those over 2 years, 7,000 or 8,000. In early mild cases, 5,000 u. is enough. Enormous doses, such as 100,000 to 300,000 u. probably are never indicated, since they would be useless even in late severe cases once the toxins have become fixed in the body tissues. Early administration is considerably more important than size of dose (with 5,000 u. as a minimum). For mild or moderate cases diagnosed early, the antitoxin is given I.M.; for severe cases and all those diagnosed late, approximately half the determined dose should be given I.V. The total calculated amount should be given in a single injection except in cases of serum sensitivity (q.v.). The former practice of giving it in divided doses over several days has no scientific basis.

Serum sensitivity: Diphtheria antitoxin is derived from the blood serum of immunized horses; hence, a skin test to rule out sensitivity to foreign serum always should precede administration. As a 1:20 dilution of the antitoxin, 0.05 cc. is injected into the skin of the anterior surface of the forearm. If after 30 minutes there is little or no erythema about the site of injection, administration of the antitoxin may proceed. (An unelevated erythema of less than 0.5 cm. usually is read as negative.) An urticarial wheal, however, indicates that extreme caution must be used in giving the antitoxin: i.e., in graduated doses, beginning with 0.05 cc. of the 1:20 dilution I.M. If, in 15 minutes, no severe local or systemic reaction has occurred, the dose may be doubled every 15 minutes thereafter until a dose of 1 cc. of undiluted antitoxin is reached. Following this, the remaining antitoxin may be given in a single injection. In the highly sensitive patient, I.V. administration is contraindicated. It is advisable to have always at hand a sterile solution of epinephrine (℞ 113) 1:1,000 for immediate hypodermic injection of 0.3 to 1 cc. (℔ v to xv) if untoward symptoms appear. A further precautionary step against dangerous serum reaction is the administration of antitoxin in the lower triceps area of the arm in older children and in the lateral midthigh muscles in young children, as circulation in these areas can be temporarily shut off by tourniquet from the rest of the body. Sensitivity to horse serum is not an indication for reduction of total antitoxin dosage; on the contrary, there is evidence that more antitoxin is needed. It is therefore suggested that the "normal" dose be at least doubled.

Supportive treatment is of great importance, second only to antitoxin. Strict rest in bed, careful nursing with emphasis on food and fluid intake, and constant observation of the dyspneic patient for signs that a tracheotomy or laryngeal intubation is needed, are imperative. Sedation (℞ 16) is indicated to allay unrest and apprehension in the dyspneic patient, and to minimize activity by the patient with myocarditis (q.v.). Tube feeding via nasal or oral tube (*see* DIETS), or parenteral alimentation may be used when the patient's local or general condition makes eating difficult or impossible. An ice collar may relieve the pain of swollen cervical lymph glands, and warm saline throat irrigations will allay sore throat in the older child. Irrigations should not be insisted on if the patient does not cooperate.

Penicillin (℞ 28, 29) should be given in all cases of diphtheria, for two reasons. First, it exerts a mild bacteriostatic effect on the specific organism (though insufficient to obviate the need for antitoxin, even in mild cases). The second and more important reason is the frequency with which other pathogenic organisms, particularly streptococci and pneumococci, are found with diphtheria bacilli in throat cultures. The pneumonia which frequently complicates diphtheria in smaller children usually is due to one of these accompanying organisms. Penicillin should be given in repository form I.M. in a dosage of 200,000 to 300,000 u./day, until recovery seems certain, usually for a minimum of 5 to 7 days. In cutaneous diphtheria, compresses of penicillin solution 250 to 1,000 u./cc. (℞ 30) should be applied to the lesions in addition to the aforementioned therapy.

Strict bed rest is the rule for all patients with evidence of myocarditis. Phenobarbital (℞ 15) and codeine (℞ 10) are useful as indicated. For falling blood pressure, 15% glucose I.V. (10 cc./lb. body wt. up to 250 cc., given very slowly) is of value but should not be given if the child is greatly disturbed by venipuncture. Posterior pituitary injection (℞ 121) 0.2 to 0.3 cc. ℳ iii to v) subcut., depending on age, every 3 or 4 hours is recommended to combat falling blood pressure. Blood pressure determinations should be made at least 3 times daily in all instances of suspected myocarditis.

Convalescence from severe diphtheria is decidedly slow, and children must be prevented from resuming normal activities too soon. Physical exertion, even normal play, may be fatal to the patient recovering from toxic myocarditis. Severe diphtheria causes anemia, which should be treated with iron. Vitamins, particularly thiamine and ascorbic acid, are indicated during both illness and convalescence: One of the current proprietary vitamin mixtures or a special prescription may be used.

SCARLET FEVER

(Scarlatina)

A common, acute, communicable, localized, hemolytic streptococcal infection characterized by a generalized toxemia and usually accompanied by a typical rash.

Etiology and Epidemiology

More than 40 different strains of erythrogenic toxin-producing hemolytic streptococci have been recovered from typical cases of scarlet fever. Other types of streptococci and occasionally *Staph. aureus,* isolated from cases resembling scarlet fever clinically, have been shown to produce an erythrogenic toxin capable of neutralizing scarlet fever antitoxin.

The disease may be transmitted by droplet spray from active cases or carriers; by contact with contaminated articles (organisms remain active in dried secretions); or by contaminated milk and food. Patients are infective until the organisms disappear from the nose and throat cultures (average 2 weeks), but a persistent sinusitis, rhinitis, tonsillitis, pharyngitis, or otitis media may prolong the period of infectivity, after apparent recovery. However, carriers—those who harbor the organisms without active infection or who have a subclinical or atypical infection—are believed to be the most common source of infection, since a relatively small percentage of case contacts become infected.

Scarlet fever occurs throughout the world, but most frequently in the temperate zones. It is endemic in densely populated areas and sporadic in rural areas. Fall and spring seasons show the highest incidence. It is rare before the age of 6 months, but more than 50% of all cases occur between the ages of 2 and 8. Young males are affected more frequently than females, and nonwhites are generally less susceptible than white persons. Epidemics of varying intensity occur.

Pathology

Two factors are involved: the local bacterial infection (septic), and the systemic or generalized reaction (toxic). The local infection is similar to any other caused by virulent organisms. Inflammation, cellular infiltration, edema, and exudation are present. The common site is the pharyngeal and tonsillar area. An exudative membrane, resembling that of diphtheria, is frequently formed and may extend either upward or downward. Other sites including abrasions, lacerations, burns, surgical incisions, or the female genital tract may be invaded by scarlet fever-producing organisms (surgical scarlet fever, puerperal scarlet fever). The systemic involvement is generally accepted as a toxic manifestation, but some believe the bacteria themselves are present throughout the tissues, while others interpret the findings as allergic phenomena. An erythrogenic toxin is produced. In addition, leukocidin, streptolysin, and fibrolysin (agents which inhibit the normal defense mechanisms) are present. The skin lesions show dilatation and engorgement of the blood and lymph vessels of the dermal layer, particularly about the ducts of the skin glands and hair follicles. Perivascular cellular infiltration, edema, and small hemorrhages may be detected. Congestion and perivascular infiltration, diffuse or focal, with occasional small hemorrhages are noted in the myocardium, liver, kidneys, spleen, and adrenals, in varying degrees of severity, depending upon the type of infection.

Symptoms and Signs

Due to the variety of infecting organisms and differences in bodily response, the clinical nature of scarlet fever varies decidedly. Any type from the very mild case without a rash to the severe, frequently fatal scarlatina hemorrhagica, may occur.

Classical scarlet fever (moderately severe) develops abruptly after an incubation period of 3 to 5 days. Sore throat, headache, vomiting, and fever (101° to 105°F.) are characteristic. Small children may have a convulsion. Lassitude and malaise are apparent. The face is flushed, but the mouth area is pale (circumoral pallor). The tongue is thickly coated, the pharynx appears reddened, raw, and swollen. A membrane-like, yellowish gray or dirty white exudate is frequently present. This may be confluent or patchy. Cervical lymph nodes are usually enlarged and tender. The pulse rate is elevated, often to 160. Within 24 hours an enanthem appears on the buccal mucosa as small scattered dark red spots (0.5 to 1.0 mm.) on an erythematous base (0.5 to 1.0 cm. in diameter). The white coating sheds from the tip and margins of the tongue revealing a raw, beefy-red color: inflamed papillae protrude through the remaining coating producing the "strawberry tongue." By the 2nd day, the rash (exanthem) usually appears on the neck and chest, and spreads to the abdomen and extremities, and is more or less characteristic. It appears as a diffuse pink-red flush of the skin with a punctate, "goose flesh" character and feel. Intradermal edema about the coil glands and hair follicles produces the tiny, but distinct, slightly raised papules. The rash, which blanches on pressure, is seen best on the abdomen, sides of chest, and where folds of skin occur: neck, axillas, elbows, wrists, knees, and groin. Dark red lines frequently appear in these skin creases, are characteristic, and are known as Pastia's lines. Variations in appearance, distribution and character of the eruption occur (scarlatina papulosa, s. miliaris, s. pemphigoides, surgical scarlet fever). In Negroes, the palms and the soles may be the only site for identification of the rash, although the tenseness and thickening of the skin and the enlarged skin papillae may aid in recognizing the eruption elsewhere.

The leukocyte count is elevated early (10,000 to 20,000, with 75 to 90% neutrophils), and over half the cases will develop an eosinophilia (4 to 20%). A reduction in both the red blood cells and the hemoglobin is common. The sedimentation rate is elevated. The urine is scanty and highly colored. Albuminuria, cylindroids and occasional hyaline casts are commonly found during the acute stage, especially when the temperature is high.

Mild cases without fever (scarlatina afebrilis), without sore throat (scarlatina sine angina), and without a rash do occur and unfortunately are frequently unrecognized. Severe types are uncommon but may occur and may be rapidly fatal, with high fever (106° to 107° F.), high leukocyte count (40,000) and profound toxemia. Petechiae and hemorrhagic phenomena may predominate (scarlatina hemorrhagica), or a septic type with a seriously inflamed, edematous throat may be seen (scarlatina angiosa).

Diagnosis

The typical case is readily diagnosed. A positive culture for one of the hemolytic streptococci in the presence of other clinical findings will confirm the diagnosis of scarlet fever. Atypical forms may be confused with measles, German measles, exanthem subitum, or drug eruptions. The mode of onset, toxic manifestations, time of appearance of rash, Pastia's lines, and the eventual desquamation (late confirmation) are distinguishing factors. Diphtheria must be ruled out by culture especially when an exudative membrane is present. (Negative cultures for *C. diphtheriae* should not influence against the injection of specific serum when doubt exists as to the diagnosis.) Scarlet fever can coexist with diphtheria, measles, chickenpox, and other diseases. Combination with diphtheria is particularly serious.

Special Tests: (1) **Dick test:** This is done by intracutaneous injection of 0.1 cc. of the Dick toxin on the flexor surface of the forearm; presence of an area of redness greater than 1 cm. in diameter in 24 hours is read as positive. A persistently positive Dick test throughout the course of the disease sheds doubt on the diagnosis of scarlet fever, but a positive test before the onset or early in the course, changing to negative, is highly suggestive of the disease. (2) **Blanching test (Schultz-Charlton test):** This is made by intradermal injection of 0.2 cc. of convalescent serum or antitoxin into an area where the rash is present; local blanching of the rash in 6 to 12 hours is positive. Positives only are significant; false negatives are frequent after the 3rd day of the rash and occasionally when a rare type of streptococcus is encountered. (3) **Rumpel-Leede test:** Constriction of the upper arm for a few minutes, as by a tourniquet, causes a shower of petechiae to appear in the skin on the volar surface of the forearm and elbow; this is commonly positive in scarlet fever but is not pathognomonic of this disease.

Course and Prognosis

The high temperature usually subsides within 24 hours of the onset, but a low grade (100° to 101°F.) septic type temperature may persist for 7 to 14 days. The throat continues sore from 4 to 14 days. The remainder of the coating on the tongue sheds in about a week, uncovering the edematous inflamed papillae (red strawberry or raspberry tongue). The rash develops for about 4 days and gradually subsides over a period of a week, at which time the characteristic desquamation begins. All these factors vary markedly in different cases. The rash may be present as a faint transient flush for but a few hours, or may persist for 10 to 12 days. Recovery is gradual over a period varying from 2 to 5 weeks.

Complications, severe and frequent in the past, are greatly lessened or prevented by modern therapy, but do occur occasionally and must be carefully watched for. Cervical adenitis, sinusitis, otitis media, or arthritis may occur. Peritonsillar abscess, mastoiditis complicating the otitis, nephritis, carditis, septicemia, and bronchopneumonia are the more serious and comparatively common sequelae. Chorea, meningitis, encephalitis, and toxic psychoses have been reported. Urticaria, eczema, and furunculosis may be skin complications. These conditions may develop at any time during the course of the disease, but usually appear as the original infection is apparently subsiding (about the 2nd week).

The mortality rate, although greatly lessened, still is significant, varying from practically nil in the mild cases to 6 or 8 per 1,000 of the severe cases.

Prophylaxis

Isolation: State laws vary in isolation and quarantine regulations. The patient should be isolated and precautions taken until the acute stage is past, and recovery evident (*see* BEDSIDE PROC.). Maintenance of partial isolation (separation from susceptible individuals and small children) for several weeks or months has been recommended by some authorities, since a carrier state frequently follows despite apparent complete recovery. Cultures of nasal and throat secretions, negative for the streptococci, are criteria for release used by others.

Contacts: Prophylactic measures are effective in direct proportion to the promptness of administration. Since relatively few contacts develop scarlet fever and the incubation period is short, preventive methods are limited. Many believe that each case should be given convalescent serum as soon as the diagnosis is suspected, but to attempt to provide prophylaxis for every known case contact is practically impossible.

Prophylactic agents: (1) Convalescent serum (human), 10 to 20 cc. I.M. (℞ 95); (2) Scarlet fever streptococcus antitoxin, 3,000 u. I.M. (℞ 96); (3) sulfadiazine, 1 Gm. twice a day for 3 days (℞ 37); (4) penicillin, 300,000 u. I.M. daily for 4 to 7 days (℞ 28, 29); (5) whole blood (human convalescent), 20 to 40 cc. I.M.

Sulfadiazine is perhaps the cheapest, most readily available, and most convenient agent to use in attempting prophylaxis, and is considered by many observers to be the best method. When using the antitoxin, the sensitivity problem must be considered.

Active immunity: The Dick toxin has been available for many years, but the value of its use has been repeatedly questioned. For immunization, 5 subcut. injections are given at weekly intervals in alternate arms. The usual doses are: (1) 650 skin test doses, (2) 2,500, (3) 10,000, (4) 30,000, and (5) 100,000.

Treatment

Although very mild cases of scarlet fever require only symptomatic treatment, all cases need bed rest, with a sufficiently long period of protected convalescence. Diet should be liquid or soft (*see* DIETS) depending upon the soreness of the throat, but nutrition must be maintained. Temperature above 103°F. should be combated by tepid water or alcohol sponge baths (*see* BEDSIDE PROC.), especially for small children. Older patients may be given acetylsalicylic acid (℞ 1). Warm saline or a medicated gargle (℞ 111), and throat irrigations (*see* BEDSIDE PROC.) are of value but should not be urged if resisted or otherwise impracticable. Either warm or cold compresses may give relief from painful cervical adenitis. Applications of cold cream or oil lotions (℞ 122, 123) are helpful for itching. Daily observation is vital for prevention of complications.

For specific treatment, the choice varies. Penicillin (℞ 28, 29), aureomycin (℞ 35), and sulfadiazine (℞ 37) combat the septic factor in the disease but have little effect upon the toxic component; while immune serum (℞ 95) and antitoxin (℞ 96) are generally effective against the toxic manifestations, with little action against the local streptococcal infection.

When convalescent serum is unavailable and antitoxin ineffective or contraindicated, multiple small transfusions, 40 to 200 cc. of whole blood, preferably from a recently recovered donor, may be given. These not only aid in combating the toxic factor, but are of some benefit for the secondary anemia usually accompanying severe scarlet fever. Responsible authorities disagree as to the "drug of choice," and many consider both factors in treatment. Treatment of complications (q.v.) is as described in the respective chapters.

RHEUMATIC FEVER

A systemic disease of inflammatory, nonsuppurative nature, protean in its manifestations, extremely variable in severity, duration, and occurrence of sequelae, and frequently followed by serious heart disease.

Etiology and Incidence

Despite the fact that rheumatic fever must still be classed as a disease of unknown etiology, it now is generally accepted that the onset of rheumatic fever bears definite relation to the occurrence of a preceding infection with a strain of group A beta hemolytic streptococci.

This association does not necessarily incriminate the streptococcus as the direct etiologic factor; rather, it is postulated that in the latent period which follows the acute streptococcal infection, a state of hypersensitivity, as yet not delineated, develops which ultimately leads to carditis, arthritis, or other manifestations of the disease.

Various other bacteria have been discarded in most quarters as possible causes of rheumatic fever, and evidence favoring a viral agent is not convincing.

Heredity may be important; children of two rheumatic parents are reported to be much more likely to have rheumatic fever than are children of nonrheumatic parents. Constitutional predisposition to rheumatic fever ("rheumatic diathesis") has been postulated, with the suggestion that children with red hair and freckles are more apt to acquire the disease.

Overcrowding, malnutrition, and dampness, all concomitants of poverty, are factors which predispose to respiratory infections and thus indirectly to rheumatic fever.

Not only do 2% of the school children in the United States have rheumatic heart disease, but it is the cause of 98% of all heart disease in patients under 20 years of age. Rheumatic fever causes more deaths during the first 2 decades of life than all other communicable diseases and pneumonia taken together, and 10 times as many deaths yearly as infantile paralysis. Rheumatic heart disease was the cause of over 50% of rejections for military service in World War II due to cardiovascular abnormalities.

Pathology

Lasègue described the disease as one which "licks the joints and bites the heart." Although the involvement in acute rheumatic fever may be widespread, the heart suffers most seriously and is the only organ subject to significant permanent structural alteration.

The pathognomonic lesion of rheumatic fever is the submiliary Aschoff nodule, usually found in association with small arteries. It represents an inflammatory reaction and consists in its early stages of small mononuclear wandering cells and a few polymorphonuclear leukocytes surrounding fragments of collagen. Later, the large Aschoff cells appear; these are characterized by basophilic cytoplasm and a large vesicular nucleus; some are multinucleated. As the Aschoff cells increase in number the other small cellular components disappear and, in the well developed nodule, only large cells are seen. As the nodule becomes older, the Aschoff cells become more nearly spindle-shaped; collagen appears and the end result is a dense avascular scar. Aschoff nodules are distributed chiefly in the myocardium but may be found in the endocardium, the valves, and the pericardium. They have been described in the adventitia of the aorta, pulmonary arteries, and the diaphragm.

The characteristic endocardial lesion of rheumatic fever is a small verrucous vegetation composed of granular material, possibly fibrin. As healing occurs, connective tissue grows into the vegetation from the valve and the mass becomes endothelialized. More important from the standpoint of permanent damage is the acute interstitial valvulitis which occurs; the healing of this process results in thickening, fusion and retraction of the cusps; similar involvement of the chordae tendineae leads to shortening, thickening and fusion and adds materially to the functional aberration.

Rheumatic pericarditis is fibrinous in character and may be widespread. Effusions of variable size may develop. Following pericarditis, the pericardial space may be obliterated.

Rheumatic pneumonitis is characterized by focal damage to the small vessels, especially the alveolar capillaries. There often is focal plugging of capillaries. In contrast to the bacterial pneumonias, the exudate in rheumatic pneumonitis is scant; therefore, the physical and X-ray signs are minimal.

Subcutaneous nodules bear some resemblance to Aschoff bodies. They consist of a center of fragmented collagen surrounded by spindle-shaped cells; at the periphery, large mononuclear cells, dilated capillaries, and prominent endothelial cells are seen.

The changes in the joints in rheumatic fever are transient; joint disability following recovery is unknown. During the acute episode, there is an increase in synovial fluid containing a little fibrin and a few polymorphonuclear leukocytes. The synovial membrane is edematous and hyperemic; in the periarticular structures may be found cellular accumulations resembling Aschoff nodules.

Peritonitis and even nephritis have been described during acute rheumatic fever. Usually, vascular lesions are found when these structures are involved. In chorea, gross examination of the brain ordinarily shows only hyperemia. Microscopic studies reveal lesions in the gray matter, the basal ganglia, the brain stem, and in the region near the aqueduct. Vascular and perivascular changes predominate, associated with thrombi, hemorrhage, and endothelial proliferation. The acute endarteritis in the brain leads to focal necrosis, especially in the cortex.

Symptoms and Signs

The onset may be acute and dramatic, but often it begins insidiously and episodes may pass unrecognized. The symptoms and signs here enumerated may appear in any combination; only rarely are all observed in a given case. Frequently, a cyclic character may be noted with recurrent attacks.

Typically, the patient is a child or young adult, often with a history of a previous episode of rheumatism and an immediate past history (1 to 3 weeks earlier) of an upper respiratory infection such as tonsillitis, pharyngitis, or scarlet fever. During the convalescent phase of the respiratory infection, the patient develops fever and arthritis. Usually, the large joints become involved first and characteristically the process is migratory. The joints become hot, red, swollen, tender, and painful. Constitutional symptoms and signs appear such as anorexia, malaise, tachycardia, and sweats. Rashes are frequent. Chief among the skin manifestations, which often are transient and thus call for close observation, are the various erythemas (e.g., marginatum, multiforme, nodosum). Likewise, subcutaneous nodules may appear, usually over bony prominences and on the extensor surfaces. Epistaxes, nontraumatic in origin, may occur at the onset of rheumatic fever in some patients.

The cardiac manifestations are of prime importance (see HEART MURMURS; MYOCARDITIS; PERICARDITIS; CARDIAC ARRHYTHMIAS). Precordial pain which may simulate the pain of coronary insufficiency is a not infrequent complaint and usually indicates the presence of carditis. Examination of the heart may reveal dilatation, embryocardia, gallop rhythm, tachycardia, arrhythmias, systolic or diastolic murmurs, or pericardial friction rubs. Cardiac insufficiency may develop. Although any one of these is presumptive evidence of acute carditis, the signs may change rapidly and a definitive prognosis as to cardiac damage cannot be given at this stage.

Cough, pleurisy, dyspnea, signs of pneumonitis or of pleural effusions may be encountered.

Abdominal pain, which may resemble that of acute appendicitis, is sometimes noted. Signs of peritoneal irritation may make differential diagnosis difficult, especially if the other signs of acute rheumatism are not striking.

Sydenham's chorea (q.v.) is characterized by purposeless, athetoid movements. Possibly 50% of all patients with rheumatic fever have chorea at one time or another, while the majority of patients with chorea develop stigmata of rheumatic fever. However, chorea rarely occurs after adolescence.

Less spectacular than the acute forms, but of equal importance, is the low grade or smoldering type of rheumatic fever seen especially in young children. Definite signs are few. The child is easily fatigued and may not gain normally. A persistently rapid pulse rate and a low grade fever are common. Mild muscle and joint symptoms, often called "growing pains," may direct attention to the joints but often are absent. If rheumatic fever is suspected, thorough and repeated search for evidence of carditis or active rheumatic disease must be made.

Laboratory Findings

No specific diagnostic laboratory test for rheumatic fever is known. Several laboratory procedures taken together may be helpful in confirming the clinical diagnosis.

At the onset of rheumatic fever the red cell count and hemoglobin usually are normal; during the course of the disease varying degrees of normochromic, normocytic anemia are found. The leukocyte count often is elevated to levels between 10,000 and 20,000; frequently, the differential count shows a shift to the left with increase in polymorphonuclears. The urinary findings are ordinarily of little importance, although in the presence of fever, albuminuria and granular casts may be reported.

The E.S.R. is of value in following the course, generally being high quite early and remaining elevated until the active process has subsided. Persistence of an abnormally rapid E.S.R., however, after signs and symptoms of the disease have disappeared, suggests the need for investigating other possible causes of acceleration.

Antifibrinolysin and antistreptolysin tests are sometimes used in diagnosis. The former is simpler to perform, but the latter more informative. A positive result with either indicates a previous streptococcic infection. A high titer (over 500) of antistreptolysin, occurring 1 month or more after the acute infection, is uncommon except in acute rheumatic fever, or following an attack of scarlet fever or acute nephritis.

Bacteriologic cultures of the nose and throat should be obtained; the presence of beta hemolytic streptococci, though not of great diagnostic import, may possibly play a role in prolonging the acute episode, and appropriate treatment is advisable.

The ECG is of definite value in the diagnosis of rheumatic fever although it may in some instances remain normal. The most common abnormalities observed during the acute phase of the disease include disturbances of AV conduction varying from prolongation of the P-R interval above 0.20 seconds to complete AV dissociation, alteration of the T-wave patterns, and findings typical of pericarditis (elevation of the R-T segments and coving of the T waves). Caution is needed in the interpretation of minor ECG changes, particularly when these involve only the T waves, in cases where the diagnosis is not clear. Such changes have been reported in a multitude of infectious diseases and thus, alone, are not to be considered specific for rheumatic fever.

Roentgenologic studies during rheumatic fever may confirm the clinical findings of cardiac dilatation or of pericardial effusion. Fluoroscopy may rarely demonstrate left auricular enlargement, but this procedure finds its chief application later, in the diagnosis of mitral stenosis. Pneumonitis may be demonstrable by X-ray examination. The joint changes are nonspecific.

Diagnosis

Rheumatic fever must be carefully differentiated from a number of diseases. Among the more important are rheumatoid arthritis, hypertrophic osteoarthritis, gonococcic arthritis, Reiter's syndrome, sickle cell anemia (in Negroes), appendicitis, tuberculosis, brucellosis, influenza, dermatomyositis, disseminated lupus erythematosus, polyarteritis nodosa, meningococcemia, gout, subacute bacterial endocarditis, serum sickness, osteomyelitis, scurvy, acute poliomyelitis, trichinosis, hemophilia, and bacillary dysentery.

In most instances, correlation of history, signs, symptoms, and laboratory data will enable the physician to arrive at the diagnosis. Recent investigations suggest that both rheumatoid arthritis and rheumatic fever often may occur in the same individual; this hypothesis is based on the finding of typical pathologic lesions of both diseases in the same patient. The exact relationship between the two diseases remains unknown.

Prognosis

The prognosis in rheumatic fever varies considerably and depends on numerous factors including age, number of previous episodes, presence or absence of valvular abnormalities, and the patient's environmental stratum. In general, permanent cardiac damage is more common when there is early onset of rheumatic fever or frequent attacks. As previously mentioned, the appearance of murmurs, either systolic or diastolic, in the acute phase of the disease does not necessarily indicate that permanent damage has been incurred. Nevertheless, persistence of such murmurs or of abnormalities of the mitral 1st or pulmonic 2nd sounds after subsidence of the acute episode must be regarded as a manifestation of permanent valvular disorder (*see* HEART MURMURS). No patient who has had rheumatic fever may be dismissed as being free of significant heart disease until he has been observed for many years. Intelligent management on the part of the physician, however, will do much to prevent the patient from becoming a "cardiac invalid." The likelihood of rheumatic recurrences in patients who live under unfavorable environmental conditions (overcrowding, dampness, poor nutrition) is definitely increased.

Prophylaxis

The prevention of rheumatic recurrences in patients who have had one attack of rheumatic fever is of great importance. As has been pointed out, the more frequent the recurrences, the more likely the development of rheumatic heart disease. The value of small daily doses of sulfadiazine to decrease the incidence of respiratory infections in susceptible patients, and thus to prevent or reduce repeated attacks of rheumatic fever, is controversial. The incidence of toxic reactions to the continued use of sulfadiazine in these doses is surprisingly low. Administration orally of penicillin for similar purposes is being studied, but final judgment must be reserved.

There is some evidence that patients subject to recurrent

rheumatic fever do better in warm dry climates such as are found in Puerto Rico and Arizona, presumably because of the low incidence of streptococcic infections. Economic considerations, however, limit the application of climatotherapy.

Treatment

At the onset of symptoms or signs suggesting rheumatic fever, complete **bed rest** must be instituted and maintained until all evidence (clinical and laboratory) of activity has subsided. During the acute, febrile phase of the illness, the patient should be kept quiet and little diversion allowed unless it affords no element of fatigue. As improvement takes place, suitable occupational therapy may be instituted. Good nursing care helps greatly to maintain the patient's morale; care must be exercised in the hygiene of the skin; the use of a "cradle," soft wrappings, or other shielding apparatus to protect involved joints is advisable.

The **nutrition** of the patient is important. A diet adequate in calories should be given; in the early stages of the illness, liquid and soft diets are preferable, especially if the patient complains of constitutional symptoms. Protein concentrates suitable for administration in liquids now are available and may be used (*see* PROTEIN DEFICIENCY). For underweight patients the caloric intake should be aimed at producing a gain in weight. On the other hand, if the patient is of normal weight or obese, no advantage accrues from a diet which causes further increase; indeed, such a diet may lead to an unnecessary circulatory burden. Fluids should be given in adequate amounts, usually 2,500 to 3,500 cc. daily; in the presence of high fever, especially in warm climates, larger amounts may be indicated. As in all febrile diseases, fluids which promote distention are best avoided. Milk and fruit juices may have to be limited on this account. Unless cardiac insufficiency is present or imminent, the salt intake should be that allowed normally. If an adequate diet is taken, supplementary vitamins are not essential, but a multivitamin preparation when necessary may be given.

The chief therapeutic effects of **salicylates** in acute rheumatic fever are to reduce temperature to normal with corresponding reduction of pulse rate and evidences of toxicity, and to relieve pain and swelling of joints. Salicylates are of greater value in the symptomatic treatment of acute attacks than in subacute or polycyclic forms of the disease.

Salicylates may be given as acetylsalicylic acid (℞ 1) or as sodium salicylate (℞ 2). Administration should begin as soon as the diagnosis of rheumatic fever is established; often these drugs are given in hourly doses of 1 Gm. (gr. xv) until mild toxic symptoms appear. Then they are withdrawn for from 6 to 12 hours and reinstituted in doses of 1 to 1.5 Gm. (gr. xv to xxiiss) every 4 hours. An alternate method consists of using 5 to 10 Gm. daily, in divided doses every 4 hours, best given after food intake. Dosage for children may be calculated on the basis of weight.

Since salicylates apparently do not affect the course or prognosis of rheumatic fever, only enough drug to achieve symptomatic relief need be given. In general, blood levels of 250 to 400 mg./100 cc. represent the necessary concentration; such levels usually can be achieved and maintained by the dosage outlined.

Salicylates are gastric irritants; in the stomach they are converted by the action of hydrochloric acid to salicylic acid, and this compound is absorbed in the upper gastrointestinal tract. Gastric irritation, which manifests itself by epigastric burning, nausea, vomiting, and anorexia, may be controlled usually by the use of enteric coated tablets of sodium salicylate (℞ 3) or by the concomitant administration of sodium bicarbonate (℞ 152), the dosage varying according to need and tolerance, from 5 to 10 Gm. in 24 hours.

Salicylic acid is rapidly excreted by the kidneys; within 24 hours after the cessation of therapy the blood usually is cleared of the drug. There is evidence to indicate that sodium bicarbonate decreases salicylic acid absorption and speeds excretion; it may, therefore, contribute to somewhat lower blood levels.

Among the other toxic effects of salicylates are tinnitus, deafness, tachypnea (salicyl dyspnea), and hypoprothrombinemia. Occasionally, salicylism may be so severe as to necessitate withdrawal of the drug, but usually a decrease in the dose suffices to control toxic symptoms. The use of vitamin K (℞ 134) usually restores the prothrombin time to normal. If administration by mouth causes vomiting, salicylates may be given by rectum. Twice daily doses of 4 Gm. (℥ i) of sodium salicylate in 60 cc. of water, by rectum, will correspond approximately to 5 Gm. (gr. lxxv) daily by mouth.

In the rare instances, when salicylates are not tolerated at all, aminopyrine (℞ 5) may be used in doses of 2 to 5 Gm. daily, divided in 6 equal portions. Although it causes none of the toxic manifestations of salicylism, aminopyrine is identified with a significant tendency to produce agranulocytosis. When used, the leukocyte and differential counts must be followed carefully and the drug stopped if leukopenia develops.

Usually, the response to salicylates is dramatic; the arthritis subsides in 24 to 72 hours, as does the fever, and the patient appears improved. Massive I.V. doses of salicylates have not proved advantageous.

Recently, para-aminobenzoic acid has been tried therapeutically, but its true effectiveness is still to be determined. Dramatic, prompt remissions of the acute attack of rheumatic fever have been obtained with the use of either the adrenocortical hormone, cortisone (Compound E), or the adrenocorticotropic hormone (ACTH). Further evaluation of these and similar agents will be necessary.

Oil of wintergreen (℞ 6) or other counterirritants may be applied locally to joints for symptomatic relief, although they usually do not add appreciably to the benefits provided by physical rest and immobilization.

In the further treatment of the case of mild or moderately severe rheumatic fever, salicylate therapy should be maintained for at least 2 or 3 weeks after symptoms have subsided. In this interval the laboratory evidence of rheumatic activity also will usually diminish or disappear. Salicylates then are withdrawn. If fever and joint symptoms recur, salicylates are resumed.

More commonly, continued low grade rheumatic activity is indicated by tachycardia with or without slight fever, persistently elevated E.S.R. or white blood count, and ECG changes.

Any evidence of rheumatic activity, especially in children, is an indication for continued rest. It may be 6 months or even a year before the active disease subsides.

Generally, the signs of rheumatic activity disappear after 1 to 3 months, following which the patient may be allowed up for limited periods each day. After 1 month of such restricted activity, he may become fully ambulatory, although strenuous exercise will be contraindicated for a minimum of 1 year. His cardiac status must be followed, at least at yearly intervals thereafter, throughout childhood and adolescence.

Digitalis is indicated for trial in rheumatic fever only when cardiac insufficiency is evident, and even then it often may not prove beneficial. Great care must be exercised to avoid toxic amounts. Many of the unfavorable effects ascribed to digitalis in the treatment of cardiac failure in rheumatic fever are attributable to the use of excess digitalis when the response to the drug has been poor.

The preparation of choice is digitoxin given orally, since I.V. preparations are best avoided (*see* CONGESTIVE HEART FAILURE). Close observation is essential; the ECG should be repeated at intervals, although digitalis effect may be masked by the changes due to rheumatic carditis.

When pericardial effusion develops, conservative measures should be used, **pericardial paracentesis** being reserved for alleviation of cardiac tamponade.

Oxygen should be administered in the presence of cardiac failure or rheumatic pneumonitis.

In cardiac failure, **diuretics** are of definite value (*see* CONGESTIVE HEART FAILURE). The xanthines are often used; theobromine-calcium salicylate or theophylline with ethylenediamine may be given. The mercurial diuretics are likewise effective but must be used with caution.

Neither **sulfonamide** nor **penicillin** therapy is indicated routinely in the treatment of rheumatic fever; nevertheless, when cultures of the nose or throat indicate the presence of beta hemolytic streptococci, penicillin (℞ 28, 29) should be given, particularly if there is a history of recent respiratory infection. The drug should be given in adequate doses for at least 7 days; if given for shorter periods of time, the streptococci are apt to reappear as soon as the drug is withdrawn.

Special emphasis should be given to the difficult and serious problem of treating a patient with the extremely active or fulminating form of rheumatic fever. Such patients are desperately ill and a fatal outcome always is imminent. The temperature and pulse are high, and often respond only partially to salicylates. The patient is prostrated, anxious, restless, and dyspneic. There is gallop rhythm or embryocardia and usually progressing congestive failure.

Absolute bed rest in a quiet room with day and night nursing care is essential. Sedatives should be given to allay anxiety and restlessness and to provide sleep. Oxygen is mandatory unless the patient cannot tolerate it. It may be given by catheter, mask or tent, whichever is most comfortable (*see* CLIN. PROC.). Fluids should be sufficient to maintain adequate hydration and normal renal function; in the presence of heart failure, fluid intake need not be limited but a salt-free diet must be rigidly enforced. Food and medications must be given with great care to prevent vomiting.

In the treatment of **chorea**, the patient should be kept in isolation if possible, and shielded from noise and excitement. If the choreiform movements are violent, side rails or nets should be used so that the patient cannot fall out of bed. The value of a ketogenic diet is controversial. Sedation is indicated, e.g., phenobarbital (℞ 15) or chloral hydrate (℞ 19). Salicylates are of doubtful value in chorea unassociated with other signs and symptoms of rheumatic fever. Hyperthermia has been used in the treatment of chorea with variable results.

Serums, vaccines, and X-ray therapy have no evident value in the treatment of rheumatic fever and should not be used. Iron and liver extracts likewise are unnecessary, except in certain subacute cases with a secondary anemia.

SYDENHAM'S CHOREA

(St. Vitus' dance, Chorea minor, Infectious chorea,
Rheumatic chorea)

An acute disease of the C.N.S. characterized by involuntary purposeless movements of the trunk and the extremities.

Etiology

Sydenham's chorea is generally considered as part of the rheumatic complex: migratory polyarthritis, chorea, and endocarditis. Approximately 72% of chorea cases are associated with evidence of rheumatic fever, and it has been stated that about 50% of young rheumatic fever patients will develop chorea. However, cases have been reported with other acute infections, particularly epidemic encephalitis and diphtheria. Sydenham's chorea is a disease of childhood, occurs more frequently in females, and is rare past 20. An association with pregnancy is recognized, and represents the majority of adult cases. It occurs most frequently in the late fall and early spring. Negroes and American Indians are relatively immune.

Symptoms and Signs

The onset usually is insidious and the first manifestation is the patient's clumsiness and tendency to drop things. The involuntary movements are rapid, irregular, jerky, and purposeless. Almost all the muscles are involved except those of the eyes. Facial grimacing is common. Voluntary movements are not impaired but are done abruptly. Muscular weakness may be fairly marked and coordination may be impaired by the involuntary movements. In severe cases, considerable dysarthria and difficulty in chewing and swallowing may occur. The muscles are hypotonic and when the arms are held vertically above the head there are irregular flexion and extension movements at the wrist, and the forearms are markedly pronated. The reflexes are present but may be somewhat diminished. The knee jerks may be prolonged. Some emotional instability is usual and occasionally there may be persistent excitement associated with insomnia or, rarely, a toxic psychosis.

Laboratory Findings

There may be a slight eosinophilia; serum calcium is frequently lowered and the sedimentation rate elevated (particularly with carditis). The spinal fluid may be normal or show a mild pleocytosis, increased pressure, increased glucose and diminished calcium. The EEG shows nonspecific dysrhythmias.

Diagnosis

Sydenham's chorea must be differentiated from habit spasm, hysteria, athetosis, epidemic encephalitis, and from chronic forms of chorea, such as Huntington's (q.v.), and a type which may appear at puberty. A history of rheumatic fever and the presence of other rheumatic manifestations are of diagnostic importance.

Prognosis

The disease is self-limited and usually runs its course in 6 to 10 weeks. About one-third of the patients have recurrences. It usually is not fatal but the prognosis may be grave in the chorea associated with pregnancy.

Treatment

General: Provide mental and physical calm, with bed rest for the acute stage. Hospitalization is recommended. Maintain nutrition; give a palatable, easily digested, high vitamin, high caloric diet by attendants or, when necessary, by tube feeding (*see* DIETS). Scrupulous cleanliness is essential, especially when involuntary evacuations occur. It is best to institute some form of occupational therapy; simple toys, jigsaw puzzles, erector sets. Massage, passive exercise, hot or cold packs (*see* BEDSIDE PROC.) and warm tub baths are of definite value. Sides of the bed should be padded to prevent injury when choreic movements are violent. Search for and care of carditis or other rheumatic manifestations are essential. Carious teeth and infected tonsils should be treated as in rheumatic fever (q.v.).

Drug therapy: Salicylates (℞ 1, 2) may be given in doses up to 4 Gm. (3 i) a day. Sedatives (℞ 15, 19, 20) may be necessary. Scopolamine (℞ 21) or morphine (℞ 11) may be required in very severe cases, but should be used only when other medications fail. Calcium and parathyroid extract may be useful. Arsenic (Fowler's solution) is outmoded; Phenylethyl-hydantoin is contraindicated. Chlorobutanol requires experience in its use, and constant supervision.

Fever therapy: Induced fever is recommended by some who use it extensively, even when a subacute carditis exists. Others consider it unnecessary or dangerous. Fever may be induced daily by the hypertherm, or similar cabinet, or by the I.V. injection of typhoid and paratyphoid vaccine (℞ 97). To be effective, a temperature from 103° to 105° F. should be produced every other day until there is a remission. It is best to give 0.1 cc. as an initial dose to determine the patient's reaction to the treatment. Succeeding doses are determined by the reaction to this 1st dose. If the 1st dose produces a temperature rise to 105° or 106° F., the same amount is given for the 2nd dose. Usually, the 3rd dose must be somewhat larger to cause an adequate rise in the temperature. The residuum of the chorea is used as a guide to continuation of treatment. Most cases need a febrile period of about a week, others may need more depending on the severity of the chorea. The injection is best given in the afternoon so that the child will not miss its dinner and so that the bout of fever will subside in time to permit a good night's sleep. When the temperature reaches 106° F., acetylsalicylic acid, 0.3 Gm. (gr. v) (℞ 1) should be given and an ice bag applied to the head. Acetylsalicylic acid is contraindicated while the temperature is going up.

Spinal tap: Repeated lumbar punctures with removal of 5 to 10 cc. of spinal fluid have been recommended for cases with initial increase in pressure or pleocytosis.

SEPSIS

Sepsis is here used in a broad sense, to describe a condition resulting from the breakdown of local defense barriers about an inflammatory process, which permits spread of infection or increased absorption of toxic material sufficient to cause constitutional symptoms. It may be manifested as **cellulitis,** resulting from local dissemination of an infection; or as **lymphangitis** and **lymphadenitis,** from spread along the lymphatic channels; or as **bacteremia** ("blood poisoning," septicemia) due to widespread distribution of infective or toxic material by way of the blood stream.

CELLULITIS

Any inflammation of the tissues that shows a tendency to spread. The skin and subcutaneous structures usually are affected, but cellulitis also may occur in the deeper tissues (e.g., pelvic cellulitis, periurethral cellulitis).

Etiology

Spread of infection from a focus may be due to inherent virulence of the infecting organism, to manipulation or other trauma of the lesion, or to lowered resistance of defense mechanisms. Streptococci and staphylococci are the most frequent infecting organisms, but any pathogen capable of invading tissue may produce cellulitis. Anaerobic bacteria, responsible for gas gangrene, may produce a characteristic cellulitis in which gas is present under the skin.

Symptoms and Signs

Evidence of sepsis, fever of varying degree, chills, malaise, and headache may be present. The intensity of symptoms varies with the nature of the cellulitis. Locally, the area is red, swollen, painful, and warm, with poorly defined borders. Leukocytosis usually develops. Deep cellulitis is characterized by generalized symptoms, local discomfort, and acute pain on palpation of the affected area. With cellulitis due to anaerobic gas-forming organisms, the outstanding features are pain and tenderness of the involved area and crepitation due to gas in the subcutaneous tissue. Cellulitis breaking down into foul-smelling purulent lesions is characteristic of anaerobic organisms such as Vincent's and other anaerobes of the oral cavity (*see* LUDWIG'S ANGINA). Colon bacilli also produce foul pus.

Diagnosis

Ordinarily, superficial cellulitis can be easily identified, although confusion with early erysipelas, erythema nodosum, and neoplastic metastases is possible. Deep (e.g., pelvic) cellulitis, however, is identifiable only by careful history, thorough physical examination and differentiation from other disorders.

Course and Prognosis

Lymphangitis, with lymphadenitis of the regional nodes, usually develops. Bacteremia occurs frequently in severe cases. Abscess formation and destruction of tissue may result. Cellulitis of the scalp may produce intracranial complications by spread through the emissary and diploic veins. Cellulitis of the floor of the mouth and neck, due to oral anaerobic organisms is the so-called Ludwig's angina (q.v.). It is a serious condition, may require surgery, but usually responds to penicillin and the sulfonamides. Cellulitis of any appreciable extent is a serious condition, especially in very young children and the elderly. Complications increase the risk; and the prognosis, especially for anaerobic infections, must be guarded.

Treatment

General: The part involved should be put at rest and elevated when possible. If severe toxic symptoms are present, bed rest is indicated. Local application of heat or wet dressings may be helpful. Sedatives (℞ 15, 23) and analgesics (℞ 10, 11) should be used when necessary.

Specific: Penicillin (℞ 28, 29), sulfonamides (℞ 37, 38), streptomycin (℞ 32), aureomycin (℞ 35), or Chloromycetin (℞ 36) will be the specific treatment in most cases, since infection with agents not susceptible to one of these drugs is uncommon. Combined therapy may be necessary. Since the beta hemolytic streptococcus is most frequently causative, penicillin usually is indicated. Treatment should be continued until all general and local signs of infection have been absent for at least 4 or 5 days. For anaerobic cellulitis due to gas-forming bacilli, gas gangrene antitoxin (℞ 98) should also be given, accompanied by prompt excision, either by single muscle or groups of muscles, of all affected tissue. Amputation is indicated only where infection is so extensive that removal of the involved tissue is inadequate to check the disease or makes loss of the limb function inevitable. For any type of cellulitis, accepted surgical methods of treatment must be applied. Prophylaxis against tetanus (q.v.) also must be considered (℞ 99, 100), especially when the initial lesion is a wound.

LYMPHANGITIS

An acute or chronic inflammation of the superficial or deep lymphatic channels.

Etiology

Lymphangitis results from spread of infection due to excessively virulent organisms, trauma, or lowered local resistance. Streptococci and staphylococci are the most common infecting agents although others, including fungi, tubercle bacilli, and spirochetes, may be responsible.

Symptoms and Signs

Acute Lymphangitis: Evidence of sepsis in varying degrees usually is present, with fever (102° to 105° F.), chills, malaise, generalized aching, and headache. Leukocytosis (15,000 to 30,-000) with a preponderance of neutrophiles is not uncommon.

Patchy areas of inflammation occurring along the path of a lymphatic vessel represent a reticular or capillary lymphangitis (e.g., erysipelas). Tubular lymphangitis is most common in the extremities, as a complication of infections (or infected wounds) of the hand or foot. This presents the characteristic irregular, pink, tender, linear streaks extending up the arm or leg toward the regional lymph nodes.

Chronic Lymphangitis: The lesion appears as a firm cord in or under the skin leading from the site of initial infection (tuberculous, syphilitic, or fungous). This cord may or may not be tender and may have abscesses, ulcers, areas of infection, or healed scars along its course where secondary foci have been established.

Course and Prognosis

Lymphangitis is almost invariably followed by lymphadenitis. Bacteremia is a constant and serious threat. Cellulitis with suppuration, necrosis, and necrotizing ulcers may occasionally develop along the course of the involved lymph channel. Prognosis is determined by the nature of the infecting organism, relative resistance of the patient, and response to treatment. The outlook often is serious for the very young, the aged, or the debilitated patient, but early adequate treatment minimizes the danger.

Treatment

Care of the original infection is of prime importance. For severe cases, bed rest is indicated. Elevation of the part is advisable. Sedatives (℞ 15, 23) and analgesics (℞ 10, 11) are used when necessary. The application of heat or wet dressings to the initial focus and along the course of the lymphangitis may help to localize the infection and relieve discomfort. Blood cultures should be made in the rapidly spreading type.

Since gram-positive organisms are the usual cause, penicillin (℞ 28, 29) is most frequently given. Sulfonamides (℞ 37, 38), streptomycin (℞ 32), aureomycin (℞ 35), Chloromycetin (℞ 36), or combined therapy, may be necessary when indicated by cultures and organism sensitivity tests. Treatment should be continued until the temperature has been normal for 72 hours and all evidence of acute infection has disappeared. Manipulation of the lesion is contraindicated, and surgery usually should be withheld until definite evidence of localization and suppuration is obtained. With chronic lymphangitis, control of the underlying infection often halts further extension, but little can be accomplished to repair the damage already done.

LYMPHADENITIS

Inflammation of lymph nodes anywhere in the body.

Etiology

Any organism capable of infecting tissue can produce lymphadenitis (e.g., bacteria, viruses, spirochetes, fungi). Streptococci and staphylococci are most frequently responsible. The infection usually is secondary but may be primary. Certain infectious diseases cause local or generalized lymphadenitis as part of their characteristic effect, and primary diseases of lymphatic tissue occur as well.

Symptoms and Signs

Lymphadenitis may appear with minimal evidence of sepsis or, conversely, mild-appearing lymphadenitis may be accompanied by severe toxic manifestations. Single nodes or groups of nodes may be affected, or involvement may be widespread, all depending upon the character of the invading organism.

A group of regional nodes become palpable and may enlarge greatly. In most types of acute lymphadenitis, they are tender and painful, and the overlying skin is inflamed; motion of adjacent structures is voluntarily inhibited due to pain. Pronounced swelling of the surrounding tissue often occurs, and suppuration with abscess formation or discharge through the skin may develop. Low grade or chronic infections may produce small, firm, nontender nodes that persist indefinitely, caseate and form cold abscesses, or erode through the surface and become chronic ulcers.

Diagnosis

The diagnosis of lymphadenitis is usually simple. A regional group or chain of enlarged nodes often provides a clue to the causal infection. For example, pediculosis capitis in children may be disclosed by the finding of enlarged posterior cervical nodes; an abscessed molar, by submaxillary lymphadenopathy; or an oral malignancy by an enlarged submental node. Enlarged postauricular nodes occur in German measles; inguinal nodes in lymphogranuloma venereum, chancroid, or syphilis; peritracheal and peribronchial nodes in tuberculosis, Hodgkin's disease, coccidioidomycosis, pertussis, nonspecific bronchiolitis, or carcinoma of the lung. Early infections may sometimes be diagnosed following the discovery of enlarged epitrochlear or popliteal nodes. Ulcerating nodes suggest tuberculosis, tularemia, anthrax, actinomycosis, or malignancy. A hard (Virchow's) node in the left supraclavicular fossa suggests metastatic carcinoma. Generalized lymph node involvement suggests such diseases as infectious mononucleosis, sarcoidosis, Hodgkin's disease, leukemia, or lymphosarcoma. The juvenile type of rheumatoid arthritis (Still's disease), secondary syphilis, plague, measles, poliomyelitis, scarlet fever, and generalized skin infections (e.g., furunculosis, impetigo, pyoderma, scabies) also may cause widespread lymphadenopathy.

Distinction between mumps (q.v.) and submaxillary or anterior cervical lymphadenitis frequently is required. In mumps, redness and pouting of the duct orifices may supply the necessary clue. In this disease the swelling develops more rapidly, and characteristically is situated over the parotid gland, while that of lymphadenitis generally is about the angle of the jaw, lower and slightly more posterior. However, if the parotitis is mild, the lymphadenitis severe, or the mumps confined to the submaxillary salivary gland, difficulty arises and the course of the disease and differential leukocyte count may determine the diagnosis. Differentiation between mesenteric lymphadenitis and appendicitis or other intra-abdominal disorders is important and often necessary. This requires a careful history, urine and blood examinations, and close clinical observation.

Course and Prognosis

Massive, acutely inflamed nodes may subside completely without sequelae, or regress to leave small firm palpable (shotty) nodes; cellulitis of adjacent tissue may develop; central necrosis may occur forming an acute inflammatory abscess or, as with tuberculous and certain fungous infections, a cold abscess. Rupture of an abscess with ulceration and sinus formation is not infrequent. Many adults exhibit unsightly scars from the drainage of infected lymph nodes in childhood. Bacteremia is a constant serious threat. The prognosis depends upon the type, virulence, and site of the infection, the patient's resistance, and adequacy of treatment. Acute massive or suppurating lymphangitis is uncommon today owing to the sulfonamides, antibiotics, and improved medical care.

Treatment

Removal of the underlying cause when possible usually results in prompt regression of secondary lymphadenitis. Penicillin (℞ 28, 29), sulfadiazine (℞ 37), aureomycin (℞ 35), Chloromycetin (℞ 36), or streptomycin (℞ 32), singly or in combination, should be given as indicated by the sensitivity of the infecting organism. Since streptococci and staphylococci are the most common secondary invaders, penicillin often is given prophylactically. Either hot, wet applications or ice packs help relieve pain. Heat may aid in localizing the infection. Sedatives (℞ 15, 23) and analgesics (℞ 10, 11) also should be given as necessary. Incision and drainage of abscesses should be done, but only when fluctuation is definitely present (never in the case of anthrax). Streptomycin (℞ 32) has proved effective in preventing chronic drainage and sinus formation when tuberculous glands are incised.

BACTEREMIA

The presence of bacteria in the circulating blood. On a clinical basis, there is a trend to include septicemia (presumed multiplication of bacteria in the blood with septic manifestations) and pyemia (bacteremia or septicemia complicated by metastatic abscesses) in the term bacteremia.

Etiology

The fundamental cause of bacteremia is the discharge of bacteria from an infected focus into the circulating blood. Continuation of this process denotes an inability of the body mechanisms to completely localize the infection, and indicates a serious clinical condition.

Pathology and Pathogenesis

Bacteremia is usually associated with certain types of infection. Bacterial infections within blood vessels, such as endocarditis, arterial or arteriovenous vegetative endarteritis, and bacterial endophlebitis can be assumed consistently to cause bacteremia. Rapidly progressing tissue infections such as osteomyelitis and cellulitis, or systemic diseases (e.g. pneumococcal pneumonia, meningitis, and typhoid) also are commonly associated with bacteremia, especially in the early stages. Likewise, apparently localized infections such as cortical abscess of the kidney, pyonephrosis, peritonitis, and carbuncle, when not adequately walled off, may be the source of bacteremia. Bacteremia also may occur with chronic, well localized infections, frequently of low grade, if local defenses are damaged by manipulation. For this reason, a transient bacteremia is frequent after extraction of a tooth, gingival surgery, or the passing of a urethral sound. Ordinarily, the defenses are quickly reestablished, but in some cases not before metastatic foci have occurred. Diagnosis may be rendered difficult when there is a nidus (which itself may be metastatic) situated within the blood stream, such as an infected thrombus or a bacterial vegetation on the endocardium. In such cases, the original infection may have been trivial and forgotten by the time the patient seeks medical aid. Here, this extremely serious form of bacteremia is the result of delivery directly into the blood of large numbers of organisms from a situation where the defense processes are mobilized with difficulty.

Symptoms and Signs

There are few symptoms or signs directly attributable to bacteremia. Fever is almost always present though variable in type. It is perhaps most often intermittent, with wide diurnal variations (septic, "spiking"), but it may be sustained at a high or low level, or be irregular. Chills are usual at the onset. Skin eruptions are frequent. These may be petechial or purpuric, but papular, pustular, or vesicular lesions are of graver diagnostic significance, since the more severe lesions indicate greater virulence of the embolic organism or lowered bodily resistance, or both. Infection of serous cavities and spaces may occur, especially in the pericardium, the larger joints, and the meninges. A complicating endocarditis (q.v.) is not infrequent. Metastatic abscesses may occur almost anywhere and, when sufficiently extensive, produce symptoms and signs

24

characteristic of inflammation in the organ affected. In severe meningococcal infections, a more rapidly overwhelming bacteremia, with hemorrhagic manifestations and collapse, part of the Waterhouse-Friderichsen syndrome (hemorrhage into adrenal glands), may develop (see MENINGOCOCCAL MENINGITIS).

Laboratory Findings

Urinalysis usually reveals albumin and, at times, erythrocytes and leukocytes. Blood counts show anemia and leukocytosis or leukopenia, depending upon the type of infection. The sedimentation rate is elevated. Other blood findings (metabolic function tests: liver, kidney) vary with the severity and organs affected.

Diagnosis

Failure of expected clinical improvement in the course of an infectious disease, exacerbation of septic manifestations, shaking chills, or increase of temperature demands a new evaluation of the patient's status. A search is likely to reveal bacteremia. Diagnosis is established by blood cultures, aimed at identifying both aerobic and anaerobic organisms (see LAB. PROC.). Anaerobic cultures and cultures under increased CO_2 and decreased O_2 tension should be made whenever the primary source and the type of infection are not obvious. Repeated examinations are necessary; a single culture cannot be relied upon to exclude bacteremia. Blood for this purpose is customarily obtained as soon after the onset of a chill as possible.

Course and Prognosis

Transient bacteremia of no clinical significance probably occurs frequently even with mild infections. Bacteremia complicating serious infections is a dangerous development. The formation of multiple embolic abscesses complicating bacteremia is far more serious and affords a poor prognosis. Untreated or unresponsive bacteremia (due to virulence of the organism or poor resistance in the host) progresses to a severe septic state, usually fatal. Metastatic abscesses may appear in great numbers throughout the body, especially with staphylococcic bacteremia. Toxemia is profound, and death results from the effects of the toxemia or the destruction of a vital organ.

Treatment

Bacteremia requires prompt treatment since it indicates lowered resistance in the patient or excessive virulence of the organism, or both. **Supportive measures** are of the utmost importance. Bed rest is imperative, hospitalization preferred. Adequate nutrition must be maintained. Fluid intake should ensure urinary output of 1,500 to 2,000 cc. a day, and blood electrolyte balance must be maintained (see ACID-BASE AND ALLIED DISORDERS). Sedatives (℞ 15, 23) and analgesics (℞

10, 11) are given when necessary. Anemia and hypoproteinemia (q.v.) must be watched for and combated with blood transfusions, plasma, or amino acids solutions, especially when the patient's food intake is inadequate.

Prompt, adequate drainage of pus is necessary, but careful protection of any developing pyogenic membrane and avoidance of unnecessary manipulation are of equal importance. Application of heat and wet compresses when indicated is of value.

Specific treatment of bacteremia is the same as that of the primary infection, but in an intensified form. Penicillin (℞ 28, 29), sulfonamides (℞ 37, 38), aureomycin (℞ 35), Chloromycetin (℞ 36), and streptomycin (℞ 32) are given singly or in any appropriate combination. Repeated blood cultures are important to determine response to therapy, to discover evidence of bacterial resistance, and as a guide to dosage. The dosage of penicillin may sometimes reach 1,000,000 u. or more a day, and of streptomycin 4 Gm./day in certain cases. Drug therapy should continue for at least several days after apparent control, as evidenced by normal temperature, progressive clinical improvement, and repeated negative blood cultures.

TUBERCULOSIS

Since pulmonary tuberculosis is predominantly the form of the disease clinically encountered, the main discussion of tuberculosis, including that of the hematogenous miliary variety, appears in the Respiratory section of the MANUAL. Special forms of tuberculosis, however, are described in appropriate sections of the book (*see* INDEX).

SARCOIDOSIS

(Boeck's sarcoid, Pseudotuberculosis, Benign lymphogranulomatosis, Schaumann's disease, Uveoparotid fever, Osteitis tuberculosa multiplex cystoides)

A chronic granulomatous disease characterized pathologically by small epithelioid tubercle-like lesions occurring in any organ or tissue, and clinically by a chronic course with few if any symptoms unless the lesions involve vital structures. (Several diseases marked by nodular lesions, previously considered as separate entities, now are included in the term "sarcoidosis.")

Etiology and Incidence

Sarcoidosis has been variously described as a type of tuberculosis, as a disease caused by acid-fast bacilli not yet identified, as a disease entity characterized by proliferation of reticulo-endothelial cells, as a systemic tumor of multicentral origin, and as the product of an unknown virus. The best supported opinion, however, is that the etiology remains unknown.

The disease is universal in distribution; numerous cases have been reported in the United States. It occurs frequently in Negroes. Most cases occur in the 2nd and 3rd decades of life, but cases also have been reported in children and the aged.

Pathology

The individual lesion of sarcoidosis is a tubercle-like structure, approximately the size of a miliary tubercle, and consists almost exclusively of large epithelioid cells which are frequently fused. Confluence of many adjacent foci frequently occurs. Langhans' giant cells are relatively rare. Lymphocytes are, as a rule, found only in the periphery, and probably belong to the normal organ structure in which sarcoid involvement has occurred and not to the sarcoid tubercle itself. In contrast to tuberculosis, caseation does not belong to the pathognomonic picture of sarcoidosis, although minute central foci of caseation are found not infrequently, provided many different foci are examined in many sections. Healing occurs spontaneously in a good many cases, either by resorption or fibrosis. Again in contrast to tuberculosis, fibrosis rarely leads to encapsulation; rather, the entire granulomatous lesion is transformed into a fibrosed nonspecific nodule, consisting of broad hyalinized fibers without nuclei or nuclear debris. Various inclusion bodies have been described, but they are not pathognomonic of sarcoidosis. They may be manifestations of the causative agent. While sarcoidosis was first described as a dermatologic disease, it has become recognized that almost any organ in the body may be involved. The sites of predilection are lymph nodes, lung, skin, bone marrow, liver, spleen, kidneys, and myocardium, approximately in the order named. Relatively rare sites are the mammary glands, adrenals, and other glands of internal secretion. As in other diseases of systemic distribution, such as lupus erythematosus disseminatus and periarteritis nodosa (q.v.), sarcoidosis may give rise to bizarre clinical manifestations. Some typical syndromes had previously been described as separate entities before the sameness of the pathologic process was realized.

Impairment of function is caused by sarcoidosis only if the seeding of a given organ is dense. Massive involvement of the bone marrow may produce calcemia. Similarly, renal impairment, diabetes insipidus, and myocardial damage have been attributed to sarcoid infiltration.

Symptoms and Signs

Many patients with sarcoidosis have no symptoms at all, and the diagnosis is made only as an accidental finding. Malaise, fatigue, and slight temperature elevation may temporarily be present. Other symptoms depend entirely upon the particular localization in each case.

Most patients with pulmonary dissemination have no respiratory symptoms, but in particularly massive involvement and in the late stages of fibrosis, dyspnea and cough may occur. Lymph node involvement usually is asymptomatic and painless unless pressure on neighboring organs is produced, for example, in massive enlargement of mediastinal lymph nodes. Involvement of bone marrow occurs most frequently in the small bones of the feet and hands, mainly in the phalanges. These may lead to local deformities with marked swelling of the involved parts. Roentgenologically, small cystlike "punched-out" areas may be seen. Isolated bone marrow involvement has been described as Jüngling's disease or as osteitis tuberculosa multiplex cystoides. Such bone lesions are more frequently associated with lupus pernio than with other forms of sarcoidosis of the skin. Skin lesions in sarcoidosis have a fairly characteristic appearance, usually described as violaceous in color, slightly raised and not itching.

Distinct syndromes in which the pathologic lesion is indistinguishable from sarcoidosis, and probably is sarcoidosis, have been described. (1) **Uveoparotid fever:** In the few cases of this disease that have come to autopsy, and in the larger numbers on which biopsies were taken, the lesions were the same as those in sarcoidosis. (2) **Mikulicz's disease:** Some, but by no means all, cases of Mikulicz's syndrome show the histologic characteristics of sarcoidosis. (3) **Regional ileitis:** Similar to (2), regional ileitis shows in some cases histologic findings indistinguishable from sarcoidosis.

A number of unclassified and ill-defined cases have been reported which showed on biopsy or at autopsy the same histologic picture. Among these may be mentioned some cases of splenomegaly, cases of undiagnosed miliary dissemination in the lung, cases of localized or generalized lymphadenopathy, and the granulomatosis occurring in some beryllium workers. However, with berylliosis (q.v.), symptoms of dyspnea usually are more severe than would be expected from the X-ray appearance because of intra-alveolar edema associated with the granulomatous lesions.

For all these cases, with the possible exception of some cases of uveoparotid fever, symptoms are much less than might be expected from the extent of the anatomic involvement.

Clinical Course

The clinical course is usually marked by very few symptoms and signs, and none is diagnostic by itself. It is always of long duration and the various separate syndromes mentioned may succeed each other. Progression is as a rule very slow. Spontaneous clearing of the lesion or healing by scar formation occurs. However, the lesions may persist for many years without showing any tendency toward progression or retrogression.

Laboratory Findings

There are no characteristic changes in the red cell, white cell, or differential count. During the active phase of the disease a moderate monocytosis or eosinophilia may be present. The urine usually is normal, although impaired renal function as manifested by azotemia and decreased urea clearance may occur. The E.S.R. frequently is elevated in patients whose disease is active. Hypercalcemia may be present in cases with bone marrow involvement. The serum phosphorus may be above normal. Increased plasma proteins with a relatively greater increase in the globulin fraction are commonly noted.

Diagnosis

A definite diagnosis can be made only by histologic examination. The typical configuration shows a tuberculoid arrangement of epithelioid cells. In later stages, the miliary granulomas may be partially or completely replaced by a coarse, fibrillar, hyaline fibrosis. In the absence of biopsy material, the following considerations may lead to a presumptive diagnosis. Symptoms are absent or slight, at least in comparison to the extent of the involvement. If pulmonary involvement is present, it usually is a fine or coarse nodular, bilateral symmetrical dissemination. With long-standing lesions there may be evidence of emphysema. Pulmonary involvement is frequently associated with considerable enlargement of the hilar lymph nodes. These may be involved even without evident pulmonary infiltration. The right upper paratracheal nodes also may be enlarged. The pulmonary nodular lesions may in part be confluent. There probably is no other disease which can produce such massive pulmonary and mediastinal involvement without producing notable symptoms.

An important diagnostic sign is failure to react to the tuberculin skin test even with high concentration of tuberculin (1 mg. OT). This occurs in about 80% of adult patients—a much higher percentage of tuberculin energy than is met with in the general population. Bone lesions, demonstrable by X-ray, may help to confirm, although their absence does not preclude, a diagnosis of sarcoidosis. The differentiation from chronic tuberculosis in an anergic phase may be difficult. Apparently, typical cases of sarcoidosis may terminate in active disseminated tuberculosis.

Prognosis

The prognosis is fair to good, depending on the organ or organs involved. Ordinarily, the patient is able to continue his accustomed work for many years without discomfort. Cutaneous sarcoidosis is a comparatively benign disease as far as prognosis for life is concerned. The eyes are affected in 25 to

40% of all cases, and blindness or impairment of vision often is a sequel. Pulmonary, visceral and bone lesions may be severe enough to be incapacitating.

Treatment

No specific treatment for sarcoidosis is known. Various forms of therapy, including X-ray treatment, have been tried without convincing results. Calciferol (R 135) has been used in a few patients with apparently encouraging results. A dose of 50,000 to 300,000 u. daily by mouth is recommended. Patients with an elevated blood calcium or BUN at the onset of treatment should receive the smaller doses and be observed more closely. Blood calcium studies are necessary at least once every 2 weeks during treatment. If the blood calcium level rises above 12 mg./100 cc., or if there is any other evidence of hypercalcemia, such as anorexia, nausea and vomiting, malaise, weakness, and dizziness, the treatment should be stopped. Early in the course of treatment the patient's symptoms may be severely aggravated.

Encouraging results also have been obtained with dihydrotachysterol (R 136). The dose used is 3.75 mg. daily for the first 3 days followed by 0.625 or 1.25 mg. daily by mouth. The same precautions are necessary as described for calciferol. Bed rest probably is advisable for as long as signs or symptoms of active disease exist, although the efficacy of such a measure has not been definitely established. Symptomatic treatment is indicated for whatever symptoms may arise.

TYPHOID FEVER

(Enteric fever)

An acute generalized infection, caused by Eberthella typhosa, *with marked involvement of the lymphatic tissues and characterized by fever, bradycardia, rose-colored eruption, abdominal signs, and splenomegaly.*

Epidemiology and Pathology

Water is the most common source of infection; food, especially milk, is the next most common. Flies may spread typhoid by carrying the organisms from infected feces to food. Direct contact infection is possible but infrequent. Healthy carriers, particularly food handlers, are responsible for many outbreaks.

The organism enters the body through the gastrointestinal tract, invading the blood stream by way of the lymphatic channels. There is hyperplasia and often ulceration of Peyer's patches, especially in the ileum and cecum. When the ulcers heal, no scar results. The kidneys and liver usually show cloudy swelling and the latter may reveal a patchy necrosis. The spleen is enlarged and soft. Rarely, the lungs show pneumonic changes.

Symptoms and Signs

The incubation period varies, averaging 10 to 14 days. The onset usually is gradual, with chilly sensations (occasionally chills), malaise, headache, anorexia, epistaxis, diarrhea or constipation, and backache. Bronchitis is present in about 40% of patients, and may lead to a mistaken diagnosis of a primary pulmonary infection.

If the course is unaltered by therapy, typically the temperature rises daily by steps and reaches its maximum in 7 to 10 days, maintaining a peak level for another 7 to 10 days, and then falling by lysis by the end of the 4th week. The pulse is relatively slow, in comparison to the degree of fever, and often dicrotic. Rose-colored spots appear between the 7th and 10th days, most commonly on the abdomen and chest. These erythematous "rose spots" are discrete, rounded, and disappear on pressure. They emerge in crops which persist for 2 to 5 days and then fade. Splenomegaly usually is noted (65%) by the end of the 1st week of the disease. Delirium and stupor are frequently observed. Leukopenia and anemia are characteristic of the disease and are most marked at the end of the 3rd week. Albuminuria, often with casts, is frequent.

Atypical clinical manifestations are common. The disease may occur with predominant pharyngeal symptoms (sore throat); with abdominal symptoms (nausea, vomiting, abdominal pain, rigidity); with respiratory symptoms (bronchitis, pneumonia); with renal symptoms (nephritis); or with nervous symptoms (meningismus, psychosis). Ambulatory ("walking") typhoid is not uncommon, especially during epidemics.

Complications

Complications occur in 25 to 30% of all cases and account for 60 to 75% of all deaths.

1. Intestinal hemorrhage may be slight or profuse, occurring most often during the 3rd week and manifesting itself by a sudden fall in temperature or an abrupt rise in the pulse rate, pallor, sweating, hypotension, and rarely abdominal pain. The mortality rate in these cases averages 25%.

2. Intestinal perforation is the most fatal (25 to 33%) complication. It is most common during the 3rd week and in adult males, especially those who have shown pronounced abdominal signs. There is sudden sharp abdominal pain, usually in the lower right quadrant, accompanied by nausea, vomiting, fall in temperature, rapid pulse, leukocytosis, and muscle spasm.

3. Less frequently, there may be pneumonia, thrombophlebitis, parotitis, myocarditis, meningitis, peripheral neuritis, alopecia, nephritis, cystitis, osteitis, and periostitis, arthritis, spon-

dylitis (typhoid spine), otitis media, psychoses, cholecystitis, or abortion.

Diagnosis

Diagnosis depends on the demonstration of typhoid bacilli in the blood, urine, or feces or the development of a positive Widal reaction. During the 1st week, typhoid bacilli may be cultured from the blood in 80 to 85% of patients; later, positive cultures are less frequently obtained. By the end of the 3rd week, the organism may be cultured from the urine or feces of 50 to 80% of patients. The Widal agglutination test becomes positive during the 2nd week of the disease; in doubtful cases, repeated tests will demonstrate a progressive rise in the agglutination titer of the patient's serum. Erroneous diagnosis may be made if the possibility of an anamnestic reaction is overlooked; that is, the reappearance of agglutinins, due to previous typhoid vaccination, as a result of nonspecific stimulation by a nontyphoid infection. Typhoid bacilli contain both H and C antigens which stimulate corresponding antibodies. It has been demonstrated that, with the anamnestic reaction, H agglutinins rise, whereas the O agglutinins rise only during a typhoid infection. Thus, the O antigen is indicated for use in diagnostic Widals, which usually remain positive for 3 to 12 months, rarely longer. Typhoid vaccination gives a positive Widal within 10 days and this may persist up to 2 years.

Typhoid fever must be differentiated from paratyphoid fever, trichinosis, typhus fever, meningitis, pyelonephritis, miliary tuberculosis, malaria, brucellosis, and abdominal Hodgkin's disease.

Prognosis

The prognosis varies greatly, the fatality rate for all cases ranging between 7 and 14%. With complications, the outlook is poorer. Recurrence of fever during convalescence is common and may be due to dietary indiscretion, constipation, physical exertion, or nervous excitement. These recrudescences last 1 to 6 days and must not be confused with a relapse. A true relapse is characterized by steplike fever, rash, and splenomegaly. One or more relapses may occur in up to 15% of all patients.

Treatment

Prophylaxis: Early recognition and isolation of patients with typhoid is essential. Stools and urine may be effectively disinfected by the use of 5% carbolic acid, 10% formaldehyde, or steam. Bed clothes, eating utensils, urinals, and bed pans must be sterilized after each use. Contact with the patient requires thorough washing of the hands with soap and water, followed by 70% alcohol, 1:3,000 bichloride of mercury, or 1:1,000 benzalkonium chloride.

Adequate purification of drinking water and pasteurization of all milk is mandatory. Typhoid carriers must not handle food intended for others.

Typhoid vaccination is of proved value. It is especially indicated for contacts, during epidemics, during travel in endemic areas, and in areas where untreated water is drunk. Children, as well as adults, should be immunized under these circumstances. Triple vaccine contains 1 billion killed typhoid bacilli and 750 million each of killed *Salmonella paratyphi* and *S. schottmülleri*/cc. The subcut. dose for an adult is 0.5 cc., 1 cc., and 1 cc. injected at intervals of 7 to 10 days. The intracutaneous inoculation of this vaccine produces effective immunity and is said to eliminate local reaction. It may, however, cause local skin necrosis and pigmented scars. The dose for this type of administration is 0.1 cc., 0.15 cc., and 0.2 cc. of triple vaccine, given at weekly intervals. The value of oral vaccine remains, at best, highly questionable.

Specific: Chloromycetin (℞ 36) and aureomycin (℞ 35) have been used orally with dramatic results in many cases. Combined oral and parenteral therapy with streptomycin has given indifferent results and its value is questionable. The precise worth of these specific agents in the treatment of typhoid fever still is to be determined.

Supportive: Skilled nursing care is most important. When possible, hospitalization is desirable; otherwise, a screened room is utilized, from which all unnecessary furnishings have been removed. If special nurses are unavailable, the family should be instructed as to isolation technic and the observance of any change in the patient's condition which might indicate a complication. In addition, members of the family should be immunized against typhoid fever. Visitors should be discouraged.

The bed should have rubber sheeting to protect the mattress from soiling and contamination. The mouth and teeth are kept clean by rinsing with saline or dilute peroxide after meals and by the use of the toothbrush and dental floss twice daily. Chewing gum tends to prevent parotitis by promoting salivation. The skin should be kept clean and dry by a tepid sponge bath daily and the frequent use of alcohol rubs and powder. Frequent turning of the patient, with passive or active exercise of the leg and thigh muscles, may prevent phlebothrombosis of the leg veins and pulmonary complications. These conditions should receive usual therapy (q.v.) except that one should hesitate to employ anticoagulants knowing that a complicating intestinal hemorrhage thereby might be aggravated.

Purgatives and laxatives are to be avoided since they cause distention. A saline or tap water enema daily will insure bowel evacuation and diminish distention. Mineral oil (℞ 139) may be given at night.

Headache may be controlled by an ice cap. Analgesics and antipyretics are not recommended because they may mask the onset of a complication. Excessive fever may be alleviated by frequent sponge baths with water at 70° F. The use of ice baths or tubs is contraindicated. Delirium may be lessened by the use of paraldehyde (℞ 18) rectally, or chloral hydrate (℞ 19).

Dietary

One of the greatest advances in therapeutics is the rational administration of food and fluids to typhoid fever patients. Formerly, restriction of diet and fluids led to dehydration, malnutrition, and avitaminosis which certainly increased the death rate. Weight loss need not be an inevitable complication in this disease. During the period of high fever, 4,000 to 6,000 cc. of fluids should be administered daily, orally or parenterally, or both. Use may be made of 10% glucose and protein hydrolysates solutions for their caloric value. Since the B.M.R. is elevated, a diet of 3,000 to 4,000 calories a day with supplementary vitamins is essential. This should consist of liquids, semisolid and soft foods (see DIETS). Frequent small feedings are preferable. The main constituents of the diet are cereal gruels, milk, cream, butter, eggs, potatoes, cream soups, gelatin desserts, custard, junket, crackers, and toast, scraped or finely ground meat, strained fruit juices, and stewed fruits. Protein hydrolysates may be given orally. Caloric intake may be increased by the addition of such foods as lactose, dextrose, jams, cream, and butter.

The patient's likes and dislikes must of course be considered and the diet varied as much as possible and served attractively so as not to affect adversely an already poor appetite. In some instances, it may be necessary to resort to tube feedings, using a liquid diet consisting of protein, dextrose, cream, egg, emulsified oil, salt, and vitamins (see DIETS). A total of 2,500 to 3,500 calories a day may be given, in feedings of 5 to 7 ounces. This diet has almost no residue, weight loss is avoided, and abdominal distention may be eliminated to a great degree. Should it develop, it usually can be controlled by an enema, reduction in the intake of carbohydrate and milk, the application of hot stupes to the abdomen, and the use of a rectal tube. If distention persists, Pitressin (℞ 120), or neostigmine (℞ 114), may be administered in the smallest effective dose. Liberal use may be made of whole blood transfusions as a supportive or therapeutic measure.

Occasionally, diarrhea may be distressing. In such patients, the diet should be reduced to boiled milk, boiled rice, and cocoa. Opium capsules (℞ 130), paregoric (℞ 128), or bismuth (℞ 129) may be administered after each diarrheal movement. As soon as the diarrhea is controlled, the high caloric diet must be cautiously resumed.

Treatment of Complications

Hemorrhage requires immediate treatment. Complete rest,

mild sedation (℞ 18, 19), temporary starvation, and frequent blood pressure readings are necessary. Small doses of morphine (℞ 11) may be used only when the possibility of perforation is excluded. When indicated, blood volume is restored by the judicious use of whole blood, plasma, protein hydrolysates, glucose, and saline. The use of coagulants has been disappointing.

Perforation demands immediate laparotomy, followed by the combined use of penicillin (℞ 28) and streptomycin (℞ 32) to combat peritonitis (q.v.).

Other complications, such as cardiac failure, phlebitis, or decubitus, must be constantly borne in mind and appropriate therapy (q.v.) instituted as indicated.

Convalescence

After 1 week of normal temperature, pulse, and blood pressure, the patient may sit up in bed. After 3 or 4 days, he may be allowed out of bed. Thereafter, as his strength returns, gradually increasing activity is permitted. The diet is slowly increased so that a full normal diet is being taken by the 10th day of convalescence. The carrier state must be ruled out by frequent stool cultures. Carriers must be educated on how to care for themselves and be forbidden to handle food for others. Rarely, cholecystectomy is advisable to eliminate a carrier focus.

PARATYPHOID FEVER

An acute generalized infection which, though usually milder, clinically and pathologically resembles typhoid fever. Paratyphoid bacilli A and B are the causative agents. Under the revised nomenclature, paratyphoid bacillus A is known as *S. paratyphi* and paratyphoid bacillus B as *S. schottmülleri*. There is no essential difference between infections with these two organisms. Epidemics of typhoid and paratyphoid fever may exist simultaneously. There is no protection against this infection, however, when immunization is carried out only with *E. typhosa*. Epidemiology is the same as for typhoid fever.

Bacteriologically, these organisms belong to the colon-typhoid-dysentery group. They grow on ordinary culture media but culture differentiation from *E. typhosa* is difficult except on special media. The most reliable test for differentiation from *E. typhosa* is the agglutination reaction.

Pathologically, there is little to differentiate paratyphoid from typhoid except that the lesions are less extensive, with less tendency to ulceration. Thus, complications of hemorrhage and perforation are uncommon.

The incubation period usually is somewhat shorter than in typhoid and the onset is much more abrupt, often with chill and severe headache. On purely clinical grounds, however, one cannot differentiate the two diseases and the laboratory procedures mentioned preceding are essential. In general, the infection is milder, diarrhea is usual, sweats may be annoying and the total duration is shorter. Rose spots may be present as in typhoid. Nausea, vomiting, diarrhea, and abdominal pain may occur at the onset and differentiation from food poisoning (q.v.) is difficult. In fact, Salmonella organisms frequently cause food poisoning but the two under consideration here are less frequently the etiologic agents than others of the group. Joint involvement may occur and various forms of arthritis must be excluded. Respiratory complications are more common than in typhoid fever but in general other complications are similar.

Correct diagnosis is made by culturing the organism from the blood stream or stool and by agglutination tests. Treatment is similar to that outlined for typhoid fever. Prognosis in general is better. Prophylaxis depends on immunization and those other measures described under typhoid fever. As in that disease, cases may occur among immunized individuals.

CHOLERA

(Asiatic cholera, Epidemic cholera, Cholera indica)

An acute specific infection, involving primarily the lower portion of the ileum, and manifested by profuse purging, vomiting, muscular cramps, dehydration, anuria, and collapse.

Etiology, Epidemiology, and Pathology

The causative organism is *Vibrio comma* (*V. cholerae asiaticae;* Koch's vibrio), a short, curved, motile, gram-negative rod, which produces a powerful endotoxin on disintegration.

Cholera is spread by the ingestion of water, milk, or other foods that have been contaminated by the excrement of patients or carriers. It is a disease of warm countries, since cold weather inhibits the growth of *V. comma* in human dejecta. It is endemic in India, China, Japan, and the Philippine Islands. Epidemics are usually caused by contamination of the water supply.

Severe generalized dehydration is present. Inflammatory changes are conspicuous by their absence, and the viscera are surprisingly normal. The principal seat of infection is in the ileum, where the lesions are superficial. They consist of minute hemorrhages and inflammation of Peyer's patches and the solitary lymph nodules. The gallbladder may become a focus of infection, as is commonly the case in cholera carriers. After death, an early and extreme rigor mortis is characteristic.

Clinical Course

The incubation period varies from 1 to 6 days, but usually is 2 to 3 days. The onset of the disease ordinarily is characterized by either a preliminary mild diarrhea, or sudden violent purging with loss of sphincter control. There is a feeling of weight and oppression, or colicky pains in the abdomen. Typical stools resemble rice water (turbid, cloudy, grayish brown liquid) or are clear and watery and contain mucous shreds. Rarely, the infection is so overwhelming that the patient dies before diarrhea begins ("cholera sicca"). Nausea and vomiting are common and follow the diarrhea.

As a result of fluid loss with the diarrhea and vomitus, severe dehydration occurs. The patient suffers from intense thirst. He exhibits a white, dry tongue; a dry, characteristically wrinkled skin; shrunken eyeballs, hollow cheeks, and cyanosis. Oliguria and anuria ensue, resulting in acidosis and uremia. The blood pressure is decreased. The temperature by mouth often is normal or subnormal, although the pulse and respiratory rates are increased. The vomiting and diarrhea continue. Death may result from asthenia, respiratory failure, acidosis, dehydration, or uremia.

Evidence of recovery becomes apparent, in nonfatal cases, about the 3rd day of illness. Reestablishment of renal secretion is the first favorable sign. The vomiting gradually ceases and the stools become formed. The temperature by mouth rises moderately, commonly reaching 101° or 103° F. The pulse rate falls to approximately normal, the blood pressure rises, the skin becomes warmer, and abdominal pain disappears.

Diagnosis and Laboratory Findings

The diagnosis of cholera is suspected on the basis of physical findings and the presence of an epidemic, and is confirmed by the isolation of *V. comma* in cultures from the stool and its subsequent identification through agglutination by immunized animal serum. Clinically, it must be distinguished from other diseases (q.v.) which may cause severe diarrhea and vomiting, such as food poisoning, bacillary dysentery, or amebiasis.

In cholera, there usually is a leukocytosis (up to 25,000). Because of hemoconcentration, the specific gravity of the blood rises above 1.058, and the red cell count is increased. A decline in CO_2 combining power reflects the acidosis which is frequently present. The daily volume of urine excreted varies from 100 to 300 cc. in most instances; albumin and casts usually are present.

Prognosis

In many instances, the outlook depends largely upon therapy. In untreated cases the fatality rate averages 50%; it may be as high as 90% early in an epidemic and decline to 15% toward the end. The fatality rate may be reduced to 5% or less by modern therapy.

Prophylaxis

In the United States, cholera has been controlled since 1873 by the purification of water supplies, the proper disposal of human excrement, and effectual quarantine methods at the ports of entry. The value of active immunization with a vaccine containing 4,000 to 8,000 killed cholera organisms/cc. is controversial, but generally required by quarantine authorities. When in endemic or epidemic regions, one must observe the usual precautions against water- or food-borne disease. These measures include the use of boiled water, avoidance of uncooked vegetables and salads, protection of food from insects, and care lest soiled hands carry infectious material to the mouth.

Treatment

It is essential to combat dehydration, acidosis, and circulatory collapse and to restore electrolyte balance by the administration of parenteral fluids. An initial infusion of 1,000 to 2,000 cc. of Isotonic Sodium Chloride Solution U.S.P. may be followed by additional quantities depending upon the needs of the patient. These may be estimated either by total fluid loss in the urine, feces, and vomitus, or by blood hematocrit and specific gravity determinations. Maintenance of normal urine volume is a good criterion of effective therapy. When acidosis (q.v.) is present or threatened (as reflected in decreased CO_2 combining power of the blood), Sodium Lactate Injection U.S.P. may be given I.V. in combination with the saline solution. (Dosage is estimated on a basis of 60 cc./Kg. body wt. as the amount necessary to yield an additional 33 volumes of CO_2/100 cc. of blood plasma.) In the event that the lactate solution is unavailable, 300 cc. of a sterile 2% solution of sodium bicarbonate may be substituted. In order to combat circulatory collapse, blood plasma may be substituted for a portion of the saline infusion. The number of plasma infusions required depends upon the individual response.

While the patient is vomiting, food and fluids should not be given. As soon as possible, 60 cc. or more of a 1% solution of sodium bicarbonate (℞ 151) may be tried every 15 minutes by mouth. This will aid in replacing the lost fluids and combating acidosis, and may have some palliative effect upon the gastric symptoms. As soon as tolerated, water, tea, and liquid food also may be given. Solid food should be withheld until vomiting has been controlled and food is desired.

Although the value of chemotherapy still is controversial, it may be useful as an adjunct to the regimen of controlled rehydration. Because of the known activity of streptomycin against *V. comma,* in all severe cases use of this drug may be advisable both orally, 4 Gm. in divided doses daily (℞ 33), and parenterally, 2 Gm. I.M. daily in 2 or more doses (℞ 32). Sulfaguanidine (℞ 44) and sulfadiazine (℞ 37) have been found to be active against *V. comma* and also may be used. Although penicillin (℞ 28) has no specific effect against the organism, it may be useful in lessening the possibility of secondary infection.

BACILLARY DYSENTERY
(Shigellosis)

An acute infection of the bowel, usually caused by organisms of the Shigella dysenteriae *and* paradysenteriae *group and characterized by frequent passage of stools containing blood, pus, and mucus, accompanied by abdominal cramps, tenesmus, malaise, and fever.*

Etiology and Incidence

About 80% of the infections are due to Flexner mannite-fermenting bacilli (*S. paradysenteriae*), and 10% to Shiga organisms (*S. dysenteriae*). *S. sonnei, S. dispar,* and Salmonella infections also occur. The organisms are disseminated by flies, contaminated food and perhaps water, and by human carriers. In many tropical areas, dysentery is endemic, and elsewhere it may occur epidemically, attacking chiefly babies and soldiers. From 15 to 80% of children, depending upon the locality, have it before the age of 5, although the incidence is rapidly decreasing through preventive measures.

Pathology and Pathologic Physiology

Dysentery bacilli, ingested with food and drink, pass directly to the intestines. There is no evidence that dysentery is, like typhoid, primarily a septicemia. Not only is the intestinal mucosa affected, but also the submucosa, the muscularis, and occasionally even the peritoneal covering. There is exudation of lymph and cells into the intestinal coats, with edema of the submucosa. The mucous membrane may be only hyperemic with excess of mucus, or it may have superficial ulcerations on the summits of the rugae. The ulcers differ from those of amebic dysentery in that the edges are not undermined. The borders are irregular, reddened, swollen, and infiltrated. A false membrane may cover the mucous membrane. In acute bacillary dysentery, practically the whole colon and often the lower part of the ileum are involved in an acute inflammatory process, which may prove rapidly fatal; in the subacute form, which is seen almost exclusively in adults, the process is usually limited to the lower half of the colon. The C.N.S. may be the seat of lesions due to prolonged absorption of exotoxin which is produced by the growth of *S. dysenteriae* in the intestine.

Symptoms, Signs, and Course

The incubation period is 1 to 4 days. In children, onset is sudden, with fever, irritability or drowsiness, anorexia, vomiting or nausea, diarrhea, abdominal pain and distention, and tenesmus. Within 3 days, blood, pus, and mucus appear in the stools. Generally, the stools increase rapidly to 20 or more daily, and weight loss and dehydration become severe. The untreated child may die in the first 12 days; if not, the acute symptoms subside by the 2nd week. There also is a rare and rapidly fatal form of dysentery with delirium, convulsions, and coma, but little or no diarrhea; death results in 12 to 24 hours.

In adults, most of the infections are afebrile with nonbloody and nonmucous diarrhea and little or no tenesmus. However, in military or asylum epidemics, and occasionally in sporadic cases, onset is characterized by griping abdominal pain, urgency to defecate, and passage of ordinary formed feces, which temporarily relieves the pain. The pain, however, soon returns and the cycle is repeated, but the stools are softer and may be streaked with blood. These attacks recur at decreasing intervals until the patient is more or less continuously at stool, frequently passing nothing but blood and pus. Tenesmus is commonly associated with dysenteric lesions in the rectum, which usually occur early in the disease. Prolapse of the rectum and consequent incontinence of feces may result from severe tenesmus. In a choleriform type of bacillary dysentery, the onset is sudden, with rice water or serous, occasionally bloody, stools. The patient may vomit and become rapidly dehydrated.

In adults, the disease usually clears up spontaneously—mild cases in 4 to 8 days, severe ones in 3 to 6 weeks. Relapses, however, are common, due to dietetic errors, exposure, and allowing the patient to leave bed or to resume a general diet too early. Reinfections, except for relapses, are rare in bacillary dysentery. However, during mixed epidemics, a convalescent from Flexner dysentery may acquire a new infection with Shiga bacillus, and vice versa. Chronic cases are rare both in adults and children, but without sulfonamide therapy, the carrier rate may be as high as 18%.

Arthritis, myocarditis, vulvovaginitis, aspiration pneumonia, otitis, mastoiditis, meningitis, pyuria, eye lesions, and neuritis are rare complications.

Laboratory Findings

The *Shigella* bacillus is found in the stools. Bacillemia and bacilluria may be present. Although the white cell count often is reduced at onset, it averages 13,000. The Schilling count is shifted to the left. Shiga toxin causes hemoconcentration. The plasma CO_2 usually is low.

Diagnosis

A presumptive diagnosis of bacillary dysentery can be made clinically in sporadic cases or during epidemics on the basis of febrile onset, frequent bloody-mucous stools, colic, tenesmus, resistance over the large bowel, palpable thickening of the wall of the colon, and pain on abdominal pressure. Tenesmus is not a constant symptom because it usually is present only with rectal involvement. The presence of pus in the stool is strongly suggestive of bacillary dysentery. The diagnosis in subacute cases, which often occur sporadically in the winter or at the beginning of epidemics, is extremely difficult.

Bacillary dysentery cannot be distinguished clinically from typhoid-paratyphoid fever and Salmonella infections. An appendicular form may simulate appendicitis. In addition, the following common conditions should be considered: digestive disturbances, diarrhea, malnutrition, dehydration, sprue, celiac disease, amebiasis, intestinal parasites, and epidemic diarrhea of the newborn. Less often it is necessary to rule out brain abscess or tumor, cholera, cirrhosis, diverticulitis, meningitis, intestinal obstruction, peritonitis, poisoning, mesenteric thrombosis, tuberculosis, duodenal, gastric or rectal ulcer, foreign body, abdominal tumor, hemorrhoids, rectal polyps, malaria, syphilis and, in adult females, pressure from uterine tumors.

Diagnosis of bacillary dysentery is confirmed by isolation of Shigella from the stools, or by a positive agglutination reaction after the 6th day. Smears of the stools should be examined for blood, pus, and parasites, as well as by darkfield for Vincent's organism, which can cause similar symptoms. Mixed bacillary and amebic infections may be present. Differentiation of amebic dysentery (q.v.), in unmixed infections, is based on the following points: In bacillary dysentery, onset usually is acute and the course brief; in amebic dysentery onset generally is gradual and the course chronic. The amebic form is not marked by toxic symptoms such as high fever, malaise, anorexia, rapid emaciation, and nervous disturbances. Liver abscess is a common complication of amebic, but not of bacillary, dysentery. A therapeutic test by daily hypodermic injections of emetine also is helpful in obscure cases. If the symptoms are not definitely improved within 2 or 3 days, amebic infection usually can be excluded and treatment for bacillary infection instituted. Since the drug is highly toxic, however, this test should be employed only when amebic infection is suspected. Proctoscopic findings also differ: the ulcers in bacillary dysentery are situated on the surface of mucosal folds and the edges are not undermined as they are in amebiasis.

Prognosis

This is good if treatment is prompt and adequate. Without therapy the mortality rate in infants is 25%, in children 5%, and in adults virtually nil. Toxemia, peritonitis, and inanition are the chief causes of death. Malnutrition not only increases susceptibility to the disease, but also increases the mortality.

Prophylaxis

Good sanitation, with elimination of flies and protection of food from contamination, is of the first importance. In endemic areas, treatment of exposed individuals with 1 to 2 Gm. of sulfaguanidine or succinylsulfathiazole by mouth daily is useful preventive therapy. Patients treated with the sulfonamides have a carrier rate of 3% as compared with the usual 18%. Three doses of 0.25 cc. Shiga toxoid will prevent Shiga infections. (Dysentery vaccines still are experimental.) Infants fed lactic acid milk rarely contract dysentery, and the use of whole lactic acid evaporated milk is recommended. The failure to recognize carriers or mild cases of dysentery in adults is responsible for many infections in children. The following precautions are necessary to prevent the spread of milk-, water- and fly-borne diseases: thorough washing of the hands before handling food for children; keeping soiled garments of dysentery patients in covered buckets of soap and water until they can be boiled; screening of houses and the use of mosquito nets.

Treatment

General: Fluid and electrolyte administration is important (*see* ACID-BASE AND ALLIED DISORDERS). Dehydrated infants who are not vomiting should be given hourly, by mouth, water with or without saccharin, 5% sucrose and 0.75% lactic acid in normal saline (1 tsp. sugar and 20 drops lactic acid/100 cc. saline), or a bouillon cube (contains 2.4 Gm. salt) dissolved in a cup of hot water and then cooled. It may be advisable to administer fluids parenterally to correct acidosis and dehydration. The patient's thirst and dehydrated appearance are adequate guides to his need for parenteral fluid. Too much fluid may cause water intoxication, with edema, pneumonia, and convulsions. If fluid therapy is prolonged supportive multivitamin therapy should be given orally or parenterally. Calcium (℞ 150) may be necessary during the acute phase of intoxication to prevent tetany. Skin turgor, determined by pinching, and the specific gravity of the blood indicate the degree of hydration. Blood or plasma transfusions often are beneficial in severe cases.

Drugs (Doses in prescriptions are for adults): Sulfonamides are effective against dysentery organisms. The average duration of the disease with sulfonamide therapy is 3 days in contrast to 18 days without it. Sulfadiazine (℞ 37) probably is the drug of choice, but sulfamerazine (℞ 38) or sulfapyridine (℞ 40) in similar dosage may prove equally effective. The nonabsorbable sulfonamides, succinylsulfathiazole (℞ 41), phthalylsulfathiazole (℞ 42), phthalylsulfacetamide (℞ 43), and sulfaguanidine (℞ 44), are of some value in reducing the bacterial content of the feces and decreasing the severity of the disease. The successful treatment of carriers, as evidenced by 9 consecutive negative stools, with full doses of sulfaguanidine or succinylsulfathiazole for 1 week has been reported. Streptomycin orally (℞ 33), either alone or combined with parenteral administration (℞ 32), may prove superior to the sulfonamides. It should certainly be used whenever the sulfonamides are ineffective. Chloromycetin (℞ 36) also has shown promise in treatment. Paregoric (℞ 128) may be necessary after each stool to allay restlessness, pain and tenesmus in patients ill with this disease.

Feeding of infants: Large amounts of fluid, but no solids, should be given for 12 to 48 hours. If the diarrhea is moderate, lactic acid whole milk without additional carbohydrate may be given as soon as nausea decreases, starting with 30 to 60 cc. (℥ i to ii) at each feeding and increasing in accordance with the infant's appetite. When the stools are "formed," the original feeding is resumed, and the amount increased so that the infant will receive 100 calories/Kg. body wt. (45/lb.). However, if the stools are very loose, 5% milk protein should be added to the milk, and the nipple hole of the bottle enlarged. Infants over 5 months old having diarrhea, but with good appetite and no vomiting, may be fed by spoon at 1 or 2 feedings daily, 30 to 60 Gm. (℥ i to ii) of junket without whey, after they have drunk their whole lactic acid milk. If a breast-fed infant has diarrhea, the breast feeding at 4-hour intervals should be continued after the preliminary fast. If the number of stools is excessive, 30 to 120 cc. (℥ i to iv) of whole lactic acid milk, with or without cane sugar or milk protein, may be substituted for the breast feedings for a few days. The mother's milk supply should be kept up by breast massage or a breast pump. If an infant vomits, the preliminary fast should be prolonged. He then may be given whole lactic acid milk, with or without cane sugar or milk protein, as outlined above. A diet consisting of 2 to 10 tablespoons of scraped, ripe apple pulp every 2 to 4 hours daily, or the equivalent amount of dried apple powder, has been recommended for mild diarrhea, especially at onset. A banana diet, salt-free diet, baked sweet potatoes, sweet foods, fruit juices, and honey also have been suggested. Yeast therapy may be harmful, but a high vitamin diet is advantageous (*see* NUTRITIONAL DEFICIENCIES). Infants who persistently refuse food, and premature infants, may be fed by gavage with a "Chetwood syringe," "Boston Feeder," or medicine dropper. If water is refused, 30 to 60 cc. (℥ i to ii) may be added to the gavage feedings. Pancreatic enzymes (℞ 138) improve digestion, reduce stool size and encourage weight gain.

Adult feeding: With adults, clear fluids may be taken as tolerated and the remainder of the fluid complement achieved with I.V. administration of 5% dextrose in saline. It rarely is necessary to resort to I.V. protein, blood or plasma therapy. When the diarrhea is controlled, a soft bland diet high in protein and carbohydrate and low in fat may be administered as tolerated (*see* DIETS).

Other treatment: Castor oil, calomel, salts, and other purgatives are harmful, and the following are of questionable value: charcoal, chalk, kaolin, aluminum gel, bismuth, tannic acid, intestinal antiseptics (except the sulfonamides and antibiotics), Flexner and Shiga antidysenteric serum, Shiga antitoxin, bacteriophage, colon and dysentery vaccines.

Infants recover from diarrhea much more quickly if kept in a cool room. Placing a tub with a large cake of ice near the bed with an electric fan blowing across it toward the patient is beneficial and does not increase the risk of pneumonia.

AMEBIASIS

(Endamebiasis, Entamebiasis; including Amebic colitis and Amebic dysentery)

An infectious disease caused by the Endameba histolytica, *frequently producing a colitis characterized by the painful passage of bloody mucoid stools.*

Etiology, Incidence, and Epidemiology

E. histolytica is the specific infective agent of amebiasis, the motile trophozoites of which live in the tissues and multiply by simple division. In most cases of the disease, the multiplication of the parasite is limited greatly by the resistive powers of the host. The infective form of the parasite is the cyst, which sometimes is seen in formed stools, and is capable of existing outside the body at room temperature for 2 to 4 weeks.

Passing through the stomach, the cysts reach the region of the ileocecal valve where excystation occurs, resulting in free trophozoites which may attack the tissues. Trophozoites appear to be especially adapted for life in the tissues. Encystment takes place only in the lumen of the gut.

Surveys indicate a general infection rate in the United States of about 10%, though in some southern localities the incidence has approached 40%. In the tropics the carrier rate generally is very high, often exceeding 50%.

Amebic infection is acquired by the ingestion of food or drink contaminated by feces containing amebic cysts. So-called carriers or infected individuals, particularly food handlers (who at the time may not have diarrheal or dysenteric stools), are the principal source. Transmission may involve direct contact with unwashed hands, or pollution of swimming pools. Where proper latrines are not used, the cysts may be carried mechanically on the legs of flies, or in their vomitus or dejecta. In many parts of the world, the use of human feces for fertilization of vegetables and fruits leads to infection when this produce is eaten raw. In highly sanitated areas, the food handler is the most important source of infection.

Pathogenesis

After ingestion the cyst passes through the stomach and small intestine, excysts in the lower ileum, and passes into the colon. Invading the mucous membrane chiefly in the regions of fecal stasis—the cecum, appendix, and ascending colon, the sigmoid colon and rectum—it penetrates the mucosa by direct phagocytosis and by the liberation of cytolysins.

The earliest lesion is a small abscess, usually in the submucosa; later, ulcers form which tend to be ragged and undermined. These lesions, focal and discrete in mild cases, may spread and become confluent. They may be associated with hemorrhage, edema, and sloughing of large areas of mucosa. The muscular coat limits the penetration of the ameba, but occasionally it is destroyed with a resulting perforation. Amebas enter the radicles of the portal vein and are carried to the liver. Most of these probably are destroyed, but if the survivors are numerous, they may cause a hepatitis, or one or more large abscesses. Many liver abscesses are secondarily infected with intestinal bacteria; most are single and are located in the right lobe. Further spread of the disease usually is by direct extension from the liver into the pleura, right lung, and pericardium. Rarely, *E. histolytica* has produced lesions in almost every other organ in the body.

Symptoms and Signs

Most cases of amebiasis are asymptomatic. Amebic ulcerations probably attain a considerable size before symptoms appear. The clinical course is variable and patients with mild or apparently cured infections may suddenly develop hepatitis or dysentery.

Amebic Dysentery: In amebic dysentery, usually over a period of 3 or 4 days, there develops increasingly severe diarrhea associated with weakness and moderate prostration. Nausea, vomiting and some right-sided cramplike pain usually are present. The stools number from 5 to 25/day and generally are brown, semifluid, and foul. Examined grossly, blood and flecks of mucus can often be seen. These probably represent the contents of individual ulcers and usually contain enormous numbers of amebas. There is little or no fever, and the leukocyte count may be as high as 20,000. Urticarial lesions have been described. Fulminating dysentery is much more commonly bacillary than amebic, and is occasionally produced by the combination of bacillary and amebic infections. After the initial attack, recurrences may occur at intervals of variable length. In the intervals between relapses, the patient experiences symptoms of colitis, with recurrent cramps and loose or very soft stools, especially after meals. If allowed to continue untreated, he may exhibit progressive emaciation and increasing though moderate anemia. Attacks often are induced by excessive alcohol intake, fatigue, emotional tension, and excess roughage or condiments in the diet. It is necessary to differentiate between true relapses with appearance of amebas in the stools, and recurrent gastrointestinal symptoms of nonspecific origin.

Amebic Hepatitis and Amebic Abscess: Involvement of the liver arises from intestinal infection. The exact frequency of amebic hepatitis and hepatic abscess is not known, but these conditions are not rarities. About a third of the patients with proved amebic liver disease give a history of dysentery. Hepatic disease may appear 1 to 3 months after an attack of dysentery or it may manifest itself directly in association with an attack. Diffuse amebic hepatitis may be an early stage of abscess formation. Abscesses are usually single and located in the right lobe of the liver but multiple abscesses and abscesses in the left lobe are not rare. Abscesses develop insidiously, although the onset of symptoms may be abrupt. The symptoms include pain or discomfort over the liver, with occasional reference to the right shoulder, irregular and intermittent fever, sweats, chills, nausea, vomiting, weakness, and loss of weight. Jaundice, except in mild degree, is unusual. If evidence of hepatitis persists after 5 or 6 days of treatment, the presence of an abscess should be suspected. When an abscess is present, the liver is usually enlarged and tender, but in some cases it is not palpable. Tenderness may be demonstrable by bimanual compression of the lower right chest wall. However, since tenderness may be well localized, it should be searched for with care. Signs of involvement of the diaphragm, pleura, or lung may be found. Fluoroscopic demonstration of fixation or deformity of the right hemidiaphragm are of value in pointing to the diagnosis. A moderate leukocytosis usually is present, but there is no eosinophilia. Amebas can be demonstrated in the stools in about 33% of the cases of hepatic amebiasis.

Liver abscesses contain a thick, semifluid material composed of more or less cytolyzed remains of tissue. This material often appears like chocolate or anchovy sauce. Motile amebas are found in it in about a third of the cases, depending largely on the part of the abscess from which the material has been derived (they may be entirely absent in the central area, where cytolysis is complete). Cysts are not present.

Complications and Sequelae

In rare instances, the lungs, brain, and other organs are infected by hematogenous spread from the intestines. Lesions of the skin are occasionally infected with amebas, especially in the region of the perineum and buttocks and particularly in association with traumatic and operative wounds. In the healing of extensive lesions of the intestine, the excessive formation of scar tissue sometimes leads to partial obstruction.

Laboratory Findings

Moderate leukocytosis may be present. Eosinophilia is not characteristic. An increased E.S.R. has been reported, especially in patients with amebic hepatitis.

The microscopic findings in the stool are important. Leukocytes and macrophages are relatively scarce. Erythrocytes are numerous in certain portions. Charcot-Leyden crystals may be present.

Motile forms of *E. histolytica* may be found in diarrheic and dysenteric stools, in exudates from lesions, and in abscess contents. Amebic infection should never be considered to be excluded as the result of a single examination. Search for motile amebas should be made only in freshly obtained material. In some cases, especially those in which cecal infection without involvement of the lower colon or rectum is suspected, it may be necessary to give a saline cathartic in order to obtain a satisfactory specimen. Blood stained flecks of mucus in the stool are likely specimens for examination. In some instances, a good specimen can be obtained in the eye of a rectal tube. When liver abscesses are suspected, material for examination may be obtained by aspiration.

Cysts of *E. histolytica* should be sought in formed and semiformed stools. They sometimes may be found even in the more fecal portions of dysenteric specimens. When stools are formed, examination of freshly passed specimens is preferable, but not essential provided the specimen remains moist. Since a single examination detects only about 20% of cyst carriers, at least 3 specimens obtained on different days should be examined. Concentration by zinc sulfate flotation is the most reliable method for finding cysts.

In cases in which parasites cannot be found on stool examination, proctoscopy following a saline enema is a valuable aid, since lesions often are readily visible. Seen through the proctoscope, amebic ulcers do not appear to be deep, ragged, or undermined, and may not suggest the presence of serious disease. While the proctoscope is in place, material for examination should be obtained through the instrument from any lesion which may be accessible. A successful method employs a heavy-walled 1 cc. pipette, the delivery end of which is bent to an angle of about 45° and inserted into a bulb from a urethral syringe. The pipette is inserted through the proctoscope, and with gentle suction, applied to a lesion.

Diagnosis

The possibility of amebic infection should be brought to

mind by the clinical picture and by epidemiologic consideration. The final diagnosis should be based on the demonstration of the etiologic agent.

Amebic Dysentery: Amebic dysentery may be confused with bacillary dysentery, balantidial dysentery, schistosomiasis, ulcerative colitis, regional enteritis, tuberculous enterocolitis, and carcinoma of the large bowel. In contrast to bacillary dysentery, the stools of amebic dysentery are relatively less frequent, less watery, less purulent and more fecal. They are characteristically colored by flecks of both fresh and altered blood and contain tenacious mucus which is not intimately mixed with the blood. In chronic cases, the stools are especially malodorous.

In an uncomplicated case of amebic dysentery, proctoscopy may be negative or may show scattered ulcerations with intervening normal mucosa. The diffuse, catarrhal colitis seen in bacillary dysentery usually is absent.

During a clinical or subclinical amebic infection, symptoms of subacute appendicitis may occur and may be associated with diffuse invasion of the appendix and cecum by amebas. Surgery upon such tissues often results in peritonitis and death. If there is a reasonable suspicion that the symptoms are of amebic origin, it may be advisable to delay operation for 48 to 72 hours in order to observe the effects of emetine.

Amebic Hepatitis and Amebic Abscess: Amebic infections of the liver must be separated from other forms of hepatitis, including abscesses due to bacterial infection. The diagnosis of diffuse amebic hepatitis can be suspected on clinical grounds. Fever, local pain, and tenderness, together with enlargement of the liver, usually are the only findings. A complement fixation test (currently under investigation) appears to be of special diagnostic significance in amebic hepatitis.

Prognosis

In untreated amebic dysentery the mortality rate may reach 20 to 40%, but when treated, the disease is fatal to less than 5% of the patients afflicted. With recurrent or chronic amebic dysentery, prolonged invalidism and a higher incidence of fatalities may be expected.

The mortality from liver abscess may vary from 1 to 100%, depending upon the number of abscesses, their accessibility for drainage, the presence of secondary bacterial infection, and the preoperative use of emetine.

Prophylaxis

Control of the spread of *E. histolytica* is not significantly different from that of other human enteric infections. The high incidence of carriers not known to have had clinical dysentery complicates the problem, but it is ultimately a matter of preventing the access of human feces to the mouths of susceptible individuals.

Treatment

The therapeutic objective in amebiasis is the eradication of all amebas from the tissue and from the lumen of the bowel.

General: In severe cases, with fever and prostration, the patient must be in bed and should receive frequent feedings of boiled milk, stale or toasted white bread, white rice, soft-cooked eggs, gelatin, and tea. An attitude of cheerfulness on the part of attendants is important to the patient. Adequate rest may be secured by use of one of the barbiturates (R 15). After the disappearance of acute symptoms in the fulminating cases there is no need to keep the patient in bed. In average cases without prostration or fever, bed rest is unnecessary—except during the period of emetine therapy, when experience dictates caution because of the demonstrated cardiotoxic nature of this drug.

Chemotherapy: Course A (for acute cases): Emetine hydrochloride (R 68), subcut. or I.M. (*never* I.V.) for 4 to 6 days is administered together with Diodoquin (R 69); the latter drug is continued for a total of 10 days, followed by carbarsone (R 70) for 10 days, and again Diodoquin (R 69) for a second course of 10 days. Total therapy thus is continued for a 30-day period. A daily retention enema in the form of either a 1% carbarsone in 2% sodium bicarbonate solution (R 71), or 2% chiniofon solution in water (R 73) may be given in the presence of extensive ulceration or X-ray deformities in the bowel. During the succeeding 12 days the patient should be given Diodoquin (R 69) or, as a second choice, carbarsone (R 70), by mouth. Since bacillary dysentery often is present as a complication, it may be of benefit to give succinylsulfathiazole (R 41), along with the emetine injections. (CAUTION! Emetine is a toxic drug, and all patients receiving it should be confined to bed. Care must be taken to avoid entrance into a vein, by retracting the plunger of the syringe before the material is injected.) Emetine may cause an increase in diarrhea, often accompanied by nausea. Pregnancy, as well as cardiac disease, is considered to contraindicate the use of emetine.

Course B (for patients who present neither acute dysentery symptoms nor indications of hepatitis): Omit the emetine injections but otherwise treat precisely as in course A.

Course C (for intractable cases that resist ordinary treatment): Cases that resist course A will frequently respond to it after a preliminary course of penicillin (R 28) and succinylsulfathiazole (R 41) has eliminated secondary pyogenic organisms which have become established in the bowel wall.

When a cure is not obtained by following the above courses, it is well to allow a rest interval of 10 to 12 days and then repeat any course of therapy.

Recent observation with certain antibiotics (aureomycin, bacitracin) which influence bacterial flora in the gastrointestinal tract indicate that in some instances *E. histolytica* may disappear during such therapy. Milibis has been used in the treatment of amebiasis with reportedly favorable results.

Amebic Hepatitis: In this condition, the results following the use of emetine are often dramatic. The favorable response to emetine (℞ 68) is so characteristic that it constitutes an important diagnostic aid.

In hepatitis the total dosage of emetine required is larger than in amebic dysentery, amounting in the average case to 1 Gm.; a daily dose of 60 mg. (gr. i) is given subcut. or I.M. for 9 days and later for 6 days, with an intervening rest period of 1 week. All cases of hepatic amebiasis should receive oral treatment, using Diodoquin (℞ 69) or chiniofon (℞ 72), during or following the initial treatment with emetine.

Chloroquine diphosphate (Aralen) (℞ 74) is equal, if not superior, to emetine in the treatment of amebic hepatitis and by far less toxic. It has the further advantage of being given orally. Since it is rapidly eliminated from the gastrointestinal tract, it should be given in conjunction with an intestinal amebacide such as Diodoquin (℞ 69).

Amebic Hepatic Abscess: All cases should receive emetine (℞ 68). In many cases, this treatment alone will suffice even in the presence of a well defined abscess. Aspiration is the surgical procedure of choice in those cases of abscess not responding to emetine therapy.

Criteria of Cure: Because of the liability of amebiasis to relapse, stools should be examined frequently. As a practical procedure, no patient should be discharged until at least 3 stool examinations, including one postcathartic specimen, have been found negative by direct smear and concentration methods. Study of the stools should be repeated weekly for 1 month, monthly for 6 months, and half-yearly for 2 years. Recurrence of gastrointestinal symptoms should not be treated with amebacidal drugs unless parasitic relapse can be proved by demonstration of *E. histolytica*.

MALARIA

An acute, or sometimes chronic, often recurrent, febrile parasitic disease characterized by periodic paroxysms of chills followed by high fever, the presence of parasites within the erythrocytes, frequent splenomegaly, and occasionally jaundice.

Etiology and Distribution

Four types of malarial parasites, each with a different biologic pattern, may affect man. These are *Plasmodium vivax, P. falciparum, P. malariae* and *P. ovale;* however, the latter two are encountered too infrequently to warrant further consideration here. Infection takes place through the bite of an infected anopheles mosquito or by the transfusion of blood from an infected donor.

In the United States, malaria is most prevalent in the Southeast although it is encountered as far north as Illinois and Indiana and as far west as California. Sporadic epidemics have been reported, rarely, in some of the Northeastern States, as in New Jersey, for example. However, most of the hyperendemic malarial areas are outside the United States, notably in the foothills of Central America, northern and northeastern South America, central Africa from the Atlantic to the Indian Ocean, northern Africa (where 90% is falciparum malaria), south and especially southeast Turkey, the Levant, Iraq and Iran, Afghanistan, India, Ceylon, Burma, China, Siam, Malaya, The Netherlands Indies, Formosa, the Philippines, and many islands of the Pacific. Curiously enough, there is a malaria-free zone in the central and south Pacific, including the islands of Galapagos, Marquesas, Fiji, New Caledonia, New Zealand, Guam, the Marshalls, and the Carolines.

Pathogenesis and Pathology

The life cycle of the malarial parasite begins when the female anopheles mosquito, feeding on a patient infected with malaria, ingests blood containing gametocytes. These are taken into the intestine of the mosquito, penetrate its intestinal wall and undergo a series of developments, to emerge as sporozoites and migrate to the mosquito's salivary glands. The parasite now is ready to complete its life cycle in man. After the mosquito delivers the sporozoites into the skin of a susceptible subject, the asexual phase of the parasite's cycle begins. In the case of *P. vivax*, it is postulated that the sporozoite may undergo a series of developments in fixed tissues of the body, probably the liver, before invading the red cells and initiating the clinical aspects of the disease. Duration of the parasite's development in the fixed tissue phase is exceedingly variable, ranging from 5 days to 3 years. This ability of *P. vivax* parasites to "hibernate" and to elaborate erythrocytic forms from time to time is responsible for the persistence of the disease and the tendency to relapses which may occur at extremely variable intervals.

In vivax malaria, the number of relapses and their spacing following a single infection probably are an expression of the biologic characteristics of the tissue phase of the particular strain of *P. vivax*. For example, the strains commonly encountered in the Mediterranean area are prone to have a long latent period (6 to 12 months) between the primary attack, or the suppressed primary infection and the first relapse, and rarely give rise to more than 4 relapses. With the southwest Pacific strains, however, the first relapse or the primary attack after discontinuance of suppressive therapy usually occurs in 3 to 6 weeks and the disease may persist through 10 or 12 relapses. Some of the strains of *P. vivax* encountered in China, Burma, and India seem to resemble the Mediterranean strains; others seem to resemble the southwest Pacific strains. As regards their response to chemotherapy, certain strains in China and India seem quite different from those encountered elsewhere. Strains met with in southern United States, like the

MALARIAL PARASITES IN THE BLOOD
(Giemsa Stain)

Plasmodium vivax		*Plasmodium falciparum*
Ring form with circle of cytoplasm interrupted by mass of red chromatin		Signet ring—½ the size of the ring form in *P. vivax* . . . .
↓		↓
Ameboid form with irregular arrangement of cytoplasm and red granular pigment (Schüffner's dots)		Ring increases in size, approaching size and appearance of vivax trophozoite. Double chromatin dots more frequent than in other species. Marginal and bridge forms are frequent. A few pigment granules give a yellowish tinge to cytoplasm . . . .
↓		
Increasing size of red cell and parasite, with increase in number of red granules (Schüffner's dots)	24–	
↓		↓
Hemoglobin replaced by a rosette of merozoites (usually 16 in number) with blue nuclei and red cytoplasm	48 hrs.	Mature trophozoite appears as solid blue mass with red chromatin near periphery . . . .
		↓
↓		The next 2 stages are rarely seen in the peripheral blood:
Rupture of the red cell; liberation of the merozoite and reinvasion of new red cells, preferably the reticulocyte form		↓
		The schizont develops as the red pigment increases and separates into dots of red surrounded by blue cytoplasm. The number of these merozoites varies between 8 and 24 . . . .
		The red cell ruptures and the merozoites invade new red cells . . . .
↓		↓
2-3 days later, gametocytes appear. They fill the red cells with chromatin and scattered pigment, paler in the male than in the female.		After acute infection has subsided, gametocytes appear in increasing numbers. These sausage-shaped crescents contain course granules of chromatin and pigment.

(48 hrs. on left side, 24–48 hrs. on right side)

Mediterranean strains, give rise to a less persistent infection than do the southwest Pacific strains and tend to exhibit long latent periods between the primary attack and the first relapse. The study of strain characteristics is proceeding, particularly with respect to the difference in response of individual strains to various antimalarial drugs.

P. falciparum does not appear to be able to "hibernate" in the fixed tissue phase and this is apparently responsible for the clinical characteristics of this infection and for the character of the response of this parasite to prophylaxis and therapy.

However, once this parasite has entered the red cell, the behavior is quite similar to that of *P. vivax*. The parasite within the red cell develops by cell division and differentiation into two forms, (1) the merozoite which, after rupture of the red cell and release into the circulating plasma, reenters a fresh red cell and begins the erythrocyte cycle again and (2) the gametocyte or sexual form, which dies unless taken into the intestine of the anopheles mosquito for completion of the sexual cycle. For a description of the microscopic appearance of the stained parasites in the blood, *see* table, "Malarial Parasites in the Blood."

Little is known of the pathologic changes accompanying the tissue phase. Recent evidence suggests, however, that this phase takes place in certain cells of the liver. In vivax malaria, after prolonged untreated infection or repeated relapses, the spleen and liver become enlarged. The spleen may become much enlarged and usually is soft and full of malarial pigment. The sinusoids are filled with numerous parasitized red cells and the macrophages contain ingested malarial pigment. The Kupffer cells may be distended with parasites and pigment. There are no characteristic changes in the other organs except the scattered presence of malarial pigment in macrophages.

In patients dying from falciparum malaria, the brain is slate gray in color and often punctate hemorrhages may be seen scattered throughout the brain substance. The capillaries are choked with parasites.

Symptoms and Signs

In vivax malaria, the primary attack begins abruptly with a shaking chill, followed by fever and sweats. Often, the initial chill is preceded by a short period of malaise or headache. The fever may last from 1 to 8 hours and, after it subsides, the patient may feel entirely well until the time of the next rigor which, in uncomplicated vivax malaria, occurs every 48 hours. In falciparum malaria, the shaking chill may be replaced by a chilly sensation; the paroxysm may last from 20 to 36 hours, there is more prostration, and headache is a prominent symptom. The temperature rises more gradually and tends to fall by lysis rather than by crisis. The intervals between paroxysms are exceedingly variable and during them the patient usually feels quite miserable and runs a low grade fever. In falciparum malaria, as in vivax malaria, the periodicity of the chills and fever varies from these patterns as a result of numerous factors, including dual infection, strain differences, and immunity. Although high fever in vivax malaria may be accompanied by delirium, cerebral manifestations are not often encountered, whereas in falciparum malaria, fever of 104° F. or the presence of severe headache, drowsiness, delirium, or confusion may be indicative of impending cerebral malaria, which usually has a high fatality rate.

Chronic malaria with "low grade" parasitemia, as seen in partially immune subjects in hyperendemic areas, may be accompanied by malaise, listlessness, periodic headache, anorexia, fatigue, and small rises in temperature. These symptoms may culminate in acute attacks of chills and fever, considerably milder and of shorter duration than in the primary attack.

Aside from the chill and high fever there are no characteristic signs at the onset of the primary attack. If the disease persists untreated, mild jaundice usually develops; the spleen and occasionally the liver become enlarged.

A fairly rare complication, termed **blackwater fever,** may be encountered in certain cases of chronic falciparum malaria treated with quinine. It also is quite possible that pamaquine (Plasmochin) may play a part in initiating the disorder. The symptoms are those of acute intravascular hemolysis with hemoglobinuria, followed by fever, prostration, varying degrees of shock, sudden anemia, and mild icterus. Prior to World War II, the mortality rate was approximately 50%. During World War II, however, blackwater fever was practically unknown, due to the fact that quinacrine (Atabrine) was used instead of quinine. If quinine is avoided in the treatment of falciparum malaria, blackwater fever will become even more of a medical curiosity. The treatment is the same as in other forms of intravascular hemolysis (see INFUSION REACTIONS).

Diagnosis

The absolute diagnosis of malaria depends on the demonstration of the parasite in the stained smear. The presence of periodic attacks of chills and fever without apparent cause always is suggestive, particularly if the individual has been in a malarious area within the past year and if splenic enlargement is found. The leukocyte count usually is normal or only slightly elevated, with an increase in the percentage of lymphocytes and monocytes. It is highly important to identify the type of plasmodium and also the geographic source, as these findings will influence both the choice of therapy and the prognosis.

Prognosis

Untreated, vivax malaria will subside spontaneously in 10 to 30 days but may recur at variable intervals. If intercurrent infection supervenes, or if the individual is in poor condition when the attack begins, the prognosis becomes less favorable. However, antimalarial therapy practically eliminates mortality in vivax malaria.

Untreated falciparum malaria, on the other hand, has a high mortality. A further hazard is the possibility of blackwater fever in patients treated with quinine.

Prophylaxis

Attempts to induce immunity artificially by the use of vaccines made of killed parasites have been unsuccessful. In persons ill with malaria, however, a gradual immunity develops which modifies the clinical course considerably. This immunity carries with it a certain degree of strain specificity. Preventive measures include the elimination, where possible, otherwise the control, of mosquito breeding places; the employment of mosquito repellents; the use of screens on doors and windows, and of mosquito netting where screens are not practicable; and the wearing of sufficient clothing, particularly after sundown, to cover the extremities as well as the body and thus to protect as much of the skin surface as possible against mosquito bites. Mosquitoes must be denied access to patients ill with malaria, otherwise the insects will become infected and capable of transmitting the disease to healthy individuals. Prophylaxis by means of chemotherapy is discussed under Treatment, below.

Treatment

1. Treatment of the acute attack: In vivax malaria, the acute attack may be effectively terminated with a variety of agents, including the cinchona alkaloids (used individually as cinchonine, cinchonidine, quinidine, or quinine, or combined as totaquine), quinacrine (Atabrine), chloroquine (Aralen), and chlorguanide (paludrine). The details of dosage and duration of therapy may be found in the table, Antimalarial Chemotherapy.

It should be emphasized that the primary attack is more resistant to therapy than are the relapses, and that each relapse responds more readily than did its predecessor. As a rule, acute attacks of falciparum malaria are more resistant to therapy than are attacks of vivax malaria and, therefore, require slightly larger doses for slightly longer periods of time. However, falciparum malaria, since it does not develop a fixed tissue phase, is invariably cured without danger of relapse if the acute attack is adequately treated. Since quinine and other cinchona alkaloids often will fail to effect a cure, they should never be used in falciparum malaria when quinacrine, chloroquine, or chlorguanide is available. Of these three compounds, chloroquine is the drug of choice in the treatment of falciparum infections. Too little is known about the relative susceptibility of different strains to the newer drugs to permit final decisions, or as to the minimum effective dose in vivax and falciparum infections. The safest rule to follow is to continue an effective dose, as listed in the table, until fever and parasitemia have disappeared and, in the case of falciparum malaria, for several days thereafter.

2. Prophylaxis or suppression: Falciparum malaria may be completely prevented by the proper use of quinacrine, chloroquine, or chlorguanide (*see* table). In the case of chlorguanide, this effect is due to a true prophylactic action resulting in a destruction of the parasite before it reaches the red cell, while with quinacrine and chloroquine the effect is one of "suppression and cure" rather than prophylaxis. Therefore, with quinacrine and chloroquine it is important to continue suppressive therapy for 2 weeks after the period of exposure.

Vivax malaria cannot be prevented by these agents but any of them can suppress the clinical manifestations of the disease and can continue to suppress them as long as the drug is taken regularly. Failure to obtain suppression is rare, even in heavy infections, if there is no diarrhea present and the drug is taken in adequate dosage (*see* table) without interruption.

3. Curative therapy: As mentioned before, cure is effected in falciparum malaria if the acute attack is properly treated with quinacrine, chloroquine, or chlorguanide, or if the disease is prevented by adequate suppressive therapy.

Vivax malaria, because of its tissue phase, is prone to periodic relapses, the periodicity of which is an expression of the characteristics of the individual strain of infecting parasite and of the immunity of the host to that strain. As time goes on, the relapses become less severe and usually less frequent, until the disease finally "burns itself out," i.e., until the reservoir of tissue forms has been exhausted. However, cure may be effected in 80% of patients after the primary attack, and in a higher percentage after relapses by the use of an 8-amino-quinoline drug such as pamaquine or pentaquine, given in conjunction with quinine for a period of 14 days. Both pamaquine and pentaquine may cause abdominal cramps, headaches, nausea, vomiting, and diarrhea, a variable degree of methemoglobinemia and very occasionally, in dark-skinned individuals, acute hemolytic anemia. With pentaquine in doses of 60 mg. (gr. i) daily, transient fevers have been encountered. Since the higher the dose the more severe the toxic manifestations are likely to be, and since cure can be effected with smaller doses if a few relapses have occurred, it usually is wiser to wait until several relapses have taken place before considering curative therapy with pamaquine or pentaquine. The red cell count and hemoglobin should be determined twice a week during therapy and each voiding observed for the presence of hemoglobinuria. The latter can be accomplished quite simply by the use of a rack and series of test tubes. At the end of each day the specimens are inspected and then discarded.

4. Gametocytocidal therapy: Gametocytes usually appear 2 to 3 days after the onset of the erythrocytic phase and may persist for long periods of time, particularly in falciparum malaria. They do not produce any symptoms and are only important as indications of a preexisting infection and as a reservoir of infection for transmission through the anopheles mosquito to other persons.

Gametocyte development can be prevented by adequate suppression with quinacrine, chloroquine, or chlorguanide, and by adequate and prompt treatment of the acute attack. Once they have developed, the gametocytes in falciparum malaria are

ANTIMALARIAL CHEMOTHERAPY FOR VIVAX AND FALCIPARUM MALARIA

Drug	Quinine	Quinacrine ("Atabrine")	Chloroquine Diphosphate ("Aralen")	Chlorguanide Hydrochloride (Paludrine)	Pamaquine ("Plasmochin")	Pentaquine
Treatment of Acute Attack: *Vivax* Malaria	1 Gm. q. 8 h. for 3 doses; then 0.6 Gm. q. 8 h. for 5–6 days.	0.2 Gm. q. 5 h. for 5 doses; then 0.1 Gm./dose t.i.d., after meals for 6 days.	1 Gm. followed in 6 h. by 0.5 Gm., then 0.5 Gm./day for 2 days.	0.3 Gm. q. 12 h. for 10 days.		
Falciparum Malaria	1 Gm. q. 8 h. for 9 days if tolerated.	Continue above dosage for 7–10 days.	0.5 Gm. q. 6 h. for 3 doses; then 0.5 Gm./day for 9 days.	....		
Curative Therapy	For recommended combinations in *vivax* malaria: see under Pamaquine and Pentaquine.	For curative therapy of *falciparum* malaria: see above. (N.B.: None of these drugs is curative in *vivax* malaria.)			*Vivax* relapses: 10 mg., plus 0.6 Gm. Quinine, q. 8 h. for 14 days.	*Vivax* relapses: 10–20 mg., plus 0.6 Gm. Quinine, q. 8 h. for 14 days.
Suppressive or Prophylactic Therapy	To suppress *vivax* malaria: 0.3–1 Gm./day. (N.B.: In *falciparum* malaria Quinine is unreliable.)	0.1 Gm./day. For the suppression of *vivax* malaria: 0.5 Gm. once/wk. To prevent *falciparum* malaria, continue the maintenance dosage for 2 weeks after last exposure.	0.5 Gm. once/wk.	0.2 Gm. twice/wk.; or 0.1 Gm./day.	Gametocytocidal Therapy. In *falciparum* malaria only: 10 mg. of either drug q. 8 h. for 3–5 days.	
Toxic or Side Effects	Tinnitus, deafness, vomiting, skin rash may occur if idiosyncrasy exists.	Nausea, vomiting, diarrhea, yellow staining of skin and sclerae, skin eruption.	Pruritus, minor visual accommodation disturbances, headache.	Virtually none.	Abdominal cramps, methemoglobinemia, hemolytic crises.	Same as for Pamaquine, with occasional transient fever.

resistant to the suppressive drugs but are susceptible to the 8-amino-quinolines. Usually, 3 days of therapy with pamaquine or pentaquine will suffice to sterilize the blood of gametocytes.

In malarious areas, it is a common practice to regard all types of fever or indisposition as due to malaria, hence the prevalence of the disease is often exaggerated. It is important to establish the diagnosis by blood smears and to adhere to the dosage outlined in the table. If fever persists after adequate antimalarial therapy, the original diagnosis was in error and other cause should be sought.

RABIES

(Hydrophobia, Lyssa)

An acute infectious disease of mammals, especially the carnivores, characterized by irritation of the C.N.S. followed by paralysis and finally death.

Etiology and Epidemiology

The etiologic agent is a neurotropic filtrable virus. It is present in the saliva of the rabid animal, which in its frenzy bites other animals or human beings, and thus transmits the infection. Although rabies now is well under control in regions where efficient public health programs are in operation, sporadic outbreaks do occur from time to time. Moreover, there are areas of the country in which the disease is endemic due to inadequate control measures. Several cases have been reported in which rabies developed following exposure of a skin abrasion or the mucosa of the mouth or nose to infected saliva.

Dogs are most commonly responsible for transmitting the virus to man, although cats, wolves, skunks, bears, and other animals may do so on occasion. Although most human cases occur during hot weather, the disease affects lower animals at all seasons.

Pathology

The virus has an affinity for nervous tissue. It travels from the site of entry through peripheral nerves to the spinal cord and thence to the brain. In the brain it multiplies and some of the virus passes through efferent nerves to the salivary glands and into the saliva. Post mortem, the gross findings are prominent engorgement of the vessels in the meninges and brain, associated with punctate hemorrhages. Microscopic examination reveals perivascular collections of lymphocytes and destruction of the nerve cells. In the cornu Ammonis, the characteristic inclusion bodies of Negri usually are found. Their presence confirms the diagnosis.

Symptoms and Signs

Rabies in man has a variable incubation period of 10 days

to an extreme of 2 or more years, with an average of 50 to 60 days. In patients who have sustained extensive bite wounds or have been bitten about the head, the incubation period usually is shorter and the infection more severe.

Infected dogs may have the disease in either the "furious" or the "dumb" form. Furious rabies is characterized by agitation and viciousness, followed by paralysis and death. Excessive salivation ("foaming at the mouth") does not always occur and, in itself, has little diagnostic value when present. In dumb rabies, the animals are quiet, salivate excessively, are paralyzed, and soon die. Even though these dogs seldom bite, their copious saliva may transmit the infection.

The disease in man is commonly heralded by a short period of mental depression, restlessness, malaise, and fever. Restlessness increases to uncontrollable excitement, with excessive salivation and pronounced spasms of the laryngeal and pharyngeal muscles. These spasms cause excruciating pain and, because they are the result of reflex irritability of the centers of deglutition and respiration, are easily precipitated by such things as a slight breeze or an attempt to drink water. Because of this, the patient refuses to drink although his thirst actually is great. Thus, the term "hydrophobia," as applied to either man or dog, is a misnomer. Death usually occurs within 3 to 5 days from asphyxia or exhaustion. In some instances, death follows general paralysis.

Diagnosis and Prognosis

Diagnosis is made from a history of the patient's being bitten by a dog (or other animal), and the characteristic clinical symptoms. These data differentiate rabies from tetanus and botulism (q.v.). Hysteria, due to fright, which occasionally occurs following a dog bite, may give the impression of rabies, but the symptoms are promptly controlled once the patient is assured that he is not in immediate danger and can be protected from rabies. Any animal that bites a human being should, when practicable, be confined and observed for 2 weeks. Dogs suspected of being infected should not be killed, but allowed to die a natural death, since this makes diagnosis easier. If the animal develops no symptoms within the 2-week period, its bite can be considered to have been innocuous. If it dies, its brain should be examined for Negri bodies; however, these may not be present in the early stages of rabies in animals.

Once symptoms of rabies develop, death is inevitable in animal or man.

Prophylaxis

Prevention and control of rabies entails the impounding and destruction of stray, ownerless dogs, and the restraint of other dogs by their owners. In many communities, mass immunization of the canine population is being actively carried out.

Treatment

Following a bite or exposure to the saliva of a mammal showing signs of rabies, the resultant wound or contaminated area should be thoroughly cleansed with a 20% solution of medicinal soft soap. Puncture wounds should be laid open to permit adequate access of the cleansing solution and to encourage some bleeding. Most authorities advise against cauterizing the wound. In dealing with bites from animals suspected of being rabid, all factors in the case should be considered and a decision made concerning the administration of antirabies vaccine. When the animal responsible is known to have the disease or cannot be examined, immediate immunization is indicated. Otherwise, a veterinarian should observe the dog for rabies for 14 days. If the dog was infective at the time of the bite, it will die during this period and immunization of the patient must then be started. However, since rabies due to bites about the face and neck tends to have a shorter incubation period, it may be advisable in such cases, to begin immunization at once and continue it until the observed animal is pronounced noninfective or until a full course of vaccine is given.

Caution should be exercised in the administration of rabies vaccine, especially in patients previously immunized, since it occasionally is followed by fatal paralysis. If the bite is made through clothing, there is less danger of rabies infection. Patients with minor bites should receive one dose of vaccine (℞ 101) daily for 14 to 28 days. Patients in whom the wounds are extensive, situated on the face or neck, or inflicted by a wild animal, should receive 2 doses daily for the first 7 days and thereafter 1 dose daily for at least 7 days. Therapy of the disease itself, once it appears, is necessarily purely symptomatic. The patient should be made as comfortable as possible (*see* CONVULSIONS, General Treatment).

TETANUS

(Lockjaw)

An acute infectious disease characterized by more or less persistent tonic spasm of voluntary muscles, plus tonic convulsions. The characteristic spasm of the masseters accounts for the name "lockjaw."

Etiology and Pathology

Tetanus is caused by an exotoxin elaborated by *Clostridium tetani*, a slender, motile, gram-positive, anaerobic, sporulating bacillus. Spore-containing cells have a characteristic drumstick appearance. Spores can remain viable for 10 years or longer under optimal conditions. They survive in many disinfectants and in steam at 100° C. for 60 minutes, although boiling may destroy them. The organism has a widespread distribution, and is especially abundant in soil and in human and animal feces. Injuries both indoors and out may result in infection, sometimes through fast-healing trivial wounds, but usually through purulent or necrotic lesions. Nail-puncture wounds, splinter injuries, blank-cartridge or other burns, infected lacerations, gunshot wounds, compound fractures, contamination of the umbilicus of the newborn, or of operation sites during dust storms, insect bites, bed sores contaminated with feces, infected sutures, and hypodermic injections, may offer ingress to *Cl. tetani*. Occasionally, the locus of entry cannot be discovered.

The exotoxin of *Cl. tetani* is one of the most potent water-soluble poisons known. It acts on the motor nerve end-plates, causing spasm of muscles near the site of infection, and also on the anterior horn cells of the spinal cord and brain stem, causing generalized tonic spasticity, upon which intermittent tonic convulsions usually are superimposed. The degenerative changes seen in the brain and cord are not specific for this disease and do not persist after recovery. It has been shown experimentally that the toxin is transported in the blood, which justifies the I.V. administration of antitetanic serum therapeutically. This finding counters an older theory that the toxin travels within the trunks of motor nerves. Once the toxin has been fixed by the gray matter of the C.N.S., its continued action cannot be checked and it must therefore be neutralized before reaching the cells.

Symptoms and Signs

The most frequent presenting symptom is stiffness of the jaw, and this must always be taken to indicate tetanus until proved otherwise. Sometimes restlessness, irritability, stiffness of the neck, or difficulty in swallowing heralds the attack. Occasionally, stiffness of the arms or legs, headache, fever, chilliness, or convulsions are the initial symptoms. Later, the patient has difficulty in opening his jaws (trismus), and spasm of the facial muscles often causes a fixed smile and elevated eyebrows (risus sardonicus). There may be rigidity or spasm of the abdominal, neck, and back muscles. Opisthotonos is not infrequent. The temperature is only moderately elevated except in cases complicated by other infectious diseases such as pneumonia, or as death approaches in fatal cases. Respiratory and pulse rates are increased. Reflexes often are exaggerated. The blood usually shows a moderate leukocytosis with an increase of polymorphonuclears. Urinary retention or constipation may result from spasm of the respective sphincters. Dysphagia may interfere with nutrition. Painful convulsions with profuse sweating are characteristic, and are precipitated by such minor disturbances as jarring the bed or a gust of wind. The patient's mind usually is clear, but coma may set in following convulsions. During convulsions, the patient is unable to speak or cry out because of the rigidity of the chest wall. Such interference with respiration, or that from spasm of the glottis, may cause cyanosis, or even asphyxia leading to death. More often, however, the immediate cause of death is not apparent. In many instances breathing ceases while the heart continues to beat for several minutes.

Local Tetanus: There is a localized form of tetanus characterized by spasticity of a group of muscles near the wound, and without trismus. Hitherto rare, this form is becoming more frequent, probably due to inadequate prophylactic doses of antitoxin. The spasticity may persist for weeks or even months and then gradually become resolved.

Diagnosis

A history of recent injury or of intestinal or bone surgery is important. The incubation period varies from 2 to 50 days, but usually is between 5 and 10 days. When prophylactic antitoxin has been given the incubation period may be lengthened to 2 or 3 weeks.

Diagnosis is made from history and symptoms, but tetanus must be differentiated from the following diseases (q.v.): acute meningitis, in which trismus is absent; rabies, in the history of which animal bite is essential; strychnine poisoning, tetany, and poliomyelitis, all of which differ from tetanus in many respects, and especially in the absence of trismus; trismus from local causes, such as peritonsillar or retropharyngeal abscess, or other local infections of the throat or around the jaws.

Prognosis

The mortality rate is influenced by the patient's age (higher in young and old), the length of the incubation period, and above all by the promptness with which treatment is begun. Those statistics available show that when treatment is delayed for 24 hours after onset of symptoms, the death rate will approach 100% for patients with an incubation period of 3 to 5 days, and 80 to 90% for those with an incubation period of 5 to 7 days. Earlier treatment may materially reduce fatalities, particularly for patients in the latter category. With yet longer incubation periods deaths are fewer, and should not total more than 30 to 40% for patients with an incubation period of 10 to 15 days, provided therapeutic intervention is prompt.

Prolonging life through the 9th or 10th day of illness considerably enhances a patient's chances for recovery. Trismus that develops early and completely is a bad prognostic sign. Lesions about the head and neck are no more dangerous than those of other regions of the body. In patients who recover, complete restoration of normal function is the rule, but moderate muscular rigidity may persist for months.

Prophylaxis

Active immunization: Persons liable to injuries, occupational or otherwise—e.g., gardeners, mechanics, industrial workers, athletes, children—should be actively immunized with tetanus toxoid. Given in appropriate dosage (*see* ROUTINE IMMUN. PROC.), this usually confers immunity from tetanus for long periods—several years or even a lifetime. However, the existence of such prolonged immunity cannot be determined except by blood titration studies; therefore, "booster" injections of 1 cc. of the toxoid every 1 or 2 years thereafter are advised. In a person not previously immunized, toxoid given at the time of injury cannot induce immunity speedily enough to protect him, and passive immunization must be used. However, if a person actively immunized within the 2 preceding years is injured, 1 cc. of toxoid generally will afford protection from tetanus, since this will boost the titer of antitoxin in his blood to an adequate level ($\mathbb{R}$ 100).

Passive immunization: Patients with severe lacerated or punctured wounds caused by objects soiled with dust, pavement brush burns and wounds, or compound fractures, should be given much larger amounts of tetanus antitoxin ($\mathbb{R}$ 99) than the customary dose of 1,500 u.; 10,000 to 20,000 u. is required, particularly when first given several days after the injury was received. The immunity following 1,500 to 5,000 u. of antitoxin does not last much beyond 10 days. Therefore, with suspicious wounds these smaller doses must be repeated, preferably at intervals of 6 days, to avoid the development of serum sensitivity. Such prophylactic serum is administered I.M. Gas bacillus antitoxin also is indicated, where there is invasion by *Clostridium welchii.* Before antitoxin is administered, the patient should be tested for serum sensitivity (*see* SERUM SICKNESS), and appropriate desensitization carried out, when necessary.

Wound prophylaxis: Splinters, wads from blank cartridges, and other foreign objects should be carefully removed, under anesthesia if necessary. Establishment of adequate drainage is imperative. With nail-puncture wounds, this may not be possible, and completely adequate serum prophylaxis must be relied upon. Meticulous attention should be given to abrasions suffered by children during outdoor play. These should be thoroughly cleansed with tincture of green soap before applying an antiseptic.

Treatment

Successful therapy depends upon four factors: early and adequate use of antitoxin; sedation; wound débridement; and competent, intelligent, continuous nursing care.

Antitoxin: Before this treatment is attempted, sensitivity to the serum (usually from equine sources) should be determined, and if it is present desensitization should be carried out (*see* ALLERGY), or tests for bovine immune serum may be made, and if the reaction is negative, this can be substituted.

The hazards of I.V. serum therapy are enormously increased in the presence of sensitivity, even after desensitization apparently is complete. In such cases, the physician may elect to use only the I.M. route for treatment, injecting two 60,000 u. doses of serum (previously heated to body temperature) at 12-hour intervals, followed, if necessary, by 5,000 u. daily. (Intraspinal and intracisternal serum therapy now is rarely recommended.) Fifteen minutes before any therapeutic injection is given, it is advisable to administer 0.3 to 0.6 cc. (♏ v to x) of epinephrine subcut. (℞ 113). Also, a syringe containing 1 cc. of epinephrine (℞ 113) and atropine sulfate (℞ 115), 0.3 mg. (gr. 1/200), is kept at hand. If an immediate reaction occurs, half of this may be injected at once, I.M. or I.V., and the remainder in 5 to 10 minutes if necessary. Every effort is made to control the symptoms of delayed serum sickness (q.v.) should they develop. Such measures include procaine injection, and appropriate doses of an antihistaminic. Otherwise, irritative phenomena, such as those associated with urticaria, may initiate disastrous convulsions.

When antitoxin therapy is instituted, some patients will have such a high concentration of toxin in their C.N.S. tissues as to be already doomed, but this cannot be known at the time. In patients capable of recovery it appears to be established that 50,000 u. of antitoxin administered I.V. in 500 cc. of Isotonic Sodium Chloride Solution U.S.P., at a rate of 15 to 60 drops/minute will neutralize the toxin in the blood stream. Twelve hours later, when the likelihood of an anaphylactic-like reaction to the previous injection is remote, an additional 50,000 u. of antitoxin is given either I.M. or I.V. Thereafter, daily injections of 5,000 u. are given I.V. These daily injections neutralize any additional toxin absorbed into the blood stream; they also maintain desensitivity to the serum, which is important in case of relapse. In addition, where a causative wound is found, an encircling peripheral infiltration of 40,000 u. of antitoxin is made 1 hour before débridement and the proximal musculature is infiltrated with another 40,000 u. There is no evidence that penicillin is effective against the tetanus bacillus; nevertheless it probaby is of value in controlling respiratory complications and secondary infections of the wound.

Wound débridement: When indicated, débridement should be prompt and thorough, following infiltration of the surrounding area with antitoxin as described above. The wound is widely opened and exposed to air, and oxidizing agents such as hydrogen peroxide are used for irrigation, in order to eradicate any anaerobes that may still be present and thus prevent further production and absorption of exotoxin. Nitrous oxide-oxygen is the anesthesia of choice. In almost all instances, however, such surgery is best deferred until satisfactory sedation has been established and the systemic injections of antitoxin have been given.

Sedation: Without satisfactory sedation, the patient may die in one of the recurrent convulsions. Ether in oil rectally, a barbiturate (℞ 23) and bromides (℞ 17), chloral hydrate (℞ 19) or paraldehyde (℞ 18) may be employed alone or in various combinations. To control convulsions, doses must be large, hence depressant drugs, particularly morphine, are to be avoided. Some clinicians use the degree of rigidity of the abdominal muscles as a guide in determining the need for sedation, since these muscles are apt to become boardlike prior to a convulsion. Or, the patient may be kept under continuous light narcosis. Surprisingly large doses of paraldehyde (10 to 40 cc. in 3 or 4 oz. of isotonic salt solution per rectum every 3 hours) can be given without harm. Paraldehyde also can be administered in Isotonic Sodium Chloride Solution U.S.P., by continuous I.V. drip. Chloral hydrate (℞ 19) in conjunction with bromides (℞ 17), 1.5 to 3 Gm. (gr. xxii to xlv) each by rectum, has been found effective. Sodium Amytal (℞ 22) may be used, either I.V. (slowly) or I.M.; the safe single dose ordinarily is 5 mg./Kg. (2.2 lb.) body wt. Sodium Amytal should be administered I.V. at a rate of 50 to 100 mg./minute, and its administration should be discontinued when the desired relaxation is observed even if the total proposed dosage has not been given. Following I.M. injection of Sodium Amytal, the maximum effects are not observed for 30 or 45 minutes. Soluble sodium phenobarbital (℞ 23), I.M. in doses of 0.15 to 0.3 Gm. (gr. iiss to v) is an effective emergency anticonvulsant, but is not to be given more often than 3 times in 24 hours.

The use of aqueous curare for its paralyzant action and amelioration of the convulsions requires special skill and should not be attempted except by an expert. However, d-tubocurarine (℞ 147) in wax and oil appears, after limited clinical trial, to be effective and much less dangerous. While the dose for an infant or child cannot be predicted on weight or age, 7 mg. (0.25 cc.) I.M. initially (CAUTION!) of a 4.8% wax-in-peanut-oil preparation containing 27 mg./cc. (180 u.) of d-tubocurarine, ordinarily is safe. The dose for an adult patient should seldom exceed 27 mg. (1 cc.) I.M. Both the dose and interval of administration must be adjusted according to the individual's clinical response, the minimal effective amount of the drug being given as infrequently as possible in every instance. In many adults, a dose of 27 mg. (1 cc.) every 24 hours is safe, and, for others, somewhat more frequent administration may be permissible. The site of injection should be protected from pressure or any manipulation that may hasten absorption of the drug. Overcurarization is treated with neostigmine (℞ 114), 1 cc. (♍ xv) subcut. of a 1:2,000 solution. If it is necessary to repeat the latter, then atropine sulfate (℞ 115), 0.4 mg. (gr. 1/150) is also given to lessen any undesirable side effects of the neostigmine. In addition, an aspiration apparatus, endotracheal tube, laryngoscope, and O_2 for nasal administration should be available for emergency use should laryngospasm occur.

Nursing and symptomatic care: Probably in no other disease is the nurse of more importance, and previous experience with tetanus cases greatly enhances her value. The patient should be isolated in a darkened, well ventilated, warm (70° F.), and quiet room. Practically all patients, under adequate sedation, can be given ample calories and fluids in a liquid diet (*see* DIETS) by tube-feeding, or with a medicine dropper if necessary, and supplemented by I.V. nutrition when indicated. Great patience on the part of the nurse is required to achieve this end. If nasal feedings do not excite convulsions, an indwelling gastric catheter via the nares may be used. It is of vast importance that the patient's fluid and electrolyte balance be maintained.

The use of an oxygen tent is beneficial in all severe cases of tetanus. Otherwise, inhalations of 5 to 10% of CO_2 in O_2 are given for 15-minute periods at frequent intervals, if this does not disturb the patient unduly. Hypostatic pneumonia is prevented by changing the patient's position frequently. If pneumonia (q.v.) does occur its treatment should be vigorous. Some deaths in tetanus are due to laryngeal spasm, and if severe stridor continues, it is wise to perform a tracheotomy and, when necessary, to maintain respiration by artificial means.

Oral and nasal hygiene, and adequate elimination are problems. Abdominal pain may be caused by severe flatulence induced by spasm of the anal sphincters, and is relieved with cleansing enemas or with suction via a Wangensteen apparatus connected to a rectal tube. Urinary retention seldom occurs, but, when present, necessitates routine catheterization.

Secretions are removed from the nose and throat by gentle swabbing, or perhaps by gentle suction, provided the latter does not serve as an excitatory stimulus. Atropine to decrease secretions is not advisable, since it makes expectoration more difficult.

All procedures that may excite convulsions must be kept to the absolute minimum. Needle-puncture therapy may fall into this category, as well as bathing. All care of patients with tetanus must be thoroughly individualized, and no procedure should be routinely followed simply because in other diseases it represents good nursing care.

ANTHRAX

(Malignant pustule, Malignant edema, Woolsorters' disease, Ragpickers' disease)

A highly infectious disease of animals, especially herbivores, which is directly or indirectly transmissible from them or their products to man. Anthrax occurs in man externally either as a **malignant pustule** or **malignant edema**; internally, as a **pul-**

monary infection (woolsorters' disease) or, rarely, as an **intestinal disease.**

Etiology and Epidemiology

The causative organism is *Bacillus anthracis,* a large gram-positive aerobic (also facultatively anaerobic), sporogenic, encapsulated rod. It sporulates rapidly outside living tissues. The spores are extremely resistant to heat, drying, and disinfectants other than oxidants. Potassium permanganate 4% kills them in 15 minutes, or hydrogen peroxide in 1 hour. In soil, the spores may remain viable for 15 years or longer.

Anthrax attacks virtually any of the warm-blooded animals, wild or domestic, but is recognized chiefly in goats, cattle, sheep, horses, hogs, reindeer, and camels. It takes the form of septicemia in animals and is practically always fatal. The bacillus is present in the organs, blood, excreta, and bodily secretions. Thus the soil becomes heavily seeded with spores. Herbivores usually become infected, not from one another, but from feeding on contaminated pasture, particularly in marshy areas where the bacilli may multiply in the soil during the summer. Dogs, cats, and swine sometimes acquire mild or latent pharyngeal infections by feeding on infected carcasses. The disease is most prevalent in Europe and Asia, particularly Siberia, China, India, and Turkey. In the United States, animal anthrax usually is well controlled, but infrequent outbreaks still occur in the following regions: southeastern South Dakota, northwestern Nebraska, the Mississippi delta region, and along a belt of Texas Gulf Coast. Except in years with such outbreaks, human anthrax is rare in the United States, only 60 to 80 cases being recognized annually, principally in Pennsylvania, New York, Massachusetts, and Texas, and chiefly from industrial sources.

Anthrax is believed not to be transmitted from one human being to another; rather it is acquired through contact with infected animals or materials, by inhaling the spores in dust, or (rarely) by ingesting infected meat or other food. A healthy person may transfer the disease to others by spores on his clothing. Insects are occasional vectors. According to the circumstances under which it is acquired, the disease is classified as "industrial" or "agricultural." Gluemakers, upholsterers, stevedores, tanners, woolsorters, leather workers, furriers, brushmakers, hunters, butchers, herdsmen, shepherds, farmers, and the families of such persons, are especially subject to infection. Agricultural anthrax is seasonal, depending on infection in domestic animals, except rarely when bone meal or fertilizer is responsible. Industrial anthrax depends on contact with animal products, e.g., waste, hide, hair—imported material usually being incriminated. Shaving brushes at one time were a notorious source of infection.

The incubation period varies from 12 hours to 5 days, with an average of 3 to 5 days.

Symptoms, Signs, and Course

Cutaneous Anthrax: This is acquired by contact with infected material, a macroscopic break in the skin not being necessary for the organism's entry. It most often takes the form of a circumscribed malignant "pustule" (so-called, but not containing pus) or multiple circumscribed pustules. The face, neck, arms, and hands are the usual sites.

Initially, the lesion may resemble an insect bite (simple erosion on an erythematous base); in a few hours it enlarges, the top turns brown and may be surrounded by a narrow, bright red ring. On the 2nd day, vesicles develop at the periphery of the papule; within 12 to 24 hours these become bluish red, rupture, and discharge a serosanguineous fluid. At the same time, the depressed center of the papule ulcerates, and on the 3rd or 4th day turns black. Occasionally, a single large vesicle is the outstanding feature of the lesion. Edema (nonpitting) develops in 12 to 24 hours after the appearance of the papule, and may spread rapidly (in one instance, from the neck to the iliac crest in 24 hours). The pustule is characterized by itching, painlessness and nonsuppuration; however, anthrax may be engrafted on a purulent base, such as impetigo.

In most instances regional adenopathy, up to walnut size, and often heralded by pain, develops on the 2nd or 3rd day. The tissues overlying these glands usually are erythematous and edematous. The adenopathy may persist for several weeks after the ulcer heals.

Under treatment, the spread of the edema is checked first, followed by its disappearance in 1 to 5 days. Also, the papule becomes flat and dry, and the black eschar sloughs away in 7 to 14 days. The ulcer then heals in 1 to 2 weeks.

In malignant edema, instead of a circumscribed lesion, there is a superficial ulceration with undermined bluish red edges, sunken in an area of extensive and spreading edema. Multiple large blisters containing serosanguineous fluid soon develop. This form is observed in the loose connective tissues of the eyelid, hand, neck, thigh, and mucous membranes.

With either of the cutaneous forms the systemic manifestations may be slight or severe, and include nausea and vomiting, headache, joint pains, and malaise. The temperature may vary from subnormal to a moderate fever, 99° to 102° F. Leukocytosis (10,000 to 13,000), or leukopenia, with 60 to 85% polymorphonuclears, may occur. Blood cultures usually are negative, but in fatal cases may become positive just before death, which may occur in 3 to 5 days.

Pulmonary Anthrax: This form usually results from inhaling the dust of animal hair containing spores. Collapse sets in rapidly and is of diagnostic significance. The picture is that of an overwhelming infection, with prostration, cyanosis, cough, hyperpnea, dyspnea, and perhaps high fever. X-ray examination of the lungs may show a diffuse patchy infiltration. Death often occurs in 18 to 24 hours. Since 99% of these patients die if not treated, the diagnosis must be established promptly. When the disease lasts for 4 to 10 days, signs of meningoencephalitis may dominate the clinical picture.

Gastrointestinal Anthrax: One epidemic (30 cases) has been described, in which signs of peritonitis, persistent vomiting, and constipation (rarely diarrhea) were displayed. Occasional patients had blood-tinged feces or discharged pure blood. The temperature usually remained normal but in some cases rose to 102.2° F., followed by excessive sweating. In most of the patients collapse, cyanosis, and apoplectic death terminated the illness in 1 to 3 days. Autopsy showed localized carbuncles in the ileum and cecum and often hemorrhages in the myocardium and brain.

Diagnosis

Knowledge of the many uses of animal hair, hide, and other products in industry and agriculture will help the physician in suspecting anthrax on the basis of the patient's occupation. The characteristic appearance of the cutaneous lesion, its painlessness and absence of suppuration, and the presence of edema, readily suggest the diagnosis, which is confirmed by the identification of *B. anthracis* in smears and cultures from the lesion. The organism is visible with a medium power lens, and is readily stained with a polychrome eosin-methylene blue stain (Wright or Giemsa). It appears as a large rod with square ends, single or in chains of two. The characteristic capsule is not always readily seen. Since anthrax-like bacilli may occur on the skin, the diagnosis should always be confirmed by animal inoculation. Meanwhile, treatment should be started without delay. In pulmonary anthrax, bacteriologic examination includes sputum or throat swabs. Since in anthrax bacteremia may be present, blood cultures also should be made, using a minimum of 20 cc. of blood. In the intestinal form of the disease, the vomitus and feces should be studied for *B. anthracis*.

Prognosis

The mortality rate averages 20% in the United States. Cutaneous anthrax from tannery and related sources usually is less virulent than that from direct animal contact. Pulmonary anthrax can be cured if diagnosis and treatment are prompt.

Prophylaxis

The chief objective is protection from spores by burying infected carcasses in quicklime; proper industrial hygiene; exclusion of insects from contact with patients; incineration of contaminated articles and excretions; and cremation of human corpses.

Treatment

Excision, incision, or cauterization of cutaneous lesions is contraindicated. The affected part is immobilized, and the patient is put on absolute bed rest. The use of local antiseptic dressings with potassium permanganate (1:1,000), mercury bichloride (1:2,000), or ichthammol (℞ 148) is advisable to prevent secondary infection. Antianthrax serum, penicillin, and the sulfonamides are effective in treatment, and are listed below in the order of probable dependability.

Before administration of antiserum (℞ 103), nonsensitivity must be determined or achieved (see SERUM SICKNESS), and epinephrine 1:1,000 (℞ 113) kept at hand during its use. Even with a nonsensitive patient, it is best to give a minute initial dose of serum, then gradually increase the dose at 15-minute intervals until 2 or 3 cc. are being given, thus minimizing possible anaphylaxis when therapeutic amounts are infused. Delayed reactions occur in virtually all patients and prolong the morbidity. From 300 to 600 cc. of antiserum diluted with 10 to 15% glucose and infused I.V. will control the majority of anthrax infections. One, 2, or 3 large doses may be given, the first consisting of not less than 150 to 300 cc. Large doses at intervals of 8 to 24 hours are more effective than repeated small doses. In cases with bacteremia, following an initial large dose, 2 to 4 daily injections of 40 to 50 cc. are recommended. Treatment is guided by the location of the lesions (those on the face and neck require the greatest amounts), the extent of the edema, toxicity, and the presence or absence of bacteremia. When the optimum dose of antiserum is given, the edema promptly decreases and disappears in 18 to 36 hours. Subsidence of the edema is a convenient therapeutic guide, and in some cases a total of more than 2,000 cc. of serum will be required.

Anthrax bacteremia is believed to be more rapidly controlled by penicillin (℞ 28) than by any other agent. In visceral anthrax or severe cutaneous anthrax, larger doses may be indicated, along with antianthrax serum.

The sulfonamides do not check the edema so promptly as does antianthrax serum, but the availability and simplicity of administration make them valuable for initial and adjuvant therapy. Sulfadiazine (℞ 37) is the drug of choice. An initial dose of 3 Gm. is given, followed by 1 Gm. every 3 to 4 hours for 2 to 3 days. Toxicity from overdosage can be avoided by frequent examination of the urine for red cells and by following the blood level. Frequent blood counts also are essential.

LEPROSY

(Hansen's disease, Elephantiasis graecorum, Leontiasis, Lepra, Lepra arabum)

A chronic, mildly contagious, infectious disease characterized by both local cutaneous and constitutional symptoms and the production of various deformities and mutilations.

Etiology

The causative organism is believed to be an acid-fast rod, *Mycobacterium leprae,* first described by Hansen in 1874. Mode of transmission is unknown. In the United States, the disease is found mostly in the Gulf States.

Symptoms and Signs

The onset is insidious, with the gradual development of lesions of the skin including macules (light red, purple or bronze, 1 to 10 cm. in diameter), infiltrated nodules (yellow or red-brown, 1 to 5 cm. in diameter), confluent nodules; diffuse infiltration (sometimes resulting in the classical leonine facies); or localized alopecia (especially of the eyebrows). Neurologic disturbances may be manifested by an anesthesia, in some instances involving only the macules, but in others an entire extremity; a painful neuritis (frequently of the ulnar, peroneal or radial nerves); various paresthesias; contractures of the hands or feet; bone absorption in the fingers and toes; trophic ulcers (most often of the lower extremities, particularly on the weight-bearing surfaces). Systemic manifestations may include lymphadenopathy, anemia, or lepra fever (an acute febrile episode, usually of several weeks' duration, accompanied by evanescent skin lesions which resemble those of erythema nodosum or erysipelas). Lesions of the eye include nodules of the lids or conjunctiva, keratitis, and iridocyclitis. Epistaxis and nasal ulcers are common.

Diagnosis

The diagnosis is confirmed by demonstration of the acid-fast organism, *Myco. leprae,* either in smears made from skin lesions or nasal septum, or in sections obtained by biopsy of suspicious lesions. Leprosy may at times be confused with erythema multiforme, lupus, multiple sarcomas, sarcoid of Boeck, scleroderma, syphilis, syringomyelia, or vitiligo (q.v.).

Prognosis

The prognosis depends upon the extent and character of lesions. Spontaneous remissions are frequently encountered in cases with predominantly neural lesions, frequently after irreversible deformities have appeared. In cases with nodular lesions, the outlook is poor. After an average period of 18 years, death comes either from intercurrent disease or from asphyxiation secondary to occlusion of the glottis by nodules. Following treatment with sulfone drugs, 15% of the patients with nodular lesions and a greater number of those with neural manifestations become arrested after 3 to 5 years of therapy. The remainder of the patients are clinically improved. Lesions in arrested patients are replaced by scar tissue and acid-fast bacilli can no longer be demonstrated.

Treatment

Institutional care: In the United States, patients in whom the diagnosis of leprosy has been confirmed should be sent to the nearest U.S. Marine Hospital for subsequent transfer to the National Leprosarium in Louisiana. Thus, danger of contagion is reduced and the patient is assured of specialized care.

Chemotherapy: At present, sulfone therapy is the treatment of choice. Three alternative drugs have been used at the National Leprosarium. Promin (℞ 75), 5 Gm., is given I.V. once a day for 2 weeks, with a rest period of 1 week after each course. Treatment is continued for several years. Promizole (℞ 76), 1 to 2 Gm., is given by mouth 3 times a day for a similar period of time. Diasone (℞ 77), 0.3 Gm., is given by mouth 2 or 3 times a day, also for a period of several years.

Chaulmoogra oil preparations (℞ 78 to 81) are of questionable value.

Streptomycin has been used in the treatment of leprosy with results sufficiently encouraging to warrant further trials. Dihydrostreptomycin, because of its lesser neurotoxicity, might be postulated as the more logical drug for a necessarily prolonged period of therapy.

Supportive treatment: Anemia may be present as a general symptom of leprosy or as a complication of sulfone therapy. In either case it can usually be successfully treated with iron therapy plus, in some instances, liver concentrate I.M. once or twice a week (*see* Anemia). The red cell count rises with improvement in the general condition of the patient. For the treatment of painful neuritis, I.V. calcium gluconate (℞ 150), 1 Gm. a day for several weeks, has appeared to effect relief in most instances. Thiamine hydrochloride, either 50 mg. I.M. (℞ 131) every day for 3 days, or 5 mg. orally (℞ 132) 3 times a day for 10 days, may be of value in relieving neuritic pains.

Local treatment: Large trophic ulcers may be treated by means of wet dressings containing either 0.5 mg./cc. of streptomycin (℞ 34); 10 mg./cc. of promin (℞ 82); or 1,000 u./cc. of penicillin (℞ 30). Smaller ulcers may be treated with 10% ichthammol ointment (℞ 148) or 5% sulfathiazole ointment (℞ 45) applied as a dry dressing. Lesions resembling those of erythema nodosum (q.v.) may appear and may be so treated.

PLAGUE

(Bubonic plague, Pestis, Black plague)

An acute febrile epidemic disease, beginning with fever and chills, quickly followed by great prostration and later by swelling of the lymph nodes, forming buboes in the femoral, inguinal, axillary, or cervical regions.

Etiology, Transmission, and Epidemiology

The causative agent is *Pasteurella pestis,* a short, plump, pleomorphic, gram-negative bacillus with a tendency toward bipolar staining.

An epidemic of plague in human beings is usually preceded by a rat epizootic, the rat being the common animal vector of this disease. Infected fleas migrate to man from dying or dead rats and, while feeding, deposit infective material (dejecta or regurgitated blood) in or on the skin. The pneumonic form of plague, which can be transmitted from man to man by droplet infection, may appear during the height of an epidemic.

Sporadic cases of plague may be due to infection from wild animals, such as squirrels, rabbits, or marmots. The disease, sylvatic plague, which also is transmitted by fleas, is endemic among these rodents in many areas of the western United States. The rodenticides, 1080 and ANTU, have been found effective in rodent control.

Pathology

From their point of entry the infecting organisms spread throughout the body via lymph channels and blood stream. In the bubonic form, the regional lymph nodes (usually inguinal or femoral) become swollen and the sinuses within them are packed with leukocytes. Hemorrhages occur; the nodes may suppurate, and may or may not discharge through the skin. Such nodes contain large numbers of *Past. pestis*. Spread to other organs often is extensive, producing foci of suppuration and necrosis in the lungs, liver, spleen, and brain.

The pneumonic form is rapidly fatal. At autopsy, lobular consolidation of a confluent type may be seen, but often pulmonary findings are limited to engorgement. Focal necrosis is less frequently encountered in distant organs, since the rapid termination prevents embolic phenomena.

Symptoms and Signs

1. Bubonic Plague: This is the more common type. Onset, which often is abrupt, is marked by a slight but definite chill, or repeated attacks of chilliness. Temperature then rises rapidly, usually to 103°F., but in severe cases may reach 106°F. Convulsions may occur in children. The facies show fear and anxiety. Vomiting, thirst, unsteady gait, generalized pains, mental dullness, and headache are the most frequent symptoms. The skin becomes hot and dry; pulse and respiration rates increase. The face becomes bloated and the conjunctiva injected. The hearing may be impaired. Mania sometimes develops. Splenomegaly often is noted. Involvement of the kidneys causes oliguria and albuminuria. Leukocytosis (90,000 to 100,000) is present. Petechiae, the "black spots" that give the disease the name "black death," may appear about the 3rd day. Gastrointestinal or pulmonary hemorrhage may occur. Buboes: Enlarged, painful, tender lymph nodes usually appear between the 2nd and 5th days, and may suppurate.

Pestis Minor: This is a mild form of bubonic plague in which the patient remains ambulant, and which is usually recognized only when known cases of plague are present in the area.

Septicemia: An overwhelming septicemia may occur as a complication. It is rapidly fatal: death may result in 3 or 4 days, even before buboes appear.

2. Pneumonic Plague: This type may occur either as a complication of bubonic plague or as a primary pneumonic invasion from droplet infection. When primary, onset is acute, with headache, anorexia, and fever, followed by dyspnea and productive cough. Pulse and respiration are rapid; temperature usually rises to 103° or 104°F. The sputum, which first is mucoid and later blood-tinged, contains *Past. pestis* in almost pure culture. The disease is rapidly overwhelming, with severe dyspnea, cyanosis, and heart failure in the later stages.

Diagnosis and Prognosis

The incubation period varies from 2 to 10 days (average 3). Sporadic cases are difficult to diagnose, and bacteriologic confirmation is necessary. Fluid from a bubo (or sputum, in the pneumonic type) contains the organism, which can be identified by culture and guinea pig inoculation. During epidemics, clinical examination alone usually establishes the diagnosis.

The prognosis for untreated patients is poor. A mortality rate of 90% has been reached in some epidemics. Sulfonamide therapy has reduced this to 20%, and observations suggest that streptomycin may reduce it still further.

Treatment

Streptomycin (℞ 32), the drug of choice, is given I.M. or subcut. at a rate of 2 to 4 Gm. daily, in divided doses of 0.25 to 0.5 Gm. every 3 to 4 hours.

Sulfadiazine (℞ 37) may reinforce the action of streptomycin. Initial dose is 4 Gm. orally, followed by 1 Gm. every 4 hours until temperature has been normal for several days and all symptoms have cleared.

BRUCELLOSIS

(Undulant fever, Malta fever, Mediterranean fever, Gibraltar fever)

An infectious disease characterized by an acute febrile stage with few or no localizing signs and a chronic stage associated with relapses of fever, weakness, sweats, and vague body aches and pains.

Etiology and Epidemiology

The causative microorganisms belong to the genus *Brucella*, of which there are 3 species primarily affecting animals: *Br. abortus* (cattle), *Br. suis* (hogs), and *Br. melitensis* (goats). Any of these species may be transmitted to man and cause brucellosis, but the disease is rarely transmitted from man to man. Human brucellosis is contracted by direct secretions and excretions, and by the ingestion of milk or milk products containing viable Brucella. Brucellosis is world-wide in its distribution. It is most prevalent in rural areas and is an occupational disease among meat-packing employees, veterinarians, farmers, and livestock producers. Children only occasionally exhibit the symptoms of brucellosis.

Symptoms and Signs

The incubation period varies from 5 or 6 days to 3 weeks or more, with an average of 2 weeks. Clinical symptoms are extremely variable, especially in the early stages of the disease. Onset may be sudden and acute, with chills and fever, severe headache, indefinite bodily pains, and general malaise. Diarrhea occurs occasionally. Typically, however, the disease is of the undulant form: onset is insidious, with mild premonitory symptoms of malaise, muscular pain, pain in the back of the neck, and headache, followed by rising temperature in the evening. As the disease progresses, the evening temperature increases to 104° or 105°F. and drops gradually to normal or nearly so in the morning, at which time there usually is profuse sweating. The intermittent fever persists for variable periods (about 1 to 5 weeks), and is succeeded by an interval of remission during which symptoms are greatly reduced or absent. After a few days to 2 weeks the febrile phase recurs, perhaps only once, but often in repeated waves (or undulations) with intervening remissions over a period of 6 to 9 months or more. In this subacute, or chronic, form of the disease constipation is usually pronounced. Other symptoms are anorexia, loss of weight, abdominal pain, joint pain, headache, backache, weakness, nervous irritability, insomnia, mental depression, and emotional instability. The only physical abnormality frequently encountered is enlargement of the spleen. The lymph nodes also may be slightly or moderately enlarged. However, these manifestations may be absent.

Complications

Complications of the respiratory tract rarely occur. Not infrequently, bone lesions, such as spondylitis, are present. Other complications include subacute bacterial endocarditis, meningitis, encephalitis, neuritis, orchitis, cholecystitis and hepatic suppuration. Brucellosis is no more likely to cause abortion in women than do other severe bacterial infections.

Diagnosis

Whenever fever of unknown origin occurs, brucellosis should

be considered whether the fever is or is not accompanied by the constitutional symptoms mentioned. The diagnosis can be established by recovery of the organism from the blood, cerebrospinal fluid or tissues. However, while it is desirable to define the disease bacteriologically in every case, this is not always possible. The agglutination test is a valuable procedure in active brucellosis, and the results are quite significant when the titers are 1:100 or higher. Intradermal tests with Brucella antigens are of little practical value in diagnosing active brucellosis. When Brucella cannot be isolated and the agglutination test is positive, correlation with a history of exposure to infected animals or their products, e.g., ingestion of unpasteurized milk; epidemiologic data; and clinical findings and course frequently will give the correct diagnosis. In brucellosis, the total leukocyte count usually is normal or reduced, and a relative or absolute lymphocytosis is present.

Before the diagnosis of brucellosis is established, the symptoms may suggest typhoid fever, tularemia, malaria, influenza, tuberculosis, and various other diseases. The presence of sweating and constipation, the intermittent character of the fever, and the absence of rose-colored spots differentiate it from typhoid (q.v.). It may be distinguished from tularemia (q.v.) by the history and the absence of a local lesion and by guinea-pig inoculation: the animals die within 7 days if the infecting organism is *Past. tularensis,* but only after weeks or months, or not at all, if it is Brucella. Pulmonary tuberculosis (q.v.) can be differentiated by demonstration of tubercle bacilli or by X-ray examination; malaria (q.v.) by the presence of malarial parasites or symptomatic response to antimalarial chemotherapy. In influenza, onset usually is more sudden and acute, the pulmonary symptoms are more pronounced, and the course is shorter than in brucellosis.

Prognosis

The prognosis in brucellosis is good, the mortality rate being below 2% for all types of cases. Patients with acute uncomplicated brucellosis usually recover completely in a short time (2 to 3 weeks), or the disease may become chronic. Chronic brucellosis may result in a state of ill health lasting for several years, although it is rarely fatal.

Prophylaxis

Since cow's milk and its products (e.g., butter, cheese) are major sources of infection and may carry the more virulent hog strain of Brucella (*Br. suis*) as well as the bovine strain (*Br. abortus*), the most important prophylactic measure is the pasteurization of milk. In addition, persons who handle animals or carcasses that are likely to be infected should wear rubber gloves, and all breaks in the skin should be protected against the possible entrance of bacteria. Every effort should be made to detect the infection in animals and curb it at its source.

Treatment

General: Until recently no specific treatment for brucellosis has given uniformly good results, and emphasis has been placed on supportive and symptomatic measures. Physical activity should be reduced to a convalescent stage in the chronic cases and bed rest enforced during the febrile period. Headaches may be alleviated with acetylsalicylic acid (R 1). Severe body pains, especially over the spine, may require codeine (R 10). For persistent insomnia, a barbiturate (R 15) may be used. Patients with chronic brucellosis occasionally exhibit a degree of mental depression and emotional instability that necessitates careful psychotherapy and, above all, reassurance that ultimate recovery will ensue.

Chemotherapy: While the sulfonamides inhibit the growth of Brucella *in vitro,* clinical results have been disappointing because of the frequency of relapse after cessation of therapy. Although the organisms are sensitive to streptomycin in concentrations that can be readily attained in the body, this drug alone has not materially altered the course of the disease in the majority of cases.

The combination of streptomycin and sulfadiazine has achieved excellent results in the treatment of both acute and chronic cases. Streptomycin (R 32), 2 to 4 Gm. daily in divided doses, is given I.M. for 14 days. At the same time, oral administration of sulfadiazine (R 37) is started with 4 Gm. initially and 1 Gm. every 4 hours thereafter for 2 weeks. Recent reports indicate that aureomycin (R 35) and Chloromycetin (R 36) also are effective in the treatment of brucellosis; these drugs should be administered for 10 days or longer.

Immune serum: Results from the administration of convalescent ("immune") serum in acute or chronic cases have been disappointing, and this treatment is not recommended.

Brucella antigens: Brucella antigen therapy is of very questionable value. Two types have been tried. One is a broth filtrate of Brucella known as brucellin (R 105). Brucellin is injected intradermally every 3 or 4 days for 3 to 4 treatments, depending upon the patient's sensitivity to it, in doses sufficient to provoke systemic reactions. The initial dose usually is 0.1 cc. Better results have been obtained in acute than in chronic cases.

The second antigen, used in chronic cases, consists of various preparations of nonviable Brucella cells, usually heat-killed (R 106). The object is to desensitize the patient to Brucella antigen. The usual procedure is to inject an amount of antigen intradermally that will produce a local reaction but no systemic manifestations. As the patient tolerates the material, increasing doses are given about every 5 days. Treatment is continued

for several weeks. Should a systemic reaction occur, discontinue
further vaccine therapy for several weeks.

TULAREMIA
(Rabbit fever)

An acute infectious disease, often bizarre in its manifesta-
tions, but usually characterized by a primary local ulcerative
lesion, profound systemic symptoms, a typhoid-like state, bac-
teremia, and not infrequently atypical pneumonia.

Etiology and Pathology

The disease is caused by *Pasteurella tularensis* (*Bacterium
tularense*), a small pleomorphic, nonmotile, non-spore-bearing,
gram-negative, aerobic bacillus. This organism can enter the
body by ingestion, inoculation, or contamination (is believed
capable of penetrating the unbroken skin). *Past. tularensis*
is widely distributed in nature with a variety of animal hosts,
the most important of which are the rabbit and the hare. The
infection is transmitted among animals by blood-sucking
arthropods. Hunters, butchers, farmers, and laboratory workers are most commonly infected. Ninety percent of cases are
traceable to contact with infected wild rabbits. The remainder
are acquired by the handling of other infected animals or birds,
or by contact with infected ticks or other arthropods, by ingestion of inadequately cooked infected meat, and occasionally by
drinking contaminated water. No case is reported of transfer
from man to man, but infection in the laboratory occurs readily.

The characteristic anatomic lesions of tularemia are areas
of focal necrosis scattered throughout the body, in various stages
of evolution. Grossly, these appear as minute (1 mm.) to large
(8 cm.) whitish yellow foci which are commonly found in lymph
nodes, spleen, liver, kidney, and lung. Microscopically, the
lesions are focal areas of necrosis surrounded by monocytes and
young fibroblasts, which in turn are surrounded by large collections of lymphocytes. The superficial primary lesions—
which may occur on the finger, eye, or mouth—are made up of
such areas of necrosis. The pneumonia and most of the gastrointestinal symptoms are produced by internal necrotic foci.
The pneumonia is a patchy lobular process. The severe toxic
systemic manifestations appear to be the result of absorption
of the organism and the by-products of its activity.

Symptoms and Signs

From 1 to 10 days after contact, usually 2 to 4, the disease
begins suddenly with headache, chills, nausea, vomiting, temperature to 103° or 104°F. and extreme prostration. Extreme
weakness, recurring chills, and drenching sweats follow. Within

24 to 48 hours an inflamed papule makes its appearance at the site of infection: finger, arm, eye, or roof of the mouth. (There may be no primary lesion in laboratory-acquired infections or when the contaminated material has been ingested.) The papule rapidly becomes pustular, then ulcerates, producing a clean ulcer crater with a scanty, thin, colorless exudate. The ulcers usually are single when on the extremities, but multiple lesions are the rule when the mouth or eye is involved. (Usually, only one eye is affected). Soon thereafter regional lymph nodes swell. These may reach large proportions, suppurate and drain profusely. By the 5th day a typhoid-like state frequently develops or the patient may show signs of an atypical pneumonia, or both manifestations may be present. A nonspecific rash (roseola-like) may appear at any stage of the disease. The spleen is often enlarged and perisplenitis may occur. There is commonly a leukocytosis of 12,000 to 15,000, but there may be no increase in number, only an increased proportion of polymorphonuclears. The temperature, either septic or typhoid-like in its manifestations, remains elevated for 3 to 4 weeks in untreated cases. The various manifestations of the disease may appear in 4 more or less distinct clinical types: ulceroglandular, 87% of cases, primary on hands or fingers; oculoglandular, 3%; glandular, 2%, regional lymphadenitis present but no primary lesion; and typhoidal, 8%. Tularemic mediastinitis, lung abscess, and meningitis have been reported as complications, but these are rare.

Diagnosis and Prognosis

Diagnosis is established by recovery of the organism from the ulcer, from enlarged lymph nodes, or from the blood. A history of even the slightest contact with a wild rabbit, plus the very sudden onset of symptoms and the characteristic primary lesion, usually are diagnostic. The intracutaneous test with the Foshay antigen is positive after the 3rd day in most cases. Agglutination tests become positive after the 10th day; probably never before the 8th day. Laboratory infections frequently are typhoidal or pneumonic, with no demonstrable primary lesion, and may be difficult to diagnose. The serums of patients with brucellosis may give positive reactions with tularemic antigens, but usually to much lower titers.

The mortality is approximately 6%. Death, when it occurs, is usually caused by overwhelming infection, pneumonia, meningitis, or peritonitis. The temperature remains elevated for 3 to 4 weeks in untreated cases and falls by lysis. Relapses are uncommon, but do occur in inadequately treated cases.

Prophylaxis

Wild rabbits and rodents should be handled with great caution especially in endemic areas. The organisms may be present not only in the animal itself but also in tick feces in the fur. Precautions include wearing protective clothing and immediate removal of ticks. Wild birds and game to be used for food must be completely cooked. Contaminated water must be disinfected by any of the usual methods before use. Foshay's prophylactic vaccine given 3 weeks in advance of probable contact is reported to prevent most cases and definitely to diminish the severity of the disease in those who do acquire it.

Treatment

The therapeutic agent of choice is streptomycin. The dosage in typhoidal and pneumonic tularemia is 0.1 to 0.2 Gm. I.M. every 4 hours (℞ 32) until the temperature has been normal for 72 hours. A total dose of 2 to 5 Gm. appears to be adequate in most cases. The response is usually prompt and recovery uneventful. The dosage in ulceroglandular tularemia is less well established. Apparently 0.1 Gm. of streptomycin I.M. every 4 hours will heal primary lesions, but will not necessarily prevent suppuration of the lymph glands. The average total dose is about 5 Gm. There is no evidence that larger amounts will produce better results. Fluid balance must be maintained, and maintenance of nutrition is of considerable importance in complicated long-standing cases. However, the whole course of the disease is remarkably shortened in duration and severity by the proper use of streptomycin. Aureomycin (℞ 35) and Chloromycetin (℞ 36) recently have been shown also to be of value in the treatment of this disease.

Continuous wet saline dressings have a beneficial effect locally on primary lesions on extremities or skin, and may diminish the severity of the lymphangitis and lymphadenitis. Large abscesses may have to be opened and drained. These will rarely develop if the diagnosis is made early and the proper therapy instituted promptly. In ocular tularemia, warm saline compresses, dark glasses, and homatropine drops (℞ 117) may be used in extremely severe cases. The intense headache usually will respond to codeine (℞ 10) given at 3 to 4 hour intervals.

YELLOW FEVER

(Fièvre jaune, Gelbes fieber, Virus amaril)

An acute infectious virus disease occurring in tropical and subtropical zones, and characterized by sudden onset, fever with relatively slow pulse, albuminuria, vomiting of altered blood, jaundice, severe prostration, and a tendency toward hemorrhage.

Etiology and Epidemiology

The filtrable virus which causes the disease is transmitted by the bite of a female *Aedes aegypti* mosquito which has previously become infected through feeding on the blood of a patient during the first 3 or 4 days of his attack of yellow fever. The infection can be transmitted by the mosquito 10 or 12 days thereafter. Jungle yellow fever is transmitted in the tropics by *Haemogogus* and other tree-inhabiting mosquitoes.

Yellow fever is endemic in western Africa and certain portions of South America, notably Brazil, Bolivia, Colombia, Paraguay, Peru, and Venezuela. Epidemics may occur following the introduction of yellow fever into an area where there are *A. aegypti* mosquitoes and open water containers for breeding near, or in, human habitations. The last epidemic in the United States occurred in New Orleans in 1905.

Pathology

Extensive necrosis of the liver cells begins in the midzonal region of each lobule and extends outward. Acidophilic-staining, hyaline masses are sometimes present. Degenerative changes in the kidneys vary from cloudy swelling to severe cellular necrosis in the convoluted tubules. In the myocardium also, degenerative changes usually are demonstrable.

Symptoms and Signs

(1) **Period of incubation:** 3 to 6 days. Prodromal symptoms usually are absent. (2) **Period of invasion:** 2 to 5 days. Onset is sudden with fever (102° to 103°F.), sometimes associated with a chill. The pulse is usually elevated correspondingly early in the disease, but later becomes slower than would be expected with the degree of fever (Faget's sign). The face is flushed, eyes injected, gums congested, and tongue red and pointed. Nausea, vomiting, and constipation are common. Jaundice usually appears on the 2nd or 3rd day. Other symptoms may include epigastric distress and tenderness; muscular pains, especially in the loins and the calves of the legs; prostration out of proportion to the degree of fever; headache, restlessness, and irritability. (3) **Period of intoxication:** 6 to 9 days. The temperature rises to 103° or 104°F. and the three characteristic clinical features of yellow fever become established: jaundice, extreme albuminuria, and hematemesis ("black vomit"). There also may be oliguria or anuria. Petechiae frequently appear and hemorrhages occur from mucous membranes as manifested by melena, epistaxis, bleeding gums. The patient is dull, confused, and often apathetic. Delirium, convulsions, and coma are common terminal manifestations. (4) **Period of convalescence:** This is prolonged. If recovery occurs, it usually begins 1 to 2 weeks after the onset, progresses slowly and usually is associated with improvement in renal function. Jaundice persists for many weeks.

Diagnosis and Laboratory Findings

A progressively increasing albuminuria is commonly noted.

The leukocyte count usually is low, but may be elevated. There is elevation of the icterus index and serum bilirubin.

During the period of invasion, diagnosis may be impossible, but it is suggested by a decline in pulse rate on the 2nd or 3rd day despite continuation of the fever, associated with a progressively increasing albuminuria, severe headache, and backache. During the period of intoxication, the diagnosis is based upon the characteristic combination of the triad: jaundice, extreme albuminuria, and hematemesis ("black vomit"). The diagnosis can be confirmed after the 3rd week of the disease by mouse protection tests. Injection of 30 cc. of blood, drawn from a patient early in the course of yellow fever, does not protect the mouse against an inoculation with yellow fever virus, whereas such a procedure 3 weeks after onset of the disease does protect the animal. Yellow fever in the early stages often is difficult to differentiate from Weil's disease. It also must be distinguished from malaria, relapsing fever, infectious hepatitis, acute yellow atrophy, influenza, and dengue.

Prognosis

The fatality rate may be as high as 85% during an epidemic, but it usually is much lower in endemic areas. Mild and even unrecognized infections are said to be common in such regions.

Control

The great reduction in incidence of yellow fever has been due chiefly to effective mosquito control measures: (1) Maritime quarantine prevents the introduction of yellow fever from ships. This includes the disinfestation of ships and their cargoes in addition to a complete quarantine of passengers for the incubation period whenever yellow fever has occurred aboard the vessel. The regulations now in force have been found effective in the United States. (2) Aerial quarantine requires immunization of persons leaving yellow fever areas, which have been delineated by the Expert Committee on Quarantine of the World Health Organization, and quarantine inspection of passengers at port of arrival, with detention or surveillance (when indicated) until probable expiration of the period of incubation. It is necessary that the airport and vicinity be free from A. aegypti. (3) Destruction of breeding places for A. aegypti (open, still water near human habitations). (4) Isolation of suspects and cases for first 4 days of fever, in rooms well screened and preferably sprayed with DDT. (5) Vaccination with attenuated yellow fever virus (such as strain 17D) is indicated for those who plan to travel where the disease is endemic. Dehydrated virus freshly dissolved within 1 hour is injected subcutaneously as a single dose of 0.5 Gm. In an endemic area, a "booster" dose of 0.5 Gm. may be given every 2 years or repeated only during epidemics. Postvaccinal jaundice sometimes occurs.

Treatment

There is no specific treatment for yellow fever. Dehydration (q.v.) may be treated by means of parenteral fluids containing dextrose, if oral intake can not be increased comfortably. Hemorrhagic tendencies may be treated by means of I.V. calcium gluconate (℞ 150), 1 Gm. once or twice a day, or oral menadione (℞ 133), 2 mg. a day. Nausea and vomiting may be alleviated by the administration of cocaine (℞ 26) by mouth with cracked ice (used with *caution!*), by codeine (℞ 10), given subcut. in 30 mg. (gr. ss) doses, or by scopolamine (hyoscine) (℞ 21) given subcut. in 0.6 mg. doses with or without sodium phenobarbital (℞ 23).

DENGUE FEVER

(Breakbone fever, Dandy fever)

An acute, febrile disease characterized by sudden onset, with headache, fever and prostration, pains in the joints and muscles, and leukopenia, and a rash that appears simultaneously with a second rise in temperature following an afebrile period.

Etiology and Epidemiology

The causative agent is a filtrable virus which is demonstrable in the peripheral blood of patients from the day before the initial fever until the 3rd or 4th day of illness.

The virus is transmitted to human beings by the bite of mosquitoes, *Aedes aegypti* and *Aedes albopictus*. The prevention of dengue, therefore, consists of controlling or eradicating the mosquito vector. Screening of buildings, spraying the buildings and screens with DDT (5% DDT in kerosene), destruction of breeding places and their routine spraying with DDT, use of a DDT aerosol bomb in living quarters, and the free application of mosquito repellents to exposed skin surfaces will diminish the chances of infection.

During this century, epidemics have occurred in the southeastern and gulf sections of the United States, and in tropical America, Spain, Egypt, Greece, Syria, India, the Indo-China coast, The Netherlands East Indies, New Guinea, and the Philippine Islands. Between epidemics, sporadic cases are seen in these areas. An attack of dengue ordinarily produces immunity for a year or more. No satisfactory vaccine against the disease has been developed.

Symptoms and Signs

Following an incubation period of 4 to 10 days, the onset is abrupt, with chills or chilly sensations, headache, postorbital pain on moving the eyeballs, lumbar backache, and severe prostration. Extreme pain and aching of the lower extremities and joints are common during the first few hours of illness. The fever rises rapidly to 102° to 104°F., with a relative bradycardia and hypotension. Anorexia is present, the bulbar and palpebral conjunctivas are injected, and a transient flushing or pale pink macular rash (particularly of the face) usually appears during this early period. A soft, slightly enlarged spleen may be palpated. The majority of cases show enlargement of the cervical, epitrochlear, and inguinal lymph nodes.

Fever and other symptoms persist for 48 to 96 hours; then there is a rapid defervescence with profuse sweating. This afebrile period is accompanied by a sense of well-being; it lasts about 24 hours and is followed by a second rapid rise in temperature, usually with a lower peak than the first. This second temperature rise is responsible for a "saddle back" type of temperature curve. Coincidentally, a characteristic eruption appears. Although this rash is ordinarily morbilliform it may be macular in character. Typically, it appears over the extremities, after which the entire body, except the face, usually becomes involved; or there may only be a patchy distribution over the trunk and extremities. Palms and soles may be bright red and edematous. Atypical cases occur without this second febrile period. Convalescence is often prolonged, lasting several weeks, and accompanied by hypotension and asthenia. Complete recovery occurs eventually in almost all cases. Uncomplicated cases are seldom fatal.

Diagnosis and Laboratory Findings

Leukopenia due to granulocytopenia is invariably found. The total leukocyte count begins falling by the 2nd day of fever and drops to a low point of 2,000 to 4,000 by the 4th or 5th day after onset. The granulocytes may drop to 20 to 40% of the total count. The urine is scanty and concentrated, sometimes containing small amounts of albumin and a few casts.

The disease may be confused with typhus or yellow fever in areas where these diseases are endemic. At the onset it may be mistaken for influenza, malaria, or measles. While there is no specific laboratory test to confirm the diagnosis, the association of fever, headache, postorbital pain, aching of lower back and extremities, saddle-back temperature curve, rash, and pronounced leukopenia, in an endemic area, usually suggests the diagnosis of dengue fever.

Treatment

There is no specific therapy; treatment is entirely symptomatic. The patient must be kept in bed under mosquito netting until the second fever has abated in order to prevent transmission of the disease to uninfected mosquitoes. Fluids should be given in large quantities, an ice cap to the head is useful in combating headache, and frequent cold water or alcohol sponging of the entire body will afford relief from high fever.

Considerable alleviation of headache and bodily aching may be obtained by the administration of analgesics (℞ 1, 4, 10). Morphine (℞ 11) in moderate doses may be required in severe cases. For nervousness and insomnia, phenobarbital (℞ 15) may be employed. For nausea, chlorobutanol (℞ 27) is said to give relief. Belladonna (℞ 118) is useful against sweating. Liniments (℞ 14) may be applied for joint pains. When itching due to the rash is severe, a dusting powder (℞ 126) will afford relief. During convalescence, when asthenia is severe, protracted bed rest is indicated. Tonics (℞ 137) are helpful.

RELAPSING FEVER

(Recurrent fever, Spirillum fever, Famine fever, Tick fever)

An acute, widely disseminated infectious disease caused by several species of spirochetes, transmitted by lice and ticks, and characterized by recurrent febrile paroxysms with intervals of apparent recovery.

Etiology, Transmission, and Pathology

Six species of the spirochete *Borrelia* are known to cause relapsing fevers; each predominates in a certain area. The various species of spirochetes are morphologically indistinguishable.

The body louse is the principal vector in Europe, Africa, and India. In America, the tick is the chief vector. The spirochetes apparently can penetrate the mucous membrane of the eye, perhaps other mucosal surfaces as well, and possibly the intact skin.

Lice become infected by feeding on the blood of a patient during the febrile period of the disease. The infected louse may then transmit the disease if crushed on the human skin so that the liberated spirochetes penetrate the skin, possibly through the site of the louse bite, or they may gain entrance through the eye via contaminated fingers. The spirochete also may be deposited on the skin in louse feces. Louse-borne relapsing fever is prevalent under those conditions which are conducive to filth and overcrowding, namely war and famine.

Ticks become infected by feeding either on a human patient or infected animals (armadillo, squirrel, chipmunk). Human transmission follows the contamination of a tick bite with the spirochete excreted in the tick feces.

In fatal cases, the spleen is enlarged and contains necrotic lesions which are laden with spirochetes. There may be hemorrhages into the skin, viscera, and mucous membranes.

Symptoms and Signs

There is a marked difference between the clinical characteristics of the different types of relapsing fevers. Only the common features are detailed here.

The incubation period averages about 7 days. The sudden onset is characterized by a chill, followed by fever up to 104° or 105°F., severe headache, vomiting, and muscle and joint pains. The fever remains high until the end of the paroxysm which may last from 2 to 7 days, when it falls by crisis. An erythematous eruption may appear early, followed by rose-colored spots and rarely hepatomegaly and jaundice. A polymorphonuclear leukocytosis is common, and the urine may contain albumin and casts. The Wassermann is positive in about 20% of patients with relapsing fever. Similar paroxysms may follow at 1- to 2-week intervals. Between bouts, the patient appears normal. Immunity develops as the disease progresses, resulting in successively milder attacks and eventual recovery. In untreated cases, the disease persists for 6 to 8 weeks.

Diagnosis

During an epidemic, the diagnosis is readily suspected. At other times, it will be suggested by the temperature chart and the clinical course.

During the febrile phase, the spirochete may at times be demonstrated by darkfield examination of the patient's blood or urine, or by examination of a thick and thin blood smear stained with Wright's stain (*see* LAB. PROC.). Mice, inoculated with the patient's febrile blood, show great numbers of spirochetes after 48 hours.

The relapsing fevers must be differentiated from malaria, dengue, yellow fever, Weil's disease, enteric fever, typhus, influenza, and early smallpox.

Prognosis and Treatment

The prognosis is good, death rarely ensuing. Untreated cases recover in 6 to 8 weeks; treated cases are cured in a short time. The arsenicals are specific for relapsing fever. Mapharsen (℞ 83) or neoarsphenamine (℞ 84) is effective. Stovarsol (℞ 85) may be given orally when I.V. arsenical therapy is impossible. Medication must be given only while the fever is rising and before the crisis in order to avoid Herxheimer-like collapse. Therapy is contraindicated between attacks and while the fever is falling. If symptoms recur, the dose may be repeated at the onset of the next paroxysm. Penicillin (℞ 28) shows considerable promise of being the drug of choice but its exact status remains to be determined.

INFECTIOUS (SPIROCHETAL) JAUNDICE

(Weil's disease, Epidemic jaundice, Spirochetosis icterohaemorrhagica)

An acute systemic infection characterized by headache, fever, myalgia, jaundice, hepatomegaly, hemorrhagic diathesis, conjunctival injection, and albuminuria.

Etiology and Incidence

This disease is caused by the spirochete *Leptospira icterohaemorrhagiae* which is a nonpathogenic parasite of rats, and is excreted in their feces and urine. Rarely, a similar disease is caused by *Lept. canicola*, a parasite of dogs. Man is infected either through the ingestion of contaminated food and water or through contact of the broken skin with materials containing the feces and urine of infected animals. Certain occupational groups such as miners, sewer cleaners, and wharfmen are especially liable to the disease. In some areas, it is classed as an occupational disease.

Symptoms and Signs

The incubation period varies from 5 to 13 days. The onset is sudden with fever, chills, severe headache, vomiting, and muscle pains, particularly in the calf muscles. Conjunctival injection is common and pronounced. Abdominal pain may be encountered. Fever varies between 102° and 104°F. for 3 or 4 days and then declines to normal. Jaundice appears by the 5th day in about 50% of patients. The liver and spleen may be palpable. Evidence of meningeal irritation may appear and the organisms have been found in spinal fluid. Oliguria is common and the urine contains albumin, casts, red cells, and bile. Uremia may occur in severe cases. Capillary hemorrhages and even purpura often are evident; massive hemorrhage rarely occurs. The leukocyte count may be normal or as high as 50,000 with a preponderance of neutrophiles.

Symptoms and signs persist for several days and nonfatal cases usually have a normal temperature by the 10th day. Relapses may occur and convalescence is prolonged if the patient is debilitated.

Diagnosis

In the presence of the above symptoms and signs, the disease should always be considered. Diagnosis is established by demonstrating the organism or by specific agglutination tests. The organism may be identified in the patient's blood up to the 10th day by darkfield examination or by guinea pig inoculation. After the 10th day, the spirochete can be isolated from the urine for periods up to 6 weeks. Specific agglutinins develop in the patient's serum after 7 days and a rapidly rising titer is diagnostic. Very high titers are reached and may persist for as long as 8 years.

Spirochetal jaundice must be differentiated from acute catarrhal jaundice, acute yellow atrophy, yellow fever, and relapsing fever. The diagnosis is often missed, especially in the absence of jaundice. Other entities that may be confused with Weil's disease are appendicitis, dengue fever, and blood dyscrasias.

Prognosis

In the absence of jaundice, the disease is almost never fatal. Among jaundiced patients, the mortality rate averages about 16%, being much higher in Japan than elsewhere. Death results from extreme toxemia, myocarditis, renal failure, pulmonary edema, or massive hemorrhage.

Prophylaxis

Exposure of human beings to water in such places as drainage ditches, sewers, and mines must be avoided; if unavoidable, such areas should be cleared of rats. Vaccines for active immunization are ineffective.

Treatment

Treatment is largely symptomatic. Penicillin (℞ 28), 400,000 to 600,000 u. daily, has been used with inconclusive results. It apparently sterilizes the urine of *Leptospirae* but otherwise seems to have no significant effect on the systemic disease. Since penicillin is practically nontoxic, it is recommended for immediate use in all cases of infectious jaundice. The sulfonamides and arsenicals are not effective. Leptospira antiserum (℞ 102) (when available) appears to exert a favorable effect on the disease. Human convalescent serum, or a transfusion from a compatible donor who has recovered from the disease within the previous year is of real benefit. All serums should be administered as soon as the diagnosis is made.

Symptomatic therapy is aimed at easing the load on the liver and kidneys (*see* HEPATITIS; NEPHRITIS). Headaches and myalgia may be relieved by acetylsalicylic acid (℞ 1) or codeine (℞ 10).

Fluid balance should be maintained cautiously at all times, parenterally if necessary, with care taken not to overburden the kidney (*see* NEPHRITIS). In cases of pronounced oliguria or anuria, high spinal anesthesia has been used beneficially. Meningitis (q.v.), if severe, is treated by repeated lumbar puncture and penicillin intrathecally in doses of 10,000 to 20,000 u. in 10 to 20 cc. of sterile isotonic saline.

RICKETTSIAL DISEASES

A group of infectious febrile diseases caused by minute microorganisms called rickettsias and transmitted to man by certain members of the arthropod kingdom. These diseases include epidemic typhus, murine (endemic) typhus, Rocky Mountain spotted fever, South American spotted fever, fièvre boutonneuse, Q fever, tsutsugamushi disease (scrub typhus), trench fever, and rickettsialpox. They are characterized clinically by a sudden onset with febrile course of from one to several weeks, a skin eruption, and involvement of the C.N.S. and lungs in the more severe forms of the disease. Certain of the diseases are further characterized by the presence of a primary lesion and the development of agglutinins for specific strains of the proteus bacillus. Brill's disease probably is a mild recrudescence of an old attack of epidemic typhus.

Etiology

Rickettsias are small microorganisms which occupy a position between the viruses and bacteria. They are visible as minute cocci or coccobacilli with the oil immersion lens of the microscope. Rickettsias differ from bacteria in that they require the presence of living cells for growth. With the exception of the causative organism of Q fever, they are retained by the Berkefeld filter, thus essentially differing from the viruses. (For further details *see* table, The Rickettsial Diseases.)

Epidemiology and Prophylaxis

Rickettsial infections are transmitted to man by the bite or attachment of lice, fleas, ticks, or mites (*see* table). In rare instances, and more commonly so with Q fever, infection may be sustained by pulmonary inhalation or conjunctival absorption of air-borne suspensions of the organisms. Prevention, therefore, essentially depends upon the eradication or control of these insects, although prophylactic vaccines are available against certain of the rickettsial diseases and play an important role in prophylaxis.

The body louse may be readily killed by the free use of 10% DDT powder applied to the undergarments and the inner surfaces of clothing. About 1 oz. is required. This treatment also is efficacious against the flea, although the use of DDT powder or a spray of 5% DDT in kerosene applied to breeding areas of this insect is advised as a supplementary measure.

The mite, or chigger as it is commonly known, is readily killed by the impregnation of clothing with dimethyl or dibutyl phthalate, or benzyl benzoate. These agents are applied by rubbing about 1 oz. of the material into clothing, taking special care to cover the socks, trouser cuffs, fly and waistband of trousers, and collar and cuffs of the shirt; undergarments should not be treated.

Satisfactory agents have not been developed for controlling ticks. Reliance must be placed upon avoidance of tick-infested areas and inspections of the body at frequent intervals (2 to 4 hours) throughout the day to discover tick attachments.

Highly effective vaccines, prepared from the embryonated chicken egg, are available for prophylaxis against typhus and spotted fever. The usual dose is 1 cc. given twice or thrice at 5 to 7 day intervals. Protection persists for 6 months; after this period, a high degree of immunity may be reestablished by the administration of a single 1 cc. dose of the vaccine.

Pathology

The pathologic findings in the rickettsial diseases are basically those of a disseminated, focal vasculitis and perivasculitis, although diffuse infiltration of organs with mononuclear cells often is encountered. In epidemic typhus fever, the endovasculitis, thrombosis, and hemorrhage are prominent and are distinctly more severe than in tsutsugamushi disease, but less so than in spotted fever where these changes are of such degree as to constitute a panarteritis with necrosis. The vessels principally involved are those of the skin, brain, heart, and kidneys, and to a lesser extent, the liver, spleen, and lungs. Little is known concerning the histopathologic changes in the human in fièvre boutonneuse, Q fever, trench fever and rickettsialpox.

The vascular lesions consist of perivascular accumulations of lymphocytes, plasma cells, and large mononuclear cells in variable proportions. When these focal infiltrations are sharply demarcated and proliferative in nature, they are known as typhus nodules. These nodules are particularly prominent in the brain and in the skin.

In addition, myocardial infiltration with mononuclear cells, and variable degrees of interstitial pneumonitis, particularly in Q fever, also are essential features of the histopathology of the rickettsial diseases. This interstitial, or rickettsial, pneumonitis may be complicated by the development of a true bacterial pneumonia due to the pneumococcus, staphylococcus, or streptococcus.

Symptoms and Signs

Following an incubation period of from 1 to 2 weeks for typhus, trench fever, and tsutsugamushi disease and from 3 to 7 days for spotted fever and fièvre boutonneuse, the onset of disease is fairly abrupt with chills or chilliness, headache, fever, and malaise. Occasionally, prodromal symptoms consisting of headache, pains in the back and legs, and general malaise may precede the actual onset by several days. During the 1st week, the fever rises steadily and is accompanied by an excruciating headache. The temperature remains elevated throughout the 2nd week of disease, following which it subsides by rapid or slow lysis. This temperature elevation usually is accompanied by a relative bradycardia, except when the course is unusually severe or when complications develop. In trench fever, the fever curve may be characterized by 2 or more febrile periods of from 3 to 5 days with 12 to 24 hours of remission between them. Conjunctival congestion, apathy, and anorexia are common. Nausea and vomiting occur infrequently.

Primary lesion: In tsutsugamushi disease, fièvre boutonneuse, and rickettsialpox, a primary lesion is commonly observed. This lesion, termed eschar in the case of tsutsugamushi disease, tache noir in fièvre boutonneuse, and initial lesion in rickettsialpox, is a small, oval or round ulcer with surrounding erythema and commonly covered by a black scab. It represents the site of attachment of the insect vector of the disease, and appears several days before the onset of disease as a small but rapidly enlarging papule.

THE RICKETTSIAL DISEASES—SALIENT FACTS

Disease and Synonyms	Principal Geographic Foci	1. Organism 2. Vector 3. Reservoir	Weil-Felix Reaction		
			OX 19	OX 2	OX K
Epidemic Typhus (Jail fever; European or classical typhus)	Balkans, China, Ukraine, Mexico, South America	1. *R. prowazeki* 2. Human body louse 3. Man	3+	2+	—
Trench Fever (Wolhynian fever)	Central Europe	1. *R. wolhynica* 2. Body louse 3. Man	—	—	—
Murine Typhus (Endemic, flea-borne, or urban typhus)	Southern U.S., Mexico, Australia	1. *R. mooseri* 2. Rat flea 3. Rat	3+	2+	—
Rocky Mountain Spotted Fever (Tick fever)	Eastern and Northwestern U.S.	1. *R. rickettsi* 2. Dog and wood tick 3. Wild rodents	3+	2+	—
South American Spotted Fever (Sao Paolo or Columbian fever)	Brazil	1. *R. pijperi* 2. Dog tick 3. Wild rodents	3+	2+	—
Fièvre Boutonneuse (Marseilles or eruptive Mediterranean fever)	Mediterranean area, Black Sea region	1. *R. conori* 2. Dog tick 3. Wild rodents	3+	2+	—
Q Fever (Nine-mile fever)	Texas and Montana, Australia, Italy, Greece	1. *R. burneti* 2. Wood and cattle tick 3. Wild rodents	—	—	—
Tsutsugamushi Disease (Mite-borne, rural, or scrub typhus; Japanese river fever)	Asiatic-Pacific area	1. *R. orientalis* 2. Chigger 3. Field mice	—	—	3+
Rickettsialpox	New York City	1. *R. akari* 2. Mouse mite 3. House mice	1+	1+	1+

Rash: With the sole exception of Q fever, a rash characteristically appears during the course of a rickettsial disease. In trench fever an eruption, consisting of red macules, usually appears during the first 24 hours, first on the chest and abdomen. Later, it may involve the whole trunk. In rickettsialpox, a generalized rash, papular and papulovesicular in character, appears on the 2nd or 3rd day. In spotted fever, fièvre boutonneuse, typhus, and tsutsugamushi disease, a macular rash appears from the 3rd to the 7th or 8th days. In the case of spotted fever, the eruption appears first on the extremities and spreads to the trunk; this is in contrast to the other rickettsial diseases where the skin manifestations first appear on the trunk, primarily the chest, and spread to the extremities. In epidemic typhus and spotted fever, the rash rapidly becomes petechial and confluent so that large areas of the skin assume a purpuric appearance. In contrast to this, the rash of tsutsugamushi disease rarely, if ever, becomes hemorrhagic while that of murine typhus and fièvre boutonneuse may become slightly petechial in nature.

Central nervous system: While the appearance of apathy, restlessness, and insomnia are characteristic of the rickettsial diseases, signs indicating progressive neurologic involvement, ranging from disorientation and delirium through convulsions to stupor and coma are frequently seen in severe cases of epidemic typhus and spotted fever.

Circulatory system: The pulse rate is relatively slow early in the disease, but with progression into the 2nd week, particularly in severe cases of epidemic typhus and spotted fever, the pulse rate rises, quality of the pulse becomes poor, and the blood pressure may drop precipitously. This hypotension is of grave prognostic significance, particularly if associated with oliguria and nonprotein nitrogen retention in epidemic typhus and spotted fever.

Respiratory system: In the severe type of rickettsial disease, such as epidemic typhus, spotted fever, and tsutsugamushi disease, cough is an early and frequently distressing symptom. The cause of this is a pneumonitis of rickettsial origin which cannot be differentiated from primary atypical ("virus") pneumonia. In Q fever, this pneumonitis is the most characteristic sign of the disease. Secondary bacterial pneumonia may play an important role as a complication.

Laboratory Findings

A normal or lowered leukocyte count is commonly found during the 1st week of the disease. As the disease progresses into the 2nd and 3rd weeks, the leukocyte count rises, particularly if bacterial complications develop. The urine is scanty and concentrated. Small amounts of albumin and a few casts are seen in the more severe forms of the disease. In many of the rickettsial diseases, agglutinins for specific strains of the proteus bacillus appear by the 2nd week of disease and usually attain a peak titer by the 3rd or 4th week. (For a summary of reactions, *see* table.) Although a titer of 1:160 is ordinarily diagnostic, a rise in titer when early and late specimens of serums are compared is more significant.

Specific complement fixation tests now are available for differentiation of the various types of rickettsial diseases. Serial specimens of serums obtained early in the disease and late in convalescence may be sent to the National Institute of Health, U.S. Public Health Service, Bethesda, Maryland. False positive Wassermann tests may be obtained early in the disease.

Diagnosis and Prognosis

The diagnosis of a specific rickettsial disease is made by consideration of the clinical signs, season of the year, geographic location, existence of epidemics, and serologic findings.

Other important diseases to be considered in the differential diagnosis are influenza, typhoid fever, infectious hepatitis, malaria, dengue, relapsing fever, meningococcemia, smallpox, chickenpox, and measles. Prior to the appearance of a rash and specific agglutinins, the differential diagnosis of a rickettsial disease from some of these other diseases may be impossible. The problem is simplified by the fact that there is a fairly sharp geographic limitation of these diseases.

The prognosis varies greatly, being very favorable in trench fever and rather grave in spotted fever. The older the patient, the more serious is the outlook.

Treatment

Nursing care and appropriate supportive therapy are extremely important in the treatment of the rickettsial diseases. Complete bed rest, avoidance of overexertion, frequent small feedings of food, a special nurse for severely ill patients, adequate fluid intake, alcohol sponges for high fever, and meticulous mouth and skin care should be stressed in nursing care.

A minimal fluid intake of from 2,000 to 3,000 cc./day in small increments is essential. From 3 to 4 Gm. of salt a day should be administered in hot climates, preferably by mouth, or parenterally in the form of normal saline supplemented with 5% glucose solution. A high caloric diet with high protein intake should be provided in convalescence. This may be supplemented with multivitamin capsules.

In the severely ill patient, the mouth should be kept moist and clean and alcohol rubs, powder, pads, and frequent changing of positions should be employed to prevent bed sores and gangrenous skin lesions. Oxygen is indicated when patients with pneumonitis become cyanotic.

Analgesics (℞ 1, 10) may be used freely for severe headache; if the headache is excruciating, Demerol (℞ 12) may be administered as a last resort. Although acetylsalicylic acid (℞ 1) is useful for general malaise, its use should be generally avoided because of marked fluctuations of temperature and profuse sweating which this drug commonly causes. Restlessness and delirium may be combated with barbiturates (℞ 23, 24) or paraldehyde (℞ 18); when delirium is exceptionally severe, it may be necessary to employ Demerol (℞ 12) though its use should be avoided in favor of paraldehyde because of possible depression of the respiratory center in critically ill patients.

Severe cough may be treated with codeine (℞ 10), expectorants (℞ 142) and inhalants (℞ 143). I.V. plasma in increments of 500 cc. once or twice a day should be used when there is evidence of peripheral circulatory failure, hypotension with oliguria and nonprotein nitrogen retention, or hypoproteinemia.

Both Chloromycetin (℞ 36) and aureomycin (℞ 35) appear to be effective against the rickettsial diseases. These drugs are given orally in daily doses of 40 to 100 mg./Kg. body wt., administered in divided doses every 4 hours for the first day. Thereafter, the daily dose and frequency of administration may be gradually reduced according to the favorable clinical response, the drug being discontinued after 2 to 14 days of therapy. Further studies are necessary to determine the optimum dose-time regimen.

Therapy with para-aminobenzoic acid (℞ 91) is of value in all patients seen on or before the 6th day of disease, and for patients of 50 or more years of age, even if seen after this period. This drug should be continued well into the afebrile period. It should be discontinued if leukocyte counts continue below 3,000 with an increasing depression of the neutrophilic fraction of the differential. The sulfonamides, penicillin, or streptomycin have no effect on the course of rickettsial diseases.

Penicillin (℞ 28, 29) or streptomycin (℞ 32) should be used to combat bacterial complications since para-aminobenzoic acid inhibits the action of the sulfonamides.

FILARIASIS

A group of diseases commonly found in tropical and subtropical countries, including Central and South America, and caused by infection with filariae.

Etiology

Infection usually is due to *Filaria* (*Wuchereria*) *bancrofti* or *Filaria malayi*. The adult worms may live in the circulatory or lymphatic systems, the connective tissues, or serous cavities. The larvae (microfilariae) may be found in the blood stream, usually at night. Infection is spread from man to man by the mosquito (Aedes, Culex). The injected larvae grow to adult worms in the lymphatics, where they may cause obstruction. In the United States, spread of the disease from infected military personnel is unlikely, since it was shown generations ago that the disease failed to become established in the general population although a large majority of Negro slaves were infected.

Symptoms and Signs

The incubation period is unknown. Clinical manifestations depend on the severity of the infestation and may include lymphangitis, lymphadenitis, orchitis, funiculitis, epididymitis, lymphvarices, chyluria, and elephantiasis. There may be accompanying chills, fever, headache, and malaise. During the acute stage, the leukocyte count may reach 40,000 with an eosinophilia up to 30%.

Diagnosis

Diagnosis is made by demonstration (during sleep or at night) of microfilariae in the patient's blood or lymph fluid. Adult worms may be found in biopsy material. An intradermal antigen, prepared from *Dirofilaria immitis,* may be useful in diagnosis.

Treatment

The prognosis is good in individuals who have not been long resident in endemic areas. Repeated infection increases the likelihood of elephantiasis. Therapy with antimonials has been disappointing. Several promising chemotherapeutic agents now are under investigation (arsenamide, cyanine dyes, Hetrazan). Surgery is indicated only for alleviation of elephantiasis, especially of the scrotum.

ONCHOCERCIASIS

Onchocerciasis is due to infection by *Onchocerca volvulus* and characterized by fibrous nodules in the skin and subcutaneous tissues, impairment of vision, and rarely (0.5% of cases) blindness. The disease is spread by the bite of black flies (*Simulidae*), and is commonly observed in southern Mexico, Guatemala, and Africa. Diagnosis depends on the demonstration of microfilariae in the fibrous nodules. Treatment consists of surgical removal of the nodules.

LOIASIS

(Calabar swellings)

Loiasis is a form of filariasis (Loa loa), found in West Africa, which is caused by the bite of a fly (*Chrysops*) and is characterized by rapid migration of the adult worms in the subcutaneous tissues. Localized transient swellings occur at the site of the migration. In the course of migration, the adult worms may wander across the eye beneath the conjunctiva or across the bridge of the nose. Microfilariae may be found in the peripheral blood, and there usually is a marked eosinophilia.

Treatment consists in mechanical extraction of the adult parasites, under local anesthesia, as they migrate across the eye or bridge of the nose.

DRACUNCULIASIS
(Dracontiasis)

Dracunculiasis is caused by the presence of the guinea worm (*Dracunculus medinensis*) in the subcutaneous tissues, producing skin ulcers through which the female discharges larvae. It is endemic in the Nile Valley, India, and Brazil. Infection follows ingestion of water containing infested crustacea (Cyclops). Local itching and burning may be intense. Diagnosis is possible only after the adult worm has reached its final destination under the skin, at which time its head may be seen in the base of the ulcer, or larvae may be demonstrated in the discharge. Treatment consists of slow mechanical extraction of the adult worm by gradual traction on its head over a period of 10 days. Septic and foreign body reactions should be treated as indicated.

LEISHMANIASIS
(Kala-azar, Oriental sore, American leishmaniasis)

Invasion of the human organism by protozoa (genus Leishmania) *transmitted by the sandfly*. Depending on the strain of *Leishmania* causing it, the disease may manifest itself as **kala-azar** (*L. donovani*), **Oriental sore** (*L. tropica*), or **American leishmaniasis** (*L. braziliensis*). The incubation period is a few days to several months.

Types, Course, and Findings

1. **Kala-azar (visceral leishmaniasis, black fever, dumdum fever)** is encountered in India, China, Africa, and the Mediterranean basin. Children are particularly susceptible. The protozoa invade the blood stream and localize in the reticulo-endothelial system with resultant fever, pronounced splenomegaly, anemia, emaciation, and leukopenia. The fever is generally irregular and recurrent, seldom sustained. Later, there may be enlargement of the liver and lymph nodes. The serum globulin is considerably elevated and the aldehyde test is indicative of kala-azar. The parasite may be demonstrated in needle biopsy of the liver, spleen, bone marrow, or lymph nodes, or in cultures from these tissues or of blood. The fatality rate is 90% in untreated cases and only 10% in the treated.

2. **Oriental sore (cutaneous leishmaniasis, tropical sore, Delhi boil, Aleppo boil, frontier sore)** is found in the Mediterranean area and is characterized by single or multiple ulcerating, granulomatous, autoinoculable lesions of the skin. The

ulcers are sharply demarcated but may fuse to involve large areas. Secondary infection is usual. Smears and biopsy of the ulcer margin reveal *L. tropica.* There are no systemic symptoms, except those due to secondary infection. Healing will occur spontaneously in 2 to 18 months, leaving a depressed scar.

3. American leishmaniasis (espundia, forest yaws, uta) occurs in Southern Mexico and Central and South America and is manifested by ulcerative lesions of the nose and pharynx. The parasites may be demonstrated in smears or biopsy material. Untreated, the disease may persist for years, death resulting from secondary infection or respiratory embarrassment.

Treatment

General: Bed rest, adequate nutrition, and fluids should be prescribed. Oral hygiene with nonirritating mouthwashes (*see* STOMATITIS) are indicated for oral lesions. Transfusions for anemia and chemotherapy for secondary infection are useful when indicated.

Specific: Pentavalent antimony compounds are preferable to trivalent preparations. Neostibosan (℞ 61) is currently the drug of choice. It is given I.V. (slowly) as a freshly prepared 5% solution in distilled water. For adults, the initial dose is 0.2 Gm. (gr. iii), followed by 0.3 Gm. (gr. v) daily until a total dose of 5 Gm. has been given. Should toxic effects (nausea, vomiting) appear during treatment, the drug should be given on alternate days, or the dosage reduced, or administration stopped, as the circumstances dictate. The response to therapy is slow, and the patient should be observed for several weeks. A second course of antimony is indicated if the parasites still are present in smears or biopsy material taken 4 weeks after the initial course. When relapses occur, they usually appear in 6 to 12 months, and are an indication for further treatment.

Leishmaniasis encountered in the Egyptian Sudan is resistant to antimony, and stilbamidine (℞ 62), when available, must be used. The dose of stilbamidine is 1 mg./Kg., body wt. freshly dissolved in 10 cc. of Water for Injection U.S.P., and administered I.V. every other day for 15 injections.

SCHISTOSOMIASIS

(Bilharziasis)

A parasitic disease with local and visceral manifestations due to infestation with blood flukes of the genus Schistosoma.

Etiology and Incidence

The *Schistosomas* belong to the class of trematodes or flatworms. The intermediate hosts are snails. Man becomes infested by bathing, wading, or other contact with the free-swimming cercariae forms of the parasite which penetrate the skin and are carried to the liver where they mature in 6 to 8 weeks. These adults then migrate to the tissues, particularly to the venules of the bladder or gut. Three species cause clinical disease: *S. haematobium,* with symptoms largely in the lower genitourinary system, though sometimes in lower colon and rectum; *S. mansoni* and *S. japonicum,* with disturbances in small intestine, colon, and rectum. Hepatic cirrhosis, splenomegaly and ascites may occur with all 3 types due to inflammation and fibrosis around eggs of the parasite in the liver. Disease due to *S. japonicum* is more severe and resistant to treatment.

The endemic distribution of the disease is as follows: *S. hematobium,* Africa, Syria, and Iraq; *S. mansoni,* Egypt, East and West Africa, West Indies, northern South America; *S. japonicum,* Japan, Formosa, central and south China, Philippines, and the Celebes.

Symptoms and Signs

Initially, there is a papular dermatitis where the cercariae have penetrated the skin. Development of the adult forms in the liver is characterized by fever, eosinophilia, and often urticaria. Later, their migration to the bladder, intestinal wall, and other tissues produces symptoms referable to these structures (cystitis, chronic dysentery). Hepatosplenomegaly is not uncommon.

Diagnosis

This is established by demonstrating eggs in the stool, urine, or biopsy of the rectum, bladder or other sites. Repeated stool examinations may be necessary and specialized concentration technics employed. Skin tests and complement fixation tests are useful, but antigens are not generally available.

Treatment

If significant constitutional symptoms or diarrhea is present, bed rest is indicated. Trivalent antimony compounds (tartar emetic, stibophen) are the only known effective agents; for maximum benefit they should be used as early in the disease as possible. Tartar emetic is more toxic but is superior to stibophen, particularly in cases due to *S. japonicum.* Stibophen should be used only when the recommended dose of tartar emetic cannot be tolerated.

Tartar emetic (℞ 66) (antimony and potassium tartrate), best tolerated 2 or 3 hours after a light meal, is administered I.V. (slowly), as a 1% solution, in an initial dose of 40 mg. (4 cc.). Since the solution is very irritating to the tissues and may cause sloughing, the needle should be wiped off with a sterile sponge and there should be no extravasation of fluid. The patient should remain recumbent for at least 1 hour after treatment. If tolerated, the dose is increased by 20 mg. (2 cc.) every 2 days to a maximum dose of 0.14 Gm. (14 cc.). This last dose is continued until a total of 18 injections has been given.

The toxic effects of tartar emetic include coughing immediately upon injection, which is not important; nausea, vomiting, stiffness of joints and muscles, sense of constriction of the chest, pain in the upper abdomen, bradycardia, dizziness, and collapse. If a toxic reaction other than coughing occurs during administration, the injection should be stopped at once. Severe coughing can be controlled or avoided by dividing future doses in half and giving the 2 portions 1 hour apart. Following any major toxic effect, the subsequent dose should be reduced or the administration of the drug temporarily or permanently discontinued, according to the circumstances.

Stibophen (Fuadin) (℞ 67) is given I.M. (slowly) as a 6.3% solution. The first 3 doses of 1.5 cc., 3.5 cc., and 5 cc., are given on successive days. Thereafter, 5 cc. is administered every 2 days for a total of 16 injections. When stibophen must be used in cases due to *S. japonicum,* the above doses should be increased to 2, 4, and 6 cc. for the first 3 days followed by 8 cc. daily until a total of 14 injections (100 cc.) are administered. The only common toxic symptoms are nausea and vomiting. Rarely, joint and muscle pains may appear. If severe toxic symptoms occur, the subsequent doses should be reduced and the administration temporarily or permanently discontinued, according to the circumstances.

Relapses are frequently encountered after 2 to 3 months. A second course of therapy is indicated, after a 3-month rest period, in all cases that continue to discharge ova or present clinical evidence of schistosomiasis.

TRYPANOSOMIASIS

A chronic systemic invasion of the human by flagellated protozoa of the genus Trypanosoma, *producing African sleeping sickness* (T. gambiense *and* T. rhodesiense) *and Chagas' disease, or South American trypanosomiasis* (T. cruzi). The African form is spread by the bite of the tsetse fly (genus *Glossina*), whereas Chagas' disease is transmitted by the bite of any one of several arthropods.

Symptoms, Signs, and Course

African trypanosomiasis is characterized by irregular fever, generalized lymphadenopathy (particularly of the posterior cervical chain), cutaneous eruptions, and areas of painful localized edema. Later, nervous symptoms predominate, such as tremors, headache, apathy, convulsions, and eventually coma and death. Rhodesian trypanosomiasis is more severe and fatal than Gambian trypanosomiasis. Chagas' disease is characterized in the early stages by fever, lymphadenopathy, hepatosplenomegaly, and enlargement of the thyroid. In the chronic phase, visceral involvement produces symptoms referable to the heart, endocrines (myxedema), and nervous system. The disease may be fatal in either stage.

Diagnosis

Diagnosis depends upon the demonstration of the trypanosomes. Early in the disease, they may be found in wet smears of the peripheral blood. Later, they can be identified in spinal fluid or in fluid aspirated from a lymph node or other tissue. In the viscera, *T. cruzi* may assume a leishmania-like appearance. Animal inoculation with tissue aspirates may demonstrate trypanosomes when other diagnostic methods fail.

Prophylaxis

This includes protection of healthy persons from the vector flies where abandonment or avoidance of endemic areas is not practicable. A single injection of 1 Gm. of suramin sodium (℞ 64) is said to confer reasonable protection for 2 to 3 months. Persons ill with trypanosomiasis should be treated in well screened buildings so as to prevent further fly infections.

Treatment

There is no effective treatment for Chagas' disease. Early cases of African trypanosomiasis (before C.N.S. involvement) should receive combined therapy with tryparsamide and suramin sodium. Tryparsamide (℞ 63) is given I.V. or I.M., dissolved in 10 cc. of distilled water, in 15 weekly injections of 1 to 1.5 Gm. initially, and then 2 to 3 Gm. (CAUTION! Optic atrophy). Suramin sodium (℞ 64) is administered I.V. or I.M., dissolved in 10 cc. of distilled water; the initial dose is 0.3 to 0.5 Gm. followed by 1 Gm. every 4 days, until a total of 10 Gm. has been given (CAUTION! Renal irritation). Recently, pentamidine (℞ 65), 0.1 Gm. I.V. daily for 10 to 20 days, has been used for early trypanosomiasis with encouraging results.

Tryparsamide (℞ 63) is the only drug of value in later stages, after the C.N.S. has become involved. The number of weekly injections should be increased to 20 and a second course should be given to all patients after a rest period of 1 to 3 months.

There are no dependable criteria of cure. The spinal fluid should be examined every 2 or 3 months for at least 2 years to detect evidence of early C.N.S. involvement.

YAWS

A chronic, nonvenereal, spirochetal (Treponema pertenue) *infection of tropical countries, which occurs almost exclusively in children*. It is spread through the discharges from the skin lesions, transmitted by body contact, clothing, or insects. Although *T. pertenue* and *T. pallidum* are morphologically similar, congenital yaws does not occur.

Symptoms and Signs

After an incubation period of 3 to 4 weeks, the "mother yaw" appears at the site of inoculation. This consists of one or more red papules which soon ulcerate. The secondary stage begins 6 to 12 weeks after the "mother yaw" and is characterized by a generalized eruption of similarly ulcerating papules, fever, headache, malaise, and arthralgia. These skin lesions may occur anywhere, but the mucous membranes are seldom involved. Spontaneous healing is usual but recurrences are frequent; some cases may develop tertiary destructive lesions in the nose (gangosa) or bone. The heart and C.N.S. are rarely involved and a fatal outcome is unusual.

Diagnosis

T. pertenue may be demonstrated in the lesions by darkfield examination of the discharge. The serologic tests for syphilis are positive. The patient's age and the usual absence of mucosal lesions are useful in differentiating yaws from syphilis.

Treatment

Primary and secondary yaws respond dramatically to therapy with arsenicals or penicillin. Three weekly I.V. injections of Mapharsen (℞ 83), 60 mg., or of neoarsphenamine (℞ 84), 0.6 to 0.9 Gm., usually are curative within a few weeks (the dose for children is reduced accordingly). The currently advocated total dose of penicillin is 1 to 3 million u., administered I.M. over a period of 6 to 8 days (℞ 28).

Tertiary yaws requires 8 or more such weekly injections of an arsenical. In addition, bismuth subsalicylate in oil (℞ 86), 0.2 Gm. weekly, is given I.M. during the first 4 weeks of arsenical therapy and for 8 weeks after its completion. The recommended dose of penicillin for tertiary yaws remains to be established, but prolonged, intensive treatment probably will be required.

The criteria for cure are the disappearance of the lesions and the development of seronegativity. The development of a negative serology is more rapid and more frequent after arsenical therapy than after penicillin. The persistence of a high titer (Kahn) or the recurrence of a positive serology is an indication for further treatment.

SYSTEMIC FUNGUS INFECTIONS

Infections caused by fungi pathogenic for man and involving various bodily systems or regions. (For fungus infections

of the skin, *see* DERMATOMYCOSES.) Fewer than 50 species of
all known fungi are capable of infecting man, and less than 12
produce fatal disease. Most pathogenic fungi attack only the
skin but others may infect any part of the body. Even the
more severe fungus infections usually develop slowly, requiring months or years to produce death. The tissues rarely react
violently, but antibody formation may be stimulated. Hypersensitivity to proteins and soluble carbohydrates of the fungi
may develop and result in asthma, hay fever, urticaria, and
other allergic manifestations. States of either hypersensitivity
or anergy, as in tuberculosis, are produced, which modify the
cytologic reactions of the tissues. The anatomic lesions of systemic fungus infections usually are granulomas in which necrosis
and pus formation may occur, producing ulcers, fistulas, and
draining sinuses. Fibrous tissue often develops in or about the
granulomatous masses.

General Therapeutic Principles

Local and systemic measures, when used selectively, may be
of benefit in the treatment of mycotic infections. These include the use of iodides, desensitization, incision or excision of
superficial lesions, chemotherapy, radiation therapy, and the
local application of fungicidal agents. In the treatment sections for the various clinically important mycoses discussed
below, specific indications and directions are given. However,
because of their relevance to the treatment of most mycotic
diseases, iodide and desensitization regimens will be considered here.

Iodides: These usually are taken orally, after meals, in the
form of a saturated solution of potassium iodide (R 48). Administration may be by the slow or the rapid method. (1)
Slow method: Starting with 3 drops in 30 cc. of water 3 times
daily, the dose is increased by 1 drop per day (not per dose)
until the patient is receiving 20 drops 3 times daily. The course
then is repeated without any interruption, again beginning with
3 drops 3 times daily and increasing it as above to 20 drops
3 times a day. Such courses should be repeated as long as
necessary, provided that no evidence of iodism is apparent. (2)
Rapid method: The initial dose is 5 drops in 30 cc. of water
3 times daily, subsequent doses being increased by 1 drop per
dose per day (i.e., an increase of 3 drops per day) to a maximum
dose of 20 drops 3 times daily. This dose may be continued
indefinitely, if still indicated and well tolerated, and may occasionally even be increased to as high as 100 drops 3 times
daily. Inhalations of ethyl iodide (R 50) or injections of
sodium iodide (R 49) may be administered to supplement or
replace potassium iodide.

Iodism may become apparent at any time, regardless of the
dose or duration of treatment, and is manifested by irritative
phenomena of the skin and mucous membranes such as rashes,

coryza, conjunctivitis, stomatitis, laryngitis, or bronchitis. Should any of these symptoms appear, the dose of iodide medication should be decreased or temporarily stopped. If iodides are discontinued, these manifestations usually disappear within a few days; after an interruption of dosage of about 2 weeks, the drug may be cautiously resumed at a lower dosage level. In some cases, it may be considered essential to continue iodide medication even in the presence of iodism; in such cases, iodide sensitivity may occasionally lessen or disappear despite continued therapy.

Desensitization: Stock or autogenous vaccines are widely used in the treatment of mycotic infections. Such vaccines are available from a variety of commercial sources, and complete details governing dosage and administration will be found in the printed instructions accompanying the package.

An intradermal skin test should be performed with 0.1 cc. of a 1:1,000 dilution of the vaccine and read after 24 and 48 hours. When this demonstrates that the patient has become sensitized to the products of the invading organism, desensitization may be beneficial. In some instances, desensitization therapy must precede the use of iodides. The initial strength of the vaccine to be used depends on the degree of sensitivity. If the skin test has produced an erythematous area of less than 2 cm. in diameter, the initial dilution should be 1:100; with a diameter of 2 to 3 cm., 1:1,000; with a diameter greater than 3 cm., 1:10,000. Injections are given subcut. 3 times a week. The initial dose is 0.1 cc., each subsequent dose being increased by 0.1 cc. over the preceding dose until undiluted vaccine is administered.

If a local or systemic reaction follows an injection (*see* Allergy), the next dose should be reduced to ½ the last tolerated amount, from which point therapy is resumed. Complete desensitization is seldom achieved and is not necessary. Some patients rapidly reach the limit of their tolerance, beyond which the size of the dose must not be increased.

ACTINOMYCOSIS
(Streptothricosis, Lumpy jaw)

A chronic, granulomatous disease, local or systemic, with a tendency to produce multiple draining sinuses.

Etiology, Incidence, and Pathology

Actinomycosis is caused by infection with *Actinomyces bovis* (the ray fungus), a gram-positive anaerobic organism that may be present naturally on the gums, tonsils, and teeth of persons with poor oral hygiene. The disease is seen most often in young adult males. (It also is widespread among cattle, being known as "lumpy jaw.") The most common portal of entry to the tissues is believed to be decayed teeth. Lung infection may result from inhaling contaminated dust of straw, hay, or grains, and primary alimentary tract infection from chewing and swallowing contaminated material.

The lesion is essentially an indurated area composed of multiple small communicating abscesses containing the parasites and surrounded by granulation tissue. It later breaks down and spreads by continuity. Mixed infection is common.

Symptoms and Signs

There are 4 clinical forms of actinomycosis. (1) **Cervicofacial** (about 50% of cases): Usually, a small, flat, hard swelling, with or without pain appears first under the mucous membrane of the mouth or throat or as a subperiosteal swelling of the jaw. Subsequently, areas of softening appear and develop into sinuses and fistulas that produce a characteristic discharge containing "sulfur granules." Other parts of the head (cheek, tongue, pharynx, salivary glands, cranial bones, meninges, or brain) may be affected primarily or by extension. (2) **Thoracic,** with involvement of the lungs resembling tuberculosis: Extensive invasion may occur before symptoms of chest pain, fever, and productive cough develop. Perforation of the chest wall, with chronic draining sinuses, may result. (3) **Abdominal,** in which the intestines (usually the cecum and appendix) and the peritoneum are infected: This form is characterized by pain, fever, vomiting, diarrhea, or constipation, and severe emaciation. First a mass of adhesions is formed, after which sinuses and fistulas develop in the abdominal wall. (4) **Generalized,** with secondary involvement of the skin, vertebral bodies, liver, kidney, ureter, and female pelvis: This may occur in untreated cases.

Diagnosis

This is based on clinical symptoms, X-ray findings, and demonstration of *A. bovis* in sputum, pus, or biopsy specimen. A dark reddish subcutaneous swelling in the submaxillary or supraclavicular region should suggest actinomycosis. Lung lesions must be distinguished from those of tuberculosis and from neoplasm. Lesions in the abdomen are most frequent in the ileocecal region and are difficult to diagnose except at exploratory laparotomy or when draining sinuses appear in the abdominal wall. Physical examination reveals a tender palpable mass suggestive of appendicitis, which must be differentiated. Secondarily infected nodules in any location may be massive and simulate malignant growths. Pyogenic infections, syphilis, blastomycosis, and sporotrichosis also resemble this disease. Diagnosis can be confirmed only by microscopic identification of the organism. In pus and tissue it appears as tangled masses of branched and unbranched wavy threads, or in the characteristic form of "sulfur granules." These are rounded or spherical granules, usually yellowish, but sometimes red or gray, varying in size up to 1 mm. in diameter. They consist of a central mass of tangled filaments, pus cells, and débris, with a midzone of interlacing filaments surrounded by an outer zone of radiating club-shaped hyaline and refractive bodies with central filaments. The true clubs are stainable with eosin. The organism can be cultured on veal infusion medium at 37° C. under anaerobic conditions.

Prognosis and Treatment

The disease persists for months or years. Prognosis depends largely upon early diagnosis and is thus most favorable in the cervicofacial form, which is most readily diagnosed, and progressively worse in the pulmonary, abdominal, and generalized forms.

Most cases of actinomycosis respond slowly to medical treatment and require extensive and repeated surgical operations, but some are cured after a few weeks with sulfadiazine (℞ 37) or penicillin (℞ 28). Potassium iodide (℞ 48), though not curative, is of considerable value as a supplement to chemotherapy in promoting resolution and absorption of granulomatous tissue. X-ray therapy is useful at times to stimulate the healing of indolent lesions, and may be repeated if necessary at intervals of 2 to 3 weeks. Aspiration is indicated for small abscesses and drainage for large ones. Iodide-iodine solution (℞ 52) may be used for irrigation; ulcers may be swabbed with this solution.

NOCARDIOSIS

A condition caused by the aerobic Actinomyces, Nocardia. This fungus is closely related to *Actinomyces bovis* but its organisms are agranular (not clubbed) and become arranged in loose clusters of interlacing, slender, branching threads rather than the true "sulfur granule" form. They are gram-positive and grow readily on 1% dextrose agar at 37° C. Some of the Nocardia are acid-fast and may be confused with tubercle bacilli. The Nocardia cause clinical syndromes which may be indistinguishable from actinomycosis. As in the case of actinomycosis, metastases may occur, with the production of abscesses in the skin, brain, or other organ, or a rapidly fatal pyemia may ensue. The lungs often are the original site of infection. Diagnosis is made by identification of the organism. Treatment is the same as for actinomycosis.

MADUROMYCOSIS
(Madura foot; Mycetoma)

A fungus infection of the feet, occasionally of the hands, characterized by chronicity, tumefaction, and multiple sinus formation, which progresses constantly until excision or amputation is performed or until the patient dies from secondary infection.

Etiology, Incidence, and Pathology

Members of the Actinomyces (Nocardia) group cause about 50% of the cases; the remainder are caused by different organisms distributed among 22 species of molds. The disease is most prevalent in the tropics and the Southern States but has occurred as far north as Canada. All races are susceptible and infection is usually contracted between the ages of 21 and 40.

The early lesion is granulomatous but is surrounded later by a dense fibrous capsule, intersected by fibrous trabeculae. In advanced cases, the foot is a mass of cystlike areas with draining sinuses and intercommunicating sinus tracts. Muscles, tendons, and bones are eventually destroyed. Characteristic granules found in the discharges are small (0.5 to 2 mm.), irregularly shaped, oval masses which may be yellow, red, white, or black. When caused by Actinomyces they resemble "sulfur granules."

Symptoms, Signs, and Diagnosis

The mode of onset varies. The first lesion may be a small papule, a deep-seated fixed nodule, a vesicle with an indurated base, or an abscess that ruptures and produces a fistula. The disease progresses slowly; 6 to 8 papules or abscesses may form in succession and then disappear. Months or years may pass before muscles, tendons, fascia, and bone are involved. The characteristic appearance is that of a swollen, deformed (club-shaped) foot with multiple fistulas discharging an "oily" or serosanguineous fluid containing the colored granules. General systemic symptoms are rare and the lesions usually are nontender until secondary infection becomes severe. The patient can walk until deformity or muscle wasting prevents it. The condition may exist, gradually progressing, for 10 to 15 years or more; the patient dies eventually from sepsis or intercurrent disease. The diagnosis is made from the clinical course and appearance and from demonstration of the characteristic colored granules in the exudate.

Treatment

Cases of Madura foot caused by Actinomyces may respond to sulfonamide therapy (℞ 37). No specific treatment is known at present for the other types. If response to medication is not prompt, the limb should be amputated to prevent death from the spread of the inevitable secondary bacterial infection.

PARA-ACTINOMYCOSIS

A somewhat varied group of conditions caused by a number of organisms belonging to the family Actinomycetaceae, *and including mycotic rat-bite fever, Haverhill fever, erysipeloid, Bacteroides infection, and botryomycosis.* The causative organisms have some superficial resemblance to Actinomyces and produce subacute and chronic infections which must be distinguished from cases of true actinomycosis.

Mycotic rat-bite fever is a systemic disease characterized by prolonged, irregular fever, arthritis and abscess formation that may resemble "true" rat-bite fever caused by *Spirillum minus*. *Streptobacillus moniliformis* (*Actinomyces muris*) has been isolated from the tissues of patients and is believed to be the causative organism. The condition rarely is fatal and usually subsides spontaneously. Arsenicals are not effective against the streptobacillus, but results with sulfonamides (℞ 37) and penicillin (℞ 28) are encouraging.

Haverhill fever (Erythema arthriticum epidemicum) is an acute infectious disease caused by *Streptobacillus moniliformis* (*Haverhillia multiformis*) and characterized by sudden onset, with malaise, headache, fever, a dusky maculopapular eruption usually limited to the extensor surfaces of the arms and legs, and polyarthritis with a duration of about 2 weeks. This disease was first reported during an epidemic in Haverhill, Mass., in 1926, and was believed to have been transmitted by unpasteurized milk. Sporadic cases following rat bites have been reported. Diagnosis is made by positive blood culture and agglutination test. The disease usually is self-limiting, the mortality is low, and treatment is symptomatic.

Erysipeloid is an infective dermatitis due to infection with *Erysipelothrix rhusiopathiae*, which causes swine erysipelas. It occurs frequently among farmers, veterinarians, and fishermen. Most of the infections remain localized on the hand, but they may appear on any part of the body and can lead to septicemia. The organism has been reported as moderately susceptible to penicillin (℞ 28) and sulfonamide (℞ 37) therapy.

Bacteroides infection: *Bacteroides necrophorus* causes necrotizing infections in animals. Human cases of meningitis, pulmonary abscess, osteomyelitis, and septicemia have been reported. The organism has been isolated in a number of cases of ulcerative colitis.

Botryomycosis (Staphylococcal actinophytosis) is characterized by chronic granulomatous lesions with the formation of definite granules resembling the "sulfur granules" of actinomycosis. However, the organisms grow as staphylococci when cultured. Treatment with penicillin (℞ 28) and establishment of drainage should suffice.

HISTOPLASMOSIS

A severe systemic fungus infection of the reticulo-endothelial system, characterized by ulcerations of the oropharynx and gastrointestinal tract, and commonly accompanied by hepatomegaly, splenomegaly, and lymphadenopathy. The severe form usually is fatal, but a benign form, affecting many thousands of persons, produces pulmonary calcifications without symptoms.

Etiology and Incidence

The infection is caused by *Histoplasma capsulatum,* a small oval budding cell 1 to 5 μ in diameter, not yet identified in nature, but which has been found in mice, rats, dogs, rabbits, and horses. The mode of transmission is unknown.

The severe form, reported in about 100 instances, mainly in the United States, also occurs in most parts of the world. Young children of both sexes are highly susceptible. After the age of 12, males contract the disease 7 times as frequently as females.

Recent chest X-ray surveys have demonstrated, in thousands of persons, symptomless, nontuberculous, calcified pulmonary lesions. Skin reactions to histoplasmin in a high percentage of these individuals suggest a benign form of histoplasmosis, or infection by some antigenically related fungus. This benign form exists throughout the United States but the highest incidence is among those living in damp, humid, rural areas, especially on the western Appalachian slope and the bordering areas west of the Mississippi and north of the Ohio rivers.

Symptoms and Signs

Evidence of infection varies according to the portal of entry, site of involvement, extent of infection, and age of the patient. Granulomatous gray or white nodules, or ulcerated areas (deep, punched-out ulcers with sharp edges), occurring on the ear, nose, lip, pharynx, or larynx are the first evidence of disease in about 30% of cases. Ulcers of the extremities may be seen. In all cases, irregular pyrexia, emaciation, leukopenia, and anemia appear and become progressively worse. Lymphadenopathy, sometimes localized to the cervical nodes, but more often generalized, is common. Eventually, splenomegaly and hepatomegaly develop. Intestinal ulceration (nausea, vomiting, diarrhea, melena) may be evident, and the bone marrow may be invaded. Primary lung involvement in the severe form of histoplasmosis is not usual, but late invasion does occur and is manifested by cough and sputum production. With children, the onset is insidious, but progression is generally more rapid. Extensive gastrointestinal ulceration is common and digestive disturbances are prominent. Lymph node involvement is less than in adults, but splenomegaly and hepatomegaly may be massive.

The benign form, usually not discovered except as a result of tuberculosis surveys, is symptomless. Chest X-rays reveal varied types of calcified pulmonary lesions, often indistinguishable from healed tuberculous lesions.

Diagnosis

Severe histoplasmosis is an insidious progressive condition, not likely to be confused with acute infectious diseases. Confusion is possible, however, with other granulomatous diseases, neoplasms, dysentery, ulcerative colitis, and that group characterized by endothelial involvement as well as the lymphadenopathies, hepatomegalies, and splenomegalies. Progressively debilitating diseases of this nature call for complete diagnostic studies and possible histoplasmosis must always be considered. Demonstration of *H. capsulatum* by culture establishes the diagnosis. The organism exists intracellularly only, producing caseation and necrosis, and is not usually found in the sputum, exudates, or feces. Specimens for culture may be obtained from lymph nodes, bone marrow, nodular lesions, or the granulomatous tissue surrounding necrotic or ulcerated areas. Characteristic growth occurs readily in 10 to 20 days on blood agar. In tissue, the organisms are seen within the endothelial cells, monocytes, and, occasionally, neutrophiles. Here they resemble and may be confused with the Donovan bodies of leishmaniasis. Skin reactions to histoplasmin are of little diagnostic value, since anergy may provide false negatives. The benign form is diagnosed by demonstrating pulmonary calcifications and a positive skin reaction to histoplasmin in the absence of bacteriologic evidence of tuberculosis.

Prognosis and Treatment

For children, the disease usually is fatal in a few weeks or several months. In adults with acute histoplasmosis the average duration of life is 5 months, but some with a less acute type may live up to 2 years or more. The benign form is apparently nonprogressive.

Since no specific treatment is known, symptomatic therapy is all that can be given. Radium has been used successfully for a few small lesions localized in the mouth.

COCCIDIOIDOMYCOSIS

(Coccidioidal granuloma, Valley fever, Desert rheumatism, San Joaquin fever, Posada-Wernicke's disease)

A highly infectious fungus disease which occurs in two forms, primary and progressive. The **primary** form usually is an acute, benign, self-limiting, respiratory disease. The **progressive** form is a chronic, malignant, often fatal infection involving cutaneous, subcutaneous, visceral, and osseous tissues.

Etiology and Incidence

The disease is caused by *Coccidioides immitis* and is most prevalent in the interior valleys of California. Since the infection may be dust-borne, individuals may possibly contract the disease by merely traveling through endemic areas, but not develop manifestations until they are in another locality. It occurs most frequently between the ages of 25 and 55, but has been reported in all age groups. Men are infected more often than women. Of those afflicted, about 12 to 20% of Negroes, Mexicans, and Filipinos, but only 1% of Caucasians, will develop the progressive form of the disease.

Pathology

The basic pathology is a granulomatous process, acute, subacute, or chronic in nature, accompanied by varying degrees of fibrosis. Central necrosis of the lesions may occur. Cavity formation or pleurisy with effusion may appear in chronic lung infection. The organisms are surrounded by lymphocytes, plasma cells, epithelioid, and giant cells.

Symptoms and Signs

Primary pulmonary coccidioidomycosis, the most common form, may give no clinical symptoms, or it may simulate a mild upper respiratory infection or produce the clinical appearance of pneumonia or acute bronchitis, occasionally with pleural effusion. Symptoms, when present, consist of fever, cough, chest pain, chills, sputum, sore throat, and hemoptysis (in that order of frequency). Physical signs may be absent or there may be occasional scattered rales and areas of dullness to percussion. Arthralgia and skin lesions resembling erythema nodosum, erythema multiforme, or a morbilliform rash on the trunk and lower extremities occasionally develop 1 to 2 weeks after onset. Leukocytosis and elevated E.S.R. usually are present. In a series of cases, X-ray findings were negative in approximately 4%, revealed fan-shaped densities extending from the hilar nodes in 39%, hilar lymph nodes without parenchymatous lesions in 24%, peripheral and sublobular infiltrations in upper and lower lobes in 26%, thin-walled pulmonary cavities in 4%, and massive pleural effusion in 3%.

A primary cutaneous (nonpulmonary) form may occur, characterized by small abscess formation and secondary lymph node involvement. A scrofulodermic type is occasionally reported.

Progressive coccidioidomycosis usually develops from the primary form and evidence of dissemination may appear a few weeks or months after the initial infection. Occasionally, it occurs several years after apparent recovery. The symptoms of progressive coccidioidomycosis are continuous low grade fever, severe anorexia, and rapid loss of strength and weight. In the pulmonary type, progressive cyanosis and dyspnea occur. Mucopurulent and occasionally bloody sputum is produced. The bones, joints, skin, viscera, brain, and meninges may be invaded as the disease progresses.

Diagnosis

Coccidioidomycosis should be suspected in every patient with an obscure illness who has been in an endemic area. Diagnosis is established by finding the characteristic spherules of *C. immitis* in sputum, gastric washings, pleural or spinal fluid, pus from abscesses, exudates from skin lesions, or in biopsy specimens. In the tissues, the organisms appear as spherules, thick-walled, nonbudding structures, 20 to 80 μ in diameter. In cultures (10 to 20 days on 1% dextrose agar at room temperature) they appear as thick-walled, rectangular arthrospores, 2.5 to 3 μ by 3 to 4 μ in size.

Sensitivity to coccidioidin develops and will produce a skin reaction 10 to 21 days after infection; this sensitivity apparently persists for life except in terminal stages of the illness, when anergy appears. Precipitins and complement-fixed antibodies are regularly present in the progressive form and in the more severe primary forms, but in the latter they disappear on recovery. The progressive form is suspected when, by X-ray, lesions are found to persist more than 5 or 6 weeks, or if new infiltrations are discovered.

Prognosis

This is excellent for primary pulmonary coccidioidomycosis; good for primary cutaneous and glandular types; but poor for the progressive type, in which the mortality rate is 55 to 60%.

Treatment

There is no specific treatment for the primary disease. The patient should be kept in bed until the temperature, leukocyte count, sedimentation rate, X-ray findings, and physical signs are normal or show progressive improvement. In about 1% of cases, thin-walled cavities persist in the lungs for months or years. Cavitation accompanied by sputum or hemoptysis may be eliminated by lobectomy or pneumonectomy.

No treatment is known for progressive coccidioidomycosis. Supportive measures, such as bed rest, nursing care, high vitamin intake, maintenance of fluid and salt balance, and correction of anorexia, hypoproteinemia, anemia, intercurrent infection, cardiac failure, and anoxia are indicated. Desensitization with coccidioidin should be attempted when hypersensitivity is present (see General Therapeutic Principles, above).

CONIDIOSPOROSIS

A peculiar type of pneumonitis, presumably allergic, which occurs in laborers in the northern forests who are repeatedly exposed to the inhalation of spores of Conidiosporium corticale *growing on the inner bark of maple logs.* The patients recover without treatment when removed from contact with the spores.

NORTH AMERICAN BLASTOMYCOSIS

(Gilchrist's disease)

A chronic, granulomatous fungus disease of the skin or lungs, capable of producing systemic involvement which is fatal.

Etiology and Incidence

The disease is caused by *Blastomyces dermatitidis,* a yeast-like fungus whose source in nature and means of transmission are unknown. Several hundred cases have been reported in the United States, chiefly from the Southeastern States and the Mississippi Valley. Other cases have occurred in Canada, Europe, Cuba, Puerto Rico, and South America. North American blastomycosis occurs most frequently in adults between the ages of 20 and 40, but can attack any age group. Males are affected 9 times as often as females.

Clinical Course

Cutaneous form: Skin lesions begin superficially on exposed surfaces as papules or papulopustules which spread slowly. Miliary abscesses containing pus and varying in size from pin point to 1 mm. in diameter develop on the advancing borders. Irregular, wartlike papillae form on the surfaces. As the lesions enlarge, central healing occurs, producing flat scars or, if bacterial infection is present, ulcerations. A fully developed individual lesion appears as an elevated verrucous patch with an abruptly sloping, purplish red, abscess-studded border, and may be 2 cm. or more in diameter. These are painless and without systemic effect. The cutaneous form of North American blastomycosis may persist for 8 to 10 years and unless treated successfully, pulmonary or systemic spread occurs. Occasionally, the cutaneous form may be secondary to the pulmonary form of the disease.

Pulmonary form: This may be primary or secondary. Primary pulmonary blastomycosis may involve the mediastinal and peribronchial lymph nodes or, more commonly, may form patches of bronchopneumonia which appear, on X-ray examination, to fan out from the hilum in the same manner as neoplastic growths. Secondary or hematogenous involvement produces widespread miliary type lesions throughout the lungs. With either type the onset usually is insidious and the first symptoms are a dry hacking cough, chest pain, fever (low grade), and dyspnea. Purulent sputum, often blood streaked, appears weeks or months later. Eventually, early symptoms become intensified, the patient loses weight, and death, usually the result of generalized spread, occurs within 1 to 3 years.

Systemic form: In this type, lungs (90% of cases), bones (especially vertebrae and ribs), liver, spleen, kidneys, or the C.N.S. are invaded and, in the seriously advanced cases, lesions are found in most tissues. Symptoms vary according to the site and extent of involvement. Bone lesions are painful, C.N.S. lesions cause paralyses, subcutaneous lesions ulcerate and resemble those of the primary cutaneous form. Once the disease becomes generalized, death is inevitable in a relatively short time (months to a year).

Diagnosis

Although comparatively rare, blastomycosis must be considered whenever a chronic progressive disease of doubtful origin is encountered. Clinically, the cutaneous, pulmonary, or systemic lesions and manifestations may be indistinguishable from those produced by other granulomatous or neoplastic diseases, e.g., tuberculosis, syphilis, sporotrichosis, coccidioidomycosis, and bronchogenic carcinoma.

A skin test, using stock or autogenous vaccine, is an aid in differentiation, since 50 to 75% of patients develop sensitivity to the organism and its by-products. However, the diagnosis can be established by identifying *B. dermatitidis* in pus, sputum, or tissue specimens. The organism appears as a thick-walled rounded body about 12 μ in diameter, occurs singly or in pairs, and budding forms are common. It grows readily in 2 to 3 weeks when cultured on Sabouraud's medium at room temperature, or on blood agar at 37° C.

Treatment

General: Supportive measures such as vitamin supplements, insurance of proper diet and rest, and avoidance of overexertion are important in the treatment of any phase of North American blastomycosis. Parenteral feeding, transfusions, and bed rest may be necessary in the advanced pulmonary form or the systemic type of the disease. Persistent treatment is indicated and may have to be continued for months, interrupted only by occasional rest periods of 1 or 2 weeks' duration.

Specific: Potassium iodide (℞ 48) by mouth is the drug of choice at present, given preferably by the slow method, but sodium iodide (℞ 49) I.V., or ethyl iodide (℞ 50) by inhalation, may be used when necessary. (CAUTION! Stop treatment at the first sign of iodism; resume at lower dosage after 1 to 2 weeks.) Since the majority of patients are sensitized to the organism or its by-products, desensitization should be begun about 2 weeks before other treatment is started (*see* General Therapeutic Principles, above). For this purpose a stock or autogenous vaccine of heat-killed *B. dermatitidis* is used (for technic *see* ALLERGY). This usually will prevent exacerbation of symptoms and the occasional dissemination of disease (therapeutic paradox) which often follows the administration of iodides.

Local: Excision of skin lesions is contraindicated, but surgical incision and drainage is necessary whenever indicated. Hot compresses, sulfonamide ointment (℞ 46), and Sopronol solution (℞ 55) used alternately have been helpful in treating skin lesions but the hazards of topical application of the sulfonamides must be considered. The judicious use of X-ray therapy in combination with iodide administration has been effective in the cutaneous form of the disease and in early cases of the pulmonary form. For advanced cases it may be palliative. Penicillin, streptomycin, or the sulfonamides are indicated whenever other susceptible organisms invade the lesions of blastomycosis.

SOUTH AMERICAN BLASTOMYCOSIS

(Paracoccidioidal granuloma, Lutz-Splendore-Almeida disease)

A severe, usually fatal, granulomatous and ulcerating fungus disease of the skin, mucous membranes, lymph nodes and internal organs.

Etiology and Incidence

The causative organism, *Blastomyces brasiliensis* (*Paracoccidioides brasiliensis*), grows on the same media and under the same conditions as the North American species, *B. dermatitidis*, but is larger (diameter 60 μ). In the tissues, it is characterized by the development of multiple small buds. The disease is limited to South America and occurs most frequently in agricultural workers in the coffee growing regions of Brazil.

The typical lesion is a slowly extending ulcer with a granular base presenting numerous pinpoint yellowish white areas in which the fungus is abundant. Regional lymph nodes enlarge conspicuously and later become necrotic and discharge through the skin.

Clinical Manifestations

There are 4 clinical forms, determined by the portal of entry of the organism: (1) **Cutaneous,** occurring most often on the face and frequently at the mucocutaneous borders of the nose and mouth. (2) **Lymphatic,** which affects the lymph nodes, usually those of the neck, supraclavicular or axillary regions, and is characterized by massive painless enlargement. Prior to the formation of abscesses and draining sinuses, it resembles Hodgkin's disease. (3) **Visceral,** usually beginning in the cecal region and producing enlargement of the liver, spleen, and abdominal lymph nodes. Abdominal pain may be the first symptom. Enlargement of the viscera is evident on palpation. Primary infection of the lungs is unusual but secondary infection occurs in 20% of the visceral cases. (4) **A mixed** type in which cutaneous, lymphatic, and visceral lesions are present simultaneously.

Diagnosis and Treatment

The diagnosis is established by identifying *B. brasiliensis* in pus or biopsy material or in cultures. Iodides are of little or no value in treatment. Recently, temporary improvement has been reported after the administration of sulfapyridine (℞ 40) or sulfadiazine (℞ 37) for 2 to 4 months, but the patients frequently suffer relapse and die within 3 to 6 months. Desensitization (*see* General Therapeutic Principles, above) followed after 2 weeks by iodides (℞ 48, 49, 50), as in the North American variety, has been suggested as a supplement to sulfonamide therapy.

CRYPTOCOCCOSIS

(European blastomycosis, Torulosis, Busse-Buschke's disease)

A chronic, frequently fatal, fungus infection which usually involves the meninges and C.N.S., but may invade the lungs, viscera, skin, or joints.

Etiology, Incidence, and Pathology

Cryptococcus neoformans (*Torula histolytica*) is the causative organism. Distribution is world-wide. In the United States, most of the cases occur in the East and in a southern zone extending from Florida to California. Adults between 40 and 60 are most frequently affected, and males twice as often as females.

C.N.S. lesions may appear as diffuse meningitis, granulomas of the meninges, endarteritis, infarcts, areas of softening, increase in neuroglia, or extensive destruction of nerve tissue. Cutaneous lesions appear as acneform pustules or granulomatous ulcers. Subcutaneous and visceral lesions are deep nodules or tumor-like masses filled with gelatinous material. Evidence of acute inflammation is slight or absent, but infiltration by lymphocytes, fibroblasts, plasma, "foam," and giant cells, is seen.

Symptoms and Signs

Four clinical types occur: (1) C.N.S. cryptococcosis, the most frequent, usually begins as a chronic, gradually progressive meningitis. Frontal headaches, dizziness, vertigo, stiffness and pain in the back, depression, disorientation, and apathy or restlessness, irritability, and delirium develop. Amblyopia, strabismus, nystagmus, ptosis, diplopia, ataxia, or hemiplegia may occur. Retinitis and papilledema are frequent. Stiff neck, positive Kernig's and Brudzinski's signs are found. No evidence of acute infection is apparent, blood pressure is normal, the temperature rarely is above 101° F. and the pulse rate seldom exceeds 100. The spinal fluid pressure is increased and a count usually reveals 200 to 800 cells, chiefly monocytes. The patient loses weight and strength, gradually sinks into coma, and dies of respiratory failure. (2) Pulmonary cryptococcosis is subacute, with low grade fever and a mild cough which produces a small amount of sputum, occasionally blood-streaked. A diffuse miliary invasion resembling tuberculosis or a localized lesion in the lungs simulating neoplasm may develop. Involvement of the mediastinum and cavity formation are rare. The pulmonary infection usually spreads to a generalized type ultimately involving the C.N.S. Frequently a mild but definite respiratory cryptococcosis precedes the meningitic form by weeks or months. (3) A cutaneous infection is characterized by scattered acneform pustules or granulomatous ulcers with multiple sinuses. (4) Subcutaneous nodules or abscesses which resemble myxomatous tumors may be produced. Invasion of the liver, spleen, and joints (usually the knees) occurs, but rarely.

Diagnosis

Diagnosis is established by finding the budding, yeastlike cryptococcus, surrounded by a large gelatinous capsule, in sputum, pus, spinal fluid, or other exudates. The capsule can be readily demonstrated by adding the sediment from centrifuged spinal fluid to a drop of India ink and examining the specimen under oil immersion. Culture requires 10 to 20 days.

Prognosis and Treatment

The prognosis is poor in all forms of this disease, and practically hopeless in cerebral and meningeal cases. Until recently, C.N.S. involvement has resulted in death within 3 to 6 months.

A few cases have apparently responded to prolonged treatment with sulfadiazine (R 37). Iodides (R 48, 49, 50), may be used cautiously with sulfadiazine, but desensitization of sensitive patients should be attempted before iodides are started (*see* General Therapeutic Principles, above). Treatment is otherwise symptomatic.

SPOROTRICHOSIS

A chronic granulomatous fungus infection, characterized by the formation of nodules, ulcers, and abscesses, usually confined to the skin and superficial lymph nodes.

Etiology and Incidence

The infecting agent is *Sporotrichum schenckii,* a saprophyte or parasite of plants. Farmers, laborers, and horticulturists—especially those who handle barberry bushes—are most often infected. Large numbers of miners also have been infected from contact with mud and timbers in the mines.

Symptoms and Signs

Seven clinical types are described: (1) **Lymphatic,** by far the most common form, begins 20 to 90 days after inoculation, as a hard, elastic, movable, nontender, spherical nodule on a finger, hand, arm, foot, or leg. It increases in size, becomes adherent, turns pink, then purple, and soon becomes black and necrotic, forming an ulcer. Within a few days or weeks subcutaneous nodules develop along the course of the lymphatic vessels that drain the area. These in turn become pink and eventually ulcerate and discharge thin pus. A single line or chain of ulcerating nodules is characteristic of sporotrichosis. The affected vessel becomes thickened and can be palpated as a hard cord. The infection may spread to the larger nodes in the axillas or groin. (2) **Disseminated form:** Hard subcutaneous nodules that rarely ulcerate are scattered over the body. There may be no primary lesion. The patient becomes acutely ill, cachectic, and usually dies in a few weeks or months. (3) **Epidermal:** Polymorphous lesions, varying from infiltrated plaques to verrucous or papillomatous weeping and fungating areas, appear on the skin, usually that of the nose, face, arms, and legs. (4) **Mucosal:** Lesions may be primary, or secondary to the disseminated form. They develop on the mucous membrane of the nose, mouth or pharynx and appear as erythematous, ulcerative, suppurating vegetative or papillomatous areas. (5) **Skeletal:** This is rare but may result from dissemination. (6) **Visceral:** Rare, but cases of pyelonephritis, mastitis, epididymitis, and orchitis have been reported. Primary lung infection is extremely unusual. (7) **Pseudoneoplastic:** Scattered, nonulcerating granulomas occur.

Diagnosis

Identification of *S. schenckii* is best made by culturing infected material or by inoculating laboratory animals (rat, mouse, or guinea pig), since this organism is rarely demonstrable in material from human lesions. The disease must be differentiated from other fungus infections and from tuberculosis, leprosy, syphilis, glanders, and tularemia.

Prognosis and Treatment

The disease usually responds to treatment, is rarely fatal, except for the fulminating disseminated form (seldom seen in the United States), but may last for months or years. Potassium iodide by mouth (℞ 48) is practically specific. Dosage should be massive (rapid method) and treatment continued for 4 to 6 weeks after apparent healing. An occasional case may require desensitization therapy (*see* General Therapeutic Principles, above). Ulcerated lesions may be painted with tincture of iodine (℞ 58) and dressed with an iodide-iodine solution (℞ 52). Abscesses into which the drug cannot penetrate should be aspirated and injected with a 1% solution of potassium iodide (℞ 51). Surgery is contraindicated.

MONILIASIS

An acute or subacute infection of the skin or mucous membranes by a yeastlike fungus, which may be localized on the skin, nails, mouth, vagina, bronchi, or lungs. Occasionally, it invades the blood stream, endocardium, or meninges.

Etiology and Incidence

The infections are caused chiefly by *Candida albicans,* but other species of Candida are sometimes responsible. The incidence of moniliasis is universal, and actual epidemics have occurred. Infants, debilitated adults, and persons with ill-fitting dentures are likely to have oral thrush. Adults whose work leads to maceration of the skin through frequent soaking in soap and water (e.g., housewives, waiters, bakers) are most apt to develop infection of the hands. Excessive sweating (*see* HYPERHIDROSIS) also favors skin infection, and pregnancy and diabetes are predisposing factors in vaginal infections.

Symptoms and Signs

Symptoms of moniliasis vary according to the site of infection. Oral infections take the form of thrush and show the typical creamy white patches. They occur as large single or small multiple plaques which leave a bright red, moist base on removal. Onychia and paronychia begin as painful reddened swellings without pus formation. Eventually, the nails become hardened, thickened and grooved, and often brownish colored. Intertrigo occurs in the axillas, inframammary areas, umbilicus, gluteal folds, and groin, and appears as well marginated, erythematous, exudative patches of varying size and shape which may be rimmed by vesicles and small pustules. Perianal moniliasis produces pruritus ani (q.v.) of the white macerative type. Severe generalized cutaneous moniliasis may have the appearance of eczematoid lesions. Mycotic vulvovaginitis (q.v.) is relatively common and is characterized by discharge, inflammation of the vaginal wall, and white scattered or confluent patches, resembling thrush, on the labia, vagina, and cervix. Bronchopulmonary moniliasis in the usual mild form produces malaise, cough, mucoid sputum, and a slight rise of temperature. Severe infection may cause physical signs of a confluent or lobar pneumonia. Fatal cases of septicemia, endocarditis, and meningitis due to *C. albicans* have been reported.

Diagnosis

The organism may be present as a saprophyte or a secondary invader in other conditions. Diagnosis of primary moniliasis is made by identifying *C. albicans* in material from the lesions, by the characteristic clinical manifestations, response to treatment, and exclusion of other or underlying diseases as a cause.

Prognosis and Treatment

Lesions generally respond readily to treatment, but recurrence is frequent, especially in individuals who have become hypersensitive to the organism. Severe pulmonary infections may cause death.

Predisposing causes, including underlying diseases, should be controlled, and desensitization (*see* General Therapeutic Principles, above) carried out in patients with positive skin tests. Acute oral lesions usually respond readily to simple alkaline mouthwashes (℞ 110), or to dilute solutions of gentian violet (℞ 53). Chronic cases may clear under simple local treatment after desensitization. Vaginitis may respond to topical application of 1% gentian violet (℞ 53) or application of a sodium propionate ointment (℞ 60) (*see* VAGINAL MYCOSIS). Bronchopulmonary forms usually are amenable to iodide therapy (℞ 48, 49, 50), following desensitization where necessary (*see* General Therapeutic Principles, above). Gentian violet I.V. (℞ 54) has produced some dramatic cures of pulmonary infections. Lesions of the skin should be treated with soaks of potassium permanganate, 1:4,000, 3 times daily (℞ 57), followed by the application of a 1% solution of gentian violet (℞ 53), or with a 5% ammoniated mercury ointment (℞ 59).

GEOTRICHOSIS

A disease caused by one or more species of Geotrichum, with lesions of the mucous membranes resembling thrush, and infections of the bronchi and lungs which may be mistaken for moniliasis, blastomycosis, or coccidioidomycosis. The organism appears to be endogenous.

The most frequent site of geotrichosis is in the bronchi. The symptoms are chronic cough, with a gelatinous type of sputum occasionally blood streaked. Coarse or medium rales are heard, chiefly at the base of the lungs. There is little or no fever, and the patient does not seem seriously ill. Pulmonary geotrichosis may be mistaken for tuberculosis: temperature and rates of pulse and respiration are increased; the blood shows leukocytosis, with increased polymorphonuclears. Coughing produces a mucopurulent sputum. Fine to medium rales are heard. Thin-walled cavities may be formed in the lungs.

Diagnosis is made by culture of oral mucus or sputum. There is a budding form of Geotrichum similar to that of Blastomyces, but it is always accompanied by the rectangular conidia which are characteristic of Geotrichum.

Prognosis and Treatment

The prognosis is good in all forms of geotrichosis under proper treatment. The bronchial form is treated with potassium iodide (℞ 48) by the rapid method, as described for North American blastomycosis (q.v.). The pulmonary form requires the same supportive measures as are employed for tuberculosis. Iodides may be given if, after careful tests, the possibility of tuberculous infection is ruled out. Geotrichum often is a secondary invader in tuberculosis. The oral lesions are treated with gentian violet, given in the same way as for those of moniliasis (q.v.).

RHINOSPORIDIOSIS

A fungus disease caused by Rhinosporidium seeberi, which produces large friable, sessile or pedunculated polyps of the mucous membranes of the nose, eyes, larynx, and vagina, and occasionally on the skin, especially of the ears and penis. The disease is seen most often in boys and young men, who apparently contract it by swimming in stagnant water. It is most prevalent in India and Ceylon but cases have been reported in the United States. The organism has not been isolated on artificial media, but the diagnosis is established by finding the ovoid spores (7 to 9 μ) in smears, or by demonstration in biopsy material of the characteristic spore-filled sporangia (200 to 300 μ).

Prognosis and Treatment

Rhinosporidiosis is rarely fatal, but the patient may die of secondary infections. Complete surgical removal of the early lesions effects a cure. The advanced cases are improved but not cured by treatment with a pentavalent antimony compound, Neostibosan (℞ 61).

CHROMOBLASTOMYCOSIS
(Chromomycosis, Verrucous dermatitis)

A fungus infection characterized by warty cutaneous nodules which develop slowly to form large papillomatous vegetations having a tendency to ulcerate. Identical clinical lesions are produced by the 3 etiologic agents: *Hormodendrum pedrosoi*, *H. compactum* and *Phialophora verrucosa*. The disease occurs throughout the world but most frequently in the tropics. It is prevalent between the ages of 30 and 50, all races are susceptible and males are infected 34 times as frequently as females.

Symptoms, Signs, and Diagnosis

The infection, usually unilateral, begins most frequently on the feet and legs, but sometimes on other exposed parts, especially where the skin is broken. The early lesion is a small, itching papule which extends out from the center and resembles ringworm. The patch is dull red or violaceous in color, sharply demarcated, and has an indurated base. New crops may appear after several weeks or months along the paths of lymphatic drainage. These areas project 1 or 2 mm. above the skin, and hard, dull red or grayish nodules may develop in the center, producing a cauliflower appearance. The infected extremities gradually become covered with these lesions. Lymphatics may be blocked, itching may or may not be present, and secondary infection may occur with resulting ulceration. Four to 15 years may elapse before the whole extremity is involved.

In late cases, diagnosis is made from the clinical appearance. Early lesions may be mistaken for dermatophytoses, and must be differentiated by finding the characteristic dark-brown septate bodies in pus or biopsy specimens.

Prognosis and Treatment

The disease is rarely if ever fatal, but is not curable except in the earliest forms. Complete surgical excision is the treatment of choice for the early lesions. Iodides (℞ 48) improve chronic cases. Iontophoresis with a 1% solution of copper sulfate (℞ 56) sometimes reduces the size of the lesions.

ASPERGILLOSIS, PENICILLOSIS, AND MUCORMYCOSIS

The molds (*Aspergillum, Penicillium,* and *Mucor*) frequently produce infections in the external ear. Occasionally, granulomatous lesions appear in the skin, in the nasal sinuses, orbit, bronchi, lungs or other internal organs. Squab feeders, fur cleaners and agricultural workers who are exposed to clouds of spores may become infected.

27

Prognosis and Treatment

The prognosis is good, except for the pulmonary and generalized infections, which are frequently fatal. Iodides are used for treatment (R 48, 49, 50), but hypersensitive patients should first be desensitized (*see* General Therapeutic Principles, above).

TRICHINOSIS

(Trichiniasis)

A parasitic disease characterized by gastrointestinal symptoms, muscular pains, and fever.

Etiology, Pathogenesis, and Epidemiology

The roundworm *Trichinella spiralis* is the causative parasite. Human infection occurs when raw or inadequately cooked pork (rarely, bear meat) containing encysted larvae is ingested. The cyst wall is digested in the stomach or duodenum and the larvae thus liberated attach themselves to the mucosa of the duodenum and jejunum. Within 3 or 4 days, the larvae mature sexually and mate, following which the smaller sized male (1.5 mm.) dies. The female (3 mm.) penetrates the intestinal mucosa and discharges living larvae by the 7th day. The minute larvae (0.1 mm.) are carried by the lymphatic and portal circulation to the systemic blood stream and thence to the various tissues and organs. Only those larvae that reach striated muscle survive; they cause a myositis, which is followed by calcification of the cyst wall of the larvae. Elsewhere the larvae are destroyed by an intense local inflammatory reaction. The diaphragm, tongue, pectoral and intercostal muscles are especially involved. Within the muscles, the larvae penetrate individual fibers and grow to 1 mm. in length. They then coil up and become encysted by the end of the 3rd month, in which state they may remain viable for several years. In animals, these encysted larvae constitute the source of infection for the next host. Early in the disease, some larvae may enter the bowel lumen and be eliminated. Later, as the adult female burrows deeper into the intestinal mucosa, few larvae fail to enter the circulation. A single adult female lives for 4 to 5 weeks, and may produce more than 1,000 larvae. Following death, the adult worms are digested and only rarely are found in the stool.

The disease is of world-wide distribution. About 17% of the adult population in the United States is said to be infected. Many cases remain asymptomatic and are discovered only at autopsy by the presence of small calcifications in the muscles.

Symptoms and Signs

The severity of symptoms depends upon the number of parasites ingested. In heavy infections there may be three clinical phases: At the stage of **intestinal invasion** (about the 1st week after ingestion), there may be nausea, vomiting, and diarrhea, with mild abdominal pain and slight fever. A maculopapular eruption may appear on the skin. **Systemic invasion** (beginning about the 10th to 22nd day) is characterized by muscular pains, edema, fever and eosinophilia. The muscles are tender, frequently swollen, tense, and painful on movement. These symptoms are especially pronounced in the muscles of respiration, speech, mastication, and swallowing. Severe dyspnea may result, sometimes causing death. Edema of the face, which causes pain on moving the eyes, is an early symptom; later it may extend to the abdomen and extremities. Fever usually is remittent, rising to 102° F. or higher, remaining elevated for 7 to 10 days, and then falling by lysis. In mild cases, fever may be absent. Eosinophilia may not appear until the 6th week but is usually present during the 2nd week. It increases rapidly, reaches its height (20 to 40% or more) in the 3rd or 4th week, and then gradually declines. It may be obscured by secondary bacterial infection. As the widely disseminated larvae outside the muscles are destroyed by inflammatory reaction, various clinical disturbances may appear, such as adenitis, encephalitis, meningitis, visual or auditory disorders, pneumonitis, pleurisy, and myocarditis. At the **stage of encystation** (about the 3rd month) most symptoms will have disappeared, although muscular pains and fatigue may persist for several months. Rarely, sequelae to previous tissue damage may become evident as neurologic disorders, myocardial weakness, nephritis, or pleuropulmonary disease, but permanent disability seldom, if ever, ensues. In very severe cases death may occur during the acute stage, or from the later sequelae.

Diagnosis

A history of ingesting raw or insufficiently cooked pork, followed by an acute gastroenteritis, is helpful in making the diagnosis. Muscle pains, edema of the face and eyelids, fever, and a rapidly increasing eosinophilia are strong confirmatory evidence, especially when an outbreak of trichinosis is in progress. Trichinae may only rarely be found in the offending pork, or in the patient's stool, blood, spinal fluid, or muscle biopsy specimen, so that negative findings do not rule out trichinosis.

Complement fixation and intradermal tests, using an antigen prepared from the larvae, are of little diagnostic value because a high percentage of the population has become sensitized through previous infection. The skin test is performed by injecting 0.1 cc. of a 1:10,000 dilution of the trichinella antigen intradermally. A positive reaction is characterized by the appearance of a blanched wheal within 5 minutes. Trichinosis must be differentiated from the following conditions: Skeletal manifestations: rheumatic fever, acute arthritis, poliomyelitis, influenza, scurvy, myositis. Febrile states: tuberculosis, typhoid fever, sepsis, undulant fever. Pulmonary manifestations: pneumonitis. Meningeal manifestations: meningitis, poliomyelitis.

Prognosis

The prognosis is good in most cases. The mortality rate is quoted as 5%. Absence of an eosinophilic response, or a sudden fall in the eosinophilic level to 1% or zero during the acute phase, is an unfavorable prognostic sign.

Prophylaxis

Trichinosis may be prevented by the thorough cooking of all fresh pork. Hogs should not be fed raw garbage since it may contain infected pork wastes.

Treatment

Purgatives have been tried early in the disease in an attempt to dislodge and expel the adult worms, but such agents are not effective since the disease is seldom diagnosed early enough and the worms are firmly attached to the intestinal mucosa. The muscular pains are usually relieved by rest in bed, but may require analgesics, such as acetylsalicylic acid (R 1) and codeine (R 10). If swelling and tenderness are severe, hot or cold applications may give some relief. Although the temperature often is high, the patient usually does not appear correspondingly ill, and tolerates the fever with relatively little discomfort.

Patients who develop bronchitis or pneumonitis should be given penicillin (R 28, 29) to prevent or treat secondary bacterial infection. Thereafter, therapy is symptomatic and supportive, aimed at assisting the patient to survive the acute toxemia, which terminates when the larvae become encysted.

SULFONAMIDE THERAPY

The sulfonamides are amides of sulfanilic acid, whose many derivatives have as their parent compound, sulfanilamide. The value of a sulfonamide for systemic therapy is dependent upon the rate of intestinal absorption, plasma binding, acetylation in the body, renal clearance, and the solubility of free and acetylated drug. These factors modify *in vivo* antibacterial activity and over-all toxicity.

Sulfonamides are principally bacteriostatic and, with the body's defense mechanisms, they act to control infection. Their bacteriostatic action depends on the maintenance of an effective drug concentration at the site of infection, and consists of interference with the enzyme systems necessary for bacterial multiplication and survival. Para-aminobenzoic acid and procaine, both somewhat similar in chemical structure to the sulfonamides, will neutralize the bacteriostatic effect through competitive inhibition. This property of para-aminobenzoic acid and procaine is used to advantage when cultures are made from blood specimens containing sulfonamides (*see* Lab. Proc.). The bacteriostatic effect of a sulfonamide also is diminished by acetylation, a process in which an acetyl group is substituted for one of the hydrogens of the para-amino portion of the sulfonamide molecule. The amount of acetylated drug present in the blood or kidneys is important not only from the standpoint of reduced bacteriostatic activity of the sulfonamide, but also because of its altered solubility. Following acetylation, many of the compounds become considerably less soluble. Free drugs as well as their acetylated products may reach oversaturation levels in the tubular urine and induce urolithiasis.

Although toxic reactions are seldom encountered with the newer sulfonamide compounds, when they do occur, they are similar to those noted with the less recently developed ones, i.e.: (1) neurologic—headache, neuritic pain, dizziness, tinnitus, depression, mania, and delirium; (2) drug fever, often simulating serum sickness (q.v.), and occasionally associated with dermatitis; (3) dermatitis, usually accompanied by severe pruritus; (4) alterations in the blood and blood-forming organs resulting in cyanosis, macrocytic anemia, acute hemolytic anemia, leukopenia, and agranulocytosis; (5) toxic hepatitis; (6) toxic nephritis and urinary complications such as urolithiasis, oliguria, hematuria, renal colic, and obstructive anuria.

Of the numerous sulfonamides that have been synthesized, only a few are of therapeutic value. These are divided into two categories, based on their absorbability which, in turn, determines their therapeutic indications.

ABSORBABLE SULFONAMIDES

Sulfonamides used for systemic treatment are readily absorbed from the intestinal tract and carried by the blood to all parts of the body. Indiscriminate use of sulfonamide drugs in minor conditions, where they have little effect and where less hazardous preparations are adequate, is not justifiable. Such injudicious use of these valuable therapeutic agents may occasionally cause sensitization and preclude their later availability for the treatment of serious infections. Topical use of sulfonamides stands in a similarly questionable position, since it is particularly prone to induce allergic reactions, confers quite limited local anti-infective action, and may actually delay healing.

Sulfamylon is unique in that on local application it has proved to be superior in antibacterial activity to penicillin, streptomycin, parachlorophenol, and tyrothricin. It is the only sulfonamide of clinical importance that is not inhibited by para-aminobenzoic acid, pus and tissue breakdown products. This drug is usually applied locally as a 5% solution.

Routine of Administration

When administering the sulfonamides it is advisable to adhere to a standard regimen as closely as possible. (1) Inquiry should be made concerning previous sulfonamide reactions; if these have occurred, a sulfonamide to which the patient is not sensitive is indicated, or it may be necessary during treatment to halt administration and use a suitable antibiotic agent instead. Occasionally, patients are able to take a sulfonamide to which they have previously reacted, when it is given in small doses. The dosage of the offending compound can be reduced and usually the same therapeutic results can be obtained by combining it with another sulfonamide compound to which the patient is not sensitive. (*See* Combination Therapy, below.) (2) Daily supervision and constant watchfulness for signs of toxic reactions are essential during the administration of sulfonamides. (3) Whenever feasible the causative organism should be isolated and its sensitivity to the sulfonamide being administered determined *in vitro*. Once this has been done the suitability of the drug and the adequacy of the dosage can be evaluated. (4) Sulfonamide blood concentrations should be determined, when possible, and the dosage regulated to provide a fairly constant level of approximately 5 to 10 mg. of free sulfonamide/100 cc. in mild infections and 10 to 15 mg./100 cc. in serious infections. It is advisable to continue administration until all symptoms have disappeared and the patient has been afebrile for at least 2 days. (5) A complete blood count and urinalysis should be done before beginning sulfonamide therapy and repeated on the 1st day and every 3rd day thereafter during administration of the drug.

Close supervision and constant observation in the previously described manner will uncover reactions promptly and reveal any tendency toward the development of drug "fastness" and "masking." Drug resistance or "fastness" exists when organisms previously sulfonamide-sensitive no longer are inhibited by a sulfonamide in therapeutic concentrations. Patients exhibiting the "masking" phenomenon appear subjectively to be improving on sulfonamide therapy although tissue destruction at the site of infection continues. This condition usually arises from inadequate dosage.

An important prophylactic measure that helps to avoid urinary complications consists of administering sufficient fluids to produce a daily urinary output of 2,000 cc. or more. Many physicians also advocate the concomitant administration of sodium bicarbonate in quantities sufficient to alkalinize the urine. The usual dosage necessary is 2 to 4 Gm. (3 ss to i) with each dose of sulfonamide. Some authorities believe that the use of sulfonamide mixtures obviates the necessity for alkalinization.

Patients receiving sulfonamides should be advised to avoid unnecessary exposure to ultraviolet rays, since photosensitivity may develop.

Although used almost exclusively for curative purposes, the

absorbable sulfonamides are occasionally given prophylactically. This has been done chiefly in rheumatic fever, during epidemics of meningitis or streptococcal infections, and pre- and postoperatively.

Sulfonamides are usually administered orally but may be given parenterally, either as an initial dose to provide a therapeutic blood level rapidly or for continuous therapy when the oral route is not feasible. The I.V. route is favored for parenteral administration and it is preferable to use 5% solutions of sodium sulfadiazine or sodium sulfamerazine, since sodium sulfathiazole is irritating in concentrations above 1%. When I.V. administration is not convenient, hypodermoclysis with a 5% solution of sodium sulfadiazine or sodium sulfamerazine may be utilized. Sterile sodium salts of the sulfonamides are employed for parenteral administration after being dissolved in Water for Injection U.S.P. or Sterile Isotonic Sodium Chloride Solution for Parenteral Use U.S.P. Glucose solutions should never be used as diluents for the sulfonamides.

The preferred systemic sulfonamides are those that are readily absorbed from the intestinal tract, have high anti-infective activity, are only slightly acetylated in the body, possess adequate solubility in free and acetylated form, cause few toxic reactions, and maintain prolonged adequate blood and urine levels. The sulfonamides meeting the majority of these criteria are sulfadiazine, sulfamerazine, sulfamethazine, sulfapyrazine, and sulfacetamide. Sulfanilamide, sulfapyridine, and sulfathiazole are falling into disuse since they do not compare favorably with the others in these respects.

Sulfadiazine is effective in the treatment of pneumococcic, hemolytic streptococcic, staphylococcic, meningococcic and gonococcic infections. The initial dose of 2 to 4 Gm. (3 ss to i) for mild infections or 4 to 6 Gm. (3 i to iss) for serious infections should be followed by doses of 1 Gm. (gr. xv) every 4 hours, day and night. In children, the initial dose is 0.1 to 0.15 Gm./Kg. body wt., and subsequent doses should be ¼ of the initial dose, given every 6 hours. For parenteral therapy, sodium sulfadiazine should be given I.V. as the 5% solution. The initial dose is based on 0.1 Gm./Kg. body wt. If subsequent doses are to be administered I.V., they should be based on 30 to 50 mg./Kg. body wt. and given at intervals of 6 to 8 hours.

Sulfamerazine has an anti-infective activity similar to that of sulfadiazine. In adults, an initial dose of 3 or 4 Gm. (gr. xlv or lx) should be followed by 1 Gm. (gr. xv) every 6 to 8 hours. Infants under 6 months may be given 0.5 Gm. (gr. viiss) initially and 0.25 Gm. (gr. iv) every 12 hours thereafter; infants 6 months to 3 years, 1 Gm. (gr. xv) followed by 0.5 Gm. (gr. viiss) every 12 hours; children 3 to 10 years, 1.5 Gm. (gr. xxii) initially and 1 Gm. (gr. xv) every 12 hours. Severe infections in all age groups may be treated with doses 50% larger than these. Sodium sulfamerazine is used for I.V. administration in a dose representing 50 mg./Kg. body wt. If subsequent doses are to be administered I.V. they should be based on 25 mg./Kg. body wt. and given every 12 hours.

Sulfamethazine closely resembles sulfamerazine in all its properties. The drug has been used successfully for similar indications and in the same dosage.

Sulfapyrazine usually is as effective as sulfadiazine in pneumococcic, hemolytic streptococcic, *Esch. coli* and *Shigella paradysenteriae* infections. The initial dose is 2 to 4 Gm. (3 ss to i) and should be followed by 1 Gm. (gr. xv) every 4 to 6 hours. Infants and children may be given doses on the scale outlined above for sulfadiazine at intervals of 6 hours.

Sulfacetamide is used particularly in the prophylaxis and treatment of urinary infections. Its high solubility obviates the danger of renal blockage. The usual dosage in adults is 1 Gm. 4 times a day. In children weighing up to 90 lbs., 40 mg./lb. body wt. is given daily divided into 4 equal doses. The drug is unique in that a 30% solution of its sodium salt is stable at the pH of tissue fluids (7.4). In this concentration it may be used as a nonirritating eye disinfectant.

Among the sulfonamides formerly more in use than at present, **sulfathiazole** was found of benefit in pneumococcic, staphylococcic, and gonococcic infections. The usual dosage is 4 Gm. (3 i) initially, followed by 1 Gm. (gr. xv) every 4 hours. **Sulfapyridine** has been used effectively in pneumococcic pneumonia. The dosage is the same as that of sulfathiazole. Because of its high toxicity, sulfapyridine is seldom used today if other sulfonamides or antibiotics are available. **Sulfanilamide** may be used for the treatment of hemolytic streptococcic infections. The dosage is 0.1 Gm./Kg. body wt. initially, with ⅙ of this amount given every 4 hours thereafter.

Combination therapy, utilizing a mixture of partial dosages of two or more sulfonamides, has proved efficacious and has minimized the occurrence of toxic reactions. Each component of the mixture acts as if present alone, exerting no influence on the solubility or toxicity of the others. Consequently, the danger of urinary complications and other reactions is sharply decreased. With triple mixtures, simultaneous administration of sodium bicarbonate usually is unnecessary. Combinations frequently used consist of sulfadiazine and sulfamerazine, or of triple combinations, containing in addition to these two compounds either sulfathiazole, sulfamethazine, or sulfacetamide. Approximately equal parts of each drug are combined to make a tablet containing 0.5 Gm. (gr. viiss) of the mixture of sulfonamides; or the same amounts may be dispensed in 1 teaspoon of a suitable vehicle. These combinations are administered in doses of 3 to 5 Gm. (gr. xlv to lxxv) initially and 1 Gm. (gr. xv) every 4 or 6 hours thereafter. In children and small adults, the doses are appropriately reduced.

Good results have been reported with the subcut. administration of an aqueous solution containing 2.5% each of the sodium salts of sulfadiazine and sulfamerazine. This may be prepared by mixing equal quantities of a 5% solution of each. For continued parenteral therapy in infants, hypodermoclysis with this combination may be given at 12-hour intervals on the basis of 0.13 to 0.2 Gm. (gr. ii to iii)/Kg. body wt. The parenteral route also may be used when the aim is to achieve a high blood level rapidly, after which oral administration can be substituted.

NONABSORBABLE SULFONAMIDES

These drugs are used predominantly for their bacteriostatic action within the bowel. Since they are only slightly absorbed they seldom cause toxic reactions and thus are suitable for long-continued administration. Sulfaguanidine compares unfavorably with the newer preparations such as succinylsulfathiazole, phthalylsulfathiazole, and phthalylsulfacetamide in respect to anti-infective action and toxicity and therefore is falling into disuse. These nonabsorbable sulfonamides often are effective in the prevention or treatment of bacillary dysenteries, cholera, ulcerative colitis, and regional ileitis. They are frequently administered preoperatively and postoperatively in patients requiring bowel surgery. The doses should be spaced at such intervals as will provide and maintain high concentrations of the drug in the stools. The optimal time-dose schedules are as follows:

1. Succinylsulfathiazole: 0.25 Gm./Kg. body wt. initially, followed by a maintenance dose of 0.25 Gm./Kg. daily in 6 equal doses at 4-hour intervals.

2. Phthalylsulfathiazole: 50 to 100 mg./Kg. body wt. daily in equally divided doses at intervals of 4, 6, or 8 hours, the total dose not to exceed 8 Gm.

3. Phthalylsulfacetamide: 3 equally divided doses to provide a total of 6 to 9 Gm./day.

4. Sulfaguanidine, for therapy of acute bacillary dysentery, 50 mg./Kg. body wt. every 4 hours day and night until the stools are reduced to 5 or less daily; then every 8 hours for at least 3 days; for prophylactic purposes, 50 mg./Kg. body wt. every 8 hours. It is not wise to continue administration for more than 14 days.

ANTIBIOTIC THERAPY

Antibiotics are anti-infective agents of biologic origin used either prophylactically or therapeutically. They are derived from bacteria (e.g., tyrothricin, bacitracin), molds and fungi (e.g., penicillin, streptomycin, aureomycin, Chloromycetin), or from other living substances (e.g., tomatin, chlorophyll).

Most antibiotics in concentrations tolerated by living tissues are bacteriostatic rather than bactericidal. Their mode of action is not well understood. The effectiveness of an antibiotic against a specific infectious agent may be measured *in vitro* and *in vivo*. The *in vitro* sensitivity of an organism to an antibiotic is not always a true index of the clinical efficacy of the substance, but generally, agents effective *in vitro*, if not toxic to the host, prove to be effective when employed therapeutically.

Organisms may develop resistance to an antibiotic. The resistance may develop rapidly, or after long or repeated courses of therapy. It is essential, therefore, that infections be brought under control as rapidly as possible by promptly (1) identifying the causative organism; (2) determining its sensitivity *in vitro*; and (3) administering adequate doses, to attain an effective *in vivo* concentration of the drug. If the patient is treated initially with inadequate amounts of the antibiotic, thus permitting the development of resistance ("drug fastness"), even greatly increased dosage later may fail to control the infection. When the emergency is such that time will not permit determination *in vitro* of the sensitivity of the infecting organisms prior to initiating therapy, it is advisable to use maximal dosage from the outset.

Clinical and experimental evidence suggests that antibiotics used in conjunction with other chemotherapeutic agents have synergistic or additive antimicrobial activity. For example, in diseases due to Brucella, *H. influenzae, K. pneumoniae, Myco. tuberculosis*, and *Ps. aeruginosa*, therapeutic activity may be enhanced when streptomycin is given in combination with one or more other appropriate chemotherapeutic agents. Penicillin and streptomycin, on the other hand, combat mixed infections caused by gram-positive and gram-negative organisms by the sum of their separate and specific actions. In addition, the combined use of at least two chemotherapeutic agents with different antibacterial spectrums will diminish the danger of "superinfection."

PENICILLIN

A highly potent anti-infectious agent, existing in several forms (F, G, K, and X), derived from species of molds belonging to the genus Penicillium. Crystalline preparations, containing chiefly penicillin G, are preferred because of their greater activity, purity and stability. Noncrystalline preparations require refrigeration in the dry state; crystalline penicillin is stable up to 3 years in the dry, unrefrigerated form. Solutions of either type of penicillin require refrigeration, and should be discarded after 3 days.

Clinical Indications

(1) Penicillin is highly effective in the following infections (q.v.): staphylococcic, hemolytic and anaerobic streptococcic, clostridial, pneumococcic, gonococcic, meningococcic, *B. anthra-*

cis, erysipeloid, syphilitic, and fusospirochetal. (2) Penicillin is moderately effective in the treatment of (q.v.) leptospirosis, actinomycosis, and diphtheria (if the drug is supplemented by antitoxin). (3) Penicillin usually is of only slight value in rat-bite fever due to *Streptobacillus moniliformis,* or mixed infections in which the predominating organism is gram-negative, e.g., ruptured appendix, liver abscess. (4) In the following conditions penicillin is not effective: viral infections, gram-negative bacillary infections, most fungus diseases, tuberculosis, amebiasis and malaria.

Administration

Inadequate dosage may result in the development of penicillin-resistant strains of at least some pathogens; therefore, sufficient amounts of the drug should be used to control the infection rapidly and to maintain a therapeutically effective drug concentration in the tissues. Duration and adequacy of treatment should be guided by the bacteriologic and clinical response to treatment. Depending on the type, location and severity of the infection, penicillin may be administered by I.M., I.V., intrathecal, or local injection, by mouth, by inhalation, or by topical application.

When oral doses are employed, these need to be 5 to 8 times the amount usually recommended for injection, and should be given between meals. However, because of the uncertainty of absorption following ingestion, oral administration is not advisable in treating severe infections. Prophylactically, ingestion of 250,000 u. of penicillin shortly after exposure to gonorrhea has been found to be effective in aborting the infection. Oral penicillin also has been used prophylactically to prevent recrudescences in patients with a history of rheumatic fever.

The I.M. route is the preferred parenteral mode of administration. Aqueous solutions may be prepared with Water for Injection U.S.P. or Isotonic Sodium Chloride Solution for Parenteral Use U.S.P. as diluents. In most cases, it will require from 30,000 to 100,000 u./cc., injected every 3 hours, to maintain a relatively constant, effective concentration of penicillin in the tissues. In severe infections dosages of 12 million u./day or more have been given. Large doses of aqueous penicillin (200,-000 to 600,000 u.) once or twice daily have been found to be as effective in treating certain infections as a dosage schedule aimed at maintaining a more or less constant blood level. Excellent results have been obtained in pneumococcic pneumonia, with injections of 200,000 to 600,000 u. every 12 hours the 1st day, and once daily thereafter until the patient has been afebrile for 48 hours.

Repository penicillin preparations are available which will maintain a therapeutic blood level for relatively long periods of time. A mixture of peanut or sesame oil and white wax, with penicillin in suspension, usually in a concentration of 300,000 u./cc., makes possible the maintenance of a therapeutic blood level for 12 to 24 hours following a single I.M. injection of 1 cc. Preparations consisting of 300,000 u./cc. of procaine penicillin G suspended in peanut or sesame oil and gelled with 2% aluminum stearate will ordinarily provide adequate blood levels for 24 to 96 hours after I.M. injection. One dose daily of 300,000 u. of a repository form of penicillin will, in most cases, suffice for infections due to penicillin-susceptible organisms. Repeated daily injections of large amounts of procaine penicillin G in oil with aluminum stearate (600,000 to 1,200,000 u.) may provide a steadily increasing penicillin blood level as treatment continues in well established or severe infections. Some physicians advocate the concomitant administration, initially, of large doses of plain penicillin to obtain a high penicillin blood level early. Because of the possibility of fatty abscesses developing after the use of penicillin suspended in oily preparations, some physicians prefer to use an aqueous suspension of procaine penicillin, or large doses of plain aqueous penicillin (*see* above). Since aqueous procaine penicillin suspensions will maintain therapeutic blood levels for 12 to 48 hours, injections once or twice daily will produce maximum therapeutic effect.

When a severe infection or a relatively resistant organism is present, penicillin injections may be given at more frequent intervals, in doses of 50,000 to 200,000 u. every 3 hours; or continuous I.M. drip or I.V. infusion of a solution of crystalline penicillin containing 25 to 50 u./cc. may be used. For intrathecal or intracisternal injection, as in the treatment of meningitis, concentrations of 1,000 u./cc. (total dose not to exceed 20,000 u.) are used, with sterile normal saline or spinal fluid as the diluent. Employing a similar concentration and sterile normal saline as a diluent, injection may be made into an empyema, abscess or joint cavity after complete aspiration of its purulent contents. Penicillin may be applied topically in powder form, in normal saline containing 250 or more u./cc., or in ointment containing 500 to 1,000 u./Gm. Incorporated into troches, penicillin is useful for treatment of infections of the oropharynx. Inhalation of penicillin often is effective against respiratory tract infections due to susceptible organisms. The penicillin may be inhaled in the form of an aerosol, made by nebulizing a solution containing 25,000 to 50,000 u./cc. (1 to 2 cc. inhaled every 3 or 4 hours), or as a finely ground powder. Vaginal suppositories containing 100,000 u. of penicillin inserted before or during the beginning of labor have been effective in reducing postpartum infections.

Penicillin may be used prophylactically as well as therapeutically. In conditions predisposing to hypostatic pneumonia, such as coma or cardiac failure, or in agranulocytosis, parenteral aqueous or repository penicillin should be given to prevent complicating infections. From 100,000 to 300,000 u. I.M. daily is the usual prophylactic dose. Penicillin alone or in combination with sulfonamides or streptomycin is frequently used prophylactically pre- and postoperatively (*see* PREOPERATIVE AND POSTOPERATIVE CARE).

Toxicity

Because of its low toxicity, there are few contraindications to the use of penicillin. Individuals who are hypersensitive to this agent may exhibit such reactions as mild malaise with or without fever, urticaria, erythematous rashes, bullous eruptions, or angioneurotic edema, or episodes resembling serum sickness. The administration of an antihistaminic, such as Neo-Antergan, may control these reactions. Certain of these allergic manifestations may be severe enough to necessitate discontinuance of the drug. Skin rashes in rare instances may persist, or recur for many weeks after penicillin therapy has been stopped. Occasionally a reaction may appear 7 to 10 days after termination of penicillin therapy. Black tongue may be seen during the use of oral troches. No harmful effects on the blood-forming organs, the liver, or the kidneys have been observed. Thrombophlebitis at the site of I.V. injection has occurred following repeated use of the same vein. Because of an antigenic structure similar to that of certain fungi, penicillin given therapeutically may cause a dermatophytid reaction in an individual who has or has had an infection due to a related type of fungus.

STREPTOMYCIN; DIHYDROSTREPTOMYCIN

Closely related antibiotics derived from Streptomyces griseus, *chiefly effective against gram-negative and acid-fast bacteria.* Dihydrostreptomycin is a chemically distinct modification of streptomycin and is considerably less neurotoxic and allergenic. Both forms are highly purified, fairly stable in the dry state, and remain potent for 1 week at room temperature. Heat accelerates loss of potency.

Clinical Indications

1. For the treatment of carefully selected cases of tuberculosis (q.v.), streptomycin and dihydrostreptomycin are recognized as the best chemotherapeutic agents available when used in combination with other approved therapeutic measures. Streptomycin is the most effective drug for the treatment of granuloma inguinale and tularemia.

2. Streptomycin is recommended in the treatment of the following: infections caused by *H. influenzae* (here combined with sulfonamide therapy) and *H. pertussis;* urinary tract infections due to susceptible strains of *Esch. coli, P. vulgaris, K. pneumoniae* (Friedländer's bacillus), *A. aerogenes,* and *Ps. aeruginosa* (*B. pyocyaneus*); brucellosis (with combined sulfonamide therapy); meningitis due to susceptible strains of Sal-

monella; endocarditis due to penicillin-resistant, streptomycin-sensitive pathogens; gonorrhea; chancroid.

3. Streptomycin frequently is of value in the following conditions: peritonitis; liver abscess; cholangitis; chronic lung infections; in empyema due to susceptible organisms; pneumonia due to *K. pneumoniae;* gastrointestinal infection caused by susceptible strains of Salmonella and Shigella. The drug also is helpful to patients undergoing intestinal surgery, since, when taken orally, it will reduce the intestinal flora preoperatively and postoperatively. Streptomycin shows promise in the treatment of leprosy.

4. In typhoid fever and most Salmonella infections, streptomycin is of questionable value. Streptomycin is ineffective in infections due to clostridia, rickettsias, *E. typhosa,* plasmodia, viruses, molds and fungi.

Administration

The preferred method of administration and dosage in a given case depends upon the type, location and severity of the infection. The aim is to secure rapidly an effective concentration of the agent in the tissues, and to maintain the desired concentration as long as possible. The sensitivity of the causative organism should be tested to determine the drug concentration theoretically necessary for therapeutic effect. Since bacteria may become resistant to streptomycin or dihydrostreptomycin, blood concentrations which inhibit the pathogen *in vitro* should be maintained.

Both drugs are most commonly administered I.M., (although they are well tolerated subcut.) in solutions containing no more than 500 mg./cc. with either Water for Injection U.S.P. or Sterile Isotonic Sodium Chloride Solution for Parenteral Use U.S.P. The optimum dose for most infections is 1 to 3 Gm. daily in divided doses of 0.5 Gm. each. Following I.M. administration, streptomycin and dihydrostreptomycin pass into the peritoneal, pericardial, pleural, intraocular, and amniotic fluids, the fetal circulation, and the bile (in the absence of hepatic or biliary damage). They do not diffuse into thick-walled abscesses or empyema cavities. Passage from the blood into the cerebrospinal fluid is variable. Since 60 to 80% of the drugs will be excreted in the urine within 24 hours after administration, therapeutically effective urinary levels may be obtained with relatively small parenteral doses. When renal function is impaired, low urine concentrations and unduly high blood levels may result.

Intrathecal injection of streptomycin or dihydrostreptomycin is of value in meningeal infections; however, concomitant I.M. administration is necessary to ensure effective blood levels. Intrathecal injections should be given slowly (10 minutes for 10 cc.) after a slightly greater amount of spinal fluid has been withdrawn. Either of the above mentioned diluents may be used, or, as some prefer, the desired dose of the antibiotic may be dissolved in 2 cc. of diluent, and the resulting solution mixed with 8 cc. of spinal fluid. The usual intrathecal dose of streptomycin or of dihydrostreptomycin sulfate is 50 to 100 mg. (not to exceed 1 mg./Kg. body wt.) every 24 to 48 hours.

Where the intrapleural or intraperitoneal route is advisable, 20 to 50 cc. of solution containing 0.5 to 1 Gm. of the antibiotic should be injected after discontinuing drainage or suction so that the drug may remain in the cavity for at least 6 hours. Similar solutions or ointments containing these concentrations may be used for topical application. Higher concentration should be used for resistant infections. (CAUTION! Sensitization frequently follows topical administration of streptomycin.)

Administration of streptomycin for local action within the respiratory passages may be accomplished by having the patient inhale, every 2 to 2½ hours, 1 to 1.5 cc. of a nebulized solution containing 50 mg. of streptomycin /cc. Concomitant parenteral administration usually is advisable.

Oral administration of streptomycin is ineffective in the treatment of systemic infections since 98% of the drug ingested is excreted in the feces unchanged. However, since oral dosage reduces the intraintestinal bacterial flora, it is of use prophylactically in intestinal surgery, and in the treatment of diarrheal diseases. A dose of 0.5 to 1 Gm. dissolved in any acceptable fluid is given every 6 hours.

Toxicity

Streptomycin, and to a considerably lesser degree dihydrostreptomycin, may cause certain toxic reactions. These reactions are more apt to develop in individuals who have become sensitized to the given drug, have impairment of renal function, or have received large doses over prolonged periods. Most patients sensitive to streptomycin may be given dihydrostreptomycin without ill effect.

Disturbances of 8th cranial nerve function occur in about 20 to 25% of patients receiving 1 Gm./day of streptomycin over prolonged periods; neurotoxicity following the use of dihydrostreptomycin in similar dosage is exceedingly rare. Prolonged treatment with doses above 1 Gm./day increases the incidence of neurotoxicity. The disturbance in 8th nerve function is manifested by vertigo, tinnitus, loss of equilibrium, and rarely by diminished auditory acuity.

Slow recovery of some 8th nerve function may occur after cessation of streptomycin administration. Vestibular incompetence is frequently permanent although compensation commonly ensues. When evidence of 8th nerve involvement is observed, the possible desirability of discontinuing streptomycin therapy must be weighed against the gravity of the prognosis if streptomycin is withheld.

Streptomycin and, less often, dihydrostreptomycin may cause

mild reactions, such as skin eruptions, eosinophilia, arthralgia, malaise, fever, and albuminuria. Some of these reactions respond to antihistaminic therapy or desensitization (see Allergy). Alkalinization of urine will decrease the incidence of renal symptoms and also increase streptomycin effectiveness for urinary infections. Since dermatitis may develop in susceptible individuals, those who must handle streptomycin should wear rubber gloves. Dihydrostreptomycin rarely causes contact dermatitis.

AUREOMYCIN

An antibiotic produced by Streptomyces aureofaciens which *appears to be beneficial in infections due to various gram-positive and gram-negative bacteria, viruses of the psittacosis-lymphogranuloma venereum group, rickettsias and* E. histolytica. Many organisms sensitive to aureomycin are resistant to penicillin or streptomycin. Among the diseases that are amenable to treatment with this anti-infectious agent are Rocky Mountain spotted fever, rickettsialpox, typhus (epidemic, murine and scrub), Q fever, pneumococcic pneumonia, brucellosis, typhoid fever, Salmonella infections, streptococcal and staphylococcal infections, meningococcemia, lymphogranuloma venereum, psittacosis, primary atypical pneumonia, and amebiasis.

Aureomycin is effective by mouth, and therapeutic concentrations usually are present in the blood 6 to 12 hours after ingestion. The average dose is 50 to 100 mg./Kg. body wt. daily; in some cases as much as 300 to 500 mg./Kg. have been given. Untoward reactions such as nausea, vomiting, and diarrhea have been reported in some patients. Moderate infections may be treated with 25 to 50 mg./Kg. body wt. daily. The drug should be administered every 4 hours the 1st day, and then every 6 hours. Dosage may be reduced after a few days, depending on the clinical response. Some physicians advocate the administration of 250 mg. every 2 hours until the patient is afebrile, then following this with a reduced dose given every 6 to 8 hours until the patient has recovered. When necessary, sterile preparations of aureomycin may be given I.V. slowly. Since I.M. injection is quite painful, other routes of administration are preferable.

Aureomycin has been successfully used as a 0.5% solution with 0.5% sodium borate in normal saline for treatment of ocular infections, e.g., dendritic keratitis, Morax-Axenfeld ulcers, and staphylococcic, influenzal, pneumococcic and inclusion conjunctivitis.

Locally, aureomycin ointment has been used for the treatment of various pyogenic skin infections.

CHLOROMYCETIN

An antibiotic produced by the soil mold Streptomyces venezuelae, *and which also can be prepared synthetically.* It is similar to aureomycin in many respects including anti-infective activity and mode of administration. Unlike aureomycin, Chloromycetin is a neutral compound which is comparatively stable. It is not affected by boiling for 5 hours nor by changes through a pH range of 2 to 9. Chloromycetin inhibits the growth of a wide range of gram-positive and gram-negative bacteria, rickettsias, and viruses. This drug may be of value in the treatment of the various types of typhus, Rocky Mountain spotted fever, lymphogranuloma venereum, atypical pneumonia, psittacosis, typhoid fever, Salmonella and Shigella infections, and bacillary urinary infections.

Chloromycetin is effective when administered orally, and therapeutic levels are present in the blood 30 minutes after ingestion. Dosage schedules have not been completely determined for all the above enumerated conditions; however, a regimen based on an initial dose of 50 to 75 mg./Kg. body wt., followed by 0.25 to 0.5 Gm. every 2 to 3 hours until the patient is afebrile, and then a similar dose every 6 hours until the patient is asymptomatic, has been widely advocated. The drug appears to be nontoxic for all practical purposes.

TYROTHRICIN

An extract obtained from B. brevis *and consisting principally of gramicidin and tyrocidin.* When applied locally it is of value in treating superficial ulcers, draining abscesses, empyema and pyodermatoses due to gram-positive organisms such as staphylococci, streptococci, and pneumococci. It is most effective when in direct local contact with the bacteria. Little effect is obtained by its use in deep-seated infections, and in the presence of excessive amounts of inhibiting body fluids, e.g., urine, saliva, and serum.

Tyrothricin should be employed locally by instillation or with compresses, and never given parenterally because of its toxicity. Before administration, the drug should be diluted with sterile distilled water to provide a concentration of 500 mcg./cc. Higher concentrations, although occasionally necessary, may prove irritating. Ointments containing this antibiotic are available.

BACITRACIN

An antibiotic obtained from a strain of B. subtilis, *having a range of activity similar to that of penicillin.* It will inhibit the growth of streptococci, staphylococci, gonococci, meningococci, clostridia, *T. pallidum,* and *E. histolytica.* Bacitracin's effect is not altered by serum, pus or necrotic tissue. For maximum benefit an effective concentration of the antibiotic must be in contact with the pathogen.

Bacitracin dissolved in Sterile Normal Saline for Parenteral Use U.S.P. in a concentration of 500 u./cc. may be applied topically, or injected into such pyogenic lesions (caused by susceptible organisms) as furuncles, carbuncles, ulcers, felons, paronychia, conjunctivitis, and pyodermatoses. Procaine, 1 to 2%, added to the solution to be used for local infiltration, will diminish the associated pain. One daily injection of 0.2 to 5 cc., depending on the size of the lesion, usually is effective. (Caution! Because the drug is nephrotoxic, it should not be administered I.M. or I.V.)

Ointments containing bacitracin 500 u./Gm. are available for ophthalmic use and for dermal application.

RECOMMENDED CHEMOTHERAPY IN MORE COMMON INFECTIONS

Disease	Causative Organism	Anti-infective Agents of Choice	Anti-infective Agents of Value
Actinomycosis	Actinomyces (various species)	Penicillin	Sulfonamides
Amebiasis	E. histolytica	Aralen Carbarsone Chiniofon Diodoquin Emetine	Aureomycin Bacitracin Milibis
Anthrax	B. anthracis	Penicillin plus sulfonamides	Bacitracin
Brucellosis	Brucella (various species)	Sulfonamides plus Streptomycin or Dihydrostreptomycin	Aureomycin Chloromycetin
Chancroid	H. ducreyi	Aureomycin Streptomycin Sulfonamides	
Cholera	V. cholerae		Sulfonamides Streptomycin Chloromycetin
Diphtheria	C. diphtheriae	[ANTITOXIN!]	Penicillin Sulfonamides
Dysentery, bacillary	Shigella (various species)		Sulfonamides Aureomycin Chloromycetin Streptomycin
Endocarditis, subacute	Streptococcus (various species) Staphylococcus (various species)	Penicillin Aureomycin	Streptomycin or Dihydrostreptomycin

RECOMMENDED CHEMOTHERAPY IN MORE COMMON INFECTIONS (*Cont'd*)

Disease	Causative Organism	Anti-infective Agents of Choice	Anti-infective Agents of Value
	Gram-negative organisms (various species)	Streptomycin Aureomycin Chloromycetin	
Erysipelas	*Str. beta-hemolyticus*	Penicillin	Sulfonamides Aureomycin Bacitracin
Gas gangrene	Clostridia (various species)	Penicillin plus sulfonamides	Bacitracin
Granuloma inguinale	*Donovania granulomatis*	Streptomycin or Dihydrostreptomycin Aureomycin	Chloromycetin Antimony compounds
Glanders	*M. mallei*	Streptomycin	Sulfonamides
Gonorrhea	*N. gonorrhoeae*	Penicillin	Sulfonamides Streptomycin or Dihydrostreptomycin
Leprosy	*Myco. leprae*	Sulfones	Streptomycin Dihydrostreptomycin
Lymphogranuloma inguinale	A virus	Aureomycin	Sulfonamides Chloromycetin
Meningitis	*N. intracellularis*	Sulfonamides	Penicillin
	H. influenzae	Streptomycin	Sulfonamides
Paratyphoid fever	*S. paratyphi et al.*	Aureomycin Chloromycetin	Streptomycin
Peritonitis	*Esch. coli Proteus vulgaris* Streptococcus (various species)	Streptomycin or Dihydrostreptomycin Aureomycin Penicillin	Sulfonamides
Pertussis	*H. pertussis*	Streptomycin	Aureomycin
Plague, human	*Past. pestis*	Streptomycin	Sulfonamides
Pneumonia	*D. pneumoniae*	Penicillin	Sulfonamides Aureomycin
	Virus	Aureomycin Chloromycetin	
	K. pneumoniae	Streptomycin Aureomycin Chloromycetin	Sulfonamides
	H. influenzae	Streptomycin Aureomycin Chloromycetin	Sulfonamides

RECOMMENDED CHEMOTHERAPY IN MORE COMMON INFECTIONS (Cont'd)

Disease	Causative Organism	Anti-infective Agents of Choice	Anti-infective Agents of Value
Psittacosis	A virus	Aureomycin Chloromycetin	Penicillin
Q fever	*R. burneti*	Aureomycin Chloromycetin	
Rat-bite fever	*S. minus*	Aureomycin	Penicillin
	S. moniliformis	Streptomycin	
Rocky Mountain spotted fever	*R. rickettsi*	Aureomycin Chloromycetin	Para-aminobenzoic acid
Scarlet fever; Streptococcal pharyngitis	*Str. beta-hemolyticus*	Penicillin	Sulfonamides Aureomycin
Sepsis, puerperal	Hemolytic streptococci	Penicillin	Sulfonamides Bacitracin
Syphilis	*T. pallidum*	Penicillin	Arsenicals Bismuth Aureomycin
Trachoma	A virus	Sulfonamides Penicillin	
Tuberculosis	*Myco. tuberculosis*	Streptomycin or Dihydrostreptomycin	Para-aminosalicylic acid Sulfones
Tularemia	*Past. tularensis*	Streptomycin Aureomycin	Sulfonamides
Typhoid fever	*E. typhosa*	Chloromycetin	Aureomycin
Typhus, epidemic	*R. prowazeki*	Aureomycin Chloromycetin	Para-aminobenzoic acid
endemic	*R. mooseri*	Aureomycin Chloromycetin	Para-aminobenzoic acid
Urinary infections	Proteus (various species) *B. pyocyaneus* *Esch. coli* *A. aerogenes*	Streptomycin or Dihydrostreptomycin Aureomycin Chloromycetin	Sulfonamides
	Streptococcus (various species) Staphylococcus (various species)	Penicillin	Sulfonamides Aureomycin
Vincent's angina	*Bor. vincentii and B. fusiformis*	Penicillin	Arsenicals
Weil's disease	Leptospira (various species)	Penicillin	
Yaws	*T. pertenue*	Penicillin	Arsenicals

PRESCRIPTIONS

(Wherever a prescribed "proprietary" is representative of a class of therapeutic agents, alternative proprietary preparations will be found listed in Part II.)

Analgesics and Antipyretics

1. ℞ Acetylsalicylic acid . . . . .   0.3 Gm. (gr. v)

   1 to 4 tablets every 3 or 4 hours.
   Rheumatic fever: 3 tablets every hour until mild toxic symptoms develop; reinstitute after 6 to 12 hours with 3 to 5 tablets every 4 hours.

2. ℞ Sodium salicylate. . . . .   0.3 Gm. (gr. v)

   1 or 2 tablets every 4 hours.
   Rheumatic fever: 3 tablets every hour until mild toxic symptoms develop; reinstitute after 6 to 12 hours with 3 to 5 tablets every 4 hours. This drug may also be administered rectally, 4 Gm. in 60 cc. of water every 12 hours being equivalent to 5 Gm. daily by mouth.

3. ℞ Sodium salicylate   (enteric
   coated) . . . .   0.3 Gm. (gr. v)

   Rheumatic fever: 3 tablets every hour until mild toxic symptoms develop; reinstitute after 6 to 12 hours with 3 to 5 tablets every 4 hours.

4. ℞ Acetylsalicylic acid . . . . .   0.2 Gm. (gr. iii)
      Acetophenetidin . . . . . .   0.15 Gm. (gr. iiss)
      Caffeine . . . .   0.03 Gm. (gr. ss)

   2 tablets every 3 hours.

5. ℞ Aminopyrine. . . . . . .   0.3 Gm. (gr. v)

   1 to 3 tablets every 4 hours.

6. ℞ Methyl Salicylate U.S.P.   (Oil
   of Wintergreen)

   Apply to affected joints.

7. ℞ Acetanilid . . . .   0.2 Gm. (gr. iii)

   1 capsule every 4 hours.

8. ℞ Acetophenetidin . . . . .   0.3 Gm. (gr. v)

   1 capsule every 4 hours.

9. ℞ Acetylsalicylic acid . . . .   0.6 Gm. (gr. x)
      Codeine sulphate . . . . . .   0.03 Gm. (gr. ss)

   1 capsule or tablet every 4 hours if necessary.

10. ℞ Codeine phosphate   15   mg. (gr. ¼)

    1 to 4 tablets orally or subcut. every 4 hours.

11. ℞ Morphine sulfate

> 8 to 15 mg. (gr. ⅛ to ¼) subcut. every 4 to 6 hours.

12. ℞ "Demerol Hydrochloride"
(ampul)

> 50 to 100 mg. I.M.

13. ℞ Benzocaine   (lozenges)

> 1 lozenge every 3 hours for sore throat, as needed.

14. ℞ Camphor Liniment, U.S.P.

> Gently apply to affected joints and wrap them in flannel cloth.

Sedatives and Hypnotics

15. ℞ Phenobarbital   15   mg.   (gr. ¼)

> 1 to 4 tablets 3 or 4 times a day.

16. ℞ Phenobarbital Elixir U.S.P. . 120.0   cc.   (℥ iv)

> 1 to 2 teaspoons every 4 to 8 hours.

17. ℞ Three Bromides Elixir N.F. . 180.0   cc.   (℥ vi)

> 1 or 2 teaspoons in water as required for restlessness and insomnia; rectally, the dose is 4 to 6 teaspoons (16 to 24 cc.) in water or saline.

18. ℞ Paraldehyde . . . . 120.0   cc.   (℥ iv)

> For delirium, 1 to 4 teaspoons in iced tea, to be followed by teaspoonful doses hourly until patient is asleep. Rectally, the dose is 0.5 cc./Kg. administered as a 10% solution in saline or cottonseed oil, repeated as necessary.
> Anticonvulsant: 3 to 6 cc. I.M., or 1 cc. (slowly) I.V.

19. ℞ Chloral hydrate. . . . . . .   0.3   Gm. (gr. v)

> 2 to 6 capsules, repeated as necessary; for rectal administration, the dose may be dissolved in water or saline.

20. ℞ Sodium bromide, 25% solution 180.0   cc.   (℥ vi)

> ½ to 1 teaspoon 1 to 3 times a day.   (Caution! Bromism.)

21. ℞ Scopolamine (hyoscine) hydrobromide   (ampul)

> 0.3 to 0.6 mg. (gr. 1/200 to 1/100) subcut. every 12 to 24 hours.

22. ℞ "Amytal Sodium"   (ampul)

> 0.5 Gm. (gr. viiss) I.V., slowly, or I.M.

23. ℞ Phenobarbital sodium (ampul)

  0.12 to 0.3 Gm. (gr. ii to v) I.M. 2 or 3 times daily.

24. ℞ Phenobarbital sodium . . . . 0.1 Gm. (gr. iss)

  1 to 3 tablets or capsules every 4 hours.

25. ℞ Pentobarbital sodium . . . . 0.1 Gm. (gr. iss)

  1 to 3 capsules as necessary.

26. ℞ Cocaine hydrochloride. . . . 0.6 Gm. (gr. x)
  Chloroform Water N.F.

       q.s. ad 15.0 cc. (℥ ss)

  5 to 10 drops (13 to 26 mg.) in water every hour for 1 to 3 doses.

27. ℞ Chlorobutanol . . . . 0.2 Gm. (gr. iii)

  1 capsule hourly for 3 or 4 doses.

Antibiotics

28. ℞ Penicillin (vial)

  30,000 to 100,000 u. I.M. every 3 hours or 300,000 u. I.M. every 12 to 24 hours.

29. ℞ Procaine penicillin (vial)

  300,000 u. or more I.M. every 12 to 24 hours.

30. ℞ Penicillin . . . . 500,000 u.
  Distilled water.. . . . . . . 500.0 cc. (℥ xvi)

  Use full strength or diluted as much as 1:4 as a wet compress.

31. ℞ Penicillin ointment (5,000
  u./Gm.)

  Apply to infected lesions twice daily.

32. ℞ Streptomycin (vial)

  For nontuberculous infections: 1 to 4 Gm. daily I.M. in divided doses.

33. ℞ Streptomycin (vial)

  0.5 to 1 Gm. orally, in water, fruit juice, or other liquid, every 6 to 8 hours.

34. ℞ Streptomycin. . . . . . . 1.0 Gm.
  Distilled water . . . . . . 2,000.0 cc. (℥ lxiv)

  Use as a continuous wet dressing.

35. ℞ Aureomycin (capsules) . . . 0.25 Gm.

  25 to 100 mg./Kg. body wt./day divided into 4 to 8 equal doses.

36. ℞ "Chloromycetin" (capsules). 0.25 Gm.

  Administer as for ℞ 35, above.

Sulfonamides

37. ℞ Sulfadiazine . . . .　0.5　Gm. (gr. viiss)

    4 to 8 tablets initially, then 2 tablets every
    3 or 4 hours.　For scarlet fever prophylaxis,
    give 2 tablets twice daily for 3 days.

38. ℞ Sulfamerazine . . . .　0.5　Gm. (gr. viiss)

    6 to 8 tablets initially, then 2 tablets every
    6 to 8 hours.

39. ℞ Sulfathiazole. . . . .　0.5　Gm. (gr. viiss)

    4 to 8 tablets initially, then 2 tablets every
    4 hours.

40. ℞ Sulfapyridine. . . . .　0.5　Gm. (gr. viiss)

    8 tablets initially, then 2 tablets every 4
    hours.

41. ℞ Succinylsulfathiazole . . . .　0.5　Gm. (gr. viiss)

    0.25 Gm./Kg. body wt. initially, followed
    by 0.25 Gm./Kg. body wt. daily in 6 equal
    doses at 4-hour intervals.

42. ℞ Phthalylsulfathiazole . . . .　0.5　Gm. (gr. viiss)

    50 to 100 mg./Kg. body wt. daily in equally
    divided doses at intervals of 4 to 8 hours.

43. ℞ Phthalylsulfacetamide. . . .　0.5　Gm. (gr. viiss)

    4 to 6 tablets 3 times a day.

44. ℞ Sulfaguanidine . . . .　0.5　Gm. (gr. viiss)

    50 mg./Kg. body wt. every 4 hours until
    stools are less than 5/day; then every 8
    hours for 3 additional days.

45. ℞ Sulfathiazole, 5% ointment. .　30.0　Gm. (℥ i)

    Apply daily to ulcer.

46. ℞ Sodium sulfapyridine . . . .　25%
    Hydrophyllic Ointment U.S.P.

                 q.s. ad 100.0　Gm.

    Apply to lesions twice daily.

47. ℞ Sulfadiazine, 5% ophthalmic
    ointment. . . . .　15.0　Gm. (℥ ss)

    Apply to lid margins several times a day.

Fungicides

48. ℞ Potassium Iodide, Saturated
    Solution N.F. . . . . . .　60.0　cc. (℥ ii)

    Slow method: 3 drops in 1 ounce of water 3
    times a day, after meals.　Increase the dose
    by 1 drop a day (not per dose) until the pa-
    tient is receiving 20 drops 3 times a day;
    then, reduce the dose without interruption

to 3 drops 3 times a day and increase again
to 20 drops 3 times a day. Continue as
long as necessary. (CAUTION! Iodism.)

Rapid method: 5 drops in 1 ounce of water
3 times a day, after meals. Increase the
dose by 1 drop per dose per day (3 drops
per day) until the patient is receiving 20
drops 3 times a day. Continue as long as
necessary. (CAUTION! Iodism.)

49. ℞ Sodium iodide (ampul)

    1 Gm. (gr. xv) I.V. once a day.

50. ℞ Ethyl iodide . . . . 30.0 cc. (℥ i)

    Inhale 0.25 cc. 3 times daily. Increase the
daily dose by 0.25 cc. every 3rd day until
1 cc. is inhaled 3 times daily.

51. ℞ Potassium iodide, 1% solution

    Sterilize by autoclaving and inject 60 cc.
(℥ ii) into abscess cavity.

52. ℞ Iodide-iodine solution

    Iodine. . . . . 1.0 Gm. (gr. xv)
    Potassium iodide . . . . . 10.0 Gm. (℥ iiss)
    Distilled water . . . . . 500.0 cc. (℥ xvi)

    For use in irrigations and wet dressings.

53. ℞ Gentian violet, 1% solution . 60.0 cc. (℥ ii)

    Clean and paint affected area once or twice
a day (about 1 hour after feeding) until
lesions have disappeared, then every other
day for 2 weeks; for vaginitis, apply daily
by swab or spray.

54. ℞ Gentian violet, 0.5% solution

    For I.V. use (filtered through Berkefeld or
Seitz filter): 5 mg./Kg. body wt. I.V. daily
or every other day for 7 to 10 days.

55. ℞ "Sopronol" (solution)

    Apply to lesions twice daily.

56. ℞ Copper sulfate, 1% solution

    Apply to lesions by means of iontophoresis
(*see* CLIN. PROC.).

57. ℞ Potassium permanganate,
1:4,000 solution

    Prepared by dissolving 0.24 Gm. (gr. iv) in
1,000 cc. (℥ xxxii) water; soak affected area.

58. ℞ Iodine Tincture U.S.P. . . . 60.0 cc. (℥ ii)

    Apply to ulcers daily.

59. ℞ Ammoniated mercury, 5%
ointment. . . . . 60.0 Gm. (℥ ii)

    Apply to skin lesions 3 times daily.

60. ℞ Sodium propionate 10%
Hydrophyllic Ointment U.S.P.
q.s. ad 120.0 Gm. (℥ iv)

> Apply to vaginal walls daily for 4 or 5 applications.

Parasiticides

61. ℞ "Neostibosan" (ampul)

> 0.3 Gm. (gr. v) I.V. every other day for 6 to 12 doses.
> *For Leishmaniasis:* administer according to directions in text.

62. ℞ Stilbamidine (ampul) . . . 0.15 Gm. (gr. iiss)

> *For Leishmaniasis:* administer according to directions in text.

63. ℞ Tryparsamide (ampul)

> 1 to 1.5 Gm. I.V. or I.M. followed by 2 to 3 Gm. weekly for 15 to 20 weeks. (CAUTION! Optic atrophy.)

64. ℞ Suramin sodium (ampul)

> 0.3 to 0.5 Gm. (gr. v to viiss) I.V. or I.M., followed by 1 Gm. every few days until a total dose of 10 Gm. is given.
> For prophylaxis of trypanosomiasis, a single I.M. dose of 1 Gm. is given.

65. ℞ Pentamidine (ampul)

> 0.1 Gm. I.V. daily for 10 to 20 days.

66. ℞ Tartar emetic, 1% solution
(ampul)

> *Schistosomiasis:* Administer according to directions in text.

67. ℞ Stibophen, 6.3% solution
("Fuadin") (ampul)

> *Schistosomiasis:* Administer according to directions in text.

Amebacides

68. ℞ Emetine hydrochloride (ampul)

> 65 mg. (gr. i) subcut. or I.M. once daily for 4 to 6 days; for amebic hepatitis, therapy is administered for 9 days, and then 6 days, with an intervening rest period of 1 week.

69. ℞ "Diodoquin". . . . . 0.2 Gm. (gr. iii)

> 4 tablets 3 times a day for 10 to 12 consecutive days.

70. ℞ Carbarsone. . . . . 0.25 Gm. (gr. iv)

> 1 capsule 3 times a day after meals for 10 to 12 days.

71. ℞ Carbarsone . . . .   2.0 Gm. (gr. xxx)
      Soda bicarbonate, 2% solution 200.0   cc.   (℥ viss)
        Administer as a retention enema once daily
        for a maximum of 5 days.   (CAUTION!
        Optic atrophy.)

72. ℞ Chiniofon . . . .   0.25 Gm. (gr. iv)
        4 tablets 3 times a day for 10 days.

73. ℞ Chiniofon . . . .   4.0 Gm. (℥ i)
      Tap water . . . . 200.0   cc.   (℥ viiss)
        Administer as a retention enema once daily
        for 7 to 14 days.

74. ℞ Chloroquine diphosphate . .   0.25 Gm. (gr. iv)
        ("Aralen Diphosphate")
        2 tablets (containing 0.3 Gm. base) daily
        for 20 days.

Antimalarials

See Therapeutic Table in Malaria Chapter.

Antileprous Agents

75. ℞ Promin   (ampul)
        5 Gm. I.V. daily as directed in text (*see*
        LEPROSY).

76. ℞ Promizole . . . .   0.5 Gm. (gr. viiss)
        2 to 4 tablets, 3 times a day.

77. ℞ Diasone . . . .   0.3 Gm. (gr. v)
        1 capsule 2 or 3 times a day.

78. ℞ Chaulmoogra oil   (ampul)
        1 to 5 cc. I.M. once or twice a week.

79. ℞ Chaulmoogra oil . . . . . .   0.3 cc.   (♏ v)
        1 to 5 capsules (enteric coated) after each
        meal.

80. ℞ Ethyl chaulmoograte   (ampul)
        1 to 5 cc. I.M. once or twice a week.

81. ℞ Ethyl chaulmoograte . . . .   0.3 cc.   (♏ v)
        1 to 5 capsules (enteric coated) after each
        meal.

82. ℞ Promin . . . .   5.0 Gm. (gr. lxxv)
      Water . . . . .q.s. ad 500.0   cc.   (℥ xvi)
        Solution for continuous wet dressings.

Other Chemotherapeutic Agents

83. ℞ "Mapharsen" (ampul)

    Yaws: 60 mg. I.V. weekly for 3 doses; for tertiary yaws give 8 such weekly injections.
    Relapsing fever: 40 to 60 mg. I.V. as fever is rising.

84. ℞ Neoarsphenamine (ampul)

    Yaws: 0.6 to 0.9 Gm. I.V. weekly for 3 doses; for tertiary yaws, 8 such weekly injections are given.
    Relapsing fever: 0.6 Gm. I.V. as fever is rising.

85. ℞ "Stovarsol" . . . . 0.25 Gm. (gr. iv)

    Relapsing fever: 6 tablets daily by mouth as fever is rising.

86. ℞ Bismuth Subsalicylate Injection U.S.P. (vial)

    0.2 Gm. I.M. weekly for 12 weeks.

87. ℞ Boric acid, 5% ointment. . . 4.0 Gm. (℥ i)

    Apply to lid margins several times a day.

88. ℞ Yellow Mercuric Oxide Ointment U.S.P. . . . . 4.0 Gm. (℥ i)

    Apply to lid margins several times a day.

89. ℞ Ammoniated mercury, 2% ointment . . . . 30.0 Gm. (℥ i)

    Apply to impetiginous areas.

90. ℞ Phenol, 1% ointment . . . . 30.0 Gm. (℥ i)

    Apply to crusts and lesions.

91. ℞ Para-aminobenzoic acid . . . 2.0 Gm. (℥ ss)

    Dissolve 1 powder in 3% soda bicarbonate solution and administer every 2 hours by mouth, followed by a half glass of water.

92. ℞ Silver nitrate, 2% solution . . 15.0 cc. (℥ ss)

    Swab the lid margins daily.

Biologicals

93. ℞ Diphtheria Antitoxin U.S.P. (vial)

    Administer according to dosage schedule given in text (*see* DIPHTHERIA).

94. ℞ Immune (Human) Serum Globulin N.N.R. (vial)

    Administer I.M. according to directions contained in the package insert or in the various treatment sections of the text.

95. ℞ Scarlet Fever Immune Serum
       (Human) N.F.   (vial)

   Prophylaxis: 10 to 20 cc. I.M.
   Treatment: 20 to 100 cc. I.M., depending on
   the patient's age and the severity of the illness.

96. ℞ Scarlet Fever Streptococcus
       Antitoxin U.S.P.   (vial)

   Prophylaxis: 3,000 u. I.M.
   Treatment: 9,000 u. I.M.; rarely I.V.

97. ℞ Typhoid and Paratyphoid Vac-
       cine U.S.P.   (vial)

   Begin with 0.1 cc. I.V. as a test dose. Repeat every other day with gradually increasing doses until symptoms of chorea subside
   or a 5 cc. dose of the combined vaccine has
   been reached.

98. ℞ Bivalent Gas Gangrene Anti-
       toxin U.S.P.   (vial)

   10,000 to 40,000 u. I.V. over 12 to 24 hours.

99. ℞ Tetanus Antitoxin U.S.P.
       (vial)

   Prophylaxis: 1,500 to 3,000 u. or more I.M.
   after skin testing.
   Treatment: Administer locally, I.M., or
   I.V., according to instructions given in the
   text (*see* TETANUS).

100. ℞ Tetanus Toxoid U.S.P.   (vial)

   For those previously immunized with toxoid, 1 cc. I.M. or subcut.

101. ℞ Rabies vaccine   (vial)

   Administer subcut. 14 to 28 doses, according
   to the manufacturer's recommendations contained in the package, and using alternately
   the tissues of the anterior abdominal wall
   and the interscapular region.

102. ℞ Leptospira antiserum (Horse)
        (vial)

   50 cc. I.M., repeated every 2 or 3 days if
   indicated.

103. ℞ Antianthrax serum   (vial)

   Administer according to directions contained in text (*see* ANTHRAX).

104. ℞ Pertussis hyperimmune serum
        (vial)

   Prophylaxis Human serum: 20 cc. I.M.
   Rabbit serum (refined): 4 cc. I.M.

(Cont'd)

Treatment Human serum: 20 to 60 cc. I.M.
or I.V. every 24 to 48 hours for 1 to 4 doses
(*see* PERTUSSIS).
Rabbit serum (refined): 4 to 8 cc. I.M. or
I.V. every 24 to 48 hours for 3 or 4 doses,
after testing for sensitivity.

105. ℞ Brucellin   (vial)

     0.1 cc. intradermally every 3 or 4 days for
     3 or 4 injections.

106. ℞ Brucella vaccine   (vial)

     0.1 to 0.25 cc. intradermally, gradually in-
     creasing the dose at 2 to 5 day intervals
     until a dose of 1 cc. is tolerated.

Mouthwashes and Gargles

107. ℞ Sodium chloride . . . . . .   4.0   Gm. (℥ i)
     Sodium bicarbonate. . . . .   2.0   Gm. (℥ ss)
     Water. . . . . .q.s. ad 500.0   cc.   (℥ xvi)

     Use undiluted as a mouthwash.

108. ℞ Alkaline   Aromatic   Solution
     N.F. . . . . 90.0   cc.   (℥ iii)

     Dilute with an equal volume of water and
     use as a mouthwash every 4 hours.

109. ℞ Potassium chlorate . . . . .   8.0   Gm. (℥ ii)
     Myrrh Tincture U.S.P. . . . 16.0   cc.   (℥ iv)
     Camphor Water U.S.P. q.s. ad 240.0   cc.   (℥ viii)

     Shake well and use as a mouthwash or
     gargle every 3 hours.

110. ℞ Sodium bicarbonate. . . . .   5.0   Gm. (gr. lxxv)
     Peppermint Water U.S.P. . . 120.0   cc.   (℥ iv)
     Distilled water. . . . q.s. ad 240.0   cc.   (℥ viii)

     Use as a spray or mouthwash as necessary.

111. ℞ Thymol . . . .   0.12 Gm. (gr. ii)
     Sodium borate . . . .   0.3   Gm. (gr. v)
     Ethyl Alcohol U.S.P. . . . .   0.6   cc.   (♏ x)
     Water. . . . . 250.0   cc.   (℥ viii)

     Use as mouthwash, gargle or spray several
     times daily.

112. ℞ Hydrogen peroxide, 3% solu-
     tion

     Dilute 1:4 and use as throat gargle 3 times
     daily.

Drugs Affecting the Autonomic Nervous System

113. ℞ Epinephrine hydrochloride,
1:1,000 solution (ampul)

0.3 to 1 cc. (℔ v to xv) subcut., I.M. or
I.V. to combat serum sensitivity.

114. ℞ Neostigmine methylsulfate,
1:2,000 solution (ampul)

1 cc. (0.5 mg.) subcut. To antagonize the
effect of tubocurarine administer I.V.; the
undesirable side effects of neostigmine may
be lessened by the simultaneous injection of
atropine (℞ 115).

115. ℞ Atropine sulfate (hypodermic
tablet)

0.3 to 0.6 mg. (gr. 1/200 to 1/100) subcut.,
I.M. or I.V.

116. ℞ "Neo-Synephrine Hydrochloride," 0.25% solution in isotonic saline. . . . . 30.0 cc. (℥ i)

1 or 2 drops in each nostril every 3 hours.

117. ℞ Homatropine hydrobromide,
1% solution . . . . . . 15.0 cc. (℥ ss)

1 drop in each eye once daily.

118. ℞ Belladonna Tincture U.S.P. . 15.0 cc. (℥ ss)

12 drops hourly for 2 or 3 doses.

119. ℞ Ephedrine sulfate . . . . . 25 mg. (gr. ⅜)

1 capsule every 3 hours if necessary.

Smooth Muscle Stimulants

120. ℞ "Pitressin" (ampul)

0.25 to 0.5 cc. (℔ iv to viii) subcut. or I.M.
every 3 to 4 hours.

121. ℞ Posterior Pituitary Injection
U.S.P. (ampul)

0.2 to 0.3 cc. (℔ iii to v) subcut. every 3 or
4 hours.

Antipruritics

122. ℞ Olive oil . . . . 96.0 cc. (℥ iii)
Glycerin . . . . 24.0 cc. (℥ vi)

Apply to skin, after bathing, for relief of
itching.

123. ℞ Peppermint Oil U.S.P. . . . 0.3 cc. (℔ v)
Olive oil . . . . 90.0 cc. (℥ iii)

Apply to skin for relief of itching.

124. ℞ Phenolated Calamine Lotion
N.F. . . . . 120.0 cc. (℥ iv)

Apply to skin for relief of itching twice daily.

125. ℞ Mercury bichloride, 1:1,000
solution . . . . 240.0 cc. (℥ viii)

Apply to skin for relief of itching.

126. ℞ Camphor . . . . 6.0 Gm. (℥ iss)
Zinc oxide . . . . 15.0 Gm. (℥ ss)
Starch. . . . . 20.0 Gm. (℥ v)

Apply freely as dusting powder.

127. ℞ Zinc oxide . . . . 8.0 Gm. (℥ ii)
Sodium bicarbonate. . . . 8.0 Gm. (℥ ii)
Starch. . . . . 24.0 Gm. (℥ vi)
Talc. . . . . 20.0 Gm. (℥ v)

Dust on lesions several times daily.

Antidiarrheal Agents

128. ℞ Camphorated Opium Tincture
(Paregoric) U.S.P. . . . . 30.0 cc. (℥ i)

1 to 2 teaspoons, repeated as required.

129. ℞ Bismuth subcarbonate. . . . 0.6 Gm. (gr. x)

2 or 3 powders as required.

130. ℞ Opium, pulverized . . . . . 30 mg. (gr. ss)

1 capsule repeated as required.

Vitamins, Tonics, and Digestants

131. ℞ Thiamine hydrochloride (vial)

50 mg. I.M. daily for 3 days.

132. ℞ Thiamine hydrochloride . . . 5 mg.

1 tablet 3 times a day, before meals.

133. ℞ Menadione. . . . . 2 mg.

1 tablet daily.

134. ℞ Menadione sodium bisulfite
(ampul)

60 mg. daily, subcut., I.M. or I.V.

135. ℞ Calciferol

50,000 to 300,000 u. daily. (Blood calcium studies every 2 weeks; if above 12 mg./100 cc., stop medication.)

136. ℞ Dihydrotachysterol (A.T. 10)   0.6   mg.

> 6 capsules daily for first 3 days followed by 1 or 2 capsules daily. (Blood calcium studies every 2 weeks; if above 12 mg./100 cc., stop medication.)

137. ℞ Elixir Iron, Quinine, and
       Strychnine N.F. . . . . . 120.0 cc.   (℥ iv)

> 1 teaspoon in water before each meal.

138. ℞ Pancreatin. . . . .   0.3   Gm. (gr. v)

> 1 tablet (crushed, if necessary) with each meal.

Laxatives

139. ℞ Liquid Petrolatum U.S.P.

> 1 or 2 tablespoons each night.

140. ℞ Milk of Magnesia U.S.P.

> 1 to 4 teaspoons at bedtime.

Cough Mixtures and Inhalations

141. ℞ Compound Benzoin Tincture
       U.S.P. . . . . 30.0 cc.   (℥ i)

> 1 teaspoon in a pint of boiling water; inhale steam 2 or 3 times daily.

142. ℞ Ammonium chloride. . . . . 10.0   Gm. (℥ iiss)
       Syrup of Glycyrrhiza U.S.P.
              q.s. ad 120.0   cc.   (℥ iv)

> 1 teaspoon in water every 4 hours.

143. ℞ Menthol. . . . . 0.12 Gm. (gr. ii)
       Chloroform . . . . 1.0 cc.   (♏ xv)
       Compound Benzoin Tincture
       U.S.P. . . . . 30.0 cc.   (℥ i)

> 1 teaspoon to a quart of boiling water; inhale vapor 2 or 3 times a day.

144. ℞ Terpin Hydrate and Codeine
       Elixir N.F. . . . . . . 120.0 cc.   (℥ iv)

> 1 to 2 teaspoons every 4 hours for cough.

Antiseptic Baths

145. ℞ Mercury bichloride, 1:10,000
       solution

> Prepare by dissolving 1⅓ to 2 teaspoons (16 to 24 Gm.) of mercuric chloride in an average tub bath (40 to 60 gallons).

146. ℞ Sodium bicarbonate (bulk)

> Add 1 cup (8 ounces) to an average tub bath (40 to 60 gallons).

Miscellaneous

147. ℞ d-Tubocurarine in 4.8% wax
in peanut oil (ampul containing 27 mg./cc.)

Administer according to instructions given
in the text (*see* TETANUS).

148. ℞ Ichthammol N.F. . . . . . 3.0 cc. (℥ xlv)
Hydrous Lanolin . . . . . . 30.0 cc. (℥ i)

Apply to ulcer once every 1 or 2 days.

149. ℞ Glucose, 50% solution
(ampul) . . . . 50.0 cc.

50 cc. I.V. as required.

150. ℞ Calcium gluconate, 10% solution (ampul)

10 cc. (1 Gm.) I.V., slowly, every 12 to 24
hours if necessary.

151. ℞ Sodium bicarbonate. . . . . 3.0 Gm. (gr. xlv)
Water. . . . . q.s. ad 300.0 cc. (℥ x)

2 ounces by mouth every 15 minutes.

152. ℞ Sodium bicarbonate (bulk
powder)

¼ to ⅓ teaspoon every 4 hours, given with
each dose of sodium salicylate (℞ 2).

LIVER AND BILIARY

LIVER AND BILIARY TRACT

The liver, the largest secreting organ in the body, possesses a major degree of reserve functional capacity, unusual resistance to damage by noxious substances, and extraordinary powers of regeneration following injury. Up to 80% of the liver cells may be damaged without producing severe symptoms, and complete recovery may ensue. The functions of the liver are many, but accurate information concerning them is far from complete.

The functional unit of the liver, the hepatic lobule, might be considered as a tube (bile capillary) whose walls are in juxtaposition with cords of liver cells; one end empties into a bile duct, while the other end is closed. Bile is excreted from small canaliculi into the larger capillary and thence into the duct. Blood from the portal vein enters the one end of this unit, filters past and between the cords of liver cells, and exits into the hepatic vein. Blood from the hepatic artery supplies the cells and also empties into the hepatic vein.

Bile is formed continuously, about 23 cc./hr. in waking hours and 15 cc./hr. during sleep (about 500 cc. in 24 hrs.), at a pressure of about 25 to 30 cm. of bile.

The bile consists of bile salts, bile pigments, mucin, fatty acids, cholesterol, lecithin, and inorganic salts. Bile salts are conjugated in the liver; bilirubin (the principal bile pigment) is modified by passage through the liver cells, and the de-esterification of cholesterol is believed to take place in the liver, the free cholesterol being passed into the bile.

Formation of urea, serum albumin, fibrinogen, prothrombin, heparin, glycogen, ketone bodies, and conjugated glycuronates is believed to occur in the liver.

Additional functions of or attributable to the liver are the deaminization of proteins, destruction of uric acid, storage of glycogen, detoxification of bacterial and mineral poisons, and the secretion, modification or absorption of foreign materials such as dyes and drugs.

Liver disease may be parenchymal, biliary, or circulatory. Damage may be patchy (scattered, localized, zonal), or diffuse (all cells affected). There are no clear-cut pathologic limitations for liver disease because of the overlapping interrelationship of the many factors.

LIVER FUNCTION TESTS

In disease, one or more of the many liver functions usually will be interfered with, but rarely all. Therefore, no single test can be expected to reveal all the dysfunctions, nor, on the other hand, can all tests of hepatic function be employed readily in the study of a single case. Tests must be selected to suit the need of the individual patient and even under well controlled conditions there often is a diversity of results because of the complex interrelationships of liver function and structure. Laboratory findings must be interpreted by careful correlation with clinical observations.

Indications for Liver Function Tests

These include such conditions as the demonstrated presence of an enlarged liver; a small liver; a liver that is tender or nodular; jaundice; either fatty or clay-colored stools; hyperthyroidism; or alcoholism. Liver function tests should be performed in the presence of a significant degree of the following conditions, especially if these are not otherwise accounted for: dark stools; dark urine; hemorrhagic phenomena; splenomegaly; pruritus; flatulence; anorexia; nausea and vomiting; or nutritional deficiency. The selection will depend upon the nature of clinical findings. The following tests are grouped according to the functional factor they are capable of assessing.

PIGMENT METABOLISM

Bilirubin is the principal pigment in blood serum and bile. It is the porphyrin fraction of hemoglobin, and is released by the disintegration of erythrocytes. Any disturbance that causes increased destruction of red cells results in an increase of bilirubin. The amount of blood pigment can be estimated by the icterus index determination.

Icterus Index

This test is made by comparing the intensity of the yellow tint in the blood serum with a standard colored solution. When used serially, it accurately determines the increase or decrease of jaundice. Values are determined by the following formula:

$$\frac{\text{Standard reading}}{\text{Unknown reading}} \times \text{dilution} = \text{icterus index}$$

Values: Normal 3 to 5; latent jaundice 6 to 15; clinical jaundice, above 15.

This is not a direct test of hepatic function; its usefulness is limited to jaundiced patients; pigments in the blood, other than bilirubin, may interfere with the readings, especially in low grade jaundice (e.g., carrots in the diet impart a yellow color of high index to the blood serum, and hemolysis of the blood specimen from careless technic deepens the color).

From 0.2 to 0.8 mg./100 cc. of bilirubin is normally present in the blood. Whether due to low concentration or from chemical attachment to some complex serum molecule, bilirubin in this form causes the delayed or indirect van den Bergh reaction. After passage through the liver into the bile, the bilirubin is either concentrated or modified (split off the complex molecule) so that it normally causes the immediate or direct van den Bergh reaction. Having passed through the bile passages, the bilirubin is converted in the intestines into stercobilinogen (urobilinogen), which is the pigment that gives normal color to the feces. Most of this is excreted in the stool, but a small portion is absorbed from the intestinal tract into the portal circulation and again passed into the liver. Most of this fraction is re-excreted into the bile or converted in the liver, but a small amount escapes into the general circulation, is carried to the kidneys and excreted in the urine as urobilinogen. Oxidation in the urine (rapid when exposed to light) produces urobilin. This cycle is termed the enterohepatic circulation of bile pigment. Interruption or augmentation of this cycle at any point will produce detectable changes which provide clues to the nature of the liver disorder.

Serum Bilirubin

Quantitative van den Bergh: This test is used to measure the amount of bilirubin in the blood serum. It is far more accurate than the icterus index in early, subclinical, or low grade disease. A concentration above 0.5 to 0.8 mg./100 cc. usually indicates the presence of disease. Values: Normal 0.2 to 0.8 mg./100 cc.; latent jaundice 0.8 to 3 mg./100 cc.; clinical jaundice above 3 mg./100 cc.

The disadvantages of this test are that it does not distinguish between various types of jaundice and is more difficult to perform than the icterus index.

Qualitative van den Bergh: Bilirubin unmodified in the

blood serum gives a delayed or indirect van den Bergh reaction. This test requires the addition of alcohol to produce the color reaction. Modified bilirubin, altered by passage through the liver unit into the bile passages, causes an immediate or direct van den Bergh reaction. In normal serum, a direct van den Bergh reaction indicates that bilirubin has reentered the blood after passage through and alteration by the liver cells. This suggests a regurgitation or backflow in the pigment cycle. A biphasic or mixed reaction may indicate the presence of both types of bilirubin. The test is useful in distinguishing between types of jaundice and in determining their origin (parenchymal, biliary, or hemolytic). However, the frequent overlapping of different factors in liver disease causes mixed results which are difficult to interpret accurately.

Urine Bilirubin

Bilirubin is not found normally in the urine. The renal threshold for normal serum bilirubin is high and is exceeded only in cases of severe hemolytic jaundice or liver damage. The modified bilirubin (prompt, directly reacting) is more diffusible than the unmodified serum bilirubin (delayed reacting type) and passes more readily through the capillary walls into the tissues and urine. Therefore, the finding of modified bilirubin in the urine is common in regurgitant or obstructive jaundice, while the presence of unmodified bilirubin is unusual except in severe retention jaundice.

Bilirubin gives the urine a greenish yellow, yellow, or brown color which is imparted to the foam on shaking the specimen. Cells, casts, and other structures in the sediment also may be stained brown or yellow.

Fecal Urobilinogen (Stercobilinogen)

From 100 to 200 mg. of stercobilinogen is excreted in the feces daily. The amount of bilirubin that reaches the intestinal tract and is there converted by bacteria into stercobilirubin determines the amount to be excreted. Increased formation of bilirubin, as in the hemolytic anemias, increases the quantity of stercobilinogen, as evidenced by dark colored stools. Decrease of bilirubin in the intestine due to bile blockage or failure of the liver to excrete the bilirubin, decreases or eliminates stercobilinogen in the feces, causing the stools to appear clay colored.

Urinary Urobilinogen (Urobilin)

Normally, 0.5 to 1.5 mg. of urobilinogen absorbed from the intestines is excreted in the urine daily. This is converted by oxidation into urobilin. A normal quantity in the urine usually signifies the presence of bile in the intestinal tract (i.e., no obstruction to bile flow). An increase suggests increased production of bilirubin or failure of the hepatic cells to convert or re-excrete that portion of urobilinogen which has been absorbed from the intestinal tract, thereby increasing the amount to be excreted by the kidneys. This indicates excessive hemolysis, parenchymal damage or partial biliary obstruction. A decrease in the amount suggests malabsorption from the colon (as in diarrhea), diminished formation of bilirubin, or complete biliary obstruction (e.g., by neoplasm).

CARBOHYDRATE METABOLISM

The liver stores glycogen and is closely concerned with its formation and utilization. Disturbances of hepatic cell function may result in a tendency to fasting hypoglycemia, diminished glucose and galactose tolerance, diminished blood sugar response to epinephrine, and occasionally glycosuria and increased blood lactic acid concentration. While each of these is a valuable diagnostic aid, disturbances of this nature appear irregularly and usually late in hepatic disease and their diagnostic value is therefore limited; i.e., liver damage may be extensive before carbohydrate metabolism is detectably altered.

PROTEIN METABOLISM

Hepatic parenchymal cells are concerned with the formation of fibrinogen, prothrombin, albumin, and globulin as well as with the deaminization of the amino acids, and the formation of ammonia; and from the ammonia, urea. Total protein and albumin-globulin ratio determinations are altered in certain forms of parenchymal liver disease (hepatitis, cirrhosis, circulatory disturbances, amyloid disease). Prothrombin is another, presumably protein, constituent of the blood which is formed in the liver in the presence of adequate vitamin K. The hemorrhagic tendency in patients with both obstructive and hepatocellular jaundice is common. Inadequate absorption of vitamin K from the intestine or hepatic cell dysfunction preventing its utilization reduces the amount of prothrombin formed. There is a wide margin of safety, however, since bleeding and the hemorrhagic tendency occur only when the prothrombin falls below 20% of its normal level.

A therapeutic test is possible in certain cases. Since bile salts in the intestine probably are essential for the absorption of vitamin K, in cases of hypoprothrombinemia due to uncomplicated common duct obstruction (bile blocked off from intestine), the I.M. administration of vitamin K will produce a prompt increase in the serum prothrombin level, but will produce little or no response if the hypoprothrombinemia is due to profound hepatocellular damage.

Cephalin-Cholesterol Flocculation Test

This test is useful in detecting parenchymal damage in hepatitis, chronic hepatic disease, and damage from biliary blockage. When certain abnormal serums are added to a cephalin-cholesterol emulsion, flocculation of certain protein elements occurs. This is a sensitive and reliable test for hepatocellular dysfunction, which can be used equally well in the study of jaundiced and nonjaundiced patients. It is roughly quantitative (readings from 1+ to 4+) and requires only one venipuncture. However, the technic must be exact. False positive reactions may occur in allergic or pregnant patients and in the newborn; also when the specimen is contaminated by heavy metals, strong acids, or bacteria. Anticoagulants in the plasma may interfere with flocculation. Strong light affects the test. The serum must be fresh. Reagents are expensive and must be freshly prepared daily. The test cannot be properly interpreted in less than 48 hours.

Thymol Turbidity and Flocculation Test

Turbidity occurs in a reagent solution when certain abnormal serums are added. The degree of turbidity is reported in arbitrary units based on comparison with a prepared standard. Flocculation, reported as 1+ to 4+, appears on standing overnight but is not an essential part of the test. Although not specific for liver disease, the test is sensitive and reliable when properly performed. With hepatitis, chronic liver disease, or biliary tract disease, a positive reaction suggests parenchymal liver damage roughly proportional to the degree of turbidity.

FAT METABOLISM

The bile salts produced by the liver are essential in the emulsification and digestion of fat. Liver cells also play a part in lipid metabolism and since concentrations of cholesterol and cholesterol esters can be measured, the following tests are useful in evaluating liver function.

Cholesterol, Cholesterol Ester Values

Repeated determinations of cholesterol partition are of considerable prognostic value. The ester fraction normally constitutes 60 to 80% of the total cholesterol. A fall in cholesterol ester value with resultant alteration of the ratio occurs in the presence of hepatocellular lesions such as acute toxemia, certain metal poisonings (e.g., bismuth and arsenicals), and acute inflammatory lesions of the liver. The fall in the ester value parallels to some extent the degree of liver damage.

In chronic hepatic dysfunctions such as uncomplicated portal cirrhosis and in long-standing common duct obstruction, both cholesterol and cholesterol ester values usually are normal, but the ester value may drop terminally. The lowering of a previously normal cholesterol ester value must be regarded as a serious prognostic sign. Elevation of both cholesterol and cholesterol esters usually occurs in conditions that prevent the bile from reaching the intestine (as in complete common duct obstruction, external biliary fistula).

DYE EXCRETING CAPACITY

This test consists of injecting into the blood stream a dye (bromsulfalein) that will be excreted almost exclusively by the liver. The amount of dye retained in the blood stream is measured after a definite length of time. Abnormal dye retention indicates hepatic dysfunction.

The 5 mg./Kg. body wt. bromsulfalein liver function test is sensitive and reliable for the detection of functional impairment of the liver and gives but few false positive reactions. It usually is positive even when liver damage is relatively minor. However, the test is useless when the patient is jaundiced. There may be occasional untoward reactions (headache, faintness, chills), but these usually are slight and transient. This test is especially useful in preoperative studies of patients with cholelithiasis, thyroid disease, and hepatocellular damage without jaundice. Normal retention is 5% or less in 45 minutes.

DETOXIFICATION CAPACITY

Another important function of the liver is the detoxification of poisons; toxic substances are converted into less toxic compounds which are subsequently eliminated in the bile and urine. The liver's ability to perform this function can be tested by giving sodium benzoate orally or I.V. Normally, this will be conjugated by the liver with aminoacetic acid and excreted as hippuric acid in the urine. A low excretion of hippuric acid (normal about 3 Gm./4 hrs.) suggests catarrhal jaundice, various types of hepatitis, cirrhosis, or liver malignancy (usually metastatic). As compared with the I.V. test, the oral method is somewhat less sensitive; it requires 4 hours instead of 1, and sometimes causes nausea and vomiting; in the presence of gastric retention there is delay in absorption. With renal damage, incomplete emptying of the bladder, or dehydration, the urinary flow is not sufficient to permit accurate estimates by either method of administration. Reading of the I.V. test is based on the normal excretion of 1 Gm. or more of hippuric acid (equivalent to 0.68 Gm. benzoic acid) in the first hour after injection.

ENZYME FUNCTION

Serum phosphatase determinations may be of limited use in differentiating obstructive from hepatocellular jaundice. These values roughly parallel the increase of serum bilirubin in obstructive jaundice and may reach 40 to 60 Bodansky u. of phosphatase activity/100 cc. In hepatocellular jaundice, the serum phosphatase rarely rises above 12 Bodansky u. even though the bilirubin increases progressively. The possibility of extrahepatic lesions, particularly certain skeletal disorders, always must be considered in interpreting high values.

The combination of a high phosphatase level with a high serum bilirubin level supports a diagnosis of obstructive (regurgitation) jaundice, while only moderately increased serum

LABORATORY DIAGNOSIS IN

TESTS	HEPATOCELLULAR DAMAGE	
	Acute	Chronic
For Pigment Metabolism		
Icterus Index	Variable, usually elevated	Variable
Quantitative van den Bergh (serum bilirubin)	Variable, usually elevated	Variable
Qualitative van den Bergh	Biphasic or mixed, variable	Variable
Urine Bilirubin	Positive	Variable
Fecal Urobilinogen (Stercobilinogen)	Variable, usually normal	Variable, usually normal
Urine Urobilinogen	Marked increase	Slight increase
For Carbohydrate Metabolism		
Glucose Tolerance	Diminished	Variable, usually diminished
Galactose Tolerance	Diminished	Variable, usually diminished
Fasting Blood Sugar	Variable, may be diminished	Diminished late
For Protein Metabolism		
Total Serum Protein	Normal unless severe or of long standing	Diminished
Albumin-Globulin (A/G) Ratio	Normal or reduced, variable	Usually reduced
Cephalin-Cholesterol Flocculation	Positive	Positive
Thymol Turbidity	Positive	Positive
Prothrombin	Usually decreased; no response to vitamin K	Usually decreased; no response to vitamin K
For Fat Metabolism		
Cholesterol	Normal or reduced	Normal
Cholesterol Ester	Low	Variable
For Dye Excreting Capacity		
Bromsulfalein	Dye retained	Dye retained
For Detoxification Capacity		
Hippuric Acid (I.V.)	Decreased	Decreased
For Enzyme Function		
Alkaline Phosphatase	Slightly increased	Slightly increased

HEPATIC DISEASE AND JAUNDICE

OBSTRUCTIVE JAUNDICE		HEMOLYTIC JAUNDICE
Partial (stone)	Complete (neoplasm)	
Increased, but fluctuating	Increased	Increased
Increased, but fluctuating	Increased	Increased
Direct, immediate reacting	Direct, immediate reacting	Indirect, delayed reacting
Positive	Positive	Negative, except in severe cases
Variable; may be increased when obstruction is relieved	Negative	Increased
Variable; may be increased after obstruction is relieved	Negative	Increased
Normal	Normal	Normal
Normal	Normal	Normal
Normal	Normal	Normal
Normal	Normal (if uncomplicated)	Normal
Normal	Normal (if uncomplicated)	Normal
Negative early	Negative early	Normal (if uncomplicated)
Negative early	Negative early	Normal (if uncomplicated)
Decreased late; responds to vitamin K	Decreased late; responds to vitamin K	Normal
Elevated	Elevated	Normal
Normal ratio	Normal ratio	Normal

(In jaundice, discoloration of the serum interferes with reading the test.)

Normal, early	Normal, early	Normal
Much increased	Much increased	Normal

phosphatase with high serum bilirubin supports a diagnosis of hepatocellular jaundice. It must be remembered that there is much overlapping of phosphatase values in both obstructive and hepatocellular jaundice.

JAUNDICE

Discoloration of tissues and body fluids with bile pigment. Although **clinical jaundice** is readily perceived, there may be a significant increase in serum bilirubin (or icterus index) detectable only by laboratory tests (q.v.). This is called **latent jaundice**.

Types

A. Retention jaundice: (1) Due to inability of the liver to dispose of abnormally increased bile pigments in the circulating blood resulting from excessive breakdown (disintegration) of erythrocytes. This type is encountered in the hemolytic anemias, sickle cell anemia, pernicious anemia, and jaundice of the newborn; also in malaria, pneumococcic pneumonia, yellow fever, and bacteremias. In these conditions, the urine contains increased urobilinogen but no free bile or bilirubin. The van den Bergh reaction is indirect, the serum phosphatase is normal, and the cephalin flocculation test negative. These tests, together with signs of anemia or of increased red cell fragility, establish the diagnosis. (2) Due to inability of damaged parenchymal cells to process and excrete normally circulating quantities of bile pigments (hepatocellular jaundice).

B. Obstructive (regurgitation) jaundice: Due to a "backing-up" or reflux of bile into the blood stream due to intrahepatic or extrahepatic biliary obstruction. With increased intrabiliary pressure there is leakage of bile from the small ducts into adjacent lymph spaces and capillaries of the liver. This type of jaundice is characterized by a direct van den Bergh reaction and the presence of bilirubin in the urine. It is seen chiefly in three conditions: (1) stone or stricture of the bile ducts; (2) neoplasm involving the head of the pancreas, gallbladder, or bile ducts; (3) encroachment upon smaller biliary radicles in parenchymal liver disease, such as acute hepatitis or cirrhosis. Clinical differentiation depends upon a careful history, physical signs, and laboratory studies. Pain and rigidity in the right upper quadrant, pruritus, and fever may occur in all three conditions but are more typical of stone in the common duct.

1. Stone in common duct (*see also* BILIARY DISORDERS): There frequently is a past history of abdominal distress and intolerance to fatty foods. Sudden colicky pain in the right upper quadrant, local spasm, fever, and jaundice are characteristic. Jaundice is obstructive in type but usually is intermittent or partial. Hence, varying amounts of urobilinogen appear in the urine and feces.

2. Neoplasm: This diagnosis should be suspected when an elderly person exhibits jaundice of steadily increasing intensity, with signs of complete biliary obstruction. Stools are acholic and urine contains no urobilinogen. Pain may or may not be present. The finding of a distended, nontender gallbladder is corroborative evidence.

3. Parenchymal liver disease: In acute hepatitis (q.v.), jaundice usually appears at onset and subsides within 10 days. In cirrhosis of the liver (q.v.), jaundice seldom is conspicuous. Other clinical features pointing to parenchymal liver disease may include splenomegaly; nodular liver; appearance of vascular "spiders" on the face, chest, and upper extremities; enlargement of collateral abdominal veins; ascites; and laboratory tests indicative of impaired liver function.

Treatment

Therapy should be directed toward the underlying disease. Surgical measures are imperative when there is evidence of extrahepatic biliary obstruction. Diligent preoperative and postoperative dietary care is essential since prolonged obstruction to bile flow may cause serious hepatic damage. The regimen is similar to that for cirrhosis (q.v.), except for moderate restriction of fat because of decreased bile flow. A suitable diet contains 125 Gm. protein, 375 Gm. carbohydrate, and 100 Gm. fat/day. Protein and fat should be derived chiefly from meat, eggs, and milk. Where evidence suggests that fat is not being properly absorbed by the intestine, absorption may be aided by the use of a wetting agent, such as the polyoxyethylene derivative of sorbitan monooleate, given as 1.5 Gm. doses with each meal (R 21).

In patients with hypoproteinemia, extra feedings of protein supplements are advisable (*see* PROTEIN DEFICIENCY). If nausea or abdominal distress prevents adequate food intake, parenteral therapy is indicated in the form of daily infusions of 10% glucose or of 5% glucose, plus parenteral amino acids mixtures, or 500 to 1,000 cc. of plasma by slow drip. The addition of 50 to 100 mg. thiamine (R 27) and 100 to 200 mg. nicotinamide (R 28) has been advocated. Concentrated human serum albumin solution I.V. is ideal therapy when there is a pronounced reduction of serum albumin.

Vitamin K, 10 mg. by mouth (R 24) or 2 mg. by injection (R 25, 26) should be administered daily to correct a prolonged prothrombin time or bleeding tendency. Bile salts (R 22) should be administered in conjunction with oral vitamin K therapy when there is evidence of obstruction to the flow of bile, but the cathartic tendency of the bile salts must be guarded against. If the prothrombin time fails to become normal after vitamin K therapy, liver damage should be suspected. In this event, transfusion is necessary if surgery is contemplated.

ACUTE HEPATITIS

Inflammation of the liver caused by infectious or toxic agents, characterized by jaundice and frequently by hepatomegaly; usually accompanied by fever and other systemic disorders.

Etiology

The infectious agents that may cause hepatitis are viruses, spirochetes, protozoa, and bacteria. The toxic agents are such substances as carbon tetrachloride, arsenicals, tetrachloroethane, and cinchophen.

Pathology

The pathologic changes may be diffuse, zonal or a combination of both.

Diffuse (common form): This is characterized by cellular infiltration, interstitial edema and necrosis of the liver cells. The cells are chaotically disarranged and the normal pattern of the liver cords is lost. The reticular framework and vascular channels usually remain intact, thereby permitting restoration of the normal architecture on healing. Jaundice is probably due to disruption of the intercellular bile canaliculi and to bile thrombi. In rapidly fatal cases, further dissolution of tissue terminates in acute yellow atrophy. The liver is shrunken and flabby, and necrotic cells interspersed with dense tissue (collapsed stroma) are seen. Fatal cases with a longer course develop healed yellow atrophy, which progresses to a coarse nodular cirrhosis (q.v.).

Zonal: The inflammation is focused chiefly at the portal radicles with resulting cellular reaction, bile duct proliferation, and increase in connective tissue. These changes are seen in recurrent hepatitis. Most patients recover completely, but a few develop hypertrophic biliary, or "cholangiolitic," cirrhosis (q.v.).

INFECTIOUS HEPATITIS
(Epidemic hepatitis; Catarrhal jaundice)

A common type of acute hepatitis which occurs sporadically or in epidemics and is caused by viruses which are introduced by fecally contaminated food or water. Young people are most frequently affected, and the peak incidence is in the late autumn. Epidemics become widespread in wartime. Crowding, poor sanitation, malnutrition, and preexisting liver damage are predisposing factors. The incubation period is 2 to 6 weeks.

Onset of symptoms usually is abrupt, with anorexia, nausea, fever and malaise. Tenderness and enlargement of the liver and pain in the right upper quadrant are usual early symptoms. Jaundice appears about 5 days after onset, at which time the fever tends to subside, while the gastrointestinal symptoms persist for about 10 days and subside with the regression of the jaundice. Lymphadenopathy is common. Splenomegaly is noted in about 15% of cases. Severe generalized pruritus, urticaria, and intermittent diarrhea occur occasionally. Many mild cases fail to develop icterus, and this fact should be borne in mind during epidemics.

Laboratory Findings

In the pre-icteric and icteric stages of infectious hepatitis, the urine may contain bile (bilirubin), and the serum reactions for cephalin flocculation and bromsulfalein retention may be abnormal. The appearance of clay-colored stools and bilirubinemia in the first days of jaundice suggests a complicating biliary obstruction. With progression of the disease there may be increased urobilinogenuria, prolonged prothrombin time, slightly decreased serum albumin, increased globulin, and decreased serum cholesterol. These revert to normal upon recovery. If a prolonged prothrombin time fails to respond to vitamin K therapy, or if there is definite change in serum protein or cholesterol partitions, a severe form of the disease should be suspected (see LIVER FUNCTION TESTS).

Diagnosis

Symptoms of fever, gastrointestinal disturbances and liver tenderness, together with laboratory signs of liver damage, should suggest the diagnosis.

Course and Prognosis

Usually, patients recover uneventfully after 6 to 8 weeks of illness. Relapses occur in about 15% and generally are due to premature resumption of activity, intercurrent infections, poor dietary management, or alcoholism. Mild residual symptoms and slight changes in liver function may persist for a year or more after recovery. These symptoms consist of right upper quadrant pain and tenderness and intolerance of fatty foods. Slight changes often are noted in cephalin flocculation, urine urobilinogen excretion, the bromsulfalein dye test, and serum bilirubin. In a small group, estimated at about 0.2%, acute yellow atrophy (q.v.) supervenes. This usually occurs within 2 weeks after onset of jaundice, but may take the form of a relapse after several months of illness. The onset of acute yellow atrophy is marked by deepening jaundice, mental confusion or torpor, hemorrhagic phenomena, pernicious vomiting, and ascites. These symptoms, together with severe functional derangement as evidenced by laboratory tests, are ominous.

Prophylaxis

Since it is known that the virus is transmitted from the feces of an infected patient, strict isolation technic (*see* BEDSIDE PROC.) should be instituted at least during the active phase of the disease. Unfortunately, there is no information at present as to the persistence of viable virus in the stools after the acute phase is over or whether a carrier state exists, which might suggest the need for continued precautions.

Treatment

The patient should remain in bed while jaundice, abdominal pain, and liver tenderness are present and until liver function tests become essentially normal. A minimum of 3 weeks' bed rest is advisable. The diet should be rich in protein and carbohydrate. The fats should be chiefly from dairy foods such as cream, butter, milk, and eggs. Where evidence suggests that fat is not being properly absorbed by the intestine, the process may be aided by the use of a wetting agent, such as the polyoxyethylene derivative of sorbitan monooleate, given as 1.5 Gm. doses with each meal (℞ 21). A satisfactory diet contains approximately 150 Gm. protein, 375 Gm. carbohydrate, and 150 Gm. fat. Thiamine (℞ 27), 10 mg. daily, may be added to stimulate appetite. In severe hepatitis, slow I.V. infusions of 10% glucose in water, or 5% glucose in saline (2,000 to 3,000 cc. daily) should be given. Patients with hemorrhagic tendencies should receive 10 mg. of vitamin K daily (℞ 24) and whole blood transfusions. After recovery, physical activity must be resumed very gradually to avoid relapse.

HOMOLOGOUS SERUM JAUNDICE
(Inoculation hepatitis; Transfusion jaundice)

Hepatitis following such procedures as blood transfusion, I.V. plasma therapy, and vaccination for yellow fever, due to inoculation with a virus similar to that of epidemic hepatitis. Although this virus may be in the blood stream long before onset of the disease, it is not recoverable from the stool as in epidemic hepatitis and there is no cross-immunity with epidemic hepatitis. Since the virus is not killed by 70% alcohol, epidemics have been traced to unsterile stylets used for taking blood counts, to unsterile syringes used in drawing blood, and to the use of a common syringe for mass inoculations. Recent experiments indicate that ultraviolet radiation of blood and plasma prior to use in transfusions may eliminate the danger of transmitting homologous serum jaundice. Where the line should be drawn between precautions which are feasible and those which will give maximum protection is an important but unsettled question.

The incubation period of homologous serum jaundice may be short (2 to 4 weeks) but usually is about 2 to 4½ months.

The onset generally is more gradual and less characterized by fever than in epidemic hepatitis, but the clinical picture is almost indistinguishable. Mortality rates have varied from 0.2 to 19% in different series. This variation probably is related to the virulence of different viral strains. The pathologic changes, clinical manifestations, and treatment are the same as those described for infectious hepatitis (q.v.).

TOXIC HEPATITIS

Hepatitis which may be caused by a wide variety of chemicals which can be taken into the system by inhalation, ingestion, skin absorption, or injection.

Etiology and Pathology

Among the responsible agents are carbon tetrachloride (most common), chloroform, tetrachloroethane, and other halogenated hydrocarbons; trinitrotoluene, arsenicals, phosphorus, and quinoline derivatives such as cinchophen. In some instances, the liver injury is directly related to the degree of exposure; in others, sensitivity to the agent (e.g., cinchophen, the sulfonamides) appears to play a part.

An important function of the liver is the detoxification of circulating poisons, which is accomplished chiefly by hydrolysis, conjugation, oxidation, and acetylation. Certain chemicals taken in excess not only injure the liver directly but also interfere with its ability to detoxify normal metabolic products. Susceptibility to such injury appears to be increased by malnutrition. A diet rich in protein and carbohydrate is believed to give partial protection against certain hepatotoxins.

Histopathologic changes in the liver consist of fatty metamorphosis, necrosis of cells, and cellular infiltration. Chronic poisoning with certain chemicals, such as carbon tetrachloride and phosphorus, leads to cirrhosis.

Symptoms, Signs, and Diagnosis

Clinical findings are similar to those in acute infectious hepatitis except that fever is less conspicuous. Jaundice may appear soon after exposure to the noxious agent, or considerably later. The diagnosis of toxic hepatitis depends upon a history of exposure to the chemical. Aside from substances given therapeutically (e.g., arsphenamine, cinchophen), the majority of liver toxins are encountered as industrial hazards.

In arsphenamine hepatitis there may be signs of diffuse parenchymatous disease or of obstructive jaundice. The latter are due to bile stasis in the small canaliculi. Some authorities believe that so-called "arsphenamine jaundice" actually is a form of homologous serum jaundice due to virus introduced by contaminated syringes.

With carbon tetrachloride poisoning both the renal tubules and liver are damaged. Therefore, the presence of hepatitis associated with signs of renal damage with or without azotemia should suggest this possibility.

Treatment

Treatment varies with the causative agent. The patient must be removed from further exposure. Alcohol should be denied. A diet rich in protein and carbohydrate, with moderately restricted fat, is advisable. For patients in stupor or coma, feeding by duodenal tube is indicated (see DIETS). Methionine (R 20) has been advocated, especially for toxic hepatitis due to carbon tetrachloride and the halogen group of chemicals. For poisoning by arsenic, selenium, and heavy metals, BAL (a compound containing SH groups) is highly beneficial (see POISONING). For severe cases of all types, I.V. glucose infusions should be given.

ACUTE YELLOW ATROPHY

(Acute necrosis; Diffuse toxic necrosis; Icterus gravis)

A widespread necrosis of the liver cells, characterized by rapid shrinkage of the liver, jaundice, hemorrhagic phenomena, neurologic symptoms and collapse, with almost invariably a fatal outcome.

Etiology and Incidence

Acute yellow atrophy may be caused by any hepatotoxic or infectious agent acting upon a liver damaged by antecedent disease. Alcoholism, malnutrition, and pregnancy are predisposing factors. The disease frequently follows unsuccessful attempts at suicide or chemical abortion by means of large amounts of poisonous drugs or chemicals. Although acute yellow atrophy is rare, statistics suggest an increasing incidence. Women are affected about twice as often as are men.

Symptoms and Signs

Early symptoms are those of the preexisting disease, or may simulate hepatitis (anorexia, nausea and vomiting, mild fever and jaundice, and generalized muscular pains often accompanied by pruritus). Within a few days these symptoms become more pronounced; severe abdominal pain centering around the liver region, intractable vomiting, intense jaundice, severe headache, mental dullness, tremors, muscular rigidity, abnormal reflexes, convulsions, and delirium or stupor develop. The abdomen is distended, pupils dilated, pulse rapid and thready, blood pressure low, temperature below normal or slightly above, tongue coated, the breath has a characteristic foul odor (fetor hepaticus), and there are widespread hemorrhagic phenomena. Death is preceded by a sharp rise in temperature and coma. The direct causes of death are acidosis, cholemia, hypoglycemia, and shock (q.v.).

Diagnosis and Prognosis

A history of liver disease and the exacerbation of jaundice, severe gastrointestinal and cerebral symptoms, hemorrhagic phenomena, and shrunken liver provide the diagnosis. Yellow fever, Weil's disease, toxic hepatitis with enlarged liver, common duct obstruction, purpura, or phosphorus poisoning may terminate in a state clinically indistinguishable from acute yellow atrophy. The cerebral symptoms may simulate those of meningitis, but jaundice, a small liver, and the absence of abnormal spinal fluid findings differentiate acute yellow atrophy.

The disease usually is fatal within 2 weeks. Rarely, enough cells escape necrosis to enable the patient to survive, in which case the disease may become either subacute or chronic ("healed yellow atrophy"). Life may be prolonged for variable lengths of time depending upon the extent of parenchymal necrosis and the ability of the cells to regenerate.

Treatment

Prompt, symptomatic treatment to combat acidosis, dehydration, hypoglycemia, and shock (q.v.) is essential. Passing a tube into the jejunum may relieve vomiting and distention, and fluids and proteins may be administered through this tube. Vitamin K (R 24, 25, 26), blood transfusions, and infusions of glucose and saline should be administered.

AMEBIC HEPATITIS
(Amebic abscess)

About 5% of patients with clinical signs of intestinal amebiasis (q.v.) develop liver complications, either focal hepatitis or liver abscess. Although the disease is prevalent in the tropics it is not limited to those regions. Amebas generally reach the liver via the portal system, where they lodge in the capillaries, invade the adjacent connective tissue, and produce areas of necrosis. Coalescence of multiple small lesions leads to abscess formation. The early stage, characterized by miliary abscesses, presents the clinical picture of hepatitis.

Symptoms and Signs

The typical patient has had intermittent diarrhea and cramps for a variable period of time, followed by pain and tenderness over the liver with occasional radiation to the right shoulder. Pain over the liver may be sharp or dull and is characteristically aggravated by movement. Fever, with or without chills and of varying degree, is frequent. Diarrhea and jaundice are not conspicuous. Jaundice occurs in about 15% of cases.

Physical examination shows a palpable, tender liver. There may be dullness to percussion in the right axilla and localized abdominal rigidity. Respiratory movements are restricted on the affected side. Fluoroscopic or roentgenographic study reveals an elevated splinted diaphragm, together with signs of pleurisy or pneumonitis at the right lung base.

Complications to be feared are secondary infection and rupture of abscesses into adjacent areas. A mortality rate as high as 16% has been reported.

Diagnosis

Clinical diagnosis is confirmed by the finding of *E. histolytica* in the stools, which is possible in the vast majority of cases, especially in fresh stools examined after a saline purge. However, since it also is possible to miss finding amebas in some instances, doubtful cases should be considered of amebic origin until every effort has been made to prove them otherwise. The sharp response to emetine or chloroquine serves as a therapeutic test.

Treatment

The time-honored use of emetine in the treatment of amebic hepatitis is being replaced by chloroquine (Aralen) given orally in daily doses of 0.5 Gm. for 10 to 14 days (℞ 6). Emetine hydrochloride is administered subcut. (℞ 1), and either form of therapy should be followed by a course of chiniofon (℞ 2), Diodoquin (℞ 3) or Stovarsol (℞ 4) to rid the intestinal tract of amebas. If the abscesses fail to respond to medication, closed drainage must be performed. The prognosis depends upon the extent and severity of the lesions and the development of complications.

INFECTIOUS (SPIROCHETAL) JAUNDICE
(Weil's disease)

A form of infectious hepatitis caused by Leptospira icterohaemorrhagiae. (*See* separate chapter on this disease.)

OTHER TYPES OF INFECTIOUS HEPATITIS

Infectious mononucleosis and chronic brucellosis (q.v.) may be complicated by fever and jaundice and thus suggest a diagnosis of epidemic hepatitis. Other clinical features of these diseases and appropriate laboratory tests serve to differentiate them.

Jaundice and fever also may be present in yellow fever, malaria, bacteremia, and pneumococcic pneumonia, and these diseases also must be distinguished from epidemic hepatitis.

FATTY LIVER

Excessive deposition of fat in the liver cells.

Etiology and Pathology

Fatty infiltration of the liver often is seen in obese persons, in whom it is due to excessive fat intake. It also can be caused by intoxicants (e.g., alcohol, carbon tetrachloride, chloroform), chronic infections (e.g., tuberculosis), metabolic disorders (e.g., diabetes mellitus, lipoid dystrophies), and anemias (q.v.). In these conditions, fatty liver probably is due to migration of fat from storage depots. In certain deficiency states (e.g., pellagra), fatty liver may result from the lack of lipotrophic factors, such as choline. As a result of fat deposition, the liver is large, pale, and smooth. It may be either soft or firm. The cells often are so distended with fat that the liver structure is barely discernible.

Symptoms, Signs, and Diagnosis

Symptoms caused by a fatty liver are not specific and cannot be distinguished from those produced by other chronic diseases such as cirrhosis, chronic passive congestion, amyloidosis, and leukemia (q.v.). Tests of liver function show but slight changes. The presence of a persistently enlarged, tender liver is suggestive, but, in most cases, discovery of fatty liver is incidental. There are occasional cases in which death occurs after an unaccountable fulminating illness with evidence of liver failure such as jaundice, ascites, and coma, and a fatty liver is revealed at autopsy. However, in such instances it seems likely that parenchymal liver injury (necrosis) also was present. Diagnosis can be made accurately by performing a punch biopsy of the liver but this procedure may be hazardous in other than skilled hands.

Treatment

The presence of fatty liver indicates that the underlying or predisposing disease is poorly controlled. There is no specific therapy except in cases related to alcoholism or some other cause of malnutrition. Where this is suspected, a high protein diet (*see* DIETS) supplemented with dried brewer's yeast (℞ 18), choline chloride (℞19), or methionine (℞ 20) should be given.

AMYLOID DISEASE

Etiology and Pathology

Amyloidosis (q.v.) occurs as a complication of certain chronic diseases, notably tuberculosis, lung abscess, bronchiectasis, osteomyelitis, and neoplasms. Tuberculosis is the most common predisposing condition. Amyloid, a substance of complex structure, contains chondroitin sulfuric acid. It forms in the tissues probably as a result of faulty endogenous protein metabolism. In the earliest lesions, amyloid deposits are found in the reticuloendothelial cells. With more extensive infiltration, the substance is seen as a homogenous mass occupying the perivascular spaces. The amyloid liver appears pale and glassy and has a firm, rubbery texture. The spleen and kidneys also are frequently involved.

Symptoms, Signs, and Diagnosis

Moderate infiltration of the liver with amyloid causes no disturbance. In advanced amyloidosis the liver and spleen are palpably enlarged, smooth, firm, and nontender. Ascites, dilated abdominal veins, and peripheral edema are characteristic symptoms, but jaundice is rare. Liver function tests remain normal. About 80% of the patients die within 2 years after onset. In differentiating amyloidosis, fatty liver, leukemia, nephrosis, cirrhosis, and passive congestion should be considered. A positive Congo red test is presumptive evidence for amyloidosis (q.v.).

Treatment

This consists of controlling, as well as is possible, the underlying disease and prescribing a protein-rich diet supplemented with vitamin B concentrates (see DIETS).

CIRRHOSIS

PORTAL CIRRHOSIS

(Laennec's cirrhosis; "Alcoholic" cirrhosis)

A chronic disease of the liver characterized by increased connective tissue that spreads from the portal spaces, with distortion of the liver architecture, and impairment of liver functions.

Etiology, Incidence, and Pathology

Portal cirrhosis occurs chiefly in late middle life, and preponderantly in males. Malnutrition is believed to be a predisposing if not a primary etiologic factor. Cirrhosis has been produced in animals by diets low in protein and specifically low in choline. The addition of choline to these diets prevented cirrhosis. It is postulated that the prevalence of cirrhosis among alcoholics is related to the associated malnutrition. Chronic poisoning with carbon tetrachloride or phosphorus produces changes similar to Laennec's cirrhosis.

The liver is diffusely nodular, scarred, and dense. Microscopic section shows parenchymal degeneration, cellular infiltration, proliferation of scar tissue, and areas of regeneration. Fatty changes are present in the early stages.

Symptoms and Signs

Cirrhosis of moderate degree may be asymptomatic. The onset of liver failure is gradual, with ill-defined symptoms. Gastrointestinal disturbances are frequent and consist of anorexia, flatulence, nausea, vomiting and abdominal pain or tenderness, usually with weight loss.

In advanced cirrhosis, the physical signs are obvious. Low grade fever, emaciation, foul breath (fetor hepaticus), jaundice, nodular liver, and splenomegaly are prominent. Portal venous obstruction is manifested by distended abdominal veins and esophageal varices (revealed by X-ray and barium contrast studies). Vascular "spiders" are seen over the face, neck, arms, and upper trunk. With progression of the disease, ascites, edema, and mental torpor supervene. (*See* table, Laboratory Diagnosis in Hepatic Disease and Jaundice, *under* LIVER FUNCTION TESTS.)

Tests of liver function invariably show impairment. In the absence of icterus the bromsulfalein dye test is perhaps the most sensitive. The cephalin flocculation test is positive in the majority of cases, especially in the presence of jaundice. Determination of the serum albumin level is helpful in gauging the trend of the disease. A low serum albumin (less than 2.5 Gm./100 cc.) is an ominous sign, whereas increased albumin suggests improvement.

Complications

Hematemesis from ruptured esophageal varices occurs in 25% of the cases. It is a dreaded event, since about 60% of these patients succumb within a year of the first episode. Intercurrent infections such as phlebitis, pneumonia, and peritonitis account for about 25% of the fatalities. Portal vein thrombosis and primary carcinoma of the liver are relatively rare but fatal complications.

Diagnosis and Prognosis

Diagnosis is made from the symptoms and signs previously described. It may be necessary to differentiate cirrhosis from Banti's syndrome, gastrointestinal carcinoma, polyserositis, and passive congestion of the liver (q.v.). When hematemesis is present, differentiation must be made from peptic ulcer (q.v.).

Active treatment of early cases often will retard progression, or possibly effect a cure, but the outlook is poor when impaired liver function and distortion of liver structure have become established. The degree of liver impairment may be estimated from three aspects: (1) Circulatory disturbances; i.e., portal hypertension as evidenced by splenomegaly, collateral venous circulation in the skin of the abdomen, ascites, esophageal varices. (2) Disturbances in biliary drainage; i.e., destruction of small or large ducts, either primary or secondary to edema or scarring. This is evidenced by serum bilirubin elevation, pigment casts, and in certain instances by phosphatase elevation. (3) Damage to the functioning liver cells, as demonstrated by positive cephalin flocculation, depression of serum albumin, bromsulfalein retention, and prolongation of prothrombin time.

A punch biopsy of the liver can furnish necessary information for diagnosis and stage or degree of involvement but should be performed only by one who is experienced in the procedure.

Treatment

During the period of liver failure, the patient should be kept in bed for at least half of each day. Emphasis is placed upon avoidance of alcohol and upon eating a diet rich in proteins but only moderately so in carbohydrates and fats (*see* Diets). An ideal diet will contain about 140 Gm. of protein, 375 Gm. of carbohydrate, and 150 Gm. (or less) of fat daily, including meat, fish or poultry at 2 meals, and at least 1 qt. of milk/day. Such a diet may be supplemented by powdered brewer's yeast, 25 Gm. twice daily (℞ 18), choline chloride, 2 to 5 Gm. daily (℞ 19), or methionine, 2 to 5 Gm. daily (℞ 20). Where evidence suggests that fat is not being properly absorbed by the intestine, absorption may be aided by the use of a wetting agent, such as the polyoxyethylene derivative of sorbitan monooleate, given as 1.5 Gm. doses with each meal (℞ 21).

When liquid diets are necessary (*see* Diets) alternate feedings of milk and fruit juices may be tried. Thiamine (℞ 27), 10 mg./day, may stimulate appetite. In patients with polyneuritis, mental changes, or impending cholemia, larger daily doses of thiamine (100 mg.) and of nicotinamide (400 mg.) (℞ 28) may be given. If oral feeding is not possible, daily infusions of 10% glucose (2,000 to 3,000 cc./24 hours by I.V. drip) are advisable.

In patients with ascites, salt intake should be reduced and fluid limited to about 2,500 cc./day. Paracentesis should be done before distention interferes with the appetite, and repeated as necessary. The intervals between punctures can be lengthened by giving mercurial diuretics and ammonium chloride (*see* Edema).

Gastrointestinal bleeding should be suspected when symptoms such as tachycardia, fall in blood pressure, abdominal cramps, or tarry stools suddenly appear. Prompt transfusion of citrated blood should be given and repeated daily until signs of bleeding disappear. Food may be withheld for several days. Sedation should be minimal. Demerol is preferable to morphine in such cases.

Intercurrent infections should be vigorously treated with penicillin, sulfadiazine, or other antibacterial agents, as appropriate to the type of pathogen present.

In liver failure, at least 2 months of intensive therapy will be needed before significant changes can occur. With the treatment described, at least 50% of the patients can be restored to a useful, active life for a period of years. Trials of concentrated human serum albumin solution and of I.V. liver extract have recently given encouraging results, and surgical measures to relieve portal hypertension and ascites are being studied.

BILIARY CIRRHOSIS

A relatively uncommon disease of the liver characterized by jaundice of long duration due to stasis of bile and inflammation within or around the bile ducts. Two forms are described: **obstructive** and **infectious.**

OBSTRUCTIVE BILIARY CIRRHOSIS

This results from obstruction of the common duct by stone, tumor, postoperative scarring, or congenital stenosis of the biliary ducts. The liver is small, firm, and deeply stained with bile. The bile ducts are dilated and surrounded by inflammatory cellular reaction. Connective tissue is moderately increased near the portal areas. The lobular structure of the liver generally is preserved.

Symptoms and Signs

There is a history of intermittent or chronic jaundice over a period of months or years. The skin has a green, bronzed appearance and frequently shows xanthomatous deposits. The jaundice is obstructive in type, with elevated serum cholesterol, elevated phosphatase, and negative flocculation test. In later stages there also may be signs of liver damage. Weakness, weight loss, flatulence, anorexia, and dull upper abdominal pain are usual symptoms. There may be occasional bouts of fever with chills, presumably due to associated cholangitis. The patient becomes progressively weaker and dies from intercurrent infection, hemorrhage, or hepatic coma.

Treatment

If the blockage is in the common bile duct, removal of the obstruction by surgery may be lifesaving. (The operative procedure obviously depends upon the nature and site of the lesion.) Symptomatic supportive therapy is indicated, and whole blood transfusions may be of value in preparing the patient for operation. If surgical repair is impossible, as in intrahepatic biliary obstruction, there is no specific therapy.

INFECTIOUS BILIARY CIRRHOSIS
(Cholangiolitic cirrhosis; Hanot's cirrhosis)

Etiology and Pathology

It is believed that certain cases of unresolved acute infectious hepatitis and cholangitis end in a chronic hepatitis involving the small bile ducts, and known as cholangiolitic cirrhosis. This resembles the hypertrophic cirrhosis first described by Hanot. The liver is large, finely granular, and of a greenish color. An inflammatory round cell reaction is found chiefly in and about the small bile ducts. Except for a moderate increase of intralobular connective tissue the liver cords and cells appear normal.

Symptoms, Signs, and Diagnosis

The disease is most common in young adults. At onset, it may simulate acute infectious hepatitis with fever, jaundice, digestive disturbances, abdominal pain, and enlargement of the liver and spleen. In the early stages, the laboratory signs are those of obstructive jaundice (q.v.). Later, signs of parenchymal liver damage appear, and the disease runs a slowly progressive, fatal course. Acute infectious hepatitis can be differentiated by the disappearance of symptoms and signs within a few days or weeks, while those of cholangiolitic biliary cirrhosis persist for many months.

Treatment

There is no specific therapy, but placing the patient on a high protein, high carbohydrate diet and administering choleretics may be of value. Careful administration of sulfonamides, penicillin, or other antibacterial agents may be attempted.

POSTNECROTIC CIRRHOSIS

(Coarse nodular cirrhosis,
Healed yellow atrophy; Toxic cirrhosis)

A chronic disease of the liver characterized by massive scarring and areas of nodular regeneration.

Etiology and Pathology

Postnecrotic cirrhosis develops as a sequel to acute infectious or toxic hepatitis. In most cases of acute hepatitis the injury is confined to parenchymal cells, the reticular framework remaining intact. In the rare cases that progress to cirrhosis destruction of the reticulum also is evident. Whether this chronic form of the disease indicates continued presence of the virus or some complicating factor is unknown.

The liver is discolored, small, and coarsely nodular. Broad bands of scar tissue surround nodular areas of regenerating liver cells.

Symptoms, Signs, and Diagnosis

The interval between antecedent hepatitis and the onset of liver failure varies from several months to 10 years or longer. Clinical signs may be indistinguishable from those of Laennec's cirrhosis. Jaundice, ascites, edema, splenomegaly, esophageal varices, and vascular "spiders" may be present. The course is unfavorable after liver failure occurs. A history of antecedent hepatitis in a young (nonalcoholic) person with these symptoms suggests the diagnosis.

Treatment

Dietary treatment has provided little if any benefit. General supportive measures are indicated, but as yet there is no specific treatment of value.

CARDIAC CIRRHOSIS

Chronic passive congestion of the liver (q.v.) may lead to cardiac cirrhosis if the congestive failure persists for more than a year. The liver usually is small, firm, and fibrotic. Fibrous markings are increased particularly about the central veins, giving rise to "pseudolobulation." The spleen is enlarged in about half the cases. Symptoms are similar to those of chronic passive congestion except that the liver tends to be smaller, whereas ascites and splenomegaly are more frequent. Treatment is that of the underlying heart failure (q.v.).

SYPHILIS OF THE LIVER

(Hepar lobatum)

The healing of syphilitic gummas produces deep scars and fissures which grossly distort the liver. The process is not finely diffuse as in Laennec's cirrhosis. Normal liver tissue may be found adjacent to broadly scarred areas. Usually, there is little functional disturbance of the liver. In the rare instances of extensive scarring, the disease may simulate decompensated Laennec's cirrhosis. Conventional therapy for syphilis (q.v.) is employed. The condition is seldom seen in present-day medical practice.

ZOOPARASITIC JAUNDICE

SCHISTOSOMIASIS

Hepatic cirrhosis may result from schistosomiasis. Early in the disease ova may be found in the stools. Fever, gastrointestinal disturbances, and eosinophilia are common findings. Chronic infestation leads to progressive fibrosis of the portal areas. Signs of cirrhosis with ascites, splenomegaly, and anemia occur in the late stage. Hematemesis is a frequent cause of death.

Treatment

The therapy in the early stage is that of schistosomiasis (q.v.). Later, there is no specific treatment of any value.

DISTOMIASIS

Several species of Distoma (liver flukes) may infest the bile ducts, giving rise to cholangitis and biliary cirrhosis (q.v.). The most common species, *Clonorchis sinensis*, is found chiefly in China, Japan, and India. Infestation occurs through eating raw fish. Diagnosis depends upon the detection of ova in the stools.

Treatment

Gentian violet is recommended for the early stage (℞ 5). Emetine (℞ 1) is of questionable value.

HEPATOLENTICULAR DEGENERATION
(Wilson's disease)

A rare familial disease of the brain, characterized by degeneration of the lenticular nuclei and a "hobnail" liver cirrhosis, similar to Laennec's cirrhosis. The liver disease usually is latent but may have clinical manifestations. The presence of (1) a Kayser-Fleischer ring (a ring of greenish pigment at the outer edge of the cornea), (2) incoordination and tremors of the extremities (*see* TREMORS), and (3) signs of hepatic disease should suggest the diagnosis. The disease is seen in young people and is fatal within a few years.

Treatment

Dietary treatment similar to that in Laennec's cirrhosis (q.v.) is said to be moderately effective.

HEMOCHROMATOSIS
(Bronzed diabetes)

A rare disease occurring almost exclusively in males and characterized by widespread systemic deposition of hemosiderin and progressive pancreatic and portal cirrhosis. It usually is accompanied by diabetes. The etiology is unknown. The diabetes is of varying severity, and presumably is related to the extent of pancreatic involvement. The diagnosis can be established by the demonstration of iron-containing pigment in biopsy material from the skin or liver. The prognosis is poor.

Treatment

To control the diabetes (q.v.) and maintain optimal nutrition (as in Laennec's cirrhosis) is the object of therapy.

CIRCULATORY DISORDERS

CHRONIC PASSIVE CONGESTION

Various pathologic conditions within the thorax, and especially cardiac disease with decompensation, may result in engorgement of the vessels and stasis of blood in the vascular bed of the liver, producing a state of chronic passive congestion. At necropsy, the liver presents a mottled, purplish red appearance. It appears swollen and its capsule seems stretched. On section, the central veins and their tributaries are seen to be engorged and the adjacent liver cords compressed. Fibrous tissue markings about the central veins and portal triads are diffusely increased.

Symptoms and Signs

The patient is disabled chiefly by congestive heart failure

(q.v.). On palpation the liver is found to be enlarged, firm and smooth, with or without tenderness. Patients usually complain of a feeling of weight or dull aching in the right upper abdominal quadrant. Ascites is present in about 50% of patients; splenomegaly and jaundice less often. Liver function tests, such as the serum bilirubin, bromsulfalein dye test, galactose tolerance test, and urine urobilinogen, may show significant changes. With return of cardiac compensation or elimination of other causative conditions, the liver edge recedes, ascites disappears, and liver function tests reveal approximately normal values.

Treatment

Therapy consists of the treatment of congestive heart failure (q.v.), with administration of diuretics, and a low salt diet (see DIETS).

PORTAL VEIN THROMBOSIS

Cirrhosis and carcinoma of the liver are the chief predisposing factors in portal vein thrombosis. It also occurs as a sequel to abdominal surgery and to infections in the biliary region, stomach, pancreas, or appendix. The diagnosis should be suspected when a patient with one of these conditions develops sudden midabdominal pain, nausea, vomiting, hematemesis, and possibly ascites. Paralytic ileus (due to infarction of the small intestines), rapid collapse and death may ensue.

When portal vein thrombosis develops slowly, or when one of the smaller branches is involved, these signs may be inconspicuous or absent, presumably owing to collateral venous circulation. Patients have been known to survive chronic portal vein thrombosis for several years.

Treatment

There is no specific treatment, therapy being supportive. The use of anticoagulants (see ANTICOAGULANT THERAPY) has been suggested as a means of preventing further propagation of the thrombus. Paracentesis for ascites, active catharsis, and administration of mercurial diuretics (see EDEMA) may be tried.

HEPATIC VEIN THROMBOSIS
(Chiari's disease)

This is a very rare condition. It may be secondary to disease of the liver, such as neoplasm, cirrhosis, pyelophlebitis, or cholangitis. Occasionally, it is seen as a complication of polycythemia. Characteristically, there is rapid enlargement of the liver and spleen, with prominent abdominal veins, ascites, edema, and terminal jaundice. Tests indicate severe impairment of liver functions. Death occurs within a few weeks or months.

Treatment

When the cause is suspected of being primarily thrombotic, a trial of anticoagulant therapy (q.v.) would appear to be indicated. Once the disease is established, however, nothing has been found to alter its fatal prognosis.

NEOPLASMS

The liver is a common site for metastatic spread of carcinoma arising in the gastrointestinal tract, pancreas, or gallbladder. The organ may become tender, nodular, and rapidly enlarged, so as to occupy the greater portion of the right abdomen. Jaundice and ascites may or may not be present. Splenomegaly usually is absent. When a neoplasm involves the common duct, obstructive (regurgitation) jaundice (q.v.) occurs.

Primary neoplasm in the liver is relatively rare. In about half the reported cases it is associated with cirrhosis. It is estimated that about 4% of patients with cirrhosis develop primary carcinoma of the liver. Symptoms may be identical with those of decompensated cirrhosis, particularly when the liver is not enlarged.

With either primary or secondary carcinoma of the liver, death follows in a few months after the above signs appear. Treatment at present is only palliative.

BILIARY DISORDERS

Biliary dyskinesia, cholelithiasis, acute cholecystitis, chronic cholecystitis, and cholangiohepatitis represent different types of biliary tract dysfunctions. However, the forms are less disease entities than they are phases of pathologic evolution, and may occur in succession or simultaneously.

BILIARY DYSKINESIA

(Biliary dyssynergia; Odditis; Postcholecystectomy syndrome)

Failure in the mechanics of bile flow due to muscular spasm or abnormal pressure relations producing pain in the biliary region, often without evidence of organic disease, and frequently following cholecystectomy.

Etiology

Spasm of the sphincter of the common bile duct (sphincter of Oddi) is directly responsible for biliary dyskinesia. Pregnancy and allergic states as well as reflex stimulation from certain intra-abdominal diseases have been suggested as causes. The term hypertonic dyskinesia refers to concomitant spasm of the gallbladder and the sphincter of Oddi, with peristaltic activity of the common duct. Atonic dyskinesia is spasm of the sphincter with passive distention of a toneless gallbladder. A similar state following cholecystectomy, especially when the gallbladder did not contain stones, may be due to abnormal spasm of the sphincter producing an uncompensated rise in intraductal pressure in the absence of the reservoir of the gallbladder.

Symptoms and Signs

Biliary dyskinesia is characterized by frequently recurring pain in the right upper quadrant, usually after eating. It is commonly associated with other neurogenic disease of the gastrointestinal tract. Hypertonic dyskinesia, the more usual type, produces nausea and a dull, spasmodic pain similar to mild colic. Atonic dyskinesia causes a continuous aching sensation. The postcholecystectomy syndrome approximates the hyperkinetic type. The presence of jaundice and fever should suggest some diagnosis other than the above.

Diagnosis

The presence of biliary dyskinesia, after the possibility of organic disease has been excluded, is suggested by the following: exacerbation of symptoms by emotional upset or anxiety; reproduction of symptoms by administering morphine sulfate (℞ 13) and their prompt alleviation with amyl nitrite (℞ 10); and evidence from duodenal intubation and cholecystography of delayed gallbladder emptying after a fatty meal. In the cholecystectomized patient, great care must be taken to rule out choledocholithiasis.

Treatment

Therapy is aimed at relaxation of the sphincter and prevention of biliary stasis. High protein diets have been shown to increase the flow of bile and bile salts. Fats should be strictly limited in the cholecystectomized patient and probably also in those with "primary" dyskinesias unless adequate relaxation can be obtained. Atropine (℞ 8), belladonna (℞ 9), and various synthetic antispasmodics (℞ 7), have proved effective. The synthetics avoid the undesirable side effects produced by atropine and belladonna. Nitrites (℞ 10, 11) may be used diagnostically and at times for relief of pain. Associated dyspeptic symptoms are occasionally alleviated by bile salts (℞ 22), especially after cholecystectomy.

CHOLELITHIASIS; CHOLEDOCHOLITHIASIS
(Gallstones; Biliary calculi)

Concretions in the gallbladder (cholelithiasis), or common duct (choledocholithiasis).

Etiology

Gallstones are present in about 10% of white adults and much more frequently in females than in males. Obesity and pregnancy are predisposing factors. Hemolytic diseases frequently give rise to calculi, but account for few of the total number of cases. The causes of calculus formation still are obscure. Biliary stasis and disturbed cholesterol metabolism have been suggested, and the onset of symptoms during pregnancy when both these factors coexist is well known. Attacks have been found at times to bear a definite relation to the menstrual cycle. Whether infection with damage to the cholecystic epithelium and subsequent changes in the pH of the bile and the cholesterol-bile acid ratio is a precursor of or a sequel to gallstone formation is debatable.

Stones in the common duct almost always are of cholecystic origin. Rarely, granular precipitation of pigment ("biliary sand") appears to form primarily in the bile ducts. Stones are mainly of 3 types: cholesterol stones, usually single (10%); pure pigment stones, calcium bilirubinate, occurring in hemolytic diseases (10%); and mixed stones, multifaceted, multiple (80%).

Symptoms, Signs, and Course

Although biliary colic is the most significant symptom of cholelithiasis, many patients are practically asymptomatic, while others have only occasional symptoms. Thus, the presence of stones in the gallbladder may be discovered only incidentally during examination for other conditions. A stone in the ampulla of the gallbladder or in the cystic duct is evidenced by pain. This is diffuse and cramping, and characteristically begins in the epigastrium after a heavy meal; later, with increasing severity it radiates to the right scapular and clavicular regions. Right upper quadrant tenderness and moderate muscle guarding are present. Nausea and vomiting are common; there may be slight fever and leukocytosis. Transient jaundice with light colored stools and bilirubinuria may occur, even if the common duct itself is not obstructed.

In choledocholithiasis there is deep jaundice. The characteristic pain is present in about 80% of cases and is associated with severe nausea and vomiting. Obstruction of the common duct is rarely complete, and stool examinations on successive days will reveal some passage of bile. Total absence of bile suggests pancreatic or ampullary tumor.

In cholelithiasis, the attacks usually subside spontaneously in a few hours, with the stone dropping back into the fundus of the gallbladder or occasionally passing into the common duct or from it into the duodenum. However, attacks of biliary colic may precede acute cholecystitis with its subsequent complications (q.v.). Repeated attacks lead to chronic cholecystitis with its complications (q.v.).

Diagnosis

The most effective procedure is competent cholecystography,

with either oral or I.V. dye administration, but this must not be used for jaundiced patients. Aspiration and examination of duodenal contents (duodenal drainage) is a valuable diagnostic aid, whether or not jaundice is present. The differential diagnoses of importance are acute cholecystitis, which is usually initiated by biliary colic and accompanied by fever, leukocytosis, and varying degrees of peritoneal irritation; acute infectious hepatitis, and homologous serum jaundice, distinguished by history of infectious contact or following the administration of serum or blood, prodromal symptoms, liver tenderness, and the course of the disease; acute pancreatitis, in which concurrent cholelithiasis is common; peptic ulcer; pneumonia; coronary artery disease; renal colic; acute appendicitis; perihepatitis, neuritis of intercostal nerves, herpes zoster. In common duct stone the differentiation of obstructive from hepatocellular jaundice is of utmost importance (*see* HEPATITIS). Once the obstructive nature has been established, a history of biliary colic, previous jaundice, a nonpalpable gallbladder, and the intermittent appearance of bile in the stools point to stone rather than tumor.

Treatment

For immediate relief of acute biliary colic due to cholelithiasis or choledocholithiasis, such drugs as amyl nitrite (℞ 10), nitroglycerin (℞ 11), atropine (℞ 8), or a synthetic antispasmodic (℞ 7), may be given. Analgesics also may be necessary. Demerol (℞ 14) often is effective and has the additional advantage of some antispasmodic action, but for severe pain either methadone (℞ 15) or morphine (℞ 13) is indicated.

Between attacks, a low fat, high protein, high carbohydrate but limited calorie diet (*see* DIETS) tends to reduce obesity, exerts a lipotropic effect on the liver (thus decreasing the operative risk in surgery), and lessens the likelihood of repeated attacks. Such diets should be supplemented with vitamins, especially the fat-soluble A, D, and K. Vitamin K (℞ 24, 25, 26) is indicated when jaundice is or has been present (*see* VITAMIN DEFICIENCIES), and especially in preoperative preparation. Where evidence suggests that fat is not being properly absorbed by the intestine, absorption may be aided by the use of a wetting agent, such as the polyoxyethylene derivative of sorbitan monooleate, given as 1.5 Gm. doses with each meal (℞ 21).

Although there is no known nonsurgical method of dissipating gallstones, surgery is not indicated for patients whose stones are large or asymptomatic and in whom there is no evidence of associated cholecystitis. Persistent pain, jaundice or other complications of stone obstruction necessitate surgical intervention. Surgery for uncomplicated cholelithiasis is indicated for the patient who shows evidence of developing hepatic, pancreatic, or cardiac dysfunction.

ACUTE CHOLECYSTITIS
(Acute angiocholecystitis)

Acute inflammation of the gallbladder, with varying involvement of the adjacent bile passages.

Etiology

Obstruction of the ampulla of the gallbladder or cystic duct is generally considered the predominant cause of acute cholecystitis. The disease usually is a complication of cholelithiasis. In the few cases without demonstrable stones in the gallbladder, stones previously present may have passed into the common duct, perhaps being discharged into the bowel. Other possible obstructing factors are kinking of the cystic duct, extrinsic pressure from tumors, adhesions, and lymph nodes, and inflammation of adjacent tissues. Obstruction causes distention, edema, and eventual circulatory compromise of the organ with resultant necrosis and gangrene. Initial tissue damage enhances the deleterious effects of the bile salts and permits bacterial invasion.

Symptoms and Signs

Acute cholecystitis occurs most frequently in the 5th and 6th decades of life, and relatively more women than men are affected. Onset is characterized by biliary colic (*see* Cholelithiasis), which is only temporarily relieved by opiates and is usually accompanied by nausea and vomiting, and less often by chills. About 25% of the patients are mildly jaundiced. There is moderate fever, rarely over 101°F., and a corresponding leukocytosis. Usually, signs of peritoneal irritation are prominent in the biliary region, though occasionally they are elicited with difficulty. The gallbladder is palpable in about 20% of cases.

Course

The disease may subside spontaneously. Complications are sufficiently frequent to warrant careful consideration of the surgical indications and close observation of the patient's course. As infection and necrosis progress, gangrene, perforation, peritonitis, subphrenic or subhepatic abscess, and inflammation of the liver or pancreas may develop. Severe inflammation of the biliary passages may occur (*see* Cholangiohepatitis).

Diagnosis

An accurate history of previous biliary disease is important, since the acute process almost invariably follows cholelithiasis. Clinical findings are fever and right upper quadrant tenderness. Moderate leukocytosis and increased sedimentation rate are usual. A significant number of cases have bilirubinemia and bile in the urine. X-ray examination of the abdomen may show opaque stones or a gallbladder infiltrated with calcium. Prothrombin determinations also may be of differential value in the jaundiced patient. Acute cholecystitis must be distinguished from pyelonephritis, perforated peptic ulcer, coronary occlusion, pulmonary disease and particularly appendicitis (q.v.).

Treatment

Spreading peritonitis or imminent rupture of the gallbladder requires immediate surgery. Most cases, however, can be observed for 18 to 36 hours for evaluation of conservative treatment. Base-line determinations of temperature, pulse, white count, differential, and liver function tests (q.v.), such as the van den Bergh, total protein, albumin-globulin ratio, prothrombin time, and liver cholesterol partition, should be performed. White counts should be repeated at 8- to 12-hour intervals, and sedimentation rates and pertinent liver function tests to determine the status of the case and to assist in differentiating cholecystitis from other pathologic conditions should be repeated as frequently as necessary.

The patient is confined to bed. Nothing is given by mouth. Nutrition and fluid balance are maintained by parenteral administration. Injection of 1,000 cc. of Isotonic Sodium Chloride Solution U.S.P. provides 9 Gm. of salt, which is adequate unless depletion by vomiting has occurred. (Blood chloride and CO_2 combining power determinations can guide therapy in respect to blood electrolytes.) A total fluid intake of 3,000 cc./day is usually required. Addition of 5 to 10% glucose to all solutions supplies some of the caloric requirements and forestalls hepatic glycogen depletion. Parenteral administration of amino acids solution may be important in maintaining nitrogen balance. Vitamin K (℞ 24, 25, 26) should be given whenever prothrombin time is increased, especially if surgery is contemplated (see VITAMIN DEFICIENCIES). Penicillin (℞ 16) in doses of 50,000 u. I.M. every 3 hours, or streptomycin (℞ 17) 0.25 Gm. every 6 hours, may be given in the hope of limiting the degree of infection.

Pain may be relieved by relaxing the sphincter of Oddi. Nitroglycerin (℞ 11), amyl nitrite (℞ 10), or one of the synthetic antispasmodics (℞ 7), often is effective. Papaverine (℞ 12) with or without atropine (℞ 8) may be sufficient. For analgesia, Demerol (℞ 14) is preferable to morphine (℞ 13), since it does not have the undesirable spasmodic effects of opium derivatives. However, methadone (℞ 15), morphine (℞ 13), or morphine (℞ 13) and atropine (℞ 8) often must be resorted to when pain is severe. Surgery is indicated for intractable cases.

If symptoms subside and the history is not of long duration, the patient may be continued on conservative treatment, i.e., low calorie, low fat, high protein, and high carbohydrate diet (see DIETS). However, the frequency of recurrences, the danger of complications, and the excellent results from modern surgery must be weighed before deciding against cholecystectomy.

CHRONIC CHOLECYSTITIS

Etiology and Pathology

Chronic cholecystitis is a sequel to repeated attacks of acute cholecystitis (q.v.) and is usually associated with cholelithiasis. Occasionally, there is no evidence of gallstones and the cystic duct probably has become partially occluded by other means. It is extremely unlikely that infection is a significant primary factor, though it often plays a secondary role. Pathologically the gallbladder appears thickened and shrunken and exhibits fibrosis of its walls with round cell infiltration. The surface loses its normal glistening blue color, and adhesions to adjacent structures are frequent.

Symptoms and Signs

Chronic cholecystitis is clinically indistinguishable from the cholelithiasis (q.v.) with which it is usually associated. The right upper quadrant tenderness is due to inflammation and distention of the viscus itself, but the biliary colic is almost invariably caused by a calculus. If cholecystography and biliary drainage fail to demonstrate stones, a diagnosis of cholecystitis should be made with great caution. The nonspecific gastrointestinal symptoms ascribed by the layman to "biliousness" ought not be attributed to a noncalculous gallbladder without direct cholecystographic evidence of dysfunction and the presence of tenderness in the biliary area.

Diagnosis

In the presence of cholelithiasis, the diagnosis is established by cholecystography reinforced by biliary drainage findings. The gallbladder fails to fill, concentrate, or empty in a normal manner. Where cholelithiasis cannot be demonstrated, cholecystography should be repeated with larger doses of radiopaque material. (The time interval between administration of the dye and filming may have been too long for that particular patient.) Biliary drainage tests may assist by indicating abnormal emptying or concentration. The presence of cholesterol crystals and a fine golden pigment (calcium bilirubinate) in the "B" fraction of bile is highly significant evidence of gallstones.

Treatment

Where the inflammatory changes are attendant upon biliary calculi, treatment is the same as for cholelithiasis (q.v.). Where diagnostic studies reveal unequivocal evidence of chronic cholecystitis without calculi or other disease of the digestive system, the same criteria for surgical intervention can be employed. Cholecystectomy for noncalculous cholecystitis is of dubious value for the alleviation of symptoms. Conservative therapy and further search for etiologic factors are preferable in most instances.

CHOLANGIOHEPATITIS

An inflammation of the biliary passages (biliary radicles, hepatic and common ducts) due to infection and often accompanied by focal abscesses of the liver.

Etiology

Although some degree of cholangitis accompanies most acute inflammatory processes of both the gallbladder and liver, ascending infection probably does not occur where there is free drainage of the biliary system. In a patient with a cholecystenterostomy, the presence of cholangitis is direct evidence of partial occlusion of the stoma. A "primary" cholangitis occurs when infection is present in the common duct, and there is an impediment to the free flow of bile into the small bowel. This is most frequently due to choledocholithiasis, less often to tumor, stricture or exogenous impingement by the biliary passages upon the lumen. Occasionally, bacteremia is the infective source, and bile stasis results from edema of the bile ducts. The organisms involved may be *Esch. coli*, *Str. fecalis*, *B. typhosus* and allied strains, *Salmonella*, or *Clostridia*. Changes in the liver range from periportal inflammation to miliary abscesses and frank suppuration, and for this reason the term cholangiohepatitis has come into more general use.

Symptoms and Signs

The patient is jaundiced and has a septic temperature characterized by a high spiking fever with severe chills. The degree of hyperbilirubinemia may vary from day to day, as may the signs of obstruction of biliary outflow (acholic stools and bilirubinuria). This is especially true when the disease is due to choledocholithiasis. Leukocytosis is present. The liver is tender, and as the disease progresses to focal abscesses, evidence of liver damage becomes prominent.

Diagnosis

Clinical differentiation from pyelophlebitis usually is impossible though, if seen early, cholangitis exhibits a more severe jaundice compared with the degree of liver dysfunction, since the jaundice is more truly obstructive. The history is of considerable diagnostic assistance. Pyelophlebitis usually is a complication of acute appendicitis or other suppurative peritoneal processes. Jaundice appears after a febrile course. Cholangitis, on the other hand, is a complication of choledocholithiasis or previous biliary surgery and, as a rule, follows the appearance of jaundice due to common duct occlusion by stone or stricture. Evidence of stones or a previous cholecystic operation is of great importance in treatment and prognosis.

Treatment

Definitive treatment must be aimed at establishing a free flow of bile. Since patients with cholangiohepatitis are acutely ill, all measures must be taken to lessen the surgical risk. If bacteremia is present, blood cultures should be made to isolate the causative organism and a chemotherapeutic agent selected according to its *in vitro* sensitivity. Since the bacteria usually are intestinal, the sulfonamides and streptomycin are the drugs commonly used (*see* SULFONAMIDE THERAPY; ANTIBIOTIC THERAPY). With the sulfonamides the usual precautions against renal and hemopoietic toxicity are of course necessary. Hydration and nutrition of the patient must be maintained parenterally, though as much food and fluid as can be tolerated should be given orally, since caloric utilization and particularly nitrogen balance are greatly enhanced by use of this route. Vitamin K, orally or parenterally (R 24, 25, 26), is given daily to promote prothrombin formation (*see* VITAMIN DEFICIENCIES), as well as supplements of vitamins B and C when parenteral maintenance must be prolonged. Preoperative transfusion is advisable, especially when long-standing liver damage has resulted in hypoproteinemia. Crude liver extract (R 23) may be of some value. When maximal benefit from conservative therapy has been attained, surgery is carried out according to the nature of the obstruction: choledochostomy for stone; reconstruction of the ducts for stricture. Nutritional and chemotherapeutic adjuncts are continued through the postoperative period. During this time when the liver should be given every chance to regenerate, diet is of great importance. It should be high in protein and carbohydrate, with sufficient fat to make it palatable. A daily intake of 3,000 to 4,000 calories is optimal for liver regeneration. Fat, in reasonable amount, is not harmful at this time.

PRESCRIPTIONS

(Wherever a prescribed "proprietary" is representative of a class of therapeutic agents, alternative proprietary preparations will be found listed in Part II.)

Anthelminthics

1. R Emetine hydrochloride   (ampul)

> 60 mg. (gr. i) daily subcut. for 6 to 9 days and repeat course after a rest period of 1 week. The patient should be at bed rest during therapy. (CAUTION! Contraindicated in organic cardiorenal diseases.)

2. R Chiniofon   (enteric coated) . .   0.25 Gm. (gr. iv)

> 3 tablets 3 times a day for 8 to 10 days.

3. ℞ "Diodoquin" . . . . 0.2 Gm. (gr. iii)
   7 to 10 tablets daily for 15 to 20 days.

4. ℞ "Stovarsol". . . . . 0.25 Gm. (gr. iv)
   1 tablet 2 or 3 times a day for 7 days.

5. ℞ Gentian violet   (enteric coated) 30   mg. (gr. ss)
   2 tablets 3 times a day before meals for 2
   weeks; repeat course after a rest period of 1
   week.

6. ℞ Chloroquine diphosphate
   ("Aralen Diphosphate") . . 0.25 Gm. (gr. iv)
   2 tablets daily for 10 to 14 days.

Antispasmodics

7. ℞ A synthetic antispasmodic
   (For available products, see dose table of AL-
   TERNATIVE PROPRIETARY PREPARATIONS.)

8. ℞ Atropine sulfate
   0.6 mg. (gr. 1/100) subcut.

9. ℞ Belladonna Tincture U.S.P.. . 30.0 cc. (℥ i)
   10 drops in water as necessary for pain.

10. ℞ Amyl nitrite   (ampul) . . . . 0.3 cc. (♏ v)
    Crush ampul in handkerchief and inhale
    fumes.

11. ℞ Nitroglycerin   (hypodermic
    tablet) . . . . 0.3 mg. (gr. 1/200)
    1 or 2 tablets sublingually; repeat in 10 min-
    utes if necessary.

12. ℞ Papaverine hydrochloride. . . 30 mg. (gr. ss)
    1 or 2 tablets as necessary for pain.

Analgesics

13. ℞ Morphine sulfate
    15 mg. (gr. ¼) subcut.

14. ℞ "Demerol Hydrochloride"
    (ampul)
    50 to 100 mg. subcut.

15. ℞ Methadone Hydrochloride
    N.N.R.   (ampul)
    5 to 10 mg. subcut.

Antibacterial Agents

16. ℞ Penicillin   (vial)
    50,000 u. I.M. every 3 hours.

17. ℞ Streptomycin (vial)
>   0.25 Gm. I.M. every 6 hours.

Nutrients, Vitamins, and Digestants

18. ℞ Dried Yeast U.S.P.
>   2 to 3 teaspoons in glass of milk twice daily
>   between meals; increase until 6 teaspoons
>   twice daily are tolerated.

19. ℞ Choline chloride . . . . 50.0 Gm. (℥ xiiss)
>   Aromatic syrup of yerba santa
>   q.s. ad 240.0 cc. (℥ viii)
>   2 teaspoons after each meal.

20. ℞ Methionine . . . . 0.5 Gm. (gr. viiss)
>   2 or 3 capsules every 6 hours.

21. ℞ Sorbitan monooleate, polyoxy-
>   ethylene derivative. . . . . 0.5 Gm.
>   3 capsules with each meal. (CAUTION! The
>   use of mineral oil during this treatment is
>   contraindicated.)

22. ℞ Ox Bile Extract U.S.P. . . . . 0.3 Gm. (gr. v)
>   1 or 2 tablets after meals.

23. ℞ Liver Injection (Crude) U.S.P.
>   (vial)
>   20 U.S.P. u. daily, I.M.

24. ℞ Menadione . . . . 2 mg.
>   5 tablets daily for hypoprothrombinemia.

25. ℞ Menadione in oil (ampul)
>   2 mg. I.M. daily.

26. ℞ Menadione sodium bisulfite
>   (ampul)
>   2 mg. daily; administered subcut. I.M., or
>   I.V.

27. ℞ Thiamine hydrochloride . . . 10 mg.
>   1 to 10 tablets daily.

28. ℞ Nicotinic acid amide . . . . . 50 mg.
>   2 to 8 tablets daily.

MUSCULOSKELETAL

ARTHRITIS; RELATED DISORDERS

Classification

A perfect classification of the arthritides and related disorders has not yet been evolved. However, the following should be a useful guide to recognition of the more important types, most of which are subsequently described in this chapter:

I. Arthritis: Possibly on an infectional basis, but etiology unproved.
   A. Arthritis of rheumatic fever (q.v.).
   B. Rheumatoid arthritis (atrophic arthritis): (1) Adult type; (2) Juvenile type (Still's disease); (3) Ankylosing spondylitis (Marie-Strümpell); (4) Psoriatic arthritis.
II. Arthritis: Infectional, e.g., gonococcal, tuberculous.
III. Degenerative joint disease (hypertrophic arthritis, osteoarthritis).
IV. Arthritis: Associated with disturbances of metabolism: Gout (q.v.).
V. Arthritis: Neuropathic origin (Charcot's joints): Tabes dorsalis; Syringomyelia.
VI. Fibromyositis.

Other conditions which may give rise to painful joints (arthralgia) include acromegaly, acute disseminated lupus erythematosus, syphilis, undulant fever, typhoid, septicemia, synovial cysts, dermatomyositis, rat-bite fever, dysentery, granuloma inguinale, lymphogranuloma inguinale, drug intoxication, erythema multiforme, erythema nodosum, actinomycosis, histoplasmosis, Gaucher's disease, intermittent hydrarthrosis, menopausal syndrome, hemophilia, hysteria, tumors, tenosynovitis, ochronosis, bursitis, herniation of subfascial fat, osteochondritis dissecans, periarteritis nodosa, psoriasis, sarcoidosis, pulmonary osteoarthropathy, Sudeck's atrophy, purpural diseases, ganglion, Raynaud's disease, Reiter's syndrome, Morton's metatarsalgia, serum sickness, and scleroderma.

I. ARTHRITIS: POSSIBLY INFECTIONAL

RHEUMATOID ARTHRITIS

A chronic systemic disease with its major manifestations involving the joints, usually polyarticularly, with morphologic changes in the synovial membrane, periarticular structures, cartilage, skeletal muscle, and perineural sheaths.

Etiology

The cause of rheumatoid arthritis is not known. A relationship to infection, allergy, metabolic disorders, or endocrine dysfunction has been postulated but not proved. Possible factors predisposing to initial or recurrent attacks include infections (particularly of the upper respiratory tract), exposure to cold, shock, fatigue, or trauma of a physical or emotional nature.

Pathology

The lesions are nonspecific in character and consist chiefly of lymphocytic infiltration and overgrowth of connective tissue. The typical pathologic lesion is the subcutaneous nodule, which occurs in various locations, e.g., over pressure points such as the elbow or along tendons or the periosteal surfaces of long bones. These nodules are found in 20% of the patients and are similar to those seen in rheumatic fever (q.v.). They range from 1 or 2 mm. to 1 cm. in diameter and are characterized by a central zone of necrosis, a zone of mononuclear cell infiltration in a radial arrangement, and an avascular zone of dense connective tissue.

1. ADULT RHEUMATOID ARTHRITIS

The disease is more common in temperate climates, 75% of the patients are women, and in 80% of cases, onset is before 40 years.

Symptoms and Signs

Onset usually is insidious, with no obvious predisposing cause, but it may be abrupt with polyarthritis, fever and prostration. Characteristically there is gradual swelling, pain and tenderness of the joints of the fingers, wrists, knees, and feet. The lesions usually are symmetrical. During the acute stage the joints are warm, occasionally red, and may contain a small amount of fluid. Constitutional symptoms of fatigue and weakness may be present but fever usually is absent. Joint and muscle symptoms are most severe when the patient wakes in the morning and usually lessen with the day's activity. Overfatigue, however, induces much joint pain the next day. The disease is notable for remissions and exacerbations, with a tendency to become chronic, with progressive deformity and limitation of activity. Remission of acute manifestations of rheumatoid arthritis is frequently associated with pregnancy or the occurrence of jaundice.

Pain in the affected joint is accompanied by splinting of the adjacent muscles, with resultant "muscle spasm." The flexors usually are the stronger muscle groups; hence, flexion deformity is the expected end result. Any joint may be involved, but the wrists, interphalangeal joints, and feet are most commonly affected. Joint swelling with muscle atrophy, proximal and distal to the swelling, causes the fusiform appearance of these joints. The characteristic subcutaneous nodules described under pathology may not always be present. The spleen may be palpable (see Felty's Syndrome) and in 50% of cases some degree of generalized glandular enlargement develops. Cardiac lesions, indistinguishable from those of rheumatic fever, have been found at autopsy in about 7% of patients so examined. An accompanying psoriasis is present in an estimated 10%. Iritis is a not uncommon complication.

As the disease progresses, joint changes become visible by X-ray. Decrease in joint space caused by destruction of the cartilage (presumably due to pannus formation) is apparent. Punched-out areas in the bone close to the joint and generalized decalcification also are present. The end result is bony ankylosis with calcified bands bridging the joint space. With continual joint pain and resultant muscle splinting, muscle atrophy and wasting occur. The skin over the joint becomes shiny, thin, and atrophied, with increased sweating.

Laboratory Findings

A moderate hypochromic normocytic anemia which does not respond to iron almost always is present. The white blood count is normal or somewhat elevated. Leukopenia and thrombocytopenia may occur in chronic cases. The E.S.R. is usually elevated during the acute stage, but may be normal. When elevated it is helpful in following the progress of the disease.

Diagnosis

Rheumatoid arthritis must be differentiated from other forms of arthritis, for some of which there is a specific treatment and an excellent prognosis, whereas rheumatoid arthritis is a severe, disabling, progressive disease requiring long and patient care, and in which heroic treatment is sometimes justified. However, it usually progresses slowly and permits adequate opportunity for arriving at a diagnosis. Doubtful cases should be observed for at least 6 months before they are labeled rheumatoid arthritis.

Differentiation of **adult rheumatic fever** is extremely difficult—often impossible clinically—and complicated serologic tests such as the antistreptolysin-O titer and the agglutination test with group A hemolytic streptococci must be done. The antistreptolysin-O titer of the serum rises after infection with group A hemolytic streptococci. In approximately 90% of patients with rheumatic fever, this titer is significantly elevated and tends to remain so while the rheumatic process is active. The agglutination test, using group A hemolytic streptococci, is positive in 50 to 60% of patients with rheumatoid arthritis, while "false positives" in other diseases are rare. A positive agglutination is strong evidence of rheumatoid arthritis, while a persistently elevated antistreptolysin-O titer points toward rheumatic fever. The joint manifestations of most patients with adult rheumatic fever respond completely to adequate salicylate therapy, whereas the response in rheumatoid arthritis is less dramatic and stiffness usually persists. ECG examination is helpful in differentiating rheumatic fever. If symptoms continue for more than 6 months, rheumatic fever is less likely to be the cause.

Gonorrheal arthritis is readily distinguished, since the gonorrheal lesion usually is monarticular and acute; the patient has either an accompanying acute urethritis or a history of it, and gonococci often can be cultured from aspirated joint fluid. Should diagnosis be difficult, however, a trial of intra-articular and parenteral penicillin should be made: if no response is obtained, a gonococcal etiology usually can be excluded.

Tuberculous arthritis ordinarily is monarticular and the joint changes seen by X-ray are much more extensive than in rheumatoid arthritis of similar clinical severity. In some cases, aspiration of the joint fluid followed by guinea pig inoculation aids in diagnosis. Biopsy of the synovial membrane may be necessary.

Osteoarthritis seldom is difficult to distinguish: the firm, fibrous nodules (Heberden's nodes) about the terminal interphalangeal joints, with mushrooming of the terminal phalanx, are characteristic of osteoarthritis, whereas in rheumatoid arthritis the proximal interphalangeal joints are involved. However, in the presence of psoriasis affecting the nails, the rheumatoid process may attack the terminal interphalangeal joints of the involved digits. With osteoarthritis alone there are no systemic symptoms such as fever or tachycardia, the E.S.R. is normal or only slightly elevated, and there is leukocytosis; the patients usually are over 40 and often are overweight; and the joints affected are those which have received the greatest amount of trauma in the course of life. Thus, in osteoarthritis, the parts most commonly affected (except for Heberden's nodes) are the knees and hips; in rheumatoid arthritis, they are the wrists, feet, and proximal interphalangeal joints.

Acute gout (q.v.) can be readily differentiated by a history of periodic episodes of acute pain with intervening remissions. The great toe is involved in 60 to 70% of cases, and the serum uric acid may be elevated. On X-ray, soft-tissue shadows of uric acid deposits and tophi may be seen. In chronic gout, differentiation may be a little more difficult, but the acute and most of the chronic cases of gout will respond to colchicine, and this therapeutic test is the final diagnostic measure to be used.

Prognosis

Of patients with rheumatoid arthritis conservatively treated over a period of 10 years, 15% are likely to be bedridden, 50% functionally capable of caring for themselves, and up to 35% ambulatory but unable to earn their living.

Treatment

Many unrelated forms of therapy have been suggested, all with some reported measure of success, which is to be expected in a condition characterized by spontaneous remissions. Prompt and dramatic remissions have been achieved and maintained during, and in many cases for considerable time after, therapy with the adrenocortical hormone, cortisone (Compound E), or with the adrenocorticotropic hormone (ACTH); further evaluation of these or similar agents, however, is necessary.

All observers agree that certain simple procedures benefit the patients. An optimistic attitude on the part of the physician is essential in these cases; every endeavor should be made to free the patient from anything producing anxiety or nervous strain.

Rest: It is highly important that the patient avoid overfatigue, hence bed rest during attacks is essential. Rest thus should range from complete bed rest in the presence of fever or other acute symptoms and signs, to a nap before dinner for the slightly ill patient, to extra hours of rest daily for patients who are in a remission stage. Fatigue of an involved joint also should be avoided, and this may be accomplished by the judicious use of simple plaster of Paris splints. Because prolonged inactivity, either general or local, may lead to disuse atrophy with loss of muscle substance and a negative nitrogen balance, rest of the joint must be carefully supervised and simple active exercises through the full range of motion, within reasonable limits of pain and fatigue, be done regularly and frequently. A patient with rheumatoid arthritis should never remain in bed for an extended period without constant medical supervision. Proper posture at rest should be stressed. If joints become ankylosed, it is important that the resultant deformity be as functionally effective as possible, with due regard for the patient's occupation or usual activities. Thus, pillows should not be placed beneath the knees, since a knee so fixed in a bent position will become unable to bear weight. In spinal arthritis, a board beneath the mattress will help prevent the development of kyphosis.

Salicylates: These are the most effective analgesics (R 1, 2) and should be given to tolerance. Enteric coating on the tablets seems to decrease the gastric irritation caused by salicylates. Recommended dosage is 0.6 Gm. after meals and again at bedtime (4 doses/day). This may be decreased or increased by 0.3 Gm./dose, depending upon the patient's tolerance. Intolerance is manifested chiefly by gastric irritation.

Transfusion: The anemia accompanying rheumatoid arthritis responds poorly to iron but transfusion of whole blood, 500 cc., may produce remission, temporary or complete, and an increased sense of well-being.

Local treatment of joints: Heat often relieves pain temporarily. It may be applied with a lamp, heating pad, or hot water bottle, but moist heat as from a flaxseed poultice (*see* BEDSIDE PROC.) is the most beneficial. More elaborate physiotherapy such as diathermy and iontophoresis usually is not of sufficient benefit to warrant its use. These patients complain of morning stiffness, which decreases with activity during the day. They can reduce this stiffness more rapidly by taking a hot bath immediately after getting up, and by exercise. Active exercises are much more beneficial than passive. Passive movements when the patient is under anesthesia should be strictly avoided, since they often cause fractures and hemarthrosis. Counterirritants such as methyl salicylate ointment (℞ 3) may be applied to painful joints. If a joint is stretched tight with accumulated fluid, aspiration may give temporary relief, but fluid usually accumulates rapidly, even when an elastic bandage is applied after the paracentesis.

Diet: No special diet is known to be beneficial. As a rule, these patients are poorly nourished and should be given a highly nutritious, balanced diet (*see* DIETS). Supplements such as a tablespoon of powdered egg in a glass of milk once or twice a day, and a tablespoon to an ounce of cod liver oil once a day may be added. Cod liver oil can be rendered less distasteful if given in tomato juice after placing a pinch of salt on the patient's tongue. A gain in weight usually accompanies improvement.

Gold compounds: Gold compounds have been used extensively in the treatment of rheumatoid arthritis for the past 10 years. Reportedly, gold produces a remission in 60 to 80% of patients with active rheumatoid arthritis. Toxic reactions appear in 20 to 40%. Most cases will relapse within 5 years. Prevention of relapses by continuous gold therapy alone or supplemented with cortisone or ACTH is being tried. Gold should not be administered to the elderly, or to patients with a history of hepatic or renal damage or blood dyscrasia.

Numerous gold preparations are available, such as Myochrysine (℞ 13). Colloidal gold has proved ineffective. Some compounds are given I.V. but most are given I.M. Myochrysine (℞ 13) contains 50% metallic gold. The drug is injected deeply into the muscle, on the following schedule: 1 injection of 10 mg. during the 1st week, 25 mg. once a week for 2 weeks, and thereafter 50 mg. a week until a total of 1 Gm. has been given. If improvement has resulted without toxic effects, the treatment may be continued indefinitely with 50 mg. once every 2 to 3 weeks. Improvement is manifested by an arrest in the activity of the disease. As a rule, pain gradually subsides, the amount of salicylates needed is reduced and, lastly, stiffness disappears. Actual joint deformity is not changed. Joint swelling, redness and heat vary, but in a complete remission with gold these should be absent.

Toxic effects include pruritus, dermatitis, stomatitis, vague gastrointestinal discomfort, albuminuria with a nephrotic syndrome, hematuria, agranulocytosis, thrombocytopenia with purpura, and aplastic anemia. When any of these manifestations appears, gold should be discontinued. Before receiving gold, the patient should have a complete urinalysis, a total and differential white blood count and an estimation of the number of platelets on the smear, with a platelet count if they seem scarce. These tests should be repeated every 2 or 3 weeks during gold therapy, and the treatment should be stopped if the total white count falls below 4,000, and especially if the polymorphonuclear count drops below 40%; or if the platelets appear scarce on the smear, and a count shows less than 90,000; or if the urine contains albumin over 2+, or any blood. Eosinophilia above 4% may precede the appearance of a rash, but since this sequence is not invariable, eosinophilia cannot be relied on as an indication of beginning toxicity. Pruritus almost always precedes the rash and is a danger signal. The dermatitis can range in severity from a single eczematous patch to generalized rash with complete exfoliation, and death. The characteristics of the rash may vary, but any pruritic eruption appearing in a patient receiving gold must be attributed to the gold until proved otherwise. Minor toxic manifestations (such as mild pruritus without a rash) may be cleared up simply by withholding treatment temporarily and in such cases the gold may be resumed cautiously, at a dosage of 25 mg./week. However, if the toxic symptoms progress, not only should gold be withheld, but the patient should be treated with BAL (2, 3-dimercaptopropanol) (R̥ 14). In toxic reactions involving the hemopoietic system—agranulocytosis and thrombocytopenia —it is not safe to temporize, as most deaths ascribed to gold have been in this group and the progression may be very rapid. In all severe reactions, BAL should be started within 2 to 3 weeks after the appearance of toxicity; otherwise the damage may become irreversible. Preferably, treatment with BAL should be given in a hospital. As it is somewhat irritating, the drug should be injected under strict sterile precautions deeply into the muscle. Using 10% BAL I.M., the dosage for a severe gold toxicity is as follows: 2 to 3 mg./Kg. body wt. 5 or 6 times the 1st day, 4 times daily for 2 days, then 3 times daily for 4 days. This usually is adequate, but some cases may require a longer period of treatment, usually with 2 doses daily. In dermatitis, the pruritus disappears first; in blood dyscrasias, the findings usually become normal within the first 3 days. Because of the high incidence of toxic reactions, gold should be used cautiously and only by a physician thoroughly familiar with all its possible effects.

Foci of infection: Any existing focus of infection, if obviously detrimental to the patient's general health, should be removed. However, a remission in rheumatoid arthritis attributable to the removal of such foci rarely occurs.

Foreign protein and vaccines: These have generally been abandoned as ineffectual and sometimes even harmful. A few dramatic remissions have been described after giving typhoid vaccine I.V., but because of the rigors of this treatment and the rarity of therapeutic results its use is hardly warranted.

Massive-dose vitamin D therapy has been advocated, but beneficial effects have not been consistent and the attendant dangers have become increasingly apparent. These dangers consist of the mobilization of calcium with elevation of serum calcium (above 12 mg./100 cc.) and deposition of calcium in the renal parenchyma with resulting impairment of the excretory function of the kidney. If the medication is continued, the changes become irreversible and renal failure with uremia and death may follow. There also is a tendency for metastatic calcification, usually in the periarticular tissues. Massive-dose vitamin D therapy is therefore not recommended.

Deformities and contractures: Flexion contractures, which are the main crippling deformities in rheumatoid arthritis, are to be prevented if possible. Once established, they require orthopedic measures, such as gentle stretching either by wedged casts or manipulation. In some instances, surgical intervention is necessary for correction. However, these patients do not respond well to operative procedure while the disease is active.

2. JUVENILE RHEUMATOID ARTHRITIS
(Still's disease)

Rheumatoid arthritis in children, similar in most respects to the adult type. The disease is modified in that it occurs in growing joints, with resultant changes in growth and development. The prevention of deformities is especially important. Characteristic is the birdlike facies due to impaired growth of the mandible. Splenomegaly and generalized glandular enlargement are frequent. Pericarditis and pleural effusion also may be encountered. The prognosis and treatment are essentially the same as in the adult type (q.v., above).

3. ANKYLOSING SPONDYLITIS
(Marie-Strümpell disease)

A chronic progressive disease of the small joints of the spine, which is classified under rheumatoid arthritis partly because

*of the peripheral joint involvement that occurs in 20% of the
cases.* Microscopically, the changes in the vertebral joints are
similar to those seen in rheumatoid arthritis. The sex distribution differs from that of adult rheumatoid arthritis in that 90%
of the patients are males (most often young men). Onset
usually is gradual, beginning with mild back pain which becomes
increasingly severe. Complete immobility of the spine due to
ankylosis eventually ensues. Diminished chest expansion resulting from involvement of the costovertebral articulations is
common. The most important diagnostic sign is a rigid back,
which may precede X-ray evidence by months. The blood sedimentation rate is almost invariably elevated. When X-ray evidence does appear, it is characteristic. The first detectable
changes usually are in the sacroiliac joints, with blurring of the
joint margin (best seen in a 35-degree angle film). The next
change is in the apophyseal joints of the spine (best seen in
the oblique view). Finally, there is calcification of the anterior
and lateral spinal ligaments which, with the generalized demineralization of the bodies of the vertebrae, gives the characteristic picture of "bamboo spine." About 20% of these patients
have peripheral joint involvement which is clinically and roentgenographically indistinguishable from typical rheumatoid arthritis, except that it shows a predilection for the hips, knees, and
shoulder girdle.

Treatment

The treatment of choice in Marie-Strümpell spondylitis is X-
radiation of the involved area, supervised by one experienced
in using this procedure. The earlier the lesion the better the
prognosis. When combined with postural exercises and a back
support such as a Taylor brace, as many as 90% of such patients
will have remission. Many cases will relapse after 1 to 2 years
but will respond to further roentgen therapy.

Salicylates (Ŗ 1, 2) are helpful in controlling pain and may
be given in the amounts advised for adult rheumatoid arthritis
(q.v.).

Cortisone or ACTH has produced beneficial effects in this disease. Gold therapy is without effect in spondylitis, but in a few
cases the peripheral joint involvement has responded to it.
However, gold should not be used for ankylosing spondylitis.

4. PSORIATIC ARTHRITIS

The etiology, pathology, symptoms, signs, and treatment are
similar to those of typical rheumatoid arthritis, except that in
the presence of psoriasis the terminal interphalangeal joints may
be involved (as previously stated) and the arthritis generally
has seemed to be more severe, less responsive to traditional
therapy, and of poorer prognosis. With the advent of treatment
employing cortisone or ACTH, however, the outlook appears
more encouraging.

II. ARTHRITIS: INFECTIONAL

The two types most commonly encountered are those due to gonococcal or tuberculous infections. (For the latter, *see* TUBERCULOSIS OF BONES AND JOINTS). However, acute suppurative arthritides can be caused by any pyogenic organism such as the pneumococcus, staphylococcus, meningococcus, or streptococcus. In these, the only worth-while diagnostic procedure is joint aspiration, with culture of the organism. An appropriate antibiotic or chemotherapeutic agent then is given intra-articularly and systemically (*see* ANTIBIOTIC THERAPY; SULFONAMIDE THERAPY).

GONOCOCCAL ARTHRITIS

An acute monarticular arthritis due to invasion of the joint by the gonococcus and usually associated with a recent or present gonorrheal urethritis.

Symptoms and Signs

Onset is generally characterized by acute multiple joint pains indistinguishable from those of acute rheumatic fever (q.v.). Usually, though not always, this stage is followed by suppuration in a single joint. Knee, wrist, and ankle are the most frequent sites, but other joints may be affected. The joint is hot, red, exquisitely tender and painful on motion and contains an excess of fluid, often accompanied by tenosynovitis near the affected area. The periarticular structures appear to be boggy due to localized edema. There usually is a concomitant urethritis or prostatitis in males, or salpingitis in females, or a history of a recent gonorrheal infection; gonococci may be isolated from the urethral discharge. X-ray changes appear rather quickly and consist of loss of joint space due to destruction of cartilage.

Diagnosis

Acute monarticular arthritis in an individual with a history of gonorrheal infection strongly suggests gonorrheal arthritis. However, paracentesis of the joint, with smear and culture of the aspirated fluid, is requisite to establish the diagnosis. The complement fixation test also is helpful, whereas the early X-ray changes and the response to penicillin therapy, while less specific for this disease, may be of supplementary value.

Treatment

Penicillin (℞ 9, 10) is specific and should be administered I.M. in doses of 300,000 u./day, or more, either in divided doses or as a single repository injection. The joint should be completely aspirated, and a single injection of 50,000 u. of aqueous penicillin in 5 to 10 cc. of saline given intra-articularly if the joint is large (e.g., the knee) or less in smaller joints. It may be necessary to give a 2nd intra-articular injection. Penicillin is so effective in gonorrheal arthritis that a lack of response casts serious doubt upon the diagnosis. However, penicillin-resistant gonococci may be present, particularly in patients who have been treated for several reinfections. In such cases, sulfonamide or streptomycin therapy may be resorted to. Sulfadiazine (℞ 11) can be given orally, 1 Gm. every 4 hours for 4 or 5 days. Streptomycin or dihydrostreptomycin (℞ 12) is given I.M. in divided doses of 2 Gm. daily for 4 or 5 days. However, penicillin-resistant gonococcal arthritis is rare—much more so than penicillin-resistant gonococcal urethritis.

Joint aspiration is important in treatment as well as in diagnosis of arthritis. If asepsis is maintained with sterile syringes and needles and with proper preparation of the field, it can be carried out as an office procedure. Infiltration with 2% procaine (see CLIN. PROC.) down to the joint capsule will reduce the pain.

III. DEGENERATIVE JOINT DISEASE
(Hypertrophic arthritis; Osteoarthritis)

A chronic arthritis usually involving multiple joints, particularly those concerned with weight-bearing.

Etiology

The etiology is unknown, but aging, obesity, and joint trauma seem to be predisposing factors. The menopause also may have some influence on the development of hypertrophic arthritis, since symptoms most often appear at that period—however, this may be due only to the accelerated aging process. More women than men are affected, and the disease occasionally is seen in young adults.

Pathology

Destruction of hyaline cartilage through wear and tear and the resultant overgrowth of bone give the X-ray picture of osteophytes and loss of joint space with sclerosis of the adjacent bone. Some degree of lipping and spur formation at the articular margins of the bone is an early characteristic. Heberden's nodes, which occur on the terminal interphalangeal joints, also are classified as degenerative joint disease because of a similar age distribution, X-ray picture and course. However, no such direct relationship to trauma or the aging process has been shown for Heberden's nodes as for degenerative joint disease in general.

Symptoms and Signs

In the absence of trauma to a given joint, symptoms rarely occur before the age of 40. Onset usually is gradual and insidious. Although there is pain, muscle spasm or joint effusion seldom occurs. Periarticular structures are not involved, and subcutaneous nodules are absent. Symptoms are not constitutional, but chiefly related to structural deformity and presumably are due to some impairment of function or elevation of the periosteum by the pathologic process. The patients frequently are obese and do not appear to be sick. Pain is the chief subjective symptom and, unlike that of rheumatoid arthritis, is most pronounced after exercise.

Laboratory Findings

The blood sedimentation rate is normal or only slightly elevated. There is no leukocytosis. The X-ray shows osteophytic formations.

Treatment

It is important to inform the patient that his arthritis is not of a progressive type that will cripple him. With this reassurance, many patients obtain pronounced relief of pain through lessening of nervous tension. Salicylates (R 1, 2) are helpful analgesics. Weight reduction should be encouraged, where indicated, in order to decrease the load on the aged joints. Support of the affected joint by an elastic bandage often is beneficial. An ointment such as methyl salicylate (R 3) rubbed into the skin over the joint by the patient before he goes to bed sometimes helps. Local heat (either radiant or from hot poultices) often affords great relief. Diathermy occasionally is effective when other forms of local heat have failed. More elaborate physiotherapy, e.g., iontophoresis (see CLIN. PROC.) with procaine, histamine or Mecholyl, may be employed. An effective method of controlling the pain of Heberden's nodes is by contrast baths. The hands are placed in hot water for 2 minutes, then in cold for 1 minute, and this alternation is continued for 15 minutes.

If these simple measures fail, and if the joint changes are advanced, surgical intervention with joint débridement may be necessary. For degenerative arthritis of the hip (malum coxae senilis), hip fusion has been of great benefit in a limited number of cases, as has cup arthroplasty. The value of infiltration of a joint with acetic acid, potassium phosphate, or benzyl salicylate has not been established. However, in the great majority of cases, weight reduction, small doses of salicylates, simple supports and simple home physiotherapy, combined with reassurance as to the prognosis, provide adequate therapy.

IV. ARTHRITIS: ASSOCIATED WITH DISTURBANCES OF METABOLISM (see GOUT)

V. ARTHRITIS: NEUROPATHIC ORIGIN
(Charcot's joints)

Charcot's joints presumably result from the loss of proprioceptive sensation associated with tabes dorsalis or syringomyelia (q.v.). The synovia is markedly distended, with many loose bodies, but there is little or no evidence of inflammation in synovial membrane and periarticular structures. The joint is typically a flail joint with hypermobility and, although said to be painless, in certain cases pain is prominent. The knee is most commonly affected in tabes and the elbow in syringomyelia, but any weight-bearing joint may be involved. The diagnosis is made by demonstrating the neurologic lesion and by X-ray evidence of increased density of the bone and narrowing of the joint space with many loose bodies.

Treatment

Therapy aimed at the neurologic condition does not help the joint and little can be done for these patients other than providing a rigid support such as a straight-knee brace, or surgical fusion of the joint.

VI. FIBROMYOSITIS

Fibromyositis includes a group of nonspecific illnesses characterized by pain, tenderness, and stiffness of the joints, muscles, or adjacent structures. It may be acute or chronic and usually is secondary to trauma, infection, strain, poisons, or exposure to damp or cold.

The term **myalgia** signifies simple muscular pain in contrast to **myositis,** which is nonsuppurative inflammation of muscle tissue. Fibrositis is a similar inflammation of the connective tissue components of the muscles and joints. These conditions are unusual as distinct entities; ordinarily they occur in various combinations ("rheumatism"). Any of the fibromuscular tissues may be involved, but those of the back (lumbago), neck (torticollis), shoulders, thorax (pleurodynia), and thighs (charleyhorse) are especially affected.

Symptoms and Signs

Sudden onset of pain, which is aggravated by motion, is usual. Tenderness may be present and even localized to small "trigger" nodules. Local muscle spasm is noted in some cases. Fever is present only if the condition is part of a general infection. Other signs and symptoms will depend on the area involved.

The condition tends to disappear completely in a few days but may occasionally become chronic or recur at frequent intervals.

Diagnosis

It is extremely important that all specific causes of fibromyositis be excluded, such as arthritis, bursitis, rheumatic fever, periarteritis nodosa, dermatomyositis, scleroderma, lupus erythematosus disseminatus, trichiniasis, and myositis ossificans. For this reason, it may be necessary to observe a patient for several months before arriving at a diagnosis of "chronic fibromyositis."

Prophylaxis and Treatment

Prophylaxis depends on avoidance or correction of any etiologic factors. When a diagnosis of fibromyositis is made, relief may be obtained from such simple measures as rest, heat, massage, salicylates (℞ 1, 2) and the use of chloroform liniment (℞ 4). Injection of a 1% solution of procaine hydrochloride into "trigger" nodules may be beneficial (*see* CLIN. PROC.). The use of splints or a bed board may sometimes be necessary.

OSTEITIS DEFORMANS

(Paget's disease)

A chronic progressive disturbance in bone metabolism, in which an initial phase of decalcification and softening is followed by calcium deposition with resultant thickening and deformity.

Etiology and Incidence

The etiology is unknown. Osteitis deformans and diabetes are frequently associated in the same family. Both sexes are about equally affected and the disease is seldom encountered in patients under 30.

Symptoms and Signs

The onset is insidious, many cases being diagnosed while the patient is under treatment for other diseases. Any bone may be involved, but the long bones and those of the spine, pelvis, and skull are chiefly affected. The early decalcification leads to softening and bowing deformities of the weight-bearing bones resulting in kyphosis, flattened vertebrae, broadened pelvis, and bowed legs. Uncontrolled recalcification leads to thickening and enlargement of the deformed bones. Spontaneous fractures are not uncommon. Enlargement of the cranial vault gives the face a triangular appearance. Impairment of hearing is a frequent complication. Bone pain and muscle cramps are common symptoms. Despite the pronounced metabolic activity occurring in the skeleton, the serum calcium is normal and the phosphorus normal or slightly elevated; however, the serum alkaline phosphatase is always strikingly elevated. X-ray of the long bones reveals increased density, loss of architecture and cortical thickening; and the pelvic bones may show areas of decalcification surrounded by areas of thickened bone, giving a punched-out appearance; the outer plate of the skull appears fuzzy, a characteristic finding in osteitis deformans. The unaffected bones appear normal.

Diagnosis

The X-ray and laboratory findings are so characteristic that diagnosis will seldom be difficult. Occasionally, osteitis deformans may be confused with other conditions that cause local or general decalcification of bone, such as multiple myeloma (q.v.), osseous metastases from prostatic carcinoma, osteomalacia, hyperparathyroidism (q.v.), and senile osteoporosis.

Treatment

There is no specific therapy. The use of aluminum acetate has been advocated by some authorities but its value remains to be determined. Parathyroidectomy is useless and contraindicated. Roentgen radiation of the bones may ease pain. During the stage of decalcification, a diet rich in calcium and vitamin D is indicated (see DIETS). Orthopedic exercises and appliances are used as needed. The outlook for life usually is good but the deformities may eventually lead to invalidism after 20 to 30 years. Sarcomatous degeneration sometimes is encountered in Paget's disease and requires radical surgery and roentgen therapy.

BURSITIS

An acute or chronic inflammation of a bursa. Bursas vary in size, may exist at birth or develop in response to repeated friction, and usually are found near joint cavities. Superficial bursas are not necessary for function, and may be readily destroyed or excised; deep bursas are functionally important and furthermore may communicate with a joint.

Etiology

Bursitis may be caused by trauma, single or repeated, or by acute or chronic infection, including syphilis, tuberculosis, gout. The following are specific and common forms of bursitis: Olecranon (miners' elbow), prepatellar (housemaids' knee), subdeltoid (subacromial), retrocalcaneal (Achilles), iliopectineal (iliopsoas), ischial (tailors' bottom, weavers' bottom), infrapatellar, trochanteric, and bunion.

Symptoms and Signs

Acute bursitis: Following an injury, unusual exercise, or acute local or hematogenous infection, there is local pain, effusion into the bursal sac, swelling, tenderness, and limitation of those motions which tend to utilize the inflamed bursa. Effusion usually is serous and rarely hemorrhagic, due to the scant blood supply of the bursal wall. The effusion is absorbed by the endothelial lining of the sac and recovery usually follows within 1 to 2 weeks. In some cases the condition may become chronic.

Chronic bursitis: There may or may not be a history or evidence of previous bursitis, repeated trauma, or foci of infection. Acute symptoms may follow unusual exercise or effort. The bursal wall is thickened, with degeneration of the lining endothelium. In late cases, the bursa may contain adhesions, villi formation, tags, and calcareous deposits, with muscle atrophy conspicuous. Depending on these preceding factors, there may be various degrees of pain, swelling, effusion, tenderness, muscle weakness, and limitation of motion. The thickened wall of a superficial chronic bursitis may be palpated readily. Sinus formation is not uncommon in syphilitic or tuberculous bursitis. Gout especially involves the olecranon and prepatellar bursas, producing degenerative changes and chalky deposits in the tissues. Subdeltoid calcareous deposits may be demonstrated by X-ray. Chronic bursitis is resistant to therapy; attacks may last for a few days or for several weeks, with recurrence the rule.

Diagnosis

Bursitis must be differentiated from periarticular tears of tendons or muscles, osteomyelitis, tuberculosis, and cellulitis. Where a bursa communicates with a joint, both structures may be involved simultaneously in a pathologic process.

Treatment

Acute bursitis: Complete rest of the extremity in a sling or splint is desirable only until diminution of pain and of protective muscle spasm will permit tolerated active motions. Pain may be relieved by suitable analgesics (℞ 1, 2, 6). Early active movements will help prevent the development of crippling adhesions and voluntary movements should be increased as the acute bursitis subsides. Diathermy, hot fomentations, and gentle massage relieve symptoms by producing a hyperemia. Deep X-ray therapy often is very effective, especially in acute subdeltoid bursitis. If effusion is pronounced, aspiration frequently is necessary, followed by a compression bandage; in acute septic bursitis, open drainage may be warranted, together with antibiotics (℞ 9, 10, 12) or chemotherapy (℞ 11).

Infiltration of the subdeltoid bursa with 1% procaine followed by passive manipulation through all arcs of motion, physiotherapy, and active motion often are effective.

Chronic bursitis: When possible, the cause of the chronicity should be determined and eliminated; the patient's occupation and sports activities must receive consideration. Gout, syphilis, tuberculosis, and foci of infection must be eliminated as etiologic factors.

Diathermy, hot fomentations, and massage may be tried, although such measures are only temporarily effective. In the presence of calcareous deposits, galvanic iontophoresis may occasionally result in reabsorption of the calcareous material.

Existent muscle atrophy must be corrected by suitable functional exercises for the involved musculature. Deep X-ray therapy often will give striking relief from symptoms of chronic subdeltoid bursitis; in some cases, even calcareous deposits will disappear following X-ray treatment.

Should the preceding conservative measures be ineffective, the following procedures must be considered:

1. Sclerosing agents: Under aseptic conditions, and following preliminary aspiration of all fluid within the bursa, 2 cc. of 5% sodium morrhuate (or other accepted sclerosing material) is injected into the sac. A compression bandage is applied for 7 to 10 days. Pain is frequent and may be severe for the first few days, requiring analgesics (R̶ 1, 2, 6). Occasionally, repeated aspirations may be required after the use of a sclerosing agent.

2. Saline irrigation: It often is helpful to irrigate the subdeltoid bursa through two 18-gauge needles in an attempt to remove calcareous material. Such needling may be immediately effective, even where no calcareous material can be washed out.

3. Manipulation: Disabling adhesions may be treated by slow but thorough manipulation of the involved joint, with or without anesthesia, followed by daily exercises through all arcs of motion.

4. Special surgery: Removal of calcareous deposits, or of the entire bursa, is indicated when other measures have failed. Excision must be followed by appropriate exercises designed to strengthen the wasted musculature. In bunion, surgical therapy is aimed at reducing the prominence of the first metatarsal head by removing a portion of that bone.

RADIOHUMERAL BURSITIS
(Tennis elbow, Epicondylitis)

Radiohumeral bursitis is discussed separately because its exact nature remains controversial. Some authorities feel it involves a true radiohumeral bursa, located between the common extensor (conjoined) muscle of the wrist and the radiohumeral joint of the elbow; other workers believe it to be a partial avulsion of the common extensor tendon from its origin at the lateral epicondyle of the humerus, with resultant periostitis. In either case, the condition can be quite disabling. It may follow effort requiring supination of the wrist against resistance (as in screwdriving) or violent extension of the wrist with the hand pronated (as in tennis).

Symptoms and Signs

Pain over the lateral epicondyle of the humerus may be severe and radiate into the outer side of the arm and forearm. Point tenderness is present just distal to the lateral epicondyle. Pain is aggravated by dorsiflexion and supination of the wrist against resistance. Weakness of the wrist in dorsiflexion is pronounced. X-ray findings usually are negative, although a periostitis has been demonstrated in some cases. In obscure cases, infiltration of the area about the lateral epicondyle with 1% procaine will completely relieve all symptoms and signs, thus establishing the diagnosis.

Treatment

Conservative: Immobilization in a splint or by adhesive strapping, with the wrist dorsiflexed and supinated, plus daily diathermy is occasionally successful. However, therapy may be required for 4 to 6 weeks and recurrence is common. Where conservative treatment fails, or symptoms recur, surgery is indicated.

Surgical: Therapy is directed toward completing any partial avulsion of the extensor muscle origin, or destroying any existent radiohumeral bursa. Surgical intervention should be attempted in the following order:

1. Manipulation: The area around the lateral epicondyle is infiltrated with sufficient 1% procaine so that all pain and tenderness disappear. With the elbow extended, the origin of the common extensor muscle of the wrist is strained by active supination and dorsiflexion of the wrist against resistance and hyperadduction of the forearm on the arm. By straining the muscle at its origin, a partial avulsion may be made complete. Manipulation is followed by daily diathermy and active motion to the limit of tolerance.

2. Curettement: Under procaine anesthesia, the periosteum of the lateral epicondyle is curetted through a stab wound, followed by diathermy and active movements as above.

3. Excision: Surgical exposure of the region about the lateral epicondyle and the radiohumeral joint will complete any partial tear and, if indicated, allow for the excision of a radiohumeral bursa.

TORTICOLLIS
(Wry neck)

A constant or transient spasm of the muscles of the neck resulting in rotated or extended attitude of the head.

Etiology and Pathology

The cause of torticollis is unknown in the majority of cases. Rarely it is due to a congenital shortening of the muscles of the neck. It may be the result of trauma to the neck, rheumatic myositis, or disease of the cervical vertebrae and adjacent soft parts. It may be a symptom of dystonia musculorum deformans or it may follow epidemic encephalitis.

Sometimes it is a symptom of an underlying psychological disturbance. The onset usually is in adult life. Males and females are equally affected. The pathologic findings in the brain are meager and inconstant. Degenerative changes in the corpus striatum have been reported.

Symptoms and Signs

Onset may be sudden but it is more likely to be insidious. The superficial and deep muscles of the neck, particularly the sternomastoid, trapezius, splenius capitis and splenius collis, are involved. As a result of the contraction of the affected sternomastoid muscle, there is rotation of the head to the opposite side and flexion of the neck to the side of the contracting muscle. The spasm may be tonic, in which case there is a sustained rotated posture, or it may be clonic resulting in repeated, jerky movements of the head to one side. After several months the sternomastoid on the affected side may become hypertrophied.

Diagnosis

Since torticollis is a symptom of many disorders, it is necessary to differentiate the various causes. Definite age of onset will eliminate congenital torticollis. A history of encephalitis lethargica and other evidence of extrapyramidal disease will be helpful in identifying torticollis of C.N.S. origin. X-rays of the cervical spine and careful examination of the cervical region will exclude torticollis resulting from local disease of the neck. Detailed psychiatric evaluation of the patient may demonstrate a psychogenic basis of the condition.

Prognosis

Torticollis is a persistent and difficult symptom to treat. Spontaneous remissions may occur but the condition usually persists for life.

Treatment

General: Whenever possible the local causes of the symptom should be removed. The value of application of collars or casts to the neck is highly doubtful. Occasionally, the torticollis can be temporarily inhibited by the patient's exerting slight pressure on his jaw on the side to which the head is being rotated. **Medical:** In cases with an organic basis, the drugs of the belladonna group may be of some value. These drugs and their dosage are given in the chapter on Paralysis Agitans (q.v.). Sedatives such as phenobarbital (℞ 8), 30 to 60 mg. 3 times a day, are occasionally of some benefit. **Psychotherapy:** Prolonged psychotherapy may bring about improvement in cases of functional origin. In addition, such patients should be taught to practice muscular relaxation.

Surgical: Section of the spinal accessory nerve and the first four cervical roots is the most effective therapy in cases of torticollis of organic origin. Both stretching of the shortened muscle and myotomy have been attempted but neither is recommended.

LOW BACK PAIN

That type of backache which commonly occurs over the lumbar vertebrae, lumbosacral area, sacrum, sacroiliac region and coccyx, and often is accompanied by pain radiating throughout the region supplied by the sciatic nerve. It varies from soreness, a dull ache, or a dragging sensation to sharp intermittent or constant agony.

Etiology

The various causes of low back pain may be classified as follows: Traumatic injury to musculoskeletal structures; infectious processes in the area; chronic destructive skeletal disorders; congenital malformations of vertebrae and pelvis; compression of spinal cord, root, or both; and referred pain from other regions.

TRAUMATIC INJURY TO MUSCULOSKELETAL STRUCTURES

Low back pain may result from injury to the musculoskeletal structures of the lumbar region by external violence, or from too hasty lifting of heavy objects, sudden standing erect after stooping, sudden turning, or even violent twisting or sneezing. Faulty posture, muscular insufficiency, increase of muscular effort (as by changing to a more strenuous occupation) also may cause muscular or ligamentous strain resulting in low back pain. The most common lesion is a sprain or tear of one of the ligaments or muscles of the lower back. Chronic relaxation often is caused by a loss of resiliency which follows recovery from acute hemorrhage within and around the musculoligamentous structures.

The pain from such injuries may be diffuse or localized. It is accentuated by pressure over certain sites, known as "trigger points." The most common of these are the lumbosacral junction; the lateral border of the tensor fascia lata and the iliotibial band; the posterior superior or inferior iliac spine; the insertion of the gluteus maximus; the transverse sacral articulation; and vague points of tenderness along the sacrospinalis muscles. Pressure over these points, in addition to producing local tenderness, often causes radiation of pain down the sciatic nerve, probably as a reflex phenomenon. Movements that put stress on the damaged musculoligamentous structures produce pain, and therefore guarding movements are prominent in these patients. They usually have no pain while at rest.

Diagnosis

Spasm of the lumbosacral and sacrospinal muscles may be noted; often there is a tendency to hold the back rigid (poker spine), and when the patient is asked to pick up an object from the floor he will not bend his body forward but will make a deep knee-bend. Observation of the movements that cause pain is helpful in localizing the area involved. The Goldthwait straight leg-raising test will elicit pain at its source. The patient lies on his back and each extended limb is raised until he complains of pain. Gaenslen's test consists of hyperextension of one hip, with the opposite knee and hip acutely flexed to fix the lumbar spine. This causes pain in the region of the sacro-iliac attachments if these have been injured. X-ray examination may reveal a fracture.

Treatment

When the painful pressure point has been located, injection of 1% procaine may give temporary relief and also serve as a therapeutic test. To control the pain, opiates, salicylates, or both, may be given (R 1, 2, 6, 7). The majority of patients will derive much benefit from elimination of weight-bearing, or immobilization through use of traction in bed, a plaster body jacket, or by a back support during ambulatory treatment. Bed boards should be placed under the mattress for back support.

After the acute phase, treatment should be directed toward removing the cause; i.e., faulty posture, scoliosis, pelvic tilt, short leg, or obesity. If the pain is due to muscular insufficiency, the back muscles should be strengthened by proper exercises.

INFECTIOUS PROCESSES IN THE AREA

Inflammatory lumbago, or **myofascitis**—perhaps the most common cause of low backache—probably is of virus origin. Other specific infections which, acting locally, may be responsible include tuberculosis, typhoid fever, brucellosis, osteomyelitis, syphilis, meningitis, poliomyelitis, dengue fever, and occasionally the contagious exanthems, in which of course other symptoms are outstanding.

The pain of myofascitis may be due to the edematous swelling of the tissues which in turn produces irritation of the nerve endings. Tuberculosis, typhoid fever, brucellosis, or other specific destructive diseases may cause actual destruction of the bone and soft tissues.

Diagnosis

Myofascitis is distinguished by its sudden onset, with mild fever and leukocytosis. Moderate elevation of the sedimentation rate may be present. Pain is diffuse over the lower back. Usually, no history of strain or injury is elicited. In diagnosing the other infectious processes that may be responsible for low back pain, the associated findings must be considered. Vertebral lesions of tuberculosis (Pott's disease) produce limitation of movement and muscle spasm; in children, night cries are characteristic. Deformity, tenderness, abscess formation and positive roentgenographic signs are to be looked for. In meningitis and poliomyelitis, the typical spinal fluid findings will aid materially in identifying the specific cause (*see* table, Spinal Fluid Findings in Health and Disease, p. 986).

Treatment

The average patient with myofascitis will show improvement after 2 weeks of back immobilization. He should be put to bed and given analgesics (℞ 1, 2, 6, 7,) as indicated. Bed boards may be placed under the mattress to prevent sagging. Local application of heat (diathermy, hot water bottle, electric pads) and of liniment (℞ 5) provide welcome relief. Full activity should be prohibited for the first few weeks after recovery. Treatment of backache due to the various other infectious processes (q.v.) depends upon controlling the causative factor. Immobilization of the back and drainage of any existing abscesses are essential in all cases.

CHRONIC DESTRUCTIVE SKELETAL DISORDERS

The skeletal structures of the lower back may be the site of any of the following degenerative processes: hypertrophic (degenerative) arthritis, atrophic (rheumatoid) arthritis, senile osteoporosis, Paget's disease, osteitis fibrosa cystica, multiple myeloma, and metastatic neoplastic lesions. Diagnosis usually rests upon a complete history, roentgen examination, and laboratory work-up, including sedimentation rate and serum phosphatase.

Pathologic findings that may be noted on X-ray examination will depend on the nature of the condition present. Hypertrophic arthritis causes gradual destruction of joint cartilage, lipping, and the formation of spurs on joint edges. Atrophic (rheumatoid) spinal arthritis (Marie-Strümpell disease) involves the ligaments and soft tissues around the joints; later, it destroys the joint and may fuse the vertebrae. Senile osteoporosis is characterized by a decrease in bone density due to loss of calcium salts, which in turn may go on to compression of the vertebrae and senile kyphosis. Paget's disease may be responsible for coarsening and loss of the normal trabeculations, with thickening of the cortex of the pelvic or vertebral bones involved. Metastatic lesions usually appear as punched-out areas in the bone, or as diffuse mottled destructive (osteoclastic) lesions. A few forms of neoplasm (prostate, breast) may have metastases with bone formation (osteoblastic). Increase in sedimentation rate or serum alkaline phosphatase indicates increased activity of the destructive process. Increased serum acid phosphatase is almost pathognomonic of prostatic cancer metastasis. Treatment is directed to the underlying disease (q.v.). The usual palliative measures are applied for local pain.

CONGENITAL MALFORMATIONS OF VERTEBRAE AND PELVIS

Maldevelopment of the spine and sacrum causes abnormal strain on the muscles and ligaments and thus predisposes to pain. Spina bifida, additional lumbar vertebrae, abnormalities of the transverse process of the 5th lumbar vertebra, difference in the shape and slant of the articular facets of the lumbosacral articulation, lumbarization of the 1st sacral vertebra, and sacralization of the 5th lumbar vertebra are the commonest developmental disturbances observed. Arthritic changes often occur as a result of the greater stress placed on the involved structures.

Diagnosis

Other than those disclosed by X-ray, the findings are similar to those noted in myofascial strain. Final confirmation of diagnosis rests almost entirely upon X-ray evidence, including anterior, posterior, lateral, and right and left oblique views up to and including the 12th thoracic vertebra.

Treatment

In some instances, conservative therapy with heat (diathermy, heat pads, infrared) and immobilization (bed rest, brace) is effective. Fixation by surgical intervention may be necessary if these measures fail to give relief.

COMPRESSION OF SPINAL CORD, ROOT, OR BOTH

Pressure upon the spinal nerves or cord may result from herniation of a ruptured intervertebral disk; tumors of the cord, cauda equina, or nerve roots; vertebral fracture or dislocation; or arthritic changes. The intervertebral disk syndrome is the most common of these.

Diagnosis

The patient with an intervertebral disk injury usually states that "something gave way" in his back during physical exertion. This was followed by back pain, perhaps radiating down the sciatic nerve on the side affected. The pain is severe and continuous in type, aggravated by cough, straining, bending forward, and long periods of standing, and is usually relieved by lying down.

Muscle spasm, guarding of movement, tenderness over lumbosacral, lower lumbar and sciatic nerve regions, and diminution of skin sensitivity over areas supplied by the affected nerve, are all typical findings when protrusion of the nucleus pulposus through a traumatic or degenerative rupture of the posterior ligaments has occurred. There may be diminution of the tendon reflexes of the involved leg. The Lasègue test, comprising flexion of the thigh with the lower extremity extended, causes pain in the back and down the sciatic nerve. Roentgenographic evidence of the herniated disk is occasionally obtainable.

Tumors, traumatic lesions, and arthritic changes responsible for pressure on spinal cord or root usually produce constant pain unaltered by change in posture and not responsive to conservative measures of immobilization. In many instances they may lead, by spinal cord compression, to paralysis below the level of the lesion. Physical signs often will establish a segmental level of the lesion. X-ray examination is most helpful in discovery of the pathologic process.

Treatment

Conservative therapy for ruptured intervertebral disk includes bed rest, with application of traction to the affected extremity. The bed should be made firm with bed boards under the mattress. Analgesics (R 1, 2, 6, 7) are useful for control of discomfort. In the ambulant phase, support with a body cast or girdle may be advisable. Such ambulant immobilization may give relief and effect a cure after several months of application. Surgical intervention is indicated for recurrence of nerve or cord damage. Removal of the offending disk often gives relief.

PAIN REFERRED FROM OTHER REGIONS

Almost any inflammatory process in the body may cause low back discomfort. Some hold that a sympathetic myofascitis is the pathologic process responsible for this condition. The most common inflammatory disorders that may be heralded by low back pain are genitourinary and gastrointestinal disturbances. Female pelvic disorders, including dysmenorrhea, malposition of the uterus, prolapse, endocervicitis, uterine and ovarian neoplasms, and salpingitis are examples. Urethritis in the female and prostatic and posterior urethral disease in the male cause identical backache. Backache from ureteral calculi, renal ptosis, cystitis, or other urinary system disorders often may be the only complaint present and must be differentiated from that caused by intrinsic back disorders.

Visceroptosis and colitis are among the many gastrointestinal disorders that may act in a similar manner. Disturbances of the hip, knee, and especially the foot, often are the source of referred pain in the back. Hence, the physican must make a thorough search, including a pelvic examination in the female, in order to determine the exact cause of low back pain.

Treatment of referred pain is directed to the causal disorder. Symptomatic relief may sometimes be obtained by immobilization of the back, by putting bed boards under the mattress, or by strapping the back. Analgesics (R 1, 2, 6, 7) may be given as indicated.

COMMONER FOOT DISORDERS

PES VALGOPLANUS
(Flatfoot)

A structural deformity in which there is outward rotation of the heel, lowering of the medial longitudinal arch, displacement of the head of the first metatarsal dorsally, pronation and abduction of the anterior part of the foot, resulting in an everted position.

Pain is present in the long arch or frequently localized in the area behind the medial malleolus. Radiation of pain to the lateral and posterior calf muscles, or up to the knee, hip, and lower back may be noted. Discomfort is increased by prolonged standing.

Treatment

This consists of correction of the anatomic deformities through use of any of the following: adhesive strappings, arch supports, external shoe corrections (i.e., Denver heel and metatarsal bars), padding of insole with felt, operative intervention. Foot exercises often are helpful.

PES CAVUS
(High-arched foot)

A condition in which the longitudinal arch is exaggerated in height, commonly associated with dorsal contracture at the metatarsophalangeal joints. The excessive pressure upon the metatarsal heads is responsible for metatarsalgia (pain in the metatarsal region) and callosities beneath the metatarsal heads. There is frequently associated shortening of the Achilles tendon, which is responsible for further increased weight being thrown on the forepart of the foot.

Treatment

The pain may be relieved by a sponge rubber bar placed across an insole just behind the metatarsal heads, or a leather bar applied similarly to the outside of the sole of the shoe.

HALLUX VALGUS
(Bunion)

Acute angulation at the medial side of the first metatarsophalangeal joint; usually caused by the wearing of pointed

30

or too-short shoes. Prolonged pressure over this angle results in the development of an inflamed bursa, which frequently becomes infected. Periostitis and formation of an exostosis occasionally occur.

Treatment

Good results may be obtained by conservative treatment. It is essential to remove all pressure from the inflamed part by enlarging or cutting away the shoe in this area. Surgical intervention may occasionally be necessary.

HALLUX RIGIDUS

Limitation of dorsiflexion at the metatarsophalangeal joint caused by arthritic changes in this joint. Because of the pain which accompanies dorsiflexion, the normal push-off phase of the gait is inhibited.

Treatment

Pain usually can be controlled by splinting the joint with a narrow metal bar inserted within the layers of the sole of the shoe.

ACHILLES TENDON CONTRACTURE

Restriction of dorsiflexion of the ankle, with a predisposition to the development of a weak foot, due to shortening of the Achilles tendon. Symptoms of metatarsalgia, calf pain, low backache, and pain along the longitudinal arch are commonly noted. In the female, the symptoms may be exacerbated by the wearing of slippers or by going barefoot. The condition usually is a result of long-continued wearing of high heels; occasionally it is a residual of poliomyelitis.

Treatment

The milder forms are treated by gradual stretching, by manipulation or exercises. In severe cases, surgical lengthening is required.

PAINFUL HEEL

This condition may be due to a variety of causes including: (1) Periostitis or plantar fasciitis resulting from undue strain on the long plantar ligaments attached to the calcaneus. (2) Bursitis at the insertion of the Achilles tendon due to poorly fitted shoes. (3) Bony spurs arising from the inferior surface of the calcaneus, which often are palpable and painful on pressure. X-ray provides definite proof of their presence.

Treatment

(1) Strain on the ligaments should be relieved by correction of the primary condition—usually pes valgoplanus. (2) Proper shoes should be worn and the bursa protected with a piece of felt cut out at the center. Heel height may be increased tempo-

rarily to relieve strain on the Achilles tendon. (3) For bony spurs conservative measures such as applying a felt or sponge-rubber pad (cut out to form a ring) will relieve pressure on the painful spot. Surgical excision has been used in some of these cases.

HAMMER TOE
(Claw toe)

A flexion deformity of one or both interphalangeal joints, usually caused by poorly fitting shoes or stockings, but occasionally a residual of poliomyelitis. The deformity results in undue pressure on the resulting knuckle and this excessive pressure also is responsible for callus (corn) formation over the affected joint.

Treatment

Conservative treatment includes the wearing of well-fitting shoes, splinting and toe-stretching. Severe cases require surgical correction.

OSTEOMYELITIS

Bone inflammation due to pyogenic microorganisms. Infection of the bone is most frequently caused by *Staph. aureus* and *Str. hemolyticus;* rarely *E. typhosa* and *Br. abortus.* Various other organisms may be found in chronic phases but they usually are secondary invaders. Among the more frequent of these is *B. pyocyaneus.* (For bone infections caused by *Myco. tuberculosis* and *T. pallidum, see* TUBERCULOSIS; *see* SYPHILIS.)

Pathology

Infection may reach the bone either by the hematogenous route, or directly, as in a compound fracture or other trauma. The hematogenous origin, more common in children, usually is secondary to an acute local infection, such as a furuncle, otitis media, or pneumonia. Usually, only one bone is involved, but two or more foci are not uncommon. Sometimes, some original foci remain dormant at first, lighting up later, to give the appearance of metastatic lesions. In heavy blood stream invasions there may be a true pyemia with multiple abscesses throughout the body, the osteomyelitis being only a part of the general infection. Often there is a history of recent contusion or local bone injury, this then acting as a point of decreased resistance.

The tissue first involved is the bone marrow; usually near the end of the shaft if it is in a long bone. There is local necrosis of tissue which soon spreads. If the center of infection is near the surface, the exudate may break through and form a subperiosteal abscess. This may spread along the surface over the shaft while, at the same time, the infection is extending along the marrow cavity. The entire shaft of the bone may thus become involved with complete necrosis, or the spread may be arrested at any point. Very soon after the death of bone, the periosteum, which has become separated from it, commences to lay down new bone over it. The necrotic bone becomes separated from the surrounding living bone in the form of a sequestrum. The tube of new bone around the old shaft is called involucrum. Through it, openings called cloacae occur and sinuses, through which pus escapes, communicate with the surface.

If the infection is in proximity to a joint, which frequently is the case, an inflammation may develop in the latter with congestion of the synovia and increase in joint fluid, but with no bacteria present. The infection may actually break through into the joint, however, especially if the latter partially surrounds the bone, as the hip joint does the neck of the femur. Then a purulent exudate forms in the joint cavity and the articular cartilage is liable to early destruction.

In the chronic stage there is a deep-seated infection around the sequestra in the depths of the bone. This is subject to periods of greater activity, which are likely to be brought on by an obstruction to drainage from closure of the sinuses. From time to time, small sequestra may be extruded through the sinuses but there usually is no opportunity for the larger ones to be cast off.

Diagnosis

Osteomyelitis is characteristically ushered in with sudden pain in the affected bone and a sharp rise in temperature. In severe cases the patient is prostrated. There is tenderness over the bone, movement is painful and is involuntarily restricted. Swelling appears later over the bone and often in an adjacent joint. Leukocytosis of some degree is almost always present. The erythrocyte sedimentation rate becomes elevated. Blood cultures occasionally are positive. If fluctuation is present over the bone or if there is an effusion in the neighboring joint, it should be aspirated and cultures and smears made to identify the causative organism. Radiographic evidence of bone involvement frequently is not present until the disease process has been present for some time and therefore it often is necessary to make a presumptive diagnosis.

Some of the conditions which may be confused with osteomyelitis at the onset are poliomyelitis, rheumatic fever, myositis, sprains, and fractures, all of which cause local tenderness, pain and limitation of motion in the extremity.

Prognosis

With the employment of chemotherapy, many of the infections which were precursors of osteomyelitis are overcome so promptly and effectively that bone infection is prevented. When acute osteomyelitis does occur, the chance of controlling it before it has spread to serious proportions is excellent, provided the treatment is started promptly. Chronic osteomyelitis, smoldering throughout a lifetime, now is fortunately uncommon.

Treatment

1. Acute osteomyelitis: The all-important factor is the prompt administration of an effective chemotherapeutic agent as soon as the presence of osteomyelitis is suspected, and without waiting for radiographic or laboratory evidence, other than a blood count. Penicillin (R 9, 10) in effective dosage is the best agent to use at the onset before the causative organism is identified, since it is effective in controlling both the streptococci and staphylococci which account for the great majority of cases. Delay in treatment militates greatly against aborting the infection, for the reason that as soon as necrosis of bone takes place, the penicillin cannot reach the dead bone and combat the organisms in it. The administration of penicillin should be continued for at least 1 week after the temperature has become normal and all local signs of swelling and tenderness have subsided. Immobilization of the affected bone by plaster or traction is indicated until all evidence of active infection has disappeared, after which early motion is desirable.

If an abscess has formed, it should be evacuated and the cavity filled with penicillin solution containing 5,000 u./cc. If there is a joint effusion with evidence of infection, daily evacuation and refilling with penicillin solution should be performed until the inflammation subsides and the joint fluid becomes clear.

Later, if there is an abscess beneath the cortex of the bone as well, this should be drained by making a window in the cortex. The question of dealing with suppurative arthritis of a joint complicating osteomyelitis requires a high order of surgical judgment. Some of these joint infections subside after simple aspiration and injection of penicillin. Hyaline articular cartilage is destroyed so rapidly by the enzymes in pus, however, that in some cases it is advisable to incise and drain early in order to prevent this. Much less harm can be done by incision and drainage in doubtful cases than by delaying this procedure too long.

Supportive treatment is important from the start in all cases. A sufficient fluid intake is especially essential and usually should be ensured by infusions of normal saline and 5% glucose solutions. In the more serious cases blood transfusions often are helpful.

2. Chronic osteomyelitis: It is probable that the lower incidence of acute osteomyelitis and the possibility of arresting the disease before serious damage has occurred will reduce greatly the number of chronic cases. The basic principles in the treatment of the chronic case are wide exposure, thorough removal of dead bone, immobilization and the use of penicillin to prevent the spread of infection and to sterilize the remaining viable bone. It cannot be emphasized too strongly that the use of penicillin or any other antibiotic is not a substitute for the thorough cleaning out of all the infected dead bone.

In cases in which organisms other than the usual streptococci and staphylococci are found, the use of other agents such as streptomycin or dihydrostreptomycin (R 12) or sulfonamide (R 11) may be indicated instead of or in conjunction with penicillin. It is well to test the susceptibility of the organism to the antibiotic periodically since there is a chance that it may become resistant.

———

TUBERCULOSIS OF BONES AND JOINTS

A chronic destructive lesion of bone or joint due to invasion by Myco. tuberculosis *from a primary focus elsewhere in the body.* This form of the disease occurs as a complication in 3.8% of tuberculous patients. Onset usually is in childhood or early adult life, and most infections are due to the bovine strain of the organism.

Symptoms and Signs

The primary focus may not be clinically evident in all cases. Any bone or joint may be attacked, but the hips, spine (Pott's disease), knees, and hands are especially prone to involvement. The infection is monarticular in about 70% of cases. There often is a history of previous trauma to the site. In addition to the constitutional symptoms of any tuberculous infection (fever, malaise, anorexia, loss of weight), there are local symptoms referable to the diseased bone or joint. These include pain, heat, swelling, limitation of motion, spasm, some tenderness, and joint effusion. The abscess may rupture through the skin, leaving draining sinuses. Occasionally, there are multiple subcutaneous "cold" abscesses in the region. The end result is destruction of the bone and cartilage, joint deformity, and ankylosis. In Pott's disease, destruction and compression of the affected vertebrae (usually only two adjacent ones are involved) produce kyphosis and often compression of the spinal cord and nerves.

Roentgenogram of the bone may be normal in the early stages of the disease, but later it is characterized by narrowing of the joint space, due to destruction of the cartilage, and by the moth-eaten appearance of bone destruction.

Diagnosis

In the presence of the symptoms and signs described above, the diagnosis is suggested by the demonstration of a primary tuberculous focus elsewhere. However, definite diagnosis depends upon finding the tubercle bacillus in aspirated pus or in a biopsy of articular tissue or of the regional lymph nodes. Tuberculous disease of the joints or bones must be differentiated from other types of arthritis and from osteomyelitis (q.v.). Lesions of the hip require further differentiation from Perthes' disease and slipped femoral epiphysis.

Treatment

A primary focus must be searched for in all cases, and should receive intensive appropriate treatment. The usual measures to increase bodily resistance and promote general health are indicated (*see* TUBERCULOSIS). Heliotherapy is useful in the treatment of sinus tracts. Prolonged immobilization of the affected bone or joint is necessary to promote healing and establish a firm bony ankylosis. Recurrence is probable unless treatment either restores full motion or provides firm ankylosis. Surgical therapy is somewhat superior to conservative methods alone. Reports on the use of streptomycin or dihydrostreptomycin (R 12) are encouraging, but definite conclusions are not yet possible. The drug should be given I.M., 1 to 2 Gm./day in divided doses, for 60 to 120 days.

NEOPLASMS

Tumors of the musculoskeletal system arise predominantly from the skeletal structures. They may be primary (benign or malignant) or secondary (metastatic). Pathologically, a benign tumor is classified as an osteoma, osteochondroma, chondroma, bone cyst, giant cell tumor, osteoid osteoma, glomus tumor, neurofibroma, fibroma, synovioma, or eosinophilic granuloma. Primary malignant tumors include osteogenic sarcoma, endothelial myeloma (Ewing's tumor), reticulum cell sarcoma, and multiple myeloma (q.v.). Bone metastases occur especially in patients with cancer of the breast, prostate, thyroid, lung, or kidney (hypernephroma).

Symptoms, Signs, and Diagnosis

Small growths may be asymptomatic, and discovered only by accident during an X-ray study for other diseases. Larger tumors, or those in an area which is subject to pressure, may be the sites of pain, swelling, tenderness, or pathologic fracture. X-ray of the involved area will demonstrate the growth but only a biopsy can be depended on to determine the type of growth. Bone tumors may occur at any age, but certain types are more prevalent in adolescents and young adults (osteochondroma, bone cyst, giant cell tumor, endothelial myeloma, osteogenic sarcoma), while others are more frequent in later life (multiple myeloma, metastatic growths). Malignant change in a benign tumor is not common, but any sudden increase in pain or rate of growth must be promptly investigated.

Treatment

Benign growths which are symptomatic or rapidly growing require surgical excision. Excision of a giant cell tumor should be followed by postoperative radiotherapy since recurrence is not unusual. All bone cysts should be treated surgically as soon as diagnosed because of the risk of pathologic fractures. Primary malignant tumors offer a poor prognosis and require radical surgery or intensive roentgen therapy, or both. The pain of multiple myeloma (q.v.) may respond to stilbamidine. Beneficial results have been reported from the treatment of Ewing's tumor with a vaccine containing erysipelas toxin and *Bacillus prodigiosus.*

The therapy of metastatic growths is that of the primary disease. Bony metastases from the prostate (q.v.) or the female breast may be benefited by the administration of estrogen or testosterone, respectively.

MULTIPLE MYELOMA

A progressive and uniformly fatal, probably neoplastic, disease, characterized by infiltration of bone and bone marrow by myeloma cells and often by the appearance in the urine of a peculiar protein (Bence-Jones protein).

Etiology, Incidence, and Pathology

The etiology is unknown. Men are more frequently affected than women, in a ratio of about 3:1. The average age at onset is in the late fifties, and the disease rarely develops before the age of 35.

The bone marrow is diffusely infiltrated by myeloma cells which are either identical with or closely resemble mature and immature plasma cells. The bony thorax and skull are most frequently involved. The process may invade soft tissues such as the liver, spleen, and kidneys. Amyloidosis may occur and hyaline masses may be deposited in the renal glomeruli.

Symptoms and Signs

Pain is the outstanding feature of the disease and often may be the only symptom. It is most commonly felt in the thorax or lumbar region, aggravated by motion or deep breathing. Other neurologic symptoms such as root pain, sciatica, or paraplegia may follow collapse of a vertebra. Pathologic fractures, not including compression fractures of the vertebrae, occur in 15 to 20% of the cases. Bleeding from the nose and gums is not uncommon. As the condition progresses, the typical signs of a malignant, wasting disease appear. Renal insufficiency is a common contributory cause of death.

Laboratory Findings

X-rays show the characteristic punched-out, osteolytic lesions and the more diffuse osteoporosis that is most pronounced in the spinal column.

Anemia is common and does not respond to the usual forms of treatment. The leukocyte count usually is within normal limits, although excessively high counts have been recorded. Eosinophilia or lymphocytosis may occur, and immature myeloid cells are commonly present. The myeloma cells also appear in the blood smear, but are frequently missed or are confused with lymphocytes, although careful studies have demonstrated these cells in as high as 73% of cases. At times they are so abundant that the cases are classified as plasma cell leukemias. The red cells may show excessive formation of rouleaux; autohemagglutination often is present, making red cell counts or blood typing difficult or impossible. The erythrocyte sedimentation rate is usually accelerated. These findings are apparently associated with a moderate to marked elevation of the serum globulin. Serum protein concentrations as high as 14 Gm. with a 1:3 albumin-globulin ratio have been recorded. The serum protein elevation occurs in about 70% of cases. Serum calcium levels frequently are high (12 to 16 mg./100 cc.) but serum inorganic phosphates usually are normal.

In the majority of patients, the urine shows evidence of renal damage. Albuminuria is the most common finding and casts and red cells may appear. Bence-Jones protein is present in the urine of 40 to 50% of cases (see LAB. PROC.).

Wright's-stained bone marrow smears (see LAB. PROC.) frequently show the typical myeloma cells, but a negative result should not exclude the diagnosis. If the infiltration is spotty rather than diffuse, the actual lesions may be missed. In some cases it may be necessary to do repeated aspirations or a biopsy of bone and marrow before a positive diagnosis can be established.

Diagnosis

The diagnosis should be suspected whenever punched-out lesions of bone are discovered by X-ray in an adult complaining of pain. The above mentioned laboratory findings will help to establish the diagnosis. In certain cases of aplastic or severe hypoplastic anemia, large numbers of plasma cells may be present in the marrow and these may be a source of confusion. The disease also must be differentiated from chronic inflammatory conditions of the mouth, nasopharynx, or bone, where the exudate may be largely composed of plasma cells.

Prognosis and Treatment

The average survival time is about 18 months and the great majority of patients die within 3 years. The results of therapy have been very discouraging. Roentgen therapy has been of no avail, and the results with radioactive phosphorus have not been encouraging. Nitrogen mustard (*see* HODGKIN'S DISEASE) will relieve pain in some patients, but its degree of effectiveness remains to be determined.

Recent reports on the investigative use of stilbamidine, pentamidine, or urethane have been more encouraging, in that pain may be lessened following treatment, although there is no X-ray evidence that the bone lesions are affected, or other indication that the prognosis is improved. Cortisone or ACTH similarly may give transient benefit.

Other treatment consists of radiation and the liberal use of potent analgesics (R 6, 7). Chordotomy or operative treatment of vertebral collapse may be considered as heroic.

ADRENOCORTICAL AND RELATED THERAPY

Because of dramatic results observed in many diseases, physicians are increasingly interested in cortisone (Compound E of Kendall; Cortone), adrenocorticotropic hormone (ACTH), and substances of related activity. The exact mode of action of these compounds is still not clear nor has the full range of their usefulness been established. However, current investigations are yielding data regarding the beneficial effects produced by these substances in an expanding variety of conditions.

Dosage and other therapeutic details remain subject to change. Therefore, the reader is referred to the scientific literature and to the latest available instructions from manufacturers of these products. In this chapter will be outlined certain fundamental guiding principles in adrenocortical and related therapy.

Description and Sources

Cortisone is one of the several crystalline hormonal substances isolated from extracts of the adrenal cortex. Chemically, it is 11-dehydro-17-hydroxycorticosterone, and it has been synthesized from a bile acid.

The pituitary adrenocorticotropic hormone (ACTH) is a purified active substance which stimulates certain adrenocortical activity. It is extracted from the pituitary glands of animals.

Metabolic Effects

It is assumed that the ultimate effects (with certain variations not yet completely explained) of the administration of cortisone and ACTH are essentially the same, since the latter stimulates activity of the adrenal cortex.

Carbohydrate metabolism is affected, in that gluconeogenesis, the storage of glycogen in the liver, and blood sugar levels are all increased, while the response to insulin is decreased. In diabetics, insulin requirements are increased during administration, but quickly revert to their original levels following its cessation.

Protein metabolism is affected in most patients, especially by high dosage. Continued large doses usually produce a negative nitrogen balance which can, however, in certain instances, be overcome by increased food intake. Where reversed albumin-globulin ratios are present, these tend to revert toward normal. Creatinuria is observed, uric acid excretion is increased and changes in the pattern of amino acid excretion occur.

Electrolyte balance is affected to varying degrees. Early retention of sodium and water is observed, usually followed by spontaneous diuresis on continued administration or following its cessation. On several occasions, however, sodium and water retention has been so great as to require lowering the dosage or discontinuing the drug because ascites or peripheral or pulmonary edema developed. High dosage often causes increased urinary excretion of potassium. In several patients such loss produced symptoms requiring replacement of potassium. These facts emphasize the necessity for constant observation of patients receiving cortisone or ACTH, so that the occasionally exaggerated and undesirable metabolic effects can be anticipated and, if possible, avoided.

Hormonal Effects

Because cortisone and ACTH are physiologically active hormones, certain excessive (but reversible) hormonal effects may follow prolonged administration or high dosage.

In some patients either cortisone or ACTH has produced rounding of the face, hirsutism, acne, striae of the skin and, in a few women, amenorrhea. However, these phenomena diminish considerably or disappear entirely after the medication is withdrawn.

In animal experiments, prolonged high dosage of cortisone often has caused a reduction in the size of the adrenal cortices; similarly, administration of ACTH has produced suppression of pituitary output of adrenocorticotropic hormone and an increase in the size of the adrenals. Muscular weakness and asthenia have been reported in patients for brief periods following the giving of these agents, which suggests that a transient period of adrenal cortical insufficiency may occur. A clinically significant degree of hypoglycemia, accompanied by decreased urinary excretion of corticoids and 17-ketosteroids, also has been observed in certain patients following cessation of dosage.

Other Physiologic Effects

With cortisone and ACTH a slight rise in blood pressure is not infrequent; a significant rise is rare.

There is evidence which suggests that, in unusually large doses, both hormones may retard wound healing through inhibition of the growth of granulation and fibrous tissues. On the other hand, wounds and ulcers have, in most instances, healed normally in patients under treatment with either hormone.

Certain mental effects have been reported. Definite improvement in the mental attitude of the patients receiving these agents usually occurs, often with acceleration of the alpha waves in the EEG. In certain instances, however, the increase in mental activity may create temporarily an exaggerated sense of well-being and, still less frequently, produce a manic state. (Conversely, mental depression has been reported in a few cases.) Insomnia occurs in some individuals. In rare instances preexistent or dormant mental derangements, such as schizophrenia, may be awakened or intensified, occasionally requiring electric shock therapy (q.v.) to halt the disturbance.

Since either of these hormones may produce euphoria, with increased psychomotor activity, it is advisable to take appropriate measures to prevent physical overexertion by patients having such cardiovascular disease as coronary insufficiency. This precaution also applies to the management of patients who have been confined to bed for protracted periods of time, even though they may have shown no evidence of cardiac disease.

Under ordinary conditions the discontinuance of therapy employing cortisone or ACTH should be gradual. In any event, continued supervision of the patient is essential. Sudden reappearance of severe manifestations of the disease for which the patient was being treated occurs in some instances.

In a few cases, following prolonged high dosage of cortisone, if treatment is withdrawn abruptly, evidence of a temporary hypoadrenal state may be observed. Weakness and hypoglycemia may occur, but return of adrenal function may be expected within 2 weeks. Likewise, a transient period of hypoactivity of certain pituitary functions may follow sudden cessation of therapy with ACTH.

Clinical Results and Laboratory Findings

Both cortisone and ACTH produce prompt relief of the symptoms of both the adult and juvenile types of rheumatoid arthritis, the improvement being noted usually within 24 hours, and sometimes as soon as 6 hours, after the initial dose. First, subjective stiffness diminishes. Next, articular tenderness and pain on motion decrease. Finally, swelling of the joints diminishes, sometimes fairly rapidly and completely, although occasionally more slowly and incompletely. The degree of improvement is limited by the amount of irreversible pathologic alteration in the affected parts, i.e., by the permanent bone, tendon, and joint changes. The appetite usually improves rapidly, and many patients, describing a loss of their previous feeling of "toxicity," experience a sense of well-being, occasionally within a few hours after the drug is first given.

An elevated E.S.R. is lowered, sometimes rapidly, usually becoming normal within 10 to 35 days after administration is begun. Occasionally, while the rate does not return to normal, it is definitely reduced. In a few instances a persistently high E.S.R. has been reduced by temporarily increasing the daily dose of the hormone. Low hemoglobin values tend to increase, and rises of 1,000,000 red blood cells/cu. mm. have been observed in anemic patients treated for 2 or more weeks.

In most patients, the beneficial effect or remission of symptoms is obtained only during the period of administration or it may last for several days or weeks thereafter. In some cases substantial relief can be provided more or less constantly for patients with conditions responding to these agents by giving one or the other in small maintenance doses, the duration of which has not been definitely established.

In patients with rheumatoid spondylitis (Marie-Strümpell's disease) the effects of these substances are, in general, essentially comparable to those observed in rheumatoid arthritis. Restoration of motion is limited, obviously, by the spinal apophyseal ankylosis and ligament calcification already present.

When one or the other of these hormones is administered to patients with acute rheumatic fever, painful, swollen, and inflamed joints become symptom-free—in most instances rapidly. Elevated temperature and E.S.R. become normal, tachycardia disappears, and in some cases, an increased P-R interval will revert to normal. Appetite usually is increased, and the patients report a sense of well-being, appearing alert instead of ill and "toxic." Relief of symptoms persists in most cases.

Cortisone is of distinct value in Addison's disease and in the adrenogenital syndrome.

Disorders such as psoriatic arthritis, lupus erythematosus (early), various allergies (bronchial asthma, hay fever, angioneurotic edema, drug sensitization, serum sickness), inflammatory eye diseases, exfoliative dermatitis, pemphigus, and panhypopituitarism often respond well to the administration of cortisone or ACTH. These or similar hormonal substances may prove of further value because of encouraging results observed in such conditions as acute gouty arthritis, ulcerative colitis, regional enteritis, nephrotic syndrome, dermatomyositis, psoriasis, retrolental fibroplasia, pulmonary granulomatosis, agranulocytosis, and certain forms of anemia.

Transient ameliorative effects have been observed in acute leukemia (lymphocytic or granulocytic), multiple myeloma, lymphosarcoma, Hodgkin's disease, chronic lymphatic leukemia, scleroderma (early), periarteritis nodosa (early), and alcoholism.

Neither substance seems to be of value in myasthenia gravis, amyotrophic lateral sclerosis, congestive heart failure, chronic myelogenous leukemia, acute monocytic leukemia, glomerulonephritis (exclusive of nephrotic syndrome), and poliomyelitis. In diabetes mellitus, the severity of the disease actually increases during their administration.

Routes of Administration; Dosage

Cortisone is effective either by oral or I.M. administration, or, in certain eye or skin conditions, when topically applied. Dosage must *always* be individualized. For example, in rheumatoid arthritis a maximal response usually requires the giving of 300 mg. the 1st day, 200 mg. the 2nd day, then 100 mg. every 24 hours for 7 to 14 days or less. Doses are given at suitable intervals, depending on whether the more rapidly absorbed oral or the more slowly utilized parenteral material is employed. When the desired response is evident, the total daily dose should be gradually reduced until an adequate maintenance level—possibly 50 mg./day or 100 mg. every 2nd day—is reached. (Failure to obtain or maintain a satisfactory response calls for an increase in dosage sufficient to produce the desired effect, after which cautious reduction may again be attempted.) With such moderate sized maintenance dosage, the development of undesirable hormonal effects is lessened.

With comparable indications, the initial doses of ACTH will average 10 to 20 mg., given I.M. every 6 hours for 7 to 21 days, after which a satisfactory maintenance level and an optimum dose interval should be sought. These usually are of the order of 5 to 10 mg. I.M. every 6 to 12 hours. As with cortisone, gradually tapering off is preferable to sudden cessation.

For suggestions concerning duration of therapy and the advisability of occasional rest periods, for dosage regimens in other diseases, and for the essential precautions to be observed in all cases, the reader should consult the latest literature and package directions issued by the manufacturers of either product.

PRESCRIPTIONS

(Wherever a prescribed "proprietary" is representative of a class of therapeutic agents, alternative proprietary preparations will be found listed in Part II.)

Analgesics

1. ℞ Acetylsalicylic acid . . . . . . 0.3 Gm. (gr. v)

   2 or more tablets after each meal and at bedtime.

2. ℞ Sodium salicylate   (enteric
   coated) . . . . 0.3 Gm. (gr. v)

   2 or more tablets after each meal and at bedtime.

3. ℞ Methyl salicylate . . . . 4.0   cc.   (℥ i)
     Menthol. . . . . 4.0   Gm.   (℥ i)
     White Petrolatum U.S.P. q.s. ad 30.0   Gm.   (℥ i)
        Rub affected parts gently and thoroughly.

4. ℞ Chloroform Liniment U.S.P. . .120.0   cc.   (℥ iv)
        Rub affected parts gently and thoroughly.

5. ℞ Methyl salicylate . . . . . . 30.0   cc.   (℥ i)
     Chloroform . . . . 15.0   cc.   (℥ ss)
     Soap Liniment U.S.P. . .q.s. ad 90.0   cc.   (℥ iii)
        Rub affected parts 10 minutes twice daily.

6. ℞ Codeine phosphate 15   mg.   (gr. ¼)
        1 or 2 tablets orally or subcut. every 4 hours
        for pain.

7. ℞ Morphine sulfate
        10 to 15 mg. (gr. ⅙ to ¼) every 4 hours for
        severe pain.

8. ℞ Phenobarbital 30   mg.   (gr. ss)
        1 or 2 tablets 3 times a day.

Antimicrobial Agents

9. ℞ Penicillin   (vial)
        30,000 u. I.M. every 3 hours or 300,000 u.
        I.M. every 12 to 24 hours.

10. ℞ Procaine penicillin   (vial)
        300,000 u. I.M. daily.

11. ℞ Sulfadiazine . . . . 0.5   Gm. (gr. viiss)
        2 tablets every 4 hours for 4 or 5 days.

12. ℞ Streptomycin or dihydrostrep-
      tomycin   (vial)
        For nontuberculous infections: 0.5 Gm. I.M.
        every 6 hours for 4 or 5 days.
        For bone and joint tuberculosis: 1 to 2 Gm.
        I.M. daily for 60 to 120 days.

Miscellaneous

13. ℞ "Myochrysine"   (ampul)
        To be given I.M. in accordance with schedule
        outlined in text (*see* Rheumatoid Arthritis).

14. ℞ BAL (2,3-dimercaptopropanol),
      10% solution in oil   (ampul)
        Give deeply I.M. in accordance with proce-
        dure outlined in text under toxic manifesta-
        tions of gold (*see* Rheumatoid Arthritis).

NERVOUS SYSTEM

PAIN

Pain may be due to a multitude of organic or psychic disturbances, and is the symptom which most often brings a patient to seek medical care.

Pain may be felt at the site of the causative lesion or it may occur in a different region (referred pain). It serves to call the individual's attention to a diseased state which might otherwise remain concealed. The location, frequency, character, radiation, and other characteristics of the pain are useful in reaching a diagnosis but are not conclusive; as always, a thorough history and physical examination are required. Local lesions usually cause localized areas of pain, whereas generalized diseases tend to produce generalized discomfort. Severity of pain may vary widely, depending on both the type and extent of the lesion and also on the sensitivity (pain threshold) of the individual.

The physician must never be content merely to control pain without also determining and treating its underlying cause. Prolonged study, including psychiatric evaluation, often is necessary before the latter can be determined.

Treatment

Therapy of the underlying causal condition (q.v.) is the prime consideration. However, when appropriate therapy of the basic disease does not or cannot afford prompt relief, symptomatic therapy is indicated. (The treatment of specific types of pain is described in many chapters throughout this MANUAL.)

Rest of the painful part, heat, cold, change in position, or counterirritants may be all that is necessary in many patients. Many useful analgesics are available to the physician. Those which act by peripheral sensory nerve depression are preferred whenever available and applicable. Thus, raw painful areas may be treated with an anesthetic ointment containing 1% dibucaine or 5% benzocaine. The local infiltration of an area with 1 to 2% procaine is sometimes useful.

When central depression is desired the *mildest effective agent* is recommended. Lesser degrees of pain usually will respond to the oral use of salicylates or salicylate combined with acetophenetidin. More severe pain requires the oral or subcut. use of codeine, Demerol, methadone, Dilaudid, Pantopon, metapon, cobra venom, or morphine, as appropriate. When very rapid relief of severe pain is desired, morphine may be slowly injected I.V. Occasionally, the I.V. use of ethyl alcohol or 1% procaine is indicated for the control of severe generalized pain. The effectiveness of these analgesics often may be enhanced by the judicious use of antispasmodics or mild sedatives. Sedatives alone are of value in controlling only mild degrees of pain. Except in such situations as during the end stages of cancer, the continued use of habit-forming analgesics is not advisable (*see* DRUG ADDICTION).

HEADACHE
(Cephalalgia)

Headache (pain in the head) is one of the most common of all symptoms and often is present in connection with a variety of conditions. The management of the problem of headache is difficult and taxes the diagnostic and therapeutic ability of the physician. The difficulty can be somewhat simplified by using

DIFFERENTIAL DIAGNOSIS OF DISEASES

Cause	Typical History

ORGANIC DISEASE
A. Intracranial (incr. press.)
  1. Expanding Lesions
    Brain tumor
	Headache: mild to severe, localized or generalized, intermittent or constant. Slowly progressive weakness on one side, convulsions, visual changes, speech difficulties, vomiting, mental changes.

Brain abscess	As above; history of ear disease, sinusitis, bronchiectasis, or lung abscess.
Subdural hematoma	As above; history of trauma, changes in state of consciousness.
2. Meningeal Irritation Meningitis, acute	Headache: severe, generalized, constant, radiates down neck; constitutional reaction, with vomiting. Preceding sore throat or upper respiratory infection.

Meningitis, chronic
    Syphilis
    Tuberculosis
	Headache: severe to dull, generalized or over vertex. History of lues or tuberculosis.

Subarachnoid hemorrhage	Headache: sudden in onset, severe and constant. Preceding history of pain in and about one eye, and of a drooping eyelid.
B. Cranial (changes in skull) 1. Paget's Disease	Headache: severe, burning type of pain, intermittent or constant, localized or generalized. History of increasing size of skull, pain in back and limbs.
2. Metastatic Neoplasms	As above; symptoms of a primary lesion elsewhere.

C. Involvement of Sensory
    Nerves of Scalp
    Supraorbital, auriculotemporal, posterior auricular, greater occipital; herpes zoster of gasserian ganglion.
	Headache: paroxysmal, radiates along course of nerve. Pain of herpes may be constant.

D. Vascular Disturbances 1. Migraine	Headache: usually unilateral, may be bilateral, throbbing sensation beginning in and about eye, spread to involve one or both sides. Prodromals: changes in mood, anorexia, scintillating scotomas. Anorexia, nausea and vomiting with headaches. Periodic attacks, each about the same, over extended period. Family history positive.

a logical, clinical approach. Attempts frequently are made to utilize the character, the severity and the localization of the head pain as differential diagnostic criteria. Unfortunately, this can be misleading. All too frequently a headache thought from its description to be of psychologic origin will be found to be due to an organic lesion and vice versa. It is important to evaluate the patient completely before any conclusion is reached.

GIVING RISE TO HEADACHE

Physical and Neurologic Findings	Special Studies That Are Indicated
Papilledema, visual field changes, aphasia, paralysis, changes in mental status.	X-ray of skull, X-ray of chest, electro-encephalography, lumbar puncture, arteriography, pneumoencephalography.
As above; evidence of local or distant infective focus; temperature may be subnormal, pulse may be slow.	As above.
As above; difference in size of pupils.	As above.
Patient usually acutely ill; may be confused, irrational, excited; may have stiff neck, positive Kernig.	Blood culture, lumbar puncture, with smear and culture of fluid.
Signs of meningeal irritation less marked than in acute form; cranial nerve signs positive.	Lumbar puncture with smear, culture and guinea pig inoculation of fluid. X-ray of chest. Blood and spinal fluid Wassermann.
Patient drowsy or comatose; stiff neck, positive Kernig, bilateral Babinski's, 3rd nerve paralysis; elevated B. P.	Lumbar puncture.
Skull tender; suggestive configuration of skull; evidence of compression of brain and cranial nerves.	X-ray of skull, serum alkaline phosphatase determination.
Evidence of a primary lesion, or of metastases, elsewhere.	X-ray of skull and other bones.
Nerve may be tender on pressure, occasionally cutaneous hyperalgesia in distribution of nerve; vesicles or scars in herpes.	
Between attacks examination entirely negative; some cases may reveal transient neurologic findings during an attack.	X-ray of skull and electroencephalography to rule out organic disease. Trial with a vasoconstrictor (dihydroergotamine).

DIFFERENTIAL DIAGNOSIS OF DISEASES

Cause	Typical History
2. Toxic States Infections; alcoholism; uremia; lead, arsenic, morphine, carbon monoxide poisoning; encephalitides.	Headache: severe, generalized, pounding, constant. History of exposure to toxins, and of other symptoms produced by the causative agent.
3. Hypertension	Headache: throbbing, paroxysmal, generalized or over vertex. History of cardiorenal-vascular disease.
4. Histamine	Headache: unilateral, involves eye, temple, neck and face, severe. Symptoms of vaso-dilatation on same side as the pain, edema below eye, running of nose, watering of eye.
E. Extracranial 1. Lesions of Eye (Eyestrain, iritis, glaucoma)	Headache: frontal or supraorbital, moderate dull pain, may be severe; frequently worse after use of eye. Pain in eye.
2. Lesions of Middle Ear (Otitis media, mastoiditis)	Headache: temporal, unilateral, intermittent, stabbing sensations. Feeling of fullness in ear, increasing deafness, tinnitus, otorrhea, general malaise with fever and acute illness.
3. Lesions of Nasal Sinuses	Headache: frontal, dull or severe, usually worse in morning, with improvement in afternoon; worse in cold, damp weather. History of preceding upper respiratory infection, pain in one part of face.
4. Lesions of Oral Cavity (Teeth, tongue, pharynx)	Headache: bilateral or unilateral, intensity varies, periodic. Pain in mouth, jaw or throat.
POST-TRAUMATIC	Headache: localized to site of injury or generalized, variable in intensity, frequency and duration. Made worse by emotional disturbances. Vertigo, worse on change of position. History of trauma, irritability, insomnia, inability to concentrate, inability to tolerate alcohol.
PSYCHOGENIC Conversion hysteria, anxiety states, and the like.	Headache: any type, frequently bizarre, vise-like, over vertex, bitemporal, generalized, constant, made worse by emotional disturbance. History of specific stresses and strains in relation to onset of headaches.

GIVING RISE TO HEADACHE *(Cont'd)*

Physical and Neurologic Findings	Special Studies That Are Indicated
Other signs produced by causative agent.	Studies applicable to the particular agent suspected; lumbar puncture, blood studies, urine examination.
Elevated blood pressure, retinal changes, cardiac findings, edema.	Blood chemistry, urine studies.
Evidence of vasodilatation, swelling of temporal vessels, tenderness on pressure of external and common carotid arteries, injection of conjunctiva, flushing of side of face.	Histamine skin test.
Changes in appearance of iris; increase in intraocular tension.	Careful and complete ophthalmic examination.
Acutely ill, tenderness over mastoid area; reddened, congested or retracted drum on affected side. Elevated temperature. May be evidence of meningeal irritation in children.	Otoscopic examination, X-ray of mastoid.
Evidence of nasal obstruction, swollen mucous membranes, tenderness on percussion over affected sinus.	X-ray of sinuses, transillumination.
Evidence of lesion in oral cavity. Tenderness on tapping affected teeth.	Dental evaluation, including X-ray study.
Usually negative physical and neurologic examination.	X-ray of skull, electroencephalography, lumbar puncture, determination of pretraumatic personality.
Frequently a bland appearance despite the most severe type of headache, but may appear tense, apprehensive, anxious. Tachycardia, elevated systolic pressure, moist palms, hyperactive reflexes. Examination often entirely negative.	Special studies as necessary to rule out organic disease. Evaluation of personality and mental status.

An accurate history is of the utmost importance. The type of pain, its location, duration and frequency should be noted, and an effort made to determine whether there are precipitating factors and prodromal and associated phenomena with the headache. In addition, an attempt should be made to evaluate the emotional status of the patient, particularly as regards his reactions to environmental stresses and strains. The physical and neurologic examinations should be thorough and complete. There are sufficient extracranial causes of headache to warrant a minute and careful physical check of the patient, including routine urine, blood and Wassermann studies. Every patient should have an ophthalmoscopic examination and, when necessary, visual field studies. When the history or examination suggests the possibility of an intracranial lesion, X-ray of the skull should be done. The films should be examined for the presence of unusual vascular markings, digital markings, areas of hyperostosis, calcifications, changes in the sella and clinoids, and for shift of the pineal. An EEG may indicate a focus and help locate the lesion. In the absence of contraindications, a lumbar puncture properly done may reveal findings of diagnostic significance. Arteriography and pneumoencephalography are hospital procedures that require the services of specialists.

Diagnosis

There is no single satisfactory classification of the causes of headache. The accompanying table is an attempt to outline a clinical approach to the problem. An awareness on the physician's part of the many conditions that can give rise to headache and a careful evaluation of the patient, with proper utilization of special studies, frequently will lead to the correct diagnosis.

Treatment

All therapeutic efforts should be directed at curing or eliminating the underlying disease process producing the headaches. Many headaches are trivial, and of such short duration as to require no special treatment. The analgesics are the safest and frequently the most effective drugs when symptomatic therapy is indicated. The management of patients with chronic headache is much more difficult. The majority of such individuals have either hypertensive, psychogenic, post-traumatic, or migrainous headaches. The general principles of treatment are the same for all four groups.

Both psychotherapy and pharmacotherapy are necessary. In many cases, **psychotherapy** need not be elaborate. A sympathetic, understanding attitude on the part of the physician and an acceptance on his part of the symptom as a real pain and not as a part of the patient's imagination will help a great deal. The patient should be seen at fairly frequent, regular intervals and should be given an opportunity to discuss his emotional difficulties. The physician should reassure the patient that there is no organic lesion, and then attempt to explain the emotional basis of the headache. Environmental readjustments, removal of irritants and stresses, and reeducation are all part of such therapy.

The **pharmacotherapy** of chronic headache includes a vast number of drugs varying from the analgesics to the hormones. In migraine (q.v.) the drugs of choice are the vasoconstrictors, particularly the ergot derivatives (℞ 42 to 45). In post-traumatic and psychogenic headache, the analgesics are the most effective. Acetylsalicylic acid (℞ 1) alone or in combination with acetophenetidin and caffeine (℞ 8) is the usual recommended basic medication. The continued use over a period of time of a mild sedative such as phenobarbital (℞ 13) once or twice a day is sometimes helpful in patients with post-traumatic or psychogenic headaches. The importance of drug therapy does not depend upon the particular medication used but rather on its combination with psychotherapy.

THE UNCONSCIOUS PATIENT

Unconsciousness: *A state of insensibility in which a patient receives no sensory impressions and has no subjective experiences; it is physiologic only during sleep.* Pathologic unconsciousness may be transitory, as in simple **syncope**, or prolonged, as in cases resulting from severe intracranial injury. It may vary in depth from semiconsciousness, or **stupor**, out of which the patient can be aroused only with difficulty, to the profound unconsciousness of **coma**, from which he cannot be aroused even by the most powerful external stimuli.

Etiology

Since unconsciousness is but one manifestation of an underlying disease or injury, its mode of onset, duration, intensity, and other characteristics will depend on the etiologic condition. The possible causes are many and various. The most common are syncope, acute alcoholism, cranial trauma, cerebrovascular accidents, poisoning (particularly by carbon monoxide or barbiturates), epilepsy, and diabetic acidosis. Other causes include cerebral anoxia (e.g., secondary to heart failure, severe anemia, heart block, or the carotid sinus syndrome), hypoglycemic and other forms of shock, infections (particularly meningeal and pulmonary), expanding lesions of the C.N.S., uremia, acidosis of any origin, cholemia, hysteria, heat stroke, exposure to extreme cold, decompression sickness, adrenal cortical insufficiency (Addison's disease), thyroid crisis, and eclampsia. During convulsions (q.v.) from any cause, the patient usually is unconscious. In aged or cachectic individuals, coma is frequent as a terminal event, regardless of the nature of the fatal illness.

It cannot be overemphasized that alcoholics are not immune to other causes of coma and that the possibility of other pathologic conditions must be ruled out before a diagnosis of uncomplicated alcoholic unconsciousness is made. Similar caution must be exercised before a conclusion is reached that oversedation is the sole cause of a patient's comatose state, or that cerebral trauma is the primary or only cause of the coma in a patient with an area of contusion or laceration of the scalp.

Diagnosis

Since the etiology will seldom be immediately evident, and an elaborate **history** usually is impossible to obtain, it is imperative that an orderly routine be followed in all cases so as to assemble all available evidence as promptly as possible. Any observers or relatives present should be questioned regarding the mode of onset or injury, the ingestion of drugs, alcohol or other toxic substances, infections, convulsions, headache and previous illnesses (e.g., diabetes, nephritis, heart disease, hypertension). Police help may be necessary to locate relatives or associates. Containers suspected of having held food, alcohol, drugs, or poisons should be examined, smelled, and saved (for chemical analysis and as possible future legal evidence). Signs of hemorrhage, incontinence, and cranial trauma should be sought. Application of painful stimuli, such as firm supraorbital or testicular pressure, often will help to differentiate coma from stupor, somnolence, or hysteria. The patient's age may be of significance, since epilepsy and infection are frequently responsible for unconsciousness in individuals under 40, whereas cardiovascular disease, especially cerebrovascular lesions, and metabolic disorders (diabetes, hypoglycemia, uremia) are more common after 40; however, there are frequent exceptions.

Physical examination should be directed toward the following: (1) Rectal temperature. (2) Skin: color, signs of trauma or of hypodermic injections (as in drug addictions, diabetes), rashes, petechiae. (3) Skull: careful examination of the scalp for areas of contusion or laceration. (4) Eyes: size of pupils and their reaction to light; corneal reflex; ocular palsy; examination of the fundi for papilledema, vascular sclerosis, or albuminuric or diabetic retinitis. (5) Ear, nose, throat: escape of cerebrospinal fluid or blood; scarred or bitten tongue. (6) Respiration: volume, rate, rhythm; breath odors, as of alcohol, acetone, paraldehyde, or bitter almonds. (7) Cardiovascular: pulse rate, volume, and rhythm; cardiac decompensation; comparative blood pressure in the two arms; sclerosis in peripheral vessels. (8) Abdomen: spasm, rigidity. (9) Extremities: cyanosis, clubbing, paresis. (10) Neurologic: stiffness of the neck; Kernig's signs; hemiplegia (as suggested by lack of spontaneous movements of one arm and leg and by the puffing out of a relaxed cheek in respiration, or by the failure of withdrawal of one arm and leg when they are vigorously stimulated); inequality of the tendon reflexes; abnormal plantar responses; muscular twitchings; convulsions.

Laboratory aids: The patient should be catheterized and the urine examined for sugar, acetone, and albumin. Blood studies should include determination of the hemoglobin, sugar, and BUN: spectroscopy will reveal abnormal blood pigments (sulfhemoglobin, methemoglobin) if present. Gastric lavage is required in suspected poisoning, both for diagnosis and treatment (*see* CLIN. PROC.; *also* POISONING). X-ray of the skull is frequently necessary, but must be deferred in the presence of shock. Lumbar puncture should be performed as soon as possible in all cases where the diagnosis is not already established.

Once this routine examination is completed, one or more clues to the cause of unconsciousness usually will have become evident. (For example, unconsciousness with convulsions, rigidity, or paralysis probably originates in the C.N.S.; irregular pulse, evidence of cardiac failure, or pronounced hypertension suggests a cardiovascular origin.) Further differentiation then can be made by focusing attention on the responsible system.

The principal diagnostic points for the more common causes of unconsciousness are as follows (for further details, *see* appropriate chapters):

Acute alcoholism: Alcoholic breath; coma, rarely deep, the patient usually responding to painful stimuli; hyperemia of face and conjunctiva; temperature normal or subnormal; pupils usually moderately dilated but equal; respirations deep and snoring, not stertorous; blood alcohol above 0.2%.

Cranial trauma: Onset of coma may have been sudden or gradual; local evidence or a history of injury, perhaps with bleeding from the ear, nose, or throat; temperature normal or elevated; pupils usually unequal and inactive; respiration variable, often slow or irregular; pulse variable, rapid initially and then slow; blood pressure variable; altered reflexes frequently present, often with incontinence and evidence of paralyses; spinal fluid may be bloody and under increased pressure; X-ray of the skull may demonstrate a fracture, or displacement of the pineal gland.

Cerebrovascular accidents: Patient usually is over 40 years of age, with a history or evidence of cardiovascular disease or hypertension; onset sudden; face flushed or cyanotic, often asymmetrical; temperature, pulse, and respirations variable; pupils usually unequal and inactive; blood pressure often elevated; paralyses commonly present; spinal fluid often bloody or xanthochromic and under increased pressure.

Epilepsy: History (e.g., from a relative) of previous "fits"; sudden convulsive onset; often incontinence; pulse, respiration, and temperature usually normal, but may be elevated after repeated convulsive seizures; bitten tongue or scars from previous attacks.

Diabetic acidosis: Gradual onset; skin dry, face flushed; fruity odor on breath; temperature often subnormal; eyeballs may be soft; air hunger (Kussmaul breathing); glycosuria, ketonuria, hyperglycemia; decreased CO_2 combining power.

Hypoglycemia: Onset often acute, with convulsions; skin moist and pale; deep reflexes exaggerated; positive Babinski; hypoglycemia during attack.

Syncope: Onset sudden; coma seldom deep or prolonged; pulse usually slow at onset, later rapid and weak.

Barbiturate poisoning: Skin often cyanotic; pupils variable; respirations shallow and slow; muscle twitchings may be present; reflexes sluggish or absent.

Treatment

The treatment of unconsciousness is essentially that of the underlying disease or injury (q.v.) but, pending its identification, certain emergency measures may be necessary, as indicated by the immediate findings. The pulse, respirations and blood pressure should be checked at frequent intervals. One or more of the following procedures may be imperative: Control of hemorrhage; maintenance of a clear airway; treatment of shock; O_2 inhalation to prevent or combat the anoxia that complicates all forms of unconsciousness except sleep; catheterization; appropriate resuscitation methods, including artificial respiration; transportation to a hospital as soon as feasible; correction of obvious fluid or electrolyte imbalance; chemotherapy. Stimulants should be avoided unless indicated specifically to combat the effects of depressant drugs (e.g., barbiturates, opiates) or heart block (as in Adams-Stokes syndrome). Morphine is contraindicated for an unconscious patient. No patient who is unconscious should be given food, fluids, or any form of medication by mouth. In protracted unconsciousness, parenteral alimentation and measures for the prevention of decubitus are essential.

MIGRAINE

A paroxysmal disorder characterized by recurrent attacks of headache, with or without associated visual and gastrointestinal disturbances.

Etiology

The exact etiology is unknown. A vascular mechanism, involving branches of the external carotid artery, may be responsible. The vascular disturbance may consist of a primary vasodilatation or an evanescent primary vasoconstriction with

secondary vasodilatation. Allergy, endocrine dysfunction, or
cerebral edema may be the etiologic factor in some patients.
Migraine attacks in any individual case may be precipitated by
the menses, ovulation, emotional strain, fatigue, eyestrain, or
the consumption of a certain food. There is a pronounced
hereditary influence.

Migraine is more common in females, particularly in conscientious, emotionally unstable individuals. The disorder usually begins around puberty and tends to diminish after the age
of 50. The incidence of both migraine and epilepsy in the same
person is significantly high.

Symptoms and Signs

A prodromal aura is common and is rather distinct for any
one patient. There may be depression, irritability, restlessness,
anorexia, scotomata, hemianopsia, paresthesias, hemiparesis, or
even hemiplegia. The aura may be transient or may outlast the
headache.

The headache is typically hemicranial and very severe, but
all variations may exist. However, like the aura, the headache
of each patient usually is specific. It may remain localized or
spread over the entire head.

Nausea and vomiting are frequently encountered along with
photophobia, and cranial tenderness. Abdominal pain is not
uncommon. The muscles of the head and neck may be contracted. Occasionally, an eosinophilia lends support to an allergic basis for the attack. Vasomotor disturbances are frequently noted.

An untreated attack may last for hours or several days. The
frequency of attacks varies from several attacks a week to 1 or
2 a year. Between paroxysms, the patient is unaffected.

Diagnosis

The diagnosis is based on the early onset, the long history of
recurrent attacks, a positive family history, and the clinical
manifestations. Migraine must be differentiated from similar
symptoms arising from such intracranial lesions as tumor, aneurysm, cerebral vascular accident, and multiple sclerosis. Pain
arising from recurrent disease of the accessory sinuses may occasionally be confused with migraine. A careful neurologic
examination must be supplemented by such diagnostic aids as
X-ray, EEG and the histamine sensitivity test.

Prognosis and Treatment

The prognosis must always be guarded. Attacks tend to
diminish during pregnancy and may cease after the menopause,
but this is not uniformly the case.

Many modes of therapy have been utilized, each with some
measure of success. This is not unexpected in a condition so
prone to be influenced by psychic factors. Treatment is di-

rected at reducing both the frequency and severity of attacks.

Prophylaxis: Psychotherapy, even mere suggestion, and environmental adjustment are important. The need for adequate rest, regular hours, personal hygiene, and proper reading habits should be stressed. Foci of infection should be eliminated. A weekly saline purge is beneficial to some patients.

Elimination diets are useful in cases of suspected food allergy (*see* DIETS). Antihistaminics and desensitization to histamine may be tried (*see* ALLERGY). A "ketogenic" effect may be achieved by the use of ammonium chloride (℞ 77) for 3 or 4 days before an expected attack (menstrual migraine). Restriction of salt and fluids, testosterone (℞ 59) and estrogens (℞ 60) have been used successfully in some patients.

Nicotinic acid (℞ 65, 66) often is effective in cases due to a primary vasoconstriction, since it has a vasodilating action; nicotinic acid amide is useless for this purpose, since it is only rarely capable of producing vasodilation.

Active therapy: Once the aura has appeared, every effort must be made to abort the attack at this stage. Bowel evacuation with an enema often is effective. Rest in a dark, quiet room is helpful, as is a tight bandage around the head at the level of the forehead. Therapy which has successfully alleviated previous headaches should be given at once, even if onset of the headache has not yet occurred. Calcium lactate (℞ 79) or the inhalation of 100% O_2 may abort an attack. Analgesics (℞ 4, 8, 10) are administered, but habit-forming drugs are to be avoided except in extreme cases.

In all established cases, ergot derivatives are the drugs of choice and should be given as early in the attack as possible. Dihydroergotamine (℞ 42) has fewer undesirable side effects than ergotamine tartrate (℞ 43, 44, 45) and is therefore superior. Ergotamine tartrate is not as effective orally as it is parenterally; much larger doses are necessary and it is poorly tolerated in the presence of nausea and vomiting. If effective, relief is obtained within 30 to 90 minutes after an injection. The toxic side effects of ergotamine include nausea, vomiting, dysmenorrhea, numbness and tingling of the extremities, and muscle pains; the drug is contraindicated in pregnancy, severe arteriosclerosis, hypertension, angina and peripheral arterial vascular disease. Undesirable side effects may largely be controlled by the addition of 0.4 mg. (gr. $\frac{1}{150}$) atropine sulfate (℞ 28) to each dose of ergotamine or dihydroergotamine. (CAUTION! Too frequent use of ergot derivatives is dangerous and may cause gangrene of the fingers and toes. Its prophylactic administration is, therefore, not recommended.)

Where ergot derivatives are contraindicated or not tolerated, prompt relief may occur in many patients following a single hypodermic injection of Octin (℞ 41). Octin is contraindicated in hypertensive individuals since it may further elevate the blood pressure. Nicotinic acid (℞ 65, 66), orally and I.V., will abort many paroxysms due to a primary vasoconstriction. Many other vasodilators and vasoconstrictors have been used, but with indifferent results.

EPILEPSY

(Falling sickness)

A chronic paroxysmal disorder of cerebral function, characterized by recurrent attacks involving changes in the state of consciousness, sudden in onset and of brief duration. The attacks often are accompanied by a convulsion in which the patient falls involuntarily. Three types of epilepsy are recognized: grand mal, petit mal, and psychic equivalent or psychomotor attacks. Each type has a specific pattern.

Etiology and Incidence

Epilepsy is of two etiologic types: **idiopathic** and **symptomatic.** In idiopathic epilepsy, no organic lesion of the brain or physiologic disturbance can be shown to cause the seizures. About 75% of all cases are of this type. In symptomatic epilepsy, an organic lesion in the brain, or some physiologic disturbance can be demonstrated as the underlying basis. The organic lesions may be tumors, abscesses, inflammatory or degenerative processes, or scar tissue formation following traumatic or vascular injury. Birth trauma to the head is of particular importance. The physiologic disturbances that may lead to or be accompanied by seizures may result from various intoxicating agents (noxious gases, alcohol), overdosage of insulin, adenoma of the pancreas (hypoglycemia), hypofunction of the parathyroid glands (tetany), alkalosis, intracranial hemorrhage (whooping cough), water retention (cerebral edema), convulsant drugs, and numerous other sources.

There is no evidence that epilepsy itself is hereditary, but disturbances (dysrhythmias) of the electrical pulsations of the brain, which are closely associated with epileptic seizures, are hereditary and have been demonstrated in an overwhelming proportion of the parents of epileptics. Such dysrhythmias probably constitute an inherited predisposition to epilepsy.

The incidence of frank epilepsy in the general population is low, having been estimated at about 0.5% or less. Males are more commonly affected than females. Most of the cases begin in childhood or adolescence, only about 30% after the age of 20.

Pathology and Pathologic Physiology

There are no specific changes in the C.N.S. The occasional

pathologic changes found are those probably caused by the seizures, e.g., dilatation of the ventricles or vascular accidents, or those of the contributory lesion or disease. Accompanying a seizure there are disturbances in the electrical activity of the cortex, which are characteristic for each of the 3 forms of seizures (*see* Diagnosis).

Symptoms and Signs

Grand mal (including jacksonian and focal seizures): In about 50% of cases, the seizure of grand mal begins with a warning (aura) that may consist of strange visceral sensations, headache, visual disturbances, vague premonitions, or bizarre, repetitive thoughts and phrases. The patient falls to the ground, in coma, unable to make any attempt to save himself or to avoid obstacles, and often receives cuts, bruises, and fractures. The fall is usually preceded by a cry or moan. Tonico-clonic spasms of the musculature with or without tongue biting and urinary and fecal incontinence then occur. There may be pronounced sweating, apnea, cyanosis, tachycardia, and excessive salivation, sometimes with bloodstained foam on the lips from tongue biting. The average attack lasts 2 to 5 minutes. On regaining consciousness, the patient is frequently dazed, drowsy and confused, and complains of headache and soreness of the muscles. He frequently has amnesia for the attack. The frequency of attacks varies from several in one day to once or twice a year. **Status epilepticus** is a serious condition in which one seizure of grand mal follows another with no intervening period of consciousness.

Jacksonian seizures are manifested by clonic convulsive movements or by paresthesias which begin in one hand or foot and then spread unilaterally upward, following the same pattern in each attack. Consciousness is retained unless the attack spreads to the opposite side of the body and develops into a grand mal convulsion. In focal seizures, the clonic convulsive movements or paresthesias originate in one part of the body, spread rapidly to involve the entire body, and are followed by coma.

Petit mal: Attacks are most common in childhood and are manifested by transient clouding of consciousness lasting from 1 to 30 seconds with or without minor movements of the head, eyes, and extremities or loss of muscular tone. The patient suddenly stops any activity in which he is engaged and resumes it when the attack is over. He may fall, without unconsciousness or vertigo. Seizures usually occur several times or many times a day.

Psychic equivalents or psychomotor attacks: Under this heading are included a group of epileptiform attacks which differ from the typical grand mal or petit mal seizures. There are disturbances of consciousness without convulsive movements. The patient does not fall to the ground unconscious.

Instead, there is a period of amnesia lasting minutes to hours during which the patient behaves in an automatic manner, with purposeless or purposeful movements, of which he is unaware. He may become violent.

Diagnosis

Idiopathic and symptomatic epilepsy must be distinguished as a guide to treatment, and to this end a careful history is important. It should include an eyewitness account of the attack, information on frequency of attacks, and the longest and shortest intervals between them; the previous occurrence of trauma, meningitis, encephalitis or whooping cough; the consumption of alcohol and its relation to seizures; the patient's birth history, especially as to birth trauma and transient paralyses or local spasms after delivery, and later history of traumatic injuries to the head which produced unconsciousness, or of severe psychic trauma. Any history of convulsions, migraine, or other neuropsychiatric disorders in the patient's family should be elicited.

Complete physical and neurologic examination should be made. Laboratory studies should include examination of the urine and blood, X-rays of the skull, lumbar puncture with complete cerebrospinal fluid studies, and whenever possible an EEG. The latter study will reveal abnormal brain waves in about 85% of the cases and give added information as to the type of seizures. With grand mal there is increased frequency of the waves, which appear as sharp spikes at the rate of 25 to 30/second. In petit mal, spikes and slow round waves alternate at the rate of 3/second. With psychomotor attacks the rate is slow, 3 to 4/second, with a flat-topped wave predominating. A normal EEG does not exclude epilepsy, since about 15% of epileptics will have a normal record if only one tracing is taken in the seizure-free interval. Pneumoencephalogram is indicated when organic disease of the brain is suspected.

Epilepsy may be confused with narcolepsy, syncope, hysteria, anxiety attacks, migraine, organic intracranial lesions, hypoglycemic seizures, hypocalcemic tetany, tetany of alkalosis, and hyperactive carotid sinus reflex. Differentiation is based on the description of the attacks and on physical and laboratory studies.

Prognosis

The prognosis is better when there is no demonstrable brain lesion. Life expectancy is slightly reduced because of the chances of external or internal injury during attacks. When mental deterioration is pronounced the outlook is poor, but this is not common in epilepsy. Death can occur during status epilepticus.

Treatment

The treatment of idiopathic epilepsy is purely symptomatic,

since the cause is unknown. In symptomatic epilepsy, it is necessary to treat the associated disease or lesion as well as the seizures. Therapy of the epilepsy component is the same in both cases.

1. Elimination of causative or precipitating factors: Physical defects (e.g., infections and endocrine abnormalities) should be corrected. Organic lesions of the brain, such as tumors and abscesses, should be removed surgically when possible. Cortical scars secondary to trauma, vascular lesions or birth injuries should be removed when the patients have focal attacks that resist medical therapy. After surgical removal of organic lesions, it usually is necessary to continue medical therapy.

2. Physical and mental hygiene: The patient should be encouraged to live as normal a life as possible. A regular diet of wholesome, simple foods including an abundance of fresh fruits and vegetables, should be followed. Alcoholic beverages must be avoided. Regular bowel habits and regular hours of sleep should be established and the patient should arise promptly on waking. Moderate physical exercise is recommended and such sports as swimming and horseback riding are permissible, with proper safeguards. Automobile driving is forbidden. Recreations such as movies, dancing, and parties should be encouraged, within reason.

Psychotherapy should be directed against feelings of inferiority and self-consciousness as well as other difficulties. Children may be kept in school and adults encouraged to work. The vocational rehabilitation facilities offered by many communities are helpful. Other members of the family must be taught a sensible attitude toward the patient's illness. Overprotection and oversolicitude should be discouraged and emphasis placed on preventing invalidism.

3. Drug therapy: For **grand mal** diphenylhydantoin sodium (℞ 19) and phenobarbital (℞ 13) are the most effective drugs and can be used alone or in combination. When seizures are infrequent (1 or 2 a year), phenobarbital alone in a daily dose of 0.1 Gm. (gr. iss) can be given at bedtime. This dose can be increased to 0.1 Gm. (gr. iss) twice daily. Diphenylhydantoin sodium in a minimum daily dosage of 0.3 Gm. (gr. v) for adults is the drug of choice for frequent seizures. This can be given in divided doses during the day or in a single dose at bedtime. If not effective in controlling seizures, the daily dose can be gradually increased by 0.1 Gm. (gr. iss) every 10 to 14 days until seizures are controlled or undesirable side effects appear (*see* below). Frequently, the combination of diphenylhydantoin sodium (℞ 19), 0.3 to 0.4 Gm. daily, plus phenobarbital (℞ 13), 0.1 to 0.2 Gm., will be more effective than larger doses of either drug alone. Mesantoin (℞ 20) in doses of 0.3 to 0.9 Gm. (gr. v to xiiiss) can be substituted when diphenylhydantoin sodium proves ineffective or produces severe side effects. Mebaral (℞ 21) is used as a substitute for phenobarbital and is given in doses of 0.2 Gm. (gr. iii) 1 to 3 times a day. Bromides (℞ 22) occasionally are more effective than the other drugs: a daily dose of 1 Gm. (gr. xv) 3 to 4 times a day is given. The chloride intake must be kept at an adequate level when bromides are being taken and symptoms of bromism must always be watched for and, if possible, avoided.

For **petit mal,** Tridione (℞ 23), 0.3 to 2.0 Gm. (gr. v to xxx) daily, is the drug of choice. Large doses of *dl*-glutamic acid (℞ 25), 8 to 20 Gm. daily, are occasionally effective. A ketogenic diet sometimes produces a good result but is difficult to maintain.

For **psychomotor seizure,** the same drugs are used as for grand mal, but frequently larger dosages are necessary.

Undesirable side effects of anticonvulsant drugs: Diphenylhydantoin sodium may produce restlessness, nervousness, nausea, vomiting, hypertrophy of the gums, unsteadiness of gait, dermatitis, and psychotic symptoms. Phenobarbital frequently causes an incapacitating drowsiness and, in less than 1% of cases, an allergic rash of a scarlatiniform or morbilliform nature. Mesantoin may produce drowsiness, fatigue, and a generalized rash; aplastic anemia also has been reported. Tridione also may cause a generalized rash and, in addition, photophobia and leukopenia or, rarely, severe anemia or agranulocytosis. Bromides frequently produce skin rashes and mental dullness. When a toxic reaction occurs, the medication should be discontinued or the dosage greatly decreased until the symptoms have disappeared, when it can be cautiously resumed. The appearance of blood dyscrasias during therapy with mesantoin or tridione is an indication for immediate discontinuance of the drug.

For **status epilepticus,** chloroform or ether will sometimes terminate the seizures. Fairly large doses of sodium phenobarbital (℞ 24), 0.4 to 0.8 Gm. (gr. vi to xii), or of paraldehyde (℞ 15), 3 to 6 cc. I.M. or I.V., are more effective and less likely to produce pulmonary complications. Paraldehyde given I.V. occasionally causes pulmonary edema or circulatory collapse. For children, smaller doses, according to weight, should be used. The full amount given in one dose gives better results than divided doses.

Treatment during a seizure should be directed toward avoiding injury to the patient. Insert some firm but reasonably soft substance between the teeth to prevent biting of the tongue and loosen the clothing about the neck. After the seizure allow the patient to sleep or remain quiet until he feels normal again.

Institutional care of patients is advisable only when there is severe mental deterioration or when the attacks are frequent and violent and cannot be controlled by medication.

CONVULSIONS

Violent involuntary contraction or repeated contractions of the voluntary muscles. Convulsions are of two main types: **tonic,** a continuous contraction accompanied by rigidity; and **clonic,** characterized by a series of spasms alternating with periods of relaxation.

Etiology

A variety of pathologic conditions may give rise to convulsions, the most frequent of which are hyperpyrexia, infectious diseases, poisoning, cerebral anoxia, tetany, hypoglycemia, cerebral edema, expanding lesions of the brain, intracranial injuries, epilepsy, hysteria, tetanus, cysticercosis of the brain, and toxoplasmosis. Diagnosis and anticonvulsant treatment in certain causative diseases are briefly outlined below; for additional details, other appropriate chapters should be consulted.

Management of Convulsions

General: The patient should be placed where he cannot injure himself by falling or by striking against hard or sharp objects. Biting of the tongue should be prevented by inserting a padded gag at the side of the mouth between the upper and lower teeth. Artificial respiration should be given whenever necessary. Convulsions ordinarily will respond to one or more of the following drugs: (1) sodium phenobarbital (R 24), 60 to 120 mg. (gr. i to ii) subcut. usually is effective within 15 or 30 minutes and may safely be repeated, even in infants. (2) Tribromoethanol rectally as a 2.5% solution in doses of 60 to 80 mg. (gr. i to iss)/Kg. body wt. often is efficacious. (The maximum dose is 10 Gm. for men and 8 Gm. for women.) (3) Paraldehyde (R 15), 1 to 6 cc. I.M., is both effective and safe. (4) Rarely, chloroform or ether by inhalation, or an I.V. anesthetic such as Sodium Pentothal in 2.5% solution, may be necessary to control seizures if other methods fail.

Hyperpyrexia: High fever is most often due to an acute infectious disease or to heat stroke. In febrile disease, the fever is associated with other evidence of acute illness; the convulsions usually are few in number. With heat stroke, there is a sudden onset of convulsions following exposure to high temperatures. Fever is pronounced and consciousness is lost early. The face is flushed and the skin dry and hot. Pulmonary congestion frequently develops and often is severe. Specific therapy is that of the underlying disease, fever being combated by the use of an antipyretic, such as acetylsalicylic acid, and sponge baths. The severe hyperpyrexia of heat stroke (q.v.) may require emergency measures. Should pulmonary edema (q.v.) develop secondary to myocardial insufficiency, it should be treated appropriately.

Cerebral infections: Infections involving the brain and most often associated with convulsions are meningitis, encephalitis, abscess, malaria, typhus, syphilis, and rabies (q.v.). The patient's history, signs and symptoms in most cases will suggest the diagnosis; spinal puncture and blood studies (including serologic) also will supply useful information. The patient usually is stuporous between convulsions. Evidence of meningeal irritation such as headache, vomiting, stiff neck, and a positive Kernig, is generally present. The underlying disease should be appropriately treated with antibiotics, chemotherapy, or specific antiserum.

Toxic agents: Convulsions may result from certain drugs or toxins, such as strychnine, atropine, picrotoxin, Metrazol, camphor, nikethamide, alcohol, lead, caffeine, or even antibiotics when administered intrathecally. The "toxic factor" of erythroblastosis (kernicterus) or of eclampsia also may cause convulsions. There is a history or evidence of ingestion of or exposure to a toxic agent. The diagnosis of eclampsia or erythroblastosis fetalis (q.v.) is seldom difficult. Plumbism requires study of the blood, urine, and spinal fluid, and X-ray of the bones. Unabsorbed toxic material should be evacuated by means of gastric lavage, colonic irrigations or emetics. The appropriate antidote should be administered immediately (*see* POISONING). Further therapy will depend on the responsible agent.

Cerebral anoxia: Convulsions due to O_2 insufficiency in the brain may complicate significant anoxia (q.v.) of any origin, but most often that caused by inhalation anesthesia, ascent to high altitudes, congenital heart disease, asphyxia, carbon monoxide poisoning, breath-holding spells, severe asthma, a hyperactive carotid sinus, or the Adams-Stokes syndrome. Cyanosis frequently is present. The history, symptoms, and signs ordinarily will make the diagnosis of the underlying cause obvious. Treatment consists of O_2 inhalation, artificial respiration (if necessary) and appropriate measures to correct the primary condition.

Tetany: This may be due to hypocalcemia, alkalosis, or (rarely) magnesium deficiency. It is infrequent in the newborn and in individuals over 2 years of age. The convulsive seizures occur frequently and are not accompanied by fever or signs of meningeal irritation. Mental clarity between seizures is characteristic. The symptoms and signs usually are so typical as to offer little difficulty in diagnosis. Blood studies will demonstrate findings indicative of hypocalcemia, alkalosis, or magnesium deficiency. Treatment of tetany (q.v.) is aimed at correcting the chemical imbalance found to be present.

Hypoglycemia: Deficiency in blood sugar may be due to hyperinsulinism (overtreatment of diabetes, or islet cell tumor), hepatic insufficiency, hypopituitarism, hypocorticoadrenalism, hypothalamic disease or ascariasis; or to functional causes (renal glycosuria, prolonged severe muscular exertion). Attacks tend to occur while the patient's stomach is empty of food and are accompanied by profuse sweating, prostration, hunger, and abdominal cramps; unconsciousness is not unusual. The decreased blood sugar level may be demonstrated during an attack. Determination of the underlying disease often is difficult, requiring prolonged laboratory and clinical studies. Immediate treatment consists of giving sugar (dextrose) orally or parenterally, to elevate the blood sugar to normal levels. Subsequent therapy of hypoglycemia (q.v.) is directed at the causative disease.

Cerebral edema: The most frequent causes of this condition are hypertension, trauma, uremia, and allergy. The diagnosis will depend on the history, symptoms, and signs of the underlying disease and should seldom be difficult to determine. Cerebral edema may be lessened by lumbar puncture (performed with caution), saline catharsis, phlebotomy, and the I.V. administration of hypertonic solutions of glucose, sucrose, and magnesium sulfate. Epinephrine is useful in allergic cases. The primary disease should be appropriately treated.

Expanding brain lesions: Tumors and hematomas are the most frequently encountered expanding lesions in the brain. There may be a history of trauma. The convulsions are focal or general, with headache, vomiting, visual disturbances, abnormal gait, or papilledema. A careful neurologic examination, together with X-ray studies of the skull and brain, spinal puncture (cautiously performed) and an EEG, usually is diagnostic. The treatment is by surgical means, whenever feasible.

Intracranial injuries and hemorrhage: These may result from birth-induced or other trauma, cerebral vascular accidents, hypoprothrombinemia, or purpura. Chvostek's sign is normally present at birth. In apoplexy, the convulsive seizure ordinarily is unilateral and most often occurs in an elderly individual with a history of hypertension or cardiac disease (emboli). The history, neurologic examination, spinal puncture (to be done only if absolutely necessary and then cautiously) and blood studies generally will establish the diagnosis. The treatment is that of the underlying disease.

Epilepsy: There usually is a history of similar attacks recurring without obvious cause, often preceded by an aura, and accompanied by incontinence and by self-injury due to falling. The seizures are first tonic, then clonic, and are followed by drowsiness. An EEG tracing may be helpful in diagnosis. Symptomatic types must be distinguished from idiopathic before treatment of epilepsy (q.v.) is prescribed.

Hysteria: Most attacks follow an emotional upset and the patient usually is an individual with a neurotic background. Superficially, the seizure resembles that of epilepsy, but the onset is generally less acute. Incontinence is not present. The patient's movements are purposeful and falling does not result in self-injury. Treatment is by means of psychotherapy (*see* THE PSYCHONEUROSES).

Tetanus: A history of a wound received 3 to 21 days before usually is obtainable. Contamination of the umbilicus with *Cl. tetani* in the newborn has occurred. The convulsions are painful, can be precipitated by minimal stimuli, and are associated with muscular stiffness, risus sardonicus, and opisthotonos. Prompt, adequate treatment with tetanus antitoxin, penicillin, sedatives, and anticonvulsants is imperative (*see* TETANUS).

Cysticercosis of the brain: This complication of infection with the larvae of *Taenia solium* (pork tapeworm) is seen most often in children, but is rare in the United States. The finding of eosinophilia in a child with recurrent epileptiform convulsions, and the X-ray demonstration of typical tumor-like lesions in the brain and muscles, usually will establish the diagnosis. The larvae may sometimes be found in subcutaneous nodules. Medical measures are useless. If the brain lesions are few in number and accessible, neurosurgical measures are indicated.

Toxoplasmosis: This disease is most frequently encountered in infants and is due to infection with *Toxoplasma gondii*. It is manifested by recurrent convulsions associated with a characteristic chorioretinitis, impaired vision and retarded mental development. X-ray of the skull may demonstrate small irregular areas of calcification. The complement fixation test often is helpful in diagnosis. Treatment consists of giving sulfathiazole, 1 Gm. (gr. xv) every 4 hours. Emetine hydrochloride, 20 to 60 mg. (gr. ⅓ to i), also may be administered daily, for 10 days.

Other conditions: Convulsions occasionally may be due to such causes as electric shock, venomous bites, overfilling of the stomach, dentition, pellagra, multiple sclerosis, diabetic coma, addisonian crisis, or status thymicolymphaticus (q.v.). The diagnosis will be made on the basis of the history and the clinical manifestations associated with the underlying disease. Treatment is that appropriate to the causal condition.

HUNTINGTON'S CHOREA

(Hereditary chorea, Chronic chorea)

A hereditary disease of adults, marked by irregular movements, speech disturbances, and dementia.

Etiology, Incidence, and Pathology

This disease is transmitted by a parent of either sex to approximately half of the offspring. Huntington's chorea never develops in individuals without such heredity. If a generation is skipped, the disease is not transmitted further. It usually becomes manifest during the 4th decade of life; minor symptoms such as clumsiness may be the first to appear.

The brain is diminished in weight, due especially to atrophy of the forebrain, the corpus striatum being affected particularly. The white matter is more reduced than the gray. A striking decrease in the number of cells of the putamen and caudate nucleus is evident. The cerebellum usually is normal.

Symptoms and Signs

Onset is insidious. Personality changes such as obstinacy, moodiness, and lack of initiative frequently antedate or accompany the appearance of the involuntary choreiform movements. These usually first appear in the face, neck, and upper extremities, and are jerky, irregular and stretching in character. Eventually, the irregular flexions and extensions may occur more often than once a second. Contractions of the facial muscles result in grimaces while those of the respiratory muscles, lips, and tongue lead to a hesitating explosive type of speech. There are irregular movements of the trunk, and the gait is shuffling and dancing. The tendon reflexes are increased. During sleep the choreiform movements usually cease. Some of these patients display a fatuous euphoria, while others are spiteful, irascible, destructive, and assaultive. Paranoid reactions are common. There is poverty of thought and an impairment of attention, memory, and judgment. As the disease progresses, walking becomes impossible, there is interference with swallowing and the dementia becomes profound. Suicide is not uncommon.

Diagnosis

A family history of Huntington's chorea is essential. A nonfamilial type of chorea occurs which closely resembles this disease, but is less often associated with mental deterioration. Such chorea may make its appearance at puberty. Lenticular degeneration, also Sydenham's chorea, must be differentiated. Neoplasm, cerebral arteriosclerosis, or cerebrovascular syphilis may cause chorea, likewise apoplexy. Usually, it is a hemichorea which results from the latter. Both hysterical and senile types of chronic chorea occur.

Prophylaxis, Prognosis, and Treatment

Individuals with a family history of Huntington's chorea should forego parenthood, perhaps by voluntarily undergoing sterilization.

Many patients with this disease eventually will require care in a mental hospital. However, no treatment is known to have any fundamental effect on this incurable disease. Following onset, the average duration of life is 15 years. Palliative drugs of the sedative type, particularly chloral hydrate (R 14) and scopolamine (R 26), may be necessary in cases showing extreme emotional disturbance.

TICS

(Habit spasms, Mimic spasms, Maladie des tics)

Sudden, habitually repetitive, purposeless movements, often localized to a particular muscle group. (To be distinguished from painful spasms such as tic douloureux, and other neuralgias.)

Etiology

Tics may occur at any age but are more common in nervous children between the ages of 5 and 12 years. It is thought that most tics begin as purposeful movements in response to definite stimuli but that eventually these same movements are carried out automatically in a purposeless fashion when the stimuli no longer are present. Rarely, some tics may be on an organic basis, such as those following encephalitis. Males and females are equally affected.

Symptoms and Signs

The movements usually are quick and abrupt, involving definite groups of muscles. Many kinds of tics may occur and involve almost any part of the body, especially the region of the head and neck. The more common types are tics manifested by blinking of the eyelids, grimacing, shaking or nodding of the head, pouting, grinning, clearing of the throat, swallowing, coughing, and a jerking of the shoulders, arms or legs. Some patients have a combination of tics which are carried out simultaneously, alternately, or following each other. Emotion or fatigue intensifies the movements. They may be voluntarily inhibited for a very short period and they disappear during sleep.

Diagnosis

Tics must be differentiated from facial spasm (clonic spasm of muscles supplied by the facial nerve) and chorea. It is with the latter condition that tics are most frequently confused. Patients with tics usually have a longer free period between movements than do those with chorea and always perform the same movement in the same stereotyped manner. Choreic movements, on the other hand, are haphazard and pointless.

Prognosis and Treatment

Frequently, the tics appearing in childhood are transient and disappear spontaneously. Some, however, persist and become chronic and progressive. Relapses are not uncommon.

In mild cases, no treatment is indicated, the tics disappearing of their own accord. Psychotherapy must be used in the more severe cases. With children it may be necessary to remove the child from the home environment for a period of time. Efforts should be made to improve the situational difficulties in which the tics developed. It usually is necessary to treat the child as a whole rather than concentrating on the tics.

Muscular drill and breathing exercises have been reported as beneficial forms of therapy. In the former, the patient is made to practice remaining immobile as long as possible. Such treatments must be carried out regularly at fixed hours. Breathing exercises are repeated frequently during the day and it is thought that the respiratory rhythm attained during the exercises tends to diminish the tics. Such a simple procedure as holding a finger steadily against the cheek is sometimes helpful in an appropriate case and posthypnotic suggestion has been useful on occasion. When possible, obvious physical defects should be corrected. Mild sedatives such as phenobarbital (℞ 13) 30 mg. (gr. ss) 1 to 3 times a day may be given as necessary.

HICCUP

(Hiccough, Singultus)

Repeated involuntary spasmodic contractions of the diaphragm followed by sudden closures of the glottis, which check the inflow of air and produce the characteristic gasping sounds.

Etiology

The condition may result from anything which produces irritation of the afferent or efferent nerve pathways, or of the centers that control the muscles of respiration, particularly the diaphragm. The cause of transient episodes may never become apparent, but with prolonged or recurrent attacks the cause usually can be determined. The afferent nerve pathways may be stimulated by swallowing hot foods or other irritating substances, and by disorders of the stomach and esophagus, such as gastric dilatation, gastritis, or esophagospasm. Other intra-abdominal causes are intestinal obstruction or ileus, pancreatitis, strangulated hernia, peritonitis, intraperitoneal tumor, or amebic, typhoid and other forms of enteritis. Liver conditions, in particular cancer metastases and hepatitis, may be causal. Attacks may occur during pregnancy or from bladder irritation. Postoperative hiccups may be so severe and weakening as to endanger life. The centers controlling the respiratory muscles which are located in the upper cervical part of the spinal cord may be affected by intracranial or cord tumors or by meningoencephalitis, as from syphilis, epidemic encephalitis, or other infections. Inflammation or tumors of the mediastinum, enlargement of the heart, and adherent pericarditis are occasional causes. Hiccups accompanying diaphragmatic pleurisy, pneumonia, uremia, or alcoholism are not infrequent. Finally, persistent hiccups may result from psychogenic causes, and it is said that in these cases the symptoms often disappear during eating.

Treatment

Numerous simple measures may be tried: a series of deep, regular respirations; drinking a glassful of water rapidly in one draught; building up the CO_2 in the body by rebreathing into a paper bag; using snuff, or tickling the nares or throat to the point of producing vomiting; forcible traction of the tongue; swallowing dry bread or crushed ice; pressure upon the eyeballs; a mustard plaster or ice bag to the epigastrium, or spraying this area with ethyl chloride or ether. Pressure on the carotid between the thumb and forefinger for 1 minute may be tried, the artery being grasped at the midpoint of the anterior border of the sternocleidomastoid. Strong digital pressure may be applied over the phrenic nerves in their course behind the sternoclavicular joints.

When irritation of the gastric mucosa is present, gastric lavage should be carried out or apomorphine administered (℞ 82), if not otherwise contraindicated. Following this a local anesthetic by mouth, such as cocaine (℞ 17) may be indicated. If necessary, a sedative is given (℞ 13, 26). Morphine usually is not very effective. Benzyl benzoate (℞ 83) or amphetamine (℞ 63) sometimes stops an attack. Galvanism of the phrenic nerves may end an attack, the anode being placed on the neck, with the cathode on the thorax at the level of the insertion of the diaphragm. Dilation of the esophagus with a small bougie may be indicated in some cases. With diaphragmatic pleurisy, tight support of the lower chest with adhesive plaster often is helpful.

Although hiccup complicating a serious disease or developing postoperatively sometimes means that a larger fluid intake is needed, it more often indicates gastric overdistention. Usually, this can be relieved quickly by continuous suction siphonage with a Levin tube and a Wangensteen suction apparatus. Inhalation therapy with 5% CO_2 in oxygen is a measure of real value in many intractable cases, particularly in postoperative patients. The inhalations should be continued until the hiccups have ceased for 1 minute and resumed if they recur. If 5% CO_2 fails, 10% may be used, but only until the patient becomes dizzy; too long continued administration may cause unconsciousness or convulsions. Some clinicians recommend trying general anesthesia if CO_2 inhalations are ineffective.

When all simpler methods have failed, temporary interruption of the phrenic nerve may be performed on the side corresponding to the leaf of the diaphragm involved, as determined by fluoroscopy. Local infiltration of the nerve may be attempted with procaine, 20 to 30 cc. of a 0.5% solution, the needle being inserted down to the anterior scalenus muscle, at a point just above the clavicle at the outer border of the sternocleidomastoid. Since the barbiturates are specific against the symptoms of procaine sensitivity, Sodium Amytal (R 18), suitable for I.V. injection, should be at hand in case of need. Not even bilateral phrenicotomy cures all cases of hiccup. When the condition is intractable and without evident cause, neurologic and psychiatric consultations are indicated.

PARALYSIS AGITANS

(Parkinson's syndrome, Parkinsonism, Shaking palsy)

A chronic disorder of the C.N.S. characterized by slowness of movement, weakness, muscular rigidity and tremor.

Etiology and Pathology

The syndrome may be produced by a variety of agents. Postencephalitic parkinsonism occurs as a sequel in a large percentage of cases of epidemic encephalitis. In older patients, the disorder often is on an arteriosclerotic basis. Toxic parkinsonism may result from poisoning with carbon monoxide or manganese. Occasionally, trauma to the head, cerebrovascular accidents, and neurosyphilis produce parkinsonism. An idiopathic form occurs in middle-aged and elderly patients. In paralysis agitans there usually is a loss of cells in the substantia nigra, corpus striatum, and other portions of the brain.

Symptoms and Signs

The patient's appearance is characteristic. He usually has a wide-eyed, unblinking, staring expression. The muscles of the face are smoothed out and almost immobile. Frequently, the mouth is held slightly open and saliva drools from the corners. The skin of the face often is unusually greasy. The patient walks with slow, short, shuffling steps, the arms flexed and adducted, and held stiffly at the sides, and the trunk slightly bent forward. He may break into a run spontaneously (festinating gait) or when pushed forward or backward (propulsion and retropulsion). There is pronounced slowness of all voluntary movements, particularly those carried out by the small muscles. Muscular rigidity is frequently present, involving opposing muscle groups equally, so that when an attempt is made to move part of an extremity, it moves with a series of jerks ("cogwheel rigidity"). Involuntary tremor, which is characteristic of the disease, frequently begins in one upper extremity and may remain there or gradually spread to the other extremities and eventually to the head. In the upper extremities, the fingers and thumbs are most frequently involved, giving rise to the characteristic pill-rolling movement. The rate of the tremor usually is between 4 and 8 movements/second. It is most severe when the extremity is at rest and may disappear temporarily on voluntary movement. It may be inhibited for a short time by conscious effort and usually disappears during sleep. Emotional excitement or fatigue intensifies the tremor.

Cramplike pains in the extremities and spine as a result of rigidity and secondary joint changes are not uncommon. There usually are no mental changes unless the condition is secondary to diffuse disease of the brain. Motor power is somewhat diminished. Sensation is intact and the reflexes are normal unless interfered with by muscular rigidity. Oculogyric crises (prolonged fixation of the eyeballs in one position), slowness and slurring of speech, and hypersalivation are not uncommon in the postencephalitic form.

Diagnosis and Prognosis

It is necessary to differentiate arthritis, multiple sclerosis, general paresis, and familial, hysterical, senile, toxic or hyperthyroid tremors. Differentiation on an etiologic basis is difficult and of little help. In many cases, it is impossible to elicit a history of encephalitis lethargica, since parkinsonism may develop many years after the original illness. A juvenile form occurs rarely and probably is the result of epidemic encephalitis.

The masklike facies, flexion attitudes of head, trunk, and extremities, loss of associated movements, rhythmic tremors and rigidity, hypersalivation, oculogyric crises, and speech disturbances, usually in the absence of pyramidal tract involvement, indicate parkinsonism.

The condition is slowly progressive but is compatible with long life. Incapacitation is gradual and increasing.

Treatment

General: A cheerful mental outlook should be encouraged. Every effort should be made to keep the patient active as long as possible. Massage and passive movement temporarily diminish rigidity.

Drugs: Analgesics (℞ 1, 8) are helpful in relieving cramplike pain, and phenobarbital (℞ 13) will frequently relieve insomnia. Amphetamine sulfate (℞ 63) decreases the frequency of oculogyric crises, helps combat lethargy, and makes the patient slightly more active and cheerful. Drugs of the belladonna group (℞ 26, 27, 28, 30) are of great value in decreasing tremor, rigidity, hypersalivation and excessive sweating. Whole belladonna, tincture of belladonna, atropine sulfate, stramonium, or hyoscine hydrobromide may be used. Frequently, the side effects of these drugs—dryness of the mouth, paralysis of the muscles of accommodation and of the genitourinary and gastrointestinal tracts—make it difficult to regulate the dose. A balance must be struck between the effective dose and that which can be tolerated. It is best to begin with small doses and gradually increase the amount until symptoms of toxicity appear, such as visual disturbances, severe nausea, constipation, pain in the throat, and excessive thirst. Sucking of hard candy may help combat dryness of the mouth. Pilocarpine (℞ 31) may diminish the paresis of accommodation and the gastrointestinal disturbances. The instillation of a drop of 0.25% physostigmine (℞ 32) in each eye daily or on alternate days may help control dimness of vision.

TREMORS

Involuntary movements in one or more parts of the body produced by alternate contractions of opposing muscle groups. They are symptoms of constitutional diseases or disorders rather than clinical entities.

Diagnosis

In differentiating tremors one should note the rate, rhythm, and distribution, and the effect of movement or rest. A rapid tremor is one that oscillates 8 to 10 times/second, while a slow tremor is one that oscillates 3 to 5 times/second. Tremors may be fine or coarse. Intention tremors are those that make their appearance or are accentuated by a volitional movement of the affected part. Rest tremors are those that are present when the involved part is kept at rest but disappear or become diminished when active movements are attempted.

Transient tremors that have no particular significance may occur in healthy individuals during periods of hunger, chilling, or excitement and after physical exertion. There is a form of tremor that is not associated with any known disease. This is a congenital tremor which occurs in several members of the same family and frequently in successive generations. It appears early in life and is present as a fine tremor involving the hands, lips, or tongue. Voluntary movement and emotion tend to make it worse. The family history and the absence of other evidence of disease are of diagnostic value in such cases.

Tremors Associated with Organic Disease

Lesions of the C.N.S., toxic states, and hyperthyroidism are the more common organic conditions with which tremor is associated.

1. Organic disease of the C.N.S. may be responsible for producing various kinds of tremors.

Paralysis Agitans: Tremor is one of the most prominent symptoms of this disease (q.v.). It is a coarse, slow, alternating tremor of about 4 to 8 movements/second, usually present during rest and tending to disappear or diminish on movement and during sleep. It is most commonly present in the fingers, forearm, head, eyelids, and tongue. In addition to the tremor, loss of associated movements, rigidity, masklike facies and slowness of movement are noted.

Hepatolenticular Degeneration (Wilson's disease): Various types of tremor may be seen in hepatolenticular degeneration (q.v.). The typical parkinsonian tremor of basal ganglia disease or the intention tremor of cerebellar disease is seen, but the characteristic, although not pathognomonic, abnormal involuntary movement of this disease is the so-called wing-beating tremor. These movements, as the name implies, are violent, rapid movements of the hand or the entire upper extremity, similar to the flapping of the wings of a bird. Wilson's disease is diagnosed by the presence of other evidence of extrapyramidal disease, cirrhosis of the liver, and a peculiar corneal pigmentation (Kayser-Fleischer ring).

Dementia Paralytica (General paresis): A fine, rapid tremor involving the face, tongue, and hands is an early symptom of this disease (q.v.). This tremor probably is due to damage to the frontal lobe and its connections with the brain stem and cerebellum. It may be increased by voluntary movement. The mental changes and spinal fluid findings are diagnostic features of this disorder.

Multiple Sclerosis: In this disease (q.v.), the tremor is of the intention type appearing only during movement of the limb and disappearing when it is at rest. Occasionally, there may be a static tremor of the head. Symptoms and signs of widespread C.N.S. involvement and the history of remissions and exacerbations are diagnostic.

Cerebral Arteriosclerosis: The tremor in this condition may either be of the intention type or resemble that of parkinsonism, depending on the part of the C.N.S. involved by the arteriosclerotic foci. The tremors associated with senility probably fall into this group. The age of the patient and other evidence of arteriosclerosis are distinguishing features in this disease.

Friedreich's Ataxia and other syndromes of the heredo-degenerative group: The tremor in these disorders resembles that of multiple sclerosis and is evidence of involvement of the cerebellum or its pathways.

2. Toxic states may contribute to the production of tremors.

Intoxication: Poisoning with a wide variety of substances frequently has tremor as a prominent symptom. Morphine and cocaine addicts show a fine tremor of the facial muscles and the fingers which becomes particularly pronounced on withdrawal of the drug. The tremor of chronic mercurial poisoning is a coarse, fairly slow one involving the muscles of the face and extremities and usually is more marked during movement. The most common toxic state in which tremor is seen is alcoholism (q.v.). In this condition there is a rapid, coarse tremor involving the fingers, tongue, limbs, and head. Frequently, it is most evident in the morning, before the intake of food or alcohol. An alcoholic drink at such times diminishes the tremor or even causes it to disappear. Alcoholic tremor is most severe during an attack of delirium tremens. In all these conditions there is other evidence of the toxin involved so that diagnosis is not difficult.

Hyperthyroidism: The tremor in this condition (q.v.) is fine, regular, and rapid and is usually confined to the outstretched fingers and hands. The associated tachycardia, exophthalmos, thyroid enlargement, and elevated basal metabolic rate are diagnostic.

Tremors Associated with Functional Disease

The tremors appearing in functional disorders may simulate those of organic disease of the C.N.S. and thus make diagnosis difficult. A psychiatric evaluation of the patient often is of considerable help in making a diagnosis.

Anxiety states: Tremor is a fairly common symptom in both chronic and acute anxiety states. In the former it resembles that of hyperthyroidism, while in the latter it is more coarse and irregular.

Hysteria: In this condition the tremor is frequently a fine, rapid one limited to an extremity or generalized. It may be a coarse, irregular shaking intensified by emotion and voluntary movement. It may be constant or appear in paroxysms.

Treatment

The treatment of tremors is that of the underlying disease. The alternating tremor of parkinsonism or other basal ganglia disease is decreased by drugs of the belladonna group (*see* PARALYSIS AGITANS). The intention tremor of cerebellar disease is not modified by drugs. Muscular reeducation makes it possible for patients to move the affected extremity with a lesser degree of tremor—in the upper extremity, for example, by performing all movements, if possible, with the arm held adducted on the chest. The tremor of dementia paralytica improves with arrest of the syphilitic inflammatory process by penicillin or fever therapy. The treatment of tremors due to various toxins is removal of the toxin and the use of general supportive measures. The latter is especially important in alcoholics where diet and vitamin therapy is important. Tremors of hyperthyroidism are alleviated by treatment of the disease (q.v.) by surgery or drugs of the thiouracil group. Psychotherapy is the treatment for patients with anxiety states or hysteria. Congenital tremor may be diminished or controlled by the use of sedative drugs such as phenobarbital ($\mathbb{R}$ 13) or hyoscine ($\mathbb{R}$ 26).

CEREBRAL PALSY OF CHILDREN

(Congenital diplegia, Little's disease, Congenital spastic paralysis)

Bilateral, usually symmetrical, nonprogressive disturbances of motility which are present from birth.

Etiology and Incidence

About 0.5% of patients admitted to pediatric hospitals have cerebral palsy. The usual cause is a developmental defect or intra-uterine cerebral degeneration. Often, a history of abnormal labor, birth trauma, or neonatal asphyxia is elicited. Though these factors may be of etiologic significance, pathologic investigation indicates that the developmental defect responsible for the cerebral palsy also is the basis of the obstetric difficulties.

Symptoms and Signs

In the more severe cases symptoms are evident from birth. Vomiting, irritability, and difficulty in nursing may be noted. The infants may be small, with delicate physical development. They are susceptible to intercurrent infections, and may succumb early in infancy. In milder cases, initial awareness of motor difficulty may not occur until the child fails to perform the expected acts at certain months. Thus, it may not sit up at 6 months or begin to talk and walk at 1 year. About 25% of cases have convulsions. The athetoid movements of the extremities usually do not appear until the 2nd or 3rd year of life.

The signs will depend on the part of the brain affected. Spastic weakness of the extremities is the most common manifestation. This usually is symmetrical, and the legs are more severely involved than the arms. A characteristic "scissors gait," exaggerated tendon reflexes, and extensor plantar responses are present. In the mild form, there may be only exaggeration of tendon reflexes, extensor plantar responses, and slight contractures of the calf muscles leading to talipes equinovarus. The most severe cases have marked spasticity of all extremities and involvement of the bulbar muscles with dysarthria and dysphagia. Involuntary or athetoid movements, cerebellar signs, or mental retardation also may be present.

About 70% of cases show some degree of mental retardation.

This often appears to be more severe than is actually the case, due to the difficulty these patients have in expressing themselves.

Diagnosis

When the symptoms and signs are present from birth, diagnosis is not difficult. When the difficulty is noted at a later date, distinction must be made from the progressive degenerative disorders such as cerebromacular degeneration (Tay-Sach's disease) and diffuse sclerosis (Schilder's disease). These are differentiated by their inexorable progression. Amyotonia congenita and the muscular dystrophies (q.v.) are distinguished by widespread flaccidity of muscles.

Treatment

Therapy will depend on the extent and type of involvement. The mild cases may proceed through a fairly normal life. In the moderately affected group, muscle reeducation, speech training, and corrective orthopedic procedures should be employed. A careful evaluation of mentality is advisable, since many patients with cerebral palsy are brighter than they appear, slowness often being due to their physical handicap. Special courses of study, and vocational guidance to fit individual capability are of great benefit. Curare has been given for the spasticity, but only transient benefit is obtained. Phenobarbital (℞ 13) or diphenylhydantoin sodium (℞ 19) should be used as needed if convulsions (q.v.) occur.

VERTIGO
(Dizziness)

A disturbance in which the individual has a subjective impression of movement in space, or of all visible objects moving about him, with resulting tendency to loss of equilibrium.

Etiology and Types

True vertigo, as distinguished from faintness, lightheadedness, and other forms of "dizziness," occurs invariably as a result of a disturbance of the equilibratory apparatus. The balancing mechanism (vestibule, semicircular canals, 8th nerve, cranial pathways and nuclei, eyes, and the sensory nerves of the muscles, joints and tendons) may be affected by any of a large variety of disorders: (1) **Otogenic:** Myringitis, otitis media, middle ear tumors, labyrinthitis, petrositis, otosclerosis, obstruction of the external auditory canal or the eustachian tube, Ménière's disease. (2) **Toxic:** Disturbances due to alcohol, salicylates, streptomycin, opiates, nicotine, caffeine, and various sedatives. **(3) Environmental:** Motion sickness, sunstroke, abrupt changes in atmospheric pressure. **(4) Ocular:** Eyestrain, glaucoma, ocular imbalance. **(5) Cardiovascular:** Hypertension, arteriosclerosis, postural hypotension, overactive carotid sinus reflex, cardiac failure. **(6) Blood dyscrasias:** Anemia, leukemia, polycythemia. **(7) Infectious diseases:** Influenza, diphtheria, typhoid fever, streptococcicosis, epidemic encephalitis, syphilis, measles, mumps, herpes. **(8) Neoplastic:** Tumors of the cerebrum, cerebellum, cerebellopontine angle, 8th nerve, and labyrinth. **(9) Miscellaneous:** Hemorrhage, psychogenic disorders, epilepsy, multiple sclerosis.

Diagnosis

In view of the multiplicity of possible causes, examination of the patient complaining of vertigo should be complete. Nystagmus (q.v.), past-pointing, poor balance when erect with the head in various positions and associated with nystagmus in sudden passive and active head movements, are all phenomena indicative of labyrinthine disease. Vestibular function may be investigated by the use of caloric, rotation, and galvanic tests.

The Kobrak caloric test consists of slowly injecting 5 cc. of water at a temperature of 40°F. (some physicians prefer ice water) into the patient's ear, with his head tilted back at an angle of 30 degrees. This usually produces horizontal and rotary nystagmus to the opposite side in 60 to 90 seconds. The test should not be performed in patients with ruptured ear drum, recent head injury, or obstruction of the canal. In the presence of a dead labyrinth or vestibular nerve paralysis, nystagmus cannot be elicited.

The rotation test is performed by revolving the patient in a special chair initially with his head upright and later flexed on his chest. In this manner, the horizontal canals are tested first and the vertical canals second. In each position, examination is made for nystagmus, past pointing, and falling to either the right or left when he stands up.

Through use of the galvanic test, differentiation can be made between disease in the labyrinth and disease in the 8th nerve. With the patient standing, feet together, eyes closed and the cathode in one hand, the anode is applied behind the ear, with a current of 5 milliamperes. Normally, there is postural deviation to the side of the anode. Absence of any response signifies a dead nerve.

Treatment

Relief of the patient's vertigo rests upon determining the specific cause of the symptom and eliminating it, if possible, by appropriate measures. Symptomatic relief may be obtained by use of Dramamine, 50 to 100 mg. every 4 to 6 hours.

CEREBROVASCULAR ACCIDENTS

Under this heading may be included apoplexy or stroke and subarachnoid hemorrhage. Cerebral angiospasm also will be discussed from the standpoint of its differential diagnostic importance.

CEREBRAL APOPLEXY
(Stroke)

The destruction of brain substance as a result of vascular hemorrhage, thrombosis, or embolism.

Etiology

Cerebral Hemorrhage: The most common cause is arteriosclerosis, usually associated with hypertension. It therefore occurs more commonly after middle life. Syphilis, congenital or mycotic aneurysm, blood dyscrasia, scurvy, or arsenical encephalitis may infrequently be responsible. Vascular hemorrhage, through the damaged vessel wall, may possibly occur due to a sudden rise in intracranial tension as a result of coitus, straining at stool or at work, vomiting, or coughing. In young persons, hemorrhage may occur without obvious cause. Of all cerebral vascular accidents, 15% are due to hemorrhage.

Cerebral Thrombosis: Arteriosclerosis is the usual cause. Less frequently, it may be due to syphilitic endarteritis, chronic lead poisoning, systemic infection in young people, and diseases which increase the coagulability of the blood (typhoid, cardiac failure, polycythemia vera). Thrombosis is most common after middle life and is responsible for 80% of cerebrovascular accidents.

Cerebral Embolism: May occur at any age and is causative in 3% of cerebrovascular accidents. The most frequent source of embolism in young people is subacute bacterial endocarditis. In middle-aged and elderly people, emboli may arise from mural thrombi in the heart, encountered in auricular fibrillation, myocardial infarction, or in the flatly dilated heart of the arteriosclerotic. Fat emboli may sometimes follow fractures. Air embolism (q.v.) may occur as a result of neck injuries or operations and in caisson disease.

Pathology

Cerebral Hemorrhage: Rupture of a damaged vessel wall results in bleeding into the surrounding brain tissue and clot formation. The hemorrhage may spread into the ventricles or into the subarachnoid space. Later, the blood and necrotic tissue are replaced by connective tissue, fibrous glia, and newly formed vessels. With large hemorrhages, part or all of the damaged area may remain as a walled-off apoplectic cyst filled with fluid. Hemorrhage usually is single but there may be two or more in some cases. The branches of the middle cerebral artery are most often affected, involving the internal capsule and the basal ganglia.

Cerebral Thrombosis: Arteriosclerosis or endarteritis of a cerebral vessel leads to thrombosis and formation of an infarct. The infarcted area undergoes softening and organization. Not infrequently, a walled-off cyst remains at the site. As in most vascular accidents, the middle cerebral artery is most often involved. Less frequently, the vertebral and basilar arteries are implicated. The cerebellum is only rarely affected.

Cerebral Embolism: Embolism is followed by thrombosis, infarction, softening, absorption, and organization. Septic emboli may be further complicated by abscess formation or the development of a mycotic aneurysm.

Symptoms and Signs

The clinical manifestations of all cerebrovascular accidents are rather similar. Premonitory symptoms are uncommon; in some cases, there may be headache, vertigo, nausea, and vomiting.

The onset usually is abrupt, except in some cases of thrombosis, where it may be more gradual. (Onset accompanied by convulsions is more likely to indicate cerebral hemorrhage.) The patient suddenly loses consciousness or falls to the ground due to a paralyzed leg. In nocturnal accidents, the patient awakens with evidence of paralysis. Coma may persist up to several hours, and may even recur after a few hours or days in some patients. Death may occur without return of consciousness.

Examination may disclose hypertension, arteriosclerosis, cardiac disease, or evidence of embolic phenomena elsewhere. Respiration often is stertorous in comatose cases. The appearance of Cheyne-Stokes respiration or the persistence of coma for more than 48 hours is a grave prognostic sign. The pulse usually is rapid, the temperature variable. The leukocyte count usually is moderately elevated, but occasionally exceeds 20,-000. Transient hyperglycemia and glycosuria are commonly encountered immediately after an attack, particularly after a hemorrhage. The urine usually contains albumin and casts as a transient disturbance, or associated with preexisting renal damage.

Neurologic findings will vary with the site and extent of the damaged area. Findings may vary from no localizing signs to a complete hemiplegia, which is flaccid at this stage. There may be conjugate deviation of the head and eyes and positive bilateral Babinski's. The corneal reflex usually is absent. Hemiplegia may be demonstrated by the puffing out of one cheek during expiration, one elevated limb falling more heavily than the uninvolved extremity, and unilateral absence of response to vigorous plantar stimulation.

The spinal fluid usually is under increased pressure and bloody or xanthochromic in patients with cerebral hemorrhage, usually normal in patients with thrombosis but there may be a mild pleocytosis, with some elevation in the protein concentration.

The differentiation as to which type of vascular accident has occurred is often impossible. Embolism is suggested in a young patient with evidence of cardiac disease and embolism elsewhere. Hemorrhage and thrombosis most commonly occur in the older age groups. Hemorrhage is indicated when the onset is characterized by convulsions, headache, nausea, or vomiting. Later evidence of hemorrhage is stiffness of the neck, Cheyne-Stokes breathing, conjugate deviation of the head and eyes, and a bloody cerebrospinal fluid.

Course and Prognosis

The outcome depends on the size and site of the lesion. Sudden death is rare. An extensive hemorrhage usually is fatal in 2 to 14 days. Death seldom occurs during an initial attack of thrombosis or embolism, and then only after the 10th day when complications (bronchopneumonia) may develop. Persistent or recurrent coma is an unfavorable prognostic sign, as is a persistent high temperature. Fatal cases usually show a progressive elevation in temperature, pulse, and respiration.

When a small vessel is involved, eventual recovery is usual. Following the initial shock, improvement occurs gradually and may continue for several months. After 2 or 3 weeks, the paralysis gradually becomes spastic, with an increase in the deep reflexes and the persistence of a positive Babinski on the spastic side. Complete recovery may occur but there usually is some permanent sequela, such as a hemiplegic gait or disturbance in voice or speech. The degree of permanent neurologic damage cannot be predicted for the first few weeks, since much of it may be due to a transient edema. At least 6 months must be allowed to elapse before improvement can be considered maximal.

Diagnosis

Other lesions of the C.N.S. usually can be excluded by a careful history. When a patient is found comatose, and no history is obtainable from an observer, the problem is more difficult (*see* THE UNCONSCIOUS PATIENT). Complete physical and neurologic examination, X-ray, and certain diagnostic laboratory procedures are then required to exclude uremia, diabetic coma, expanding brain lesions, alcoholism, subarachnoid or extradural hemorrhage, drug poisoning, and epilepsy. In particular, one should note evidence of trauma, the state of the eyeballs, pupils, and fundi, the odor of the breath and character of respiration, the blood pressure, and evidence of neck stiffness.

Cerebral Angiospasm: Localized brain tissue ischemia may be due to a transient spasm of an intracranial artery usually occurring in association with hypertension or a rise in blood pressure from a previously normal level. Allergy and sensitivity to tobacco may be the etiologic factors responsible. Transient and varied neurologic syndromes may result. A diagnosis of angiospasm must be avoided until all possibility of organic pathology has been excluded. Therapy consists in the detection and correction of allergic sensitivities and complete abstinence from smoking. Suspected angiospasm may be corrected or ruled out in a given case by the I.V. injection of 30 to 65 mg. of papaverine hydrochloride (℞ 39), repeated in 2 hours if indicated.

Prophylaxis

Arteriosclerosis and hypertensive vascular disease (q.v.) should be managed in the usual way. Physical and emotional activities require moderation. Smoking should be discontinued or at least decreased. Sedatives (℞ 13, 15) may be used to lessen nervousness. When indicated, antisyphilitic therapy (q.v.) must be instituted. Cardiac conditions are treated in the prescribed manner.

Treatment

During coma: The patient should not be disturbed or moved except when essential, such as to loosen clothing and to avoid the development of decubitus (q.v.) or hypostatic pneumonia (q.v.). If the patient must be transported, gentle handling is required to avoid further damage. Whenever hypostatic pneumonia is threatened because of the degree of immobility, the presence of cardiac failure or the general debility of the patient, penicillin should be given prophylactically in doses of 300,000 u. I.M. every 12 hours (see ANTIBIOTIC THERAPY).

Phlebotomy for hypertensive patients remains of unproved value, but may be done to lower the blood pressure temporarily. Lumbar puncture must be done for diagnostic purposes and should be repeated every 24 to 48 hours until the fluid is almost clear and the pressure normal. Intracranial tension and edema may be reduced by the I.V. use of 50% glucose (℞ 78), repeated as needed. An ice cap to the head probably is useless, but also is harmless. Bladder overdistention must be avoided by frequent catheterizations or the temporary use of an indwelling catheter, and precautions taken to avoid infection (q.v.). If angiospasm is suspected, 30 to 60 mg. (gr. ss to i) of papaverine hydrochloride (℞ 39) may be given I.V. and repeated in 2 hours. Aminophylline (℞ 40) may be used in place of papaverine.

The administration of sedatives or stimulants is not advised since they are useless at this time and may actually be undesirable. The value of anticoagulants (q.v.) in definite cases of thrombosis or embolism remains to be established. Where septic embolism has occurred or is suspected, the use of appropriate antibiotics or chemotherapy is indicated.

During convalescence: When consciousness returns, fluids and nourishment should be given orally if possible, otherwise parenterally or by rectum, in order to maintain fluid balance. The physician should encourage the patient at all times until recovery is certain. Daily visits should be made to avoid giving the patient a feeling of hopelessness and despair. The bladder and bowels are controlled by catheterization and enemas as indicated. Continued effort must be directed at the prophylaxis of decubitus (q.v.) and hypostatic pneumonia (q.v.). Mild sedatives (℞ 13, 15) may be used cautiously but opiates are to be avoided at all times. Phlebotomy may be repeated in the presence of marked hypertension.

As the clot is slowly absorbed, it may act like a tumor and manifest itself by increasing intracranial pressure, progression of signs, and deepening or recurrent coma. In all such cases, neurosurgery is indicated. Surgical intervention has been life-saving in some patients and has lessened the neurologic sequelae in others.

Functional restoration of paralyzed limbs must be attempted as soon as coma lightens. Passive motion through all arcs and light massage several times daily are useful in promoting circulation, maintaining muscle nutrition, and avoiding joint stiffness. The patient should be coaxed to use the paralyzed muscles, aided initially with passive movements. However, fatigue is to be avoided at all times. When indicated, splints should be applied between exercises to prevent contractures.

As soon as his general condition and strength permit, the patient should be allowed out of bed for gradually increasing periods. When muscle strength permits (usually after 6 to 8 weeks), walking may be attempted, first with assistance and then with the use of a cane. Unsupported ambulation (hemiplegic gait) usually is possible by the 6th month.

The therapy of speech disorders is long and tedious, requiring the constant attention of both the physician and the patient. Fortunately, recovery of speech may be expected in most cases.

SUBARACHNOID HEMORRHAGE

Sudden bleeding into the subarachnoid space.

Etiology and Pathology

The most frequent cause of subarachnoid hemorrhage is the rupture of a congenital intracranial aneurysm. Less frequently, it may be due to mycotic or arteriosclerotic aneurysm, hemorrhagic diseases, and syphilis. It is most frequent between 25 and 50 years of age and a migraine history is common in patients with subarachnoid hemorrhage.

Hemorrhage usually arises at the bifurcation of a vessel, where the muscular coat is poorly developed and an aneurysm is likely to be present. The majority of aneurysms are located along the middle or anterior cerebral arteries or the communicating branches of the circle of Willis. With healing, adhesions produce a pachymeningitis or an adhesive arachnitis.

Symptoms and Signs

Before rupture, an aneurysm may be asymptomatic or may manifest itself as a result of pressure on adjacent structures. There may be ocular palsies, diplopia, squint, and pain in the face due to pressure on the 3rd, 4th, 5th, and 6th cranial nerves. Visual loss and a bitemporal field defect signify pressure on the optic chiasm. Pressure on the optic tract produces a homonymous hemianopsia.

With rupture, there is a sudden onset with severe head pain, nausea, and vomiting. Consciousness may be lost, but more often the patient is semicomatose. Mixture of the escaping blood and cerebrospinal fluid irritates the cerebral cortex, producing evidence of increased intracranial pressure (headache, vomiting, dizziness, papilledema, seldom convulsions, and alterations in pulse and respiratory rates). There is marked stiffness of the neck, Kernig's sign, and bilateral Babinski's. The temperature may be elevated but usually returns to normal by the 3rd day. Focal signs are rare, unless the vessel has ruptured into the brain substance. Later, the extravasated clot may act as an intracranial tumor. The cerebrospinal fluid is bloody and under increased pressure.

Diagnosis

Subarachnoid hemorrhage must be differentiated from other cerebral vascular accidents. Arteriography is useful in distinguishing an unruptured aneurysm from a brain tumor. X-rays of the skull may reveal calcification in the wall of an aneurysm.

Course and Prognosis

With the cessation of active hemorrhage, the spinal fluid gradually clears and the pressure returns to normal in about 3 weeks. Occasionally, organization of the blood clot may produce a pachymeningitis and simulate a tumor. Adhesive arachnitis also may develop. About 60% recover from a first attack, but recurrence is not unusual.

Prophylaxis and Treatment

Treatment should be directed at any underlying vascular disease, blood dyscrasia, cardiac disease, and syphilis. Severe exertion should be avoided. In some cases of aneurysm, ligation of the afferent artery may be indicated.

Bed rest is indicated until 4 to 6 weeks after bleeding has ceased. Fluid balance and nutrition should be maintained, parenterally if necessary. Chloral hydrate (℞ 14) or paraldehyde (℞ 15) may be used for restlessness. Opiates and anticoagulants are contraindicated.

A diagnostic spinal tap is always indicated. The desirability of further taps to reduce intracranial pressure will depend on the patient's reaction to the initial puncture. If the patient's condition improves after lumbar puncture, repeated taps may be performed at intervals until bleeding ceases, slowly reducing the intracranial pressure to half its original level with each tap. In some instances, cisternal puncture may be necessary as an emergency procedure, but should be done by someone experienced in this technic.

INTRACRANIAL NEOPLASMS

(Brain tumors)

Neoplasm, metastatic or otherwise, tuberculoma, gumma, hemorrhage, aneurysm, and abscess are among the conditions which may create expanding lesions within the skull. For clinical purposes, all of these may be regarded as tumors, but this text is primarily concerned with neoplasms that arise from intracranial tissues. These are more common than is generally supposed and are frequently misdiagnosed.

Intracranial neoplasms are of 5 classes: (1) gliomas (e.g., spongioblastoma, astrocytoma); (2) tumors of covering cells of nervous system (e.g., meningioma, sarcoma); (3) hypophyseal tumors (adenoma; craniopharyngioma); (4) dysembryomas (e.g., teratoid cyst, pinealoma); (5) vascular tumors (e.g., hemangioma). Some of these possess true malignancy, infiltrating contiguous tissues (but never metastasizing outside of the C.N.S.), while others are benign and of circumscribed growth. However, any progressively expanding intracranial lesion may exert malignant physiologic effects through increasing the general intracranial pressure, or by interfering with the functioning of the brain area involved and, by direct pressure, affecting contiguous areas, nerves, or vessels. Supratentorial tumors occur chiefly in adults and infratentorial in children. Some gliomas are highly vascular; rarely, cerebral trauma produces hemorrhage within them. In such instances an initial misdiagnosis is almost inevitable. Repeated subarachnoid hemorrhages should always suggest tumor.

General Symptomatology

Headache, vomiting, and papilledema in the absence of cardiorenal disease are the classic symptoms of increased intracranial pressure and constitute presumptive evidence of an intracranial expanding lesion. Transient dizziness and diplopia, or transient palsy of one or both 6th nerves are other symptoms. Traction or pressure on the spinal roots may cause diminution in deep tendon reflexes, prefaced in some instances by sharp pain in root areas. Drowsiness, lowered mental acuity, hypertension, perhaps with increased pulse pressure, slowed pulse, and shallow, irregular respirations, may appear later. In some instances, focal diagnostic signs never appear but in others irritative (localized or generalized convulsions) and paretic phenomena will become evident before intracranial pressure is greatly increased.

TUMORS OF THE CEREBRUM

Frontal: Here the most common types of tumors are meningioma and astrocytoma. Because of the paucity of information about definite physiologic centers in the frontal lobes, personality changes and evidences of pressure exerted backward on the pyramidal tracts or their cortical origins usually must be depended upon for diagnosis. Symptoms such as inappropriate jocosity and diminishing power of attention often appear, also petit mal characterized by sudden attacks of mental confusion. Later, there may be periods of stupor. A partial or complete loss of smell (anosmia) may occur unilaterally or bilaterally, secondary to encroachment on one or both olfactory nerves; and involvement of the precentral gyrus may cause interference with speech emission. Ipsilateral retrobulbar neuritis with a central scotoma and optic atrophy often occurs; concurrently there may be contralateral papilledema. (With uncomplicated papilledema visual acuity may remain unaffected for a relatively long period.) In some instances, papilledema may appear first on the affected side. Right frontal lobe and left cerebellar lobe tumors are frequently difficult to differentiate. Staggering backward on the heels and gradual paresis characterize the right frontal; wide base and dysrhythmic movements, the left cerebellar.

Parietal: Oligodendroglioma and glioblastoma are the most common tumors here. Motor weakness with early focal epilepsy is presumptive evidence of a parietal lesion. Objective contralateral sensory changes may or may not appear, but numbness or tingling in the affected part—face or body—may precede the focal fit. Perception of pain and temperature are not altered. Contralateral astereognosis (loss of power to recognize objects by touch) may be present. Disturbances of speech, either of phonation or of recall (aphasia), may occur; in certain instances a high degree of word blindness (alexia) may result. Defects in the contralateral visual field also may develop.

Subcortical: Occurring in the motor areas, subcortical tumors may never cause focal seizures, or may cause them late, and only after a considerable degree of paresis has occurred in the contralateral limb. A thalamic syndrome may occur, with inability to register emotion in the contralateral side of the face. Contralateral alterations of response to all forms of sensory stimulation may appear, also athetosis, i.e., wormlike movements of the hands and feet. Deep burning pain may result from contact with sharp or cold objects. Ipsilateral quadrantic or complete hemianopsia for form or color, or both, may develop.

Temporal: Glioblastoma multiforme and oligodendroglioma are the most common forms at this site. Temporal lobe tumors are extremely difficult to diagnose (as are otitic abscesses). There is one known bilateral center here, that of smell and taste, and one unilateral center for storage of auditory memories. Reduction may be noted in the ability to recollect names of persons, places, and things. However, the correct word is recognized when heard. Dramatic and sudden dreamy mental states, with hallucinations of vision and explosive sensations of taste and smell, due to uncinate irritation, may occur; this is the so-called uncinate fit. In rare instances the pupils will be fixed, or a thalamic syndrome—as previously described—will occur.

Occipital: Glioblastoma multiforme is the most common. A contralateral homonymous hemianoptic defect is characteristic. Visual jacksonian fits, which are crude and lacking in formulation—perhaps a twinkling or flashing—may preface the field defects. Angiomas characterized by subarachnoid hemorrhage at times occur in this location.

Corpus callosum: Glioblastoma multiforme is the most often occurring tumor of this region. A progressive quadriplegia is characteristic; this is sometimes preceded by an extraordinary loss of control and power, the patient flopping like a baby when unsupported. Some loss of ability to perform purposeful movement (apraxia) is seen. Slurred speech, changed intelligence, and involuntary sphincter relaxation are common. General intracranial pressure signs may appear late or not at all.

TUMORS OF THE BASE OF THE SKULL

These tumors may arise from such areas as the olfactory groove or the wall of the cavernous sinus, or from persisting cells of the primitive notochord, and are characterized by involvement of cranial nerve function. Unilateral primary optic atrophy may occur. Increased intracranial pressure may appear late; its absence plus a series of cranial nerve palsies is suggestive of a tumor in this location.

TUMORS OF THE BRAIN STEM

Cranial nerve palsies and quadriplegia constitute the general picture of tumors of that portion of the brain stem which extends from the subthalamic region to the inferior level of the medulla. The level at which the tumor occurs of course determines the symptoms. In medullary involvement there may be interference with vocal cord and soft palate functions, together with hemiparesis and hemianesthesia.

TUMORS OF THE PONS

Combinations of 5th, 6th, and 7th nerve palsies may be seen, together with contralateral pyramidal paralysis. Disturbances of urinary secretion and temperature control may occur. A tumor of the anterior crus cerebri will cause an ipsilateral 3rd nerve paralysis, with dilatation of the pupil (mydriasis), ptosis of the eyelid, and contralateral hemiplegia. In many cases, papilledema never appears; when it does, it is a late symptom.

TUMORS OF THE PINEAL BODY

Ordinarily, these tumors occur in children. They often produce signs of precocious puberty, especially in males. There may be periods of tonic extensor spasm, resembling decerebrate rigidity. Bilateral tremor (red nucleus involvement) and bilateral pyramidal tract signs appear. Pupillary response to light may be lost (Argyll Robertson pupil), and later even the reaction to accommodation. These tumors necessarily give rise to the quadrigeminal plate syndrome: interference with conjugate upward eye movements, and later with conjugate downward eye movements.

VENTRICULAR TUMORS

Third and lateral ventricles: These tumors may be either primary or invasive. Intermittent blocking of interventricular drainage may occur. Choroid plexus adenomas ordinarily produce intense hydrocephalus; ballooning of the floor of the 3rd ventricle may cause sudden blindness. Pressure on the tuber cinereum and hypophysis may produce symptoms of somnolence, irregular fever, increased weight, and polyuria. Midbrain compression may give rise to such symptoms as occur with pineal body tumors.

TUMORS OF THE CEREBELLUM

Midline or vermis: These tumors, which in children often are medulloblastomas, present a rather typical picture. Vomiting, papilledema, and other compression signs appear early. The legs are ataxic, and there is difficulty in walking and staying erect. Nystagmus may be absent. The head may be violently retracted during "cerebellar" tonic fits.

Lateral lobes: Astrocytoma cystica and angioblastoma are the most common tumors of this region. Increase in intracranial pressure is prompt and severe. The ipsilateral limbs become hypotonic, with disturbance in their rhythm of movement. Not infrequently the head is tilted toward the affected side, and the patient tends to fall toward that side. Nystagmus is usual.

TUMORS OF CRANIAL NERVES

Optic nerve: Gliomas of the optic nerve itself and of the optic chiasm occur. The former can often be detected with the ophthalmoscope; the latter often is part of a generalized neurofibromatosis.

Acoustic nerve: These tumors grow from the sheath of the nerve at the cerebellopontine angle. In rare instances they are bilateral. Usually, there is unilateral tinnitus followed by diminution of hearing and loss of all reaction to caloric tests for labyrinthine function (see VERTIGO). Power in the ipsilateral facial muscles may be reduced, and the patient may have attacks of dizziness, postural ataxia, and cerebellar ataxia of the ipsilateral arm. Nystagmus may be present.

Trigeminal nerve: Neuromas of the gasserian ganglion are distinguished from tic douloureux by an objective depression of sensation in the areas of distribution of the 5th nerve.

TUMORS OF THE HYPOPHYSIS

Hypophyseal adenomas are of 3 types, chromophile, chromophobe, and basophile. In chromophile adenoma the clinical picture is that of hyperpituitarism and acromegaly (q.v.). The blood sugar is increased, and there may be glycosuria. Increased hairiness is usual. The male may become impotent. Chromophobe adenomas are the most common. They produce symptoms of hypopituitarism, with obesity, decreased hairiness, and impaired sexual function. The B.M.R. is lowered, and sugar tolerance rises. Both these types lead to characteristic erosion and expansion of the sella turcica. Deep-seated frontal headache is common. Bitemporal hemianopsia occurs from pressure on the optic chiasm. Later, the nasal fields also may be involved. The 3rd and 6th nerves may be compressed; trigeminal neuralgia often occurs; typical uncinate fits are not unknown; rarely, pyramidal tract symptoms are seen. Basophile adenomas are rare. They are seen as a rule in young women of excessive overweight. Pressure symptoms are less frequent in this type of tumor.

Diagnosis

Removing spinal fluid usually is a dangerous procedure when an expanding intracranial lesion exists. Generally, the pressure is normal with brain stem tumors, and may be so with supratentorial tumors. In cord tumors complete or partial subarachnoid block practically always exists, as demonstrated by concurrent lumbar and cisternal puncture. Spinal fluid protein and cells may be increased, according to the site and nature of the lesion; in brain tumors such changes are merely confirmatory, not diagnostic. Flat-plate X-rays of the skull may furnish valuable leads; the following changes may be seen: (1) calcification within the tumor; (2) evidence of increased intracranial pressure (atrophy of sella turcica; increase in convolutional impressions; diffuse atrophy of the skull bones; separation of sutures); (3) displacement of the pineal shadow; (4) erosion of bone adjacent to the tumor. Encephalography and ventriculography (X-ray studies after introduction of air) give information about displacement, enlargement, or decrease in size of the ventricles. These data often are diagnostic, but such procedures are for the expert only. The EEG often is helpful in adding supportive evidence. The differentiations necessary with suspected brain tumor are too numerous to detail. In the main, the characteristic phenomena of brain abscess, however, are slow pulse, low fever, and focal signs. The successful diagnosis of neoplastic lesions generally depends upon repeated examinations, an appreciation of the significance of quite small functional defects, and their correlation with the known facts of intracranial anatomy and physiology.

Treatment

Prompt neurologic or neurosurgical consultation is obligatory if a brain tumor or other expanding intracranial lesion is suspected. Treatment is primarily surgical, but some of the tumors are sensitive to X-rays—including the medulloblastomas, which occur as cerebellar growths in children. The latter are mentioned because, in emergency, X-ray therapy pending operative intervention may be lifesaving. It must be remembered, however, that X-ray may cause hemorrhages in some varieties of brain tumor, particularly the gliomas. When a long journey to a neurosurgeon is necessary, a qualified general surgeon may, as an emergency measure, perform a ventricular tap and thereby reduce an otherwise fatal intracranial pressure. Glucose (R 78), 25 to 50 cc. of 50% solution I.V., often is lifesaving, and can be repeated as necessary. In some instances, artificial respiration and oxygen therapy are indicated. Because of its depressant action on respiratory function, morphine should never be used to control any pain in these patients, but codeine sometimes is given in amounts up to 60 mg. (gr. i) subcut. (R 2), and repeated every 3 to 4 hours when necessary. Some neurosurgical clinics, however, prohibit even the use of codeine for pain in the presence of increased intracranial pressure, depending instead upon caffeine plus acetylsalicylic acid (R 9), or aminopyrine and caffeine (R 10).

ENCEPHALITIS

Any one of a number of uncommon clinical conditions characterized by inflammatory and degenerative lesions of the brain and cord. Poliomyelitis and rabies (q.v.) logically come under this general head, but because of their special importance they are described separately.

Classification

   I. Arthropod-borne Virus Encephalitides
  II. Von Economo's Encephalitis
 III. Postinfectious Encephalomyelitis
 IV. Miscellaneous Viral Encephalomyelitides
  V. Guillain-Barré Syndrome

ARTHROPOD-BORNE VIRUS ENCEPHALITIDES

A filtrable virus has been found responsible for St. Louis encephalitis, equine encephalomyelitis (Western and Eastern types), louping ill, Japanese B, and Russian forest-spring encephalitis. Only the first two of those diseases have been identified in this country. St. Louis and Western equine encephalomyelitis are primarily diseases of wild and domestic animals. Mosquitoes, fowl mites, and other arthropods serve as vectors of the virus: ticks may harbor it from season to season. Eastern and Western equine encephalomyelitis cause epizootics in horses, while St. Louis encephalitis causes inapparent infections in horses. The St. Louis and Western forms are widely distributed in the United States, especially in the West and Middle West. Man is an accidental host, and the exact mode of transmission to him still is unknown: there is no known case-to-case spread, and isolation of patients is not required. Nevertheless, the disease often appears in a number of persons in the same community at approximately the same time. Such human outbreaks of equine encephalomyelitis have occurred locally in Massachusetts and Texas. Cases of St. Louis encephalitis and Western equine encephalomyelitis and of poliomyelitis may occur in human members of the same community at the same time. The incidence is highest in warm weather, and all age groups are affected. Sporadic cases sometimes appear.

Symptoms and Signs

St. Louis encephalitis and Western equine encephalomyelitis have essentially the same clinical features. In infants, the onset is abrupt, with high fever, convulsions, bulging fontanel and generalized rigidity. Temperatures of 103° to 106°F. persist for 1 or 2 days and may become normal within a week. In older children and adults onset is more gradual, with headache, chilliness, muscle pains, and gastrointestinal or respiratory symptoms. Within a day or two severe headache, somnolence often progressing to coma, disorientation, and delirium develop. The face is flushed and swollen, and there may be tremors of the tongue, lips, and hands. The neck and back are somewhat stiff but not rigid as in purulent meningitis. Abnormal reflexes are common but transient. Nystagmus is uncommon and ocular palsies are rare. Flaccid paralysis of extremities (unlike poliomyelitis) is infrequent. The average temperature is 102° to 103° F. and returns to normal by the 10th day. There often is relative bradycardia. Some of the symptoms and signs may outlast the pyrexia. Eastern equine encephalomyelitis is more severe and fulminating than the other varieties.

VON ECONOMO'S ENCEPHALITIS

(Epidemic encephalitis, Encephalitis lethargica)

This disease affects human beings and is presumed to be of virus origin but the causative agent has not yet been identified.

Beginning in central Europe in 1916, it spread throughout the world and was epidemic in the United States from 1919 to 1925. Occasional sporadic cases of encephalitis currently seen resemble von Economo's disease. All age groups are affected. The disease is most prevalent in cold seasons. Direct person-to-person transmission is assumed to occur.

Symptoms and Signs

This type of encephalitis is characterized by an acute stage of fever, lethargy, somnolence, ocular palsies, and hyperkinetic phenomena. This may be followed by a chronic progressive stage in which occur symptoms of basal ganglia involvement, ocular crises, personality and behavior disorders, and disturbances of the vegetative nervous centers. Extreme variability of symptoms and signs in different patients or in the same patient from time to time is characteristic. The diverse manifestations are explained by the extent and character of the lesions in the brain. Onset may be sudden or gradual, and is sometimes preceded by respiratory symptoms, headache, and fever. Some cases primarily exhibit rigidity and other hyperkinetic phenomena, or tremors, choreo-athetoid, myoclonic, and other dyskinetic movements. Emotional disturbances and delirium may alternate with stupor or coma. Weakness, paralysis, tendon reflex changes, pain, and sensory disturbances often are transient. Fever is variable and in some instances absent altogether. The acute stage may be brief or greatly prolonged, often with sharp exacerbations.

Recovery is complete in approximately 50% of patients surviving the acute stage; the remainder exhibit a variety of chronic, often progressive symptoms. The chronic phase begins immediately after the acute stage, or after intervals up to 15 years. It may appear after an abortive or unrecognized acute attack.

POSTINFECTIOUS ENCEPHALOMYELITIS

Postinfectious encephalomyelitis is characterized by focal perivascular demyelination, and may follow measles, German measles, chickenpox, smallpox, vaccination (vaccinia), and antirabic treatment. No infectious agent has been recovered from the brain. Strong indirect evidence points to allergic sensitivity in the pathogenesis of this disease. Considering the frequency of the conditions which may lead to it, postinfectious encephalitis is extremely rare. Onset usually is during convalescence from acute viral exanthems; or 9 to 13 days after vaccination; or during the second half of a course of antirabic injections, or shortly after their completion.

The disease may attack primarily the brain, cord, or peripheral nerves. In the encephalitic type the illness begins with fever, headache, and somnolence. There may be convulsions, delirium, paralysis, or weakness of extremities, loss of sphincter control, and impairment of sensation. In myelitic and neuritic cases, flaccid paralysis, reflex and sensory changes in the extremities, and signs of transverse myelitis are seen. The severity and course of the illness are variable and may be mild, acute, chronic, or fatal.

MISCELLANEOUS VIRAL ENCEPHALO-MYELITIDES

A number of other known viruses may produce encephalitis. Among these are the viruses of herpes simplex, lymphogranuloma venereum, lymphocytic choriomeningitis and mumps. Proved cases of encephalitis due to herpes simplex and lymphogranuloma venereum are rare. The clinical syndrome is that of a febrile illness with headache, nausea, vomiting, delirium or irrational behavior, somnolence, stiff neck, pupillary abnormalities, tremors, and transient disturbances in tendon reflexes.

The clinical illness caused by the virus of lymphocytic choriomeningitis generally consists of a prodromal febrile period of 1 to 3 weeks, followed by headache, chilliness, muscle aches, and continued fever with stiff neck. Usually, the neurologic examination is otherwise negative (*see* MENINGITIS). In a small number of cases, symptoms and signs of encephalitis also occur, manifested by confusion, delirium, pain, and other sensory disturbances, weakness of the extremities, loss of sphincter control, cranial nerve palsies, and reflex changes.

Mumps meningoencephalitis occurs as a complication of epidemic parotitis. It may precede or follow clinical involvement of the salivary glands, testes, ovaries, breasts, or pancreas; or it may occur without any sign of mumps. Clinical meningoencephalitis is an infrequent complication, although abnormalities in the spinal fluid can be found in one-third of the patients with mumps. When the encephalitis develops, onset of symptoms is fairly abrupt, with headache, nausea, vomiting, somnolence, and stupor or apathy. Nuchal rigidity is present, and there may be reflex disturbances; cranial nerve palsies or paralyses of extremities are rare. The course usually is brief and the prognosis excellent.

GUILLAIN-BARRE SYNDROME

This myeloradiculoneuritis of unknown cause, with symptoms of proximal motor weakness and distal sensory disturbances of the extremities, often follows acute infections. It is characterized by exceedingly high spinal fluid protein content without increase in cells. In some instances, cranial nerve palsies (facial weakness) and mental disturbances indicate involvement of the brain as well. The disease usually is self-limited, lasting from a few weeks to several months.

Diagnosis

Encephalitis is to be considered when a patient has an acute onset of fever and headache with signs and symptoms of diffuse or focal involvement of the brain. Clinical diagnosis is substantiated by the demonstration of abnormal elements in the spinal fluid. Arthropod-borne encephalitides occur in epidemic form during warm weather. Equine encephalitis may be contemporaneous with an epizootic in horses. Von Economo's encephalitis should be suspected when ocular palsies, general muscular rigidity, and abnormal involuntary movements are outstanding findings. The demyelinating encephalitides are recognized by a history of preceding illness or prophylactic treatment (e.g., vaccines).

Leukocytes in the blood generally are normal in number or moderately elevated; other routine laboratory studies are not diagnostic. The spinal fluid is abnormal (see table, page 986) in most instances but not diagnostic of a specific etiologic agent. By appropriate means specific viruses may be isolated from blood, spinal fluid, or nervous tissue. Complement fixation or neutralization tests employing acute and convalescent phase specimens of blood can be used for specific diagnosis of the arthropod-borne virus encephalitides as well as the miscellaneous group of viral encephalitides, including those caused by the viruses of herpes simplex, lymphogranuloma venereum, lymphocytic choriomeningitis, and mumps. Negative results of such laboratory tests in many cases suggest that other, as yet unknown, agents also cause encephalitis. (Such examinations are performed by the U.S. Public Health Service.)

Differential diagnosis (see table, p. 986) requires consideration of bacterial meningitis, tuberculous meningitis, fungus infections, neurosyphilis (luetic meningitis, paresis), encephalopathy due to uremia, hypoglycemia, porphyria, heavy metal poisoning (lead, arsenic), hypertensive and cerebrovascular disorders (hemorrhage, embolism, thrombosis), brain tumor, brain abscess, typhus fever, typhoid, Weil's disease, botulism, toxoplasmosis, poliomyelitis, rabies, psychosis, encephalopathy following whooping cough, pneumonia, and other infectious diseases; multiple sclerosis, status epilepticus, and nutritional deficiency states (q.v.).

Prognosis and Sequelae

The arthropod-borne encephalitides have an over-all case fatality rate of 20%, which is higher in infants and the aged. Eastern equine encephalomyelitis in infants and children has a fatality rate of 50%. Recovery is complete in those who survive the acute attack, except in infants, who may later show mental deterioration, spasticity, and recurring convulsions.

Von Economo's encephalitis has a fatality rate of 20 to 40%. Among survivors of the acute stage a large number manifest

SPINAL FLUID FINDINGS

Condition	Pressure	Appearance	Cells
Normal	100 to 200 mm. H$_2$O	Clear	0 to 10/cu. mm.
Meningismus	Normal or increased	Clear	Normal
Meningococcic meningitis	Increased	Turbid or purulent	500 to 20,000, mostly polymorphonuclears.
Tuberculous meningitis	Increased	Clear to slightly cloudy	50 to 500; polymorphonuclears may predominate early; lymphocytes, later.
H. influenzae meningitis	Increased	Purulent	500 or more, mostly polymorphonuclears.
Pneumococcic meningitis	Increased	Purulent	500 or more, mostly polymorphonuclears.
Esch. coli meningitis	Increased	Purulent	500 or more, mostly polymorphonuclears.
Torula meningitis	Normal or increased	Cloudy	Polymorphonuclears and lymphocytes increased.
Lymphocytic choriomeningitis	Increased or normal	Clear to cloudy	500, but varies; almost all lymphocytes
Acute syphilitic meningitis	Normal or increased	Clear to turbid	25 or more; mostly lymphocytes.
Dementia paralytica	Normal or increased	Clear	15 or more, mostly lymphocytes.
Poliomyelitis	Usually normal	Clear	10 to 1,000: late, mostly lymphocytes.
Von Economo's encephalitis	Normal or increased	Clear	0 to 100 lymphocytes.
Arthropod-borne (St. Louis & equine) encephalitis	Increased	Clear or turbid	10 to 2,000; early, polymorphonuclears; later, lymphocytes.
Mumps meningo-encephalitis	Normal or increased	Clear to slightly cloudy	Up to 2,000, mostly lymphocytes.
Rabies	Normal or increased	Clear	Normal or slightly increased.
Postinfectious encephalitis	Normal or increased	Clear	0 to 100 lymphocytes.
Meningomyeloradiculitis (Guillain-Barré syndrome)	Normal or increased	Clear or turbid	Normal.
Lead encephalopathy	Increased	Clear or slightly xanthochromic	Increased; mostly lymphocytes.
Cerebral thrombosis	Normal or increased	Clear	Usually normal.
Cerebral hemorrhage	Usually increased	Xanthochromic or bloody	Red cells predominate.
Brain tumor	Often increased	Clear; occas. xanthochromic	Usually normal.
Cord tumor	Normal or low	Clear; may be xanthochromic	Normal; may be slightly increased.

IN HEALTH AND DISEASE

Protein	Sugar	Miscellaneous
15 to 45 mg./100 cc. Pandy −	40 to 60 mg./100 cc.	Spinal fluid sugar level varies with blood sugar level.
Normal Pandy −	Normal	Spinal fluid essentially normal. No pathogenic organisms present.
Increased Pandy +	Decreased or absent	Gram-neg. intra- and extracellular cocci; only intracell. diagnostic.
Increased Pandy +	Decreased	Cultures and guinea pig inoculation +. Delicate web forms on standing. Acid-fast bacilli in stained sediment.
Increased Pandy +	Decreased or absent	Stained smear: gram-neg. pleomorphic rods, often short, cocci-like.
Increased Pandy +	Decreased or absent	Stained smear contains gram-pos. lancet-shaped cocci in pairs.
Increased Pandy +	Decreased or absent	A disease of infants. Stained smear reveals gram-neg. rods.
Increased Pandy +	Decreased	Positive culture on Sabouraud's media. Budding yeasts seen on smear of spinal fluid sediment.
Slightly increased Pandy + or −	Normal	Cultures negative.
Increased Pandy +	Normal	Wassermann + (in 85%±). Colloidal gold: first or midzone.
Increased Pandy +	Normal	Wassermann +; colloidal gold, first zone reaction.
Normal or increased Pandy + or −	Normal	Cultures negative
Slightly increased Pandy +	Normal	
Increased Pandy +	Normal	Serum complement fixation and virus neutralizing tests are positive for this specific type.
Usually increased Pandy + or −	Normal	Lymphocytes found if cells are present. Colloidal gold: midzone.
Normal or slightly increased	Normal	
Normal or slightly increased Pandy +	Normal	
Greatly increased (above 300 mg./100 cc.) Pandy +	Normal	Albumino-cytologic dissociation is diagnostic.
Increased. May be very high. Pandy + or −	Normal	Lead is present (also in urine).
Normal or slightly increased	Normal	
Usually increased Pandy + or −	Normal	Xanthochromia increases for first few days and decreases thereafter.
Increased Pandy +	Normal	
Increased Pandy +	Normal	May clot spontaneously. Block may be confirmed by combined lumbar and cisternal puncture, and by Queckenstedt test.

serious sequelae. Children may show behavior disturbances or mental retardation. Adolescents and adults often develop the Parkinson syndrome. Among the wide variety of sequelae are rigidity, tremors, disorders of speech and respiration, blepharospasm, diplopia, oculogyric crises, masklike facies, increased salivation and perspiration, obesity, diabetes insipidus, narcolepsy, and cataplexy. At differing rates, most patients exhibit progressive neurologic involvement.

The postinfectious or demyelinating encephalitides have a fatality rate of 5 to 30%; the majority who survive recover completely. In those with myelitis, recovery is less complete.

In most instances, choriomeningitis and mumps encephalitis have a good prognosis. In other sporadic cases of encephalitis, mortality rates range from 10 to 20%, but recovery usually is complete in survivors.

Prophylaxis

Vaccines have been prepared for active immunization against St. Louis encephalitis, Eastern and Western equine encephalomyelitis, and Japanese B encephalitis, but are not commercially available. The actual protective value of vaccines in man is not known.

Treatment

There is no specific treatment. Convalescent serums may be used but there is no evidence of benefit; the same can be said of a herpes rabbit vaccine for von Economo's encephalitis. Rest in bed in a quiet environment and good nursing care are essential during the acute stage. Careful attention to bowel and bladder function is important. Urethral catheterization may be necessary. Patients should be turned frequently from side to side to prevent decubitus ulcers. Stuporous patients may require parenteral or tube feeding with liquid nutrients until they are able to eat. A respirator may be necessary if the respiratory mechanism is impaired.

Carefully performed lumbar punctures to relieve increased intracranial pressure are considered valuable. Stuporous or comatose patients should receive penicillin (℞ 52, 53) prophylactically against pneumonia.

For hyperpyrexia and restlessness, tepid baths, alcohol sponges, and an ice cap are useful. Disturbed insomnic or delirious patients may be given paraldehyde (℞ 15), Sodium Amytal (℞ 18), chloral hydrate (℞ 14), or phenobarbital (℞ 13). For rigidity, tremors, and spasm, scopolamine (℞ 26) is of value. Narcolepsy is effectively controlled with amphetamine (℞ 63).

Prolonged convalescence is essential; patients should not return to work for several months after apparent recovery. (For treatment of the postencephalitic Parkinson syndrome, see PARALYSIS AGITANS.)

MENINGITIS

An acute inflammation of the meninges of the brain or spinal cord, or both.

General Considerations

The disease may be caused by viruses, bacteria, protozoa, yeasts, or fungi, which usually are introduced into the meninges from foci elsewhere in the body. It is a complication especially to be feared in cases of otitis media, mastoiditis, and ruptured brain abscess. Infections of the sinuses, tonsils, and orbit also may spread by extension to the meninges. Generalized infections may attack the meninges, or the pathogens may be carried by the blood stream from foci in the lungs, heart valves, bones, or even the skin, to metastasize in the brain or meninges.

Bacterial meningitis, with the exception of that caused by tubercle bacilli, usually is characterized by a purulent exudate which may cover the entire brain and cord. Dilatation of the ventricles and flattening of the convolutions frequently occur, and the infection may extend into the ventricles. Late in the course of the disease, especially in staphylococcal and pneumococcal infections, adhesions may form and obstruct the flow of cerebrospinal fluid. An obstructive internal hydrocephalus may be present. The meninges and perivascular spaces of the cortex are diffusely infiltrated with leukocytes, mostly polymorphonuclears, and often contain large numbers of bacteria.

Meningitis should be suspected in the presence of fever with severe headache accompanied by pain and stiffness in the neck and back, and positive Kernig's and Brudzinski's signs. Changes in the sensorium and in emotional response are first noted. These range from subtle alterations in behavior or slight irritability at the beginning of tuberculous meningitis to the deep coma of established purulent meningitis. An elevated leukocyte count is present in purulent cases.

Diagnostic Procedures in the Meningitides

Lumbar or other puncture: Although the combination of signs and symptoms pointing to meningeal infection and indicating the need for examination of the spinal fluid usually is fairly clear, lumbar puncture should not be done until examination of the optic fundi has been made and the presence of papilledema ruled out. Cisternal or ventricular puncture is the preferred procedure in the presence of papilledema. Fluid obtained by lumbar, cisternal, or ventricular puncture should be subjected to gross inspection, cell count (including type of cell), Pandy test, quantitative spinal fluid protein determination, quantitative sugar determination, culture in nutrient broth and on blood agar plates (one of which is incubated under decreased O_2 tension), and to examination of the stained smear of centrifuged sediment. Manometric pressure determination should be done in the course of obtaining the spinal fluid. Specific etiologic diagnosis may have to await the results of culture, but information obtainable from immediate clinical observation and examination of the fluid usually allows a relatively early tentative diagnosis (*see* table, p. 986).

A clear spinal fluid under increased pressure and containing fewer than 100 cells/cu. mm. practically rules out all forms of bacterial meningitis except tuberculous. Finding a normal sugar content is strong evidence against any form of bacterial meningitis and leaves the signs of meningeal irritation to be explained on another basis, e.g., meningismus, brain tumor, brain abscess without meningeal infection, lead poisoning, syphilis, mumps meningoencephalitis, or subdural hematoma.

If the spinal fluid is opalescent, showing lymphocytes predominantly, and with reduced sugar content, tuberculous meningitis is suggested. In meningococcic infection such findings might appear for a few hours early in the disease, but the case history should be helpful in differentiation. If the spinal fluid is essentially unchanged 6 to 12 hours later, meningococcic infection is unlikely. (Chest X-ray and tuberculin test aid in diagnosis when positive, but are of little significance when negative.) Poliomyelitis or, more exactly, polioencephalitis, may produce a spinal fluid difficult to distinguish from that of tuberculous meningitis, but the normal or elevated sugar in the former and its reduction in the latter is indicative. Also, the sensorium of the tuberculous meningitis patient is clouded; that of the poliomyelitis patient, clear. Lymphocytic choriomeningitis may yield a fluid suggesting tuberculous meningitis, but the onset is much more rapid and the cerebrospinal fluid sugar is normal.

If the fluid is frankly purulent but organisms cannot be found on smear, appropriate treatment should be started and the fluid cultured. If organisms are found, their appearance and staining qualities will be diagnostic.

Smears: If the spinal fluid is frankly purulent it may be smeared directly onto clean slides, spread evenly, and the films air-dried. Gentle heating will fix the film. One film may be stained with methylene blue, and one by Gram's method (*see* Lab. Proc.). Organisms may be numerous, or scarce and difficult to find. In tuberculous meningitis, organisms are never abundant in the spinal fluid. They may be identified in the sediment obtained from prolonged centrifugation of 5 cc. or more of fluid, or by examination of the filmy web (pellicle) which often forms when tuberculous spinal fluid stands 12 to 24 hours undisturbed. If tubercle bacilli are suspected, Ziehl-Neelsen's method of staining for acid-fast bacteria should be used (*see* Lab. Proc.). The meningococcus is gram-negative, which distinguishes it from the other three coccal organisms that commonly cause meningitis, and it has the further distinction of being the only one of these found inside pus ˙cells.

H. influenzae is characterized by pleomorphic forms, some of which are so small as to resemble cocci. It is gram-negative and unlikely to be found inside pus cells. If *H. influenzae* is abundant in the spinal fluid, it is sometimes possible to mix a drop of the fluid directly with a drop of *H. influenzae* type B antiserum and observe the diagnostic swelling of the capsule surrounding the organisms. Ordinarily, the spinal fluid will contain so few organisms that the test for capsular swelling will have to await culture of the organism.

Spinal fluid culture: Tubercle bacilli are so slow of growth on laboratory media (Petroff's) or in inoculated guinea pigs that prior to the advent of streptomycin therapy these means of culture rarely revealed the diagnosis while the patient still was alive. Because growth on Dubos' medium is so much more rapid than on previous media, diagnosis now can be made more quickly. Meningococci will grow only on blood-enriched media, and most readily in an atmosphere of reduced O_2 tension. (This latter may be achieved by placing the inoculated petri dish and a lighted candle or a ball of burning cotton in a jar with an airtight top. While the flame is burning, the top is quickly secured in place. Burning continues for a few seconds—long enough to replace some of the O_2 with CO_2.) Such cultures may be removed for examination at 24 hours and replaced, if no growth has occurred, for another 24 to 48 hours. Spinal fluid should always be inoculated into previously warmed nutrient broth or onto prewarmed blood agar plates as soon as possible after it is obtained (directly from the spinal needle, if possible). Meningococci are not very hardy and therefore great care must be taken in culturing them.

Blood culture: In cases of suspected meningitis, and particularly in purulent meningitis, blood cultures should be taken. It is true that a positive blood culture seldom alters the treatment except to intensify it, but the known presence of bacteremia puts the physician on the alert for possible septic complications other than the meningitis.

MENINGOCOCCAL MENINGITIS

(Cerebrospinal fever, Epidemic meningitis, Spotted fever)

Meningococcal meningitis is due to infection of the meninges with *Neisseria intracellularis* and is the most common purulent meningitis. Four types of this organism may cause the disease in man. Until recent years, this form of meningitis has occurred irregularly in major epidemics in densely populated areas, especially during the winter and spring. It is spread by droplet spray from the nose and mouth of carriers, who may be persons apparently healthy or who have a mild upper respiratory meningococcal infection but have not yet developed meningitis. Carriers may be present in urban areas even where no clinical cases of meningitis exist, and during epidemics they may include 10 to 30% of the population.

Meningococcal meningitis is preceded by a stage of meningococcemia although this may not be clinically evident. On the other hand, meningococcemia of a highly fulminating type may be rapidly fatal with little or no evidence of meningitis. In such cases, autopsy often reveals hemorrhages in the adrenal cortex (Waterhouse-Friderichsen syndrome).

All pathologic changes significant of meningococcal meningitis are confined to the C.N.S. and consist of an intense purulent meningeal inflammation. At autopsy, the brain is swollen and covered, particularly at the base, with a purulent exudate. There is intense congestion and noticeable flattening of the gyri due to increased intracranial pressure. If the patient survives a severe attack, internal hydrocephalus may develop as a result of obliteration of the subarachnoid space by the infection. Deafness and less frequently other evidences of cranial nerve damage may follow.

Symptoms, Signs, and Diagnosis

The disease is ushered in by severe headache, projectile vomiting, high fever, and rapidly developing confusion, delirium, and coma. Neck and back rigidity become pronounced, and convulsive twitchings or frank convulsions are frequent. In severe cases, an extensive purpura may precede the meningitic symptoms by several hours as a result of profound meningococcal bacteremia. The small irregular spots, which give rise to the name "spotted fever" contain meningococci and should be aspirated (with a 24- or 25-gauge needle and a tuberculin syringe) for microscopic examination and culture. Cases of meningococcemia may display high fever, prostration, hemorrhagic phenomena and little or no evidence of meningeal irritation.

In small infants, the manifestations of mild meningeal infection may be masked for several days, the symptoms suggesting upper respiratory infection or perhaps pyelitis. It is important that any infant with fever, high leukocyte count, and noticeable changes of behavior, without definite signs of disease elsewhere, should have a lumbar puncture (see CLIN. PROC.).

Principles to be observed in diagnosing this or other forms of meningitis are described under Diag. Proc. in the Meningitides (above).

Prophylaxis

During epidemics the incidence of the disease and the carrier rate may both be greatly reduced by oral administration of 2 or 3 Gm. of sulfadiazine a day for 2 or 3 days (℞ 56).

Treatment

General: Supportive care is the same as for any other serious infectious disease, and includes adequate fluids, nourishing diet, sedation, and special nursing care. If vomiting occurs, I.V. injections of physiologic saline and 5% solution of dextrose are indicated. A daily urine output of 1,000 to 1,500 cc. should be maintained while the patient is under chemotherapy. Sedation should be minimal but adequate to ensure sufficient rest (R 13, 15, 16, 24). Analgesics (R 1, 2) may be used for headache but morphine (R 5) should be prescribed only if absolutely necessary and then in minimal dose. Adrenal cortical extract (R 62) has been recommended for use in cases that exhibit severe shock resulting from extensive hemorrhage into the adrenal cortex (Waterhouse-Friderichsen syndrome). Catheterization, cathartics and enemas may be necessary during the early stages. Diet should be dictated by the patient's tolerance but should be increased as rapidly as possible.

Chemotherapy: The sulfonamides are specific against the meningococcus, and of these sulfadiazine is the drug of choice because of its low toxicity and proved effectiveness. Adequate treatment usually results in great improvement within 48 hours. The initial dose should preferably be given parenterally (R 57) to ensure a prompt bacteriostatic concentration in the blood. The subcut. or I.V. route may be used, but the former is simpler and less dangerous. As an initial dose sodium sulfadiazine 30 to 60 mg. (gr. ss to i)/Kg. of body wt. may be given I.V. as a 5% solution. Oral sulfonamide medication (R 56) may be begun as soon as tolerated, but if not retained, parenteral therapy may be resumed, giving the same total amount daily in 2 or 3 equally divided doses at 8- or 12-hour intervals. Sulfadiazine blood levels should be determined frequently, at least every 24 hours, during the early stages, to ensure adequate dosage and to guard against overdosage. Levels of 10 to 15 mg./100 cc. are necessary, but concentrations exceeding these levels may produce complications. When oral sulfadiazine is tolerated, the total daily dose is given in equally divided amounts at 4-hour intervals. Maintenance of an alkaline urine to prevent precipitation of acetylsulfadiazine in the urinary tract is advisable (see SULFONAMIDE THERAPY). Sulfonamide therapy should be continued for 2 to 5 days after complete clinical recovery. Penicillin should be used for those patients who are sensitive to sulfonamides or who fail to respond to them, and in cases of overwhelming infection, such as meningococcemia. The suggested dosage is 30,000 to 100,000 u. every 3 hours I.M. (R 53), and, when indicated, intrathecally in doses of 10,000 u. daily for 1 or 2 days. Lumbar puncture should be done for the relief of increased intracranial pressure, or when there is no response to treatment, or on the appearance of a relapse, and always as a final check before the patient is discharged. The period of convalescence is generally about a month for complete recovery but may be longer in the severe cases.

TUBERCULOUS MENINGITIS

This is the most common form of meningitis except during epidemics of meningococcal meningitis. It is invariably associated with tuberculous infection (gross or microscopic) elsewhere in the body, and has its greatest incidence in children between the ages of 1 and 5 years. In the child, the initial symptoms are irritability, drowsiness, constipation, anorexia, vomiting, and slight fever. As the disease advances the fever increases, drowsiness deepens to stupor, and convulsions occur as the intracranial pressure mounts. In older patients, change in behavior and complaints of headache are prominent (*see* Diag. Proc. in the Meningitides, above). The discovery of choroid tubercles during ocular fundal examination is of great diagnostic significance. While a positive chest X-ray or tuberculin test gives important confirmation of the etiology, negative findings cannot be relied upon to rule out tuberculosis.

Treatment

The primary tuberculous focus should be identified, and treated at the same time as the meningitis. Streptomycin (℞ 54) (or dihydrostreptomycin) I.M. is indicated in an average daily dosage of 2 Gm. I.M. every 4 to 6 hours, each dose not larger than 0.5 Gm. Therapy must be continued for 4 to 6 months if indicated. It is recommended that 25 to 50 mg. of streptomycin (not dihydrostreptomycin) in 10 cc. of Water for Injection U.S.P., spinal fluid or normal saline be given intrathecally, over a period of 10 minutes after a slightly greater amount of spinal fluid has been withdrawn. Administer this daily or every other day for 2 to 6 weeks in addition. Both promizole and para-aminosalicylic acid combined with streptomycin have been tried with some favorable results; further observation is necessary before the value of this type of therapy can be determined. Supportive treatment includes gavage feedings, sedation as needed for convulsions, and repeated lumbar puncture to relieve intracranial pressure (*see* CLIN. PROC.).

INFLUENZAL MENINGITIS

Only the type B strain of *H. influenzae* is a common cause of meningitis in man. Nothing about the onset of influenzal meningitis clearly sets it off from other purulent meningitides. It is most frequent in infants and children in whom it often exists for several days as an apparent respiratory infection; however, the presence of irritability, unexplained elevation of temperature, and elevated leukocyte count should suggest the possibility of meningitis. Some nuchal rigidity is usual but a lumbar puncture should be done in all doubtful cases (*see* Diag. Proc. in the Meningitides, above). Occasionally, onset is stormy, with high fever, delirium, and convulsions.

A presumptive diagnosis of *H. influenzae* meningitis can be made when gram-negative pleomorphic rods are found in smears of the spinal fluid. The spinal fluid may be centrifuged (about 2,500 r.p.m.) for 15 to 20 minutes, if organisms are hard to find, in order to obtain enough for the capsular swelling test. A positive test is highly important, since the immediate administration of specific antiserum may make the difference between uncomplicated recovery and permanent C.N.S. damage or death. If typing cannot be done directly, the spinal fluid should be cultured in broth and on blood agar plates and typing again attempted as soon as colonies are noted— usually 12 to 24 hours.

Treatment

A combination of 3 agents—specific antiserum, streptomycin, and sulfadiazine—gives the best results, although recovery sometimes can be effected with any one of these. An immediate dose of sodium sulfadiazine (℞ 57), 30 mg. (gr. ss)/lb. body wt., and not exceeding 3 Gm., should be given parenterally, followed by oral sulfadiazine (℞ 56). Measures to relieve dehydration and alkalinize the urine also should be started promptly (see SULFONAMIDE THERAPY). Specific antiserum (rabbit) (℞ 58) must be given at the earliest possible moment. The dose is calculated on the basis of spinal fluid sugar levels (the more severe the infection the greater the depletion of spinal fluid sugar; see table, p. 986). Antiserum, whose potency is expressed in terms of precipitable antibody nitrogen, is supplied in vials containing 25 mg. of such nitrogen. It is suggested that patients having over 40 mg. of sugar/100 cc. in the spinal fluid receive one vial of antiserum I.M. (after skin test reveals nonsensitivity to rabbit serum); those with 40 to 25 mg./100 cc., 2 vials; those with 25 to 15 mg., 3 vials; and with less than 15 mg., 4 vials. On the day following administration of serum one should obtain some of the patient's serum in order to test whether it contains enough antibody to cause swelling of the *H. influenzae* capsule. The serum doses suggested are for initial administration; additional serum may be given 48 hours later if the patient's condition is not improved. Streptomycin (℞ 54) in average doses of 2 Gm. daily I.M., in divided doses, and, depending on age, 25 to 50 mg. intrathecally, should be given for 10 days. Recent reports indicate that intrathecal therapy may be unnecessary. If sulfadiazine (℞ 56) cannot be given by mouth, injections (℞ 57) should be made every 8 hours so that the total daily dose is 60 mg. (gr. i)/Kg. of body wt. Sufficient glucose solution (5 or 10% in distilled water) should be given to relieve dehydration and ensure normal urinary flow. Sodium bicarbonate by mouth, 6 to 15 Gm., may be given daily to ensure alkalinity of the urine (see SULFONAMIDE THERAPY).

The patient may be remarkably improved after several days' treatment but relapses are almost certain to occur if treatment is stopped too soon. To forestall any relapse, streptomycin should be administered for a minimum of 10 days, and sulfadiazine for at least 3 weeks, after which sulfadiazine may be continued in reduced dose, depending on the patient's condition, for 2 to 3 months.

ESCHERICHIA COLI MENINGITIS

Purulent meningitis due to Esch. coli, *or to* Salmonella *organisms, and rarely encountered except in newborn or young infants* (see Diag. Proc. in the Meningitides, above).

Treatment

As a rule, the prognosis is good if treatment is started promptly. In purulent meningitis of the newborn it is advisable to start treatment at once with sulfadiazine (℞ 56, 57), 60 mg. (gr. i)/lb./day in divided doses, and penicillin (℞ 53) 30,000 to 50,000 u. I.M. every 3 hours. If cultures reveal *Esch. coli* or *Salmonella*, penicillin should be stopped in favor of streptomycin (℞ 54) given by combined I.M. and intrathecal routes. Streptomycin should be continued for a minimum of 10 days or until spinal fluid cultures have been negative for several successive days. Sulfadiazine (℞ 56, 57) should be given simultaneously with streptomycin throughout the illness and should probably be continued in reduced dosage for at least 1 or 2 weeks after apparent recovery. Blood transfusions also are a definite part of the treatment of *Esch. coli* meningitis, not only as supportive therapy, but also because transfused blood is thought to convey some specific antibodies (found in blood of adults but not in that of newborn infants). General care and feeding of infant patients consists of parenteral fluids including glucose solution and amino acids solution if vomiting prevents feeding by mouth. Often, the infant will eat fairly well throughout the disease; if not, gavage may be resorted to, in the absence of vomiting.

PNEUMOCOCCAL MENINGITIS

A purulent meningitis caused by the pneumococcus and especially common in infants and young children. It usually follows pneumococcal infection of the paranasal sinuses, middle ear, throat, or lungs, or a skull fracture. Diagnosis is made by finding the lancet-shaped gram-positive coccal form (usually in pairs) in spinal fluid smears and is confirmed by culture of the organism and typing with type-specific antipneumococcal serum (see Diag. Proc. in the Meningitides, above).

Treatment

Therapy consists of sulfadiazine (℞ 56, 57) and penicillin (℞ 53) in full dosage plus blood transfusion. Whether to give penicillin intrathecally is not settled but many feel that following spinal drainage, up to 10,000 u. in 5 or 10 cc. of normal saline should be injected. This undoubtedly provokes some additional meningeal reaction but probably is worth while and justifiable. Supportive treatment consists of parenteral fluids and gavage feeding and usually is necessary for part of the course of the disease. Penicillin and sulfadiazine (in reduced dose) should be continued for a minimum of 2 weeks after apparent recovery. Relapse and subsequent chronic meningitis occur not infrequently.

STREPTOCOCCAL MENINGITIS

An uncommon form of meningitis usually due to a primary streptococcus infection in the sinuses, mastoids, or upper respiratory tract. The cord stump in newborn infants, or breaks in the mother's skin in the genital or breast area, often provide entrance to streptococci with resultant septicemia and meningitis (*see* Diag. Prog. in the Meningitides, above).

Treatment

Streptococcal meningitis responds well to sulfadiazine (℞ 56, 57) and penicillin (℞ 53) when treatment is started early. Both should be continued until recovery and for at least a week thereafter. Eradication of any foci elsewhere is of course indicated. Blood transfusion is given in all cases along with other supportive treatment. Gavage feedings usually are necessary for a few days. If response to therapy is slow, intrathecal injection up to 10,000 u. of penicillin in 5 to 10 cc. normal saline may be given daily.

STAPHYLOCOCCAL MENINGITIS

Formerly, staphylococcal meningitis was almost always fatal. It was not uncommon in the newborn as a sequel to staphylococcal infection (e.g., furuncle, bacteremia). Recoveries now are reported with increasing frequency. The prognosis is fair provided the diagnosis is made early and vigorous sulfadiazine (℞ 56, 57) and penicillin (℞ 53) therapy begun at once.

ACUTE SYPHILITIC MENINGITIS

A relatively rare type of meningitis, generally occurring in young adults as a result of a primary infection with T. pallidum; *or as a complication of congenital syphilis.* Symptoms of meningitis usually develop within 1 or 2 years of the primary infection but may appear at any time or may complicate parenchymatous neurosyphilis. Its incidence is increased at least tenfold by inadequate treatment of early, but not of late, syphilis.

Symptoms, Signs, and Diagnosis

Onset may be acute or subacute, and symptoms usually are present for 2 to 4 weeks before the patient seeks medical aid. Clinically, the disease manifests itself in 3 forms: (1) Acute syphilitic hydrocephalus characterized by headache, nausea and vomiting, choked disks, and signs indicating involvement of the meninges of the posterior fossa. (2) Acute vertical menin-

gitis with headache, nausea and vomiting, and convulsions or
mental symptoms indicating involvement of the meninges over
the vertex.   (3) Acute basilar meningitis with cranial nerve
palsies indicating involvement of the meninges of the base of
the brain.

The blood serology is positive in more than half the cases.
Cerebrospinal fluid pressure is increased; 25 to 2,000 cells may
be present, with polymorphonuclear forms composing 5 to 15%;
protein content elevation reaches 50 to 200 mg./100 cc. and the
sugar and chloride may be normal or decreased (see table, p.
986).   The colloidal gold curve usually is of a midzone or 1st
zone type.   The cerebrospinal fluid Wassermann is positive in
about 85% of·cases.   Spirochetes have been found in the fluid
(see also Diag. Proc. in the Meningitides, above).

Treatment

A total dosage of at least 9.6 million u. of penicillin (℞ 53)
should be given I.M. in divided doses at 3-hour intervals over
a period of 12 days.   The results generally are dramatic, with
clearing of signs and symptoms in a few days.   Rarely are there
residuals.   Prior to the proved effectiveness of penicillin the
arsenicals were used with good results.

BENIGN LYMPHOCYTIC CHORIOMENINGITIS

*An acute, grippelike virus C.N.S. disease which may result
from direct or indirect contact with mice harboring the virus.*
Apparently it can also be transmitted from dogs to human
beings by blood-sucking insects.   Transmission from man to
man is unknown.

Symptoms, Signs, and Diagnosis

Fever, malaise, headache, generalized aches and pains, drowsiness, nausea, vomiting, stiff neck, Kernig's sign, bradycardia,
and changes in the deep tendon reflexes occur 15 to 20 days after
exposure.   Cough and pharyngitis may be present.   Spinal fluid
examination reveals increased pressure, slightly elevated protein, normal sugar, and 100 to 1,500 cells/cu. mm., mostly lymphocytes (see Diag. Proc. in the Meningitides, above).   Meningeal symptoms usually last about a week.

Prognosis and Treatment

Most patients recover completely.   Treatment is entirely
symptomatic.

MISCELLANEOUS FORMS OF MENINGITIS

Numerous other organisms occasionally may be responsible
for meningeal infection.   When due to gram-negative bacilli,
such as Friedländer's bacillus, or *B. pyocyaneus*, streptomycin
(℞ 54) parenterally and intrathecally is the treatment of
choice, although sulfadiazine (℞ 56, 57) may at times be effec-

tive. Aureomycin (℞ 55), 25 to 50 mg./Kg. body wt. daily in divided doses, may be used with benefit in Friedländer's bacillus infection (*see* ANTIBIOTIC THERAPY). Actinomyces (*see* SYSTEMIC FUNGUS INFECTIONS) may invade the C.N.S. and should be treated vigorously with sulfadiazine (℞ 56, 57) and penicillin (℞ 53). *Torula histolytica* has a predilection for the brain and meninges, but as yet there is no specific therapy for this infection. Viral meningoencephalitides (*see* ENCEPHALITIS) may be due to such conditions as mumps, infectious mononucleosis, herpetic infections, poliomyelitis, and lymphogranuloma venereum.

Cocci, other than those mentioned previously, e.g., the gonococcus and *Micrococcus tetragenus,* are rare causes of meningitis and call for the use of penicillin or sulfadiazine or both. Therapy of the unusual forms of the disease is not as a rule entirely successful.

MENINGISMUS
(Meningism)

A complex of meningeal symptoms often encountered at the onset of acute febrile disorders, especially in children. Mumps, measles, acute upper respiratory infections, pneumonia, sinusitis, otitis media, and bacillary dysentery are the most common diseases in which it has been observed. In most instances, onset is abrupt and is preceded by high fever and prostration. The symptoms and signs are similar to those of meningitis, including severe headache, stiffness of the neck and back, positive Kernig's sign, and vomiting. Convulsions and coma also may occur. These symptoms appear singly or in combination. Lumbar puncture is necessary for differentiation from meningitis. In meningismus the cerebrospinal fluid pressure usually is elevated, the fluid is clear, colorless, and the cell content usually normal. Occasionally, there may be a mild pleocytosis (10 to 50 cells/cu. mm.) and a moderately increased protein content (*see* table, p. 986).

Treatment

Measures for control of the causal disease should be instituted. The diagnostic spinal puncture of itself often relieves the meningeal symptoms in 3 to 24 hours. Fluids (glucose and electrolytes) should be given in large quantities, parenterally if not tolerated orally. In the presence of vomiting, severe illness, or coma, oral therapy is not feasible. Sedation with paraldehyde (℞ 15) or barbiturates (℞ 13, 16, 24) is often helpful in the acute stage. Sponging the entire body with 35% alcohol or tepid water may allay restlessness by reducing fever. Acetylsalicylic acid (℞ 1) is useful in relieving headache and

general discomfort and in reducing high fever. An ice bag
applied to the head also is helpful.

POLIOMYELITIS

(Infantile paralysis, Acute anterior poliomyelitis)

*An acute viral infection which attacks the C.N.S. and some-
times results in flaccid paralysis of various muscle groups.* It
occurs both as an endemic and epidemic summer disease.
Children are more susceptible than adults.

Etiology and Epidemiology

The causative agent is one of the smallest and sturdiest of
the filtrable viruses, estimated to be 10 to 15 millimicrons in size.
It is a stable virus and remains viable in aqueous suspensions
of human feces kept at ice-box temperatures for months. In
infected spinal cord preserved in 50% glycerin it has remained
active for years. Strong oxidizing agents such as potassium permanganate and hydrogen peroxide, heating at temperatures of
55° to 65° C. for a short period of time, and ultraviolet radiation destroy the virus, but it can withstand concentrations of
chlorine that kill enteric bacteria in water.

The natural mode of transmission is unknown. The virus
is thought to enter the body by way of the upper gastrointestinal tract (including the oral cavity and pharynx). In fatal
cases it is found chiefly in the C.N.S. and in the walls of the
upper intestinal tract. It is known to be present in the pharynx
just before onset of the disease and during the week following
onset, and it is excreted in the feces for 4 to 6 weeks or more
after an acute attack. Healthy human carriers are frequently
discovered during epidemics.

There are several theories as to how the virus is disseminated
throughout a community. These include spread by direct
human contact, or contact with contaminated objects, including
food. During an epidemic the virus has been isolated from
sewage, flies, and fly-contaminated food.

Contrary to earlier teachings, multiple cases within families
are common, although usually not more than one member of a
family becomes paralyzed. In contrast to other infections,
severe forms of the disease tend to occur in robust and well
nourished children as well as in less fortunate ones. Recent
tonsillectomy is a predisposing factor in bulbar poliomyelitis.
There is some evidence that severe exercise may precipitate the
paralytic disease in individuals who might otherwise have remained healthy carriers.

Pathology

The characteristic lesions of poliomyelitis are found in the
gray matter of the spinal cord, in the motor cortex, the

vestibular nuclei, and the cerebellar centers. In the cord, the ganglion cells in the anterior horns at the cervical and lumbar levels are most frequently attacked. Widespread damage at these levels is responsible for paralysis of the extremities. The lesions in all parts of the C.N.S. consist of destruction of neurons, neuronophagia, and perivascular and interstitial round cell infiltration. Although the virus probably is not so neurotropic as was once thought, demonstrable lesions in other parts of the body are scanty. Nevertheless, lymph node hyperplasia is common.

Symptoms and Signs

The clinical forms are extremely varied. Cases are usually classified as "abortive," nonparalytic, and paralytic. In the abortive type (which is estimated to account for 80 to 90% of cases) the illness may be so mild as to go unnoticed. In many abortive cases, however, there is a sudden onset of fever, malaise, headache, sore throat, and sometimes vomiting. The physical examination and spinal fluid are negative and there is no clinical indication of C.N.S. involvement. The symptoms disappear after 24 to 72 hours and the patient remains well. Paralytic cases in which there is a "dromedary" or diphasic course often have a similar onset, i.e., a brief, mild, nonspecific illness of short duration, followed by apparent recovery. But in these cases there is a recurrence of fever and headache after 4 to 7 or more days, accompanied by signs of C.N.S. involvement—restlessness, stiff back, stiff neck, spasm of the hamstrings and various other muscles, muscle pain, loss of reflexes, muscle weakness, and paralysis. In nonparalytic cases the signs stop short of actual muscle weakness, although muscle spasm may be prominent. Only about half the cases with C.N.S. signs have such a diphasic course. In the others, the disease begins with "second phase" signs, and muscle spasm and paralysis may develop rapidly. The site of paralysis depends on the location of lesions in the spinal cord or medulla. If the cranial nerve nuclei are involved, the bulbar form of the disease develops and paralysis of the pharyngeal, laryngeal, facial, and other muscles innervated by cranial nerves may occur. Difficulty in swallowing, nasal regurgitation, and nasal voice are common early signs of bulbar poliomyelitis. The spinal fluid during the second phase usually shows an increased cell count (largely lymphocytes) and increased protein. Average cell counts range from 25 to 150, and protein levels from 60 to 100 mg./100 cc. However, any cell count over 8 to 10 or protein over 45 mg. is considered abnormal. The blood count during the early acute stage may remain normal, or may show a moderate leukocytosis (10,000 to 14,000) with 30 to 55% lymphocytes.

Diagnosis

Diagnosis of the full-blown paralytic case is relatively easy, especially during an epidemic of poliomyelitis. The characteristic history and the physical findings of stiff neck and back, reflex changes, and paralysis (or bulbar signs), together with an abnormal spinal fluid, usually leave little doubt. In mild nonparalytic and abortive forms, and in the preparalytic stage, the problem is more difficult. Here, epidemiological features—the summer season and the presence of an epidemic—are of considerable importance. Any child with fever who complains of headache, vomiting, sore neck or back, or muscle tenderness, should be suspected of having poliomyelitis. He must be observed carefully, for there is no way of knowing which cases will remain mild and which will go on to severe paralytic disease. Positive spinal fluid findings are helpful but not essential to diagnosis, since the spinal fluid is normal in abortive cases during the acute illness, and may remain normal in nonparalytic and sometimes even in fatal paralytic cases.

In the differential diagnosis, the arthropod-borne encephalitides—equine and St. Louis encephalomyelitis (q.v.)—are important in areas where these diseases flourish. It may be impossible clinically to distinguish between them and poliomyelitis, but specific serologic reactions will establish the diagnosis of encephalitis. Mumps meningoencephalitis, which may occur in the absence of parotitis, and lymphocytic choriomeningitis may closely resemble nonparalytic poliomyelitis. Since these diseases tend to occur in the winter, they offer diagnostic problems chiefly in connection with isolated interepidemic cases of poliomyelitis. Both mumps meningitis and lymphocytic choriomeningitis, unlike poliomyelitis, can eventually be diagnosed by serologic means.

In addition, the postexanthem encephalitides, purulent meningitis, and tuberculous meningitis (q.v.) should be kept in mind in differential diagnosis, as well as more remote possibilities such as rheumatic fever and acute osteomyelitis.

Prognosis

In the early stages of poliomyelitis it is impossible to predict the outcome. Extreme restlessness and apprehension seem to indicate a poor prognosis, as do rapidly ascending paralyses which eventually involve the bulbar centers. Although the degree of fever is not related to the severity of paralysis, the duration of fever is of some prognostic significance, for paralysis does not usually progress after fever has subsided.

Recent statistics indicate that less than 25% of patients with the paralytic form of the disease suffer severe permanent disability from poliomyelitis. About 25% have mild disabilities, and over 50% recover with no residual paralyses. With changing concepts of diagnosis, particularly the inclusion of nonparalytic cases in any series, there is some difficulty in comparing current statistics with earlier ones. The case mortality rate is 1 to 4%—sometimes as high as 10%. Mortality figures are influenced largely by the number of bulbar cases in a given epidemic. The mortality rate in bulbar poliomyelitis usually is over 50%.

Prophylaxis

Since the manner in which poliomyelitis infection spreads is unknown, there are no clear-cut rules for avoiding it. However, during epidemics the following measures are recommended. Local public health authorities may modify these to suit specific needs of a community.

(1) Patients known to have poliomyelitis, whether in the mild nonparalytic or severely paralytic form, should be isolated. There is no difference in the amount of virus excreted or in the duration of its excretion in mild or severe cases. The period of isolation usually is 3 weeks. (2) Contact with persons suffering from unexplained minor illnesses should be avoided. (3) If excreta are to be disinfected, the disinfectant should be well mixed with the feces and allowed to stand for several hours. Chlorinated lime or 5% cresol may be used. (4) Personal cleanliness should be carefully observed: washing the hands before eating is of particular importance. (5) All elective operative procedures, especially tonsillectomy and tooth extraction, should be postponed until the epidemic is well over. (6) Overexertion and extreme fatigue are to be avoided: violent exercise frequently precedes the onset of paralytic poliomyelitis. (7) Swimming in polluted water should be avoided. (8) Flies must be kept away from food, since they are known to carry the virus of poliomyelitis. (9) High standards of community sanitation, particularly as to water and milk supplies, must be maintained.

Treatment

There is no specific treatment for poliomyelitis. No drug is known which destroys the virus or controls its spread within the body. None of the sulfonamide compounds is efficacious, nor is penicillin or streptomycin. The usefulness of convalescent serum therapy has not been demonstrated, and administration of gamma globulin in the preparalytic stage has proved ineffective. Clinical management of poliomyelitis thus resolves itself into supportive and protective measures during the acute stages and special physical therapy and orthopedic care throughout convalescence. Certain forms of the disease, e.g., bulbar cases and those with respiratory muscle paralysis, require special types of treatment.

As a rule, patients with abortive or mild nonparalytic poliomyelitis need no treatment beyond bed rest and light diet. Rest is important, since there is statistical evidence that undue physical activity in the early period of infection may precipitate paralysis. In a recent study it was observed that severe permanent paralyses occurred in 90% of patients who persisted in their usual physical activities during the first 2 days of preparalytic symptoms. In contrast, mild paralyses persisted in only 15% of patients who were put to bed immediately when symptoms appeared. Bed rest for 7 to 10 days is recommended for all mild cases and for all young patients with suspicious febrile illnesses occurring during poliomyelitis epidemic.

In the early febrile stages of more severe poliomyelitis, symptomatic treatment is similar to that for other acute infectious diseases. Mild analgesics and sedatives may be beneficial (R 1, 2, 24). It is best to hospitalize a patient in whom a definite diagnosis has been established. If the patient is acutely ill and has traveled a long distance to the hospital in hot weather, dehydration and salt depletion are apt to be present. It is important to correct these promptly by parenteral administration of isotonic salt solution.

During the stage of active myelitis, emphasis should be on rest and avoidance of strain or unnecessary procedures. Bed boards beneath the mattress, and a board at the foot of the bed, are recommended to help maintain a favorable position. In the acute stage when fever is high and paralyses are developing, the patient often exhibits restlessness that is not readily controlled by sedatives. At this time he may be allowed to assume any position he finds comfortable. But as early as possible he should be kept in a position best suited to protect his weakened muscles. Here, nursing vigilance is of extreme importance. The immediate application of splints to all paralyzed extremities has been abandoned since the advent of Miss Kenny's teachings. Relief of muscle spasm and pain and protection of weakened muscles are the objectives of early treatment. These are best accomplished by the application, several times a day, of hot, moist packs kept in place for about 20 minutes. Prostigmine, physostigmine, and curare have been used in attempts to relieve muscle spasm, but their value has not been established.

Urinary retention is a frequent complication of paralytic poliomyelitis. It may be treated successfully with parasympathetic stimulating drugs such as Urecholine (R 37) or Doryl (R 38). If drug therapy fails and repeated catheterization becomes necessary, sulfadiazine should be administered as a prophylactic against urinary tract infection (R 56).

Constipation is not uncommon and may be troublesome to control. It usually subsides spontaneously after a week. Strong purgatives are contraindicated but warm saline enemas, or a mild laxative (R 84) may be tried.

Respiratory failure is one of the most serious complications in poliomyelitis. It may be due either to paralysis of the muscles of respiration or to involvement of the respiratory centers in the medulla. In respiratory muscle paralysis, the Drinker respirator may be lifesaving, but patients kept in it for a long time are particularly subject to pneumonia, massive pulmonary collapse, and sudden death. Penicillin (℞ 53) is sometimes given prophylactically against pneumonia.

Respiratory failure due to involvement of vital medullary centers is treated with continuous oxygen inhalation, employing a mixture of humidified 95% O_2 and 5% CO_2. This type of respiratory failure occurs in bulbar poliomyelitis usually along with paralysis of the pharyngeal and laryngeal muscles. Such paralysis adds an obstructive element to the respiratory difficulty: the patient is unable to cough and raise bronchotracheal secretions, which therefore tend to pool. In order to prevent drowning, these secretions must be removed by frequent swabbing out or, better, by the use of a suction apparatus such as is employed with surgical patients. Postural drainage also is effective. Atropine may be useful in diminishing the quantity of secretion (℞ 28, 30).

The Drinker respirator is of little help in bulbar cases with respiratory failure and may even be harmful. The respiratory center is functioning irregularly and the respirator cannot, therefore, be synchronized with the patient's own respirations. Furthermore, the application of negative pressure adds another obstacle to the raising of secretions and may increase the danger of drowning. An artificial respirator and mask, providing intermittent positive-pressure respiration, has been used over periods of 6 to 24 hours with some success. Among the simplest devices is that developed by the Army Air Force, operating from an oxygen tank through a demand valve (e.g., the pneumatic balance resuscitator). This has the advantage that the patient's own respiratory activity takes over the rate and volume of breathing automatically whenever spontaneous respiration occurs. A lightweight plastic respirator now is commercially available, while a device to provide electrical stimulation of the diaphragm has demonstrated its effectiveness in selected cases.

A recently popularized treatment for bulbar poliomyelitis is by tracheotomy and insertion of a tracheal tube as soon as signs of central respiratory failure—such as recurrent cyanosis, pooling of tracheal secretions, or inability to cough—appear. Continuous O_2 (adequately humidified) is given through the tube and the airway is kept free with a suction apparatus. Oxygen concentrations of 40 to 60% are used, although in emergencies it may be necessary to use 100% O_2 for brief periods. If the O_2 is under a positive pressure of 2 to 6 cm. of water, the exchange of gas at the alveoli is increased, and the danger of pulmonary edema (q.v.) is lessened. The effectiveness of O_2 therapy may be followed by means of an oximeter, or by arterial O_2 determinations, and the concentration of O_2 altered accordingly. Penicillin (℞ 53) is given as a prophylactic against pulmonary infection during the acute phase. These procedures seem to have been lifesaving in some instances.

The general care of patients with bulbar poliomyelitis requires special attention to fluid and nutritive requirements. If there is difficulty in swallowing, all fluids and nutriment should be given parenterally. Proctoclysis is a satisfactory way of administering saline. A liquid diet high in calories—protein and carbohydrate—may be given by gavage, but extreme watchfulness is necessary to prevent aspiration following vomiting or regurgitation.

The treatment of paralytic poliomyelitis, in early convalescence and later, requires the combined efforts of orthopedist, pediatrician or internist, physical therapist, and nurse. In early convalescence, as soon as the acute febrile stage is over and pain has subsided, it is essential that everything be done to maintain the blood supply and tonus of affected muscles. This is accomplished by hot packs, massage, passive and active motion, and early reeducation of muscles. Such measures ensure maximum restoration of muscle function and help to preserve weakened limbs in optimal condition for possible late orthopedic surgery.

General care during convalescence should include attention to diet, correction of nutritional anemia if present (R 70), occupational therapy, and understanding and amelioration of the psychological difficulties that beset the handicapped child. The problem of late convalescence in paralyzed individuals requires special orthopedic attention.

MULTIPLE SCLEROSIS

(Disseminated sclerosis, Insular sclerosis, Sclerosis en plaques)

A chronic, slowly progressive disease of the C.N.S. characterized pathologically by disseminated patches of demyelinization in the brain and spinal cord, and clinically by multiple symptoms and signs and by remissions and exacerbations.

Etiology and Incidence

The cause is unknown. The disease has been variously attributed to infection by a spirochete or a virus; toxic factors, such as metallic poisons; metabolic factors, such as a myelin-splitting ferment in the blood; trauma; allergy; and vascular lesions as a result of an abnormality of the clotting mechanism of the blood. The two sexes are about equally affected. In two-thirds of the cases onset of symptoms occurs between the ages of 20 and 40. The disease is rare in warm climates.

Symptoms and Signs

The onset usually is insidious and the disease is characterized by the variety of complaints and findings with remarkable remissions and persistently recurring exacerbations. Occasionally, the onset is sudden; but commonly, minor visual disturbances, a fleeting ocular palsy, transient weakness, slight stiffness or unusual fatigability of a limb, minor interference with walking, vague difficulties with bladder control, occasional dizziness or mild emotional disturbances—all evidence of scattered involvement of the nervous system—occur months or years before the existence of disease is recognized. However, on recognition of a disease process, the most frequent presenting symptoms are paresthesias involving one or more extremities or one side of the face, definite weakness or heaviness of the limbs, or visual disturbances such as partial blindness in one eye, double vision, dimness of vision, or a homonymous field defect.

The well known Charcot's triad—nystagmus, intention tremor and scanning speech—is found late, and is uncommon in the early stages. There are many clinical syndromes, but the three most common are: **Cerebral,** characterized by mental symptoms, emotional lability, convulsive seizures, hemiplegia, aphasia, and hemianopsia; **brain stem–cerebellar,** manifested by nystagmus, scanning speech, intention tremor and ataxia; **spinal,** with cord involvement being evidenced by transient paresthesias, weakness and ataxia of one or more of the extremities. These and other types are not clear-cut and there is frequent overlapping. Euphoria and precipitate urination usually are common with all types.

Objective findings in multiple sclerosis are many and varied:

Mental: Milder changes are commonly found as euphoria, apathy, lack of judgment, or inattention. The severe forms, mania or depression, are uncommon. Suicidal thoughts are frequent. Sudden weeping or forced laughter may be evidence of involvement of pathways of emotional control.

Speech: There is no difficulty in finding words, but slow enunciation with a tendency to hesitation at the beginning of a word or syllable (scanning speech), is common.

Eyes: One or more of the following eye signs usually are present sometime during the course of the disease: nystagmus; transient paralysis of external ocular muscles with diplopia; partial atrophy of the optic nerve with increased temporal pallor; changes in the visual fields (central scotoma for color and form or general narrowing of the fields). Choked disks and total blindness occur, but are rare, as are pupillary changes and Argyll Robertson pupils (diagnosis doubtful when pupillary changes are seen).

Cranial nerves: These are not usually affected directly. Deafness occurs rarely but facial paralysis is not uncommon. Bulbar signs are paralysis of the vocal cords and disturbances of phonation, chewing and swallowing.

Motor: Deep reflexes (pyramidal tract signs) are generally increased; increased knee jerks, positive Babinski, and frequently clonus, are present. Superficial reflexes, particularly upper and lower abdominals are diminished or absent. Tremor is commonly present and occurs when a purposeful motion is attempted. Continuation of this effort accentuates the tremor. The motion is shaky, irregular, tremulous, and ineffective (ataxic), and is described as an intention tremor. Other effects are muscular weakness and spasticity producing a stumbling, weaving (drunken) gait.

Sensory: Paresthesias, sensations of numbness, blunting of sensation, disturbances of sense of position, and an occasional hemianesthesia occur. The changes are transient and fleeting and require careful study to elicit them.

Autonomic: Mild disturbances of bladder function (difficulty in micturition, partial retention, slight incontinence) are frequent but usually transitory. Vesical and rectal incontinence are signs of severe and advanced involvement. Sexual impotence in the male and anesthesia in the female are not uncommon. Priapism is rare.

Muscular atrophy: Uncommon, although atypical types of the disease may occur in the form of persisting spastic paraplegia (often associated with optic atrophy).

Diagnosis

The cerebral type must be differentiated from expanding intracranial lesions such as brain tumors or abscesses and from cerebrovascular accidents. When the brain stem is involved it is necessary to rule out acoustic neuroma, cerebellar tumors, gliomas of the brain stem and tumors outside of the brain stem. In the presence of spinal cord symptoms, cord tumor, syringomyelia, amyotrophic lateral sclerosis, syphilis, subacute combined system degeneration and the hereditary ataxias must be considered.

A definite diagnosis rarely can be made during the first attack. History of remissions and exacerbations is most important confirmation. The spinal fluid is normal in over 50% of cases. The most characteristic abnormality is a first-zone (paretic) gold curve. A slight increase in cells (lymphocytes) may be seen but the spinal fluid findings are not characteristic. Late spinal fluid findings may include a slight increase in cells and a positive globulin. The triad of intention tremor, nystagmus and scanning speech occurs late in the disease.

Prognosis and Treatment

Although the average duration of life is 10 to 15 years following the onset of the disease, many patients live much longer. The course is variable. Some patients have frequent attacks and are rapidly incapacitated, while others have remissions for as long as 25 years.

There is no specific therapy. Spontaneous remissions make it difficult to evaluate any form of treatment.

General management: Efforts should be made to keep the patient as near a normal level of activity as is consistent with his physical state. Overwork and fatigue should be avoided. Bedridden patients should be watched carefully to prevent the development of decubitus (q.v.) and efforts made to avoid urinary tract infections. Urinary frequency may be lessened by the use of tincture of belladonna, 10 drops 3 times a day (℞ 30). Belladonna should be used for as long as there is evidence of urinary frequency and evidence that the belladonna is effective. The presence of dryness of the throat, slight delirium, severe nausea, and constipation should lead to either a discontinuance of, or a reduction in, the amount of the drug.

Physiotherapy: Massage and passive movement of the weakened, spastic limbs are of some value. Muscle training is beneficial to the patient both physically and psychologically.

Psychotherapy: Encouragement and reassurance are essential, and the hopeless outlook should be minimized. Invalidism should be postponed as long as possible, and some form of therapy maintained constantly.

Pharmacotherapy: None of the recommended modes of drug therapy has proved to be of definite value. However, for their psychotherapeutic and tonic effects, drugs such as arsenic and quinine may be worth a trial. Arsenic may be given in the form of one of the arsphenamines (℞ 71), I.V. at weekly intervals for a period of 4 to 6 weeks. The course may be repeated every few months. Fowler's solution (℞ 72) can be given by mouth, beginning with 1 drop in water 3 times daily and gradually increasing the dose to 10 drops 3 times a day for a period of 6 weeks. There should be a rest period of at least equal extent before the course is repeated. Arsenic also may be given in the form of sodium cacodylate (℞ 73) up to 60 mg. (gr. i) daily for 1 month; subsequent monthly courses of therapy may be given every other month for an indefinite period. Quinine (℞ 74) usually is given as the hydrochloride in a dose of 0.3 Gm. (gr. v) once or twice a day for several weeks. Use of anticoagulants such as dicumarol and heparin still is in the experimental stage and may cause severe hemorrhages. Massive doses of all the vitamins have been given, particularly vitamin B and its components.

Climatotherapy: Since multiple sclerosis is relatively uncommon in the subtropics, it has been recommended that patients with this disease move to such a climate if possible.

Miscellaneous: Fever therapy, produced artificially or by the use of typhoid vaccine, is sometimes followed by a remission of symptoms. However, this treatment is debatable, since an acute exacerbation may follow it, or the condition of the patient may become worse.

SYRINGOMYELIA

A chronic, progressive disease of the spinal cord and medulla (syringobulbia) characterized pathologically by cavitation and gliosis, and clinically by a dissociated sensory loss, muscular atrophy, and spasticity.

Etiology, Pathology, and Pathologic Physiology

The cause of true syringomyelia is unknown. It is thought to be a developmental anomaly. Localized cavitation may occur as a result of necrosis secondary to vascular lesions, syphilis, intramedullary tumors, tuberculosis, or trauma to the cord. Males are more commonly affected than females. It usually occurs between the ages of 10 and 30 years.

The disease process involves primarily the central gray matter of the cord in the cervical and lumbar regions. There is gliosis and cavitation which may be localized to one area or may involve the entire length of the cord and spread into the medulla, giving rise to syringobulbia. The early loss of pain and temperature sense with retention of touch (dissociated sensory loss) is the result of the destruction of the fibers of pain and temperature as they cross in the gray commissure. Involvement of the anterior horn cells, pyramidal tracts, and the posterior columns produces atrophy, spasticity, and ataxia.

Symptoms and Signs

The onset usually is insidious. Atrophy and weakness of small muscles of the hands may be noticed first. Painless burns or injuries may first attract attention. Pain in the extremities is not uncommon. On examination, a loss of pain and temperature sensation usually is found in a shawl-like distribution over the arms and shoulders. Atrophy and fibrillation may be noted in the muscles of the hands. Charcot's joints and painless felons may be present. There may be spasticity, hyperactive reflexes, and a Babinski response in the lower extremities. Scoliosis is not uncommon. Involvement of the medulla (syringobulbia) is indicated by nystagmus, atrophy of the tongue, difficulty in swallowing and talking, Horner's syndrome, and by loss of pain and temperature sensation in the face.

Diagnosis

It is necessary to differentiate the muscular atrophies and dystrophies, brachial neuritis, spinal cord tumors, multiple sclerosis, and subacute combined degeneration. The dissociated sensory loss, the atrophy and weakness of the muscles of the upper extremities, spasticity in the lower extremities, scoliosis, trophic changes, and the presence of heredodegenerative stigmas, such as webfeet, clubfeet, cervical ribs, all point to a diagnosis of syringomyelia.

Prognosis and Treatment

The disease is slowly progressive but it may remain stationary for many years. Some patients live for as long as 40 years.

Death usually occurs as a result of aspiration pneumonia following bulbar paralysis, or from some intercurrent infection.

A cheerful and encouraging attitude on the part of the physician, family, and attendants should be maintained. Avoid invalidism of the patient as long as possible. Protect his hands, feet, and joints by appropriate orthopedic appliances when trophic disturbances are present. Surgical drainage of the cystic cavity after laminectomy is sometimes beneficial, particularly in cases where a complete subarachnoid block exists. X-ray treatment is not always successful but is the best therapy available at present. Diffuse exposure should be given over the entire spinal cord with concentration over the affected sites, always administered by an experienced radiologist.

MUSCULAR DYSTROPHIES; ATROPHIES

These disorders of the neuromuscular apparatus, many of which are heredofamilial, can be divided into the following classifications:

    I. The Dystrophies
        A. Progressive muscular dystrophy
            The several subgroupings are differentiated according to distribution of the muscular wasting and the presence or absence of hypertrophy or pseudohypertrophy: 1. Pseudohypertrophic (Duchenne) type. 2. Hypertrophic (Spiller) type. 3. Facioscapulohumeral (Landouzy-Dejerine) type.
        B. Myotonia dystrophica and myotonia congenita
    II. The Atrophies
        A. Peroneal muscular atrophy (Charcot-Marie-Tooth)
        B. Hypertrophic interstitial neuritis (Dejerine-Sottas)
        C. Amyotrophic lateral sclerosis (including progressive muscular atrophy and progressive bulbar palsy)
        D. Amyotonia congenita
        E. Infantile muscular atrophy
    III. Myasthenia Gravis
    IV. Familial Periodic Paralysis

I. MUSCULAR DYSTROPHIES

PROGRESSIVE MUSCULAR DYSTROPHY

A heredofamilial disorder of unknown cause which affects males more commonly than females. The pathologic changes are limited to the somatic muscles in most cases but occasionally the cardiac muscles are involved. These changes consist of atrophy of some of the muscle fibers, swelling of some of the others, increase in the sarcolemmal nuclei, increase in connective tissue septums, and deposition of fat between the hypertrophied fibers.

Symptoms and Signs

The onset usually is gradual. The child begins to walk clumsily, tends to fall, and then has difficulty in getting up unaided. On examination it will be noted that there is pseudohy-pertrophy of some muscles and wasting of others. The pseudo-hypertrophy frequently involves the calves which, though they appear large, are weak and feel rubbery on palpation. The atrophy tends to involve the pelvic musculature. Atrophy around the shoulder girdle produces winging of the scapula. In rising from a supine position on the floor, the patient will first roll over on his abdomen, rise to a kneeling position, and then help himself to the erect position by "climbing up" his own legs. The disease usually is slowly progressive and the patient eventually becomes bedridden, although in most instances the affliction itself does not shorten life.

Diagnosis

Progressive muscular dystrophy is differentiated from the atrophies by its onset at an early age, absence of fibrillations in the atrophic muscles, the lordosis, the waddling gait, and the characteristic method of rising from the ground.

Treatment

It is best to keep the patient fairly active and encourage him to live a life as close to normal as possible. Massage delays the development of contractures. There is no specific medica-tion that will retard the progress of the disease. Glycine (R 81) has been given in doses of 10 to 20 Gm. daily. The vita-mins, particularly vitamin E, have been tried in large doses without any beneficial effect.

MYOTONIA DYSTROPHICA; MYOTONIA CONGENITA
(Myotonia atrophica; Thomsen's disease)

Heredofamilial disorders of unknown cause, once thought to be separate entities, now known to represent different stages of an essentially degenerative process spread over several gen-erations, appearing as cataract in the earlier and eventually as the full-blown disease in the later generations. The myotonia has its onset in childhood but the muscular atrophy does not usually appear until late in the 2nd decade or in the 3rd decade of life. Males are more commonly affected than females. The pathologic changes in the muscles are similar to those seen in muscular dystrophy.

Symptoms and Signs

The only symptom of myotonia congenita is an abnormal contractibility of the muscles. Characteristically, the patient is unable to relax his grip, but the myotonia may be present in any of the muscles. Emotion and sudden forced effort will aggravate the myotonia. Mechanical excitability of the muscle is exaggerated and contraction is unduly prolonged on elec-trical stimulation.

In myotonia dystrophica there are characteristically distributed muscular atrophy, cataracts, early baldness, and atrophy of the endocrines, especially the testes, in addition to the myotonia. Usually, the neck musculature is most severely affected, so that the patient is unable to flex his head on his chest when he is in a recumbent position. The atrophy involves the facial musculature, producing the typical hatchet face, and late in the disease may extend to the muscles of the extremities and trunk. The disorders are slowly progressive but are compatible with fairly long life.

Diagnosis

The myotonia, the endocrine factors and the cataracts differentiate these conditions from the atrophies and from the other forms of muscular dystrophy.

Treatment

General measures are similar to those for progressive muscular dystrophy. Quinine (℞ 74) relieves the myotonia but has no effect on the muscular weakness and atrophy.

II. MUSCULAR ATROPHIES

PERONEAL MUSCULAR ATROPHY
(Charcot-Marie-Tooth disease)

A heredofamilial disorder of unknown etiology in which males are more commonly affected, characterized by interstitial neuritis of the peroneal nerves, and degeneration of the anterior horn cells, the dorsal columns, and the nerve roots. The affected muscles show a simple atrophy secondary to the nerve involvement.

Symptoms and Signs

The disease begins insidiously and progresses slowly. Symptoms usually appear when the patients are between 15 and 30 years of age. Atrophy characteristically begins in the peroneal and tibial muscles and gradually spreads to involve the gastrocnemius, and eventually the small muscles of the hands. The patients have a characteristic "stork leg" appearance because the atrophy is limited to the muscles below the knees. Clubfoot is almost always present. The most incapacitating symptom is foot-drop. There usually is a complaint of numbness, tingling, and paresthesias in the lower extremities. Examination will reveal impairment of position and vibration sense and occasionally some loss of cutaneous sensation. The deep tendon reflexes usually are absent, the ankle jerks being the first to disappear. This disorder is the least incapacitating of all the muscular atrophies and dystrophies. It is slowly progressive but the patients are able to remain active for many years and may live an average life span.

Diagnosis

Peroneal muscular atrophy is differentiated from the other forms of muscular atrophy and dystrophy by the hereditary factors, the characteristic appearance of the legs and the evidence of neuritis.

Treatment

There is no specific treatment. Patients should be encouraged to live as normal a life as possible. Massage and exercises will maintain the nutrition of the wasted muscles for a long time. It will be necessary eventually for the patients to wear a brace to correct foot-drop.

HYPERTROPHIC INTERSTITIAL NEURITIS
(Dejerine-Sottas disease)

A rare disease of unknown etiology in which there is hypertrophy of the peripheral nerves, roots, and ganglia due to a proliferation of the cells of the sheaths of Schwann. The age incidence is between 10 and 30 years and males are more commonly affected.

Symptoms and Signs

The clinical picture is very similar to that of peroneal muscular atrophy and it is thought by some that the two diseases are really one entity. Earliest complaints are of numbness and paresthesias in the lower extremities. Weakness and wasting of the muscles appear early. There may be abnormalities of the pupils and disturbances in the gastrointestinal tract as the result of sympathetic nerve involvement. The deep tendon reflexes usually are absent or diminished. Occasionally, the hypertrophied nerves can be palpated. The disease usually is slowly progressive with rare remissions and the patient's life usually is not endangered.

Diagnosis

Hypertrophic interstitial neuritis must be differentiated from the muscular atrophies, dystrophies, and other forms of neuritis. Microscopic sections of a biopsied nerve will reveal the characteristic onion-peel swelling of the nerve fibers.

Treatment

There is no specific treatment. The general measures recommended for peroneal muscular atrophy are applicable here.

AMYOTROPHIC LATERAL SCLEROSIS; PROGRESSIVE MUSCULAR ATROPHY; PROGRESSIVE BULBAR PALSY

The three disorders represent descriptive subdivisions of one disease. The definite etiology is unknown. Trauma, syphilis, and lead poisoning have been advanced as possible causes. The disease usually occurs after the age of 40 and males are more frequently affected than females. Although some patients have lived for 5 years or more, the prognosis is grave and death usually occurs in 2 to 3 years. There is degeneration of the motor neurons in the spinal cord, medulla, and motor cortex. When the pathologic changes are limited primarily to the anterior horn cells of the spinal cord, the condition is known as Aran-Duchenne progressive muscular atrophy. When the changes are maximal in the motor cranial nerve nuclei in the medulla, the resulting clinical picture is known as progressive bulbar palsy. Amyotrophic lateral sclerosis represents a combination of one or both of the above mentioned forms with signs of involvement of the long motor tracts. There are atrophic changes in the fibers of the wasted muscles.

Symptoms and Signs

Amyotrophic Lateral Sclerosis: The disease begins insidiously, the earliest complaint being that of weakness and atrophy of the muscles of the hands. The weakness and atrophy spread to involve the muscles of the forearms and shoulder girdles. In the beginning, only one upper extremity may be involved but there is gradual spread to the other. The atrophy may begin in the shoulder girdles and spread down to involve the arms. Fibrillations are almost always present. The lower extremities usually are weak and spastic. The deep tendon reflexes are frequently hyperactive throughout and there is ankle clonus and a positive Babinski's sign. For a long time the clinical picture may be one of weakness and spasticity with little evidence of atrophy. The spasticity may involve the bulbar muscles.

Progressive Muscular Atrophy: The clinical manifestations are similar to that of amyotrophic lateral sclerosis, except that there is no evidence of long tract involvement. Instead of spasticity in the lower extremities there may be atrophy and weakness. The deep tendon reflexes are usually preserved until the atrophy is far advanced.

Progressive Bulbar Palsy: As a result of involvement of the motor nuclei of the medulla, there is difficulty in chewing, swallowing, and talking. Frequently, there may be involuntary outbursts of laughing and crying. Atrophy and fibrillations of the tongue are usual.

Diagnosis

These conditions must be differentiated from the muscular dystrophies and other forms of muscular atrophy, syringomyelia, cord tumor, and multiple sclerosis. The diagnostic features include the relatively late onset, the evidence of involvement of both upper and lower motor neurons, the fibrillations and the absence of sensory findings.

Treatment

There is no specific treatment and no drug or vitamin has

proved to be of definite value. General supportive therapy is indicated. Rest and avoidance of fatigue are recommended. Physiotherapy will maintain the nutrition of the wasted muscles and relieve the spasticity for as long as possible. When the bulbar nuclei are affected, a soft diet is recommended and in advanced cases it may be necessary to resort to nasal feedings.

AMYOTONIA CONGENITA

There is no known cause of this disease, which is not inherited but may affect more than one child in a family. It is equally common in males and females and appears at birth or shortly thereafter. There is a reduction in the number of motor cells in the spinal cord and medulla. The remaining cells usually are abnormal or malformed. There is demyelinization of the anterior roots and peripheral nerves. The muscles are composed of small fibers with many sarcolemmal nuclei and there is an increase in the connective tissue and fat.

Symptoms and Signs

The infant makes very few movements although none of the muscles is completely paralyzed. The bulbar and respiratory muscles are usually spared and the orbicular muscles of the eyes and mouth have relatively normal strength. The involvement is otherwise generalized, the legs being usually more affected than the arms. The movements of the extremities are feeble and the baby is unable to hold the head up or to sit erect. The muscles are small, feel soft, and frequently are difficult to palpate. There is a marked hypotonicity of all the muscles. The deep tendon reflexes are diminished or absent. The mild cases occasionally improve but it is rare for patients to live to adult life. In the severe cases, death occurs in a few months as a result of respiratory complications.

Diagnosis

Amyotonia congenita must be differentiated from infantile muscular atrophy and the rare cases of progressive muscular dystrophy occurring in infancy. The generalized weakness, the hypotonia and the absent reflexes appearing very early in infancy are diagnostic.

There is no specific therapy. Massage and passive exercise will help maintain the nutrition of the muscles and prevent contractures until muscle training can be instituted to develop the voluntary use of the weakened muscles.

INFANTILE MUSCULAR ATROPHY
(Werdnig-Hoffmann's disease)

This disease is considered to be identical with amyotonia congenita (q.v.) except that it develops at a somewhat later age, the first symptoms generally appearing when the child is 6 to 8 months old.

III. MYASTHENIA GRAVIS

*A disease characterized by progressive weakness of the muscles
due to impairment of conduction at the myoneural junction.*

Etiology, Pathology, and Pathologic Physiology

The cause is unknown. The disease is occasionally associated
with tumors of the thymus and with hyperthyroidism. Females
are more commonly affected than males and it occurs most frequently between the ages of 20 and 50 years.

There are lymphoid cellular deposits, termed lymphorrhages,
in the skeletal muscles. In about 50% of cases there is an enlargement of the thymus. Abnormalities have been noted occasionally in other endocrine glands. The physiologic derangement is the impairment of conduction at the myoneural junction of striated muscle. This is thought to be due either to a
lack of acetylcholine or an increase of cholinesterase at the
myoneural junction preventing the transmission of the normal
impulse.

Symptoms and Signs

Abnormal fatigability and weakness of the muscles are the
outstanding symptoms. Characteristically, the weakness of the
involved muscles is increased by their use. After a period of
rest, their strength returns and it is for this reason that the patients feel strongest in the morning and become tired and weak
toward evening. The muscles of the neck, throat, lips, tongue,
face, and eyes are the ones primarily involved. The muscles of
the trunk and extremities are occasionally involved.

The onset usually is gradual. The patients begin complaining
of double vision, difficulty in swallowing, chewing, and talking.
These symptoms are always worse in the evening. An expres-
sionless facies and unilateral or bilateral ptosis will be noted
on examination. Atrophy is rare but may be present occasionally, as may weakness of the muscles of the trunk or extremities. There are no sensory changes and the deep tendon reflexes are preserved though quickly exhausted. The course is
variable and there may be prolonged remissions. Some cases
end fatally in a very short time as a result of choking, but in
80% the disease is compatible with a normal life span.

Diagnosis

Myasthenia gravis is differentiated from amyotrophic lateral
sclerosis, syringomyelia, pseudobulbar palsy, the dystrophies,
multiple sclerosis, diphtheritic and infectious polyneuritis and
the neuroses by means of the history of variation in strength of
the muscles in the morning and in the evening, the increased
fatigability after use with improvement after rest, the neostigmine test, and the myasthenic reaction of Jolly. (When faradic
stimulation is applied to a muscle, the first few stimulations will
produce brisk contractions which are followed by a gradual
diminution of the response on subsequent stimulations.)

The best method of confirming the diagnosis is by means of the neostigmine test. This may be done as follows: The amount of weakness is first determined and then the patient is given an I.M. injection of 1.5 mg. of neostigmine (R 35) and 0.6 mg. (gr. 1/100) of atropine (R 28). A positive response is characterized by a rapid abolition of the weakness 1/2 to 1 hour after the injection, with return of the symptoms in 4 to 8 hours. Administration of 0.5 mg. of neostigmine I.V. is reported to give prompter, more complete and more easily interpreted results than does the I.M. test.

Treatment

General measures: A life of restricted activity is necessary. During acute exacerbations, complete rest is essential. In most instances, the patient may have a general diet but in the severe cases a soft or a liquid diet should be given and it may be necessary to resort to tube feedings. Anesthetics should be avoided.

Drug therapy: Neostigmine (R 35) is the drug of choice. In severe cases it is given I.M. in a dose of 0.5 mg. with 0.6 mg. (gr. 1/100) of atropine (R 28) 3 to 4 times a day about an hour before meals. In milder cases it may be given orally in the form of a 15 mg. tablet (R 36), several to many times a day. Atropine (R 28), 0.4 mg. (gr. 1/150) or tincture of belladonna (R 30) 0.6 to 1.5 cc. (♏ x to xxv) should be given orally 3 times a day to prevent the untoward reactions of neostigmine on the intestinal, respiratory and cardiovascular systems.

Potassium chloride (R 75) may be given as an adjuvant to the neostigmine. Ephedrine sulfate (R 64) also can be used either alone or in combination with the other drugs. Guanidine (R 80) is sometimes beneficial, and usually is given in combination with neostigmine. Guanidine can be given indefinitely as long as it seems to be of some benefit and toxic symptoms do not appear—e.g., nervousness, gastrointestinal and circulatory disturbances, decrease of plasma volume, and blood sugar changes. A test dose of 10 mg./Kg. body wt. (in capsule form) should be given and subsequent dosage determined from the patient's reaction to the initial amount. The occurrence of toxic symptoms necessitates reduction in dosage, and further relief follows the use of atropine (R 28). Glycine (R 81) in a dosage of 15 Gm. 2 or 3 times a day may be tried alone or in combination with neostigmine.

Surgical therapy: Surgical removal of an enlarged thymus has been beneficial in some cases but the operation has a high mortality rate. Improvement may follow X-radiation of the thymus.

IV. FAMILIAL PERIODIC PARALYSIS

A rare heredofamilial disorder of unknown etiology characterized by intermittent paralysis of somatic muscles. Rarely, it may occur as a complication of thyrotoxicosis. Disturbance of potassium metabolism occurs, with the serum potassium decreased during attacks and normal between attacks. Onset usually is about the time of puberty. Attacks may be precipitated by high carbohydrate intake, exposure to cold, excessive fluid intake, constipation, menstruation, overexertion, fatigue, and mental excitement. No definite pathologic changes have been demonstrated.

Symptoms and Signs

Prodromal symptoms may occur the day before the attack. These consist of excessive hunger and thirst. Just prior to the attack, there may be increased sweating, dryness of the mouth, and a feeling of stiffness in the extremities. The attack comes on rather rapidly with the paralysis reaching its height in about an hour. The severity of an attack varies from a complete paralysis of all of the somatic muscles to a moderate weakness of the arms and legs. The muscles of the extremities and trunk are chiefly involved, the proximal more than the distal, in a symmetrical fashion. The eye muscles and the bulbar muscles usually escape. During an attack, there are no sensory changes but the deep tendon reflexes are lost and the electrical excitability of the muscles disappears. The attacks last anywhere from 2 to 48 hours. The frequency varies from several a week to one attack every 2 or 3 years. Consciousness is retained throughout the period of paralysis and there is no clouding of the sensorium. Changes in the ECG usually are present at the onset of an attack. Death may rarely occur during an attack as the result of respiratory paralysis. The attacks tend to become less severe and less frequent after the age of 30. With adequate treatment, individuals with this disease may look forward to a normal life span.

Diagnosis

The disorder must be differentiated from cataplexy, epilepsy, Landry's paralysis, and hysteria. The familial history, the loss of reflexes and the loss of electrical excitability of the muscles during an attack and the transient recurrent nature of the attacks are of diagnostic significance.

Treatment

The patient must avoid anything that might precipitate an attack. Rarely, it may be necessary to place the patient in a respirator to tide him over a period of respiratory paralysis. Potassium chloride (R 75) is used both to prevent and to abort attacks. Potassium chloride 12 Gm. should be given orally at the onset of an attack. For emergency use, 1 Gm. of potassium chloride in 50 cc. of solution can be given I.V. (R 76). This should be injected slowly. In doses of 3 Gm. 3 to 4 times a day, potassium chloride prevents attacks.

NEURITIS; NEURALGIA

NEURITIS

Inflammation of a single nerve (mononeuritis), of 2 or more nerves in separate areas (mononeuritis multiplex), or of many nerves simultaneously (polyneuritis). The term has come to mean a syndrome of sensory, motor, reflex, and vasomotor symptoms, singly or in combination, produced by lesions of the nerve roots or the peripheral nerves.

Etiology

The agents producing neuritic lesions may be grouped into the following categories: (1) mechanical, (2) vascular, (3) infectious, (4) toxic, and (5) metabolic.

Mechanical agents are the usual cause of mononeuritis, and sometimes of mononeuritis multiplex. They consist of direct blows, penetrating injuries, contusions, compression, or avulsion due to fracture or dislocation of bones. Pressure paralysis usually occurs during sound sleep or anesthesia, especially in thin individuals, and is most likely to affect superficial nerves at bony prominences such as the ulnar at the elbow, the radial at the mid-humerus, and the peroneal at the knee. Tumors, bony hyperostosis, casts, and crutches also may cause pressure palsies. Violent muscular activity or forcible overextension of joints will sometimes produce mechanical neuritis. Repeated small traumas may be causative; e.g., those encountered by engravers through tight gripping of small tools, or by air-hammer operators through excessive vibration of the tools. The prolonged cramped postures necessary in some occupations (e.g., gardening) may be responsible.

Mononeuritis multiplex is seen most often in **vascular** diseases, because of the disseminated nature of vascular lesions. Periarteritis nodosa, arteriosclerosis, hemorrhage into nerves, refrigeration, and radium exposure all may produce neuritic lesions. Involvement of several nerves with a common blood supply occurs in Volkmann's ischemic paralysis or in the occlusion of a major artery.

Localized **infectious** neuritis may be caused by direct invasion of the nerve by pyogenic organisms; e.g., the facial nerve in mastoiditis. It also occurs in syphilis, leprosy, tetanus, and tuberculosis. Acute febrile diseases usually are the cause of polyneuritis, and occasionally of mononeuritis or mononeuritis multiplex. Such diseases include herpes, diphtheria, typhoid, malaria, septic sore throat, measles, and Guillain-Barré's disease.

Toxic neuritis generally takes the form of polyneuritis but sometimes involves only one nerve. Poisoning by heavy metals (lead, arsenic, gold, thallium, mercury, bismuth, copper, antimony, zinc, tin, silver, and manganese) is a common cause. Hydrocarbons and organic solvents figure heavily among nonmetallic toxins. These include alcohol, carbon monoxide, carbon disulfide, carbon tetrachloride, tetrachloroethane, benzene, emetine, Evipal, barbital, chlorobutanol, orthodinitrophenol, and the sulfonamides.

Metabolic neuritis is almost always a polyneuritis. Nutritional deficiency, in which lack of thiamine presumably is the chief factor, is seen in alcoholism, pellagra, beriberi, gastrointestinal dysfunction, hysteria, psychoses, and other chronic diseases. Polyneuritis also is seen in diabetes, pernicious anemia, acute porphyria, and gout.

Pathology

When a peripheral nerve is mildly damaged, the axone and myelin become swollen and tortuous. These changes are reversible. With severe (irreversible) damage, the axone and myelin become fragmented and phagocytes remove the debris. Connective tissue sheaths show focal or diffuse proliferation. In infections there is infiltration with inflammatory cells. Vascular changes include endothelial proliferation, vascular occlusions, and hemorrhages. In focal neuritic lesions the nerve peripheral to the injured area degenerates. Damage to the C.N.S. may be associated. Regeneration of nerve varies with the cause, type, and severity of the lesion. It progresses at the rate of 2 to 4 cm./month.

Symptoms, Signs, and Clinical Forms

Sensory symptoms are outstanding. Tingling, pins and needles, burning, boring, stabbing are some of the descriptive adjectives patients use. Pain often is worse at night and may be aggravated by touching the affected area or by temperature changes. Numbness and objective loss of sensation occur in severe cases. The nerve trunks are tender.

Motor symptoms of weakness may progress to complete paralysis. Affected muscles become tender, atonic and atrophic. Fasciculations or fibrillations may be seen. Muscular responses to electrical stimuli are altered. Tendon reflexes are diminished or absent. Deformities occur, especially in untreated cases.

Vasomotor symptoms of hyperemia, sweating, and bullae are more common in partial and irritative lesions. Complete lesions generally produce pallor and dryness of the skin, and osteoporosis. Trophic changes are common in severe, particularly prolonged, cases.

Clinical forms: Mononeuritis, both single and multiple, is characterized by symptoms of pain, weakness, and paresthesias of the affected part. Bell's palsy, with its characteristic distortion of the face due to a lesion of the facial nerve, is a special form of mononeuritis. Multiple mononeuritis is asymmetrical, and involvement of the various nerves may be simultaneous or spread over a considerable period of time.

Polyneuritis, or multiple peripheral neuritis, occurs as a bilaterally symmetrical, simultaneous involvement of sensory, motor, and vasomotor nerves. Manifestations begin in the fingers and toes and progress up the extremities. The sphincters and trunk commonly escape. Subjective numbness, tingling and other paresthesias precede actual anesthesia. Pain, often burning in character, is prominent and poses a difficult problem. Muscular weakness begins peripherally and is associated with muscle tenderness, atrophy, and diminished tendon reflexes. Sympathetic involvement is indicated by hyperhidrosis, edema, and livid discoloration of the skin.

Associated symptoms and signs: Cerebral symptoms of confusion, delirium, and headaches occur with C.N.S. involvement. In such cases, cerebrospinal fluid findings include increased protein, pleocytosis and serologic changes. Any C.N.S. signs strongly suggest generalized damage from some toxic, metabolic, or infectious disease.

Physical examination may reveal hypertension, arteriosclerosis, weight loss, or signs of infection, anemia, or malignancy. Scars, fractures, and bony callus are present in many traumatic cases. The nerve trunks may show areas of enlargement.

Laboratory Findings

Examination of the blood may reveal evidence of anemia, usually pernicious, stippling of red cells in lead poisoning, or eosinophilia in periarteritis. Urinalysis may show porphyrins in porphyria, heavy metal poisoning, and some infections. A positive urine sugar test may disclose diabetes as being an underlying cause. X-ray of the bones in many cases will reveal changes due to trauma, malignancy, or hypertrophic arthritis.

Diagnosis

Neuritis is a symptom rather than a specific disease entity, and the underlying cause must be sought (*see* chapters on the various diseases named below). If neuritis is the presenting symptom, this requires an adequate history, general physical examination, neurologic evaluation, and laboratory tests. The etiologic agent is usually found in the general work-up rather than the neurologic examination. In cases of mononeuritis, attention should be directed toward a mechanical or traumatic etiology, although infectious agents may be responsible. Mononeuritis multiplex usually is due to vascular disease but occasionally results from toxic substances. Guillain-Barré's disease, Boeck's sarcoid, lupus erythematosus, brucellosis, and other infections all may cause a mononeuritis multiplex. Neuritis with intractable pain strongly suggests metastatic malignancy. In polyneuritis, the etiology is most commonly toxic, infectious, or metabolic. Poliomyelitis, tabes dorsalis, multiple sclerosis, progressive muscular atrophies and dystrophies must be considered. Arthritis, fibrositis, and dermatomyositis may simulate neuritis. In differential diagnosis, psychoneurosis often is a confusing factor.

Causalgia (q.v.) is a persistent burning pain aggravated by sensory stimulation and associated with vasomotor and trophic changes. This symptom may persist long after the acute process has subsided. The term "neuralgia" (q.v.) should be limited to severe, lancinating, recurrent pains of brief duration which can be produced by a trigger mechanism.

Prognosis and Treatment

Under appropriate treatment recovery usually is rapid in mild cases, but a repetition of the original causes may produce recurrence. Recovery may be incomplete, and severe cases may result in chronic muscular atrophy and sensory, motor, and vasomotor disturbances.

Specific therapy is directed toward the etiologic agent. Further mechanical trauma must be avoided. Surgery for tumors or protruded intervertebral disk, for nerve suture or neurolysis, and for nerve transplant must be done when indicated. Vascular diseases present a difficult problem but vasodilating drugs (R 33, 34) may be tried. Diabetes and pernicious anemia require careful control. Specific therapy must be employed (q.v.) for heavy metal toxicity (e.g., lead, arsenic) and for infectious diseases.

The acute stage of neuritis should be treated with rest of the affected parts. Salicylates (R 1, 3), barbiturates (R 13), codeine (R 2), or some of the newer analgesics (R 6, 7) may be required for relief of pain. When the neuritis is the result of vasospasm, flushing doses of niacin (R 65), 100 mg. I.V. 3 times a day, are sometimes remarkably helpful. Tetra-ethyl-ammonium chloride (R 11) will occasionally give temporary relief if the sympathetic ganglia are involved. (CAUTION! This drug may cause severe fall in blood pressure, weakness, nausea, abdominal distention especially with I.V. use.) Considerable relief of pain may be obtained by repeated local anesthetic block of the appropriate sympathetic ganglion in neuritis with burning pain or vasomotor signs.

In the intractable case, radiotherapy over the offending nerve may give prolonged and occasionally permanent relief. Morphine should be avoided. The extremities should be protected from pressure from bedclothes and trauma. Rigid immobilization is to be avoided because of the danger of ankylosis of joints. Heat in the form of hot packs or soaks assists in relief of pain and permits early physical therapy. Daily passive movement of all joints through the full range of motion is an absolute essential and should be started immediately. This includes muscle stretching when shortening threatens. Active movement of severely affected parts is contraindicated. A high protein, high vitamin diet is important, especially in infectious, toxic, and metabolic neuritis. Protein hydrolysates by mouth or parenterally are indicated in cachectic patients, and supplements of thiamine (℞ 67), ascorbic acid (℞ 68), and brewers' yeast (℞ 69) are advisable.

When acute symptoms subside, active exercises are substituted for passive. Resistive and reconditioning exercises help speed return of muscle power. During convalescence, a standard diet with decreasing vitamin supplements may be resumed.

Chronic atrophy and other permanent residuals may probably be avoided in many cases by proper early treatment. Motor residuals are amenable to retraining, orthopedic appliances, or corrective surgery. Persistent pain will sometimes require procaine or alcohol nerve block or, rarely, a nerve root section. Radiotherapy is worthy of a trial. Causalgia presents a difficult problem that may necessitate sympathectomy, section of posterior roots, or interruption of the spinothalamic tracts of the spinal cord. Prefrontal lobotomy has been resorted to with good results in carefully selected cases.

NEURALGIA

Paroxysms of acute pain in the distribution of a peripheral sensory nerve, usually for which no etiologic basis or morphologic changes can be found. (The term often is used incorrectly as a synonym for "neuritis.")

TRIGEMINAL NEURALGIA
(Tic douloureux)

A syndrome marked by brief attacks of severe pain in the course of one or more of the branches of the trigeminal nerve, usually without evidence of organic changes in the nerve. The cause of the condition remains unknown. It may occur at any age after puberty, but usually begins about the age of 50. Women are affected somewhat more frequently than men.

Symptoms and Signs

The characteristic symptom is intense pain usually described as a stabbing, lightning-like, or shooting sensation of short duration in the distribution of one of the divisions of the trigeminal nerve. The superior maxillary and mandibular branches are most often involved; the ophthalmic branch usually becomes affected secondary to superior maxillary involvement. The pain usually is unilateral, although spread to the opposite side may occur. In the early stages, the attacks rarely last more than 1 or 2 minutes, with periods of freedom from pain as long as weeks or months. As the disease advances, the symptom-free intervals become shorter. Many patients describe hypersensitive areas most common about the nose and mouth. These "trigger zones," when touched, excite an attack. Attacks also are often precipitated by exposure to cold, washing the face, talking, eating, and drinking. There is no reduction in acuity of sensation over the distribution of the nerve.

Diagnosis

In patients with tic douloureux the history usually is typical enough to be diagnostic. In neuritis involving the trigeminal nerve, however, there usually is a history of acute onset, the pain is prolonged, the nerve is tender on pressure, and there may be analgesia or hyperalgesia over the cutaneous distribution of the nerve. Tumors or other lesions involving the nerve produce persistent pain and sensory impairment. Post-herpetic pain is accompanied by a history of a herpetic eruption.

Treatment

Analgesics (R 1, 3, 6, 7) offer only temporary relief. Trichloroethylene inhalation 3 times daily frequently results in significant if not lasting relief. From 20 to 25 drops of trichloroethylene (R 12) are poured on gauze and inhaled until the odor no longer is present. Peripheral avulsion of the involved branch as it leaves the skull may give relief up to 8 months. Injection of 98% alcohol into the branch at its exit from the skull may abolish the pain for as long as 18 months. Permanent cure can be obtained only by injection of alcohol into the gasserian ganglion or by section of the sensory root of the nerve proximal to the ganglion.

GLOSSOPHARYNGEAL NEURALGIA

A rare syndrome characterized by recurrent attacks of severe pain in the back of the throat, tonsils, back of the tongue and the middle ear. The cause is unknown. Rarely, the condition may occur as the result of a tumor in the cerebellopontine angle. Males are more commonly affected than females. The syndrome usually appears after the age of 40. There is no organic pathology demonstrable in the nerve or its ganglia. Life expectancy is unaffected. Occasionally, there are long remissions.

Symptoms and Signs

The pains occur paroxysmally and are severe and excruciating, similar to those of trigeminal neuralgia. They usually begin in the throat and the base of the tongue and radiate to the ears. They may radiate down the side of the neck in front of the ear. The pain may occur spontaneously or be precipitated by chewing, swallowing, talking, sneezing, coughing, or yawning. The attacks usually are brief, lasting seconds to a few minutes. The paroxysms occur intermittently and may be separated by long free intervals.

Diagnosis

Glossopharyngeal neuralgia must be distinguished from trigeminal neuralgia involving the mandibular division. This can be done by the location of the pain and by the precipitation of an attack on swallowing or touching the tonsils. Tumors involving the tonsils and the pharynx must be excluded.

Treatment

Medical therapy usually is of no value. Cocainization of the pharynx and the tonsils may lessen the paroxysms. Analgesics are useless since the attacks are over in a few seconds. The treatment of choice in severe cases is surgery. Surgical avulsion of the nerve in the neck should be performed when the pain is primarily in the pharynx; the nerve should be sectioned intracranially when the pain is more widespread.

SCIATICA

Severe pain in the lower extremity over the region innervated by the sciatic nerve and its branches.

Etiology

The sciatic nerve is the longest in the body. It sends off branches into the upper thigh muscles and into the joints, skin, and muscles of the leg. Because of its peculiar course and distribution, it is more exposed to internal and external trauma and inflammation than any other nerve. Hence, the causes of sciatica are many and varied. For convenience they may be divided into the following categories: (1) Compression or trauma of the sciatic nerve; (2) toxic, metabolic, or infectious disorders involving the sciatic nerve; and (3) pain referred to the sciatic nerve from other lesions.

Compression or trauma of sciatic nerve: Mechanical pressure upon the nerve or its spinal roots is the chief cause of sciatica. Compression may result from a herniated intervertebral disk, hypertrophied ligamentum flavum, spondylolisthesis, cauda equina tumor, arthritis involving the vertebral foramen (spondylitis), pregnancy, nearby focal infections with tissue swelling, and neoplasms such as fibroids, metastases from tumors of prostate or breast, and retroperitoneal tumors. Pressure upon the nerve often is due to continuous reflex spasm of the overlying piriformis muscle, owing to irritation of the sacroiliac joint. Fibrositic lesions of adjacent musculature and fascia (i.e., psoas, glutei, piriformis, tensor fascia lata, or iliotibial band) may cause pain by traction upon the nerve. Trauma to the sciatic nerve often occurs in the course of walking, running, bicycling, prolonged standing with poor posture, or sitting (particularly on one side) on the edge of a chair. It also may be induced by continued strenuous use of a lower extremity such as occurs in driving a car for long periods of time.

Toxic, metabolic, or infectious diseases: Sciatica may be due to lead poisoning, alcoholism, vitamin B deficiency, viral infection, syphilis, or any lesion producing an inflammatory change directly in the nerve tissue. The sciatic neuritis that sometimes complicates diabetes mellitus has been attributed to a vitamin B deficiency, but is more probably of vascular origin. On the other hand, sciatica complicating alcoholism often is the result of an accompanying vitamin B deficiency.

Referred pain: Anal lesions often are the cause of sciatica, due to the persistent, intense nervous impulses which are generated and conveyed to the sciatic nerve by the sympathetic and parasympathetic nerve fibers from the anus. Joint disease such as arthritis of the hip or lumbosacral joint often gives rise to referred sciatic nerve pain. Sacroiliac injuries frequently are responsible for acute or chronic sciatic symptoms.

Symptoms and Signs

Pain of sciatica is variable in onset and character (gnawing, shooting, lancinating, or dull). It usually begins in the leg, and may be absent or only slight in the back. Some patients experience numbness along the lateral aspect of the foot. Sciatic pain generally is constant although it may be spasmodic; if due to spinal root involvement it is usually aggravated by coughing, sneezing, or defecation. If the cause is a ruptured intervertebral disk the onset frequently is acute with lancinating pain and an associated sensation of something having given way in the back. In some instances, patients with sciatica do not recall any acute onset and give no history of preceding injury. Frequently, the pain experienced after the acute attack disappears with bed rest, only to return some months later when a slight injury causes recurrence.

Diagnosis

The patient with sciatica should be examined thoroughly since the possible causes are so numerous. In evaluating the history, attention should be given to any injuries, toxins, or infectious or metabolic disturbances that may be present. Injuries causing a tear or sprain of contiguous structures or disk rupture often occur in the course of heavy lifting, falling heavily on the buttocks, or bending far forward. The possibility of excessive exposure to lead also is to be considered. A complete physical examination should include the vagina and rectum to rule out pelvic and anal pathologic conditions. A neurologic examination will aid in establishing the extent and character of the nerve involvement. For example, absent or depressed ankle jerk or hyperesthesia of the lateral aspect of the foot indicates root involvement of the 5th lumbar and 1st sacral nerves. Orthopedic examination should be thoroughly inclusive to determine the presence of muscle atrophy, trigger points, limitation of motion, postural deformities and muscle spasm (*see* Low Back Pain). The Patrick test is useful in determining whether the pain is referred from a hip lesion. The patient lies in the supine position, and is instructed to place the heel of the affected limb above the patella of the other limb and attempt to touch the table with the knee of the affected limb. If the hip is injured the knee remains "hung up" in the air. Injection of trigger points with an anesthetic helps to rule out reflex pain as the cause.

The spine, pelvis, and lower extremities should be X-rayed to discover any abnormalities such as congenital defects, metastatic lesions, or signs of a ruptured disk. Laboratory studies including urinalysis, sedimentation rate, alkaline phosphatase, serologic tests for syphilis, and spinal fluid examination may assist materially in establishing the clinical diagnosis.

Since herniated intervertebral disk is so frequently responsible for sciatica, it should be given immediate consideration. The findings in cases of ruptured disk are extremely variable because the amount of extrusion varies greatly as does the position of the rupture.

Examination of the patient reveals tenderness near the sacroiliac joint and along the course of the sciatic nerve in the buttock, with muscle spasm, absent or reduced Achilles tendon reflex, and a limping gait. Lasègue's sign is positive, i.e., there is no pain on flexing the leg at the knee and the thigh on the abdomen, but pain occurs when an attempt, usually unsuccessful, is made to extend the leg from this position. Scoliosis with convexity to the affected side also is often noted. Patients may have paresthesias and anesthesias along the lateral aspect of the leg and foot, alone or associated with other symptoms. Atrophy of thigh muscles may be detected.

The typical patient with a ruptured intervertebral disk walks with an unnatural flexion of the articulations of the affected limb. Sitting may be more uncomfortable than standing, which he therefore prefers. Upon arising from a sitting position he usually places one hand on the small of his back, keeps the affected extremity flexed, balances on the normal limb, and stands up cautiously (Minor's sign). When attempting to pick up an object, the involved extremity is kept flexed to avoid exacerbation of pain (Neri's sign).

Roentgenographic studies often are helpful, but not completely reliable, since findings may be negative in the early acute stage of ruptured disk, and even in later stages. A positive sign is a decrease in the intervertebral space, with or without a protruded disk as seen on myelographic study.

Treatment

Removal of the cause is basic to the cure of sciatica. Where etiology is undetermined or where conservative therapy is being tried prior to more radical procedures, the following measures are recommended: Strict bed rest on a firm mattress with fracture boards; analgesics (R 1, 2, 6, 7) given temporarily to control pain, with caution to avoid the risk of habituation; immobilization accomplished by adhesive strapping or a well-fitted, properly padded pelvic support or brace; local heat over the course of the nerve applied with electric pad, diathermy, heat lamp, hot water bottle, or sitz bath; a high vitamin diet, with added B complex (*see* Diets). Some benefit may be derived from frequent spraying of the painful area, as often as every 3 hours, with ethyl chloride.

When recent herniation of a disk is suspected, the following manipulative procedure may be cautiously tried a few times since it sometimes causes the disk to be drawn back into its intervertebral position. The thigh is flexed with the knee bent and then the extremity is suddenly pulled straight. If the procedure is successful, bed rest should be maintained for at least 1 week thereafter.

Conservative management of long-standing herniated disk consists of immobilization through continued bed rest, adhesive strapping, or a body brace. Heat in the form of diathermy, heat pads or infrared lamp may be comforting. Surgical excision may finally be required for permanent relief. Excision also is indicated for hypertrophied ligamentum flavum and tumors impinging on or involving the sciatic nerve in its origin or course. Myofascitis and articular strains may be treated by immobilization, application of heat, and, if necessary, infiltration with a local anesthetic. Surgery usually is necessary for spondylolisthesis and congenital anomalies of the spine. Transsection of the muscle or aponeurosis often is necessary to relieve pain caused by pressure from the piriformis muscle or tensor fascia lata. Faulty posture should be corrected by exercises and proper shoes. (For details of treatment *see* chapters devoted to toxic, metabolic, or infectious diseases that may cause a sciatic "neuritis," such as syphilis, tuberculosis, arthritis, vitamin deficiency, diabetes mellitus, multiple sclerosis, lead poisoning, poliomyelitis, pernicious anemia.)

Many therapeutic modalities have been tried with variable success in resistant sciatic pain. Some physicians have reported good results with manipulative procedures, with or without anesthesia. Epidural (caudal) injection of 30 to 60 cc. of a 0.5% solution of procaine has benefited some patients. Other measures that have been tried are block anesthesia of the greater and lesser sciatic nerves, intraneural or perineural injection of 0.5% procaine, and neurolysis or liberation of the nerve.

MULTIPLE NEUROFIBROMAS

(Von Recklinghausen's disease, Neurofibromatosis, Molluscum fibrosum, Multiple neuroma)

A developmental disease, of unknown etiology, which is characterized by multiple tumors of the skin (sometimes localized as a plexiform neuroma), and associated with circumscribed patches of pigment, café au lait spots. The disease often is familial, with the incidence in males slightly greater than in females.

Pathology

The tumors, usually multiple, are soft, pedunculated, sessile, or occasionally plexiform. They occur as localized swellings sometimes in relation to, but not always in the precise course of, the peripheral nerves, spinal roots, cranial nerves, or the cauda equina. The basic tumor is a fibrous new growth initiated by a schwannoglial cell of multiple embryonal potentialities. This parent cell induces the formation of a whorl of fibroblastic cells more or less concentrically around itself.

Symptoms and Signs

Despite the involvement of the nerves, pain, paresthesia, anesthesia, or loss of function is infrequently found, but when present is the result of pressure of the tumors on adjacent organs. Congenital deformities of the skeletal system often are associated with this disease, such as spina bifida, giant growth of limbs, and kyphoscoliosis. Bone lesions may exist in which there is X-ray evidence of central rarefaction and disappearance of bone structure. Cutaneous pigmented areas, ranging from light brown to deep brownish black (*café au lait* spots) are pathognomonic of this disease and represent melanin deposition in the basal cells of the epidermis. These never extend across the midline of the body and may be present without any other manifestations of neurofibromatosis.

Prognosis and Treatment

The disease is essentially benign and the patient usually dies from some other condition; the prognosis should be guarded, however, since complications occasionally may occur from strategically situated tumors or from sarcomatous degeneration. In such instances, and when the tumors are large, painful, or invasive, surgical excision is necessary. No beneficial or prophylactic treatment exists for the general systemic aspects of this developmental disease.

HERPES ZOSTER

(Shingles, Zona, Acute posterior ganglionitis)

An acute infection of the C.N.S. involving primarily the dorsal root ganglia, and characterized clinically by a vesicular eruption and neuralgic pain in the cutaneous areas supplied by peripheral sensory nerves arising in the affected root ganglia.

Etiology, Incidence, and Pathology

Herpes zoster may be primary, in which case the causative

agent is believed to be a virus closely related to that of varicella. However, it occasionally occurs as a complication of poisoning with substances such as carbon monoxide, arsenic, or bismuth. It also may appear in the course of pneumonia, tuberculosis, Hodgkin's disease, or uremia, and sometimes as a complication of other lesions in the vicinity of posterior root ganglia, such as fracture-dislocation of the spine, neoplasms, carcinoma, syphilis, the meningitides, and subarachnoid hemorrhage.

Herpes zoster is more frequent in males than in females, and while it may occur at any age it is most common after the age of 50. It usually appears in early summer and late autumn.

Inflammatory changes occur in the sensory root ganglia, the posterior horn of the gray matter, the meninges, and the dorsal and ventral roots. The cutaneous eruptions are caused by an inflammatory infiltration of the epidermis and dermis, with vesicle formation resulting from serous exudate beneath the stratum corneum.

Symptoms and Signs

In the primary infections, there usually are prodromal symptoms of chills and fever, malaise, and gastrointestinal disturbances for 3 or 4 days, with or without pain along the site of the future eruption. On about the 4th or 5th day the characteristic lesions appear as crops of vesicles on an erythematous base in the cutaneous distribution of one or more posterior root ganglia. The eruptions most often occur in the thoracic region, and spread unilaterally. About the 5th day after their appearance the vesicles begin to dry and scab. One attack apparently confers immunity. Post-herpetic neuralgia may follow, with persistence of pain for months to years. This is most frequent in elderly people. Secondary herpes zoster has no prodromal symptoms, usually shows a bilateral distribution of lesions, and the attack is not followed by immunity.

Geniculate herpes (Ramsay Hunt syndrome) results from involvement of the geniculate ganglion. It is manifested by pain in the ear and vesicular eruptions in the external auditory canal, on the auricle, the soft palate, and anterior pillar of the fauces. There is facial paralysis on the involved side.

Ophthalmic herpes results when the gasserian ganglion is involved. It is manifested by pain and a vesicular eruption in the distribution of the ophthalmic division of the 5th nerve, which may result in ulcerations and opacities of the cornea. Occasionally, there is a 3rd nerve palsy.

Diagnosis

The diagnosis is readily made after the vesicles appear in characteristic distribution, but is difficult in the preeruption stage. The zone of involvement usually is hyperesthetic. It is necessary to distinguish pleurisy, trigeminal neuralgia, Bell's palsy, and in children, chickenpox (q.v.). According to the location of the nerve involved, the pain may resemble that of appendicitis, renal colic, cholelithiasis, or colitis.

Prognosis and Treatment

Most patients recover without any residuals except for scarring of the skin. Post-herpetic neuralgia may persist for years. The facial paralysis usually disappears in geniculate herpes.

There is no specific therapy. Some success has been reported following the use of aureomycin (R 55). Soothing powders or lotions locally are useful. Boric acid or zinc oxide powders (R 46, 47) may be dusted on the lesions and covered by a dry dressing. Collodion dressings (R 48) or application of tincture of benzoin (R 49) are frequently helpful. For ophthalmic herpes the use of a collyrium (R 50), castor oil instillations (R 51), atropine (R 29) and a protective pad are indicated. Recent results with cortisone or ACTH are most encouraging.

Acetylsalicylic acid, alone (R 1) or with codeine (R 4) can be used to relieve pain. The administration of 0.5 to 1 cc. (℔ viii to xv) of posterior pituitary injection (R 61) subcut. during the acute stage sometimes shortens the attack. Procaine block of the nerves supplying the hyperesthetic area may bring relief, and aid in diagnosis. The treatment of post-herpetic neuralgia is difficult. The analgesics usually are unsuccessful and morphine is absolutely contraindicated. X-radiation of the spinal cord and nerve roots or of the gasserian ganglion, by a physician experienced in this procedure, may be effective.

The sensory root of the ganglion may be sectioned as in the treatment of trigeminal neuralgia. In spinal cord involvement, the affected posterior roots may be cut or the spinothalamic tract may be sectioned on the opposite side above the level of the lesion.

PRESCRIPTIONS

(Wherever a prescribed "proprietary" is representative of a class of therapeutic agents, alternative proprietary preparations will be found listed in Part II.)

Analgesics

1. R Acetylsalicylic acid . . . . . 0.3   Gm. (gr. v)
      1 to 3 tablets every 3 or 4 hours.

2. R Codeine phosphate 30   mg. (gr. ss)
      1 or 2 tablets orally or subcut. every 4 hours.

3. R Sodium salicylate (enteric coated) . . . . 0.3   Gm. (gr. v)
      2 tablets 3 or 4 times daily.

4. ℞ Acetylsalicylic acid . . . . . 0.6 Gm. (gr. x)
   Codeine sulfate. . . . . . . 0.03 Gm. (gr. ss)
   1 capsule every 4 hours.

5. ℞ Morphine sulfate
   8 mg. (gr. ⅛) subcut. every 4 to 6 hours as necessary.

6. ℞ Methadone Hydrochloride
   N.N.R. . . . . 5 mg.
   1 tablet every 6 hours.

7. ℞ "Demerol Hydrochloride" . . 50 mg.
   1 tablet every 4 hours.

8. ℞ Acetylsalicylic acid . . . . . 0.22 Gm. (gr. iiiss)
   Acetophenetidin . . . . . . 0.16 Gm. (gr. iiss)
   Caffeine . . . . 0.03 Gm. (gr. ss)
   1 to 3 tablets or capsules every 4 hours for 4 doses.

9. ℞ Caffeine . . . . 0.06 Gm. (gr. i)
   Acetylsalicylic acid . . . . 0.3 Gm. (gr. v)
   1 or 2 capsules every 4 hours for pain.

10. ℞ Caffeine . . . . 0.06 Gm. (gr. i)
    Aminopyrine. . . . . 0.3 Gm. (gr. v)
    1 capsule every 4 hours for pain.

11. ℞ Tetra-ethyl-ammonium chloride
    (vial)
    0.1 to 0.5 Gm. I.V. or I.M.

12. ℞ Trichloroethylene
    20 to 25 drops by inhalation 3 times daily.

Sedatives and Anticonvulsants

13. ℞ Phenobarbital . . . . 30 mg. (gr. ss)
    1 to 3 tablets 1 to 3 times a day.

14. ℞ Chloral hydrate. . . . . . 0.3 Gm. (gr. v)
    3 capsules for restlessness, repeated as necessary.

15. ℞ Paraldehyde . . . . 60.0 cc. (℥ ii)
    Orally: 1 to 2 teaspoons.
    Rectally: 0.5 cc./Kg. body wt. as a 10% solution in cottonseed oil.
    I.M. or I.V.: 1 to 6 cc. (CAUTION! Pulmonary edema.)

16. ℞ Pentobarbital sodium . . . . 0.1 Gm. (gr. iss)
    1 or 2 capsules at bedtime for sleep; may be dissolved in a small amount of water and administered rectally.

17. ℞ Cocaine hydrochloride. . . . 0.09   Gm. (gr. iss)
     Water. . . . . 20.0   cc.   (℥ v)
        1 teaspoon in a glass of water every hour for
        3 or 4 doses if required.

18. ℞ "Amytal Sodium"   (ampul)
        0.5 Gm. (gr. viiss) I.M. or I.V., slowly.

19. ℞ Diphenylhydantoin sodium. . 0.1   Gm. (gr. iss)
        1 capsule 3 to 5 times a day.

20. ℞ "Mesantoin". . . . . 0.1   Gm. (gr. iss)
        1 to 3 tablets 3 times a day.

21. ℞ "Mebaral". . . . . 0.2   Gm. (gr. iii)
        1 tablet 1 to 3 times a day.

22. ℞ Three Bromides Elixir N.F. . 180.0   cc.   (℥ vi)
        1 teaspoon 3 or 4 times a day.

23. ℞ "Tridione". . . . . 0.3   Gm. (gr. v)
        1 or 2 capsules 1 to 3 times a day.

24. ℞ Sodium phenobarbital   (ampul)
        0.06 to 0.8 Gm. (gr. i to xii) subcut., I.M., or
        I.V.

25. ℞ *dl*-Glutamic acid   (bulk powder)
        4 to 10 teaspoons daily in milk given in 3 or 4
        equal doses.

Drugs Affecting the Autonomic Nervous System

26. ℞ Scopolamine (hyoscine) hydro-
        bromide . . . . 0.3   mg.   (gr. 1/200)
        1 to 4 tablets orally or subcut. 3 or 4 times
        daily.

27. ℞ Stramonium Tincture U.S.P. . 60.0   cc.   (℥ ii)
        10 drops 3 times a day, gradually increasing
        the dose to 1 to 1½ teaspoons 3 times daily.

28. ℞ Atropine sulfate . . . . . 0.4   mg.   (gr. 1/150)
        1 or 2 tablets orally or subcut. 3 or 4 times
        daily.

29. ℞ Atropine sulfate, 1% solution . 8.0   cc.   (℥ ii)
        1 or 2 drops in the affected eye once or twice
        a day.

30. ℞ Belladonna Tincture U.S.P. . 60.0   cc.   (℥ ii)
        10 to 25 drops 3 or 4 times daily.

31. ℞ Pilocarpine hydrochloride . . 0.6   mg.   (gr. 1/100)
        1 tablet daily.

32. ℞ Physostigmine (eserine) salicyl-
       ate, 0.25% aqueous solution 15.0   cc.   (ℨ ss)
       1 drop in each eye daily or every other day.

33. ℞ "Mecholyl Chloride"
       Administer by iontophoresis (see CLIN.
       PROC.).

34. ℞ "Mecholyl Chloride" . . . . 0.06   Gm. (gr. i)
       White Petrolatum U.S.P. . . 30.0   Gm. (ℨ i)
       Apply to affected parts without rubbing.

35. ℞ Neostigmine methylsulfate,
       1:2,000 solution   (ampul) . 1.0   cc.   (ℳ xv)
       Contents of 1 ampul subcut. or I.M. 1 to 4
       times daily before meals. Atropine 0.4 mg.
       (gr. 1/150) may be added to the injection to
       lessen the undesirable side effects of neo-
       stigmine.

36. ℞ Neostigmine bromide 15   mg. (gr. ¼)
       1 tablet as necessary.

37. ℞ "Urecholine Chloride" 5   mg.
       2 or 3 tablets as required.

38. ℞ "Doryl"   (ampul)
       0.25 mg. (gr. 1/250) subcut. (never I.V.).

Antispasmodics

39. ℞ Papaverine hydrochloride
       (ampul)
       30 to 60 mg. (gr. ss to i) I.V., repeated in 2
       hours if necessary.

40. ℞ Aminophylline   (ampul)
       0.24 to 0.5 Gm. (gr. iv to viiss) I.V., repeated
       in 2 hours if necessary.

41. ℞ "Octin"   (ampul)
       100 to 150 mg. subcut. or I.M. (never I.V.).
       (CAUTION!   Octin is contraindicated in hy-
       pertensive patients because it may produce a
       further elevation in blood pressure.)

Vasoconstrictors

42. ℞ Dihydroergotamine   (ampul)
       1 mg. (gr. 1/60) subcut., I.M., or I.V., re-
       peated in 1 or 2 hours if necessary.

43. ℞ Ergotamine tartrate   (ampul)
       0.25 mg. (gr. 1/250) subcut. or I.M., repeated
       once in 30 minutes if necessary.

44. ℞ Ergotamine tartrate.   1   mg.   (gr. 1/60)

    5 tablets immediately and 2 tablets every ½ hour if necessary until a total of 9 to 12 tablets has been taken.

45. ℞ Ergotamine tartrate. . . . . .0.002   Gm.   (gr. 1/30)
    Atropine sulfate . . . . . .0.0004 Gm.   (gr. 1/150)
    Cocoa Butter U.S.P. . .q.s. ad 2.0   Gm.   (ℨ ss)

    Insert 1 suppository rectally at onset of attack; repeat in ½ hour and again after 1 hour if necessary.

Emollients and Protectives

46. ℞ Boric acid   (powder)

    Dust on affected area 2 or 3 times a day.

47. ℞ Zinc oxide   (powder)

    Dust on affected area 2 or 3 times a day.

48. ℞ Flexible Collodion U.S.P. . . 15.0   cc.   (ℨ ss)

    Paint on affected areas.

49. ℞ Compound Benzoin Tincture
    U.S.P. . . . . 15.0   cc.   (ℨ ss)

    Paint lesions at angle of mouth.

50. ℞ Boric acid, 2% solution . . 30.0   cc.   (ℨ i)

    Instill several drops in the affected eye as necessary.

51. ℞ Castor Oil U.S.P. . . . . . .   8.0   cc.   (ℨ ii)

    1 drop in the affected eye daily.

Antimicrobial Agents

52. ℞ Procaine penicillin   (vial)

    300,000 u. I.M. daily.

53. ℞ Penicillin   (vial)

    30,000 to 100,000 u. I.M. every 3 hours; for syphilitic meningitis, a minimal total dose of 9.6 million u. is administered I.M. in divided doses every 3 hours over a period of 12 days. For nonsyphilitic meningitis, also, administer 10,000 u. intrathecally once a day (see ANTIBIOTIC THERAPY).

54. ℞ Streptomycin   (vial)

    0.5 Gm. I.M. every 6 hours; the intrathecal dose is 25 to 50 mg. once daily.

55. ℞ Aureomycin   (capsules) . .   0.25   Gm.

    25 to 100 mg./Kg. body wt./day in 4 to 8 equally divided doses.

56. ℞ Sulfadiazine . . . . 0.5   Gm. (gr. viiss)

> 8 tablets initially, followed by 2 tablets every 4 hours until the patient is afebrile for 2 to 5 days. For prophylaxis of meningitis: 4 to 6 tablets daily for 2 or 3 days.

57. ℞ Sodium sulfadiazine   (ampul)

> 30 to 60 mg. (gr. ss to i)/Kg. body wt. daily, administered I.V. in divided doses every 8 or 12 hours as a 5% solution in Water for Injection U.S.P., or subcut. as a 1 to 3% solution.

58. ℞ Anti-Hemophilus Influenzae
     Type B serum (rabbit)   (vial)

> 25 to 100 mg. antibody nitrogen I.M., depending on severity of the disease (see INFLUENZAL MENINGITIS).

Hormones

59. ℞ Testosterone propionate   (vial)

> 25 mg. I.M., 3 times weekly.

60. ℞ Ethinyl estradiol . . . . . . 0.05   mg.

> 1 tablet daily.

61. ℞ Posterior Pituitary Injection
     U.S.P.   (ampul)

> 0.5 to 1 cc. I.M.

62. ℞ Adrenal cortex extract   (vial)

> 500 to 5,000 dog u. subcut., I.M., or I.V.

Analeptics

63. ℞ Amphetamine sulfate 10   mg. (gr. ⅙)

> 1 tablet before breakfast and lunch.

64. ℞ Ephedrine sulfate 25   mg. (gr. ⅜)

> 1 capsule 4 to 6 times a day.

Vitamins and Hematinics

65. ℞ Nicotinic acid (Niacin)   (ampul)

> 100 mg. I.V. 3 times daily. Migraine: Gradually increase the dose from 25 mg. to 100 mg. daily, I.V. After 1 month, replace with ℞ 66.

66. ℞ Nicotinic acid (Niacin) . . . 50   mg.

> 2 to 4 tablets daily (preceded by ℞ 65).

67. ℞ Thiamine hydrochloride . . . 10   mg.

> 3 tablets daily.

68. ℞ Ascorbic acid 50   mg.

> 3 tablets daily.

69. ℞ Dried Yeast U.S.P. . . . . . 0.5 Gm. (gr. viiss)
    1 tablet 3 times a day.

70. ℞ Ferrous sulfate . . . . 0.2 Gm. (gr. iii)
    2 or 3 tablets 3 times daily after meals.

Tonics

71. ℞ Neoarsphenamine (ampul)
    0.4 Gm. (gr. vi) I.V., slowly, at weekly inter-
    vals for 4 to 6 months.

72. ℞ Potassium Arsenite Solution
       U.S.P. (Fowler's Solution) 60.0 cc. (℥ ii)
    1 drop in water 3 times daily, gradually in-
    creasing to 10 drops 3 times a day for 6
    weeks.

73. ℞ Sodium cacodylate . . . . . 60 mg. (gr. i)
    1 capsule daily for 1 month; courses may be
    repeated every other month for an indefinite
    period.

74. ℞ Quinine hydrochloride. . . . 0.3 Gm. (gr. v)
    1 capsule 1 to 6 times daily.

Agents Influencing Fluid and Electrolyte Balance

75. ℞ Potassium chloride, 25% solu-
       tion. . . . . 180.0 cc. (℥ vi)
    For myasthenia gravis: 1 teaspoon 3 to 6
    times a day.
    For familial periodic paralysis: 3 tablespoons
    at onset of attack, then 3 teaspoons 3 or 4
    times daily.

76. ℞ Potassium chloride . . . . . 1.0 Gm. (gr. xv)
       Water for Injection U.S.P. . 50.0 cc. (℥ iss)
    Sterilize by boiling or autoclaving for 30 min-
    utes. Inject slowly I.V.

77. ℞ Ammonium chloride (enteric
       coated) . . . . 0.5 Gm. (gr. viiss)
    12 to 16 tablets daily, in divided doses, for 3
    or 4 days before an expected attack of men-
    strual migraine.

78. ℞ Glucose, 50% solution (ampul)
    25 to 50 cc. I.V.

79. ℞ Calcium lactate. . . . . . . 0.3 Gm. (gr. v)
    6 tablets every 2 hours.

Miscellaneous

80. ℞ Guanidine hydrochloride. . . 0.12   Gm. (gr. ii)

>   Orally: 10 mg./Kg. body wt. initially; sub-
>   sequent doses depending on the patient's
>   needs and the reaction to the last dose.

81. ℞ Glycine (aminoacetic acid)

>   For progressive muscular dystrophy: 3 to 7
>   teaspoons daily in orange or grape juice.
>   For myasthenia gravis: 5 teaspoons 2 or 3
>   times daily.

82. ℞ Apomorphine hydrochloride

>   8 mg. (gr. ⅛) subcut.

83. ℞ Benzyl benzoate . . . . . . 4.0   Gm. (ℨ i)
     Alcohol U.S.P. . . . . 20.0   cc. (ℨ v)

>   1 teaspoon in a glass of cold water, repeated
>   every 2 hours if necessary.

84. ℞ Cascara Sagrada Extract U.S.P. 0.3   Gm. (gr. v)

>   1 or 2 tablets at bedtime.

NEUROPSYCHIATRIC AND PSYCHOSOMATIC

PSYCHOSOMATIC ASPECTS OF MEDICAL PRACTICE

"Psychosomatic" is a relatively new term, coined in an attempt to reunite in medical thinking those inseparable components, psyche and soma, that have somehow suffered an artificial dichotomy. In a limited sense, a psychosomatic disorder is one that can be analyzed and understood only when psychologic as well as physiologic factors are taken into consideration. The functions of the nervous system are unitary and integrated, and while we are accustomed to the concept of voluntary and involuntary nerve reactions, we are not as yet adequately indoctrinated with the fact that a psychic parallel exists; namely, conscious and unconscious ideation. We accept various derangements of the involuntary nervous system as normal accompaniments of conscious fright and worry, such as examination-period anorexia, diarrhea, or vomiting. But we are not oriented to the idea that unconscious emotion, which by its nature is chronic, may exert long-continued similar effects. The fact to be assimilated is that every psychic tendency, i.e., all psychic energy, seeks adequate bodily expression.

Nineteenth-century medical thought was dominated by the concept of cellular disease as leading to structural alteration and thus to physiologic or functional disturbance. This idea has become modified in some situations, namely, essential hypertension and vascular disease. Here, it appears that functional disturbances result in cellular disease and structural change. Now there is a concept that psychologic upset may sometimes antedate and cause functional impairment, which, in turn, may progress to pathologic changes in the cells. As yet we do not understand the functioning of our brain as it receives, retains, and later reactivates impulses transmitted to it from the environment through receptor organs such as the eye and ear. However, that these external impulses result in a more or less permanent functional alteration in the cellular structures within the brain cannot be questioned. To what extent internally originating nervous impulses reaching somatic cells can alter the latter is a question still to be answered.

It is estimated that one-third of a general practitioner's caseload, excluding psychotics, will consist of persons in whom no definite bodily disease can be found to account for their illnesses. Another third will have symptoms that are not explained by, or are out of proportion to, any organic disease that may be discovered. Thus, in two-thirds of his patients the physician must take into account and rectify the mechanism whereby psychic tension finds bodily expression. When the patient has been assured either that he has no physical disease, or that his disability is out of proportion to the disease present, it usually is easy to make him understand that emotional disturbance may be responsible for his physical symptoms. This is best accomplished by citing as examples such psychogenic physiologic disturbances as blushing, goose flesh, palpitation, and diarrhea. The greater the success in switching the conversation from symptoms to personal affairs, the sooner will the real problem disturbing the patient come to light. He should be encouraged to talk about himself as a person rather than as a medical case; to express his fear of cancer or heart disease, or his worry over inability to concentrate, as the case may be. Brought into the open, and with reassurance given, these fears and worries may disappear, and the symptoms with them. Since psychosomatic concepts are merely an extension and application of current knowledge about neuroses to the psychopathology of other conditions previously thought to be in the realm of purely physical medicine, reference to the chapter on the psychoneuroses may be helpful.

NERVOUSNESS AND FATIGUE

Nervousness: *A state of restlessness, mental or bodily, or both.* **Fatigue:** *A subjective state arising from a variety of conditions, not always accompanied by an actual decrease in the body's capacity for work.* Not all patients with fatigability are nervous, and vice versa, but the two symptoms frequently are coexistent.

While the patient may complain that he is easily upset, often he cannot put into words what he means by feeling "nervous."

To him it is an unpleasant, sometimes frightening, experience making it difficult to work or concentrate and causing him to feel anxious and apprehensive. Often he will be restless, fidgety, and easily startled. His facies may reflect irritability, worry, or bewilderment. He may display mannerisms, nail-biting, or tics.

In fatigue, the patient usually reports a disinclination and partial inability to work or even play, and may complain of flagging ambition and interests. His tiredness may come on after little or no exertion. Some patients even after a full night's sleep feel more tired on waking than later in the day.

Etiology, Physiology, and Diagnosis

Like nervousness, susceptibility to fatigue depends on the degree of stability and integration of the whole person. The normal body possesses a comfortable margin of metabolic reserves and develops symptoms of fatigue only after unusually prolonged exertion. Rarely does the fatigability seen in patients result from exhaustion of metabolic reserves. Therefore, pathologic fatigue must be distinguished from normal fatigue. In normal fatigue, rest alone restores the feeling of well-being and capacity for work.

Some of the biochemical disorders that produce pathologic fatigue are recognized (*see* below, and elsewhere in the MANUAL). Normally, the blood constituents are maintained within a narrow range and any variation may cause a patient to feel fatigued and actually reduce his ability to work. The brain is particularly dependent on a continuous and stable supply of O_2 and glucose. Congenital defects of the heart that impair circulation can be responsible for chronic easy fatigability, even without other evidences of circulatory failure. Likewise, anemia or other causes of anoxia may be responsible. Disturbances in carbohydrate metabolism are commonly encountered, e.g., the hypoglycemia due to hyperinsulinism, and the hyperglycemia associated with diabetes mellitus. Disturbances of hydrogen ion concentration, as in acidosis, the amount and character of serum calcium, gross examples of which may be seen in tetany and parathyroid disorders, also are important causes. Deficiency of food proteins in the blood is not infrequent. The accumulation of waste products in the body, such as ketone bodies in diabetes and the protein residues in kidney disorders, may cause chronic fatigability. Chronic alcoholism or the prolonged use of drugs—in particular morphine, cocaine, bromides, and barbiturates—may produce the symptom. Sensitivity to drugs, tobacco, or other substances may be contributory.

Endocrine imbalance often produces pathologic fatigue. Disorders of the thyroid, ovaries, pancreas, and adrenals are the best known causes. Addison's disease is a dramatic example. The role of the pituitary probably is extremely important, but its mechanism in this respect is incompletely known.

Emotional conflicts may produce fatigability and nervousness. Conversely, the physical states causing fatigability may cause nervousness. Both elements may be intermixed. For example, there are apparently healthy people who develop symptoms of fatigue and nervousness if they postpone a meal for as much as an hour or exceed their usual range of physical activity. Often, their symptoms can be relieved by ingesting small amounts of carbohydrate, although such patients do not necessarily have remarkable hypoglycemia when their symptoms occur.

The first problem in diagnosis of nervousness and fatigue is to determine which symptom appeared first. If nervousness clearly appeared before fatigue, the cause probably is psychologic; if fatigability appeared first, tuberculosis, brucellosis, malaria, or other chronic conditions such as dietary deficiencies —lack of vitamins, proteins, or perhaps of saturated fatty acids —must be looked for. An insidiously developing hypothyroidism may produce (without signs of myxedema) insomnia, great fatigability and nervousness, the latter sometimes making it difficult to determine the metabolic rate accurately. In hyperthyroidism, nervousness and myasthenia are characteristic symptoms. A functional disorder of the pancreas or an adenoma involving overgrowth of the islets of Langerhans must be considered, particularly if the symptoms come on before breakfast or 2 or 3 hours after meals. In typical cases it will be found that at these periods the blood sugar falls much below normal. Artificial premature menopause practically always produces nervousness and many of these women never completely recover their former stability or capacity for work. Liver dysfunction usually causes extreme fatigability, which is especially marked in viral hepatitis.

Psychologic components: Mental and emotional difficulties are responsible for nervousness and fatigability in the majority of patients. Neurocirculatory asthenia (q.v.), or effort syndrome, is a striking example. In general, lack of specific goals or plans for the future, and lack of the sense of belonging to a social or family group, can be basic sources. Symptoms may arise only in specific situations. For example, some people will be free of nervous symptoms while on vacation; others may have symptoms only when at home, or when another person, such as an "in-law," is in the home. On the other hand, it may come to a point where there are practically no life situations in which the patient is not nervous. The symptoms in such instances usually are a psychoneurotic (q.v.) response to a situation unconsciously resented.

Each component of the person's development should be investigated to determine whether psychologic conflicts are the leading factor. A normal adult will have passed through or have expected to pass through the following stages of development: (1) independence of his parents, both psychologic and economic; (2) the achievement of a personal status in the community in keeping with his age, family and cultural background, and reasonable ambitions; (3) marriage and parenthood. Failure or frustration in any of these may cause him to be chronically nervous, perhaps without recognizing the source.

Situations under which human beings may become frustrated and maladjusted are too numerous to recount here. Obtaining a pertinent history is something of an art. If a major frustration can be found to have occurred about the time the symptoms first appeared, it is probable that the nervousness and fatigability are largely due to this event. The patient who has unresolved conflicts (sometimes arising in earliest childhood), or has been severely hurt by failure, frequently represses memory of the causative events. Such "forgotten" experiences may virtually become a deep-seated psychic "abscess," filled with emotional tension that finds its only outlet in making the patient feel vaguely uneasy, anxious, tense, guilty, and leading him to compensatory forms of ineffective behavior. He knows there is something wrong, but does not know what. Leading the patient to recall (when this is possible), and freely to discuss the traumatic events may bring remarkable relief from fatigue and nervousness.

All the major psychoses (q.v.) may begin with symptoms of nervousness. Abortive forms of the pathologic depressions in particular must be kept in mind, since these may be manifested only by nervousness, taciturnity, early morning waking, and inability to make decisions. Often, and especially in a manic-depressive psychosis, there will have been similar episodes. The patients may be unaware of their mood swings and, whenever they are unable to work normally, will endeavor to establish a physical reason. To this end, minor and previously symptomless physical disharmonies may be magnified into definite ailments. Nervousness and fatigue may be prominent in the symptomatology of certain neurologic conditions, particularly postencephalitis, the sequelae of head injuries, cerebral syphilis, multiple sclerosis, subacute combined sclerosis, and brain tumors. Except where the physical signs and the laboratory findings are unequivocal, an estimate of the significance of nervousness and fatigue cannot be made without detailed history. Much loss of time and misdirected treatment can be avoided by obtaining one initially.

Prognosis

The prognosis varies with the cause of the upset. When the primary disorder has been relieved, young people usually recover readily while older people may continue to be somewhat nervous and easily fatigued. In patients with constitutional inadequacy (a diagnosis which should be made only after careful deliberation), and in cases where the etiology remains obscure, the probability of improvement is slight.

Treatment

The first step is to relieve the primary disorder. In many mild cases of psychoneurosis the physician can give adequate psychotherapy without help from a specialist. Symptoms often can be relieved by helping the patient to understand the source of his trouble and aiding him in resolving a difficult home situation or making other environmental readjustments.

In patients with nervousness and fatigue, who also have actual or suspected organic disease, it should not hastily be concluded that the organic condition is the sole cause of symptoms. Errors are easily made in connection with suspected or actual minor endocrine disorders: most adolescents with nervousness and fatigue have normal endocrines; malposition of the uterus rarely is an important causative factor, and menstrual irregularities are less commonly caused by endocrine dysfunction than by neurotic disorders. In persons over 35, possibly deficient ovarian or testicular secretions often are mistakenly considered the cause of nervousness and fatigue. The male menopause, as a symptom-producing syndrome, is rare. Therapeutic trials with testosterone are difficult to interpret, except by the use of long alternating control periods with placebos. Ovarian hormone therapy often will afford great relief to those women in menopause who experience nervousness, fatigue, and vasomotor symptoms (flashes, sweats, chills). Except in Addison's disease and hypothyroidism, adrenal cortical extract and thyroid are contraindicated.

Few drugs increase energy without undesirable side effects. The amount of caffeine necessary to relieve fatigue usually increases the nervousness. Amphetamine (℞ 13) may be helpful, particularly in patients who feel most fatigued in the morning or those with moderate nervousness and mental depression. Amphetamine should not be administered before meals or after midday, since it tends to decrease appetite and cause insomnia.

Protracted loss of sleep induces fatigue. Insomniacs often are helped by being told they probably are fighting sleep because of unconscious fear of losing control of self. Certain individuals are benefited by a mild hypnotic (℞ 1) for 2 or 3 successive nights to aid in re-establishing their sleep pattern. However, dependence on hypnotics or sedatives should be avoided if possible.

For nervousness in a high-strung "jittery" person, or during periods of stress in otherwise stable individuals, moderate doses of phenobarbital (℞ 2) may help. Because of the dangers of intoxication (bromism) bromides should not be administered over prolonged periods, in either large or small doses. Older persons may benefit from pre-dinner wine, cocktail, or highball, and perhaps an ounce of whisky at bedtime. In patients with capricious appetite, or on eccentric diets, a therapeutic trial of thiamine (℞ 7), 100 mg. daily, plus a multivitamin preparation (℞ 9) for a minimum of 4 to 6 weeks, may prove beneficial.

THE PSYCHONEUROSES

A group of relatively benign mental disorders that are substitutive reactions in which the symptoms play some concealed but protective role within the mental life of the patient. The term "neurosis" was formerly reserved for certain of these disorders in which the causes of the symptoms were supposed to contain vaguely defined physical components. Such a differentiation is being gradually discontinued, as it now is believed that none of these reactions arises in the absence of troublesome but often unrecognized psychologic factors. The psychoneurotic's external behavior is not upset by his inner experiences in the abnormal manner or to the extent that occurs in the psychoses, in which the capacity for discriminating between reality and subjective experiences may be gravely impaired. Ordinarily, this capacity is not seriously weakened in the psychoneuroses; i.e., the patient's **ego** remains relatively sound. However, the conscious portion of his ego is subjected to emotions, thoughts, or impulses to act, or combinations of these, that to the patient himself seem strange, foreign, and unintelligible, and over which he may be able to exert relatively little control. While the symptoms in the psychoneuroses are for the most part subjective, there may be objective physical manifestations as well. In conversion hysteria, for example, involuntary movements or changes in various bodily functions or sensations may occur. One seldom sees pure hysteria, however, or pure compulsions, or pure phobias, but rather syndromes in which there is a little of each, although one particular phase may predominate sufficiently to warrant a classification. And conscious anxiety is seldom absent from the symptomatology. (The significance of anxiety is discussed under Anxiety Hysteria.) When appraising these reactions, one must remember that borderline and transition cases exist, not only between the various psychoneuroses, but between the neuroses and the psychoses as well.

Classification

The Freudian school's present concept of the symptomatology that characterizes each of the psychoneuroses is in general adhered to in this text. Following an introductory statement, the text will deal with the more common and important psychoneuroses. Treatment of each is not described individually; instead, a brief discussion of psychotherapy and other treatment appears at the end of the entire chapter.

In Freud's original formulation, the instincts were divided into two main groups: the **sex instincts,** which energized all impulses pertaining to love, sex, and procreation; and the **ego instincts,** which were concerned with self-preservation. However, since the ego, which serves as the outer sense organ for the psychic life, is only gradually differentiated after birth, both from internal and external perceptions, the aims formerly assigned to ego instincts now are thought of as derivatives. The energy derived from primitive impulses, thus essentially from the sex instincts, is known as the **libido.** This libidinal energy in particular permeates the **unconscious,** which Freud believes to constitute the most important part of psychic life. The unconscious is not merely a repository for memories tracing back to earliest infancy, but a self-sufficient motivating system which constantly influences behavior. It leads a life of its own in fantasy and is not bound by the facts of reality, thus permitting the existence within it of illogical and totally contradictory ideas, both facts and fantasies, some of which may be in absolute conflict one with the other. The restless libidinal energy gives dynamic force to the unconscious, colors conscious activity and character, and accounts for the emergence of symptoms. Any unconscious idea or **fantasy** that is surcharged with energy constitutes a **complex.** The portion of the **ego** that is conscious stands between the unconscious realm of fantasy and the outer world of reality. Censorship imposes a **resistance** to the emergence from the unconscious of ideas that may engender conscious conflict. The same censorship mechanism may force conflictual conscious ideas into the unconscious, i.e., they undergo **repression.** Such ideas cannot be recalled by any conscious act of will, except with the aid of special technics, thereby differing from ideas that have undergone **suppression.** In evolving his nomenclature, Freud called the unconscious energy system the **id,** and that part of the mind subserving the censorship function the **superego.** The latter derives its attributes from identification with the parent's ideas of behavior, which become incorporated as an actual part of the child's developing personality. Since the greatest portion of the superego is unconscious, these ideas determine the pattern the individual thereafter is more or less obliged to follow. The **ego-ideal,** also a portion of the superego, is an idealized image of what one would like to be. A small conscious portion of the superego is experienced as **conscience.**

The primitive psychic energy, or libido, not only pervades the unconscious, but may be projected outward onto persons or things **(object libido),** or it may invest the ego as an object **(narcissism),** or remain fixed at certain levels of development. In the last phase of development (the **genital),** the libido comes to invest the procreative organs. By the **Oedipus com-**

plex is understood a hostile genital desire to replace the parent of the same sex in the affections of the parent of the opposite sex. By **castration complex** is meant the infantile idea that a genital, or phallic, loss has been sustained, or the fear of such loss, generally tinged with feelings of guilt.

Arrest of the libido at certain stages of development is known as **fixation.** Such a fixation, usually only partial, may take place at the **oral, anal,** or **urethral** phases of infantile development, which collectively are called **pregenital** stages. Any later shifting back of the libido in the unconscious to points of infantile fixation is called **regression,** a state in which the more recently acquired, or more adult, points of view are left somewhat deenergized, while concepts that existed in infancy or childhood become suffused anew by the libido and may again become dominant.

To a large extent, every neurotic person presents traits characteristic of a child. He is sensitive, suggestible, introspective, likes to indulge in fantasy, and may be difficult to get along with. He feels inadequate and inferior although his attempts to compensate for this may create an opposite impression. He is afraid to be alone, brooks little interference, craves attention, and is closely attached to his family even though he quarrels with them. He wants to talk of his illness constantly, and resents his sufferings being taken lightly. Having rather intense likes and dislikes, he forms either strong attachments or none at all. Most often the daughter is tied to the father, and the son to the mother. Frequently, these patients are ceremonious about food or other things. Although ostentatiously ardent in courtship, the male often is impotent, the female anesthetic or even frigid. In brief, the unconscious conflict resulting from persistent infantile trends and immature psychosexual development, when acted upon by the environment, may lead to severe frustration and thus to neurosis.

Usually, an adult's neurosis has been preceded by a prolonged or evanescent neurosis in childhood or adolescence. Suggestive symptoms in childhood are enuresis, disturbances of speech, nightmares over a prolonged period, crying out during sleep, food idiosyncracies, delirium accompanying slight rises in temperature, destructiveness, temper tantrums, excitability, undue phobias or compulsions, shyness, nail-biting and sleepwalking. Most children exhibit some of these symptoms at one time or another and many of them will escape a later neurosis. Nevertheless, such symptoms always constitute a danger signal.

Most, but by no means all, adult neuroses begin between late adolescence and age 35, a period which a vulnerable personality may find laden with reminiscent disappointments and frustrations. To understand and treat these illnesses it is necessary to know the events within the family that can be traumatic in the life of a child, and to search for current life experiences which the adult patient unconsciously interprets as a repetition

of them. A universal repugnance against recognizing that the
husband or wife, on deep unconscious levels, represents a substitute for the father or mother creates difficulties for the physician and patient alike in comparing similarities between adult
and childhood experience. But one can in no other way ap-
preciate, for example, that a married woman's illness may arise
because the husband does not fulfill her fantasied demands
based on some childhood love image, usually the father; or that
an unmarried person's neurosis following a parent's second marriage may arise because of unconscious disappointment. The
unconscious hostility and subsequent feelings of guilt engendered by such disappointments, neither consciously knowable
nor expressible, are potent forces in continuing the reactivated
conflicts. An unwanted pregnancy, a husband's temporary displacement in the wife's affection following the birth of a child,
actual or threatened financial insecurity, or a job demanding
aggressiveness, diverse as such factors are, may echo real or
fantasied deprivations in childhood. Society, or a boss, or a
spouse can to all appearances deliberately let one down, frus-
trate one, make unreasonable demands, no less than one's
parents ostensibly did in childhood. One mechanism deserves
special emphasis: an unconscious longing for continuation of
the infant-like passivity and dependency is readily awakened
during physical incapacitation, even in a normal individual.
On the other hand, a person in whom such unconscious long-
ings have always been strong but disavowed, and who has
developed conscious reactive character traits to deny their
existence (such as extreme self-sufficiency or contempt for
weakness) may, under the same circumstances, display fool-
hardy disregard for his symptoms.

The physician is not justified in considering symptoms as
psychoneurotic unless psychogenic factors sufficient to explain
them are discovered. In other words, merely being unable to
discover any "physical" explanation for the patient's complaints does not necessarily mean that a psychoneurosis exists.

ANXIETY HYSTERIA

(Anxiety states; Anxiety neurosis)

*A condition characterized by more or less constant appre-
hensive expectations, tension, sometimes fatigue, with acute
panic-like exacerbations of anxiety, perhaps accompanied by
sweating, palpitation and other physical manifestations of acute
fear.*

Etiology; Personality Structure; Mechanisms; the Sig-
nificance of Anxiety in the Neuroses

The problem within the psyche of handling anxiety is becoming increasingly recognized as the basis of psychogenic illnesses.
This anxiety is of 3 main types: (1) that of the infant, due

34

to his psychic helplessness; (2) that occurring later in life when some environmental situation threatens a return to this state of infantile helplessness (e.g., economic distress), designated as ego-anxiety; (3) that resulting from fear of bodily harm or mutilation, called castration anxiety. Anxiety occurs when an individual finds himself trapped between two opposing forces—an increase of unrelieved instinctual tension and a fear that something disastrous will happen if he attempts to relieve that tension, even though an opportunity to do so exists. When the personality becomes organized into an adult-like pattern, at about 6 years of age, the ego thenceforth defends itself against any recognition that unconscious impulses exist, much less the rigidly prohibited ones. (All memories that are of any actual significance concerning the first 5½ to 6 years of life undergo repression into the unconscious.) If certain unconscious impulses remain unduly energized, however, their insistent demand for recognition usually creates a forewarning conscious tension and anxiety. The various psychic symptoms of the several types of psychoneuroses in particular represent the mechanisms of defense available to the ego against suffering this anxiety. In addition, the average psyche does not tolerate other than nominal anxiety without regression, i.e., a shift of the libido back to earlier stages of personality evolution. This shift usually succeeds, however, only in awakening even less manageable conflicts.

It is the child's nature, no less than the adult's, to react to frustrations with aggressive and hostile fantasies, which in turn awaken fears of reprisal and consequent anxiety, since the child believes that the world operates according to the Mosaic law, "an eye for an eye, and a tooth for a tooth." Forbidding him to explore his genitals, for example, may be considered by the child as a threat of genital mutilation (castration anxiety), or merely ignoring his curiosity or aggressiveness may cause him to believe that these traits are considered "bad." The child's task is threefold: simultaneously to cope with his instinctual energies, to retain the love of those around him, and to keep his resultant anxiety within a limit he can tolerate without using psychopathologic methods to control it. Thus, he requires a parental definition of limits, sketched with tolerance and good will, whereby he learns that thoughts and fantasies, of themselves, are not dangerous, and what latitude of actual aggressiveness he is allowed. (A child feels great anxiety when his aggressiveness is unrestrained; under these circumstances his own aggressive and other instinctual impulses are perceived as a threat even to himself.) Otherwise he must define his own limits for himself and, having no other recourse, may impose too rigid concepts of behavior upon himself in forming his superego structure, accepting as a guide his own perhaps fantastic ideas of "good" and "bad." He thus becomes a candidate for a subsequent anxiety neurosis, and this is perhaps the most common type of personality organization that underlies such neuroses. (Paradoxically, an opposite situation also is found in anxiety neuroses; namely, a too lenient superego. However, this idea will not be developed in this text.)

Individuals such as the above develop into overconscientious persons who are afraid to make mistakes or otherwise compromise their self-imposed high standards. Imbued with a sense of insecurity and inadequacy, and inclined toward tenseness and uneasiness, they are particularly sensitive to financial insecurity, to disturbances in interpersonal relationships, and to sexual difficulties, such as premature ejaculation, coitus interruptus, or marital infidelity. These frustrations readily awaken their old unconscious conflicts and prohibited impulses, e.g., hostile or aggressive wishes.

In attempting to deflect anxiety from consciousness, many patients with anxiety neuroses sooner or later adopt the mechanism of phobia formation, of course without realizing it. In dreams, animals often represent those human beings whom the dreamer conceives to be all-powerful and hence dangerous in relation to himself; a relationship that even adults may believe in their unconscious to exist between themselves and persons of authority—a heritage from their childhood fantasies about their parents. By a similar symbolization, and by the mechanism of projection, an animal (e.g., horse, dog, cat), or object (e.g., germ, brass, silver), or situation (e.g., crowds, closed or open spaces, heights), may come to represent for the patient his insistent unconscious desires and wishes, which have been condemned by his superego. If the phobic animal or situation now is avoided, the fear and dread of retaliation for those wishes is magically circumvented. If a phobia's protective magic gradually lessens, additional phobias may be necessary; their gradual numerical increase in anxiety hysteria is not unusual.

Symptoms

Anxiety attacks frequently occur in childhood, also around the time of puberty, or may appear at any subsequent time. Nocturnal attacks may be preceded by nightmares, the content of which may or may not be remembered. Attacks also may occur in daytime, without warning. Unformulated dread, or fear of an impending calamity such as death or insanity, may be the dominant ideation. These episodes sometimes last only a few minutes. Any of the physiologic accompaniments of fear may be manifest, including vomiting, diarrhea, urinary urgency, and widespread vasomotor disturbances. Unconscious conflicts and anxiety sometimes play an important role in aggravating or possibly initiating organic disorders, particularly bronchial asthma, peptic ulcer, chronic colitis, enteritis, and heart disease, especially coronary artery disease. As previously stated, the patient may gradually acquire many phobias, including erythrophobia (the fear of blushing).

Diagnosis

Anxiety is prominent in many psychotic disorders (particularly latent schizophrenia), often is associated with somatic illness or toxic states, and is frequent in all the psychoneuroses. The differentiation usually is not difficult if the attacks are circumscribed. If there are phobias, an obsessive-compulsive neurosis also must be considered. A patient may misinterpret attacks of anxiety as indicating heart disease, although his heart is functionally sound.

Prognosis

This tends to vary according to the duration of symptoms before the institution of adequate psychotherapy. No one (child, adolescent, or adult) outgrows a pathologic anxiety state. Although phobias sometimes disappear spontaneously this usually occurs only at the expense of a personality reorganization of a type that jeopardizes future adjustments. Some of these patients require months of intensive psychotherapy, while others respond more rapidly.

NEURASTHENIA

A term reserved for a triad of complaints: fatigue, somatic discomfort, and mild mood disturbances. **Hypochondria,** classified by Freud as a separate psychoneurosis, is the insistent and protracted preoccupation with organs or functions which the patient may believe incurably diseased. It is closely akin to neurasthenia in etiology, and will not be discussed separately. As a descriptive term, hypochondria is commonly employed in a much less specific sense, referring to a tendency to show mild symptoms of this nature.

Etiology; Personality Structure; Mechanisms

The neurasthenic's abnormal preoccupation with self probably extends back to earliest infancy. A baby's physical care may be excellent, yet be carried out with a lack of interest, e.g., absence of warm fondling, which communicates itself to him. His libido, or instinctual energy, can at first have no object other than himself; he is totally narcissistic, incapable of interest in others, and largely occupied with pleasure in himself. Normally, his libidinal energies gradually invest the images of persons in his environment, particularly the parents'. If the infant is frustrated in making these transfers in the ways normal for him—one of which is believed to be his infantile "masturbation" and its accompanying fantasies (an impulse toward a repetitious self-manipulation of the genitals regularly occurs in infants, especially during the nursing period and the years from 3 to 6)—then the majority of his libidinal energy remains centered on himself. In later years, his own moods and bodily sensations (muscular, visceral and cutaneous) not only receive his careful ideational attention, but also may be intensified through being unduly suffused with libidinal energy. Since these individuals continue to be incapable of finding normal pleasure in environmental objects, in a very real sense they are early deprived of any pleasure in living.

Many neurasthenic patients are shy, awkward, and lack self-confidence, exhibiting irresolution, indecision and irascibility. Others are critical, dissatisfied, envious and resentful. Not uncommonly a tendency to projection is noted, i.e., the patient unjustly blames contemporaries for his misfortunes. Many patients develop a complaining attitude and take pleasure in finding fault with and annoying others.

Symptoms

Neurasthenia often is described as a state of irritable weakness. Fatigue, a subjective sense of weakness and exhaustion, is the most common symptom; it paralyzes efficiency and may be a strong factor in making the patient believe that he is organically ill. Psychic tensions express themselves as worry about physical organs and processes. Disturbances in the vasomotor functions (e.g., blushing, sweating, cold extremities) and cardiac functions (e.g., palpitation, tachycardia, extrasystoles) result from instability of the vegetative nervous system. The somatic discomforts may be many and varied. Frequent symptoms are anorexia, discomfort after meals, gaseous eructations, and constipation, which may alternate with diarrhea. Gastric secretions and motility may be altered. Mucous colitis frequently occurs. There may be various types of headache or a sensation of bandlike cranial pressure, backache, dizziness, or spots before the eyes. Impaired potency, premature ejaculations, nocturnal emissions and failure at coitus alarm and distress the male, who magnifies the significance of these symptoms. Masturbation is common and may or may not be accompanied by conscious conflict.

Irritability and mild depression are the most frequent mood disturbances. The patients may be unable to concentrate or make decisions. Many are introspective and gloomy. Anxiety may or may not be conspicuous. Disturbing dreams and broken sleep are common.

Diagnosis

Neurasthenia must be differentiated from all the conditions discussed under Nervousness and Fatigue (q.v.). The syndromes most important to exclude are psychotic depressions, schizophrenia, early paresis or tuberculosis, hypo- and hyperthyroidism, blood dyscrasias, peptic ulcers, neoplasms, Addison's disease, and chronic brucellosis, although there are many others. In the psychotic depressions, the depression usually is more intense, the patient's ability to test reality may be seriously impaired, and he may believe that he is ill because he has sinned, hence is worthless and doomed (especially in involutional melancholia). Many mild cases of manic-depressive psychosis are misdiagnosed as neurasthenia. In this psychosis the periods of depression are episodic, while depression in neurasthenia tends to be more continuous, with the patient concerned about his health even when comparatively happy. The schizophrenic usually does not have so many physical complaints, and sooner or later some of these can be recognized as obviously delusional. In addition, the schizophrenic displays poverty of affect; i.e., the emotions accompanying his ideations are inappropriate in degree and sometimes in kind. For instance, he may display apathy toward objectively distressful circumstances in his life.

Prognosis

Some neurasthenic and hypochondriac individuals approach the psychotic in psychic structure, which makes the prognosis grave. All are serious psychotherapeutic problems. Certain so-called "acute" cases, occurring in individuals who previously were without symptoms and fairly efficient socially, may become readjusted with a minimum of psychotherapy.

CONVERSION HYSTERIA
(Major hysteria)

A condition characterized by a tremendous variety of physical or psychic symptoms, or both, that serve to defend the ego from recognition of unconscious instinctual wishes which threaten to erupt into consciousness, and also act as substitute gratifications for those wishes. (The patient thus manages to retain self-respect while accomplishing his unconscious wish or purpose.)

Etiology; Personality Structure; Mechanisms

The individual who later may develop conversion hysteria seemingly never is able completely to relinquish all unconscious possessive (incestuous) love for the parent of the opposite sex. Such persons are apt to return in fantasy to this attachment when they meet with some environmental situation that frustrates them libidinally. And in so doing, their infantile wishes, hostilities, and guilt feelings are re-energized. The deprivations that precipitate the conversion hysteric's symptoms usually are much more readily detected than in the other neuroses. With women these will most often be connected directly with the sex life, while with men other factors may be more apparent, particularly threats to self-esteem such as may arise from the economic struggle.

Exhibitionistic and other infantile character traits often characterize these individuals. Frequently, they are given to histrionic poses and pathos, even to suicidal gestures, and often are abnormally suggestible. They remain egocentric, although on the surface they may be open, friendly and, particularly with the opposite sex, seductive, since usually they are voracious for attention and love. They are changeable, however, in their own affections because of their inability to love in an adult altruistic way. Sensitive to frustrations, they often feel inferior and may occupy much of their time with daydreams that serve to bolster their own sense of importance but which obviously partially disregard reality.

In conversion hysteria, conscious perception of anxiety sometimes is completely prevented because of the effectiveness with which the unconscious conflictual energy is discharged either through a dissociated portion of the personality, as in some variety of automatism, or through its canalization along lower nervous pathways, i.e., the somatic (*see* Symptoms, below). This absence of conscious anxiety probably accounts for the serene indifference displayed by some conversion hysterics toward their various neurotic symptoms.

Symptoms and Signs

Gross simulation of virtually any pathologic state may occur with hysteria, hence only representative phenomena will be outlined here. (1) **Sensory:** Perversion of sensations (e.g., tingling, formication) and anesthesia are common. Bilateral contracture of the field of vision may occur; or complete blindness, usually unilateral. Pains simulating the various types of headache, structural diseases of the spine (sometimes followed by actual curvature), peptic ulcers, appendicitis, joint diseases, or peripheral neuritis can occur. (2) **Motor:** Either spastic or flaccid monoplegia, hemiplegia, or paraplegia may develop, with or without contractures. Astasia-abasia, or inability to walk or stand, no longer is a common symptom in hysteria. The occupational neuroses, such as writer's cramp, are hysterical reactions; also some tics, tremors, and spasms, viz., certain instances of blepharospasm or torticollis. Hysterical convulsive seizures may occur, as well as aphonia and mutism. Hyperventilation leading to tetany sometimes is seen. (3) **Visceral:** Nausea, vomiting, hiccups, and dysmenorrhea may be conversion symptoms; also boulimia (excessive appetite); pseudocyesis (simulated pregnancy, with amenorrhea); aerophagia (air swallowing); constipation, diarrhea, and urinary retention. (4) **Vasomotor:** Local or generalized vasoconstriction and vasodilatation are common. Areas of edema have been described, but rarely. Anal and genital pruritus are occasionally of hysterical origin. (5) **Psychic:** Hysterical dissociations of personality are frequent. When a motor activity is carried out in the waking state without the patient's awareness it is called an **automatism.** When a secondary portion of the personality assumes motivational control of the organism either for moments or years, with subsequent amnesia for the episode, this is called a **fugue.** Closely akin to the fugue is **somnambulism,** except that the patient is sleeping. In addition **cataleptic** (i.e., trance) **states** may occur, either spontaneously or following a hysterical convulsion. These simulate profound sleep and may last for weeks, during which the deep reflexes may be absent, and involuntary micturition and defecation may occur. Impotence, frigidity, and vaginismus (q.v.) frequently are of hysterical origin, as are hallucinations. Amnesia, either circumscribed, retrograde, or anterograde (continuing since some particular date), may be present. The so-called traumatic or war neuroses usually represent hysteria. Frequently in these the original trauma is relived partially or totally in dreams, and often with distortions. In addition, the patients display irritability, impairment of memory, and depression, and many complain of headache and dizziness.

Diagnosis

Conversion hysteria must be differentiated from organic disorders, malingering, the other neuroses, and schizophrenia. Usually, the hysterical person's motor or sensory disturbances are not consistent with anatomic structure; e.g., an anesthesia stopping exactly in the midline or with "glove" distribution. There is no true clonus or Babinski reflex with hysterical spastic paralysis, nor are there bladder symptoms or tendency to bedsores with hysterical paraplegia. With hysterical flaccid paralysis, the maintenance of normal muscular electric reactions is diagnostic. In hysterical mutism, the patient cannot whisper, which differentiates it from aphonia (also not rare in hysteria), but he can communicate by writing, which the aphasic patient cannot do. Total blindness of hysterical origin can be differentiated by the EEG. The organically ill patient readily accepts a suggestion that his symptoms are of emotional origin, and hopes it is true, while the hysterical individual resents and rejects it. In the malingerer, obvious contradictions, discrepancies, and exaggerations of the symptoms are usual. The schizophrenic does not show the easily shifting emotions displayed by the hysteric. Also, with schizophrenia (q.v.) there is a tendency toward disturbances in associations (flow of ideas) and deterioration of habits; e.g., of dress or cleanliness. The onset of hysterical symptoms coincidental with an acute emotional state is significant, as is the hysteric's customary indifference to his symptoms.

Prognosis

The symptoms of conversion hysteria usually can be rapidly relieved, but they tend to recur either in the same or another form. Intensive psychotherapy for weeks or months may be necessary to preclude these recurrences. The prognosis for actual cure is better than in any of the other neuroses.

COMPULSION NEUROSES
(Compulsive states, Obsessional neuroses, Obsessive-Compulsive neuroses, Psychasthenia)

A condition in which the patient feels compelled to think, feel, or do something that he recognizes as irrational. When the neurosis is so severe as to verge on the psychotic, this recognition may be partially lost. An urgent impulse to think certain thoughts is an **obsession;** to perform certain acts, a **compulsion.** With this psychoneurosis, in contrast to the others, the manifestations are limited almost entirely to phenomena in the psychologic (i.e., mental) realm.

Etiology; Personality Structure; Mechanisms

The partial fixations of libido that serve as the groundwork for these neuroses appear to result from traumas during the period when the child's interests are focused on anal functions. At a certain point it is demanded that he voluntarily control his defecations. In order to retain and even increase love from his mother, he attempts to do so. This demand may be made before the child is physiologically capable of complying, or during a period when he feels that his psychologic recompense (i.e., love from his mother) is insufficient. At this stage the child's thoughts are to him magical, omnipotent things, and to wish that his mother would "go away," i.e., desist from her demands, also is to fear that she will do so. (Later, this child's first concept of death will be that a person "goes away," and thus retroactively his earlier wishes may assume for him a new and guilt-laden significance. During psychoanalysis, obsessions and compulsions often are found to aim at the protection of persons whose death the patient unconsciously wishes.) Consequently, any defiance of this bowel training by the child creates enormous anxiety for him, as does the hostility he feels when reproved for lack of control. Normally, his hostility and anxiety are not greater than he can tolerate if this training is properly handled, but otherwise he is forced to utilize pathologic efforts to control it. He may develop a neurosis forthwith, or he may "fix" his anxiety through evolving reactive, i.e., opposite, character traits, and thus become the antithesis of an aggressive-sadistic and uncontrolled individual.

A large portion of compulsive neurotics are meticulous, precise, self-conscious, overconscientious, and perhaps shy, individuals. Usually, they are orderly, penurious, feel inadequate and insecure, and clutch at reassurance and support. Often of superior intellectual capacity, they rarely attain their highest possible efficiency because so much psychic energy is dissipated in their mental conflicts. In any executive capacity, in the home or elsewhere, it is difficult for them to delegate work or authority since they must meticulously review all details.

Both obsessions and compulsions serve an identical purpose

—the partial expression of an unconscious wish and, simultaneously, a magic expiation for it. **Ambivalence** (the urge to do versus the urge not to do) is at its height in this neurosis. This is because these patients' harsh superego, the internalized parental image, makes the ego miserable in the effort to discharge any unconscious instinctual energy, however "normal" or innocuous may be the impulses it motivates. Isolation and undoing are two other mechanisms seen in this neurosis. **Isolation:** Ideations that otherwise would be extremely objectionable, such as murder and incest wishes, may become conscious as obsessions, because the patient is able to feel them as mere thoughts. Through isolation the emotions concerned with them have been displaced onto other material. **Undoing:** With repetition compulsions, one purpose is to reverse or deny the secret unconscious meaning of the compulsive act. By repeating the act there is a magical undoing of its meaning. As the neurosis progresses the patient may have to repeat the act several times to accomplish this.

Symptoms and Signs

This neurosis may become the most torturing of neurotic illnesses. Although the patient may regard his obsessive thoughts, doubts, or compulsive acts as silly, needless and purposeless, he suffers intolerable tension if he does not carry them out. A woman may be obsessed by the idea that she may murder her child, or a man that he may infect his family with deadly bacteria. Obscene thoughts may horrify a prudish person; or blasphemous thoughts or obsessive doubts about the existence of God, a religious individual. Another patient may have an idea that he is changing in appearance, which necessitates constant scrutiny of himself in a mirror. These or other compulsive ceremonials may occupy much of a patient's time. One individual may have to undress in a certain way; another to sleep in a certain position; others must touch all telegraph poles and step on all twigs on the sidewalk.

Kleptomania (impulse to steal), pyromania (to set fires), dipsomania (to drink), and exhibitionism (to expose the body), may be compulsive in nature. Almost any thought or act can become compulsive, including sexually perverse ones. Phobias are also encountered in this neurosis.

A compulsion neurosis may occur at any age, and is not infrequent in young children and the aged. The neurosis tends to be episodic, but may fluctuate only in intensity. However, remissions that last for moments to months are not uncommon.

Diagnosis

Schizophrenia, manic-depressive psychoses and certain organic nervous illnesses that may release compulsive phenomena, such as paresis or encephalitis lethargica, must be differentiated. Sometimes what initially was considered only an obsessive-compulsive tension state becomes recognizable as a frank schizophrenia, usually of paranoid type. A patient's failure to regard his thoughts or acts as absurd, as well as a tendency to attribute them to outside influences, indicates schizophrenia; less rumination (reweighing some idea endlessly) and greater tension indicate the neurosis. The fact that the neurosis may undergo remissions and may be accompanied by depression, and that a patient with a manic-depressive psychosis may display obsessions, makes this differentiation important. Obsessions almost always precede the depression in a neurosis, while the reverse is true in a psychosis.

Prognosis

Types of therapy that leave the unconscious processes untouched have no effect on a compulsion neurosis and the prognosis always is serious. Nevertheless, these patients often derive considerable relief merely from discussing their symptoms with their physician, since they unconsciously interpret this as a parental absolution of their guilt. The acute cases beginning in adolescents or adults may be modifiable by means of psychoanalysis, while those existing from childhood often are unchangeable. With this neurosis, spontaneous remission should not be mistaken for cure.

TREATMENT OF THE PSYCHONEUROSES

When adequate tests have excluded organic disorders as a cause of the patient's illness, and where history-taking interviews have yielded information to justify it, the patient may be told that his symptoms probably are due to psychic conflicts, perhaps mostly unconscious, and that anxiety and other emotions are interfering with his bodily functions and straight thinking. For many reasons important to both physician and patient, it will be wise to secure a psychiatrist's opinion of the case and to turn over to him the treatment if he concurs in the diagnosis. Where such arrangement is impracticable, however, the physician's only recourse is to deal with the case as best he can, and often he will be able to do a creditable job, particularly if the neurosis is of recent onset and not too severe. In order to do this, however, he must be able to listen to the patient sympathetically and uncritically, at once with detachment and acute awareness, and to maintain an attitude of courtesy and benevolence. Furthermore, he should neither resent nor fear the patient's feelings of hostility, discouragement, or dissatisfaction toward him, for if he does it will be intuitively recognized by the patient, who will be unable to cope with this counterhostility. It must be remembered that the neurotic individual fears not only his own but other people's emotions and thoughts, since he retains feelings of omnipotence in his own mental life from his childhood fear that to think is to act. Yet it is essential for effective psychotherapy that he freely express his thoughts and thus re-experience his fears, so that as his insight increases he can see that his unconscious hates, desires and loves are not a danger to himself or others except as they influence his own ego, call forth within it abnormal mechanisms of defense and attitudes that disturb his interpersonal relationships, and thus rob him of his rightful zest in living. That psychotherapy may be and usually is painful for the recipient should be kept constantly in mind by the physician and made clear to the patient at the beginning.

In brief, unsatisfactory, haphazard interviews, perhaps scattered over a period of years, a physician probably will spend more time with the patient than if he adopts a regular plan of treatment at the outset. With a planned schedule, the patient can be encouraged not only to review between sessions his patterns of reaction, including attitudes toward himself and others, but also to jot down material for discussion with the physician during the next interview. In the early phases of therapy, when the physician's aim is to gain an estimate of the total personality, such a routine is particularly helpful. However, thereafter unrehearsed productions are usually encouraged, and significant material will eventually come to light if the patient is allowed sufficient time and a tactful atmosphere in which to talk.

The objective of any psychotherapy a general physician attempts to give will be simply to aid the patient toward an easier and more comfortable adjustment to his environment. Although in a sense such therapy is superficial, one can capably guide it only by understanding the ego's mechanisms of defense, and by realizing the nature of the conflicts (some of which have been outlined) that may underlie the patient's symptoms. Otherwise the physician attempts to navigate without sextant, radar, or rudder. Only with an occasional and most unusual patient will he meet a situation in which it will be desirable for him to explain to the patient the deeper unconscious conflicts that cause the symptoms, even though these may be obvious. For, merely to outline (i.e., verbalize) these to the patient probably would do him little good (and might do irreparable harm), since in general it is one's emotional response to the environment that determines adjustment, rather than reason, i.e., intellectualization. Our feelings are what cause us to label events as dangerous, desirable, or pleasurable, and thus they dictate what we are to believe or disbelieve concerning both our own inner impulses and the world outside. Thus an interpretation in therapy that the patient rejects or ignores today may be accepted within 1, 2, or even 6 months. This occurs because the emotions responsible for its initial rejection are no longer conceived by the patient to be the only possible response he can make to the situation. The therapist's role, therefore, is to serve as a trusted point of reference as the patient gradually acquires beliefs more in keeping with an adult's concept of reality, and thus ceases to permit his own infantile ideas and emotions to guide him. Therefore, the therapist should do any mental probing only with great caution, and should for the most part let the patient take the lead in the discussions. At the same time, the patient should be constantly encouraged to make comparisons between ever earlier ideas and emotions relating to significant persons in his past environment and his present-day reactions. (A psychoanalyst often accurately estimates the trend and perhaps the actual content of a patient's conflicts months before touching upon it in therapeutic sessions, which he usually does only when the patient himself begins to discern these factors. In the interim, however, the patient's emotional reorientation to situations at ever deeper mental levels has been progressing.)

Some of the material necessary for the physician and patient to review together, so that each may gradually discover the source of the patient's illness, are: (1) family background, including temperaments of parents or parental substitutes; (2) history of early development; (3) past and present attitudes about all family members; (4) school adjustments, such as attitudes toward teachers, schoolmates, and extramural activities; (5) sexual adjustments, including fantasies, fears, worries about sex; (6) mood reactions, whether serious or cheerful, placid or quick-tempered; how the patient reacts to success or failure in others; how he works best, whether in seclusion or in company; (7) social adaptability, including patterns of friendships; reaction to criticism or losing; whether overmodest or overconfident, egoistic or altruistic; (8) general neurotic tendencies, including circumstances that bring on uneasiness; whether the individual is a constant user of drugs; whether he is insistent about order and routine and is overconscientious, superstitious, or overfond of gambling; if there are any thoughts, acts, or habits that act as sources of remorse, doubt, or worry; what his reaction to illness has been; and whether the patient has special interest in some particular philosophy or cult.

By the time this review has been completed, the physician will have discerned certain of the patient's habitual idiosyncratic responses, and can ask for more detail as to the circumstances that call them forth. In some sessions the patient may seem unwilling to talk, and it is wiser not to prod him. These silences usually are motivated unconsciously, although the patient probably will secretly rationalize that he is deliberately holding back. He may thus unconsciously test whether his therapist is "really" interested in him; i.e., whether he really must fear the therapist, or really can depend on him. Sometimes the patient's more significant ideas will be suddenly divulged after 2, 3, or more of such apparently sterile sessions, meaning that he has gradually overcome specific inner resist-ances and fears. On the other hand, he may talk continuously for many sessions before he begins to recognize that his glibness represents a flight from the ideas that are of true significance in his illness.

The force that operates in all psychotherapy (even in the so-called "bedside manner") can be appreciated only through understanding the transference mechanism, which is the intrinsic tool of psychoanalysis. (It is because the physician usually is identified in the patient's unconscious with the magical, all-powerful, and inherently protective father-image, that the physician's attitudes often produce significant differences in the response of a patient even in physical illnesses; e.g., extreme ineptitude in handling a specifically sensitized individual could awaken and reinforce his dormant aggression against himself and suicide-like desires for death.) Almost all of us are inclined to misinterpret the present in terms of the past; i.e., we "transfer" past attitudes to the present. The patient with a neurosis, though not recognizing his motivation, strives to relive his past, and particularly his childhood, more satisfactorily. Thus he is prone to identify persons in his environment with pivotal persons in his childhood; consequently, his adult associates may be startled, for example, by his incongruous dependency, love, or hostility toward them. In psychonalysis, an identical phenomenon occurs, the patient transferring his love and hostilities onto his analyst, whom he may concomitantly or alternately identify unconsciously as his father, mother, brother, or other person, especially one intimately associated with his childhood. An analyst's reaction to such emotional demands by the patient should be identical with his reaction to the patient's attitudes toward others: he interprets these to the patient at propitious moments and attempts to point out the unconscious impulses from which they spring. When the patient can gradually begin to feel that the analyst's interpretations are true (i.e., can accept them emotionally), these emotions will become detached from their infantile associations, which thus will lose all power to motivate him. Once this has been accomplished, the patient will no longer need his symptoms as a defense against these childhood impulses. Although the general physician seldom, if ever, explains to the patient the similar emotional transfers onto himself, his own knowledge of them will minimize his vexation when the patient displays apparently unjustified anger, fear, or love toward him.

The neurotic patient cannot realize, of course, that his symptoms constitute a "primary gain" for himself by saving him from facing up to his inner disturbing fantasies and desires. What usually precipitates his illness is this: Some adverse external event occurs which he unconsciously interprets, not as a transient frustration, but as the beginning of a constant frustration of some unconscious longing. In other words, the patient was already unduly vulnerable to his environment (a normal person can also become ill if he undergoes too much stress) solely because of his own demands upon it. This may be an unconscious demand for attention, or a longing for dependency, or an aim to "incorporate" and thus enslave, a loved one, or a fear of responsibility or of aggression. Also, it is well to recall that the average psyche does not tolerate anxiety without regression, i.e., a shift of the libido back to earlier stages of personality evolution, which usually succeeds, however, only in awakening even less manageable conflicts (*see* introduction to the PSYCHONEUROSES; *also*, Anxiety Hysteria). With many neurasthenic individuals, one may readily sense their longing, almost demand, for dependency, which is understandable when the basis for their illness is recalled; as is the hysteric's sensitivity to the normal stresses and strains of marriage. Probably all physicians have seen hysterical paralyses relieved by suggestion, perhaps with the adjunctive use of faradic sparks or other noisy mechanical device which, of course, is resorted to only as a face-saving expedient for the patient's ego.

Hypnotism is useful to alleviate hysterical symptoms and can be safely attempted by any physician who will limit himself to giving therapeutic suggestions about symptoms and not attempt deep probing for information. Experienced psychotherapists sometimes use hypnotism, or drugs such as Sodium Amytal (R 6), to procure not-readily-recallable information from a patient. This method was particularly useful with some of the acute war neuroses, but only an expert should attempt it.

For the analyst the patient's dreams constitute an extremely valuable means of discovering his unconscious mentation (through his "free associations" about them), but considerable study and experience are necessary before a general physician can utilize the patient's dreams therapeutically. However, asking the patient routinely to describe his dreams is an excellent method for convincing him, by analogy, that strata of meaningful activity operate beneath his conscious awareness, and also for gaining experience about the language of dreams.

Freud's *Introductory Lectures,* summarizing the types of observational data upon which the psychoanalytical theory rests, can be of assistance to the physician in understanding both normals and neurotics. That man in the aggregate and individually is difficult to civilize was a conclusion Freud's observations forced upon him. The fact is inescapable that each human being contains within himself the same potentials for aggression as are inherent in the race, as reflected in man's dominance over all other forms of life, and in his wars, prejudices, and other aptitudes for intersocial conflict. Impulses toward matricide, patricide, fratricide, incest, and the like, and the mental and social conflicts engendered by them, constitute the theme of much of our classical literature. These themes we can accept and enjoy for the reason that such impulses within ourselves, as heritages from our formative years, are so stringently repressed from our own conscious awareness. And further, our secular laws, in prescribing punishment for actions but not for thoughts, recognize (1) that we feel free to fantasize doing many things we dare not express in action and (2) that we could hardly prevent these thoughts even though we would wish to do so. On the contrary, an individual's superego may interdict and proceed against certain of his unconscious fantasies without such discrimination. In psychotherapy, therefore, it is necessary to accept the philosophy that a patient's spontaneous wit, "free associations," slips of tongue, behavioral attitudes, and inexpedient acts usually reveal more about his unconscious motivations than do his conversation and other premeditated verbal expression, in which these unconscious impulses are inevitably concealed from self-discernment.

Self-centeredness is the infant's natural condition, and human beings learn to conform and to give only through first learning that in no other way can they consistently receive environmental support and approval. Thus, the therapist must recognize that a man may unconsciously resent his children because he is immature and has not progressed beyond his original self-centered condition; that the death-wish against her child which causes a pregnant woman to attempt abortion may in some form continue to operate after the child is born, one possible outcome being to create a ruinous maternal overprotectiveness; and that a daughter-in-law and mother-in-law antipathy may be merely a revival of Oedipal jealousies. The physician must realize that such situations are not unique, and further that our outstanding traits often are directly opposite to our unconscious drives. This comprehension is necessary if he is to lead the patient to see the relationship of his unconscious mental life to his symptoms.

Drugs, at least those currently available, have no place in treatment of neuroses, except occasionally to relieve insomnia or temporarily to allay anxiety. Indiscriminately used, they tend to ally themselves with the neurosis. That is, they prevent the patient from taking the step of recognizing that psychotherapy is not a passive experience and that he must aid himself, with the physician's help. Also diets, periods of rest, and other management devices that may be necessary for the patient's physical well-being during psychotherapy should be unmistakably labeled for the patient as not being treatment for his neurosis, but merely palliative and supportive measures. Finally, it should be remembered that associated but unrelated physical ills may exist concurrently with the neurosis, and must receive appropriate treatment.

Some psychiatrists occasionally use electroshock therapy (q.v.) as an emergency measure in a severe neurosis, but administer only 1 or 2 treatments and these usually only in preparation for psychotherapy, the purpose being to allay the patient's anxiety temporarily. Electronarcosis (by allowing a small current to flow continuously for several minutes following the convulsion) is another experimental therapeutic approach in mental illness, especially in the psychoses. Needless to say, only an expert should decide upon and conduct such technical procedures.

THE PSYCHOSES

Any mental disorder, including the psychoneurotic reactions, involves the total personality and extends to its depths. In the psychoses, however, the disturbance is of such magnitude that the mind is distorted more or less in entirety. The conscious portion of the **ego** no longer functions efficiently in its role of recognizing the source of at least some of the impulses that reach and pervade it. In one degree or another, therefore, it accepts as environmentally authentic material that actually is ideational. Thus the psychotic displays inability to correct his misconceptions about what is real and what is unreal.

Except that it includes the senile, presenile, and arteriosclerotic psychoses, this section deals only with those psychoses that are presumed to arise solely from intrapersonality conflict: schizophrenia, paranoia, and paranoid conditions, the manic-depressive psychoses, and the involutional psychoses. Numerous other causes for psychoses exist, such as specific infections, including syphilis, epidemic encephalitis, acute chorea, and tuberculous, epidemic cerebrospinal, or other forms of meningitis. Other causes are alcoholism, convulsive disorders (e.g., epilepsy), brain tumor, metabolic disease, trauma, and drugs and other exogenous toxins. This last group of substances includes mercury, manganese, carbon disulfide, carbon monoxide, opium and its derivatives, bromides, cocaine, the barbituric acid group, peyote, mescaline, belladonna, chloral, and paraldehyde. Many of these reactions are adequately described elsewhere in the MANUAL (q.v.). Delirium is a temporary psychosis. Patients with mental deficiency or a so-called psychopathic personality may develop a psychosis, often displaying atypical manic-depressive or schizophrenic reactions. There is little doubt that in most instances the "psychopath" is as he is because of his environment, and he and the feebleminded individual may become psychotic because of continuing environmental stress.

SCHIZOPHRENIA
(Dementia praecox)

The term "schizophrenia" means *splitting of the mind,* which is more descriptive of this condition than early or precocious dementia, as implied by the term "dementia praecox." Dementia, an irreparable impairment of cognitive and intellectual functions, does not occur with this condition. Rather, schizophrenia may be considered as a psychobiologic reaction that arises on the basis of personality inadequacies, and results in an inability to meet the demands of adult adjustment. The reaction is characterized by progressive withdrawal from contact with persons and activities in the environment and regression to a childlike or infantile type of feeling or acting. An inferior affective capacity is one of the important results when the personality becomes disorganized or split in schizophrenia. This is displayed as an inadequate and inappropriate emotional response to situations, and represents a deterioration of emotional expression.

Etiology, Incidence, and Predisposing Factors

Schizophrenia constitutes from 15 to 20% of the first admissions to public mental hospitals, and 60% of their permanent population. The age of onset ranges from childhood to late middle life, but the psychosis is most frequent in adolescence or early adult life.

No constant or characteristic structural or biochemical change has yet been established in this condition. That the causes of schizophrenia are to be searched for in the individual's basic personality and the extent or limit of its adaptive power is the most generally accepted concept today. Childhood conditioning experiences, intrapsychic conflicts, persistent but consciously rejected instinctive urges and drives, feelings of insecurity or guilt, and other long-standing troublesome problems and frustrated purposes, in one combination or another, must be considered as potent precipitating forces.

Schizophrenia often represents only an extreme expression of the patient's previous schizoid type of temperament and personality. The contrasting poles of this type are sensitiveness on the one hand, and dullness or coldness on the other. The sensitive schizoid is timid and shy, self-conscious, perhaps stubborn and suspicious, and often dissatisfied; he is constantly being wounded. Reserved and socially inept, he may find in books a substitute for human companionship. The subjects he chooses usually are not of concrete objective type, but rather of abstract nature. He frequently is ambitious, conscientious, particular, and perfectionistic. Other schizoids lack the finer sensibilities of the group above. Many of these lack spontaneity and appear colorless personalities. This group varies from kindly, honest, but emotionally dull, unsociable and uncompromising individuals, to cold, reserved, and callous types.

Prodromal Stage

Frequently there is no abrupt transition, but rather an in-

sidious change in mood and outlook. Long-existing disharmonies of thought, habit and interest become accentuated. The
individual may seem preoccupied, be considered lazy, and may
begin to believe others are talking about him or do not care for
him. Such **ideas of reference** are common. He may become
restless, taciturn, or ill at ease, yet appear unworried about odd
mannerisms that make their appearance. Some ruminate on
sexual topics and others on hypochondriacal ideas. At this
stage the conflicts are not greatly disguised and may often be
discovered without difficulty.

The Manifest Psychosis

An apparent poverty and increased disharmony in the feeling
tone of the individual now may appear. However, some patients show not an absence of mood, but a prevailing one, such
as euphoria or depression. But these moods will generally be
found to have little or no relation to conscious mental content
and none to external circumstances. Not infrequently, the
opposite emotional response will be evoked by an idea or experience—an **emotional dissociation** or **disconnection.**

Since schizophrenia may be considered as a reaction characterized by introversion, or the direction of the individual's
energy and interests upon himself and his subjective life, and
by the expression of rejected material through symbolism,
one expects and finds no disturbance in consciousness or memory, and so none of orientation. The patient's intellect is inert
rather than impaired.

The affect, or feeling tone, having been withdrawn from conscious mental assets and attached to complexes and other material in the unconscious, and being therefore inaccessible to
the individual, the patient often feels changed throughout.
He may come to feel he observes, as a spectator, his own actions
which seem to him impersonal and mechanical. Such states of
depersonalization are not uncommon. In his attempt to rationalize this sense of the loss of the limits of his own personality, his **nihilistic ideas** may increase until he feels he is dead,
or no longer has a body, or that there is no world.

Paralogia, a condition in which the reply to one's question
indicates that it has been understood, although the answer because of defective reasoning, is erroneous, is due to the **dereistic
thinking** which occupies much of the schizophrenic's attention. Symbols and associations, molded by unconscious instinctive drives and affects, rise into consciousness and constitute **dereistic,** or **dreamlike thinking,** a pleasurable thinking that disregards realistic, logical, and scientific concepts and
thus tends to falsify reality.

Often, the dominant ideational content of the schizophrenic
is delusional in nature. The **delusions** tend to center around
themes of persecution, or grandiosity, and of sex. While these
often appear grotesque, apparently they always are specific and

adapted to the peculiar psychologic needs of the individual.

Normally, associations and ideas progress with logical connection on to ultimate completeness of thought, but in the schizophrenic they may be so fragmented and shortened, or otherwise distorted, as to appear illogical. In early schizophrenia, a **flight of ideas** may occur; this later tends to develop into incoherence. **Neologisms,** or coined words, probably represent extreme condensations and symbolizations of complexes, conflicts, and other unconscious material highly charged with affect. **Blocking,** or sudden cessation of a thought—and its verbal expression—is one of the hallmarks of schizophrenia, and presumably occurs when the patient's thoughts approach affectively overcharged and forbidden psychological ground. The train of thought abruptly terminates and cannot be reinitiated.

Hallucinations, the projection of inner experiences on to the external world, are frequent, and in no other mental disorder appear so frequently in the presence of clear consciousness. These are most frequently auditory. Visual hallucinations tend to be limited to the acute phase of the disease.

The capricious, impulsive behavior of the schizophrenic probably is to be looked upon as an **ambivalence of impulse.** His conflicting impulses, some conscious, some unconscious, control behavior in erratic sequence, or even struggle simultaneously to direct it. This conflict may result in acts directly opposite to those suggested to the individual. This reaction, as well as **increased suggestibility** whereby the individual follows out each suggestion immediately, **echolalia,** and **echopraxia,** the latter two meaning, respectively, repetition of words spoken to him and repetition of the acts of another person—all common in varying degrees in schizophrenics—may be interpreted as defense reactions against the intrusion of the disavowed environment.

Activity mannerisms may occupy a large place in the clinical picture. They consist of stereotyped (without variation) affectations of manner, speech, and gait; of grimaces, tic-like movements, puckering out of the mouth or wrinkling the forehead, and, in many instances, of elaborate and ritualistic routines of behavior.

With such disorder and disequilibrium manifest in the mental life of the patient, it is not surprising to find a certain physical disequilibrium often accompanying schizophrenia. This may be manifested in cold, cyanotic extremities, or blotchy skin and widely dilated pupils. Seizures may occur, especially in the early stages. Some patients show a lowered metabolism. During acute phases, many schizophrenics lose weight.

Clinical Types

As transitions from one type to another often occur during different phases of the psychosis, the present tendency among psychiatrists is not to attempt to divide schizophrenia into the various classic types. However, these are descriptively important.

1. Simple: Manifested by a gradual and insidious change in personality, with increasingly pronounced disturbances in emotion, interest, and activity. If hallucinations occur they are fleeting. Delusions play no important role. Interest is withdrawn from the external world and there is a diminished response to social demands. Varied degrees of this deviation may appear. Many such persons become tramps, vagrants, delinquents, or prostitutes. Apathy, preoccupation, and inactivity characterize many hospitalized individuals of this type.

2. Hebephrenic: There is a tendency to include under this classification cases not readily fitting into other groups. The ideational content of the hebephrenic tends toward fantasy, with fragmentary rather than elaborate or systematized delusions. Hallucinations are frequent, associations are markedly loose, speech is incoherent, emotional reactions are shallow and incongruous, and regressive features (soiling, wetting), and a certain silliness of response and action, often predominate. The patient becomes bafflingly inaccessible. The disintegration of personality is perhaps greater than with any of the other types.

3. Catatonic: Characterized by phases of stupor and excitement, frequently alternating suddenly, although any given catatonic episode may consist of only one phase. The catatonic form frequently has its onset, which may be acute, between the ages of 15 and 25; and more often than the other types is precipitated by an emotionally disturbing experience. The prognosis for recovery and reintegration of personality is more favorable than in other types, but after several episodes the condition tends to become chronic.

Patients in **catatonic stupor** show increasing inattention, preoccupation, emotional poverty, dreaminess, and frequently progress to mutism. Inattention to their bodily needs, refusal to eat, and retention of saliva, urine, and feces are common. Negativism, gesturing, grimacing, and immobility may supervene and extend for a period of extremely variable duration. The patient slowly or at times suddenly emerges from this stuporous phase. He then may become virtually normal or may pass into a state of catatonic excitement.

A form of catatonia characterized by impulsive, often stereotyped, overactivity so largely motivated from within as to appear purposeless is called **catatonic excitement.** The patient may appear delirious or be sleepless and thus rapidly exhaust himself. Negativism and destructiveness may be observed. The speech may vary from mutism to a rapid pressing flow.

4. Paranoid: Delusions which are illogical and unrelated to reality, hallucinations, and the usual schizophrenic disturbances in associations and affects, together with negativism, are the most prominent symptoms in this group. This type tends to make its frank appearance in persons 30 to 35 years of age. Delusions of persecution are the chief manifestation, but depressive, hypochondriacal, or fantastically expansive, obviously wish-fulfilling, ideas are common.

Prognosis

A permanent disorganization of personality does not invariably result from a schizophrenic episode. Not only the catatonic, but also the other forms may be episodic in character; frequently, however, the course of the disease ultimately becomes uninterrupted. Patients may recover with little "scarring," but careful observation generally detects slight losses in spontaneity, in sense of humor or elasticity of personality, and a dulling of affectivity. If the psychosis represents an insidious development from a previously distorted personality and its inherent characteristics, the prognosis usually is poor. Consequently, the "mildness" of early symptoms bears no relation to ultimate outcome. In the simple type, the prognosis is not good, and the course of the hebephrenic form tends to be progressive. In the catatonic type many of the patients are restored to their prepsychotic level for varying lengths of time. The paranoid type is considered particularly malignant, although remissions which may be looked upon as social recoveries do occur.

Diagnosis

Schizophrenia in its initial stages must be differentiated from hysteria, compulsion neurosis, and manic-depressive psychosis (q.v.). Various conditions such as thyrotoxicosis, fevers, kidney or heart disease, toxemia of pregnancy, may precipitate a latent schizophrenia or a delirioid state resembling this disorder. Carefully appraising the patient's prepsychotic personality often helps in such differentiations.

In hysteria, the patient's psychologic motive more often is apparent, the symptoms are paroxysmal and more sudden in onset; and, unlike the schizophrenic, where normal and psychotic elements exist side by side, the hysteric shows an alternation of normal and psychotic. In hysteria, the symbolization is conventional and intelligible, while in schizophrenia the use of symbols is individualized and archaic.

Compulsion neurosis: A patient with a compulsion neurosis consciously strongly resists his obsessions and compulsions, while the schizophrenic tends to display increasing apathetic unconcern. (The schizophrenic's hypochondriacal complaints lack the dramatization seen in the psychoneuroses.)

Manic-depressive psychosis: This frequently is most difficult to differentiate. The onset of schizophrenia tends to be more insidious, and the excitement paroxysmal rather than sustained as in the manic. The quality of infectiousness about the mood of the manic is lacking. The schizophrenic's delusions are more grotesque and create less tension. More often than the reverse, a psychosis at first thought to be a manic-depressive episode subsequently proves to be schizophrenic.

Treatment

Psychotherapy: According to some authorities a schizophrenic illness is to be viewed as a repudiation by the patient of an imagined hostile environment. To demonstrate that his conception rests on an unreal basis, it is necessary that the schizophrenic be supported by sincere and patient friendliness until he can gain insight into the fact that his illness has arisen because of his own misinterpretations. The objective is to stimulate his attention, detach his emotions from subjective material, redirect his interests to things outside himself, inculcate healthful social habits, and abstract him from his spiritual isolation. Important aids are occupational therapy, congenial companionships, and a carefully planned recreational program. The patient's distorted ideas should not be refuted, but accepted without critical comment or perhaps with an observation that they probably will change or have a different significance to him as he recovers from his illness. As the patient improves he may be allowed to interpret his own ideas, but this is not specifically encouraged. For, except by a skilled therapist, only extremely superficial interpretations can safely be given, since the psychologic significance of his psychotic ideas might be overwhelmingly traumatic to the patient.

Insulin therapy: This treatment is suitable only for institutionalized patients, since constant supervision is required. Insulin (℞ 14), 10 to 20 u., subcut. is given on the first day and increased by 5 to 10 u. on each succeeding day until signs of severe shock appear. (Food, of course, is withheld during the preceding several hours.) Coma is occasionally produced by a dose of 40 u., but most patients require 80 to 90 u. Subsequently a smaller amount may have the same effect, and it is wise to reduce the dose by 5 to 10 u. from time to time to test the effect. Shock treatments, at a rate of 5 to 6 times a week, may have to be continued until 65 or 70 have been given, but favorable cases often respond by or before the 50th treatment. In discontinuing the therapy, the dose is tapered off by a reduction of 20 to 40 u./day.

Wet, dry, and convulsive types of insulin shock are encountered. (1) Wet shock, the most common, starts with sweating, hunger, sleepiness, slurred speech, and confusion. Coma follows and a Babinski sign appears, to be replaced later in case of extreme shock by a general areflexia that includes loss of the pupillary light reflex. (2) Dry shock is practically the same except that the patient perspires very little. (3) In the convulsive type generalized clonic movements are characteristic.

Extreme caution must be observed when patients characteristically respond with convulsions, which may occur at any
time between the onset of hypoglycemia and full waking. Provided the total period of hypoglycemia has not exceeded 6
hours, an uncomplicated shock may be continued for 2 to 3
hours.

Shock is terminated by administering glucose. If the patient
is in light shock and able to swallow, he is given 2 Gm. of glucose by mouth for each unit of insulin previously administered
that day. Otherwise, 300 Gm. or more of glucose in a 25%
solution is given by nasal tube; or in extreme cases, 25 to 50
cc. of 50% glucose I.V. (R 19). Epinephrine (R 20), 0.3 to 0.5
cc. of a 1:1,000 solution subcut., occasionally is administered to
speed arousal after the glucose is given. Upon regaining consciousness, the patient must immediately take additional carbohydrates by mouth (usually several slices of bread). A car-
bohydrate-rich meal is given as soon as the patient is fully
conscious. Throughout the course of therapy a high caloric
(4,000 to 5,000 C. daily), high vitamin diet is prescribed (see
DIETS).

Insulin shock therapy is attended by many dangers, among
which are after-shock (a relapse into unconsciousness, perhaps
many hours later), prolonged coma, severe convulsions, and extreme vasomotor or circulatory collapse.

Convulsive shock therapy: Electroshock has largely supplanted Metrazol for producing these therapeutic convulsions,
as it is less terrifying to the patient, is equally or more efficacious therapeutically, and produces fewer fractures. Further
electroshock treatments are usually contraindicated if a patient
has not improved with 20 convulsions. Schizophrenic patients
often become extremely disturbed after several convulsions,
which ordinarily precludes the use of this form of therapy unless
the patient is hospitalized. The relative value of insulin and
electroshock therapy in schizophrenia has not yet been statistically determined, but there is some indication that insulin
may prove to give lasting benefit more frequently, especially in
the paranoid type. (For details about electroshock therapy see
Involutional Melancholia.)

PARANOIA AND PARANOID CONDITIONS

Classic paranoia, which is rarely if ever seen, is a psychosis
in which a circumscribed delusional system exists without
dilapidation of conation, affect, or associative processes. (By
conation is meant the instinctually motivated striving aspects
of the personality that are more or less beyond volitional control.) In its less strict and more modern sense, paranoia also
describes any personality reaction characterized by the mechanisms of projection and compensation. To understand many
normal as well as psychotic manifestations, familiarity with
the nature of these mechanisms is necessary. They may be

employed to excess in practically all psychoses, but usually are only incidental or transitory except in classic paranoia, paranoid conditions, and paranoid schizophrenia. The paranoid conditions range by imperceptible gradations from classic paranoia on to the state of disorganization seen in paranoid schizophrenia. Step by step, from patient to patient, a greater admixture of schizophrenic features is seen. This is reflected in inadequate affective responses, increasingly disorganized associations, and the symbolization and projection of mental material as hallucinations. In all of these reactions there is a tendency for what is troublesome within to be projected outward in ideational and verbal form. A patient with paranoid psychosis carries to extremes the normal methods of maintaining self-esteem; i.e., by blaming others for his own failures, denying the possession of those of his traits that he dislikes, and by overcoming his feelings of insecurity with various compensatory strivings.

Etiology

The personality aspects from which paranoia arises are: the need to shield particularly sensitive portions of thought-life, hunger for a recognition that cannot be achieved, and the fears and guilt feelings these conflicts and strivings evoke. Character anomalies become continuous with the psychosis; both are based on the habitual way in which the patient reacts to his inner conflicts and outer adversities. Sexual conflicts, often unconscious, usually are operative. Homosexual tendencies, normal at certain ages and stages of development, either reawakened or never fully relinquished and unconsciously craving expression, are perhaps basic. Freud's description of this mechanism is that the man cannot admit to conscious recognition the existence of his unconscious "I love him"; to be admissible he could only say "I hate him," but this does not solve the conflict. Eventually, the unconscious thought is projected and finally enters consciousness—as a subjectively valid interpretation of environmental happenings—in the distorted form "he hates me," to which later is added "he persecutes me." It is then but one further ruminative step to the patient's conscious belief that he is important else he would not thus be singled out for attention. Grandiosity begins. (Grandiose and persecutory ideas almost always go hand in hand.) Perhaps the more rigid the personality and therefore the less possible the recognition that conflicts exist in any part of the psyche, the nearer the symptoms will approach those of classic paranoia. Conversely, the nearer the conflicts come to conscious recognition, and hence more dangerous to the ego, the nearer will the symptoms approach those of schizophrenia. (Sometimes an individual's intellectual and emotional acceptance of and coming to terms with his homosexuality may prevent—with proper psychotherapy—a schizophrenic dissolution of personality.) In a woman, conscience-dictated frustrations of heterosexual urges may cause discontent, tension, and a general sense of dissatisfaction to such an extent that regression takes place and homosexual conflicts are awakened. She may either believe she is persecuted by women or, working out her conflict on a heterosexual plane, by men; or else that some important man—perhaps her physician—loves her and their union is being prevented only by her enemies.

Symptoms

The history may reveal that as a child the patient was especially needful of appreciation; was moody, resentful of school and parental discipline; was unable to form good play adjustments, and perhaps suspicious. A compensatory striving toward superiority may have resulted. In the growing-up stage, the rigidity and tendency toward pride may have increased, as well as the patient's inherent sensitiveness to the attitude of others toward him. Before the psychosis becomes manifest, prodromal symptoms sometimes occur. Perhaps numerous situations have caused the patient to react with wounded and bitter pride. He analyzes his moods and sensations, may become hypochrondriacal, is more reserved, and withdraws from attempts to discuss his problems. He displays sullen quietness, behind which lurks haughty disdain. Periods of moody dreaminess occur. Suddenly or gradually the conception may be born that his failures have been due to the enmity of others. Now he sees new and hidden significance in commonplace events: people deliberately slight him; his situation is endangered; he experiences vague fears and becomes increasingly resentful. All suspicions are vigorously defended. Hallucinations may or may not occur; however, either through hallucinations or ideation, he comes to feel important. Perhaps now he assumes the caricatured mien of the individual he thinks himself to be. The exalted paranoic may believe himself a chosen one of God —perhaps a reincarnation of Christ. He may develop a humble air, grow a beard, exhibit idiosyncrasies in clothing, and picture himself as tolerant and understanding. He believes he would be serene were he not constantly molested. Affect determines his logic. He reinterprets past events through retrospective falsification and these falsifications consolidate his new evaluations. The litigious type, probably an individual who always had been defensive about his "rights," after some legal action having resulted unsatisfactorily, may launch further lawsuits. His drive is to prove himself right and others wrong, rather than the desire for justice he expresses. By these activities sensitive insecurity is protected.

Another patient may believe himself loved by some wealthy or powerful woman. He writes to her; her failure to reply is to test his love. He may see symbols in the sky, or birds may chirp in an unusual fashion to show him he is loved. In other cases, sexual impotence may represent a paranoid defensive pattern; this shields the patient from conscious knowledge of his fundamental conflicts. Or dissatisfactions with self may be projected as the wife's discontent, and thus lead to delusions of her infidelity. Deafness in insecure persons often facilitates paranoid reactions. Their seclusiveness, suspiciousness, and proneness to misinterpret others' actions often are overcompensated by extreme aggressiveness. *Folie à deux,* a mental disorder in which two intimately associated persons develop the same paranoid ideas, is explained by the responsiveness of the weaker and more submissive to the stronger. Generally the "infected" individual relinquishes his delusions when separated from the other. *Folie à deux* is not infrequent between man and wife, but is more frequent between sisters or brothers, or any two individuals with the same background.

The paranoiac usually has superior intellectual endowments, which in fact are necessary for his rationalizations. Excessive use of this mechanism almost is a hallmark of the condition. His prolonged tense and expectant affective state stimulates attention, he sees connections where none actually exist, and at times his concepts are rationalized into an extensive delusional system.

Diagnosis

So-called **acute paranoia** is discussed under the manic-depressive psychoses (q.v.). In paranoia the ideas are more sustained and are supported by a less changeable affect, in contrast to the usual vacillations in the manic. Since the mental operations are only exaggerations of normal mechanisms, at times it is difficult to differentiate the nonpsychotic paranoiac from the psychotic paranoiac. The patient must be deemed psychotic if the reaction is continuous, if his beliefs cannot be corrected, if they tend to spread, and if they are completely illogical. Classifying these reactions as approximating either the paranoic or the schizophrenic pole is aided by evaluating the degree of disturbance in the individual's contacts with reality. The more the repressed material comes into consciousness as hallucinations and the more archaic the form of adjustment, the nearer the reaction approaches schizophrenia.

Prognosis

Patients with classic paranoia or those with reactions closely approximating it, probably never recover; however, they may not require hospitalization. The patients' conduct often remains within bounds, society looks upon them as "cranks," they rarely act without reflection, and therefore avoid commitment more often than patients with schizophrenic-like reactions. Remissions may occur in the latter types, but the ultimate prognosis nevertheless is poor.

Treatment

Whether the patient is to remain free in the community is determined by his potential danger to others. If delusions are directed against specific persons, confinement is probably necessary; the greater the expressed hatred the more imperative is commitment. In all dealings with paranoid patients—schizophrenic or otherwise—scrupulous honesty and truthfulness are necessary. Often the patient will follow reasonable suggestions and greatly modify his behavior. The physician may become his one confidant. Despite contrary appearances, the paranoiac and schizophrenic crave love, as they live inwardly in a cold and colorless solitude to which they have withdrawn not through choice but from unconscious motivation. Healthy human companionships have come to appear unattainable and, through fear of their own aggressiveness, dangerous. They withdraw to their citadel only after—to them—endless frustrations. Hence, tolerance on the part of the physician, a philosophic detachment combined with a justified humility, a sense of humor about his own ineptness as well as the patients' peccadillos, discretion, understanding, and warmth, are the tools used to ease the paranoiacs' tensions, to help them achieve calmer environmental adjustments, and to bring some serenity, transient though it may be, into the lives of these sometimes turbulent and always troubled individuals. Even slight deafness in a paranoid individual should be corrected, if possible; otherwise the use of a hearing aid should be insisted upon. Help in unraveling the family problems or irritating work situations are representative ways by which the physician may be able to aid his patient.

Drugs play only an incidental and not a curative role in managing and treating these patients. Extreme tension may be somewhat allayed with phenobarbital (R 2), 30 mg. (gr. ss) 3 times daily, and occasionally a mild hypnotic such as Amytal (R 3), 0.1 to 0.3 Gm. (gr. iss to v) at bedtime, may be indicated if the patient suffers from protracted insomnia.

MANIC-DEPRESSIVE PSYCHOSES

The term **affectivity** means the basal tone of the feeling life, and the manic-depressive psychoses are called **affective psychoses** because the patient's ideas, actions, and feeling tones are in harmonious agreement. Classically, the disorder is characterized by alternating periods of mania and depression, but some patients exhibit only one phase, which may be either depression or elation. An occasional patient may have only 1 or 2 attacks during his lifetime, but periodic recurrences are the rule.

Etiology and Incidence

If the disease is initiated by a manic episode, it most frequently occurs between the ages of 15 and 25; if by a depressive episode, between 25 and 35. Its incidence is greatest among the higher social and professional group, and twice as great in women as in men. An estimated one-third of siblings of patients with the disorder become affected; thus, presumably heredity plays a role. However, factors of environment may be of primary importance, as a child can incorporate his parents' traits through emulation and identification. The psychosis usually occurs in individuals with a "cyclothymic" temperament, which may be described under 3 subdivisions. The **hypomanic** is outgoing, vivacious, optimistic, and easily swayed by new impressions. His superficial judgment often leads to failures; for these he has ready excuses. Some hypomanics are hypercritical, domineering, and argumentative. The **syntonic** is the "normal" cyclothyme. He is genial, sociable, uncomplicated, and a practical realist. He radiates a certain warmth and ease. The **melancholic** often is quiet, kindly, solemn; but may be gloomy, submissive and self-depreciatory; his hesitation and indecision betray his feelings of insecurity. He often is preoccupied with his work.

Symptoms and Signs

The manic phase: Excitement is the cardinal symptom. It may be **mild** (hypomania), **acute,** or **delirious.** There is a quickening of the individual's entire tempo, which is reflected in an apparent wealth of mental associations (verbosity), tireless overactivity, and feelings of elation. The patient may be mischievous, playful, and have fleeting delusions of grandeur. Irritability and anger may punctuate his elation when his requests are denied. If "impure" affects are present—as seen in a manic with a paranoid-like reaction—he may be haughty, arrogant, and demanding and become abusive toward those who momentarily annoy him. Close observation reveals that his apparent wealth of ideas actually represents a limited range of associational products, and his wordiness is a flight from, rather than a product of, thinking. He is preoccupied with the phonetics instead of the meanings of words. Everything around him distracts his attention. Since he is not concerned with its ideational content, his talk assumes a character not unlike that of free associations, and thus often affords clues to his unconscious motivation.

The manic's increased psychomotor reactions range from simple overactivity to sustained and frenzied busyness. He may tear his clothing, decorate himself bizarrely, disarrange his room, smear the wall with feces—all without malice. He sings, shouts to any passer-by, makes obscene sexual proposals, is too excited to eat, sleep, or pay attention to any physical illness, mild or serious. Particularly when his excitement is not extreme he may not appear fatigued, yet in other instances these patients rapidly exhaust themselves. Actual hallucinations are rare, but illusions that simulate hallucinations are not uncommon. While these patients usually retain correct orientation, their poorly sustained attention may disturb this. A short mild depression often precedes a manic episode.

The depressive phase: In a considerable number of patients the episodes are confined to depressions, and often these patients' prepsychotic personality has been of the melancholic type. Manic-depressive depressions may be mild, acute, or stuporous. Many mild manic-depressive depressions are not recognized as such. They usually take the form of inertia and staleness or of hypochondriasis. In either case, the patient will be downhearted, and a patient with hypochondriacal complaints will consider these the cause rather than the result of his depression. These mildly depressed patients may be fearful, quiet, indecisive and have feelings of inadequacy. If "impure" affects exist, they may be irritable, sensitive, and morose, or peevish, stubborn, and faultfinding instead of sad. The more severe depressions often begin thus, but profound affective distress rapidly supervenes. This is reflected in a stooped posture and an immobile, or perplexed and troubled, facial expression. The patient sleeps poorly, wakes early, perhaps becomes constipated, and his sexual desires decrease. Because of psychomotor retardation, all physical activity becomes a great exertion. Subjectively, the patient may feel that his usual environment is strange or that a disaster is impending from which he cannot escape, and his outlook becomes hopeless. If the feelings of distress are projected, his ideas become delusional. A complaining, or a suspicious persecutory, paranoid trend may exist; or his thought life may be concerned with hypochondriacal ideas, self-accusations, ideas of guilt, remorse, and self-depreciation. His intense fear may create clouding of consciousness; however, unless a patient's attention is thus impaired by affective distress, orientation is not disturbed. Illusory misinterpretations are common, but hallucinations are infrequent. The psychomotor retardation, alone or augmented by some belief the patient holds—for instance, that he is unworthy of food—may make spoon- or tube-feeding necessary. Suicidal attempts or self-mutilations are not uncommon.

Stupor is the most intense form of these depressions: the patient makes no response to external stimuli, his sensorium is clouded, he is mute, and his face is masklike or wears a fixed expression of anxiety; spontaneous motor activity is slight or absent. A short hypomanic period often terminates the depressive episode.

Diagnosis

The psychosis must be differentiated from schizophrenia, paresis, so-called acute paranoia, and such psychoneurotic states as compulsion neuroses, neurasthenia, and hypochondriasis (q.v.). Paresis may be differentiated by history, neurologic signs, and laboratory tests. Acute paranoia is a misnomer for a hypomania in which exuberance is replaced by anger, resentment, irritability, irascibility, and perhaps delusions and litigious tendencies. Because of the obsessive ideas which a depressed patient may express, a compulsion neurosis sometimes is simulated; the differentiation is made by determining whether the obsessions or the depression came first. The patient's solicitude about his health is continuous and prolonged in neurasthenia. In hypochondriasis, mild symptoms usually will have existed for a considerable time, and the attack does not come on abruptly as in the depressive state.

Prognosis

The prognosis for individual episodes is good and there is no residual "scarring" of the personality. However, the disease may assume a certain chronicity in which the intervals between episodes are brief or nonexistent. The duration of manic-depressive episodes cannot be predicted with certainty, but on the average, manic attacks last six months and depressive attacks nine months. If a first episode is a depression, it may be the last; if it is manic, others are apt to follow. The probability of future attacks varies inversely—to a degree at least —with the age when the disease first appears; if before 20, the prognosis is poor. Recurring episodes may occupy a large portion of some patients' lives; normal periods tend to become shorter as age advances. Chronic mania is uncommon before the age of forty, and the melancholia is more apt to become chronic. Repeated attacks usually leave the mind unchanged in basic functionings, but occasionally a patient may show some impairment of initiative and judgment.

Treatment

Only an occasional patient with manic-depressive psychosis can be cared for at home, and then a psychiatric consultant must be available and psychiatric nurses kept on 24-hour duty. It often is difficult to persuade the family to commit the patient to a hospital, as they do not realize to what extent the defective judgment of these patients constitutes a risk to themselves and others. When relatives are told that electroshock therapy may be indicated, and if so, that it may put an end to the episode, they may more readily agree to the patient's commitment.

The manic phase: Manic patients want to be constantly occupied and outlets for their energy must be supplied, but not to the point of producing exhaustion. Arguments and contradictions should be avoided and the patient allowed to do as he wishes within safe limits. The patient's distractibility sometimes makes spoon-feeding or tube-feeding necessary (*see* Melancholia). A high caloric diet is imperative. The treatment of choice for excitement and insomnia is the use of prolonged neutral baths in tubs especially designed for the purpose ("continuous" tubs). These baths may be given for several hours daily, or continuously up to several weeks. Hypnotics are used as little as possible and repeated only when absolutely necessary. The most suitable are paraldehyde, chloral hydrate, and the barbituric acid derivatives. Chloral hydrate (℞ 4), 2 to 2.6 Gm. (gr. xxx to xl), alone or combined with barbital (℞ 1), 0.3 to 1 Gm. (gr. v to xv), may be used. Paraldehyde (℞ 5) is given in doses of 4 to 12 cc.

If the patient is in good physical condition, and constant nursing attention, which is absolutely essential, is available, partial narcosis, prolonged for a period of days, occasionally will terminate a manic episode. Sodium Amytal (℞ 6) is the drug usually employed for this purpose, and the treatment is begun by giving 0.2 Gm. (gr. iii) by mouth, or rectally, every 3 or 4 hours. The doses are gradually increased during the first 3 or 4 days, until the patient is kept asleep or deeply somnolent for 15 to 20 hours daily. He is kept continuously on his side to prevent aspiration of mouth contents or strangulation, and turned at regular intervals. At least two periods of wakefulness are allowed each day for feeding and nursing care. The physician sees the patient during each of these periods. Pulse, blood pressure, and temperature are periodically determined; cyanosis is watched for, and the narcosis immediately terminated if any untoward signs or symptoms develop. If its course is uneventful, the narcosis sometimes is continued for 10 days, after which the dose of Sodium Amytal is gradually decreased over a period of 3 or 4 days. The effectiveness of this therapy is thought to depend on a partial dissolution of psychotic resistance to psychotherapeutic leverage. The psychotherapy used at this stage is entirely supportive. The constancy of the nurse's attentions and regularity of the physician's visits have supportive value. No interpretive psychotherapy is attempted at this time. After the patient has recovered from the episode, psychotherapy by an expert may decrease the probability of recurrence, but this is at best uncertain.

The depressive phase: General care is the same as for involutional melancholia (q.v.). Electroshock convulsions, 8 to 10, will terminate many of these depressions, but since this is a recurrent disease and because of the amnesic features associated with the therapy, experienced judgment is required to decide to what extent and with which patients it is to be used.

In managing mildly depressed patients, an organized program which fills the day is desirable. None of the activities should be strenuous or exhausting. Repetitive, and what the patient may consider as mildly degrading occupations—such as sorting and counting the various types in a keg of mixed nails, or weeding a lawn—may arouse resentment against the environment, and thus deflect the patient's aggression away from himself. Also, the patient may respond better to an attitude of cool kindness than to a warmly sympathetic approach. As the depression recedes, the danger of suicide increases, since there is less psychomotor retardation and the patient has more energy to carry it out. This fact (which relatives find difficult to understand) calls for doubled precautions during convalescence. Indecision is characteristic of all depressions, and is a cardinal symptom in some of the milder cases; therefore, the patient should not be required to make decisions until he has fully recovered, and in many cases should not resume his usual business occupation for weeks or months thereafter. At least in the psychotic depressions, the use of stimulative drugs such as amphetamine is of questionable value and in some instances may be harmful.

INVOLUTIONAL PSYCHOSES

Whether involutional psychoses are related to manic-depressive psychoses is debatable, but for practical purposes considering them as separate entities is justifiable. They generally occur after the age of 40: in women most often in the late 40's, and in men in the late 50's. At these ages, the woman's child-bearing potential, the symbolized source and end of energy and womanliness, is failing; and the man's physical and mental vigor, and hence the symbolized ability to coerce fate, is waning. In this psychosis, the patient's anxiety is tremendous and is accompanied by agitation, hypochondriacal and nihilistic ideas, delusions and hallucinations. The psychodynamics probably are similar to those outlined under the manic-depressive depressions (q.v.), but with an involutional psychosis fearsome delusions are more frequent, and lacking are the manic-depressive's psychomotor retardation and history of earlier attacks of mania or depression.

Etiology

The patient often will have exhibited such pre-morbid traits as intolerance, stubbornness, penuriousness, oversensitivity; a tendency to self-punishment as manifested by avoidance of pleasure, a rigid moral code for himself and others, and over-conscientiousness. Worrying, fretfulness, apprehension, and compulsive meticulousness may have further reflected his insecurity. At the age when the psychosis occurs a sense of frustration is perhaps usual. The time may appear to have passed when earlier errors can be repaired and when unfulfilled ambitions can be achieved. Hence, old conflicts often become stronger and threaten the ego with their accompanying anxiety. This ceaseless anxiety may bring the patient to a preoccupation with thoughts of death. In some but not all instances the psychosis is precipitated by loss of position, the death of an individual upon whom the person was dependent, or breaking up of the home.

Symptoms and Signs

Insidious changes in attitude and behavior may precede the manifest psychosis by weeks or months. Spells of weeping, dis-

35

inclination for effort, pessimism, peevishness, irritability, and insomnia are common prodromal symptoms. This drastic variation from his accustomed affects is recognized by the patient, and he perhaps states that he is beginning to lose his mind. When the manifest psychosis begins, depression, anxiety and agitation are seen, and delusions of sin, unworthiness, and impending death occupy his mind. Guilt feelings may cause the patient retroactively to interpret some earlier indiscretion as an "unpardonable sin." He perhaps insists that he is to be butchered, or that he is damned and God cannot forgive him. He states that he deserves his fate, yet begs for reassurance, only to refute any that may be offered as illogical and ridiculous. He may rationalize that his inner distress results from organic changes and disease; that his brain has dried up, that his intestines are rotting away, or that he has no stomach. Hallucinations are common; God may talk to him, or a deceased parent reprove him. Although the patient's consciousness probably will be clear, the subjective absorption of attention may cause him to appear confused, perplexed, and bewildered. His fear of death, projected in symbolic forms and delusions, possibly accounts for the insomnia. (Characteristically, depressed patients wake up early in the morning.) Food may be refused because the patient believes it is poisoned, or because of nihilistic ideas about the absence of his stomach, or because he thinks himself unworthy. In no other psychosis is suicide so frequently attempted. This may represent an attempt to destroy rejected portions of the personality, and thus put an end to gnawing conflicts and troublesome desires. The patient loses weight, becomes dehydrated, and picks at his skin; his respirations are shallow, and his extremities cold and cyanotic. In some cases the psychosis has a distinct paranoid coloring, and these patients often will have shown prepsychotic traits somewhat like those observed in the paranoid psychoses (q.v.).

Diagnosis

In manic-depressive depressions, hallucinations are less common, and the apprehension, fear, and ideas of impending destruction are less marked. Also stereotypies (unvarying repetition) of behavior or speech, or other schizophrenic-like symptoms less seldom occur. The latter are more in keeping with involutional melancholia. Patients with arteriosclerotic psychosis who are depressed seldom exhibit the profound, sustained fear seen in the involutional psychotic, and slight loss of memory is usual rather than preoccupation. In the psychoneuroses hallucinations are rare and there are no true delusions. Any fear these patients may have is paroxysmal, although they may exhibit sustained anxiety. In contrast to the psychoneurotic, a patient with melancholia strives more against his sensed danger, and as well may display gross misinterpretations of reality relationships.

Prognosis

With the advent of convulsion therapy, recoveries have been enormously increased; 80 to 90% of these patients are benefited by electroshock convulsions. Previously about 40% recovered, but frequently only after an illness of 2 or 3 years. The prognosis for the paranoid type is less favorable. With the latter, insulin may be indicated if electroshock fails to cure (*see* Schizophrenia).

Treatment

The danger of suicide is too great to permit these patients to be cared for outside a mental hospital. A high caloric diet is essential, and refusal to eat for longer than 24 hours is an indication for tube feedings (*see* DIETS). Aspiration pneumonia should be guarded against through careful technic. Paraldehyde (℞ 5) in amounts up to 8 to 16 cc. (ℨ i to iv) is particularly useful for the insomnia. In aged infirm patients, sedatives must be used with extreme caution. Because these patients are so fearful, all changes in routine should be carefully explained beforehand.

Electroshock therapy: Absolute contraindications to the use of electroshock therapy are few; they include extreme hypertension, severe arteriosclerosis, cardiac decompensation, coronary disease, intracranial disease, pregnancy, and skeletal deformities. Deaths attributable directly to shock therapy are rare. The occurrence of fractures can be reduced to a negligible point by proper technic. Electroshock treatments should be administered only by a physician well trained in the procedure.

Curare is a helpful adjunct. By reducing muscular spasm, it minimizes skeletal trauma during the convulsions. (The drug is contraindicated in patients with myasthenia gravis, since they are unduly sensitive to it.) A preparation suitable for I.V. injection must be used (℞ 15). The customary dose of standardized curare is 3 mg./17.7 Kg. (40 pounds) body wt., but ¾ of this amount is safer, particularly for the first administration. Oxygen and an intratracheal airway must be at hand, as the larynx may become paralyzed from overcurarization. Overcurarization is treated with neostigmine (℞ 16), 1 cc. subcut. of a 1:2,000 solution. If it is necessary to repeat the latter, then atropine (℞ 17), 0.4 mg. (gr. 1/150) also is given to lessen any undesirable side effects of the neostigmine. Curare should be allowed sufficient time to take full effect, usually several minutes, before the convulsion is induced.

Shock treatments are given with the patient lying on a firm, smooth, resilient surface, such as a litter with a firm pad. No metal should touch the patient; hairpins, jewelry, and false teeth are removed. After the patient is lying in correct position upon the litter, he is asked to sit up. An ordinary pillow then is placed lengthwise across the litter and against the patient's buttocks; when the patient again lies down, the necessary hyperextension of the spine is effected. Six assistants are needed. Two stand on opposite sides and apply pressure on the patient's shoulders, each with his other hand grasping the wrist of the patient's arm nearest him. The patient's arms then are flexed and held firmly but not immovably against his chest during the convulsion. Another assistant applies downward pressure on the pelvis. Two others hold the patient's legs, with one hand above, and the other below, the knee. The sixth attends to the mouth gag. This may be an applicator thickly padded at one end with gauze, which is placed between the patient's molars on one side; or a firm gauze-covered roll of cellulose may be placed in such position that the canines bite on it as the mouth closes during the convulsion. The mouth opens widely when the convulsion begins, and during this phase the sixth assistant applies upward pressure on the jaw to prevent its dislocation and keeps the gag in position to prevent biting of the tongue or lips when the jaws close.

Before the electrodes are applied, the patient's temple areas are washed with warm soapy water, and an electrolytic-conducting jelly is rubbed on. The amount of current and length of application necessary to produce a convulsion vary: representative figures are 70 to 150 volts; 300 to 1,200 m.a.; 0.1 to 0.5 second. More than 1 application may be required, but not more than 3 or 4 should be attempted on any one day. The patient is allowed a few deep breaths between each. Ordinarily, the operator will increase the current, or time, or both with each subsequent passage of current until the convulsive threshold is reached. Once this is determined, the same settings on the machine usually will be used initially on the next treatment day. Convulsions begin with a tonic stage affecting the extensor muscles, and end—the longer phase of the two—with clonic contractures of the flexors. A convulsion may last for 1½ minutes. When it ends, the patient is kept on his back until he has taken at least one deep respiration. Then he is turned on his side and a pillow is so arranged under his head that free drainage of mucus from his mouth and throat is assured. Massaging and pinching the abdominal muscles may aid in initiating respirations and, if necessary, artificial respiration can be given. An experienced person must stay with the patient until full consciousness returns. Immediately after convulsions, patients may be so overexcited as to require restraints.

Patients develop varying degrees of amnesia if a sufficient number of convulsions are given. This usually is at first an inability to recall familiar names, and it may progress until after recovery the patient may remember few of his psychotic ideas. Severe and lasting impairment of memory may be produced if more than 20 convulsions are administered in a consecutive series. With fewer than 15, usually only a transitory amnesia results. Customarily, electroshock treatments are given 1, 2, or 3 times a week. Each patient's schedule should be individualized, taking into account his physical condition and particular needs.

On an average, patients with involutional melancholia recover after 6 to 8 convulsions. After the depression is lifted, most of these patients pass through a 15- to 20-day period of euphoria before they "level out."

PRESENILE, ARTERIOSCLEROTIC, AND SENILE PSYCHOSES

Each of these psychoses is a dementia caused by organic changes in the cortical brain cells. Except in the arteriosclerotic psychoses, there is an uninterrupted deterioration of the patient's mental powers, which may begin as a simple inability to make fine ethical discriminations, and increase until almost all mental capacity is lost. The contents of consciousness are reduced both in quantity and quality: impressions are taken in slowly; associations are tardy or nonexistent; memory is defective; disorientation and confusion may exist; the capacity for integrating past and present experience is lost; and the personality may appear desiccated through lack of its usual affective responses. The presenile psychoses—Alzheimer's disease and Pick's disease—are relatively rare forms of dementia which may occur in the 40's, the arteriosclerotic dementias may be seen from 50 upward, while uncomplicated senile dementias seldom appear before the age of 60. Clinically, the senile and arteriosclerotic dementias are often difficult to differentiate, except in the 50's.

PRESENILE PSYCHOSES

ALZHEIMER'S DISEASE

In an individual exhibiting symptoms of dementia during the 40's, this disease should be suspected. It is characterized by fairly rapid mental deterioration, memory defects, disorientation, delirium, speech disturbances, restlessness, hallucinations, and apprehensive delusions. The ability to perform purposeful movements may be impaired or lost. The most conspicuous pathologic lesion is the development of tangled threadlike fibrillary structures in the cortical ganglion cells. There also is nerve cell atrophy and neuroglia proliferation. Dementia becomes pronounced in the later phases of the disease, and spasticity and epileptiform seizures may occur. The typical atrophic changes usually are visible by means of air encephalography.

PICK'S DISEASE

This disease usually occurs between the ages of 45 and 60, and is twice as frequent in women as in men. In most instances dementia is well established within a year, although the memory usually is retained until the disease is far advanced. However, the fundamental dementia is revealed by the patient's inability to utilize the recalled material in forming new concepts. The symptoms arise from a relatively diffuse cortical atrophy, plus circumscribed, localized, bilateral areas of atrophy chiefly in the frontal and temporal lobes. The white matter atrophies early and the loss of ganglion cells is pronounced. The brain may be reduced in weight by 200 to 300 Gm. The pupillary and other reflexes and the spinal fluid findings are not disturbed. Some patients with the disease are depressed, irritable, and suspicious, while others are euphoric. Stereotyped purposeless activity is common. A gradual aphasia occurs, but is not accompanied by the spontaneous logorrhea so frequently seen in aphasia due to vascular disease. Echolalia, apraxia, alexia, and agraphia are common. The patient becomes asthenic, requires bed care, is helpless, develops sphincter incontinence, loses all capacity for speech, and dies within 4 to 6 years, usually from some intercurrent infection.

ARTERIOSCLEROTIC PSYCHOSES

Any pronounced personality change in a person over 50, if paresis is excluded, should arouse suspicion of arteriosclerotic psychosis. Characteristic syndromes are produced if the arteriosclerosis is predominant in either the larger basal vessels or the finer arteries supplying the cortex, but any differentiation between these two conditions often is difficult. (After age 60 the picture of senile dementia may be complicated by a concurrent cerebral arteriosclerosis.) Onset of the diffuse small-vessel form often is insidious, and may first be manifested by easy mental fatigability, anxiety, irascibility, decreased initiative, loss of ability to concentrate, and perhaps a tendency to depression. Dizziness, headaches, and other unpleasant cerebral sensations may occur. The capacity for quick and accurate thinking is gradually lost, and the finer sentiments become blunted. The affections may change, and the patient may become obstinate, childish, and willful. Memory impairment, which may at first be only inability to recall a word, becomes general as time passes. Fluctuations are characteristic: memory and general alertness may be particularly bad one day and fairly good the next. Unlike the person with senile dementia, the patient usually is aware of and distressed by his disabilities. As the disease progresses, episodic outbursts of excitability, bewilderment, and confusion may occur, particularly at night. The patient may become meddlesome and quarrelsome; dress may be neglected; defective judgment and decreased inhibitions may result in sexual indiscretions or offenses. Panic states may be seen. Ideas of jealousy and hypochondriasis, as well as delusions of persecution, and sometimes of grandeur, are not uncommon. Speech is laborious and coordination of finer movements impaired.

The first evidence that the larger vessels are sclerosed may be an apoplectic stroke or an aphasic attack. However, there may be premonitory symptoms, such as morning headaches, mental and physical fatigability, vertigo, emotional lability; short periods of confusion, especially at night; fleeting aphasias or apraxias, and momentary loss of power in arm or leg. As the disease develops, the patient often weeps at trifles. The facies become immobile, and coarse muscular tremors sometimes appear. Heart and kidney disease may be associated. Occlusion or rupture of a vessel may cause focal destruction of nervous tissue, with resultant upper motor neurone paralysis and various aphasias and apraxias. These focal lesions, and especially those causing the serious aphasias, hasten the deterioration and dementia. Epileptiform attacks, either jacksonian or general, may occur and sometimes are the most prominent symptoms. Intercurrent mild infections usually exacerbate the symptoms.

SENILE DEMENTIA

Waning mental capacity sufficient to warrant a diagnosis of a senile dementia seldom appears before the age of 60, and it often is difficult to draw the line between such dementia and the mental state common to old age. An exaggerated tendency to reminisce frequently precedes both the characteristic amnesia for recent happenings and the concurrent recession of ready recall to ever earlier life periods. Recognizing none of this, the patient's personality characteristics are displayed in accentuated form as he attempts to overcome the new frustrations he naturally meets. Egocentricity, irritability, and resentment of any imagined interference by younger persons are common. Various compensations are attempted; exaggerated sexual activity or sexual indecencies may result; there may be ideas of marital infidelity; pride of appearance may be lost. The patient may be distrustful, prying, and suspicious. He may become disoriented and wander about aimlessly, particularly at night. Defective judgment may cause him to disregard traffic hazards, leave gas jets open, and become victimized by unscrupulous persons. Many patients hoard useless articles. Both hallucinations and delusions are common. These symptoms often are accompanied by conspicuous physical signs of senility.

The senile psychoses may be divided into types and certain of these are adequately described by their names: viz: **simple deterioration** (the most common); **delirious and confused; depressed and agitated. The paranoid type** is distinguished by delusions of persecution. With this type, orientation usually remains unimpaired and defects of memory may be comparatively insignificant for a long time; as these increase the delusions become more absurd (*see* Paranoia). **The presbyophrenic type** usually occurs in individuals whose prepsychotic personality was characterized by adaptability, vivacious activity, and cheerfulness. This warmth of personality is retained but the patient vacillates between friendliness and irritability. Severe memory defects exist, of which the patient is unaware.

Characteristically, these voids are filled by confabulations (fantasies related as realities). These patients are loquacious, restless, and constantly busy in purposeless and sometimes destructive ways. Presbyophrenia is seen somewhat more commonly in women than in men.

Diagnosis

Certain differentiating features have been touched on in the preceding text and will not be repeated. On grounds of sheer probability, a diagnosis of arteriosclerotic dementia is given preference over that of senile dementia. The depressed and agitated type both of senile and arteriosclerotic dementia occasionally must be differentiated from involutional melancholia and from manic-depressive depression (q.v.). Differentiation is based on the patient's age and evidence of organic mental impairment or beginning vascular disease.

Prognosis

The prognosis in any of these forms of mental disease is uniformly bad. However, an arteriosclerotic psychosis is not always uninterruptedly progressive. Particularly if there is an associated cardiac or renal disease, these patients may have periods of confusion which clear after a few weeks of simple hospital regimen. Subsequently, they may retain considerable, though impaired, mental capacity for several years before either an increasing dementia or a vascular accident produces permanent disability.

Treatment

Patients with a mild form of senile or arteriosclerotic dementia may be cared for at home, but life must be carefully regulated, particularly for the arteriosclerotic. Any condition that causes mental strain must be eliminated, and light pleasant occupations encouraged. Alcohol is contraindicated. For patients subject to arteriosclerotic convulsions, phenobarbital (R 2) not exceeding 0.27 Gm. (gr. ivss) daily in 3 equal doses is recommended. During disturbed episodes, other sedatives also are indicated. Paraldehyde (R 5) probably is the most useful; it is given in doses of 4 to 16 cc. (3 i to iv), repeated every 4 hours if necessary until the desired degree of sedation is obtained. In the aged, all sedation must be used with caution.

If the patient's judgment becomes defective, it may be necessary to appoint a legal guardian. If the patient talks of or attempts suicide, or shows any other tendencies dangerous to himself or others, he should be hospitalized.

ANOREXIA NERVOSA

Food aversion, self-induced, which attempts to serve as a solution of psychic conflicts. Severe emaciation is usual. More common in women, the condition is frequently accompanied by amenorrhea.

Etiology

Some psychiatrists believe that the syndrome arises against a schizophrenic background. Others consider it a hysterical manifestation.

These patients seem incapable of the ideational adjustment necessary to assume an adult sex role. The years from puberty through the thirties see most cases develop, and marriage may be a precipitating event. Psychoanalytic case reports indicate that on deeply unconscious levels, oral impregnation or related fears and fantasies often operate. The ego's repression of such mental contents from conscious awareness is bolstered through the disavowal of hunger. It seems established that Simmonds' disease (hypophyseal emaciation) and anorexia nervosa are unrelated etiologically.

Symptoms and Signs

The somatic symptoms, including the low B.M.R. (perhaps minus 35 or 40), reflect the depressant effects of starvation. Fewer than 1,000 calories may have constituted the daily food intake for many months. Vomiting may be complained of but the amount usually is small since these patients habitually limit the volume of their food intake below that creating gastric distress. Besides the usual constipation, there may be other gastrointestinal complaints, often vague and indefinite. Patients sometimes weigh as little as 65 or 70 pounds, usually have an appearance of senescence, pallor without anemia, intolerance to cold, dryness of the hair and skin, low blood pressure, subnormal temperature, and slow pulse rate. There may be edema of the ankles, generally of slight degree. Despite dietary inadequacy, there usually is no recognizable avitaminosis. Hairiness of the arms and legs may be seen.

The psychic symptoms vary. Frequently, these patients continue capable of occupations, interests, and efforts astonishing in such frailty. They may insist that they eat amply; or if not, that they can eat no more. Oddly, they often have the notion that some other family member is not eating enough. Under observation they may resort to various subterfuges to dispose of food. This reflects a frequent rationalization: that their emaciation is not a matter for serious concern.

Diagnosis

Laboratory tests give limited aid in establishing the diagnosis. Besides the low B.M.R., there is a tendency toward depression of the gastric acid and blood sugar values. The glucose tolerance curve usually is flat.

Tuberculosis and other wasting diseases must be excluded. In some instances, uncharacteristic symptoms arising from regional or terminal jejunoileitis will closely simulate anorexia nervosa. In hypothyroidism, increased blood cholesterol is common.

The cardinal symptoms of Simmonds' disease may be mimicked exactly. The following points are helpful in the differentiation: (1) In young unmarried women, consider as anorexia nervosa until proved otherwise. (2) Occurrence in the male sex favors a diagnosis of pituitary cachexia. (3) Occurrence in women with onset following parturition, particularly if delivery is associated with much hemorrhage, is strongly suggestive of a true pituitary lesion. (4) Onset following an acute, severe infection suggests true pituitary disease. (5) Loss of sexual hair (axillary and pubic), occurs much more frequently in Simmonds' disease. (6) Patients with Simmonds' disease rarely display energetic activity. Apathy is characteristic. (7) Sensitivity to insulin (prolonged hypoglycemic shock), and to thyroid is common in Simmonds' disease. (8) Any remarkable improvement due to adequate food intake favors a diagnosis of anorexia nervosa.

Prognosis and Treatment

Treatment will succeed in many cases although some patients unavoidably succumb to intercurrent infections. Progression to chronic mental illness will occur in others.

Since these patients may actually fear to gain weight, curbing their activities often is a serious problem. Hospitalization in the early phases of therapy usually is imperative. The physician must receive total authority in the situation from the family, limit their visits to the minimum, particularly at mealtime, and assign duties to carefully selected nurses; without such authority the physician cannot carry out effective treatment. Psychiatric consultation is advisable in all cases, and absolutely necessary in some. Often, however, the family physician can "turn the trick" unassisted. The physician's appraisal is explained frankly to the patient. A concrete demonstration is good psychotherapy, therefore an immediate weight gain becomes the objective. However, this may be defeated by thyroid medication. Because the B.M.R. returns to normal with improved nutrition, thyroid extract is contraindicated in the usual case. First, a calculation of the patient's customary daily caloric intake is made. To this amount, 300 calories are added, the diet being of the high protein, high vitamin variety. At 5- or 6-day intervals, similar 300 calorie additions are made until the daily intake is 3,400 to 3,600 calories. For 2 or 3 days after each increase, the patient will experience gastric distress which gradually subsides. When leaving the hospital, the patient is instructed to record the body weight carefully 2 or 3 times a week. If gain is not progressive, it may mean that without realizing it the patient has decreased the food intake.

Medication to increase the appetite is inadvisable for psychologic reasons.

Six months or more of a high caloric diet may be necessary before an entirely satisfactory state of nutrition is achieved. Where evidence suggests that fat is not being properly absorbed by the intestine, the process may be aided by the use of a wetting agent, such as the polyoxyethylene derivative of sorbitan monooleate, given as 1.5 Gm. doses with each meal (℞ 22).

Diethylstilbestrol 0.5 mg., daily by mouth, may be administered cyclically 3 weeks out of 4 to aid in priming the uterus for subsequent return of ovarian function (*see* AMENORRHEA), and to shorten the period of uterine inactivity often encountered. In many instances, the menstrual function returns to normal without specific treatment.

Psychiatric consultation is indicated when the dietary regimen is without immediate benefit. Depth therapy will be neither essential nor desirable with some patients, while others will require either narcoanalysis or psychoanalysis. In order to prevent recurrences, all patients should receive psychiatric help if possible.

ALCOHOLISM

Alcoholism: *The morbid effects of excessive ingestion of ethyl alcohol.* **Acute alcoholism:** *Acute intoxication; a temporary mental disturbance with muscular incoordination.* **Dipsomania:** *"Spree" drinking; periodic urges to drink, such desire usually being absent between episodes.* **Chronic alcoholism:** *The pathologic results of the habitual use of alcohol in toxic amounts.*

Etiology, Psychology, Incidence

The psychic effects from alcohol occur secondary to its narcotizing action on the C.N.S. During the initial phases of that action exhilaration is experienced, since ideation and emotions are less inhibited. The perceptual senses are dulled, and the ability correctly to observe both self and others is impaired. Thus ego-pleasant semi-illusions temporarily distort reality. In pursuing exhilaration, many normal persons occasionally drink until intoxicated, but seemingly have no psychic need for "addiction." In contrast, modern studies indicate that, with few exceptions, only individuals with serious personality maladjustments become chronic alcoholics. They are immature, insecure, oversensitive, and anxious. Without alcohol they are unable to meet and enjoy people socially, and suffer from marked feelings of inferiority. Theirs is a neurotic pattern; a sickness, and not a depravity.

"Alcoholics Anonymous," composed of former drinkers, is in many instances successful in helping an individual give up liquor. The alcoholic's associations within the group—their solitude for him and his in turn for other habitués—probably play important roles. Such associations may allow expression for unconscious strivings that otherwise could not find acceptable outlets.

Approximately 10% of the first admissions to hospitals for mental disease in the United States belong to the alcoholic group.

Physiology, Pathologic Anatomy

Following a single experimental ingestion of alcohol, a maximum level in the blood is maintained for about 5 hours. Its distribution throughout the body is fairly uniform, except that in the brain and spinal fluid the rise and fall in concentration occur more slowly. Ordinarily, exhilaration is experienced with blood levels of 100 to 200 mg./100 cc.; depression and severe ataxia, with levels of 200 to 300 mg.; and death is apt to result from levels above 500 mg. "Addicts" generally tolerate larger amounts of alcohol in the body than do others. The reason for this is not completely understood. From 5 to 10% of ingested alcohol is excreted, and the remainder oxidized to CO_2 and water, at a rate of 5 to 10 cc./hr., each cc. furnishing about 7 calories. Since its oxidation rate cannot be accelerated in response to energy demands, alcohol cannot serve as an adequate food. There are conflicting theories about the roles of insulin and thiamine in the metabolic mechanisms when both alcohol and other carbohydrates are available in the body, but probably the frequent and symptomatically important B vitamin complex deficiency seen in chronic alcoholics is due more directly to inadequate intake than to specific disturbances in intermediate metabolism. Thus, impaired nutrition probably is caused by the reduced food intake usual in heavy drinkers, and furthered by the gastritis commonly present in this group. The gastritis may be partly due to the effect of alcohol on the gastric secretions, which are increased in amount and acidity, while the pepsin content remains low.

The relationship between cirrhosis of the liver (q.v.) and alcoholism is not a simple, direct one. However, the disease is relatively frequent among alcoholics, and possibly depends on specific nutritional deficiencies and disturbances. Some impairment of liver function is usual, perhaps preventing adequate glycogen storage and accounting for a tendency to develop hypoglycemia, since a compensatory mobilization of glucose may be impossible. Additionally, there is a sharp diminution of sugar tolerance, as measured by the ease with which glycosuria can be produced.

After death in alcoholism, either acute or chronic, no gross or microscopic lesions are found which are limited to this etiology alone. In chronic alcoholics, the common findings are visceral fatty degeneration, particularly of the liver and heart. Both alcohol's direct action and nutritional deficiencies, particularly of thiamine, are considered mainly responsible for the peripheral nerve degeneration and brain changes often found. A chronic leptomeningitis is not infrequent, as manifested by localized opaque and edematous areas; this is called "wet brain" when the pia-arachnoid edema is pronounced. ("Wet brain" is a pathologic, not a physiologic, diagnostic term; clinically, these patients usually benefit from increased fluids.)

SYNDROMES IN ACUTE ALCOHOLISM
ACUTE INTOXICATION

Symptoms and Signs

The symptoms and signs depend upon the progressive depressant action of alcohol, particularly on the nervous system. The uncomplicated psychic phenomena require no description. As concentrations mount, reflex irritability decreases, muscular incoordination develops, and sensory disturbances appear, such as diplopia, tinnitus, and numbness. Usually, the pupils are dilated, but may be constricted or unequal. At this stage, the skin may be flushed, arterial pressure moderately lowered, the pulse rapid and full. As a rule, impairment of consciousness is gradual, but coma may occur with unexpected rapidity. Circulatory collapse, disturbance of heat regulation with lowered temperature, acute urinary retention, or incontinence of urine and feces may develop. Convulsions are sometimes seen. Death may occur suddenly or following many hours of deep coma.

Complications and Sequelae

As indicated, the signs of shock may supervene during coma; later, pneumonia due to aspiration, hypostasis, or exposure may develop. Occasionally, a debauch is followed by intractable vomiting. Lacerations at the junction of the esophagus and cardia from retching may lead to severe or fatal hemorrhage. Jaundice, accompanying acute changes in the liver parenchyma; acute pancreatitis, presumably secondary to regurgitation into the pancreatic duct; and nephritis, perhaps related to impurities in the liquor, may be encountered. Acute distention of the abdomen imitating peritonitis or intestinal perforation can complicate the picture.

Diagnosis

The usual diagnostic errors are fractured skull, subdural or subarachnoid hemorrhage, cerebrovascular accident, uremia, and diabetic or insulin coma.

PATHOLOGIC INTOXICATION

An occasional unstable individual, particularly one of hysterical or epileptoid temperament, will, on drinking even a small amount of alcohol, exhibit a transitory psychotic state. This usually commences with dramatic suddenness. The patient is disoriented, confused, and has hallucinations and delusions. The disorder lasts from a few minutes to a day or more, usually ending in profound sleep, with subsequent amnesia for the episode.

ALCOHOLIC TRANCE OR AUTOMATISM

Rarely, after a moderate amount of alcohol, an individual, while not appearing drunk, will develop a trance state, frequently with subsequent amnesia, during which he may either go about his daily tasks in an automatic fashion, or wander away.

SYNDROMES IN CHRONIC ALCOHOLISM

SOMATIC MANIFESTATIONS

Chronic alcoholics may appear to be overweight, due to a bloated appearance. Facial telangiectases are frequent. Liver dysfunction, vitamin deficiency, and gastritis concomitantly cause a multiplicity of phenomena, including gastric and intestinal atony, eructation, and anorexia. The patients are prone to develop nutritional edema, pellagra, and occasionally "beriberi" heart. Scurvy is rare, but vitamin C deficiency sometimes plays an etiologic role in the subdural hematomas occasionally seen, although trauma frequently is an associated factor.

Commonly, the principal functional damage is to the nervous system. Even without other manifestations, tremors of the hands and tongue are common, and loss of muscular power may be progressive. Neuritis is not infrequent. Alcohol probably bears more than an indirect relationship to this, but a vitamin B_1 deficiency appears to be constantly associated. Severe pain and burning are at times the sole complaints. The onset may be gradual, with paresthesias of the hands or feet, or rapid, with motor manifestations. The paralysis, not necessarily symmetrical, is apt to involve the feet, hands, and arms. Cord involvement may be evidenced by varying degrees of sphincter dysfunction. Tachycardia (vagus neuritis) is frequent, and a mental syndrome (Korsakoff's psychosis) may accompany alcoholic neuritis. Optic and retrobulbar neuritis alone may develop, with nicotine sometimes acting as a synergist.

PERSONALITY DETERIORATION

Numbers of alcoholics ultimately suffer a disintegration of personality, ranging from impairment of emotional control to dementia. Experimental work suggests that the oxidative metabolism of the brain is disturbed by thiamine deficiency. Because of an increasing incapacity for inhibitory control, the patient becomes more impulsive, untruthful and unreliable, and displays a growing tendency to gloss over discreditable behavior. Money may be squandered, responsibility evaded, and feelings of affection lost; the patient is touchy, irritable, critical. His unwarranted euphoria readily gives way to profane outbursts or tears. He may be congenial with cronies, but at home surly and brutal. His own maladjusted sexuality, perhaps now including organic impotence, may cause him to suspect his wife's fidelity. Poverty of ideas and incapacity for attention increase, and as memory becomes impaired, the dementia becomes recognizable, and later perhaps extreme. Actual dementia is irremediable, but if alcohol is discontinued when the first character changes appear, the process is largely reversible.

KORSAKOFF'S PSYCHOSIS

This psychosis may or may not be preceded by delirium tremens. If so, the hallucinations and delirium gradually are replaced by amnesia, disorientation in time and place, and falsification of memory. The mood usually is one of joviality. When questioned, fictitious episodes (confabulations) are related, to the extent that the severity of the amnesia may not at first be apparent. Polyneuritis often is associated, and nystagmus and ocular paralyses may occur (due to thiamine deficiency). The syndrome is more frequent in women than in men. Some patients recover after 6 to 8 weeks; some after several months, with only slight memory impairment; and some, never.

ACUTE HALLUCINOSIS

In contrast to delirium tremens, this psychosis never merges into a Korsakoff's, and there is no subsequent amnesia for the episode. The hallucinations are usually auditory—accusatory, threatening, or both—and cause great fear. Hallucinatory homosexual accusations are common, and a delusional system may be rapidly acquired. In his panic, the patient may attempt suicide. Recovery usually occurs in 5 days to a month; however, the condition occasionally ends in schizophrenia.

ALCOHOLIC PARANOIA

Paranoia is discussed elsewhere (q.v.), and the recognition of an "alcoholic" paranoia as a true alcoholic psychosis is hardly justified. However, such classification is clinically convenient, simply because so often seen. Since the patient imputes to his wife the interest he fundamentally feels for other men, delusions of jealousy and marital infidelity are the common manifestations. The prognosis is bad. When separated from home and alcohol, the patient may quickly deny that he continues to entertain these ideas, but they usually recur promptly when he no longer is restrained.

DELIRIUM TREMENS

This is an acute psychosis characterized by delirium, confusion, tremor, and vivid, predominantly visual, hallucinations. The syndrome seldom is seen before 3 or 4 years of chronic alcoholism. It often is precipitated by injury or acute illness.

Patients frequently stop drinking before the frank delirium commences, due both to their physical and mental state. It is thought that sudden withdrawal of alcohol will not precipitate the syndrome. In the prodromal period, there often is aversion to food, with irritability and sleeplessness. Vitamin B deficiency probably plays a role in the anorexia, nausea, and other gastrointestinal symptoms. At onset, the patient may suffer only occasional illusions and hallucinations, but these gradually increase. Frequently, the hallucinations are of fantastic moving animals—often colored, and large or small. Added tactile hallucinations may cause the patient to feel as well as see small animals on his skin. Auditory and olfactory hallucinations are less frequent. The mood usually is one of irritability, apprehension and fear. Occasionally, it is one of euphoria, silliness, or such as reflects amusement. Preposterous confabulations may be narrated. Consciousness is clouded, and the patient is confused, disoriented for time and place, and often misidentifies his friends and acquaintances. Motor restlessness may be great. Sleeplessness is characteristic.

Usually, the face and conjunctivae are congested, the skin moist, and there is a coarse tremor of the hands; the tongue is tremulous and, in many instances the muscles of the lips and face also. The pulse often is irregular, weak, and rapid. The temperature generally is elevated and may be high. Except when neuritis prevents it, the tendon reflexes usually are increased, and epileptiform convulsions may occur. Albuminuria is common.

The psychosis lasts from 2 to 10 days, and frequently terminates with a profound sleep. Mortality is about 15%, with heart failure and pneumonia as the most common causes of death.

WET BRAIN

After several attacks of delirium tremens, a different syndrome, "wet brain," may develop. It is characterized by coma, muttering, delirium, fixed facies, and purposeless picking movements of the hands. This condition may run a protracted course, and emaciation can become extreme unless tube feeding is promptly resorted to (see BEDSIDE PROC.). The prognosis is grave.

TREATMENT OF ALCOHOLISM

Most of the mental syndromes in chronic alcoholism require treatment in a closed ward or institution, especially alcoholic deterioration, Korsakoff's psychosis, acute hallucinosis, and alcoholic paranoia. Many cases of delirium tremens also need institutional care, but an occasional mild case can be treated at home, provided competent nursing and adequate auxiliary care are constantly available. Similar provisions are necessary in the home management of pathologic intoxication, alcoholic trance, and acute intoxication — all potentially catastrophic states, even if brief.

Acute Intoxication: There is evidence that, with the use of insulin and glucose, drunkenness or alcoholic stupor can be more readily relieved than with other methods. However, this therapy is specifically contraindicated except in a hospital with 24-hour laboratory service where, if necessary, blood sugar and CO_2 levels can be frequently determined. General technics are detailed under schizophrenia (q.v.). It must be remembered that alcoholics may spontaneously exhibit symptoms of hypoglycemia, meaning that insulin must be used cautiously in every instance. Suggestions concerning dosages are included at appropriate points in the text below.

CAUTION! If a patient, after drinking, is stuporous or comatose, it is essential that other possible causes be ruled out (*see* THE UNCONSCIOUS PATIENT). Too often patients with an alcoholic breath are adjudged drunk, are treated expectantly, and preventable deaths ensue. Among conditions to be excluded are: cerebral concussion or contusion, with or without fractured skull; status epilepticus; apoplexy; cerebral embolism, thrombosis, or tumor; subdural hematoma; toxic delirium, as from infection; uremic or diabetic coma; and other intoxications, as from carbon monoxide or morphine. Hysterical trance states also must be excluded. These differentiations are accomplished by history, X-ray of the skull, neurologic check-up, urine examination, blood chemistry determinations, and by lumbar puncture. The latter is contraindicated if choked disks or other findings suggest the presence of an intracranial tumor.

To prevent aspiration pneumonia, the stuporous or comatose alcoholic should be turned from side to side at regular intervals, and receive penicillin I.M., 30,000 u. every 3 hours. Also, the patient's head should be lowered. In addition, temperature, pulse, respiration, and blood pressure are determined every half hour until the patient's exact status is certain, according to the above differentiation. For patients with depressed respirations or in coma, O_2 is indicated, either by tent or nasal catheter.

Patients with uncomplicated acute intoxication ordinarily recover spontaneously but, in some cases, circulatory collapse or shock (q.v.) may supervene. Vigorous treatment, in addition to the measures already outlined, is indicated. This includes gastric lavage, external heat, strong coffee enema, and I.M. caffeine sodium benzoate (℞ 21), 0.5 to 1 Gm. (gr. viiss to xv) every hour until respirations are increased or the patient is alert. In addition, 100 cc. of 50% glucose is immediately given I.V. and is repeated every hour as necessary (℞ 19). Shortly after the first glucose injection—if no specific contraindication exists—insulin 30 u. is given subcut. (℞ 14). Thiamine hydrochloride (℞ 8), 100 mg. I.V., also is indicated. A conscious patient is allowed both water and orange juice by mouth.

If unconscious, and no other factors complicate the alcoholic stupor, 250 cc., or more, of I.V. Isotonic Sodium Chloride Solution U.S.P. every 3 to 4 hours will perhaps be indicated. Lumbar puncture as a therapeutic measure may be desirable (*see* Treatment, Delirium Tremens). In the treatment of postalcoholic headache and dehydration, fluids containing sodium chloride by mouth are useful.

Delirium Tremens: The patient should be placed in bed and alcohol withheld. Exhaustion must be prevented. Imaginative attendants usually can control these patients without physical restraints, thus preventing much struggling. Morphine and depressing hypnotics are contraindicated. Paraldehyde, 12 to 16 cc. (℞ 5), may be given 1 to 3 times in 24 hours. If not tolerated by mouth, paraldehyde may be given rectally, or 2 to 8 cc. (ʒss to ii) may be given I.M.; it should not be given I.V. In addition, Sodium Amytal (℞ 6), 0.5 to 1 Gm. (gr. viiss to xv) may be administered once daily by vein (1 cc./minute, discontinuing when relaxation is secured). To combat acidosis and dehydration, 500 cc. of ⅙ molar sodium lactate solution (℞ 18) and 500 cc. of Isotonic Sodium Chloride Solution U.S.P. are given subcut., or preferably I.V. The patient perhaps can be persuaded to drink such solutions also. The daily fluid intake should approximate 3,000 cc. If the spinal fluid pressure is increased, 30 to 50 cc. should be drawn off; otherwise, 15 to 20 cc. This is repeated in 48 hours if the acute delirium continues. Thiamine, 20 to 50 mg. or more, I.M. or I.V. is given daily (℞ 8); also nicotinamide (niacinamide) in 100 mg. doses I.V. (℞ 10). The former tends to relieve cardiac involvement secondary to B_1 deficiency; the latter, to clear up certain types of spastic muscular manifestations that occur in delirium tremens. After several days, a vitamin B preparation by mouth (℞ 7, 12), or yeast (℞ 11), in iced milk is substituted. (In Korsakoff's psychosis, which may commence as delirium tremens, large vitamin B dosage also is indicated.) If immediate stimulation is necessary, caffeine sodium benzoate, 0.5 Gm. (gr. viiss) every 4 to 6 hours for 4 to 6 doses, may be given (℞ 21). Saline laxatives should be used to promote intestinal elimination. At first, only milk and eggnog may be tolerated. Sometimes not even these will be; then glucose I.V., 5 to 15% in Isotonic Sodium Chloride Solution U.S.P., is indicated. If the patient tolerates but refuses alimentation, tube feedings are given (*see* BEDSIDE PROC.). If insulin-glucose therapy is utilized (*see* 1st paragraph, Treatment, Acute Intoxication) extreme caution is necessary. Insulin, 10 to 15 u. 2 to 3 times daily, may be deemed advisable, each unit being simultaneously covered by 2 Gm. of glucose I.V., as a 20% solution in Isotonic Sodium Chloride Solution U.S.P.

Chronic Alcoholism: In the opening paragraph under treatment, the institutional and other measures indicated for the mental syndromes associated with chronic alcoholism are briefly discussed. However, in treating chronic alcoholics who do not exhibit such derangement, psychiatric consultation is advisable; in some instances treatment by one of the conditioned reflex methods may be recommended. Many alcoholics will profit by being guided into Alcoholics Anonymous. From the physical standpoint, correction and prevention of deficiency states (q.v.) such as pellagra, beriberi, and scurvy, and also cirrhosis (q.v.) is highly important. A prophylactic vitamin B complex preparation (Ŗ 11) is justified, plus a multivitamin preparation (Ŗ 9). An attempt must be made to enforce a balanced diet, rich in B vitamins; e.g., whole grain breads and cereals, legumes, lean pork, liver, heart, kidney, and milk. If neuritis develops, bed care is indicated, with daily parenteral injections of 100 mg., or more, of crystalline vitamin B_1 (Ŗ 8). Nicotine should be eliminated. Liver extracts and niacinamide (Ŗ 12) are beneficial if lesions of pellagra are present.

DRUG ADDICTION

(Chronic intoxication with drugs; Pharmacopsychosis;
Morphine, or other drug, habit; Morphinism, Cocainism,
Barbiturism)

A condition in which an individual has become so accustomed to the repeated, daily use of a drug, that he is dependent upon it for his sense of well-being and, if forced to abandon it, suffers a psychic craving and may, though not necessarily will, develop a characteristic "abstinence syndrome" due to alteration of certain physiologic processes.

Among the drugs that may cause addiction are the opiates (morphine, heroin, Dilaudid, metopon, Dicodid, eukodal, and codeine), the synthetic analgesics (Demerol, and methadone), sedative drugs (bromides, barbiturates, chloral, and paraldehyde), marihuana, peyote (mescaline), alcohol, and cortical stimulants (cocaine and amphetamine). Chronic alcoholism and chronic bromism (q.v.) are discussed elsewhere.

Certain characteristics—tolerance, which means a diminishing effect on repetition of the same dose of a drug; physical dependence, an altered bodily state brought about by prolonged taking of a drug which necessitates its continued use to prevent the appearance of abstinence symptoms; and emotional, or psychologic dependence—are more firmly established in addiction to the opiates than to other drugs. Emotional dependence is the most important characteristic of all habit-forming drugs. Tolerance and physical dependence are not developed following the use of cocaine, amphetamine, marihuana, or peyote, yet they are addicting drugs. Little tolerance to the sedative drugs is acquired, but physical dependence on barbiturates can occur. The opiates, the synthetic analgesics, cocaine, and marihuana, are all subject to Federal control, under the Harrison Narcotic Act, while the sedative drugs, peyote, and the stimulant, amphetamine, are subject to legislative control in certain states.

The Harrison Narcotic Act was passed to provide Federal control of opiates and their derivatives as well as many other habit-forming drugs. The physician is warned concerning the writing of prescriptions for drugs falling under the scope of the Federal regulations. Habit-forming drugs should be prescribed only when absolutely necessary. Patients who demonstrate evidence of emotional instability are particularly vulnerable to addiction; hence great care should be exercised in prescribing for them.

Etiology

Drug addiction results from two factors, the presence of a personality disorder and the availability of an addicting drug. Physical illness seldom is an important factor. The most common personality defects underlying drug addiction are the psychoneuroses (q.v.) and constitutional psychopathic inferiority. Contact with the drug may be made through a physician's prescription during an illness, through self-medication, or by deliberate experimentation with the drug through association with persons already addicted. Psychoneurotic individuals ordinarily take drugs to relieve their emotional or physical distress, while psychopathic individuals take them in order to enjoy their intoxicating effects.

Symptoms and Signs

1. Opiate drugs and synthetic analgesics: There are no characteristic signs of addiction to opiate drugs. However, addicts frequently spend their entire income on drugs, do not eat, and therefore become emaciated. Needle marks and scars over the veins of the arms and legs are commonly seen. Miosis is not a reliable sign. Persons habituated to morphine or methadone do not appear to be intoxicated. Demerol addicts usually take so much of the drug (2.5 to 5 Gm. daily) that they show signs of toxicity—mydriasis, muscle tremor, and epileptiform seizures.

1a. The opiate abstinence syndrome: In the early stages of addiction, withdrawal of morphine results in restlessness, depression, and mild disturbances in the autonomic nervous system. These symptoms are not unendurable and they disappear within a few days. If the drug is suddenly withdrawn from a patient strongly addicted to it, a characteristic self-limited, acute illness develops. In the first 8 to 16 hours of abstinence no signs are noticeable except drowsiness. After 16 hours, slight restlessness, yawning, perspiration, rhinorrhea and lacrimation are seen. After 24 hours, patients become progressively more restless and show mydriasis, goose flesh, and uncontrollable muscle twitching. They stop eating, may vomit frequently, develop diarrhea, suffer severe muscular aches in the back and legs, and cannot sleep. Considerable weight may be lost in one day. Body temperature is slightly elevated and blood pressure, heart rate, and respiratory rate are increased. Blood sugar and blood lactic acid values are augmented, and leukocyte counts elevated. Increased red cell counts, hematocrit levels, and hemoglobin values reflect dehydration due to vomiting, sweating, increased respiratory rate, and decreased fluid intake. The symptoms reach maximum intensity 48 hours after the last dose, continue intense until the 72nd hour, and thereafter gradually decline. In 7 to 10 days after withdrawal, all the acute manifestations subside, but patients complain of weakness, insomnia, and nervousness for several months. The abstinence syndrome is due to a disturbance in the spinal cord and other parts of the C.N.S., and is not psychogenic in origin. Patients frequently exhibit emotional reactions during withdrawal, but true abstinence signs can be differentiated from these. Hysterical and anxiety reactions are common, but psychotic episodes seldom occur. The abstinence symptoms seen after withdrawal of heroin, Dilaudid, Dicodid, and eukodal are qualitatively identical with, and just as severe as, those of abstinence from morphine. Abstinence symptoms from metopon, codeine, or Demerol are qualitatively similar to those from morphine, but milder. Abstinence from methadone differs in that few signs of disturbed autonomic function are seen, the onset is slow, intensity mild, and the course prolonged.

2. Barbiturates: Barbiturate addiction is increasingly prevalent in the United States and is the commonest complication of opiate addiction. The short-acting barbiturates are the most popular among addicts. Barbiturate addicts may ingest as much as 2.4 Gm. (gr. xxxvi) of these drugs daily. A high degree of tolerance is not developed. The symptoms are intoxication, mental confusion, ataxia, slurred speech, drowsiness, amnesia, diminished reflexes, and nystagmus. Consequently, addicts frequently incur serious injuries from falls or other accidents, and may commit crimes, yet retain no memory of them. Addiction to other sedatives, such as chloral or paraldehyde, may produce similar behavior and clinical manifestations indistinguishable from those of barbiturate addiction.

2a. Barbiturate abstinence syndrome: If a person has been taking as much as 0.75 Gm. (gr. xii) of a potent barbiturate daily for as long as 2 months, and the drug is abruptly withdrawn or the dose suddenly reduced, epileptiform seizures are likely to occur 2 to 7 days later. In the first 2 or 3 days of abstinence, patients usually are restless and sleep poorly. Most patients have 2 or 3 convulsions and then recover. Psychotic episodes, which may resemble any psychiatric entity, frequently follow abrupt withdrawal of barbiturates.

3. Marihuana: Smoking marihuana produces a mild state of intoxication which is popular among maladjusted adolescents. The usual symptoms are giggling, reddened conjunctivae, drooping of the eyelids, and a characteristic odor on the breath resembling that of cubeb cigarettes. Apparently it is difficult, by smoking marihuana, to obtain enough of the active principle to cause gross intoxication. Habitués enjoy the delusions of time and space which the drug produces. Sex offenses and crimes attributed to marihuana are largely due to the personalities of the users rather than the effects of the drug. Occasionally, psychotic episodes occur in persons with borderline psychotic personalities after smoking a marihuana cigarette. No tolerance is developed and there is no abstinence syndrome in the case of marihuana.

4. Peyote consists of the buttons of certain varieties of cactus found in the arid Western States and Mexico. The effect of peyote is due to its content of mescaline, which produces hallucination of all the special senses, particularly sight. The drug is used by some Indian tribes as part of their religious ceremonies. Nothing is known concerning tolerance and physical dependence.

5. Cocaine and Amphetamine: Pure cocaine addiction now is almost nonexistent. The effects of large amounts of the drug are so unpleasant that most drug addicts avoid cocaine except in conjunction with a physiologic antidote—usually morphine. Cocaine was originally popular among addicts as a snuff but now is taken almost entirely by vein. The drug produces a short-lived feeling of ecstasy. The injections sometimes are repeated every few minutes to recapture this sensation and with this repetition toxic effects, such as tachycardia, hypertension, mydriasis, muscle twitching, formication, sleeplessness, and extreme nervousness appear. Hallucinations and delusions of a paranoid nature may develop, and in this state such people are dangerous and may commit murder. No tolerance develops to cocaine, and there is no abstinence syndrome.

Amphetamine might be termed the modern cocaine. It has been abused largely by morphine addicts, inmates of penal institutions, and thrill-seeking adolescents. Addicts formerly were able to obtain the drug readily by buying the amphetamine-type inhalers then being sold for symptomatic treatment of colds. They removed, chewed and swallowed the paper strips containing the amphetamine. Habitués might take as much as 1,500 mg. daily. The effects, though similar to those of cocaine, are milder. The users experience anorexia, insomnia, and a sense of exhilaration and increased muscular efficiency. Mydriasis, tachycardia, and hypertension are always present. Muscle tremors and twitches may be seen. Various confused states and psychotic episodes may occur in individuals with personalities that border on the psychotic. Very little tolerance is developed and there is no abstinence syndrome.

Diagnosis

The majority of addicts seeking medical aid readily admit their addiction. If they do not, diagnosis must be made from the signs and symptoms. Needle marks and abscess scars are particularly significant. A definite diagnosis of morphine addiction may have to be made on the occurrence of withdrawal symptoms when access to the drug is prevented. Tests are available for the detection of morphine, barbiturates, and amphetamine in the urine, but these are not readily available to most physicians.

Prognosis and Treatment

The prognosis of drug addiction usually depends on that of the personality defect underlying the addiction and therefore must always be guarded. The prognosis for any case and with any type of drug addiction becomes progressively worse with the duration of addiction and the number of relapses following treatment.

Three basic facts should be understood: (1) Drug addicts must be treated in a rigidly controlled environment, as in institutions. (2) Withdrawal of drugs is not synonymous with treatment, but is only the first, simplest, and easiest step. (3) Psychotherapy offers the only hope of relief for drug addiction, and it must be carried out continuously for several months or even years if good results are to be expected.

Institutional care: Attempts at out-patient or in-patient treatment in general hospitals are almost never successful. The Federal Government maintains two institutions for the treatment of narcotic drug addicts. (Persons addicted exclusively to barbiturates are not accepted.) Information concerning admission to these institutions can be obtained from the Surgeon General, U. S. Public Health Service, Washington, D. C.

Withdrawal therapy: (*a*) **Morphine and related analgesics:** Withdrawal of morphine with the substitution of hyoscine, belladonna, insulin, or heavy sedation is irrational and dangerous. Abrupt withdrawal of morphine is unnecessarily cruel. The best methods of treatment are reduction of the dose the patient is using, or substitution of methadone in gradually decreasing doses. Methadone, 1 mg., should be substituted for each 4 mg. (gr. $\frac{1}{15}$) of the accustomed dose of morphine. No more than 90 mg. (gr. iss) of methadone should be given in one day, since this dose will suppress all symptoms of abstinence regardless of the dose of morphine the patient has been using. It is best to give both morphine and methadone on the 1st day and to maintain the original dosage of methadone for 2 days before reduction is begun. When substitution is first effected, the patient should be watched for signs of excessive sedation or of sensitivity to methadone. In patients with serious organic disease, the withdrawal period should extend over

30 days or more. (For a typical methadone withdrawal schedule for uncomplicated cases, covering 15 days, *see* Table.)

Methadone Withdrawal Schedule

Day	Stage	Drug	Amt./Dose (mg.)	No. Doses
1st	Addiction	Morphine	90	4
2nd	Substitution	Morphine	45	4
		Methadone	15	4
3rd & 4th	Substitution	"	22.5	4
5th & 6th	Reduction	"	10	4
7th & 8th	Reduction	"	5	4
9th	Reduction	"	4	4
10th	Reduction	"	2.5	4
11th	Reduction	"	2.5	3
12th	Reduction	"	2.5	2
13th	Reduction	"	2.5	2
14th	Reduction	"	2.5	1
15th	Abstinence	None	0	0

Reduction of morphine on a similar schedule gives almost as good results. Only mild signs of abstinence develop on either morphine or methadone reduction schedules. Minor emotional disturbances are to be expected regardless of the withdrawal method used. The physician must adopt a reassuring but uncompromising attitude. A light, soft diet with ample fluids should be prescribed. Pentobarbital 0.1 Gm. (gr. iss) may be given at night from the 11th to the 20th days. Excessive sedation should be avoided.

(*b*) **Barbiturates:** Withdrawal of barbiturates from persons accustomed to taking large amounts should be individualized. A slow, cautious reduction of the daily allowance, by not more than 10% daily, should be made over a period of 2 to 4 weeks. If insomnia and restlessness develop, the reduction in dosage should be stopped for a day or so, as these symptoms often herald the onset of convulsions.

(*c*) **Marihuana, Peyote, Cocaine, Amphetamine:** No withdrawal treatment is required in cases of addiction to these drugs.

Psychiatric treatment: The psychiatric therapy of drug addiction does not differ from that indicated for a nonaddict with a similar personality structure. The drug involved has no bearing on the problem. In brief, the therapy must be highly individualized according to the patient's psychic needs. The majority of addicts are severely neurotic. Therefore, the section on the psychoneuroses (q.v.) may prove helpful as a general orientation to psychotherapy.

PRESCRIPTIONS

(Wherever a prescribed "proprietary" is representative of a class of therapeutic agents, alternative proprietary preparations will be found listed in Part II.)

Sedatives and Hypnotics

1. ℞ Barbital . . . . 0.3 Gm. (gr. v)
   1 to 3 tablets as required.

2. ℞ Phenobarbital. . . . . 30 mg. (gr. ss)
   1 to 3 tablets 3 times daily.

3. ℞ "Amytal". . . . . 0.1 Gm. (gr. iss)
   1 to 3 tablets at bedtime.

4. ℞ Chloral hydrate . . . . 0.3 Gm. (gr. v)
   6 to 8 capsules as required.

5. ℞ Paraldehyde. . . . . 60 cc. (℥ ii)
   1 to 4 teaspoons, orally or rectally, repeated
   every 4 hours if necessary. The I.M. dose
   is 2 to 8 cc.

6. ℞ "Amytal Sodium"
   For Manic-Depressive Psychoses, administer
   orally as tablets, rectally as a suppository, or
   I.V. as a sterile solution, according to dosage
   schedule given in text.

Vitamins

7. ℞ Thiamine hydrochloride. . . . . 10 mg.
   10 tablets daily.

8. ℞ Thiamine hydrochloride (ampul)
   20 to 100 mg. daily, I.M. or I.V.

9. ℞ Hexavitamin Tablets, U.S.P.
   2 tablets daily.

10. ℞ Nicotinamide (ampul)
    100 mg. I.V. daily.

11. ℞ Dried Yeast U.S.P. . . . . . . 0.5 Gm. (gr. viiss)
    10 tablets or capsules daily.

12. ℞ Nicotinamide . . . . 50 mg.
    1 or 2 tablets daily.

Miscellaneous

13. ℞ Amphetamine sulfate. . . . . . 5 mg.
    1 tablet after breakfast.

14. ℞ Insulin Injection U.S.P. (vial)
    For Insulin Shock Therapy: Administer ac-
    cording to schedule given in text (see PSY-
    CHOSES: Schizophrenia).

15. ℞ d-Tubocurarine chloride (vial)
    3 mg./17.7 Kg. (40 lbs.) body wt. adminis-
    tered I.V.; the initial dose should be only ¾
    of this calculated dose.

16. ℞ Neostigmine methylsulfate,
　　　1:2,000 solution　(ampul)

　　　　1 cc. subcut., repeated if necessary to antag-
　　　　onize the effect of tubocurarine.

17. ℞ Atropine sulfate . . . . 0.4 mg.　(gr. 1/150)

　　　　Administer subcut. to lessen the undesirable
　　　　side effects of neostigmine.

18. ℞ Sodium lactate, ⅙ molar solution
　　　(sterile bottle). . . . . . . 500.0 cc.　(℥ xvi)

　　　　Administer subcut. or I.V., drops at a rate
　　　　not exceeding 60/minute.

19. ℞ Glucose, 50% solution　(ampul)

　　　　25 to 100 cc. I.V. as required.

20. ℞ Epinephrine hydrochloride,
　　　1:1,000 solution　(ampul)

　　　　0.3 to 0.5 cc. (℔ v to viii) subcut.

21. ℞ Caffeine and Sodium Benzoate
　　　Injection U.S.P.　(ampul)

　　　　0.5 to 1 Gm. (gr. viiss to xv) I.M. every
　　　　hour until respiratory rate is normal.

22. ℞ Sorbitan monooleate, polyoxy-
　　　ethylene derivative. . . . . 0.5 Gm.

　　　　3 capsules with each meal. (CAUTION! The
　　　　use of mineral oil during this treatment is
　　　　contraindicated.)

PHYSICAL AND CHEMICAL

BURNS

Burns of the skin or mucous membranes may be due to thermal, electrical, radioactive, or chemical agents. During combustion, irritating gases may be liberated and inhaled. These, rather than heat, usually are the cause of damage that may occur in the lower respiratory tract (trachea, bronchi, and alveoli) and accompany the external burns.

Pathology and Pathologic Physiology

The essential effect of a burn is the destruction of cells. In thermal burns the depth of destruction is proportional to the intensity and duration of the exposure to heat. In chemical burns where the toxicity of the chemical is not promptly neutralized by body fluids, as in the case of phenol, phosphorus, and mustard gas, there may be slow extension of the area of necrosis for several hours.

The predominant feature of many electrical burns, particularly those from an arc of high voltage, is the depth of destruction. The lesion may be circumscribed on the surface and penetrate deeply through muscle to bone. If the burn overlies a large vessel, necrosis of the vessel walls with delayed hemorrhage may result.

Severe burns produce shock. The primary syncopal shock is due to disturbance of the autonomic nervous balance and its control of the vascular system. Secondary, or true, burn shock develops more slowly and is due to loss of plasma into the wound. Heat, chemicals, and electricity damage capillaries and increase their permeability. These damaged but still functioning capillaries lie beneath the zone of necrosis in both partial and full-thickness burns. Plasma, water, electrolytes, and approximately ⅔ of the dissolved protein pour freely into the wound area. Although return of much of this protein-rich plasma transudate to the blood stream is accomplished by flow through the lymphatic trunks, its formation exceeds its return for the first 36 to 48 hours and the wound becomes distended with edema. After 48 hours, with healing of the capillaries, resorption gains on formation, and subsidence of edema is prompt provided there is no wound infection. Thereafter, substances soluble in the body fluids, such as the sulfonamides, when applied to the wound surface are absorbed into the general circulation.

The lesions usually become infected only if the epidermis is broken. Bacterial growth is enhanced by dead tissue. Staphylococci and streptococci predominate in infected wounds of the upper part of the body. In those of the lower part, particularly the buttocks and thighs, various fecal organisms also are found. Long-standing open wounds of full-thickness burns tend to become bacterial quagmires with deep-rooted infections.

Symptoms and Signs

Thermal and electrical burns are extremely painful. If, as is usual in most burns of full-thickness, the sensory nerve endings of the skin are destroyed, the acute pain is promptly followed by numbness. The pain plus anxiety frequently causes acute syncope or primary shock. Thermal burns of 10% or more of the body surface, particularly in children, are followed in a few hours by secondary or burn shock (see Pathology). Patients who have received thermal burns, especially around the mouth and nose, while in enclosed spaces, should be watched for signs of irritation in the respiratory tract. There sometimes is a latent period of several hours between the inhalation of noxious gases and onset of bronchial occlusion and pulmonary edema. Chemical burns due to acids, alkalis, or phosphorus usually are apparent within a few minutes; there is pain and visible tissue destruction. The sensory disturbance and visible changes induced by certain chemicals, such as mustard gas, may not appear for several hours.

Electrical burns, particularly those of high-voltage origin, may be followed immediately by cardiac standstill and loss of consciousness. Artificial respiration often is effective in maintaining life and should not be abandoned until it is certain that the victim is dead.

Since the treatment of a wound is based upon its depth, the latter should be determined when the lesion is first seen. Mild damage results only in vascular dilatation, localized edema and tenderness—a so-called "first-degree" burn. Deeper damage but still of partial-thickness, in addition to the visible dilated, functioning, vascular bed, causes blebs of the epidermis. This is a "second-degree" burn. "Third-degree" burns are those that involve the full-thickness of the skin. Deep, partial-thickness wounds are often confused with those of full-thickness. The full-thickness wound is usually coagulated, sometimes charred, and seldom blebbed. There is no visible circulation. Sometimes, the red cells are coagulated *in situ*, revealing a normal vascular pattern, but the red pigment cannot be displaced by pressure. In the partial-thickness wound with intact circulation, pressure causes blanching, and release of pressure is followed more promptly than normally by return of the circulating red cell pigment. The full-thickness wound is insensitive to touch or prick, while the partial-thickness wound is hypersensitive.

A diagnosis of shock is based on the presence of anxiety, restlessness, confusion, somnolence, a rapid pulse rate, sweating, fall in blood pressure, and cessation of renal output. Anuria (q.v.) is most significant. Not infrequently, advanced shock exists with normal, or even elevated blood pressure.

Treatment

The treatment of burns will vary somewhat, depending on the cause of the burn. In all burns, however, therapy includes strict asepsis, care of the wound, prevention or relief of shock, control of infection, correction of anemia, and maintenance of nutrition. Since all these factors are intimately related, therapy must be carefully integrated. Circumstance may dictate the order of treatment in such a manner that subsequent complications have to be accepted, e.g., proper surgical care may have to be postponed because of impending shock; this forced neglect of the wound may lead to additional infection and resulting destruction of residual viable epithelium.

In the following outline of therapy, unless specifically stated otherwise, the local measures are intended to apply to thermal burns. The general measures recommended, however, are valid in the treatment of all types of burns.

Care of the wound: In the local treatment of most chemical burns, oils or greasy salves are contraindicated during the first 24-hour period. After a thorough cleansing with water of the contaminated and burned areas, a wet dressing should be applied. This is kept wet continuously during the first 24 hours with saline, water, or preferably a mild oxidizing-reduc-

ing agent such as saturated solution of sodium thiosulfate
(℞ 59). Following the expiration of this period, the burned area
should be treated in the same manner as a thermal burn.

In injuries due to thermal burns, bacterial contamination is
lessened by thorough cleansing with bland soapy water, irrigation with sterile normal saline, and prompt application of a
sterile protective dressing. Blebs should be protected from
rupture by an adequate amount of gauze, and the part should
be immobilized by splinting and a firm pressure bandage. If
the blebs are broken or the epidermis cracked, the firm, immobilizing dressing is also indicated to limit the spread of infection from contaminating bacteria already present on the wound
surface. Dry sterile gauze may be used for the initial dressing,
but vaseline gauze will be more comfortable over wounds of
partial thickness. Penicillin ointment in an inert, water-miscible base also is acceptable (℞ 6). Because of rapid absorption,
sulfonamide ointments (℞ 5) should not be used in large
wounds. (The possibility of sensitization to antibiotics or the
sulfonamides used topically must always be kept in mind.)

Cytoxins such as tannic acid, silver nitrate, picric acid, and
the vital dyes, including gentian violet, should not be applied
to wound surfaces, since they destroy viable cells and thus
deepen the wound.

In partial-thickness wounds without signs of infection (i.e.,
increasing local tenderness, lymphangitis, fever, and rapid
pulse), the initial dressing is not disturbed until the wound has
had time to heal. Changing the dressings on unhealed wounds
invites bacterial contamination and also may dislodge regenerating and spreading epithelium. The dressing may therefore
be left in place for 2 weeks, or longer, if the wound is of deep
partial-thickness.

In full-thickness wounds, bacterial contamination may be lessened and healing hastened by early surgical débridement and
immediate grafting. If the burn involves more than a small
area, and especially if there are additional areas of partial-thickness injury, it is wise to delay surgical excision and grafting
until the patient's fluid balance and physiologic equilibrium are
assured. If equilibrium is initially precarious or not restored,
surgical procedures are best postponed and the slough removed
by the chemical method or left to separate spontaneously, with
grafts eventually laid on a granulating surface. Spontaneous
sloughing may be accelerated by wet dressings of saline or
Dakin's solution.

Chemical sloughing: This is accomplished by the application of a pyruvic acid-starch paste prepared as follows: To
1 liter of distilled water add 7 cc. of chemically pure pyruvic
acid. Add 80 to 100 Gm. cornstarch to 200 cc. of this stock solution and mix thoroughly. Heat the remaining 800 cc. of stock
solution almost to boiling, mix with the previously prepared
paste, and allow to cool. Since pyruvic acid-starch paste works

by separating the slough at its margins, additional margins are created by cross hatching the insensitive slough with a scalpel and opening any overlying blisters. A thick layer of paste then is applied and covered with vaseline gauze or a waterproof dressing to prevent drying. Re-dressings are indicated every 2 or 3 days, or before the paste has dried out. At the time of re-dressing, separation of the slough may be hastened by judicious sharp dissection. With chemical sloughing usually at least 8 days must elapse before grafting is possible.

General treatment: Patients in primary shock or collapse should be placed in recumbency, reassured, and given suitable medication. The excitability due to pain must be differentiated from that of hysteria or anoxia. Pain is frequently less than is suggested by the first impression; it may be relieved by a small dose of morphine sulfate I.V. (℞ 36). (I.V. injection eliminates the variability in rate of absorption encountered in the circulatory deficiency of shock and tends to prevent eventual overdosage.) Hysteria can be relieved by a barbiturate I.M. (℞ 37). Anoxia due to pulmonary irritation and injury should be treated with oxygen (*see* PULMONARY EDEMA). Pain should be controlled by the use of suitable analgesics (*see* PAIN) and anesthetic ointments such as benzocaine (℞ 10), which may be applied to the mucous membranes as well as the skin. If mucous membranes of the mouth or vagina are involved, vaseline gauze packs should be used to keep apart opposing surfaces. Soothing mouthwashes (*see* STOMATITIS) are useful for oral lesions. Burns of the eye are discussed in the chapter on EYE INJURIES; Burns (q.v.).

Burn shock due to plasma loss may develop rapidly after extensive burns, and prompt preventive therapy is imperative. If 10% or more of the body surface is burned, plasma diluted with sterile physiologic saline solution should be given I.V. immediately in an amount equal to the estimated loss of plasma into the wound (*see* below). In addition, fluid must be given for the normal requirements of kidney function and for insensible water loss, and food to prevent starvation acidosis. As much as possible should be given by mouth, but if nausea is present, as is usual in extensively burned patients, this may cause vomiting, and I.V. administration must be resorted to.

The amount of plasma and fluid to be given a patient may be estimated by either (1) the surface area formula, (2) the interstitial space expansion formula, or (3) a combination of both. The efficacy of either formula must be judged by careful observation of the renal output. An inlying catheter and hourly measure of the urinary excretion is mandatory in all extensively burned patients during the first 48 hours.

1. The surface area formula is based upon the theories that the demands of the wound for fluid are proportionate to its extent; that the rate of edema formation will decrease with time after injury; and that the fluid requirement for normal metabolism, including kidney function, must be met in addition to those of the wound. In the average-sized adult, for each estimated 1% of the body surface burned, 75 cc. of plasma and 75 cc. of colloid-free isotonic electrolyte fluid are given in the first 24 hours. These fluids will fill the expanding spaces and keep up with seepage from the wound surface. For oral administration, an isotonic solution of sodium is prepared, with ⅓ of the sodium as bicarbonate and ⅔ as chloride, and flavored with fruit syrup. For I.V. administration, isotonic sodium chloride solution may be used, but a physiologically balanced solution (e.g., Ringer's) is preferable. Of the calculated amount of plasma and electrolyte fluid, ½ is given in the first 8 hours and ½ in the subsequent 16 hours, thus adapting the rate of the therapy to the expected rate of transudation into the wound.

In keeping with the decreasing rate of edema formation, the plan for the second 24 hours provides a fluid ration equal to ½ that given in the first 24 hours. In addition to the above, 2,000 cc. of fluid is given in each 24-hour period to maintain urine flow. This is preferably given by mouth and consists of palatable liquids, those containing sugar and potassium, such as fresh fruit juices, being offered freely. If I.V. administration is necessary, glucose in water is used. The volumes of each of these 3 fluids are subject to alteration according to the exigencies of the case, the continued presence of hemoconcentration, or cessation of renal output indicating need for accelerated intake. Whole blood may be substituted for some of the plasma in extensively and deeply burned patients.

2. The interstitial space expansion formula, based on the anticipated wound expansion, is suggested for patients with burns involving 30% or more of the body surface. The following amounts of fluid are to be given during the first 48 hours: (a) For wound edema, a volume equal to 10% of the body weight. (b) For external loss, an amount varying according to the area of wound: 25 to 30% of body surface, 1,000 cc.; 35 to 60%, 2,000 cc.; 60% or more, 3,000 cc.

Add (a) and (b): ⅔ of this combined volume is given as plasma and ⅓ as noncolloid isotonic electrolyte solution. This 48-hour ration is divided into 4 equal parts: 2 for the first 12 hours, 1 for the second 12, and 1 for the following 24-hour period. The time intervals are, of course, calculated from the time of the burn and, if the patient is first seen 6 hours later, the full 12 hours' ration must be given in the first 6 hours. Thus, for a 150 lb. (70 Kg.) man with a 50% burn, the volumes for the first 48 hours would be as follows: For 10% weight, 7,000 cc. of fluid; for external loss, 2,000 cc., totaling 9,000 cc., ⅔ of which (6,000 cc.) is given as plasma, and ⅓ (3,000 cc.) as saline.

(c) For renal excretion, 1,500 cc./24 hours, 3,000 cc. total of noncolloid fluid, ½ as isotonic electrolyte I.V. and ½ as glucose in water I.V., or as palatable fluids by mouth.

(d) For insensible loss, 1,500 cc./24 hours, 3,000 cc. total, of noncolloid, nonelectrolyte solution, as glucose in water I.V. or as palatable low salt fluids by mouth.

In total, therefore, the patient, with 50% of his body surface burned, would receive 9,000+3,000+3,000=15,000 cc. of fluid in 48 hours.

The renal output is a guide to the adequacy of the fluid therapy. Hourly outputs of 50 to 200 cc. indicate a sufficiency and warn against increasing the fluid intake. A falling or low hourly output (30 cc./hour down to 5 cc./hour for 3 hours or more) calls for immediate increase of fluids. The earlier a low urine output appears after the burn, the more pressing is the need for increased therapy. Hourly urine outputs of over 200 cc. for more than 6 hours during the first 48 hours signify overtreatment and, after the 48th hour, spontaneous diuresis. Such an hourly volume calls for a drastic cut in fluid administration in order to avoid plethora, pulmonary edema, or congestive heart failure.

Against infection, both local and systemic measures should be taken. The importance of débridement in controlling the spread of infection already has been discussed. Adequate débridement of partial-thickness wounds without injuring viable epithelium is difficult to achieve. Radical débridement is indicated for full-thickness wounds. Tetanus antitoxin 1,500 to 3,000 u., or more (℞ 7), or a booster dose of tetanus toxoid (℞ 8) in an individual so immunized within the preceding 2 years, should be given to all patients having burns of full- or partial-thickness.

Immediate systemic chemotherapy is indicated for all burned patients except those with minor partial-thickness lesions. Even for these patients, chemotherapy is advisable in case the blebs rupture and admit infection, or in preventing the occasional infection that occurs with intact blebs. Penicillin (℞ 1, 2) is the drug of choice, especially for burns on the upper part of the body. Because of its low toxicity it can be given when shock is present or impending. When the wounds are on the lower half of the body, streptomycin (℞ 3) also is given to combat gram-negative bacilli. A sulfonamide (℞ 4) may be added but, in extensively burned patients, not until adequate renal function is assured (*see* SULFONAMIDE THERAPY).

Sulfonamides used locally are inadequate, and undesirable because of their rapid absorption from wound surfaces and possible ill effect upon the kidneys. However, they may be applied sparingly to small burns (℞ 5). Penicillin in a water-miscible ointment base (℞ 6) is harmless and may reach the necrotic tissues more effectively than that given systemically.

Anemia develops rapidly in patients with extensive full-thickness wounds and is progressive and severe. Its early cause is hemolysis resulting directly from heat. As much as 8% of the circulating red cells may thus be lysed in an extensive, severe burn. Whole blood transfusion should therefore replace part of the plasma in the early treatment of severe burns, even in the presence of hemoconcentration. Adequate fluid must be supplied to the kidneys to enable them safely to excrete the excessive products of hemolysis.

The later, progressive anemia, presumably related to the infection and occurring in deeply and extensively burned patients, should be treated vigorously with whole blood transfusions, as it develops. As much as 600 cc. of whole blood daily has been required in the first 10 days after injury. Neglect of the anemia encourages the infection and malnutrition.

Malnutrition, like the anemia, develops rapidly in severely burned patients in response to the trauma and subsequent infection. There is a precipitous and prolonged rise in oxygen consumption and nitrogen excretion and an increased rate of utilization of vitamin C and perhaps of other specific food substances. Protein deficiency, edema, muscular wasting, and inanition appear. Loss of appetite is common. Every effort should be bent, through food and supplementary I.V. therapy, toward maintaining an adequate balance of proteins, calories, and vitamins. Protein hydrolysates or amino acids mixtures may be given I.V. Although it is not proved that they are an adequate substitute for plasma in the maintenance of the serum protein level, they may be helpful in maintaining protein intake for a few days, until the patient can ingest an adequate diet.

SUNBURN

(Erythema solare)

A common affection characterized by a superficial inflammation of the skin caused by actinic rays from the sun or artificial sources.

Etiology and Predisposing Factors

The ultraviolet rays ranging between 2,800 and 3,100, with the maximum effect of 2,967 angstroms are responsible for the reaction.

Persons vary greatly in their reaction and sensitivity to ultraviolet rays. Blondes and the rufous type generally are more susceptible than brunettes, men more reactive than women, and young infants more than adults. Women have increased photosensitivity during the first days of the menses and the 2nd to the 7th months of pregnancy. Active tuberculosis, hyperthyroidism, and perhaps other diseases increase sensitivity, as also may occur with sulfonamide therapy. There is some variation in the sensitivity of different parts of the body.

Clouds do not necessarily remove ultraviolet rays, and reflection from snow, sand, water, or ice greatly increases exposure. High altitudes and more perpendicular sun rays (seasonal variation) also increase exposure, other factors being equal.

Symptoms and Signs

Mild to moderate exposure results in a simple erythema of the skin, while severe exposure produces vesiculation and bulla formation. If large areas are involved by erythema, edema, vesiculation, and bullae, in addition to burning, pain, and smarting, there may be moderate to severe constitutional symptoms including insomnia, chills, fever, weakness and even delirium and collapse. The reaction usually commences several hours following the exposure and reaches its maximum within 12 to 24 hours. Peeling and itching of the skin ensue as the reaction subsides. Varying degrees of temporary pigmentation or tanning occur. In susceptible persons, a severe reaction is often followed by persistent and extensive freckling.

Diagnosis

History of exposure and the resultant erythema and vesiculation, confined to exposed areas, are characteristic. There may be associated conjunctivitis and cheilitis. Furunculosis, impetiginized eczematoid dermatitis, and contact dermatitis due to local medicaments may complicate the condition. Varying degrees of exposure may precipitate true light sensitivity dermatoses or initiate lesions in such basic diseases as pellagra or lupus erythematosus.

Prognosis

Generally good. Very severe sunburn associated with heat prostration and shock (q.v.) has at times been fatal.

Prophylaxis

Prevention of sunburn can be accomplished by sensible gradual exposures and is a wise yet seldom practiced precaution. Avoidance of prolonged initial exposure is most important. The average brunette will tolerate, as a maximum, two 15- to 20-minute exposures to strong sunlight the 1st day, two 30- to 45-minute exposures the 2nd day, with successive gradual increase. The individual's tolerance must determine the schedule. Increased tolerance is developed by thickening of the keratinous layer of the epidermis and by development of melanin, the latter creating "tanning." Blondes, redheads, and others with known low tolerance should begin their schedules with 5 or 10 minutes of exposure, and use protective hats and clothing otherwise, and creams, lotions, or oils. Petrolatum (℞ 11) or zinc oxide ointment (℞ 12) often is sufficient to prevent undue evaporation from the skin, and to filter the rays.

Persons receiving, or who recently have received, sulfonamide therapy should be warned against undue exposure to sunlight, because of the photosensitivity induced by these drugs.

Precautions outlined above with respect to sunlight should be exercised correspondingly with ultraviolet ray therapy.

Light-protective preparations contain chemicals which filter out the ultraviolet rays; included among the chemicals used are quinine, titanium oxide, methyl or phenyl salicylate, para-aminobenzoic acid, or certain glycosides (esculin). Greasy or oily "antisunburn" preparations may cause pyodermas or furuncles and usually are less desirable. The following preparations are useful: Protective cream (℞ 13); protective lotion (℞ 14) (this lotion washes off easily and so must be reapplied after each swim); protective ointment (℞ 15). The latter resists removal by water, and is especially useful for small areas which repeatedly burn, such as nose, chin, and malar prominences. Women may prefer a protective enamel (℞ 16) that effectively protects from sun and wind, persists for a long time, and acts as a substitute for "make-up." All of these protective preparations permit gradual tanning.

Treatment

Treatment of sunburn depends on the degree and extent of involvement. A generalized mild erythema is treated by "powder baths," several times daily and before retiring, with a powder containing equal parts of zinc oxide, talc, and boric acid (℞ 17). Rose water ointment (℞ 18) is soothing, cooling, and counteracts excessive drying of the skin. Sedatives or hypnotics will aid in preventing miserable and sleepless nights. If extensive vesiculation and bulla formation have occurred, hydrolyzed cornstarch baths (1 lb. to tubful of water) may prove soothing. Any lesions secondarily infected should be treated with wet compresses or soaks (℞ 19, 20). During the intervals between such treatments, a soothing drying lotion (℞ 21) may be used. Large bullae should be opened aseptically. After the acute edema, redness, vesiculation, and oozing have subsided, the application of soothing cream (℞ 22) or rose water ointment (℞ 18) is indicated. Patients suffering from shock and prostration should be hospitalized and treated, both locally and systemically, as for severe burns and heat prostration (q.v.).

HEAT DISORDERS

HEAT PROSTRATION

(Heat collapse, Heat exhaustion, Heat syncope)

A syndrome resulting from exposure to excessive heat, characterized by prostration and varying degrees of circulatory collapse.

Etiology

Heat prostration results from failure of the peripheral circulatory system and represents a different response to the environmental conditions that cause heat hyperpyrexia (q.v.). Vasodilation is the usual response to exposure to high temperature and if there is no compensatory increase in blood volume, peripheral failure occurs.

Symptoms and Signs

The victim is listless, apprehensive, may be semicomatose or, in severe cases, unconscious. Usually, the skin is ashen, cold, and wet, perspiration is profuse, blood pressure lowered, and peripheral vascular failure evident. Premonitory symptoms— weakness, dizziness, vertigo, headache, dim or blurred vision, irritability, and mild muscular cramps may precede the attack by several hours or days. The pulse rate usually is less than 100, but tachycardia has been observed. There is no significant elevation of the body temperature. Onset may occur at night or during the course of another illness. This condition frequently complicates surgery in the tropics.

Diagnosis and Prognosis

Heat prostration is distinguished from food or chemical poisoning and malaria by history and rapid response to treatment. The prognosis is excellent. Heat prostration usually is transient, and the mortality rate is very low, although death can occur from circulatory failure.

Prevention

Prevention of heat prostration is readily accomplished by avoiding undue exertion and excessive exposure, by maintaining adequate salt intake (℞ 24), and by wearing light, loose, well ventilated clothing when conditions of high environmental temperature exist. Proper acclimation to heat is essential.

Treatment

Place the patient in a reclining position in a cool environment when possible. Loosen tight clothing. Cool water containing 0.5 Gm. sodium chloride/pint may be given by mouth (℞ 25). The essential problem is management of acute circulatory failure. Patients in profound collapse should be given 1,500 cc. of isotonic saline solution I.V. (℞ 24), slowly and cautiously in order to avoid overloading an already embarrassed circulation. Cardiac stimulants (℞ 51), plasma, and oxygen may be given for support. Sodium bicarbonate is contraindicated.

HEAT CRAMPS
(Stokers' cramp, Firemen's cramp, Miners' cramp, Cane-cutters' cramp)

A condition resulting from physical exertion in high temperatures, characterized by sudden development of severe cramps of the abdominal or skeletal muscles.

Etiology

Heavy muscular work when atmospheric temperature is above 100° F., associated with profuse perspiration and failure to replace resultant salt loss.

Symptoms and Signs

The patient usually is found on the floor or ground with legs drawn up, or threshing about, grimacing and occasionally crying out from the excruciating pain. The cramps occur in paroxysms, most frequently of the flexors of the arms and legs, with relative comfort between spasms. Examination reveals palpable spasms or knots of muscles, pale, wet skin, rectal temperature 98° to 100° F. and normal blood pressure. The onset usually is acute; occasionally, symptoms are mild the first day but become severe within 24 hours. An untreated attack may last hours or days.

Prevention

Prevention may be effected by adequate salt intake. Sodium chloride added to drinking water (℞ 25), or plain or enteric coated salt tablets may be taken (℞ 23).

Treatment

Administration of sodium chloride and water is specific. Place patient in recumbent rest in a cool place. Give sodium chloride in water by mouth unless gastric distress is evident (℞ 23, 25); if so, give isotonic saline solution I.V. (℞ 24). Hot packs and saline cathartics are contraindicated.

HEAT HYPERPYREXIA

(Sunstroke, Heatstroke, Thermic fever, Siriasis)

A profound disturbance of the heat-regulating mechanism characterized by high fever and collapse, and sometimes by convulsions, coma, and death.

Etiology

Prolonged exposure to excessively high temperature or the direct rays of a hot sun, combined with high humidity and lack of air circulation are the responsible factors. Individuals past 40 and those with systemic disease are most susceptible.

Symptoms and Signs

The onset usually is sudden and acute. Diminution or cessation of sweating may precede the attack by several hours. The patient is flushed, the skin hot and dry. Weakness, headache, vertigo, anorexia, nausea, and precordial distress are the usual complaints. Muscular twitching or cramps may occur. Pyrexia is apparent on physical examination. The patient appears anxious and listless, pupils are contracted early but dilate later, tendon reflexes are diminished, pulse rate may be 160 or more, respiration 20 to 30, and the blood pressure may be slightly elevated with a wide pulse pressure. The temperature rises rapidly to 105° or 106° F. or higher. Convulsions and projectile vomiting may develop and are of serious import. Profound shock and circulatory collapse may follow and usually persist until death. The leukocyte count may be increased and disturbances of the clotting mechanism may occur.

Diagnosis

A presumptive diagnosis of heat hyperpyrexia should be made when any person exposed to high temperature has pyrexia without other apparent cause. Meningitis, malaria, or pneumonia may be suspected, but heat hyperpyrexia represents an acute emergency and when a history of undue exposure to heat is obtained, treatment must not be postponed while awaiting a positive diagnosis.

Prognosis

Hyperpyrexia is a serious threat to life. Mortality may be as high as 20% and depends partially upon the duration of the acute condition prior to treatment. A rectal temperature exceeding 106° F. is a grave prognostic sign; a temperature above 108° F. produces irreversible changes in the brain. Old age, cardiac disease, renal disease and chronic alcoholism lessen the possibility of recovery.

Treatment

Heroic measures are indicated and must be instituted immediately. If the rectal temperature is 106° F. or over, an ice-water tub bath is given, and the skin massaged vigorously until the temperature falls below 103° F. Rectal temperatures must be checked every 10 minutes and constant attendance by a nurse or physician is necessary. Hypothermia may occur during or after the bath and, if severe, requires the application of heat, and treatment for collapse. When the temperature has been reduced, the patient is placed in a cool, well ventilated room with an electric fan directed toward the bed. Massage is continued since it combats the vasoconstriction induced by the cold bath, aids in acceleration of heat loss, and stimulates the return of cooled peripheral blood to the overheated brain and other viscera. If high temperature tends to recur, resume the ice-water bath. The use of wet sheets with forced ventilation, ice-water sponge baths, and rubbing with ice are inadequate except for mild cases. Sedative drugs (R 37, 38, 39) are contraindicated except to control convulsions. Morphine or epinephrine should not be given. I.V. fluids may be indicated for collapse or as supportive measures. Injections of 1,500 cc. of isotonic saline solution may be given twice a day (R 24), but not before the temperature falls below 102° F., and then only slowly and cautiously in order to avoid pulmonary edema or cardiac failure. The patient should remain in bed several days and a further convalescent period is advised, especially if organic disease is present.

DECOMPRESSION SICKNESS

("The bends," Caisson disease, Compressed-air illness,
"Altitude bends," Aeroembolism)

*A clinical disorder caused by a too rapid change from a higher
to a lower atmospheric pressure, with resultant gaseous desaturation of the body tissues and the formation therein of gas
bubbles.* **Aeroembolism** is that special form of decompression
sickness which occurs following sudden change to a gaseous
pressure less than atmospheric, as in rapid ascent to high altitudes.

Etiology

This condition is encountered in tunnel workers and others
who work under increased atmospheric pressures (e.g., "sandhogs," divers), and in occupants of rapidly climbing nonpressurized aircraft (*see* MEDICAL ASPECTS OF FLYING). Ages over
40, obesity, chronic diseases, alcoholism, and fatigue are predisposing factors. Physiologically inert gases—nitrogen when air
is involved, and helium in helium-oxygen diving—are the responsible agents.

Symptoms and Signs

Following too rapid decompression from pressures above 1 atmosphere, or from atmospheric pressure to lower pressures, liberated gas bubbles act as air emboli occluding small veins, capillaries and arteries, and collecting in the tissues, especially fatty
tissue. The resultant symptoms depend on the part of the body
involved and the degree of embolization. Onset usually is
within 30 minutes after the rapid change to a much reduced
pressure but it sometimes may be delayed for several hours.
In decompression from greater than atmospheric pressure, localized sharp pains in the abdomen, or about the joints of the
extremities ("the bends"), vertigo ("the staggers"), nystagmus,
tinnitus, nausea, vomiting, pulmonary edema, and such neurologic manifestations as paralysis of the bladder or rectum, monoplegia, or diplegia may be present. Shock and collapse may
occur in severe cases.

The symptoms of aeroembolism due to decompression to
lower than atmospheric pressure, as in high-altitude flying, differ
somewhat from those encountered following exposure to increased atmospheric pressures. For unknown reasons, the spinal
cord escapes injury. Muscle and joint pains are frequently
present, whereas girdle pains are seldom noted. Respiratory
symptoms ("chokes") varying from substernal distress and
paroxysmal cough to tachypnea or even asphyxia, and cutaneous

manifestations (tingling, formication, numbness, pruritus, rashes, temperature sensations, aeroemphysema) are common complaints, as are visual disturbances (lacrimation, burning, diplopia, scotomas) aero-otitis media, sinus pain, toothache, and abdominal distress due to expansion of intestinal gases.

Diagnosis

The diagnosis usually is easy if the victim's occupation is known. Exposed workers are customarily provided with an identifying badge or card for the information of police officers and physicians and to indicate where they are to be sent in case of emergency.

Prognosis

In severe untreated cases, circulatory failure, coma, and death quickly ensue. With prompt and efficient treatment, the chances of complete recovery are excellent. In patients untreated for several hours, sequelae are likely to develop, particularly neurologic disorders; bladder or bowel paralysis usually is temporary, but weakness of an involved extremity may persist.

Treatment

Therapy consists of prompt and adequate recompression in a "medical lock," up to a maximum pressure of 165 pounds, or 1 atmosphere (15 pounds) above that at which symptomatic relief becomes evident, whichever pressure is lower, followed by controlled decompression to normal atmospheric pressure. This decompression may be accomplished by reducing the pressure in the "lock" by steps or by a uniformly constant decrease in pressure. "Locks" of this type (with tabulated directions concerning the rate of decompression) are available in areas where this particular occupational hazard is likely to be encountered. Inhalation of 100% O_2 during decompression will hasten the elimination of nitrogen from the body. Obese individuals require more prolonged decompression because 5 times as much nitrogen is dissolved by fatty tissue as by nonfatty tissue. In the presence of shock, O_2 inhalation and absolute bed rest are indicated until the pulse and blood pressure have remained stabilized for a minimum of 2 hours.

Aircraft occupants suffering from minor degrees of aeroembolism need only be brought down to and kept at a lower altitude in order to effect recovery. For severe cases, O_2 therapy and absolute rest are indicated, as above.

RADIATION REACTIONS AND INJURIES

The harmful effects, acute or delayed, produced on body tissues by exposure to the ionizing radiations from radium, radon, other radioactive substances, and to X-rays.

Etiology

X-rays and gamma rays differ from each other only in wavelength, gamma radiation being shorter and more energetic. Modern, high-voltage X-ray machines are capable of producing radiation of wavelengths comparable to gamma radiation. These are true electromagnetic radiations and their effects on tissue probably are due to the ionization set up in the cells. Radium and radioactive substances in addition to producing gamma rays produce particles commonly spoken of as alpha and beta rays which also cause ionization in tissues. These particles travel a much shorter distance but ionize rather heavily in this distance. Alpha particles are stopped by a single sheet of paper and the most powerful beta particle rarely travels more than 2 cm. in tissue. Very energetic X- and gamma radiation will penetrate several feet of lead.

Pathologic Physiology

General: The exact mechanism of action of the radiations is not known but it is believed to be a disturbance in cellular activity resulting from chemical changes caused by ionization. It is known, for example, that the sulfhydryl enzyme systems are adversely affected by ionizing radiations.

In the order of decreasing sensitivity, the various tissues affected are: (1) Lymphoid cells; (2) red cell precursors; (3) polymorphonuclear and eosinophilic leukocytes; (4) epithelial cells: (*a*) basal epithelium of secretory glands, especially the salivary glands; (*b*) basal epithelium of the gonads (spermatogonium, follicular epithelium); (*c*) basal epithelium of the skin and mucous membranes, particularly the stomach and intestine; (*d*) epithelium of the lung alveoli and liver bile ducts; (*e*) tubular epithelium of the kidneys; (5) endothelium of the blood vessels, pleura, and peritoneum; (6) connective tissue cells; (7) muscle cells; (8) bone cells; (9) nerve cells.

Acute: In mild acute radiation sickness following overexposure to X-rays or radium there often are no detectable histologic changes. If vomiting is severe and protracted, the usual findings of alkalosis are present. Long-standing diarrhea may produce dehydration and acidosis.

In severe acute radiation sickness, as after large doses of any penetrating radiation such as occurred at Hiroshima and Nagasaki, pathologic examination of individuals who died showed extensive hemorrhages throughout the body, aplastic bone marrow, and general destruction of lymphatic tissue. In addition to thrombocytopenia and increased capillary permeability, and thus an increased bleeding time, and petechiae, massive doses of penetrating radiations produce an increase in blood heparin which may be sufficient to render the blood incoagulable. All these factors add to the danger of death from hemorrhage. Added to these hematologic changes and the disturbances in water balance, infection played an important role in the death of many of these individuals.

Delayed: Long-continued or repeated mild exposures to ionizing radiations may result in amenorrhea, loss of testicular function, anemia, leukopenia, agranulocytosis, and may produce leukemia. Experience during World War II on atomic energy projects indicated that large groups of individuals exposed repeatedly to low doses (e.g., 0.1 roentgen/day) while working with radioactive isotopes developed as the only manifestation a mild reduction in total leukocyte count. More severe or localized exposure causes loss of hair, skin atrophy and ulceration, telangiectasia, keratoses, and ultimately skin carcinomas. Any difference in the effect of the different types of radiation beyond a quantitative effect has not yet been proved.

Very large doses in limited areas will produce fibrosis of the tissues such as is seen in the underlying lung following massive radiation for breast carcinoma. Bone structure may be damaged so that pathologic fracture occurs, or as a late result, sarcoma may arise.

Internal absorption of radioactive materials may lead to serious consequences. Most of the naturally occurring radioactive materials are deposited in bone after absorption. Bone tumor formation and necrosis are the result of alpha radiation emanating from these materials over long periods of time. A good example of this is the jaw necrosis and sarcoma seen in radium-paint workers who were in the habit of touching the paint brush to their tongues. Such cases are rare now but may again become prevalent if workers with radioactive isotopes are allowed to become careless. Overdosage with radiophosphorus used in the treatment of leukemias, and the like, may produce aplasia of the bone marrow with leukopenia and other blood dyscrasias, followed by death from infection.

Symptoms and Signs

Acute Radiation Sickness: This is a systemic reaction which often follows the administration of fairly large doses of roentgen or gamma radiation. The onset is gradual, usually occurring within several hours after the treatment. It usually is self-limited with or without treatment and lasts from 24 to 36 hours if no further irradiation is given. It consists of various degrees of malaise, lassitude, anorexia, and often progresses to vomiting that may be persistent and require treatment. It may be so severe as to require abandonment of radiation therapy. Bloody diarrhea may occur. These disorders are most often seen when the viscera, especially the stomach, spleen, and liver, are overly radiated. This is especially true in the case of a debilitated patient. There is considerable individual variation in sensitivity.

With huge doses of radiation, either external or internal, the reaction may be so severe as to produce death in a moderately short time. Fatalities usually result from severe anemia, hemorrhage, or infection secondary to a pancytopenia due to bone marrow aplasia. Severe radiation burns may at times be fatal.

Delayed Radiation Sickness: This form of the systemic reaction usually is seen in workers who are subject to long-continued small exposures of radiation. The onset is insidious and the patient rarely is aware of the danger until severe damage has been done. Lassitude and easy fatigability are early symptoms. Amenorrhea also may be early. After months or years of chronic exposure symptoms associated with anemia, leukopenia, and thrombocytopenia appear. Hemorrhages, bone necrosis and sarcoma may occur in the advanced forms. Death eventually results from severe anemia, hemorrhage, or terminal sepsis.

Where only local exposure has occurred, such as of the hands or face, the skin may become dry and scaly with loss of hair and atrophy of the underlying connective tissue. This may be followed by keratoses, cutaneous carcinomas, or chronic painful ulcers with sharply defined margins.

Diagnosis

When a patient is receiving X-ray therapy and the acute form of radiation sickness occurs, the diagnosis usually is obvious. Some difficulty may arise when the patient already has some of the symptoms by virtue of the established disease process.

In the chronic forms where the exposure is either unknown or neglected, diagnosis may be extremely difficult, and often may be reached only after very painstaking search into the past history for possible sources of exposure. Occupation and history of medication are cardinal points to be carefully studied.

Treatment

The management of the patient who is receiving a full course of X-ray therapy frequently requires much care and close cooperation between radiologist and referring physician. Often, the size of dosage and interval between treatments must be adjusted so that the patient's condition does not progressively deteriorate. Supportive therapy should be started before the condition develops and should be continued between treatments in an effort to avoid or ameliorate this complication of therapy.

Acute Radiation Sickness: No specific remedy for the acute forms has yet been found. Supportive measures are in order and should consist of a bland high caloric diet (*see* DIETS), increased sugar intake, and vitamin B (℞ 46). Recent evidence has shown that administration of desoxycorticosterone (℞ 47) may be of benefit as may also a trial of pyridoxine (vitamin B_6) (℞ 48, 49). Bed rest and sedation (℞ 37) are important. If the reaction is more severe parenteral fluids may be used (5% glucose or 5% glucose in saline) and plasma or whole blood may be required. In the event the exposure has been extreme, the patient is managed much as is one with a major thermal burn. If the blood becomes incoagulable as a result of a heparin increase, toluidine blue (℞ 34) or protamine sulfate (℞ 35) may be given I.V. at 24-hour intervals if necessary.

Chronic Delayed Radiation Sickness: The most important consideration is diagnosis and removal of the patient from the offending radiation. In chronic radium poisoning such as seen in workers in radium paint, the mobilization of the material by means of decalcification regimens using low calcium diet (*see* Diets) and high doses of ammonium chloride (℞ 26) has been used. This form of treatment may be effective in the early stages, but is of little value in removing any appreciable amount of the radium deposited in the bone in the later stages when the deposits are fixed in the cortex. Appropriate regimens probably will be worked out if poisoning by other newer radioactive substances occurs. Use of a radon ointment, supervised by a radiotherapist, has proved successful in the treatment of chronic skin ulcers, although surgery may later become necessary. In the event of bone necrosis (e.g., jaw, head of the femur) or bone sarcomas, surgery may be indicated.

For anemia, the usual symptomatic therapy including blood transfusions is indicated, but response may be poor if the marrow has been permanently damaged. If amenorrhea or testicular dysfunction has occurred, there is no effective treatment and there is little chance for the restoration of normal gametogenesis. Many geneticists believe that there is danger of gene alteration in later generations if men or women who have been temporarily sterilized by radiation are allowed to have children. No concrete evidence to support this theory is yet available.

MOTION SICKNESS

Nausea and vomiting induced by irregular or rhythmic movements. Depending upon the circumstances, the syndrome is termed: seasickness, air sickness, car sickness, train sickness, swing sickness, and the like.

Etiology and Physiologic Mechanisms

The common denominator in motion sickness is exposure to acceleration, which may be purely angular as in a Barany chair, or linear as in an elevator, or radial as in a swing. More frequently it is encountered as a mixture of various forms and degrees as in a ship which rolls, pitches, yaws, and scends.

Irritation of the vestibular apparatus (electrical, caloric, inflammatory, or degenerative) is apt to induce nausea and vomiting, and destruction of the vestibular apparatus produces complete immunity from the effects of motion. It has become possible to localize more accurately those structures of the C.N.S. essential to the development of motion sickness since the discovery that extirpation of the cerebellar nodulus in dogs produces complete immunity to the effects of swinging.

The vestibular and cerebellar mechanisms are not the sole factors involved in the production of motion sickness in man. Other factors appear to be contributory, such as disturbances in visual orientation occurring when an individual views rapidly moving surroundings, as from a train window, or when positional orientation is impaired, as when viewing a moving horizon aboard a ship or aircraft. Fatigue, dietary or alcoholic excesses, mild disease of the gastrointestinal tract or mild infections of the upper respiratory tract may cause individuals usually free from motion sickness to become ill.

Certain other environmental factors may contribute to the sensitivity of man to motion: high temperature and humidity, inadequate ventilation, perceptible concentrations of fumes and odors of, for example, gasoline, engine exhaust, paint, food, dejecta, and vomitus.

The gastrointestinal tract is a common site for bodily expression of emotional stresses, and a familiar response is nausea and vomiting. Hence, much emphasis has been placed on the psychologic bases of motion sickness. Fear and anxiety attending travel by aircraft undoubtedly contribute to some instances of motion sickness (*see* MEDICAL ASPECTS OF FLYING). Furthermore, conditioning may develop so that susceptible individuals become nauseated before any motion is experienced. Thus, prevention of motion sickness is as important as its treatment.

Symptoms and Signs

Cardinal symptoms are nausea recurring in waves and culminating in violent emesis. Premonitory signs are yawning, hyperventilation, salivation, a greenish pallor, profuse cold sweating, somnolence, waning of attention, depression and, more rarely, hiccuping. Once nausea and vomiting have developed the motion-sick individual may experience generalized weakness, be unable to perform tasks requiring effort or concentration. Some patients complain of giddiness but the absence of sustained vertigo or nystagmus is noteworthy. With prolonged exposure to motion many individuals experience adaptation and gain "sea legs" with gradual return of well-being. However, such adaptation may fail with exposure to more severe motion, or disappear during a short period away from the accustomed motion. Prolonged motion sickness, while not fatal, may produce an alarming condition marked by arterial hypotension, profound weight loss, dehydration, starvation with acidosis, and depression.

Treatment

General: Individuals susceptible to motion sickness should be advised to minimize motion by selecting positions least likely to expose them to scending motion, e.g., amidships or between the wings in aircraft. They should avoid alcoholic or dietary excesses before or during a trip. Reading, or any unusual visual stimuli (watching a rolling horizon) should be avoided. A supine or semirecumbent position is advised. During the first period of exposure, fluids and only the simplest of foods should be taken in small amounts at frequent intervals.

Drugs: Of the belladonna alkaloids, scopolamine (Ŗ 40) has gained widespread use because of its tranquilizing effect without marked mydriasis, cycloplegia, tachycardia, or suppression of salivation or sweating. Some prefer to use extract of belladonna (Ŗ 41). In patients over 40 years repeated doses of these drugs may produce a mild cycloplegia and rare instances of excitement have been reported. If maintenance of normal alertness is not required many individuals may be made more comfortable during shorter exposures by moderate sedation sufficient to induce light sleep. Sedation may be used in combination with scopolamine. The barbiturates (Ŗ 39, 42) or chloral hydrate (Ŗ 43) are admirable for this purpose. Chlorobutanol (Ŗ 44) has been used for many years as a specific, but its effect seems to rest solely upon its sedative action. Amphetamine sulfate (Ŗ 52) may sometimes prove useful in combating the depression that accompanies motion sickness. In intractable vomiting with starvation and dehydration, the parenteral administration of physiologic fluids (saline and glucose) may become necessary as a general supportive measure. Dramamine (Ŗ 45) has recently been shown to be quite effective in the prophylaxis and treatment of motion sickness; usually, the drug is administered orally, after meals and at bedtime, in doses of 50 to 100 mg.

MEDICAL ASPECTS OF FLYING

With increasing civilian air travel, the physician will be called upon more frequently to advise his patients whether an existing disorder contraindicates flying, or how it may be affected by high altitudes. Most of the large, modern air liners have sealed cabins in which barometric pressure can be partially controlled, thus making it feasible for most persons to fly in comfort. All passenger planes, however, are not so equipped and, even in those that are, individuals may experience some discomfort from unavoidable changes in air pressure during rapid ascent or descent. The rare, but possible failure of a pressure system must also be kept in mind, particularly with respect to the safety of persons already handicapped by certain disabilities.

Physical Aspect

The physician should first consider the changes that take place in the body with alterations of atmospheric pressure (*see* DECOMPRESSION SICKNESS). On ascending rapidly to high levels, the lowering of barometric pressure causes a progressive decrease in the partial pressure of oxygen in the lungs and the hemoglobin is consequently less adequately oxygenized. At an altitude of 18,000 feet the air contains about 10% oxygen instead of the normal 21%. Oxygen deprivation may result in a mental disturbance similar to that of alcoholic intoxication, an increase in the heart and respiration rates, and a rise in systolic blood pressure.

In persons with congenital defects of the respiratory tract, changes in air pressure may cause the development of a pneumothorax. In tuberculous patients under treatment with artificial pneumothorax or pneumoperitoneum, overexpansion of air in these regions during ascent may lead to serious results through shifting of viscera and the breakdown of adhesions. It may be advisable to reduce the amount of air in the pleural or abdominal cavity before the patient is allowed to ascend in a plane, and to limit the ascent to moderate altitudes. Patients with other pulmonary conditions which restrict the functioning of the lungs, such as severe diffuse fibrosis or emphysema, do not tolerate air travel well.

In the cardiac patient, the most important consideration is the degree of cardiac reserve present. Patients with low cardiac reserve, who suffer congestive failure from mild exertion at sea level, or those with known coronary disease should not be subjected to low atmospheric pressures.

The auditory mechanism is especially sensitive to changes in air pressure. In the presence of acute upper respiratory infection, the opening into the eustachian tube or accessory sinuses may be constricted by inflammation, exudate, or edema of the mucous membranes. If the eustachian tube is not patent (*see* EUSTACHITIS), the ear drum is subjected to distortion due to the unequal air pressures on either side, which may result in inflammation (aero-otitis). This often can be avoided by the preflight use of nose drops (℞ 54) or an inhaler (℞ 53), containing a vasoconstrictor. No damage is caused in an ear drum which is already perforated. In persons with deafness due to adhesions, sharp changes of air pressure have been reported occasionally to break up the adhesions with beneficial effect. In patients with infected sinuses, ascent usually causes evacuation of the sinus contents; during descent the narrow ostia of the sinuses may close, with resultant pain over the affected area and in the adjacent teeth. These effects may be prevented by the use of vasoconstricting nose drops (℞ 54) or inhalers (℞ 53) at the beginning of a descent. The use of chewing gum, repeated swallowing or yawning, and closing the nostrils and mouth during forced expiration of the breath may help to open the eustachian tubes and equalize the pressures on the ear drums. Sometimes, individuals may sleep through ascent or descent, frequently as a result of having taken some medication, with resultant ear discomfort.

Allergic patients sensitive to air-borne allergens usually find relief in air travel because of the absence of excitants. Occasionally, an asthmatic patient may have an attack precipitated by the nervous tension associated with travel of any sort.

Anemic patients may experience discomfort at high altitudes in planes without air pressure control. Tissue anoxia is likely to occur, even in slightly rarified atmospheres, in those with a red cell count of 2,500,000/cu. mm. or less. Blood transfusion before flight is advisable for these patients.

Normal pregnancy up to the end of the 8th month does not contraindicate air travel, but during the 9th month flight should not be undertaken without examination of the patient and approval by an obstetrician of all the details of the trip.

Normal infants usually tolerate air travel without discomfort.

Air sickness is similar to motion sickness (q.v.) from other causes, and is usually induced by excessive motion of the plane. "Stratosphere" flying usually is much smoother than low altitude flying, and larger planes are less affected by atmospheric disturbances than are small planes. There also seems to be a contributory emotional factor in many cases of air sickness. The nausea often may be overcome to some extent by keeping the eyes fixed on an object inside the plane and by not allowing them to shift with the plane's movements or to follow a rolling horizon. There also are numerous preparations available which will prevent or ameliorate air sickness (℞ 40, 41, 42). Dramamine (℞ 45) has shown great promise in the relief of motion sickness.

Psychic Aspect

Because civilian air travel is still relatively new, it often produces some degree of fear in passengers, especially on their first flight, and in some instances even on subsequent flights. This may exacerbate disease processes already present. In nervously unstable individuals it may result in hysteria, fainting, or even fatal shock. Sedative therapy is indicated in such cases. Alcoholic liquors are best avoided before and during flight, especially if the individual is prone to easily induced upsets of equilibrium.

Public Health Aspect

The great speed and range of travel provided by the airplane have important implications in the field of epidemiology. Persons in the incubation stage of a contagious disease may easily be the means of carrying the infection from an area where it is endemic to one in which it can take root easily and spread to epidemic proportions. Because of this possibility, persons who actually have a communicable disease or are known to have been recently exposed to infection should not be approved for air travel until all danger of contagion is past.

————————

WOUNDS

Tissue injuries accompanied by a break in the skin or in the mucous membranes.

1. Abrasions (scuff burns, mat burns) are caused by rubbing or scraping off the outer layers of the skin or mucous membrane. These lesions are easily infected by bacteria-laden foreign bodies ground into the abraded surface. They require thorough cleansing with soap and water, gentle removal of foreign particles, and the application of a sterile dressing with pressure for the control of hemorrhage.

2. Incised wounds tend to bleed easily since the vessels have been cut cleanly across by a sharp cutting object such as a knife, razor, or broken glass. These wounds are less likely to become infected because very little tissue is destroyed, usually little foreign material is carried into the wound, and the profuse flow of blood tends to wash out most of the infective material. If the wound is fresh (less than 8 hours old) and uncontaminated, it can be closed after inspection for the presence of foreign bodies (and where necessary, for the identification of severed nerves and tendons), cleansing of the surrounding area with soap, water, alcohol, and ether, and copious irrigation of the wound itself with normal saline solution. Closure by suture is done without tension or drainage, and should be followed by complete immobilization of the affected part. When the length and depth are not great, closure may be effected by the use of one or more butterfly adhesive tape dressings. If the incised wound is contaminated, or is more than 8 hours old, a sterile sponge should be placed in it while the tissues around it are cleaned. All foreign material should be removed and dead, crushed tissue excised. Irrigation of the lesion with normal saline solution, followed by closure, as in an uncontaminated wound, is next carried out. If closure is not indicated, because of the serious nature of the tissue damage, the wound should be packed loosely with fine mesh gauze and the part immobilized. Delayed closure or skin grafting may be performed 4 to 7 days later, when the clinical signs (healthy, clean, uninflamed tissues) indicate that the wound is surgically sterile.

3. Lacerations or tears usually are produced by blunt instruments, shell fragments, or falls against sharp objects. Such wounds have torn and uneven edges. Hemorrhage is seldom severe since the blood vessels are irregularly torn across. Foreign matter frequently present in the wound, sluggish bleeding, and damage to surrounding tissues causing necrosis are all characteristic of lacerated wounds and are conducive to infection. Care of lacerated wounds is similar to that of contaminated incised wounds (*see* above).

4. Puncture wounds are made by penetrating instruments such as nails, needles, and knives. Such lesions are excellent sites for the development of infection since they usually do not bleed freely and the point of entry seals over quickly, making the depths of the wound ideal for the propagation of infective agents. The wound should be cleansed and if foreign bodies have entered the tissues the tract should be laid open and excised. Once the foreign bodies have been removed and débridement carried out in the manner described under contaminated incised wounds, the lesions should be dressed without suturing.

General Prophylactic and Therapeutic Measures

Hemorrhage usually is easy to control in a minor wound through the application of a pressure dressing. This procedure may be supplemented by elevation of the involved extremity. Bleeding from an isolated visible blood vessel, when not arrested by pressure, is best controlled by ligation of the vessel. Only when blood continues to gush from a wound despite these measures should a tourniquet be applied proximal to the wound and a search made for the severed vessels. The tourniquet should be released every 10 to 15 minutes for a brief period of time. Once these vessels have been identified and ligated the tourniquet can be removed.

In order to prevent infection, all wounds should be treated as aseptically as possible, and patients with contaminated wounds should receive prophylactic administration of a chemotherapeutic agent (*see* Antibiotic Therapy; Sulfonamide Therapy), coupled with immunotherapy. Tetanus antitoxin (℞ 7) 3,000 u. should be given after preliminary testing of the patient for sensitivity (*see* Tetanus). A booster dose of tetanus toxoid (℞ 8) may be given to an individual who has been actively immunized to tetanus within the preceding 2 years. Some physicians advocate the prophylactic administration of polyvalent gas gangrene antitoxin (℞ 9) to patients with severe lacerations or deep puncture wounds that are heavily contaminated. Once a wound has become infected, the patient should be treated locally and systemically as described in the chapter on Sepsis (q.v.).

ELECTRIC SHOCK

Injury produced by the passage of electricity through the grounded body. The source of electricity may be lightning or "live" wires. Touching defective electrical equipment with wet hands or while in a bath tub or shower is a frequent cause.

Symptoms and Signs

The clinical manifestations usually depend on the amount of current that passes through the body. Conductivity is greater when the skin is wet or the body thoroughly grounded. Lightning bolts leave the victim unconscious and rigid in the position held at the moment he was struck. Respiratory paralysis is common; other findings may include tremors, vomiting, and severe burns. Death may be instantaneous, but recovery can be expected in over 50% of cases. Contact with high-tension currents produces muscular contraction and unconsciousness, with severe burns at the point of contact. If the contact is made with the hands, the victim may be "frozen" to the wire. Respiratory arrest is frequent and is responsible for a fatal outcome, although the heart remains strong until the end. Low-tension currents usually are not dangerous but, rarely, may cause death by ventricular fibrillation.

Treatment

Any contact of the victim with a "live" wire must be broken by shutting off the power (when possible) or by forcible separation, using a nonconducting material (dry wood or rope). The rescuer must not attempt to pull the victim from the "live" contact unless he first protects his own hands and arms with insulated gloves or a thick, dry, woolen garment. Artificial respiration by the prone pressure (Schaefer) method (see RE-SUSCITATION METHODS), using O_2, if available, should be started as soon as the contact is broken and continued until the return of normal respiration or the onset of rigor mortis (3 to 4 hours). Caffeine and sodium benzoate, 0.5 Gm. (gr. viiss) I.V., may safely be given and repeated in 30 minutes if necessary (℞ 50). Epinephrine 1:1,000, 0.5 cc. I.V. (℞ 51), may be injected slowly in cases of peripheral vascular collapse. Mechanical respirators must be used cautiously to avoid the danger of pulmonary rupture. If burns (q.v.) are present, they should be treated appropriately.

DROWNING

Drowning is essentially respiratory obstruction due to laryngeal spasm that results from the compulsion to breathe while the respiratory orifices are submerged in a liquid. The acute anoxemia which results may be followed by respiratory arrest. Only a small amount of liquid enters the trachea, but large amounts may enter the stomach. The victim loses consciousness; eventually his pulse fails, and death ensues unless he is promptly rescued and appropriately treated.

When seen immediately, the patient is found to be unconscious, his skin is cold and cyanotic, pulse imperceptible, and heart sounds inaudible.

Treatment

Place the victim in a prone position (*see* RESUSCITATION METHODS), with the head slightly lower than the thorax, and ensure a free airway by removing any dentures or other foreign matter from the mouth. Clothing should be loosened or removed and the patient kept warm by blankets. Since the signs of death are not reliable in cases of drowning, artificial respiration, using O_2 if available, must be carried out in all cases of respiratory arrest and continued until normal respiration returns or evidence of rigor mortis appears.

The preferred manual maneuver is the rocking method, since this is less tiring to the operators. The patient is placed face down on a stretcher or table and see-sawed to an angle of 40° at a rate of 12 to 15 times/per minute. The Schaefer prone pressure method should be used if a tilting device is not immediately available. Rolling the victim over a barrel is useless, since there is little or no water in the lungs, and the procedure serves only to waste precious moments before artificial respiration can be started.

Commercial respirators of the suck-and-blow type, with controlled maximum and minimum pressures for inspiration and expiration, are excellent if used properly. Even better, if available, are the newer (e.g., U.S. Air Force models) intermittent positive-pressure respirators, which blow air into the lungs at gentle pressures, and allow passive expiration. These can be used continuously for hours. Mechanical respirators that force air in under high pressure should be used, if at all, with extreme caution.

Caffeine and sodium benzoate (℞ 50), 0.5 Gm (gr. viiss) I.V., may be given and repeated in 30 minutes. The patient should receive penicillin (℞ 1) prophylactically for 3 or 4 days in doses of 50,000 u. I.M. every 3 hours or 300,000 u. every 8 to 12 hours, to prevent pneumonia.

INFUSION REACTIONS

Undesirable phenomena which may accompany or follow the I.V. administration of blood or various solutions. Infusions have come to be considered minor procedures, yet the potential dangers accompanying them are great.

Infusion reactions are not yet completely understood, so that any attempt at classification is necessarily inadequate. However, the following grouping is acceptable at the present time: hemolytic, allergic, physical, chemical, transmission of disease, and cardiovascular.

HEMOLYTIC REACTIONS

Reactions precipitated by intravascular hemolysis in the recipient of his own or the donor's red blood cells—usually the latter—during or following a whole blood transfusion.

Etiology

Hemolysis results from (1) blood group incompatibility, (2) "abnormal" hemagglutinins, or (3) rarely from the use of a universal donor.

1. Incompatibility: Despite recent advances in blood grouping, incompatibility still is a frequent cause of hemolysis, with many resultant fatalities. Poor technic in cross matching or the use of old and weak typing serums may be responsible. Poor technic includes failure to evaluate completely the Rh status, where an Rh-negative patient may have been previously immunized by the blood of an Rh-positive donor.

2. Abnormal hemagglutinins, including irregular isoagglutinins, cold agglutinins, and blood subgroups not yet understood.

3. Universal donor: This refers to the use of any group O donor (group I Jansky, IV Moss) whose serum contains both A and B agglutinins which if present in very high titer, may not be sufficiently diluted and suppressed during administration to prevent a reaction. The use of a universal donor is common, and, only rarely, is a mild or moderately severe reaction encountered.

Symptoms and Signs

The severity of the hemolytic reaction varies and depends upon the degree of incompatibility, the amount of blood administered, the rate of administration, and the integrity of the kidney, liver, and heart.

The onset is acute and may occur during or immediately following a blood transfusion, rarely later. The patient complains of discomfort, anxiety, and a generalized sensation of tingling. There may be difficulty in breathing, precordial oppression, a bursting sensation in the head, flushing of the face, and severe pain in the neck, chest, and especially the lumbar area. Evidence of shock appears with a rapid feeble pulse, cold clammy skin, dyspnea, fall in blood pressure, nausea and vomiting. Occasionally, urticaria is present. A severe chill quickly follows and is accompanied by a sharp rise in temperature. The acute phase develops within an hour, seldom longer, and is usually followed by an elevated serum bilirubin or icteric index and hemoglobinuria, with or without oliguria or anuria and clinical jaundice. At times, onset is with severe chill and fever, followed later by hemoglobinuria.

In severe cases, the hemoglobinuric phase with oliguria may last for 24 hours, followed by anuria, uremia, and coma. When a comatose state is reached, the patient rarely recovers. When recovery does occur, it is usually initiated by copious diuresis with elimination of retained nitrogenous wastes. In fatal cases, death usually ensues during the 2nd week.

The exact cause of renal failure is not known. Many explanations have been offered, including mechanical blockage of the renal tubules by hemoglobin precipitated in the presence of acid urine, anaphylaxis due to renal sensitivity to some component in the incompatible blood, and inadequate renal blood flow due to vascular spasm and shock.

Prognosis

This depends on several factors, e.g., amount of blood injected, degree of incompatibility, functional capacity of the kidneys, and general condition of the patient.

Prophylaxis

Hemolytic reactions may be avoided by a careful history of previous transfusions, the use of freshly drawn or properly stored blood, careful cross matching, the use of unheated blood, and allowing 15 minutes for administration of the first 50 cc., with close observation for untoward reactions. Routine alkalinization of the urine before transfusing will not prevent a hemolytic reaction but will counteract precipitation of hemoglobin in the renal tubules. The use of group-specific A and B substance is recommended for group O blood to suppress the agglutinins.

Treatment

Stop transfusion. Alkalinize the urine as soon as hemolysis is suspected and maintain by parenteral administration of sterile solutions of sodium bicarbonate (℞ 27), sodium lactate (℞ 28), or sodium citrate (℞ 29), followed by potassium citrate orally (℞ 30) until hemoglobinuria ceases. This procedure may not always be effective, but it is harmless if not carried to the point of severe alkalosis. The physician must watch for evidence of alkalosis (q.v.), and if it occurs, discontinue alkalis for 6 hours, or longer if necessary.

A total of 6,000 to 7,000 cc. of fluids should be given daily by all routes until the hemoglobinuria ceases. Diuresis is encouraged by hypertonic glucose (℞ 31) given I.V., to which may be added the alkalinizing agents listed above. If the patient is anuric, fluid administration should be carefully regulated (see ANURIA).

For unknown reasons, remarkable improvement has followed a transfusion of 200 to 300 cc. of compatible blood given as soon as possible after a reaction. Renal decapsulation has been attempted, with indifferent results.

For medicolegal reasons, existent specimens of both the donor's and the patient's blood should be retyped and again cross matched. When possible, fresh samples also should be tested to rule out any possible mislabeling of the initial samples.

ALLERGIC REACTIONS

Reactions due to hypersensitivity of the patient to an unknown component in the donor's blood. These are frequently observed and are thought to be due at times to a food allergen recently ingested by the donor.

Symptoms and Signs

Allergic reactions usually are mild, with urticaria, eosinophilia, and slight angioneurotic edema. Less frequently, there may be difficulty in breathing, asthmatic rales, and incontinence, indicating a generalized spasm of smooth muscle. Very rarely, a rapidly fatal anaphylactic shock may be encountered.

Prophylaxis

Advise donors to report after at least 3 or 4 hours' fasting.

Treatment

Discontinue transfusion. Epinephrine, 0.5 to 1 cc. (m viii to xv) of 1:1,000 solution ($\mathbb{R}$ 51), usually gives complete relief. The antihistaminics are of value in some cases (*see* ALLERGY).

PHYSICAL REACTIONS

Reactions due to extraneous physical changes in donor's blood before infusion. Such changes may result from inadequate citration, excessive handling, or undue exposure to air. The recipient's reactions will vary with the etiologic factor responsible. The use of hypotonic sodium citrate solution may cause hemolysis of the stored blood, with a resultant hemolytic reaction (q.v.) following its administration. Insufficient citration or improper handling of the blood may result in formation of small clots, which will act as minute emboli. These emboli rarely produce symptoms, however, since only very small clots can pass through the infusion needle. Freezing of blood will result in hemolysis and overheating blood will cause denaturation. Bacterial contamination is a serious hazard.

Prophylaxis

Adequate citration is obtained by the proper use of sodium citrate ($\mathbb{R}$ 32) or ACD solution ($\mathbb{R}$ 33). Blood containing sodium citrate may be used for 7 days after withdrawal; that containing ACD solution, up to 21 days. All blood must be stored at 3° to 5°C. prior to use. Blood should be drawn under aseptic measures in a closed system.

CHEMICAL REACTIONS

Reactions due to faulty technic and materials, such as impure anticoagulants, pyrogens, and unclean apparatus.

Symptoms and Signs

Chemical reactions are manifested by a severe chill followed by fever, usually occurring within 1 hour after an infusion. The chill lasts for 15 to 30 minutes, whereas the fever may persist for several hours. The icteric index and urine are not affected.

Prophylaxis

Use of proper technic, clean apparatus, and fresh pyrogen-free solutions.

Treatment

The patient should be kept warm; if possible, hot fluids should be administered orally.

DISEASE TRANSMISSION

1. Syphilis may be transmitted through the use of a luetic donor, especially one in the primary (seronegative or seropositive) or secondary stage. Infection transmitted in this fashion usually manifests itself in 1 to 4 months by secondary lesions without any preceding chancre or, at times, merely by the development of a positive serologic test. (For treatment, see SYPHILIS.)

Prophylaxis: The donor's skin and genitalia should be examined routinely for evidence of primary or secondary syphilis (q.v.), serologic tests should be made, and a careful history taken for possible recent exposure. Storing citrated blood for 4 days or more destroys the spirochete. The use of treponemicidal drugs in stored blood is recommended by some.

2. Malaria is easily transmitted by infected donors. Many such persons are not aware that they have malaria; it may be latent for as long as 10 to 15 years and still remain transmissible. The effect of time and antimalarial drugs on the malarial parasites in stored blood has not been established, so that storage cannot be depended upon to render blood safe. If malarial symptoms appear, they should be treated appropriately (see MALARIA).

Prophylaxis: Ask all prospective donors if they have ever had malaria or lived in a region where malaria is prevalent. Do not use such donors if others are available. Blood smears should be examined for parasites, but it must be emphasized that a negative smear is not proof that malaria is absent.

3. Other diseases: Infectious hepatitis (q.v.) not infrequently follows the infusion of whole blood, plasma, serum, or other products prepared from human blood or contaminated with it. Rarely, other diseases may be transmitted by blood transfusion, among which are influenza, relapsing fever, measles, smallpox, and septicemia.

CARDIOVASCULAR ACCIDENTS

Cardiac failure due to overloading the circulation rarely occurs unless the cardiac reserve is diminished by some form of organic heart disease. In the presence of heart disease or long-standing anemia, where the cardiac musculature and cardiac reserve are likely to be deficient, infusion should be given slowly. The patient should be observed for evidence of increased venous pressure or pulmonary congestion. If apparatus is available, direct observation of venous pressure during the course of the infusion is a useful precaution. Should untoward symptoms appear, infusion should be stopped and the patient treated appropriately (*see* PULMONARY EDEMA).

Air 'embolism of sufficient degree to cause symptoms is very rare, since sufficient air does not enter the circulation except under extremely unusual circumstances.

Retinal and intracranial hemorrhages may follow an infusion, for reasons not yet understood.

POISONING

The general principles to be followed in treating poisoning, usually acute, caused by the more frequently encountered chemicals and drugs are discussed first. (In lead poisoning, both acute intoxication and chronic plumbism are described.) The special toxicology for individual agents or groups of substances having related action or similar antidotes follows. Throughout the chapter, the names of toxic substances appear in alphabetic order for ready reference.

Poisoning due to bacterial or other toxins in food is covered in the chapter on GASTROENTERITIS AND FOOD POISONING. Another important group of poisonings is dealt with in the chapter on VENOMOUS BITES. The reader will find separate chapters on ALCOHOLISM, DRUG ERUPTIONS, and DRUG ADDICTION, which also are forms of poisoning but in a different category.

In the diagnosis of poisoning, the history and related circumstances, plus significant objects in the immediate vicinity of the patient, are of vital importance. Remnants of food, drinking glasses, bottles, or other containers nearby may provide evidence of the kind of poison that has been taken. Accident, suicide, or even murder, may be involved; therefore, it is necessary to make a careful record of all relevant data, since legal questions later may have to be answered. (*See also* chapter on THE UNCONSCIOUS PATIENT.)

ACUTE POISONING AND ITS TREATMENT

The treatment of poisoning involves the following principles and procedures: (1) Evacuation of the bulk of the poison from the stomach and intestinal tract by gastric lavage, emetics, or cathartics. (2) Inactivating ("antidoting") the residuum not removed by gastric lavage. When stomach tube is used, introduce antidote and other remedies into the stomach before removing the tube. Occasionally, systemic administration of an antidote may be required. (3) Elimination of the poison that has been absorbed. (4) Symptomatic treatment as indicated.

Evacuation of the stomach: Caution must be exercised to prevent aspiration, which often results in pneumonia. It is best to have the patient in head-low posture during lavage. (1) Stomach tube: Large amounts of water must be introduced into the stomach and siphoned off repeatedly until washings return free from the poison. The stomach tube must not be used when strong mineral acids, caustic agents, or ammonia have been swallowed, for fear of esophageal or gastric perforation; it also is contraindicated in strychnine poisoning because convulsions may be induced by attempts to pass it. (2) Emetics usually are less effective, but the following may be tried: Mustard (1 tbsp. to 1 cup of warm water), repeated in 15 minutes if not effective; powdered ipecac 2 Gm. (gr. xxx); syrup of ipecac (1-2 tsp. every 10-15 min.); zinc sulfate 1.3 Gm. (gr. xx) in water; copper sulfate 0.3-1 Gm. (gr. v-xv); apomorphine hydrochloride 6 mg. (gr. 1/10) subcut. or I.M. (Caution! In narcotic poisoning, apomorphine may not act.) Do not give emetic to patients vomiting profusely (merely giving water will suffice to wash out stomach) or to comatose or greatly depressed patients, for it will not act and constitutes an added injury. (3) Cathartics in the form of magnesium sulfate, 30 Gm. (℥ i), or senna, 2 Gm. (gr. xxx) with magnesium sulfate, 120 cc. (℥ iv) may be given in the absence of diarrhea. (Caution! In irritative poisoning, emetics and cathartics are contraindicated.)

Antidotes: These should be specific whenever such are available (*see* Special Toxicology). When alkaloids have been swallowed, give tannic acid 0.6-2 Gm. (gr. x-xxx) in ½ glass water immediately, followed by another glassful of water; or strong tea, or potassium permanganate (0.2% sol.). In heavy metal poisoning, give raw egg white or milk. BAL (British Anti-Lewisite) is highly effective in many cases of heavy metal poisoning (*see* below). When a specific antidote is not available, activated charcoal may be given in liberal doses (tsp. to tbsp.) frequently repeated. For irritative poisoning use demulcents: egg white; milk; oil; flaxseed tea; acacia; starch water; barley or oatmeal gruel; gelatin sol.; flour and water; crushed bananas; mucilage of acacia.

Elimination: This is favored by forcing fluids—by mouth if possible, parenterally if necessary. Glucose in saline is generally preferred. Elimination sometimes demands venesection followed by blood transfusion.

Symptomatic treatment: Poisoning due to drugs exerting a primary C.N.S. depressant action should be treated with stimulants. If the depression is not great, a mild stimulant such as caffeine and sodium benzoate 0.5 Gm. (gr. viiss) I.M., or ephedrine 25 mg. (gr. ⅜) I.M. or subcut., repeated as necessary, will usually suffice. If the depression is severe, so as to cause deep coma with loss of reflex activity, more vigorous therapy with the stimulants is required: amphetamine I.V., 40 mg. initially followed by 20 mg. every 30 min. until the patient is conscious (total dose not to exceed 400 mg.); picrotoxin 1 mg. (gr. 1/60) I.V. every minute until return of corneal reflexes, with care to avoid convulsions; or Metrazol 0.1 Gm. (gr. iss) I.M. or I.V., repeated as necessary. When respiratory center failure is present or appears imminent, artificial respiration and O_2 inhalation (with CO_2, 5%, if this results in deeper breathing) are indicated as well. A respirator should be used if prolonged artificial respiration is necessary (*see* RESUSCITATION METHODS, p. 1183, 1185). Pulmonary edema is treated in the usual manner (q.v.). Circulatory failure, peripheral or cardiac in origin, also should be treated in the usual fashion (*see* SHOCK; CONGESTIVE HEART FAILURE).

BAL (British Anti-Lewisite) **therapy for heavy metal poisoning:** During World War II, 2,3-dimercaptopropanol (BAL) was developed as a method of treatment for lewisite poisoning. It has proved effective clinically in poisoning by the heavy metals, arsenic, cadmium, gold, and mercury, and experimentally in poisoning by antimony, bismuth, nickel, chromium, zinc, and copper. In order to be beneficial, BAL should be used as promptly as possible after symptoms of toxicity appear. The drug is administered I.M. (never I.V.) as a 10% solution in peanut oil containing 20% benzyl benzoate (commercially obtainable in ampuls). The optimal dosage has not been established and may vary with the degree of symptoms and the nature of the poison (*see* Special Toxicology, under the various heavy metals). Relief of symptoms usually is prompt (i.e., within 3 days).

Treatment with BAL should be reserved for severe cases of poisoning, since it may of itself produce untoward reactions. Abscesses may develop at the site of injection, and dermatitis from external contact. The most frequent reactions to treatment are pain in the extremities, abdomen, and head. Others are malaise, nausea, vomiting, salivation, urticaria, lacrimation, paresthesia, perspiration, sense of warmth, tachycardia, and increased blood pressure. These symptoms usually disappear within 1/2 to 3 hours, and are amenable to symptomatic treatment with barbiturates, epinephrine, or ephedrine.

SPECIAL TOXICOLOGY

ACETANILID

Acetophenetidin
(Phenacetin)

Aniline Dyes
Aniline Inks

Symptoms and Signs

Cyanosis, due to formation of methemoglobin; dyspnea;

weakness; vertigo; weak and irregular pulse; anginal pains;
rashes or urticaria (particularly with acetophenetidin); occasionally vomiting, delirium, followed by depression; death from
circulatory or respiratory failure.

Treatment

When substance has been **swallowed**: Gastric lavage or
emetics; sodium bicarbonate; recumbent posture; O_2 inhalation; external heat; analeptics, such as Metrazol 0.1 Gm. (gr.
iss) I.V., or caffeine and sodium benzoate 0.5 Gm. (gr. viiss)
I.M.; artificial respiration; blood transfusions. When aniline
has been **inhaled**: Proceed as above except for enteral treatment.

ACETONE

Nail Polish Remover

Symptoms and Signs

Inhalation of significant amounts of acetone fumes causes
bronchial irritation and pulmonary congestion. Absorption of
large quantities via either the respiratory or gastrointestinal
tract results in decreased respiration, pulse, and temperature,
dyspnea, stupor and, in extreme cases, death by ketosis.

Treatment

If acetone was recently ingested use gastric lavage or an
emetic. If required, give a stimulant I.V., such as Coramine
5 to 10 cc. or caffeine and sodium benzoate 0.5 Gm. (gr. viiss),
every 15 to 30 min. (For further details of treatment *see*
KETOSIS.)

ACIDS AND ALKALIS

Acids	Alkalis
Acetic	*Ammonia Water*
Hydrochloric	*Potassium Hydroxide*
Nitric	*(Potash)*
Nitrohydrochloric	*Sodium Hydroxide*
Phosphoric	*(Caustic Soda, Lye)*
Sulfuric	*Carbonates of the*
	above

Symptoms and Signs

Corrosion of mucous membranes of mouth, throat and
esophagus; pain in digestive tract; intense thirst; dysphagia;
nausea and vomiting ("coffee ground")—parts of gastric
mucous membrane may be present in vomitus; diarrhea; collapse with rapid feeble pulse; clammy skin; shallow, difficult
respiration. Later effects: Inflammation, intense swelling and
ulceration of mouth, throat, esophagus; mediastinitis; gastritis,

duodenitis, enteritis; jaundice; albuminuria; ulceration of stomach; perforation; peritonitis; strictures; fatty degeneration of heart, liver, kidneys.

Treatment

With corrosive poisons, avoid stomach tube (may cause gastric or esophageal perforation); avoid emetics (may cause gastric rupture). With concentrated acids avoid chalk and alkaline carbonates (liberated CO_2 may cause gastric distention or rupture); give magnesium oxide, milk of magnesia, milk, egg albumin, lime water, or soap in copious amounts of water; demulcents.

Against caustic alkalis, give 500 cc. (℥ xvi) of vinegar and water (equal parts), diluted citrus fruit juice, or citric or tartaric acid 2-4 Gm. (℥ ss-i); give olive oil or melted butter to protect irritated mucous membranes. Use recumbent position; external heat, especially over cardiac region; stimulants (caffeine, atropine, camphor, Metrazol, strychnine). For pain, morphine, 8-15 mg. (gr. ⅛-¼). Later, if cardiac failure develops, a digitalis preparation. If perforation of esophagus or stomach with the development of mediastinitis or peritonitis occurs, antibiotic therapy (q.v.) is necessary.

For after-treatment in any corrosive poisoning, bismuth subcarbonate in 2 Gm. (gr. xxx) doses. For esophageal pain, give 1 tsp. of mixture of orthoform (4 cc.), epinephrine 1:1,000 sol. (4 cc.) and mucilage of acacia (52 cc.) preceding liquids. Later, soft diet. Glucose I.V. Early and regular passage of esophageal bougies (starting the 6th day) has been advocated to prevent esophageal stricture.

ACID, ACETYLSALICYLIC: *See* SALICYLATE

ACID, BORIC

Symptoms and Signs

Nausea, vomiting, diarrhea; headache; dysphagia; cold sweats; dyspnea; muscular debility; scarlatinal eruptions; subnormal temperature; cardiac weakness; collapse.

Treatment

Gastric lavage; symptomatic therapy.

ACID, CARBOLIC: *See* PHENOLS

ACID, CHROMIC

Chromates   *Dichromates*

Symptoms and Signs

Gastrointestinal corrosion; intense pain in throat and stomach; colic; leg cramps; bloody vomiting and purging; mouth and throat stained yellow; dilated pupils; great depression; collapse.

Treatment

Gastric lavage or emetics; give magnesium oxide or milk of magnesia freely; chalk; lime water, stimulants; demulcents; morphine 15 mg. (gr. ¼) for pain; external heat.

ACID, HYDROCYANIC: *See* CYANIDES

ACID, OXALIC

Binoxalates   *Oxalates*

Symptoms and Signs

Gastrointestinal irritation; severe pain in throat and stomach; intense thirst; extreme muscular weakness; vomiting (usually bloody); twitching of muscles (particularly of face); cold, cyanotic skin; intense headache; feeble fluttering pulse; dilated pupils; oliguria; collapse, sometimes convulsions; coma.

Treatment

As soon as possible give magnesium oxide or chalk, or a soluble magnesium or calcium salt, with a very small amount of water, followed by stomach tube if mucosa has not been deeply corroded (corrosion indicated by burning pain and collapse); or, in unaggravated cases, by emetic. Injection I.V. of 10-20 cc. of 10% calcium gluconate or 5% calcium chloride to counteract the production of tetany by hypocalcemia. Later, magnesium sulfate purge. Avoid alkalis or their carbonates or bicarbonates, which may form soluble poisonous salts. Give stimulants for collapse; recumbent position; external heat; demulcents.

ACONITE

Aconitine   *Larkspur*
Delphinine   *Veratrine*

Symptoms

Tingling and numbness in mouth and throat, extending to stomach and body, particularly the finger tips (of diagnostic value for aconite), followed by numbness and anesthesia of skin; chilly sensation; salivation; gastric and abdominal pain; vomiting, diarrhea, and colic (tending to be more pronounced with veratrine); restlessness; staggering; dizziness; pupils first contracted then dilated, impaired vision; low temperature; pulse first slow and feeble, then irregular and very rapid; fall in blood pressure; respiration slow, shallow, and irregular; great prostration; cold livid skin; staring eyes; syncope; death from cardiac or respiratory paralysis.

Treatment

Horizontal position. **Avoid emetics!** Use stomach tube with tannic acid 0.6-2 Gm. (gr. x-xxx) or animal charcoal 1 tbsp., or iodine 50 mg. (gr. ¾) with potassium iodide 0.12 Gm. (gr. ii) and 30 cc. (℥ i) water, or 0.1% potassium permanganate solution; respiratory and cardiac stimulants; atropine; O₂; heat to body with head lower than feet; artificial respiration.

ALCOHOL, ETHYL (ETHANOL) (*See also* ALCOHOLISM)

Brandy, Whisky, and other Liquors

Symptoms and Signs

Incoordinated movements; excitement and exhilaration followed by depression; abdominal pain; nausea; vomiting; headache; muscular weakness; vertigo; ataxia; delirium; weak rapid pulse; subnormal temperature; dyspnea; cyanosis; unconsciousness; circulatory collapse; coma; death from respiratory paralysis.

Treatment

Gastric lavage with 1 to 3% solution sodium citrate or carbonate or bicarbonate, or magnesium oxide, or weak soapsuds; or emetics (avoid apomorphine because of the added C.N.S. depression); cathartics, such as magnesium sulfate 60 Gm. (℥ ii); stimulants, such as caffeine rectally as strong coffee, or 0.5 Gm. (gr. viiss) with sodium benzoate I.M.; ephedrine, 25 mg. (gr. ⅜) I.M. or subcut.; inhalation of aromatic spirit of ammonia; artificial respiration (95% O₂, 5% CO₂); keep patient warm and change posture frequently to prevent pneumonia.

ALCOHOL, METHYL (METHANOL, WOOD ALCOHOL, COLUMBIAN SPIRIT)

Symptoms and Signs

C.N.S. depression and muscular incoordination; violent gastric and abdominal pains, emesis; headache; disturbed vision and pain in eyes (sudden blindness may occur); delirium, cerebral edema; low body temperature; cyanosis, dyspnea, weak and irregular pulse, fall in blood pressure; acidosis; coma; death from respiratory or circulatory failure.

Treatment

Combat acidosis (q.v.), due to formation of formic acid from methyl alcohol, by lavage with 1-3% sodium bicarbonate, or magnesium oxide or weak soapsuds; I.V. injection of 5% sodium bicarbonate (ampul) not over 6 cc./Kg. body wt. given slowly, over a period of at least ½ hr. Sodium lactate sol. (ampul) diluted with sterile water to ⅙ molar concentration, given I.V. in similar amount, instead of the sodium bicarbonate, may be preferable. Cathartics, such as magnesium sulfate

30-60 Gm. ($\tilde{3}$ i-ii) also should be administered. If cerebral edema is present, use I.V. glucose or sucrose (50-100 cc. of 50% solution). Supportive treatment: stimulants, artificial respiration, and other methods as for ethyl alcohol poisoning (q.v.).

AMMONIA, GAS

Symptoms and Signs

Conjunctival and corneal irritation; salivation, nausea, vomiting, purging, abdominal pain; choking sensation, cough, bronchial irritation, respiratory arrest, pulmonary edema.

Treatment

Wash eyes thoroughly with water for at least 5 minutes; dilute solution of citrus fruit juice or other weak acid for gastrointestinal irritation; artificial respiration, inhalation of O_2 under positive pressure for prevention of pulmonary edema (q.v.), respiratory stimulants. (CAUTION! Avoid respiratory depressant narcotics.)

AMMONIA, WATER: See ACIDS AND ALKALIS

AMYL ACETATE (ISOAMYL ACETATE, BANANA OIL, PEAR OIL)

Symptoms and Signs

Conjunctivitis; laryngeal irritation or edema; nausea; vomiting; headache; incoordinated movements; C.N.S. depression; albuminuria.

Treatment

Gastric lavage if ingested; stimulants as in ethyl alcohol poisoning. If signs of pulmonary edema develop, O_2 under positive pressure (see BEDSIDE PROC.).

AMYL NITRITE: See NITRITES

ANILINE: See ACETANILID

ANTIMONY COMPOUNDS
Tartar Emetic
Fuadin

Symptoms and Signs

Metallic taste; nausea, violent vomiting; purging (rice-water stools); severe abdominal pain; severe coughing; joint pains and acute arthritis; cramps in calves; depression; pulse first rapid then slow and imperceptible; salivation; slow shallow respiration; cyanosis; cold sweat; great thirst; subnormal temperature; profuse perspiration; muscular weakness; cyanosis; coma; death from cardiac failure.

37

Treatment

Gastric lavage with tannic acid, 2 Gm. (gr. xxx) in water; later magnesium oxide; saline cathartics (30 Gm. magnesium sulfate); recumbent position; respiratory and circulatory stimulants; O_2 artificial respiration; external heat; demulcents; morphine 10-15 mg. (gr. $\frac{1}{6}$-$\frac{1}{4}$) to control violent pains; I.V. injection of 5% glucose or isotonic saline to counteract dehydration.

ANTIPYRINE

Aminopyrine

Symptoms and Signs

Granulocytopenia, which may lead to agranulocytosis (q.v.); skin eruptions; excitement, delirium; convulsions.

Treatment

Counteract stimulation by I.V. injection of short-acting barbiturate, such as pentobarbital sodium 0.5 Gm.

ARSENIC

Cobalt Salts	*Paris Green*
Donovan's Solution	*Rat Poisons*
Fly Paper	*Scheele's Green*
Fowler's Solution	

Symptoms and Signs

Metallic taste; burning pain in esophagus and stomach; colicky pains; vomiting and profuse diarrhea with "rice-water" stools followed by bloody discharges; depression; intense thirst; dryness of mouth and throat; constricting sensation in throat; garlicky odor of breath and stools; vertigo; frontal headache; muscular cramps; cold, clammy skin; small, rapid, feeble pulse; cold extremities; cyanosis, sighing respiration; stupor, circulatory collapse; convulsions; coma; skin eruptions.

Treatment

Gastric lavage. To delay absorption of poison prior to gastric lavage, use hydrated iron oxide (from dilute ammonia and tincture iron chloride, washing the precipitate with water), give it moist, 2-3 tbsp. every 10 min. or, preferably, with equal parts of magnesium oxide, until symptoms are improved. Promptly evacuate stomach, and give copious lavage. Also, administer BAL (British anti-lewisite), 2 to 3 mg./Kg. as a 10% solution in peanut oil with benzyl benzoate, I.M. every 4 hrs. for several days; this now is the treatment of choice. Demulcents; morphine 15 mg. (gr. $\frac{1}{4}$) subcut. for pain; stimulants; spirit of nitrous ether; external heat. Later, saline cathartics and castor oil; combat dehydration by I.V. infusion of 5% glucose (500-1,000 cc.). Sodium thiosulfate, 20-30 cc. of 10% solution I.V., or 1 Gm. orally.

ASPIRIN: *See* SALICYLATE

ATROPINE: *See* BELLADONNA

BARBITURATES (*See also* DRUG ADDICTION)

> *Barbital*
> *Phenobarbital*
> *Other Barbituric Acid derivatives*

Symptoms and Signs

Headache; mental confusion; ataxia; twitching of muscles; ptosis of eyelids; sleep (sometimes preceded by excitement and delirium), at first quiet, then deepening rapidly into coma; respiration at first slow and quiet, then slow and shallow, then noisy; cyanosis; moderately dilated pupils; absence of corneal and other reflexes; nystagmus; occasional hippus (rapid spasmodic change in size of pupil); temperature may be elevated or subnormal; skin eruptions may occur; cyanosis; anuria; circulatory collapse. Respiration stertorous, irregular. Pulse in severe cases small, soft, irregular. Blood pressure low. Death from respiratory failure within a few hours exceptional; usually occurs after several days' unconsciousness, from pulmonary edema or inflammation, the pneumonia being accompanied by fever and other classic signs.

With smaller doses, excitation, delirium, exaggerated reflexes, muscular rigidity (lockjaw), and tonic cramps may predominate. Urine should be tested for barbiturates if the diagnosis is in doubt, or for medicolegal purposes.

Treatment

Adults usually recover without treatment from oral doses of less than 2 Gm. Examine patient frequently for evidence of deepening narcosis or recovery as a guide to subsequent need for therapy. Absorption usually complete by 8 hours, after which gastric lavage is useless and may cause aspiration pneumonia. When indicated, lavage with potassium permanganate, 0.2% solution. Combat anoxia by assuring a patent airway, aspiration of mucus, O_2 inhalation, and artificial respiration if indicated. Drug therapy depends on specific needs and indications. For respiratory depression give caffeine and sodium benzoate, 0.5 Gm. (gr. viiss) I.V. or I.M. every 15-30 min. if necessary. Circulatory collapse requires fluids I.V. (*see* SHOCK) and such stimulants as Neo-Synephrine, 10-20 mg. I.M. every 30 min. if indicated; epinephrine 1:1,000 sol. is less useful for this purpose since it produces marked cardiac acceleration and secondary vasodepression. Analeptics also are respiratory stimulants but they are dangerous and should be used only if one is unable to elicit such signs as pupillary reflexes, knee jerks, or breath-holding response. Picrotoxin, 10 mg. (gr. ⅙) I.V., or Metrazol, 0.1-0.3 Gm. (gr. iss-v) I.V., are administered intermittently every 10-20 min. or in similar doses by continuous

I.V. infusion until any evidence of muscle excitation appears; thereafter, maintain this stage of stimulation by somewhat less frequent I.M. injections of this same dose. Overdosage of analeptics produces convulsions, which should be combated with an inhalation anesthetic such as ether or a rapidly eliminated I.V. barbiturate such as pentobarbital sodium, 0.3 Gm. (gr. v). Alternative analeptics include ephedrine sulfate, 30 mg (gr. ss) I.M. every 30 min.; amphetamine sulfate, 40 mg. I.V., followed by 20 mg. I.V. every 30 min.; or Coramine, 5 to 10 cc. I.V. every 5 min.

Supportive measures are very important and include maintenance of fluid balance, catheterization every 8 hours, and the prevention of pneumonia by the prophylactic use of penicillin, 30,000 u. I.M. every 3 hours.

BARIUM COMPOUNDS

Symptoms and Signs

Vomiting, violent abdominal pains, diarrhea; tremors, convulsions; great rise in blood pressure, extrasystoles. Death from cardiac arrest.

Treatment

Give 30-60 Gm. (℥ i-ii) sodium or magnesium sulfate orally; 0.3-0.5 Gm. (gr. v-viiss) Sodium Amytal I.V., or 2 Gm. (gr. xxx) chloral hydrate, to counteract convulsions; 15 mg. (gr. ¼) morphine, subcut., if necessitated by violent pains.

BELLADONNA

Atropine	*Scopolamine (Hyoscine)*
Daturine	*Solanine*
Duboisine	*Stramonium*
Hyoscyamine	

Symptoms and Signs

Dryness and burning in mouth and throat; great thirst; pupils dilated and unresponsive to light; photophobia and blurring of vision; weakness; giddiness; headache; nausea, vomiting; delirium, great excitement and confusion (simulating acute psychosis); stupor; twitchings; dysphagia; husky voice; rashes, particularly in children; breathing slow and stertorous; pulse first slow then rapid and small; elevation of temperature and of blood pressure; convulsions; skin usually dry, hot and flushed, but in fatal cases livid, with cold extremities; pulse rapid and intermittent; deep coma; death from respiratory paralysis. In scopolamine poisoning the depressant action predominates, with coma rather than delirium, skin cyanotic instead of flushed; tachycardia is rare.

Treatment

Give as antidote 2 Gm. (gr. xxx) tannic acid in 120-240 cc. (℥ iv-viii) of water, followed immediately by another glassful of water; copious gastric lavage or emetics 5-10 min. later; activated charcoal, pilocarpine hydrochloride, 10 mg. (gr. ⅙) subcut., repeated if necessary until mouth is moist; morphine, 8-15 mg. (gr. ⅛-¼) subcut. (with caution, and not in scopolamine poisoning). For excitement or delirium, ice cap to head; short-acting barbiturates, e.g., 0.3 Gm. (gr. v) pentobarbital sodium I.V. (CAUTION! Avoid long-acting barbiturates.) In stage of depression, strong coffee, caffeine, stimulants; external heat; artificial respiration; alternate hot and cold sponge baths. Enemas rather than cathartics (which may fail). Catheterize.

BENZENE (BENZOL)
Toluene (Toluol)   Xylene (Xylol)

Symptoms and Signs

Nausea, vomiting, headache; rapid irregular pulse; ataxia; dizziness; excitement (restlessness, delirium), followed by depression and coma. Death from respiratory or cardiac failure. In subacute and chronic poisoning, damage to the hematopoietic organs (hypochromic anemia, diminution of granulocytes, hemorrhagic diathesis due to thrombopenia).

Treatment

When the substance has been **swallowed,** use gastric lavage or emetic; mineral oil; alternate hot and cold water to chest; ammonia by inhalation (with caution!). When the poison has been **inhaled,** fresh air; artificial respiration; no emetic, oil, or stomach tube; otherwise as when swallowed.

BENZINE
Gasoline   Naphtha
Kerosene   Petroleum Ether

Symptoms and Signs

After inhalation: Giddiness, flushed face or cyanosis. With concentrated fumes, narcosis or deep coma and labored respiration, cyanosis, dilated pupils, and death from respiratory failure. **After swallowing:** Burning in mouth and stomach; headache; nausea, vomiting; inebriation; cold skin; great thirst; tremors; feeble pulse; fall of temperature; dyspnea; convulsions; unconsciousness. Kerosene causes less coma and more local irritation, with vomiting. Aspiration pneumonia a common complication.

Treatment

When the poison has been **swallowed:** Gastric lavage or emetic; morphine 15 mg. (gr. ¼) subcut. for pain; stimulants; external heat; artificial respiration; inhalation of 95% O_2 and 5% CO_2.

When the substance has been **inhaled:** Fresh air; no emetic or stomach tube; otherwise as when swallowed.

BICHROMATES: *See* Acid, Chromic

BISMUTH COMPOUNDS

Symptoms and Signs

Nausea, vomiting, abdominal pain; headache; fever; stomatitis, bluish line on gums; agranulocytosis with angina; dermatitis.

Treatment

Gastric lavage, high enemas, respiratory and cardiac stimulants when necessary. BAL, while not as specific as in gold or arsenic poisoning (q.v.), should be employed in severe cases.

BLUESTONE: *See* Copper Salts

BROMATES: *See* Chlorates

BROMIDES

Symptoms and Signs

Acute poisoning (rare): Profound C.N.S. depression and stupor.

Chronic poisoning (Bromism): Mental dullness, apathy, memory and speech disturbances; somnolence; hallucinations, delirium, manic excitement; anorexia, nausea, foul breath; rashes (round, elevated, hard nodules resembling acne); conjunctivitis and coryza.

Treatment

Discontinue bromide medication. In acute poisoning, stomach tube or emetic; caffeine, strong coffee, or camphor for stimulation. In chronic bromide intoxication, sodium chloride 8-12 Gm. (℈ ii-iii) daily as iced salt solutions or bouillon (1 cube of 3 Gm. may contain 2.4 Gm. NaCl). Force fluids (daily intake should be at least 4,000 cc.). In severe cases, continuous aspiration of gastric juice, as long as bromide is contained in it, materially aids in removing bromide ions from the body. Sedative hydrotherapy (warm baths) but not medicinal sedatives.

BRUCINE: *See* Strychnine

CADMIUM

Symptoms and Signs

When swallowed: Violent gastric and abdominal cramps, vomiting, diarrhea. **When inhaled:** Dryness of throat, cough, sensation of constriction in chest; brown color of urine (cadmium oxide); severe dyspnea; cold skin; shock; coma.

Treatment

BAL, 2 to 3 mg./Kg. body wt. I.M., as a 10% solution in peanut oil with benzyl benzoate, every 4 hrs. for 2 days. Gastric lavage with milk or albumin; external heat; stimulants; artificial respiration if breathing is labored. Combat dehydration by I.V. infusion of 0.9% saline, 500-1,000 cc.

CAFFEINE

Symptoms and Signs

Burning pain in throat; faintness, giddiness; insomnia, restlessness, excitement; headache; ringing in ears; nausea, abdominal pain, vomiting; thirst; fatigue; muscular tremors; cold skin; numbness; diuresis; palpitation, extrasystoles, tachycardia; rapid and deep respiration. In very severe cases, violent choreic tremors, collapse; weak, small, irregular pulse; cold extremities.

Treatment

Gastric lavage or emetics if patient is seen within 30 min. after ingestion; 0.3 Gm. (gr. v) pentobarbital sodium or other short-acting barbiturate I.V.; morphine 15 mg. (gr. ¼) subcut.; external heat. In collapse, 5% glucose I.V.

CAMPHOR

Symptoms and Signs

Characteristic odor present in breath and urine; mental excitement; dizziness; restlessness; headache; nausea, vomiting, colic; tinnitus; clammy skin; weak rapid pulse; face first flushed then pale; narcosis; delirium, hallucinations; uncoordinated movements; convulsions; circulatory collapse. With large doses, burning pain in stomach.

Treatment

Gastric lavage or emetic, if patient is seen early after ingestion; 0.3 Gm. (gr. v) pentobarbital sodium I.V. (avoid long-acting barbiturates). If no short-acting barbiturate is available, give ether inhalations or 2 Gm. (gr. xxx) chloral hydrate for convulsions (avoid opiates); external heat; alternate hot and cold douches; coffee by mouth or rectum; artificial respiration; saline cathartics.

CANNABIS (*See also* DRUG ADDICTION)
Hashish
Marihuana

Symptoms and Signs

Exhilaration, pleasurable intoxication; sense of prolongation of time; hallucinations, delirium, mania; drowsiness; muscular weakness (especially in legs); dilated pupils; rapid pulse; slow respiration; sometimes increased sexual desire; convulsions.

Treatment

Copious gastric lavage with warm water; emetics; tannic

acid; 0.6 mg. (gr. 1/100) atropine subcut.; 0.3 cc. (♏ v) amyl nitrite by inhalation; strong coffee; artificial respiration; external heat. If inhaled, omit gastric lavage and emetics.

CANTHARIDES (SPANISH FLY)
Cantharidin

Symptoms and Signs

Burning pain in throat and stomach; swelling and blistering of tongue; dysphagia; severe gastroenteritis, salivation, nausea, vomiting, bloody diarrhea, severe colic; tenesmus; burning pain in back, bladder, and urethra; strangury; thirst; heart and respiration briefly stimulated then greatly depressed; syncope; may be delirium and tetanic convulsions; collapse; coma. (No aphrodisiac effect in human beings.)

Treatment

Apomorphine, 5 mg. (gr. 1/12) subcut. (CAUTION! Do not use other emetic or stomach tube.) Demulcents. (CAUTION! Avoid oils!) Stimulants; 15 mg. (gr. 1/4) morphine subcut. for pain; anesthetics for convulsions; external heat. Treat acute nephritis and cystitis in the usual manner (q.v.).

CARBOLIC ACID: *See* PHENOLS

CARBON DIOXIDE

Symptoms and Signs

Exposure to atmosphere containing 2% carbon dioxide causes discomfort, which increases with advancing concentration until a fatal level of 10-15% is reached. Symptoms include: inflamed throat; sensations of heaviness and pain in head; rise of blood pressure, giddiness; ringing in ears; loss of muscular power; dyspnea; generalized lividity of skin; violent heart beats; fall of blood pressure; coma, generally without convulsions.

Treatment

Fresh air; O_2 inhalation. If respiration has ceased, dash cold water on face and chest, and give artificial respiration; ammonia or amyl nitrite inhalations; strong coffee enema; stimulants; friction and heat to extremities. Maintain treatment continuously (recovery has occurred after a long period of unconsciousness).

CARBON DISULFIDE

Symptoms and Signs

Incoordinated movements; headache; flushed skin; sore throat; nausea; hiccup; severe vomiting; congested face; bloodshot eyes; dizziness; partial loss of consciousness; dilated pupils; dyspnea; stuporous sleep passing into coma.

Treatment

Gastric lavage or emetic; fresh air; O_2 inhalation; stimulants; bromides or chloral hydrate for sedation if necessary; ammonia inhalation; artificial respiration.

CARBON MONOXIDE

Acetylene Gas	*Automobile Exhaust Gas*
Illuminating Gas	*Furnace Gas*
(Coal Gas)	*Marsh Gas (contains CO)*

Symptoms and Signs

Dizziness; intense headache; weakness; sometimes vomiting; muscular twitchings; full bounding pulse; throbbing in temples; elevated blood pressure; dilated pupils; drowsiness; stupor; respiration accelerated and stertorous; skin dusky, lips blue, pale, or pink; tetaniform convulsions, and marked muscular rigidity, particularly of the jaw; anesthesias and paralyses; bluish red patches on skin; apnea; coma.

Treatment

Immediate removal of patient, with least possible exertion on his part, from contaminated air; avoid chilling; artificial respiration; inhalations of O_2 containing 5% CO_2. Phlebotomy is of doubtful value, and must always be followed by blood transfusion. Apply external heat, keeping patient warm and at complete rest for many hours; stimulants; Coramine, Metrazol, saline injections rectally or I.V. If headache persists (cerebral edema), give 50 cc. of 50% glucose or sucrose I.V.

CARBON OXYCHLORIDE (CARBONYL CHLORIDE; PHOSGENE GAS)

Diphosgene	*Trichloronitromethane*
Dichlorethyl Sulfide	*(Chloropicrin)*
(Mustard Gas)	*Chloracetophenone*
	(Tear Gas)

Symptoms and Signs

From Carbon Oxychloride: Onset of symptoms often delayed for up to 24 hours. Cough; lacrimation; dizziness; intense dyspnea; eyes, nose, mouth irritated; pulse very slow; subnormal temperature; respiration first slow then rapid; pulmonary edema. From Chloropicrin: Weak, irregular heartbeat; gastritis. From Tear Gas: Temporary blindness. From Dichlorethyl Sulfide: Erosion of cornea and mucosa of pharynx, trachea, and bronchi. Hyperemia, edema, vesication, and even necrosis of skin.

Treatment

Remove clothing immediately (gases adhere to them and continue their effects); wash skin with soda bicarbonate, 2% solution; absolute rest; phlebotomy to combat pulmonary

edema and cardiac failure—withdraw about 500 cc. of blood
if patient is not in shock, and give caffeine and sodium benzoate, 0.5-1 Gm. (gr. viiss-xv) I.M.; O_2 under positive pressure; boric acid sol. to eyes; external heat; cardiac stimulants;
abundant fresh air.

CARBON TETRACHLORIDE
Cleaning Fluids, noninflammable

Symptoms and Signs

After inhalation: Symptoms like those of chloroform inhalation (q.v.), but of slower development and with more
prolonged after-effects. Otherwise, like those which occur
after swallowing; i.e., persistent headache; drowsiness; confusion; unconsciousness; hallucinations; abdominal pain; slow,
irregular pulse; thick speech; sometimes vomiting; dilated
pupils. Later (1-3 days after exposure): jaundice; cirrhosis or
acute yellow atrophy of liver; renal failure (acute toxic nephrosis).

Treatment

After inhalation: Stimulants (Avoid alcohol!); high carbo-
hydrate-high protein diet and large doses of methionine 3-5
Gm. daily I.V. to protect liver. **After swallowing:** Gastric
lavage or emetic; stimulants, avoiding alcohol; saline cathartics.
Diet and methionine as after inhalation.

CHLORAL HYDRATE
Chloralamide

Symptoms and Signs

Nausea; vomiting; headache; lessened reflexes; profound
sleep; muscular relaxation; cold extremities; slow, feeble respiration; very weak, slow pulse; low blood pressure and temperature; cyanosis; cold sweat; collapse; coma; asphyxia; often
pin-point pupils.

Treatment

Stomach tube, using tea or coffee for lavage; stimulants by
mouth or rectum; picrotoxin I.V., 6 mg. (gr. 1/10) every 10 min.
or 1 mg. (gr. 1/60) every min. until corneal reflexes return;
ephedrine sulfate, 30 mg. (gr. ss) I.V.; or amphetamine sulfate,
40 mg. I.V., every 30 min. until consciousness reappears. Place
patient in Trendelenburg position; electroshock for stupor;
O_2; external heat; cold to head; artificial respiration; 50-100
cc. of 25% glucose I.V.

CHLORATES
Bromates   Nitrates

Symptoms and Signs

Nausea; vomiting; salivation; headache; abdominal pain;

weakness; diarrhea; diuresis; dyspnea; jaundice; cyanosis; quick, feeble pulse; fall of blood pressure; anuria; extreme dyspnea; circulatory collapse; delirium; coma; terminal convulsions.

Treatment

Gastric lavage or emetics; 15 mg. (gr. ¼) morphine subcut. for pain and nervous irritability; demulcents; external heat. (CAUTION! Avoid anything that may increase renal congestion, such as croton oil.)

CHLORINE

Bromine	*Javelle Water*
Chlorinated Lime	*Labarraque's Solution*
Chlorine Water	

Symptoms and Signs

After inhalation: Severe irritation of respiratory mucosa and of eyes; spasm of glottis; distressing spasmodic cough; choking; vomiting; pulmonary edema; dyspnea; asphyxia; acute congestive heart failure; cyanosis. **After swallowing:** Intense irritation and corrosion of mouth, throat and stomach; possible perforation of esophagus and stomach; severe abdominal pain; anxiety; rapid pulse; prostration; circulatory collapse.

Treatment

After inhalation: Ammonia by inhalation; fresh air; artificial respiration; inhalation of O_2; phlebotomy (500-700 cc.); caffeine and sodium benzoate 0.5-1 Gm. (gr. viiss-xv) I.M. **After swallowing:** Gastric lavage; ammonia water, 1 cc. (♏ xv) in 60 cc. (℥ ii) water, repeated in 10-30 min.; stimulants; sodium thiosulfate, 1.3 Gm. (gr. xx); demulcents; 15 mg. (gr. ¼) morphine sulfate subcut., for pain and restlessness.

CHLOROFORM

Ether	*Nitrous Oxide*

Symptoms and Signs

Chloroform: Stertorous, shallow, irregular respiration; dilated pupils; cold clammy skin; pulse slow and weak; deep narcosis; lowered blood pressure; cardiac and respiratory failure.
Ether: Stertorous, shallow, labored respiration; lowered temperature; weak, rapid pulse; cyanosis, respiratory failure.
Nitrous Oxide: Delirious laughter preceding coma.

Treatment

After inhalation: Lower patient's head and pull tongue forward to assure patent airway; give artificial respiration, O_2; alternate hot and cold water to face and chest. **After swallowing:** Gastric lavage or emetic; sodium bicarbonate; stimulants: (if epinephrine or ephedrine is used, doses should be smaller than usual because of possible ventricular fibrillation); O_2; amyl nitrite 0.2-0.3 cc. (♏ iii-v) by inhalation; artificial respiration.

CHROMIUM TRIOXIDE; CHROMATES: *See* ACID, CHROMIC

COAL GAS: *See* CARBON MONOXIDE

COBALT SALTS: *See* ARSENIC

COCAINE (*See also* DRUG ADDICTION)

Symptoms and Signs

Stimulation, then depression; fullness in head; sometimes nausea and vomiting; loss of self-control; excitement, anxiety, hallucinations; sweating; choreiform movements; dry, numb throat; dilated pupils, exophthalmos; rise in temperature; numbness in hands and feet; failure of sight and hearing; vertigo; pulse first slow then rapid; blood pressure first elevated then lowered; labored respiration; clonic and tonic convulsions; narcosis; cyanosis; coma or delirium; respiratory paralysis.

Treatment

Tannic acid (5 Gm.) with stomach tube, or emetics; stimulants; external heat; mustard over heart; pentobarbital sodium 0.2-0.5 Gm. (gr. iii-viiss), or other short-acting barbiturate, I.V. to relieve nervous excitement or delirium. (CAUTION! Avoid morphine.) O_2 inhalation; artificial respiration; chloroform or ether inhalations. Nitroglycerin, 0.6 mg. (gr. 1/100) subcut. sometimes valuable.

CODEINE: *See* OPIUM

COLCHICINE
Colocynth   *Elaterin*

Symptoms and Signs

Gastric pain; nausea; violent vomiting; profuse watery and bloody diarrhea; profuse salivation; burning of throat and skin; dilated pupils; hematuria, oliguria; pulse rapid then slow; respiration first slow and full, then shallow; great prostration; cold, pale, sweaty skin; consciousness retained; muscular pains, convulsions; paralysis, first of limbs, then extending until muscles of respiration are paralyzed; collapse; asphyxia.

Treatment

Gastric lavage with tannic acid, or emetic; morphine 15 mg. (gr. 1/4) subcut. for pain and nervous irritability; stimulants; heat to abdomen and extremities. Calcium gluconate, 1 Gm. (gr. xv) I.V., if griping is pronounced.

CONIINE
Conium (Poison Hemlock)
Gelseminine   *Gelsemium*

Symptoms and Signs

Frontal headache; giddiness; weakness; muscular relaxation; staggering; burning in mouth and throat; nausea; vomiting; salivation; dysphagia; cold moist skin; gradual loss of muscular power; somewhat dilated pupils; pulse first slow, then rapid and feeble; respiration first rapid and deep, then slow and labored; spasms; foaming at mouth; coma; paralysis, beginning at feet and ascending to cause asphyxia from paralysis of respiratory muscles.

Treatment

Recumbent position; stomach tube with tannic acid, or emetic; strong tea, or 60 mg. (gr. i) iodine and 0.6 Gm. (gr. x) potassium iodide in tumblerful of water followed by gastric lavage or emetic; stimulants; demulcents; external heat; friction; artificial respiration.

COPPER SALTS
Zinc Salts

Symptoms and Signs

Both metals produce metallic taste; nausea; vomiting; purging which may become bloody; severe abdominal pains; salivation; kidney irritation; weak, soft pulse; shallow, rapid respiration; headache; giddiness; cold sweat, clammy skin; unconsciousness; delirium; coma; convulsions; collapse. Concentrated solution of zinc chloride corrodes lips and mouth. In copper poisoning, vomitus and stools have a green color.

Treatment

Gastric lavage; potassium ferrocyanide in 0.3-1 Gm. (gr. v-xv) doses in water, or as gastric lavage; or milk, albumin, or magnesia; cathartics; demulcents; morphine 15 mg. (gr. ¼) subcut. for pain and nervous irritability; stimulants; external heat; artificial respiration if breathing becomes labored; potassium iodide, 30 Gm. (℥ i); strong coffee.

CORROSIVE SUBLIMATE: *See* MERCURY COMPOUNDS

CREOSOTE; CRESOLS: *See* PHENOLS

CROTON OIL

Symptoms and Signs

Severe gastroenteritis and abdominal pain; vomiting; purging; small thready pulse; moist skin; pinched face; prostration; burning in mouth, throat and stomach; collapse.

Treatment

Gastric lavage with copious quantities of water and milk or oil, or emetics; 15 mg. (gr. ¼) morphine subcut. for pain; demulcents; stimulants; external heat; flaxseed poultice to abdomen; 5-10 drops spirit of camphor in milk or on sugar, repeated as required; combat dehydration.

CURARE
Curarine

Symptoms and Signs

Agitation; complete paralysis of voluntary muscles, starting with those of the face and neck, spreading to extremities and finally to the diaphragm and the intercostal muscles; elevated temperature; heart slowed; diuresis; respiration gradually diminished; consciousness not affected; death by asphyxia. (When curare or curarine is swallowed, the action is similar, but much less severe.)

Treatment

Physostigmine, 1-2 mg., or neostigmine methylsulfate, 0.5 mg. subcut.; spirit of nitrous ether (1-2 tsp. repeated in 10-20 min.); artificial respiration; catheterize frequently to prevent reabsorption of toxin; stimulants; external heat. If due to poison arrow, treat wound locally as for snake bite (see VENOMOUS BITES).

CYANIDES
Acid Hydrocyanic
Bitter Almond Oil   Cherry Laurel Water

Symptoms and Signs

With large doses death is almost instantaneous. With small doses there is vomiting, diarrhea; mental confusion; vertigo; headache; extreme dyspnea and violent respiration; slow, imperceptible pulse; weakness; glassy, protruding eyes, dilated pupils; characteristic odor (peach blossoms, bitter almond) of breath; pale face; mouth may be covered with foam, sometimes bloodstained; asphyxia; unconsciousness; violent convulsions; paralysis; stupor, coma; respiration becomes extremely slow and ceases while heart continues to beat for some time.

Treatment

Amyl nitrite immediately 0.3 cc. (♏ v), inhaled for 15-30 sec. every 2-3 min., followed by sodium nitrite 0.3 Gm. (gr. v) in 10 cc. of water I.V. at a rate of 2.5-5 cc./min., followed immediately through the same needle by 25-50 cc. of a 50% solution of sodium thiosulfate. (This treatment requires at least 2 operators.) One hour later give half-doses of those antidotes, repeating this latter procedure after another hour if signs persist or reappear. Epinephrine 1:1,000 sol. should be at hand to combat possible collapse. Medicinal methylene blue, 50 cc. of 1% in Ringer's sol. I.V., is not so effective as nitrite. Immediate artificial respiration. Gastric lavage with 3% hydrogen peroxide or 0.2% potassium permanganate sol. Recumbency is imperative; external heat and O_2 inhalation may be required.

DATURINE: *See* BELLADONNA

DICHLORETHYL SULFIDE: *See* CARBON OXYCHLORIDE

DIGITALIS

Digitalin	*Squill*
Digitoxin	*Strophanthin*
Scoparin	

Symptoms and Signs

Headache; giddiness; precordial distress; nausea, vomiting; abdominal pain, purging; great muscular weakness; salivation; disordered vision; pupils usually dilated, may be contracted; protruding eyeballs, blue sclerotic coat; pulse slow and irregular, rapid and weak on arising, yet heart may beat violently; extrasystoles, cardiac arrhythmias; low temperature and cold extremities; face pale; consciousness not impaired until late; finally lethargy followed by delirium and convulsions; coma; sudden death from cardiac paralysis.

Treatment

Horizontal position, continued for several days after improvement (slightest exertion may produce circulatory failure and sudden death); gastric lavage if indicated, best with tannic acid; saline cathartic; atropine subcut.; nitroglycerin subcut.; stimulants; artificial respiration. Avoid diuretics, if possible, if patient is edematous.

DIPHOSGENE: *See* CARBON OXYCHLORIDE

DONOVAN'S SOLUTION: *See* ARSENIC

DUBOISINE: *See* BELLADONNA

ELATERIN: *See* COLCHICINE

ERGOT

Ergotin	*Ergotoxin*

Symptoms and Signs

Tingling, itching, and coldness of skin; great thirst; vomiting; diarrhea; burning pain in feet; cramps in extremities; dilated pupils; dizziness; rapid, small, feeble pulse; weakness; cold skin; sometimes convulsions; hemorrhages; abortion during pregnancy; gangrene of extremities, or cataract may be secondary effects.

Treatment

Recumbent positions; tannic acid with stomach tube, or emetic; castor oil, 30 cc. (℥ i) or magnesium sulfate 30 Gm. (℥ i); stimulants; friction; external heat; nitroglycerin 0.6 mg. (gr. 1/100) subcut. and amyl nitrite 0.3 cc. (♏ v.) by inhalation are physiologic antidotes; papaverine 60 mg. (gr. i) I.V.

FLUORIDES
Ammonium Fluoride
Sodium Fluoride (Soluble Fluorides generally)

Symptoms and Signs

Salivation; lacrimation; weakness; somnolence; nausea, vomiting, abdominal cramps; muscular weakness; excitement; tremors; blood pressure falls; respiration first deep and rapid, then shallow; epileptiform convulsions; dyspnea; deep coma; respiratory failure.

Treatment

Give immediately calcium gluconate, 1 Gm. I.V.; gastric lavage with chalk and water, or lime water, or copious amounts of milk; emetic; demulcents, particularly milk. Keep patient warm and quiet.

ESERINE: *See* PHYSOSTIGMINE

ETHER: *See* CHLOROFORM

FLY PAPER: *See* ARSENIC

FORMALDEHYDE

Symptoms and Signs

After inhalation: Intense irritation of eyes and nose: dyspnea; headache; sense of suffocation; edema of glottis; bronchitis; pneumonia. **After swallowing:** Irritation of mouth and throat; gastric pain; nausea; vomiting (may be bloody); dyspnea; vertigo; intense anxiety; small rapid pulse; albuminuria, hematuria, oliguria, anuria; diarrhea; stupor; convulsions; collapse; coma.

Treatment

After inhalation: Fresh air; inhalation of ammonia; gentle stimulation if necessary. **After swallowing:** 240 cc. (℥ viii) of 0.2% ammonia water internally (considered best); or diluted aromatic spirit of ammonia; egg white or milk, then gastric lavage with 0.1% ammonia or emetic; stimulants and demulcents. Combat acidosis (q.v.), due to oxidation of formaldehyde to formic acid, by giving sodium lactate or bicarbonate I.V.

FOWLER'S SOLUTION: *See* ARSENIC

FUNGI, POISONOUS (*See* GASTROENTERITIS; NON-BACTERIAL FOOD POISONING, p. 490)

GAS
Acetylene, Automobile Exhaust, Furnace, Illuminating, Marsh: See CARBON MONOXIDE
Mustard, Phosgene, Tear: See CARBON OXYCHLORIDE
Sewer: See HYDROGEN SULFIDE

GASOLINE: *See* BENZINE

GELSEMININE: *See* CONIINE

GOLD SALTS (*See* RHEUMATOID ARTHRITIS, p. 902, for details of toxic manifestations to gold compounds and procedure for treating these with BAL.)

GUAIACOL: *See* PHENOLS

HEROIN: *See* OPIUM

HYDROGEN SULFIDE
Alkali Sulfides   *Sewer Gas (contains H_2S)*

Symptoms and Signs
Breathed in concentrated form rapidly causes unconsciousness and death. With lower concentrations, violent irritation of mucous membranes occurs, causing conjunctivitis, pharyngitis, bronchitis, pulmonary edema, and pneumonia. After absorption through the lungs, central depression (sometimes preceded by stimulation) takes place, resulting in violent headaches, dyspnea, muscular weakness, feeble pulse, fall in temperature and blood pressure, convulsions, coma, and respiratory failure.
Long exposure to diluted gas causes nausea, headache, confusion, excitement, insomnia; sneezing, coryza, cough, laryngitis, bronchitis; giddiness; dyspnea; lacrimation; dryness and burning in mouth and throat; dilated pupils; muscular and cardiac weakness; cramplike abdominal pains; epigastric distress; livid face; anemia; dermatitis. Sulfides have a corrosive action on mouth, throat, and esophagus; cause severe pain in throat and stomach.

Treatment
Fresh air at once; inhalation of 95% O_2 with 5% CO_2; friction to extremities; external heat; cardiac and respiratory stimulants; artificial respiration for respiratory embarrassment. Keep patient horizontal and absolutely quiet to prevent cardiac failure.

HYOSCINE; HYOSCYAMINE; HYOSCYAMUS:
See BELLADONNA

IGNATIA: *See* STRYCHNINE

INK, ANILINE: *See* ACETANILID

IODINE

Symptoms and Signs

Disagreeable metallic taste; brown color of lips and oral mucous membranes; burning pain in throat and stomach; intense gastroenteritis; vomiting (yellow vomitus; or blue if starch is present in stomach or added); purging (may be bloody); intense thirst; marked cardiac depression; face pale; strangury or anuria; may be albumin or blood in urine; small, rapid, feeble pulse; skin cold and clammy; cyanosis; dyspnea; convulsive movements; collapse.

Treatment

Gastric lavage with solution of soluble starch (if not available, use 1 to 5% sodium thiosulfate solution or egg white). Prompt and frequent administration of starch as such, or rice or barley in water or as gruel; demulcents and stimulants; 15 mg. (gr. ¼) morphine subcut.; external heat. Maintain acid-base balance by parenteral fluids.

IODOFORM

Symptoms and Signs

Discomfort, anxiety, restlessness; characteristic odor and taste in mouth; headache; drowsiness; delirium; hallucinations; mental confusion; rapid weak pulse; high temperature; prostration; coma; respiratory failure.

Treatment

Gastric lavage or emetic, and respiratory and cardiac stimulants; if iodoform has been absorbed from a wound, wash wound with sodium bicarb. sol., or with oil of eucalyptus or sponge with alcohol or ether; morphine 15 mg. (gr. ¼) subcut. to control delirium.

JABORANDI: *See* PHYSOSTIGMINE; PILOCARPINE

JAVELLE WATER: *See* CHLORINE

LABARRAQUE'S SOLUTION: *See* CHLORINE

LARKSPUR: *See* ACONITE

LAUDANUM: *See* OPIUM

LEAD POISONING, ACUTE AND CHRONIC
(Plumbism)

Acute lead poisoning is rather rare and usually occurs accidentally, whereas chronic lead poisoning is a common industrial hazard. The two conditions will therefore be considered separately.

ACUTE LEAD POISONING

Symptoms and Signs

Sweetish metallic taste; dry throat; burning pain in mouth, pharynx and stomach; great thirst; cramps in stomach, bowels and legs; constipation followed by diarrhea; stools may be bloody or black (lead sulfide); vomiting (may be bloody); intense vomiting and diarrhea may produce severe dehydration; muscular weakness and even paralysis of limbs; livid face; cold sweats; headache; dizziness; convulsions; stupor; coma; collapse; rapid, tense pulse becoming weaker and relaxed.

Treatment

Gastric lavage with magnesium, sodium, or aluminum sulfate sol., followed by plain water to remove lead sulfate thus formed; demulcents and stimulants; calcium gluconate 1 Gm. I.M.; chloral hydrate or papaverine for spasms; 15 mg. (gr. $\frac{1}{4}$) morphine and 0.5 mg. (gr. 1/120) atropine subcut. for pain; external heat.

CHRONIC LEAD POISONING

Etiology and Incidence

Chronic lead poisoning may result from inhaling pathogenic quantities of lead, i.e., more than 1 mg./day, in contaminated dust, fume, or spray; from swallowing lead dust adhering to the nasopharyngeal structures, or from eating food from hands contaminated with lead or leaded materials (paint). Lead may be absorbed through breaks in the skin but only volatile lipoid soluble organic lead preparations, such as tetraethyl lead, can be absorbed through intact skin. By these avenues lead poisoning may occur in more than 150 industrial occupations, including lead industries, plumbing, painting, glazing, auto body finishing, mining (lead sulfide in deep mines, sulfates and carbonates in shallow workings), lead smelting (fumes of lead oxide and sulfates), white-lead working, zinc smelting, lead roasting in air to form oxides, storage battery manufacture (red lead and litharge), enameling bathtubs and similar fixtures, rolling sheet lead, shot making, lace making, calico printing (oxides—red lead), vulcanizing of rubber, brass polishing, printing trade (e.g., type founding, lithography), tinning, sandpapering dried paint, glass trade (mixing and grinding); working with lead-dyed artificial flowers, yarns, wallpaper, or with insecticides; also in manufacture of tetraethyl lead (*see* below) and mixing with gasoline; but not in working with tetraethyl lead gasoline, where the lead is too diluted.

Chronic lead poisoning may occur, but rarely, from drinking

water passed through lead pipes or from ingesting foods stored in lead-lined or lead-contaminated containers or wrapped in lead foil, or acid foods kept in glazed pottery; or acid foods which have reacted to solder in tin cans; or fruits that have been sprayed with lead-containing insecticides (lead arsenate). Hair dyes and other cosmetics containing lead are other sources of poisoning, and children may contract it by chewing paint off cribs, toys, or other objects.

Certain persons are more susceptible than others to lead poisoning. Predisposing conditions are unhygienic environment, hepatic or renal disease, alcoholism, infections, and malnutrition.

Symptoms, Signs, and Diagnosis

Lead absorption must be distinguished from lead intoxication, in which there is actual injury to the tissue cells. A diagnosis of lead poisoning is certain when there are at least 1 of the following signs of lead absorption and 2 of lead intoxication.

Lead absorption: (1) "Lead line" on the gums, a blue line that cannot be rubbed away. (Mercury and bismuth produce similar lines.) It may be absent, especially in clean, healthy mouths. (2) Urinary elimination, under controlled conditions, of more than 0.1 mg. lead/liter; average, 0.15 mg. This may be absent for several days. (3) Fecal excretion of over 0.6 mg. /day, under controlled conditions. (4) Lead in blood above 0.1 mg./100 cc. (5) In children, X-ray shows heavy opaque lines along bone epiphyses.

Lead intoxication: (1) Preceding a toxic episode, the skin is pasty, sallow, subicteric. The pallor seems disproportionate to the anemia resulting from destruction of red blood cells (which probably is due to their increased fragility): count rarely less than 3,500,000. (2) Basophilic aggregation in more than 2% of erythrocytes (modified Manson's stain), or punctate basophilia of erythrocytes, a stippling of the red cells which, when it occurs in large numbers (at least 5 in 50 average fields) practically is pathognomonic of plumbism. The number of stippled cells may vary greatly from day to day, and repeated counts are often necessary to determine any substantial increase in their number. The stippling can be brought out by simple staining of unfixed blood smear by hypotonic saline methylene blue sol.

Premonitory symptoms of lead intoxication: Anorexia, indigestion, heavily coated tremulous tongue, foul breath, joint pains, mild transitory generalized abdominal pain. Protracted constipation alternating with diarrhea; malaise, fatigue, and weakness.

After prolonged exposure, these symptoms may develop into toxic episodes consisting of the following: **(1) Colic:** severe agonizing paroxysms of abdominal pain, with dull pain between attacks; almost always preceded by constipation. Abdomen hard and retracted. This retraction, plus slow pulse, rise in blood pressure, and temporary relief of pain on inhalation of amyl nitrite, differentiates lead colic from acute intra-abdominal inflammation. Fever is rare; no leukocytosis, but a relative mononucleosis. **(2) Palsy:** occurring in part most used, usually preceded by weakness and dull, localized muscle pains. Weakness of extensor muscles of middle and ring fingers is characteristic; followed by wrist drop; rarely, foot drop and steppage gait. Extensor muscles of forearm and the shoulder muscles are sometimes affected. Very little sensory disturbance; no pain when palsy is fully developed. **(3) Encephalopathy:** this occurs in massive exposures and often results from tetraethyl lead poisoning. Onset may be explosive and often is preceded by restlessness, headache, tremors. Epileptiform convulsions may appear first, followed by coma and delirium often ending in death; sometimes there is partial recovery with mental deterioration, blindness, deafness, or paralysis. (CAUTION! Always examine urine, feces, and blood, and X-ray bones of children with unexplained colic, paralysis, or convulsions.)

Special manifestations of lead intoxication are encountered in pregnant women, who may abort or give birth to infants who soon die. Patients with chronic plumbism occasionally develop optic neuritis and deafness; they frequently show mental dullness. It has been claimed though not proved that lead poisoning predisposes to arterial hypertension, arteriosclerosis, cardiac hypertrophy, chronic nephritis (especially contracted kidney), liver cirrhosis, and gout.

Prophylaxis and Treatment

The risk of lead poisoning in lead industries may be reduced by installing exhaust systems, vacuum cleaning, thorough ventilation, and the use of moist instead of dry processes. Respirators or "snouts" worn by the workmen are helpful in avoiding contamination via the air passages, but air-supplied helmets are better. Paints should be rubbed down with waxed or wettable sandpaper that can be used on moistened surfaces. Scrupulous personal cleanliness should be insisted upon—particularly of the hands, nails, face, and lips before eating. Food and utensils should be protected from contamination (no food should be eaten where work is conducted). Workmen should change their outer clothing when leaving work. There is no satisfactory antidote against chronic lead poisoning, although 120 cc. (℥ iv) sulfuric acid lemonade 2 or 3 times daily has been recommended, prepared by adding 4 cc. (℥ i) of dilute sulfuric acid to 1,000 cc. (℥ xxxii) of lemonade. Regularly exposed persons should have frequent physical, urine, and blood examinations.

After recovery from chronic plumbism, the patient should not be further exposed to lead, as slight contact will bring a recurrence of symptoms. The use of calcium-poor, acid-forming diets, acids, alkaline salts, and iodides, advocated by some, has been proved ineffective in prevention or treatment of lead poisoning, and so has vitamin C.

Treatment of the condition consists of the following: For lead colic: (1) calcium chloride or calcium gluconate 1 Gm. I.V. (2) Antispasmodics (oral) such as atropine, 0.5 mg. (gr. 1/120), nitroglycerin 0.6 mg. (gr. 1/100), papaverine 30-60 mg. (gr. ss-i), or erythrol tetranitrate 30 mg. (gr. ss). (3) Alum, either in 6% solution (100 cc.) or as the curd which forms when 6 Gm. alum is added to 500 cc. (℥ xvi) boiling milk. (4) Morphine 10-15 mg. (gr. ⅙-¼) subcut. should be used only when the previously named remedies fail to give relief; it usually is rendered unnecessary by the I.V. administration of calcium. (5) Cathartics usually fail during an attack; enemas and mineral oil might be tried; and magnesium sulfate after the antispasmodics have acted.

Angiospastic cerebral manifestations demand immediate and energetic spasmolytic and blood-pressure lowering medication: amyl nitrite inhalation; papaverine, 30-60 mg. (gr. ss-i) I.V.; hot packs; and phlebotomy. Reduction of cerebral edema, in convulsions, by repeated I.M. injections of small doses (0.1 cc./Kg.) of 25% magnesium sulfate sol. or 50 cc. of 50% glucose or sucrose sol. I.V. Cerebral decompression.

Paralysis requires treatment with massage, active movements, and galvanic stimulation. Do not use strychnine.

LEAD, TETRAETHYL

Symptoms and Signs

Insomnia; nausea, vomiting; vertigo (particularly in the morning); headache; pallor; low blood pressure and temperature; tremors; sometimes delirium or mania; colic frequent, but neuritis and "lead line" rare.

Treatment

Fresh air; artificial respiration; aromatic spirit of ammonia; ammonia by inhalation; isotonic salt sol. I.V.; cardiac and respiratory stimulants; blood transfusion.

LOBELIA; LOBELINE: *See* TOBACCO

LYE: *See* ACIDS AND ALKALIS

MATCHES: *See* PHOSPHORUS

MERCURY COMPOUNDS

Symptoms and Signs

Metallic taste; severe gastroenteritis, with corrosion if taken in concentrated form; burning pain in mouth, throat, and stomach; salivation; colicky pains; nausea; severe vomiting (vomitus often containing blood and mucous membranes); profuse watery and bloody diarrhea; severe fluid loss may produce shock, and possibly early death. Usually, patient improves and develops severe colitis 1 or more days later, with diarrhea, melena, abdominal cramps, tenesmus; thirst; face pale and shrunken; cold clammy skin and extremities; small, thready, feeble, irregular pulse; shallow, irregular, rapid respiration subnormal temperature. With the colitis severe stomatitis develops which may make swallowing impossible. After 1 or 2 days, severe nephrosis, with first increased then diminished quantity of urine, which contains albumin, blood, and casts. Finally, anuria and uremia with convulsions; coma; collapse.

Treatment

Whites of several raw eggs followed by gastric lavage, or emetic if lavage cannot immediately be performed; follow by 1 pt. egg albumin water and again wash out stomach. As promptly as possible administer 2,3-dimercaptopropanol (BAL), 2 to 3 mg./Kg. body wt., I.M., as the 10% sol. in peanut oil with benzyl benzoate; repeat this dose of BAL every 2-4 hours for several days. (Such striking results are obtained with BAL that it has superseded the older antidotal methods of treatment.) Other measures are Murphy drip with potassium acetate, 6% sol., and 500 cc. of 20% glucose I.V. once or twice daily, possibly with 0.5 Gm. (gr. viiss) of aminophylline added, but keeping the fluid intake low during the period of anuria. Protein should be given freely at first, but restricted later; salt intake also should be restricted. Iodides are contraindicated. Kidney decapsulation has been recommended but is dangerous. X-radiation of kidney has been advised. Morphine 15 mg. (gr. ¼) subcut. for pain; stimulants; external heat. Combat acidosis (q.v.) by I.V. administration of sodium bicarb., or lactate.

MORPHINE SALTS: *See* OPIUM

MUSHROOMS, POISONOUS (*See* GASTROENTERITIS; NONBACTERIAL FOOD POISONING, p. 490)

Muscarine
Phalloidin

MUSTARD GAS: *See* CARBON OXYCHLORIDE

NAPHTHA: *See* BENZINE

NAPHTHALENE

Symptoms and Signs

Restlessness; depression; twitchings; convulsions; strangura; urine dark brown to black; coma with stertorous breathing.

Treatment

Gastric lavage or emetics; demulcents; stimulants.

NICOTINE: *See* TOBACCO

NITRATES: *See* CHLORATES

NITRITES

Amyl Acetate	*Potassium Nitrite*
Amyl Nitrite	*Sodium Nitrite*
Nitroglycerin	

Symptoms and Signs

Flushed face with violent, then diminished heart action; excessively severe, throbbing headache; dizziness; faintness; great muscular relaxation and tremors; pallor; dilated pupils; irregular respiration; at times vomiting; colics; bloody diarrhea; convulsions (rarely); cyanosis (methemoglobinemia); syncope; circulatory collapse. Death from respiratory or cardiac failure.

Treatment

Horizontal posture and abundant fresh air; stomach tube (when poison has been swallowed), or apomorphine hydrochloride, 6 mg. (gr. 1/10) subcut.; in all cases, stimulants; alternate cold and hot applications to chest; artificial respiration. Trendelenburg position. If cyanosis is pronounced inhalation of oxygen, and blood transfusions.

NITROBENZENE (OIL OF MIRBANE; ARTIFICIAL OIL OF BITTER ALMONDS)

Symptoms and Signs

Characteristic odor of bitter almonds; mental dullness; drowsiness; headache; nausea, vomiting; ataxia; nystagmus; brown urine having characteristic odor; convulsive movements; weak respiration; irregular pupils; dyspnea; delirium; extreme cyanosis; coma; respiratory arrest.

Treatment

After swallowing: Gastric lavage or emetic; ammonium carbonate, 0.12-0.6 Gm. (gr. ii-x); stimulants; alternate hot and cold applications to chest; O_2; artificial respiration; blood transfusions if cyanosis is severe. After inhalation: Treat as above except for gastric lavage and emetics.

NITROGLYCERIN: *See* NITRITES

NITROUS OXIDE: *See* CHLOROFORM

NUX VOMICA: *See* STRYCHNINE

OPIUM (*See also* DRUG ADDICTION)

Codeine	*Laudanum*
Heroin	*Morphine*

Symptoms and Signs

Initial mental exhilaration and physical ease; then headache, weariness, drowsiness; pin-point pupils; respirations slow and shallow. Pulse at first rapid and forcible, later slower, then more feeble; mouth and throat dry; gradual onset of unconsciousness, from which patient at first can be aroused, though with difficulty, but later cannot; muscles relaxed and reflexes lost; jaw falls; respirations become very slow (sometimes 3-4 /min.), irregular and stertorous; Cheyne-Stokes breathing; pulse becomes rapid and feeble, then slow; temperature low; progressive fall in blood pressure; skin rashes; constipation; urinary retention; cyanosis; extreme prostration; skin pale, with cold sweat; convulsions may occur in later stages, especially in children; pupils begin to dilate; coma, death.

Treatment

Copious gastric lavage with 0.1% solution of potassium permanganate. Introduce 30 Gm. ($\frac{2}{3}$ i) magnesium sulfate in solution through stomach tube before removing it (morphine is excreted to a large degree into the intestines); copious administration of activated charcoal. If respiration is depressed: 0.5 Gm. (gr. viiss) of caffeine and sodium benzoate I.V. or enemas of strong coffee; 30 mg. (gr. ss) ephedrine sulfate I.M. or 40 mg. amphetamine sulfate I.V.; to be repeated every 30 min. to 1 hr. until consciousness and normal rate of respiration are restored. (Avoid strychnine, picrotoxin and Metrazol because morphine is a spinal cord stimulant and convulsions might be precipitated.) Inhalation of 95% O_2 and 5% CO_2. If patient can be aroused, keep him awake by making him walk, by slapping with cold towel, or other method; maintain body temperature by external heat. Change patient's posture frequently to prevent hypostatic pneumonia. If coma is prolonged catheterize bladder and repeat high enemas and laxatives.

OXALATES: *See* ACID, OXALIC

PARALDEHYDE

Symptoms and Signs

Paraldehyde odor on breath; excitement; incoherence; muscular relaxation; rapid pulse; contracted pupils, insensitive to light; slow respiration; unconsciousness; collapse; respiratory failure.

Treatment

Gastric lavage or emetic; stimulants; picrotoxin 0.6 mg. (gr. 1/100), or amphetamine sulfate 40 mg. (gr. 2/3) I.V.; external heat; artificial respiration; O_2.

PARATHION (ORGANIC PHOSPHATE INSECTICIDE)

Symptoms and Signs

Poisoning may follow inhalation, swallowing, or absorption

of parathion through the skin. Principally due to inactivation of cholinesterase. Headache, blurred vision, miosis, weakness; nausea, colic, diarrhea; hyperhidrosis, lacrimation, salivation; pulmonary edema.

Treatment

Do not give morphine. Atropine 0.5 mg. (gr. 1/120) subcut. or I.V., followed by 1–2 mg. (gr. 1/60-1/30) every hour up to a total of 10–20 mg. in a day, if necessary to control symptoms. O_2 and artificial respiration may be needed if respiration is embarrassed.

PARIS GREEN: *See* ARSENIC

PETROLEUM: *See* BENZINE

PHENACETIN: *See* ACETANILID

PHOSGENE GAS: *See* CARBON OXYCHLORIDE

PHENOBARBITAL: *See* BARBITURATES

PHENOLS

Carbolic Acid
Creosote
Cresols

Guaiacol
Phenols in general

Symptoms and Signs

Burning pain from mouth to stomach; characteristic odor on breath; patches, first white then brown, on lips and in mouth (local necrosis); great depression and weakness; headache; nausea; salivation; vomiting (rarely); abdominal pain; vertigo; pulse and respiration first accelerated, then irregular, feeble and intermittent; urine black after standing; albuminuria, hematuria, oliguria; fall in blood pressure and body temperature; pale, livid, clammy face and skin; collapse; coma; death from respiratory failure, or possibly edema of glottis or lungs. Large doses may cause immediate unconsciousness, rapidly followed by death. Esophageal stenosis, rarely. Aspiration pneumonia not uncommon as a complication.

Treatment

It is essential to remove the poison from the stomach before extensive absorption occurs. Olive oil, which has the property of dissolving phenol without hastening its absorption, should be given at once in large quantities by mouth. Stomach tube should be passed as soon as possible and extensive lavage given with olive oil, leaving some clean oil in the stomach at the end. (If olive oil is not available, cottonseed oil or water may be used.) If the toxic product is not recovered, it acts on the C.N.S., causing convulsions. Alcohol, mineral oil, and fats and oils in general other than those mentioned above should be avoided, since they either fail to dissolve the phenol sufficiently or promote its absorption. (CAUTION! If the gastric wall has become corroded, passage of the tube or emetics may be dangerous. The presence of corrosion may be assumed when the phenol has been taken in a relatively pure state, in considerable quantity, and when the patient is seen late and is suffering severe gastric pain.) Give 15-30 Gm. (ʒ ss-i) magnesium or other soluble sulfate; lime water; soapsuds; egg albumin or other demulcent; copious amounts of isotonic saline sol. I.V. to promote diuresis; stimulants; caffeine and sodium benzoate 0.5 Gm. (gr. viiss) in 500 cc. of 20% dextrose sol. I.V. Recumbent position; cold to head; O₂; artificial respiration; external heat. Soft diet may be given next day, general diet on 3rd or 4th day. Esophageal analgesic 4 cc. (ʒ i) (to lessen pain on swallowing), consisting of a mixture of orthoform (4 cc.), epinephrine 1:1,000 sol. (4 cc.), and mucilage of acacia (52 cc.).

When phenol has been applied to the skin or mucous membrane, it can be successfully neutralized with 50% alcohol or castor oil. If large areas of skin are involved, systemic poisoning may result from absorption.

PHOSPHORUS
Matches (containing   Certain Rat Poisons
yellow phosphorus)

Symptoms and Signs

Gastrointestinal irritation, pain and burning; garlicky taste and breath odor; vomiting (vomitus bloody or coffee-colored, luminous in dark, garlicky odor); bloody diarrhea. If the patient survives, there may be a quiescent period of 1-3 days followed by: nausea and vomiting; great hunger; tender, enlarged liver; skin eruptions; pruritus; jaundice; ecchymosis and petechiae; headache; vertigo; great prostration; pulse weak, thready, intermittent; heart sounds obscure; greatly reduced blood pressure; irregular temperature; hematuria, albuminuria, oliguria; dyspnea; collapse; coma or delirium; convulsions.

Treatment

Copious and repeated gastric lavage, with 1% copper sulfate (which envelops phosphorus particles with an insoluble coating of copper phosphide), followed by 0.1% potassium permanganate, 1-3% sol. of hydrogen peroxide or normal saline; then catharsis with 50 Gm. (ʒ iss) magnesium sulfate and also liquid petrolatum to coat stomach; high colonic irrigations with warm water. (CAUTION! For several days, in subsequent diet avoid all edible oils and fats, or substances containing them, e.g., milk, since these promote absorption of phosphorus.) Oil of turpentine (old, ozonized oil best), 1-2 cc. floated on hot water or in gelatin capsules or in mucilaginous emulsion, 3-4 times at

15-30 min. intervals; magnesium oxide, or chalk (in gruel); morphine 15 mg. (gr. ¼) subcut. to relieve pain; 1-3% hydrogen peroxide internally; blood transfusions, if necessary; external heat; sodium bicarb. or alkaline drinks freely to maintain and increase alkalinity of blood. During quiescent period high carbohydrate, high protein diet, with I.V. amino acids or protein hydrolysate supplementation.

PHYSOSTIGMINE (ESERINE); PILOCARPINE

Calabar Bean	Pilocarpus
Neostigmine (Prostigmine)	(Jaborandi)

(NOTE: Substances are different, but are grouped because of similar symptoms and signs and identical treatment.)

Symptoms and Signs

Dizziness, vertigo; muscular weakness; vomiting; violent and persistent purging; cramplike pains; pupils first dilated then contracted, sometimes to pin-point (miosis often absent); nystagmus; sweating; salivation and lacrimation; heart slow; respiration first accelerated, then slow and weak; fall of blood pressure; pulmonary edema; muscular twitchings; collapse; dyspnea; death from respiratory failure or cardiac paralysis.

Treatment

At once, 0.6-1 mg. (gr. 1/100-1/60) atropine sulfate subcut., or in severe cases I.V. repeated in 30 min. if necessary; this is the best physiologic antidote. Gastric lavage with tannic acid or potassium permanganate, 0.1% solution repeated in ½ hr.; or emetic (CAUTION! Do not use apomorphine); 1 tsp. spirit of nitrous ether every ½-2 hrs.; stimulants; chloral hydrate; if other treatment ineffective, artificial respiration.

PICROTOXIN: *See* STRYCHNINE

PILOCARPINE: *See* PHYSOSTIGMINE; PILOCARPINE

POTASH: *See* ACIDS AND ALKALIS

POTASSIUM CHROMATE: *See* ACID, CHROMIC

POTASSIUM CYANIDE: *See* CYANIDES

POTASSIUM DICHROMATE: *See* ACID, CHROMIC

POTASSIUM HYDROXIDE: *See* ACIDS AND ALKALIS

POTASSIUM NITRATE: *See* CHLORATES

RAT POISON: *See* ARSENIC, *see also* PHOSPHORUS

RESORCINOL (RESORCIN)

Symptoms and Signs

Vomiting; dizziness; tinnitus; chills; faintness; sweating;

salivation; tremor of hands; low temperature; delirium; convulsions; feeble respiration; cyanosis; unconsciousness.

Treatment

Olive oil, followed at once by gastric lavage or emetic; cardiac and respiratory stimulants; demulcents; external heat; recumbent position; friction.

SALICYLATES

Acetylsalicylic Acid (Aspirin)
Methyl Salicylate (Oil of Wintergreen)
Phenyl Salicylate (Salol)
Salicylic Acid
Sodium Salicylate

Symptoms and Signs

Vomiting; epigastric pain; profuse perspiration; headache; dizziness; tinnitus; visual disturbances; delirium; restlessness, excitement, and hallucinations; pulse rapid and feeble; blood pressure low; pallor; skin eruptions; dyspnea, even Kussmaul's respiration (air hunger) due to acidosis. Urine shows salicylate reaction: ferric chloride produces port-wine color (not affected by boiling); occasionally; evidence of nephritis, more rarely glycosuria.

Treatment

Lavage with sodium bicarb. sol. Saline cathartic. Sodium bicarb. by mouth or rectum to antagonize acidosis (q.v.). Glucose I.V.; stimulants.

SALOL: *See* SALICYLATE, PHENYL

SANTONIN

Symptoms and Signs

Objects appear first blue, then yellow; blindness frequently follows and may last a week or more. Convulsions a prominent symptom; headache; vomiting, abdominal pain, diarrhea; hematuria. Consciousness preserved until late, when delirium, stupor and coma with slow feeble heart, diminished frequency and depth of respiration, and profound prostration set in.

Treatment

Gastric lavage or emetic; saline cathartics. Counteract convulsions by I.V. injection of short-acting barbiturate, e.g., pentobarbital sodium 0.3 Gm. (gr. v); or chloral hydrate 2-3 Gm. (gr. xxx-xlv) by rectum (CAUTION! Avoid opiates); cardiac and respiratory stimulants.

SAVIN OIL

Tansy Oil

Symptoms and Signs

Savin Oil: Acute abdominal pain; vomiting; tenesmus,

bloody stools; dyspnea; sometimes stranguria and bloody urine; uterine hemorrhage; abortion in pregnancy; convulsions; collapse; coma.

Tansy Oil: Convulsions; dilated pupils; weak pulse; respiration hurried; anuria; hematuria; pulse gradually weakens; unconsciousness.

Treatment

Gastric lavage or emetic; castor oil, or 30 Gm. (℥ i) magnesium sulfate; demulcents and stimulants; external heat; cold to head; pentobarbital sodium 0.2 Gm. (gr. iii) I.V., or chloroform or chloral hydrate, or bromides to relieve pain and nervous irritability. Treat nephritis (q.v.) in the usual manner.

SCOPOLAMINE: See BELLADONNA

SEWER GAS: See HYDROGEN SULFIDE

SILVER SALTS

Symptoms and Signs

Stained patches on lips, first white and then black. Burning pain in throat and stomach; acute gastroenteritis; nausea, vomiting (white and cheesy, turning black in sunlight); cramps, purging; dizziness; weak thready pulse; shallow respiration; convulsions; circulatory collapse; paralysis; coma.

Treatment

Sodium chloride or tannic acid followed by stomach tube or emetic, and repeated; plenty of milk or other demulcents; pentobarbital sodium 0.2 Gm. (gr. iii) I.V. for pain and nervous irritability; stimulants.

SNAKE BITE (See VENOMOUS BITES, p. 1177)

SODA, CAUSTIC: See ACIDS AND ALKALIS

SODIUM CYANIDE: See CYANIDES

SODIUM HYDROXIDE: See ACIDS AND ALKALIS

SQUILL: See DIGITALIS

STINGS OF INSECTS, SCORPIONS, AND THE LIKE (See VENOMOUS BITES, p. 1180)

STRAMONIUM: See BELLADONNA

STROPHANTHUS: See DIGITALIS

STRYCHNINE

Brucine	*Nux Vomica*
Ignatia	*Picrotoxin*

Symptoms and Signs

Restlessness, excitement; stiff neck; muscular twitchings; sense of suffocation and dyspnea; sudden muscular rigidity;

muscles jerk when any part of the body is touched; tetanic painful convulsions every 3-30 min., lasting 1-5 min.; opisthotonos; jaws rigidly shut; face livid; eyeballs rolled up and prominent; pupils dilated; risus sardonicus; respiration suspended, pulse feeble and rapid during paroxysm; relaxation with exhaustion, shallow respiration and small tense pulse, followed by another paroxysm, which may be spontaneous or caused by a jar, touch, or noise; attack follows attack, and exhaustion deepens to paralysis; death from asphyxia or exhaustion.

Treatment

Administer immediately a short-acting barbiturate I.V., such as pentobarbital sodium 0.3-0.7 Gm. (gr. v-xii); if not available, inhalation anesthetic may be given during paroxysm; or 1-4 cc. paraldehyde I.M. Avoid long-acting barbiturates or morphine (morphine increases reflex irritability). Gastric lavage with 0.1% potassium permanganate or 1-2% tannic acid, or emetics, but only after convulsions have stopped. Horizontal position in darkness and absolute quiet. If muscle twitchings recur, repeat I.V. injection of short-acting barbiturate. Give O_2, respiratory stimulants (ephedrine, amphetamine, caffeine), artificial respiration.

SULFUR DIOXIDE

Symptoms and Signs

At first, sneezing, coughing, choking, lacrimation, and bronchial irritation; then headache; drowsiness; giddiness; tinnitus; loss of muscular power; violent heart action; dyspnea; respiration first increased then irregular and convulsive; inspiration shallow and weak, expiration powerful and prolonged; unconsciousness; cyanosis; pupils first contracted then dilated; convulsions; coma.

Treatment

Fresh air at once; O_2 under positive pressure, if necessary; artificial respiration; inhalations of ammonia or amyl nitrite; if respiratory movements cease, throw cold water on face and chest; if heart stops, strike chest a few sharp blows with open palm; friction and heat to extremities; stimulants; warm, strong coffee enema (1 pt.).

SULFONETHYLMETHANE (TRIONAL)
Sulfonmethane (Sulfonal)

Symptoms and Signs

Giddiness; confusion; ataxia; weakness; prolonged profound sleep; hematoporphyrinuria; anuria; ptosis of eyelids; partial paralysis; sometimes convulsions; nervous depression; may be gastric pain, vomiting; stupor; collapse; coma; respiratory and circulatory failure.

Treatment

Gastric lavage or emetic; spirit of nitrous ether, 4-8 cc. (ℨ i-ii) every ½ hr.-2 hrs.; magnesium sulfate, 30 Gm. (ℨ i); sodium bicarb. in 4 Gm. (ℨ i) doses; stimulants; artificial respiration.

TANSY OIL: *See* SAVIN OIL

TARTAR EMETIC: *See* ANTIMONY COMPOUNDS

THALLIUM SALTS

Symptoms and Signs

Gastric irritation; salivation; stomatitis; diarrhea; debility; drowsiness; pain in legs; neuritis; paresthesias and paralysis, particularly in lower extremities; retrobulbar neuritis; alopecia; diuresis; dyspnea; delirium; convulsions; heart first stimulated then depressed.

Treatment

Gastric lavage with 1% sodium or potassium iodide; or emetics; stimulants and demulcents. Later, sodium iodide, 0.3-1 Gm. (gr. v-xv) I.V. daily may hasten elimination of thallium.

TIN SALTS

Symptoms and Signs

Metallic taste; gastroenteritis; colic; vomiting; diarrhea; general weakness; diminished heart action; motor paralysis leading to ataxia, stiffness, irregular movements; occasionally convulsions.

Treatment

Gastric lavage or emetics; magnesium oxide freely, followed by demulcents; morphine 15 mg. (gr. ¼) subcut. for pain; stimulants.

TOBACCO

Lobelia   *Nicotine*
Lobeline

Symptoms and Signs

Excitement; confusion; restlessness; muscular twitchings and weakness; abdominal cramps; clonic convulsions followed by severe depression and prostration; salivation; nausea; violent vomiting and diarrhea; cold, pale, clammy skin; sweating; pulse generally slow at first, then rapid, weak and irregular; blood pressure at first elevated, then lowered; respirations quick, deep and labored. With large doses this order may be reversed: tremors (lobelia causes no tremors or convulsions except with asphyxia); palpitation; pupils first contracted then dilated; headache; vertigo; disturbed hearing and vision; confusion; collapse; coma. With excessive toxic doses, paralysis of C.N.S.; heart continues to beat; death due to respiratory paralysis.

Treatment

Tannic acid and gastric lavage, or emetics; activated charcoal; artificial respiration to counteract paralysis of muscles involved in respiration; O_2; 4-8 cc. (3 i-ii) doses of spirit of nitrous ether; ephedrine sulfate, 30 mg. (gr. ss) I.M., or amphetamine sulfate, 40 mg. I.V. (CAUTION! Avoid strychnine); cold to head; external heat.

TRIONAL: *See* SULFONETHYLMETHANE

TURPENTINE OIL

Symptoms and Signs

Characteristic odor of breath; giddiness; restlessness, excitement; ataxia; insomnia; intoxication; gastrointestinal irritation; nausea, vomiting; may be purging; stranguria; albuminuria; bloody, scanty urine (violet odor); dilated pupils; cyanosis; dry or moist skin; stertorous breathing; feeble, rapid pulse; delirium; collapse; coma.

Treatment

Stomach lavage or emetic; 30 Gm. (3 i) magnesium sulfate; stimulants; demulcents; copious amounts of water; enema if bowels have not moved freely; morphine 15 mg. (gr. ¼) subcut. for pain and nervous irritability. Treat acute nephritis (q.v.) in the usual manner.

VERONAL: *See* BARBITURATES (Barbital)

WINTERGREEN OIL: *See* SALICYLATE, METHYL

WOOD ALCOHOL: *See* ALCOHOL, METHYL

WHITE PRECIPITATE: *See* MERCURY COMPOUNDS

ZINC SALTS: *See* COPPER SALTS

VENOMOUS BITES

POISONOUS SNAKES

Varieties, Distribution, and Habits

Two principal groups of poisonous snakes are found in the U.S.A., the coral snakes and the pit vipers, a differentiation which is essential to the choice of appropriate therapy for snake bite. The harlequin coral snake is found from North Carolina to Florida and through Southern Louisiana and Texas, while the sonoran coral snake is distributed from Western Colorado and Utah southwestward to Mexico and Southern California.

The pit vipers include the following: Copperhead (Eastern and South Central U.S.); cottonmouth moccasin (Virginia to the Rio Grande); massasauga, a variety of rattler (Western New York to Kansas, and from Kansas to Mexico); pigmy rattler (Virginia to the Rio Grande); timber rattler (across the plains from Canada to Mexico), and the diamondback rattlers (the eastern type from North Carolina to Florida and westward to Louisiana, and the western type from Louisiana to California).

Coral snakes seldom attack man unless provoked. However, pit vipers, especially the copperhead, cottonmouth moccasin, and diamondback rattlers, will strike promiscuously.

Wound Characteristics

The coral snakes inflict inconspicuous fang marks, which later may be entirely obscured by edema. A pit viper's bite is more evident; it may bleed, and hemorrhagic edema may cause a red currant-like infiltration about the wound which spreads along the lymphatics as the venom is carried through them into the circulation. A necrotic ulcer usually develops locally after the bite of a pit viper but seldom after that of a coral snake, except through a secondary pyogenic infection.

Toxicology

The principal constituent of coral snake venom is a neurotoxin which is said to have a special affinity for the cells of the respiratory center, although it also affects cells elsewhere in the cord and brain. The chief constituents of viper venom usually are hemorrhagin, cytolysins, and thrombase, although in the case of the tropical rattlesnake of Mexico and Central America (*Crotalus terrificus*), a neurotoxin is the important constituent. Cytolysins and hemorrhagin dissolve the endothelial cells lining the blood and lymph vessels, and especially those of the capillary walls. Intravascular thrombosis may result from the action of thrombase. Snake venom frequently causes hemolysis.

Symptoms and Signs

Coral snake bite: There is immediate intense burning and pain at the site. Somnolence, prostration, nausea, vomiting, incontinence, and paralysis ensue, especially paralysis of the respiratory muscles. Ptosis, diplopia, and ultimately pupillary dilatation are usual eye symptoms. Terminal phenomena are coma and convulsions; death may occur in a few hours from respiratory failure.

Pit viper bite: Characteristically, there is intense pain in the wound, which later becomes excruciating and tends to radiate. Weakness, tingling and numbness of the extremities, cold perspiration, and feeling of suffocation are experienced. Within an hour, generalized urticaria may appear, with intense itching and burning. Meanwhile, hemorrhages into the kidney cortex, intestinal wall, mesentery, pericardium, adrenals, skin and mucous membranes may occur, sometimes with frank bleeding from the conjunctiva and lips. Except in the case of *Crotalus terrificus* venenation, neurologic symptoms usually are inconspicuous and death results from circulatory collapse.

Prognosis

Coral snake bite: Death may occur in a few hours from respiratory paralysis or, if the amount of the venom is sublethal, the symptoms may rapidly abate and the patient recover. **Pit viper bite:** Because the amount of venom may be lethal even for the largest individuals, bites from the bigger varieties of viper are especially dangerous to persons of small physique, particularly children.

Treatment

Local: A tourniquet should be applied proximal to the wound (only tightly enough to impede venous and lymphatic drainage) and released for 1 minute every 30 minutes to prevent gangrene. The tourniquet is reapplied each time farther from the wound if the swelling progresses. Cruciform incisions are made over the bite, each at least ½ inch long and ¼ inch deep. The wound is flushed with saline solution to help in removing the venom. Suction then is applied, either by mouth if the oral mucosa is intact, or with a mechanical pump. Any venom accidentally swallowed by the operator will be inactivated by the gastric juice.

Systemic: This is the same as for any potentially necrotic and infected wound, i.e., a sulfonamide or penicillin in adequate dosage. Tetanus antitoxin also should be given, since the snake's mouth may have transmitted tetanus bacilli or spores.

Supportive: It is essential to prevent exertion, reassure the patient, prohibit alcoholic beverages, and order complete rest in bed. To relieve nervousness and pain, phenobarbital 0.1 to 0.2 Gm. (gr. iss to iii) by mouth (℞ 39) may be given and repeated as necessary; or instead sodium phenobarbital, 0.15 to 0.25 Gm. (gr. iiss to iv) I.M., repeated in 6 hours if necessary (℞ 37). Or, except for coral snake poisoning, in which respiratory depressants must specifically be avoided, morphine 10 to 15 mg. (gr. ⅙ to ¼) subcut. may be used (℞ 36). For threatened peripheral vascular failure, either strychnine 1 to 2 mg. (gr. ⅟₆₀ to ⅟₃₀) subcut. or by mouth (℞ 55), or caffeine and sodium benzoate I.M. or I.V., 0.2 to 0.5 Gm. (gr. iii to viiss) (℞ 50), or both simultaneously, may be indicated. To combat collapse, physiologic saline with 10% glucose and either whole blood or human blood plasma, I.V. should be given. In every instance, the patient must be kept under close observation for at least 24 hours, as symptoms may suddenly become worse after 15 hours, and relapses several days later are not unknown. In coral snake poisoning artificial respiration may be necessary, perhaps in a respirator.

Specific: No antivenin for coral snake poisoning is available. However, Nearctic Crotalic Antivenin, for pit viper poisoning, is procurable from the Antivenin Institute of America through Wyeth Incorporated. It is available in a syringe (equipped with sterile needle) containing 10 cc., the average initial dose for systemic administration. In addition, an injection of 2 to 3 cc. or more around the wound is advisable to minimize tissue necrosis; subsequently, similar injections proximal to the wound as the tourniquet is shifted also may be advisable. After adequate doses of the serum have been injected, the tourniquet can be removed. For systemic treatment, the dosage and route of administration will depend upon the age, size, and clinical condition of the patient. If the patient is a child, or in shock, I.V. administration may be indicated, provided he is known or is demonstrated beyond doubt, not to be allergic to horse serum. Otherwise, I.M. injections are to be preferred. The intraperitoneal route occasionally must be used in small children, when I.V. administration is difficult or impossible. Children, because of the higher concentration of venom in their smaller bodies, may require 2 to 3 times the adult dosage of antivenin. The injections of 10 cc. are repeated every 1 to 2 hours until symptoms are significantly diminished; they should be continued at the same rate as long as the swelling, paralysis, or other symptoms are progressing. The doses are gradually reduced in frequency and amount according to the patient's clinical improvement. It must be remembered that overtreatment is the lesser error in snake venenation; 50, or 100, or even 150 cc. of antivenin may be required.

Crotalus terrificus antivenin is available in Mexico and Central America; a probable source in Mexico is the same as for scorpion antivenin (*see* Scorpions, below).

GILA MONSTER

A lizard, limited to the region of Arizona and New Mexico, which inflicts a wound with multiple lacerations. Its venom is neurotoxic. Symptoms of local pain and numbness, particularly in the affected extremity, generalized perspiration and vertigo develop. Subsequently, necrosis of the wound may occur.

Treatment

This consists of the same local and supportive measures (if necessary) as in snake venenation, excluding incision of the wound. No specific antivenin is available.

SPIDERS

Several varieties are poisonous; however, only the female black widow causes frequent fatalities, which are estimated at

5% of the persons bitten. This spider is found throughout the U.S. It has a coal-black body ½ inch long. The mature female has 1 red or orange hourglass marking on its belly, while the immature female has in addition 3 similarly colored spots on its back. Men are the most frequent victims, and two-thirds of the bites (2 puncture points) occur on the genitals, buttocks, and thighs. The sting produces a sharp pain, which generally disappears fairly rapidly (but may last for 4 or 5 hours), and the patient may feel quite comfortable until local muscular cramps begin 15 to 30 minutes later. The venom is neurotoxic and causes an ascending motor paralysis, also destruction of peripheral nerve endings. Weakness, tremor, and excruciating pain in the limbs usually develop, together with abdominal cramps, and boardlike rigidity of the abdominal musculature. Later, reduced heart beat, feeble pulse, labored breathing and speech, and stupor and delirium may supervene. Convulsions may occur, especially in small children. The prognosis depends on the amount of venom introduced, the age and physique of the patient, how soon the diagnosis is made, and how promptly treatment is begun.

Treatment

Local treatment of the wound usually is ineffective and unnecessary. Since expert nursing care is needed, the patient should be hospitalized if possible. Supportive treatment similar to that outlined for snake poisoning is indicated. In attempting to control the excruciating pain, it may be necessary to give both morphine (℞ 36) and phenobarbital sodium (℞ 37) simultaneously. Calcium gluconate, 10 cc. of a 10% solution I.V. (℞ 56), injected slowly, is given immediately and repeated as necessary to control muscle pain; prolonged warm baths also may aid in allaying the pain. Specific antivenin, *Latrodectus mactans* antivenin, which is distributed by Sharp & Dohme, Inc., in 2.5 cc. ampuls, should be given I.M. immediately, and repeated as recommended in the package insert. Convalescence may be prolonged for weeks, with residual muscular weakness, and numbness and tingling in the limbs. Repeated calcium gluconate injections usually abolish these symptoms.

BEES, WASPS, HORNETS, ANTS

The toxin common to this group is in some respects similar to snake venom. Certain individuals are profoundly sensitive to it and may exhibit symptoms of anaphylaxis (for treatment of which, *see* SERUM SICKNESS). Bee venom extract is available for subsequent desensitization of such persons.

The common lay practice of applying mud packs to wounds of this nature, which already are potentially infected, is to be deplored. In some stings, especially those of the honeybee, the stinger is left behind in the wound; this should be carefully removed. Discomfort can be reduced by prompt application of fairly strong household ammonia solution, or, if the pain is intense, by infiltration of the area with a 2% procaine solution. Antihistaminics, administered orally or applied locally in ointment form, may relieve discomfort in these patients, as in cases of bites by mosquitoes or other insects (*see* below).

BLOODSUCKING FLIES, FLEAS, LICE

These include mosquitoes, sand flies, horse flies, deer flies; the various fleas; head and pubic lice; and bedbugs. Their saliva contains an anticoagulant agent and a sensitizing agent; certain individuals, therefore, exhibit reactions similar to serum sickness (q.v.), and require similar treatment. In these persons the wound may vesiculate after a few hours, and itching may be intense. In mosquito bite, especially, a mixture of equal parts of camphor and chloral hydrate, triturated (℞ 57), relieves the itching; or a camphorated phenol in oil preparation (℞ 58) may be employed.

CENTIPEDES

Scolopendra morsitans, habitat southern U.S., is the only centipede dangerous to man in N. America. The toxin is a cytolysin. The bite, a 2-puncture wound, causes local inflammation, erythema, edema and, at times, purpura involving an entire limb. The burning, aching, local pain, and the other symptoms usually disappear in 4 to 5 hours, and fatalities probably never occur. Treatment consists of cool wet dressings of a saturated magnesium sulfate solution, and phenobarbital (℞ 39) or morphine (℞ 36) for sedation or to relieve pain.

SCORPIONS

The bites of several varieties in the Southwest are dangerous, and the severity of the symptoms depends largely on the age (i.e., the size) of the victim. Among the toxins in the venom are neurotoxin, cardiac toxins, and agglutinins. Locally, the symptoms consist of pain, numbness and weakness of the affected limb, and lymphangitis and lymphadenitis proximal to the wound. The systemic symptoms simulate those of strychnine poisoning. In patients under 3 years of age, fatalities are frequent. Adults usually recover.

Treatment

A 2% procaine-epinephrine solution infiltrated locally will relieve the pain. Supportive measures as for snake venenation may be indicated; however, no morphine should be given. In the treatment of children especially, an antivenin is indicated, and can be procured from the Biological Institute of the Department of Health, Mexico, D.F.

TICKS

The wood tick, *Dermacentor andersoni* (*see also* ROCKY MOUNTAIN SPOTTED FEVER), and the dog tick cause toxic manifestations in man, their venom producing hyperemia and hemorrhage, particularly in the C.N.S. The sites of their attachment may become reddened and indurated and exhibit petechial hemorrhages. The wood tick may cause "tick paralysis," which occasionally culminates fatally. It is an ascending motor paralysis, and any unexplained muscular weakness, particularly in a child, calls for careful search for ticks on the patient's body. The most common sites of attachment are the pubic region, axillas and especially the back of the neck, or scalp.

Treatment

Removal of the tick by gentle traction usually causes disappearance of all but major symptoms. The application of oil to the body of the tick interferes with its respiration and facilitates its complete removal without leaving the head embedded in the skin. More severe cases will require appropriate emergency and supportive treatment.

MITES

Among those varieties causing toxic manifestations are the chigger, or "red bug," the rat mite (Southern U. S.), fowl and straw itch mites, and *Sarcoptes scabei*. Their venom is similar to that of ticks and causes a local pruritus, with or without a sensitization reaction similar to serum sickness. Mites are almost never a threat to life unless they serve as vectors of pathogenic organisms.

Treatment

Therapy of scabies (q.v.) is outlined elsewhere; for the local treatment of other mite-induced lesions, camphorated phenol in mineral oil (℞ 58) is effective in asphyxiating the mites and simultaneously reducing the itching and pain. (For the treatment of allergenic reactions, *see* SERUM SICKNESS.)

RESUSCITATION METHODS

Interference with, or arrest of, spontaneous respiration may be due to a variety of causes. Since it constitutes a threat to life, the situation demands immediate measures designed to secure adequate oxygenation of the blood. In cases of respiratory arrest, where the heart continues to beat, artificial respiration is indicated. Laryngeal obstruction from foreign body, edema, or any other cause requires immediate tracheotomy (*see* ACUTE LARYNGOTRACHEOBRONCHITIS). Asphyxia neonatorum will be considered independently, as a special form of asphyxia.

Artificial Respiration

This may prove to be lifesaving in such conditions as drowning, strangulation, electric shock, undue inhalation of smoke or other poisonous gases, and drug poisoning. Treatment by one of the methods described below should be started instantly and continued until normal breathing is definitely reestablished or until death is certain; recovery has occurred after as long as 8 hours of artificial respiration. Even when spontaneous breathing returns, the victim must be closely observed for recurrence of respiratory arrest. The technic is designed to increase and decrease the capacity of the thoracic cavity rhythmically and continuously by manual or mechanical means. The chest must be given ample time to expand; artificial respiration is sometimes rendered ineffectual by being done too rapidly. A free airway is mandatory and must always be assured by loosening the victim's clothing and removing any dentures, fluids, or debris from the mouth and nose. It may be necessary to grasp and hold the tongue forward. O_2 (by mask) is indicated, if available, and the victim should be protected against chilling by the use of blankets, coats, or other means. Heat, externally applied, may be necessary. Should spasm of the epiglottis prevent gaseous exchange, a tracheal catheter may be passed through the epiglottis, if possible, or through a tracheotomy opening, if necessary. Respiratory stimulants (℞ 50) are useless except as a supplement to artificial respiration where the respiratory center is depressed by such agents as morphine or barbiturates. When normal breathing returns, the patient must be kept lying quietly until recovery is well established, to avoid undue strain on the heart.

Schaefer (prone pressure) method: This maneuver requires no equipment and may therefore be instituted immediately and anywhere. The victim is placed face down, with his head preferably 6 inches lower than his feet. The operator straddles the victim's thighs, places his palms flat on the back over the lower ribs, then alternately, in cadence at the rate of 12 to 15 times a minute, he gradually throws his weight forward on his hands, compressing the lowest ribs to produce the expiratory movement of breathing. He then rapidly assumes an erect position, thus releasing the ribs to allow for inspiration. Since one operator rapidly tires, others may be substituted as needed, but the regularity of the rhythm must not be lost.

Other methods: Where the Schaefer method is precluded by injuries of the spine or thoracic cage, or for other valid reasons, one of the following procedures may be employed for artificial respiration:

Rocking method: This is less fatiguing to the operator, but requires a long, wide, flat object (board, door, stretcher) on which to lay the patient, and a sawhorse or other support at the middle to make a seesaw. With the patient face down on the board and with his extremities (not his chest) bound to it with bandages, he is seesawed to an angle of 40 degrees, 12 to 15 times/minute. The rocking motion shifts the abdominal viscera alternately toward and away from the diaphragm, which is thereby moved up and down, and this results in respiration.

Silvester method: This is indicated only when the patient cannot be turned face down. It is more tiring to perform than the Schaefer method, the patient's tongue tends to fall back, and the secretions cannot drain out. A firm cushion, 3 inches thick, is placed under the shoulders of the supine patient so as to raise the chest and extend the neck. The operator kneels at the head, grasps the forearms, and then brings the arms upward, outward, and toward himself, pressing the victim's elbows firmly against the ground; this maneuver expands the thorax. After 2 seconds it is reversed, ending with the forearms flexed and pressed firmly against the ribs at the side of the chest (expiration). The cycle is repeated 12 times/minute.

Laborde method: With the patient supine, his chin is depressed, the tongue is grasped with the fingers (using gauze to prevent slipping) and alternately pulled forward and upward and released at the rate of 15 cycles/minute. The object is to stimulate the phrenic nerve, and thus cause contraction of the diaphragm.

Mechanical devices: Respirators should be operated only by persons well acquainted with their use. These appliances alternately increase and decrease (within safe limits) the atmospheric pressure about the chest, thereby compressing and expanding the thoracic cage. Recently, a method has been introduced which compresses and expands the atmosphere to which the airways (and therefore the bronchial tree) are exposed, thus leading to a gaseous exchange within the lungs without any movement of the thorax itself.

ASPHYXIA NEONATORUM
(Apnea neonatorum)

Failure of the newborn infant to start breathing may occur despite all precautions. However, a high quality of obstetric care is an essential prophylactic. During labor, opiates, anesthetics, and oxytocics must be used with extreme caution and in the minimal effective doses. Anoxia (q.v.) in the mother should be corrected by appropriate means. When fetal asphyxia is suspected from the character of the fetal heart beat (i.e., a rate above 160 or below 100, or an irregular beat) appropriate measures to ascertain and remove the cause or to hasten delivery are indicated. Undue pressure of forceps on, or the sudden decompression of, the oncoming fetal head is to be avoided so as to lessen the risk of intracranial injury.

Prophylaxis

Routinely, immediately after delivery of the head, and preferably before the infant's first inspiration, the airways should be gently cleared of any fluid or mucus, using the finger or suction through a tracheal catheter. This often will initiate spontaneous respiration by stimulating the gag reflex, which is present in all newborn infants except those suffering from extreme degrees of asphyxia. Gentle stripping of the neck toward the mouth, with the infant held up by the ankles (contraindicated in suspected intracranial hemorrhage), will frequently bring up into the mouth where it can then easily be removed, any foreign material aspirated during intra-uterine respiratory movements. The infant should be kept warm with warm towels or blankets, particularly if born prematurely. Once respirations begin, the infant is best left undisturbed in an atmosphere of about 40% O_2 as long as he continues to improve.

Treatment

Should the above measures be unsuccessful, one of the following methods of inducing respiration is indicated, even in the absence of an audible or palpable heart beat, and should be continued until spontaneous breathing occurs or death is certain. (1) **Mouth to mouth:** A sterile face mask or gauze pad is interposed to prevent exchange of microorganisms between the operator and the infant. Only one puffed mouthful of air at a time is blown into the infant, lest emphysema or even alveolar rupture of the lungs develop. This is repeated at a rate of 30 times/minute. Gentle compression of the baby's chest after each insufflation will allow the air to escape. (2) **Mouth to lung:** A tracheal catheter (No. 14 F.) is introduced into the larynx and air is blown into the infant's lungs as in the mouth-to-mouth method, but only at a rate of 15 times/minute. (3) **Silvester method,** or a **mechanical method** of artificial respiration (q.v.), with O_2 if available.

Although widely used, such respiratory stimulants as Metrazol, caffeine, alpha-lobeline, and Coramine are ineffective, even in convulsive doses, in the presence of anoxia, and may be dangerous. Attempts to stimulate the respiratory center by such irritating stimuli as alternate hot and cold plunges, dilation of the sphincter ani, ethyl chloride spray to the skin, or traction on the tongue are shocking to the infant and should be avoided except as a last resort when other methods have failed.

Children surviving asphyxiation are highly susceptible to sepsis and the development of secondary asphyxia, and must be watched carefully for several days, using O_2 freely. Other complications of birth or the neonatal period that may develop should be treated promptly in the usual manner.

PRESCRIPTIONS

(Wherever a prescribed "proprietary" is representative of a class of therapeutic agents, alternative proprietary preparations will be found listed in Part II.)

Antimicrobial Agents

1. ℞ Penicillin   (vial)

   50,000 u. I.M. every 3 hours or 300,000 u.
   I.M. every 8 to 12 hours.

2. ℞ Procaine penicillin (vial)

   300,000 u. I.M. every 12 to 24 hours.

3. ℞ Streptomycin   (vial)

   0.5 Gm. I.M. every 4 to 6 hours.

4. ℞ Sulfadiazine . . . . 0.5 Gm. (gr. viiss)

   8 tablets initially, followed by 2 tablets every
   4 hours.

5. ℞ Sulfadiazine, 5% ointment . . . 30.0 Gm. (℥ i)

   For local application to minor burns.

6. ℞ Penicillin ointment (1,000 u./Gm.)

   Apply locally to lesions.

Antitoxins

7. ℞ Tetanus Antitoxin U.S.P.   (vial)

   1,500 to 3,000 u., or more, subcut. after first
   testing for sensitivity.

8. ℞ Tetanus Toxoid U.S.P.   (vial)

   1 cc. subcut. as a booster dose to previously
   immunized individuals.

9. ℞ Pentavalent Gas Gangrene Anti-
     toxin U.S.P.   (vial)

   Contents of 1 or more vials, I.M. or I.V.

Dermatologic (Sunburn) Preparations

10. ℞ Benzocaine, 5% ointment . . . 60.0 Gm. (℥ ii)

    Apply to burned surfaces.

11. ℞ White Petrolatum U.S.P. . . . 60.0 Gm. (℥ ii)

    Apply before exposure to sun.

12. ℞ Zinc Oxide Ointment U.S.P. . . 60.0 Gm. (℥ ii)

    Apply before exposure to sun.

13. ℞ Methyl salicylate . . . . 15.0 cc. (℥ ss)
      Sodium borate . . . .   1.8 Gm. (gr. xxvii)
      White Wax U.S.P. . . . . 20.0 Gm. (℥ v)
      Light Liquid Petrolatum U.S.P.. 20.0 cc. (℥ v)
      Water. . . . . 28.0 cc. (℥ vii)
      White Petrolatum U.S.P. . . . 15.0 Gm. (℥ ss)

    Heat water and dissolve borax. Melt bees-
    wax, petrolatum, and mineral oil together.
    Add liquid to fats, constantly stirring, with
    temperature down to 45° C. Apply before
    exposure to sun.

14. ℞ Tannic acid . . . . 4.8 Gm. (gr. lxxii)
    Isobutyl-p-aminobenzoate . . . 8.0 Gm. (℥ ii)
    Glycerin . . . . 24.0 cc. (℥ vi)
    Ethyl alcohol 70% . . . q.s. ad 240.0 cc. (℥ viii)

> Sunburn protective and treatment lotion.
> Apply before exposure to sun.

15. ℞ Titanium oxide . . . . 20.0 Gm. (℥ v)
    Zinc oxide . . . . 10.0 Gm. (℥ iiss)
    Talc . . . . 10.0 Gm. (℥ iiss)
    Bentonite . . . . 2.0 Gm. (℥ ss)
    White Petrolatum U.S.P. q.s. ad 120.0 Gm. (℥ iv)

> Sunburn protective ointment (resists water).
> Apply before exposure to sun.

16. ℞ Tragacanth (powder) U.S.P. . . 0.3 Gm. (gr. v)
    Zinc oxide . . . . 13.0 Gm. (℥ iii)
    Talc . . . . 8.0 Gm. (℥ ii)
    Magnesium carbonate . . . . . 0.3 Gm. (gr. v)
    Quinine sulfate . . . . 10.0 Gm. (℥ iiss)
    Glycerin . . . . 8.0 cc. (℥ ii)
    Water . . . . 38.0 cc. (℥ ixss)
    Neutracolor q.s. for natural skin
       tint

> Protective enamel; washed off easily with
> soap and water. (CAUTION! In some individ-
> uals, quinine may act as a skin-sensitizing
> agent.)

17. ℞ Zinc oxide
    Boric acid
    Talc . . . . āā 60.0 Gm. (℥ ii)

> Dust on skin several times daily and at bed-
> time.

18. ℞ Rose Water Ointment U.S.P. . . 60.0 Gm. (℥ ii)

> Apply to erythematous areas.

19. ℞ Potassium permanganate . . . 0.12 Gm. (gr. ii)

> Dissolve 1 tablet in 1½ quarts of warm water
> (1:11,000 dilution) and use for wet com-
> presses or soaks for bullous sunburn, for 20
> minutes 2 or 3 times daily.

20. ℞ Aluminum Acetate Solution N.F.
    (Burow's Solution) . . . . 240.0 cc. (℥ viii)

> Dilute 1:10 or 1:20 with water and use as
> wet compresses 3 or 4 times daily.

21. ℞ Zinc oxide . . . . 20.0 Gm. (℥ v)
    Talc . . . . 20.0 Gm. (℥ v)
    Bentonite . . . . 5.0 Gm. (gr. lxxv)
    Glycerin . . . . 10.0 cc. (℥ iiss)
    Water . . . . 35.0 cc. (℥ ix)
    Alcohol U.S.P. . . . . 35.0 cc. (℥ ix)

> Drying shake lotion. Apply to affected
> areas. (Where such may be necessary or desir-

able, a wetting shake lotion can be made by
simply substituting equal amounts of water
for alcohol in above prescription.)

22. ℞ Aluminum Acetate Solution N.F.
    (Burow's Solution) . . . . 10.0 cc. (℥ iiss)
    Anhydrous Lanolin U.S.P. . . . 20.0 Gm. (℥ v)
    Zinc Oxide Paste N.F. . . . . 30.0 Gm. (℥ i)

    Soothing cream. Can be used on inflamed
    areas even if some oozing is present.
    NOTE: Many effective commercial sunburn
    preparations are available which the phy-
    sician may also prescribe.

Fluids and Electrolytes

23. ℞ Sodium chloride . . . . 0.5 Gm. (gr. viiss)
    2 tablets with each drink of water.

    For heat cramps: 2 tablets dissolved in glass
    of water every hour until relieved.

24. ℞ Sterile Isotonic Sodium Chloride
    Solution for Parenteral Use
    U.S.P.
    1,500 cc. I.V. 2 or 3 times a day as indicated.

25. ℞ Sodium chloride . . . . . . 0.5 Gm. (gr. viiss)
    Water. . . . . 500.0 cc. (℥ xvi)
    Use as cooled drinking water to combat heat
    cramps.

26. ℞ Ammonium chloride (enteric
    coated) . . . . 0.5 Gm. (gr. viiss)
    4 tablets 3 or 4 times daily.

27. ℞ Sodium bicarbonate, 5% solution
    (ampul)
    6 cc./Kg. body wt. I.V.; repeat as necessary
    to maintain an alkaline urine.

28. ℞ Sodium lactate, ⅙ molar solu-
    tion (ampul)
    25 cc./Kg. body wt. I.V. or subcut.; repeat as
    necessary to maintain an alkaline urine.

29. ℞ Sodium citrate, 3% solution
    (sterile bottle)
    450 cc. I.V.; repeat as necessary to maintain
    an alkaline urine.

30. ℞ Potassium citrate (powder)
    2 teaspoons at once, followed by 2 tablespoons
    daily with 3 ounces of lemon water or other
    fluids.

31. ℞ Glucose, 10% solution (sterile bottle)

> 1,000 cc. I.V. as needed to maintain diuresis.

32. ℞ Sodium citrate (ampul)

> Each ampul contains 1.5 to 2 Gm. of sodium citrate as a 2.5 to 5% solution in Water for Injection U.S.P. or Sterile Isotonic Sodium Chloride Solution for Parenteral Use U.S.P. One ampul for each 500 cc. of blood to be withdrawn.

33. ℞ ACD solution (sterile)

Citric acid	0.8 Gm.	(gr. xii)
Sodium citrate	2.2 Gm.	(gr. xxxiii)
Dextrose (anhydrous)	2.45 Gm.	(gr. xxxvii)
Distilled water ....q.s. ad	100.0 cc.	(℥ iiiss)

> Use 15 cc. for each 100 cc. of blood to be withdrawn for indirect transfusion.

Antihemorrhagic Agents

34. ℞ Toluidine blue (medicinal)

> 2 mg./Kg. body wt., dissolved in 250 to 500 cc. of Sterile Isotonic Sodium Chloride Solution for Parenteral Use U.S.P. given I.V. every 24 hours for overheparinization.

35. ℞ Protamine sulfate, 1% solution (ampul)

> 5 to 10 cc. (50 to 100 mg.) I.V. every 24 hours for overheparinization.

Analgesics and Sedatives

36. ℞ Morphine sulfate

> 10 to 15 mg. (gr. ⅙ to ¼) subcut., or 5 mg. (gr. 1/12) I.V., injected slowly.

37. ℞ Phenobarbital sodium (ampul)

> 0.12 Gm. (gr. ii) I.M.

38. ℞ Sodium bromide .... 8.0 Gm. (℥ ii)
    Chloral hydrate........ 4.0 Gm. (℥ i)
    Water........ .q.s. ad 60.0 cc. (℥ ii)

> 1 tablespoon in milk by mouth, or in starch water by rectum, every 4 to 6 hours as required.

39. ℞ Phenobarbital .... 30 mg. (gr. ss)

> 1 to 3 tablets as required.

40. ℞ Scopolamine (hysocine) hydrobromide .... 0.3 mg. (gr. 1/200)

> 2 tablets 30 minutes before embarking or enplaning, followed by 1 tablet every 4 hours for 4 doses. Then 1 tablet every 6 hours.

41. ℞ Belladonna Extract U.S.P. 15   mg.   (gr. ¼)

> 1 or 2 tablets or capsules before embarking or enplaning, then 1 three times a day. Moderate mouth dryness indicates full dosage.

42. ℞ Pentobarbital sodium . . . . . 0.1   Gm.   (gr. iss)

> 2 capsules 1 hour before embarking or enplaning, and repeat with 1 capsule after 12 hours if necessary.

43. ℞ Chloral hydrate, 10% solution . 60.0   cc.   (℥ ii)

> 3 teaspoons 1 hour before embarking or enplaning, and repeat with 1 teaspoon every 4 hours when awake.

44. ℞ Chlorobutanol . . . . 0.3   Gm.   (gr. v)

> 1 to 3 capsules, repeated once if necessary.

45. ℞ "Dramamine" . . . . 0.1   Gm.

> ½ or 1 tablet 4 times daily, after meals and at bedtime.

Vitamins and Hormones

46. ℞ Vitamin B complex   (vial), containing in each dose:

> Thiamine hydrochloride . . . 10   mg.
> Riboflavin 5   mg.
> Nicotinic acid amide . . . 100   mg.
> Pyridoxine hydrochloride . . 5   mg.
> Administer I.M. twice daily.

47. ℞ Desoxycorticosterone acetate   5   mg.
     (ampul)

> 5 mg. I.M. 3 times daily.

48. ℞ Pyridoxine hydrochloride
     (ampul)

> 100 mg. I.V. daily.

49. ℞ Pyridoxine hydrochloride . . . 50   mg.

> 2 tablets daily.

Miscellaneous

50. ℞ Caffeine and Sodium Benzoate
     Injection U.S.P.   (ampul)

> 0.2 to 0.5 Gm. (gr. iii to viiss) I.M. or I.V. as indicated.

51. ℞ Epinephrine hydrochloride,
     1:1,000 solution   (ampul)

> 0.3 to 1 cc. (♏ v to xv) subcut. or slowly I.V.

52. ℞ Amphetamine sulfate . . . . . . 5 mg.
    2 tablets on arising and 1 tablet at noon.

53. ℞ Nasal inhaler
    (Various vasoconstrictor-type inhalers are commercially available.)
    Inhale as necessary before and during plane flights.

54. ℞ Ephedrine sulfate, 1% solution . 30.0 cc. (℥ i)
    3 to 5 drops in each naris as necessary.

55. ℞ Strychnine sulfate (hypodermic tablet) . . . . 1 mg. (gr. 1/60)
    1 or 2 tablets subcut. or by mouth for threatened peripheral vascular failure.

56. ℞ Calcium gluconate, 10% solution (ampul) . . . . 10.0 cc.
    Contents of 1 ampul I.V., injected slowly, and repeated as often as necessary to relieve the pain and muscular spasms.

57. ℞ Camphor
    Chloral hydrate . . . . āā 8.0 Gm. (℥ ii)
    Triturate and apply locally to bite of insect; In individuals with a particularly sensitive skin, dilute in mineral oil or olive oil before applying.

58. ℞ Phenol . . . . 0.5 Gm. (gr. viiss)
    Menthol . . . . 0.5 Gm. (gr. viiss)
    Camphor . . . . 0.5 Gm. (gr. viiss)
    Liquid Petrolatum U.S.P. q.s. ad 100.0 cc. (℥ iiiss)
    Apply locally to skin areas infested with mites, and to relieve pruritus.

59. ℞ Sodium thiosulfate, saturated solution
    Apply to chemical burns as a continuous wet dressing for 24 hours.

RESPIRATORY

THE COMMON COLD

An acute catarrhal infection of the respiratory tract, usually with major involvement of its upper portions, but frequently involving the entire tract; often referred to as "upper respiratory infection," or "coryza."

Etiology

Infection by a filtrable virus usually is the initiating factor of this most common of all diseases. The causative agent is

readily transmitted to susceptible hosts, especially those whose
resistance has been lowered by environmental or constitutional
factors. The common pathogens normally present in the nasopharynx infect the weakened mucosa following the initial viral
invasion. Occasionally, these common pathogens alone may be
responsible for coryza, when local resistance has been lowered.
The following factors, alone or in combination, may so decrease
the immunity of the upper respiratory tract as to facilitate viral
or bacterial infection: (1) general debility; (2) structural abnormalities, such as hypertrophied adenoids; (3) foci of chronic
infection; (4) allergic disorders of the nasopharynx; (5) vasomotor instability, productive of prolonged ischemia of the nasopharyngeal mucosa following exposure to cold or emotional
strain; (6) injury to mucous membranes due to inhalation of
noxious fumes.

Symptoms and Signs

The onset is characteristically abrupt. There may be initial
malaise, sneezing, rhinorrhea, or a scratchy sensation in the
throat. There may be no fever at any time during an uncomplicated cold. Many patients experience chilly sensations or a
definite chill followed by fever (100° to 102° F.), however. Headache and a tickling sensation in the nose are almost universal
symptoms. The feeling of fullness in the nose and throat and
of burning and smarting of the eyes that is often experienced is
quite discomforting. The senses of smell, taste, and occasionally hearing, are impaired. Patients frequently complain of
vague aches and pains in the back and extremities.

As the disease progresses, the nasopharyngeal mucosa becomes engorged and the nares obstructed. A profuse serous
discharge is produced, necessitating almost constant sniffling
and nose blowing. Examination of the nasopharyngeal mucosa
reveals it to be hyperemic, swollen, and covered with serous
discharge. In the later stages the discharge thickens and becomes mucopurulent. Repeated nose blowing and the profuse
flow of secretions from the nose often cause excoriation of the
external nares and upper lip.

The disease may be limited to only a portion of the upper
respiratory tract but usually the process extends so as ultimately
to involve the entire tract. The sinuses and eustachian tubes
are almost invariably affected from the earliest stages of the
disease, and frequently their involvement may become more
pronounced so that a true sinusitis (q.v.) or eustachitis (q.v.)
develops. With extension of the inflammatory process to the
pharynx and larynx, cough and hoarseness become prominent.
Involvement of the trachea is associated with retrosternal pain
and a feeling of tightness. A hacking, nonproductive cough,
usually worse at night and interfering with sleep, is common.
Bronchial involvement often may be so extensive that all the
features of bronchitis (q.v.) are observed.

Diagnosis

Many serious disorders, including measles, diphtheria, streptococcal pharyngitis, meningitis, and whooping cough (q.v.), cause catarrhal upper respiratory symptoms at their onset and therefore may be confused with coryza. Definite differentiation of these entities from the common cold depends on the characteristics that later develop. Influenza (q.v.) and grippe bear a great similarity to the common cold and often these terms are loosely used interchangeably. Although the influenza virus may at times cause the same symptoms as those of the common cold, the two are usually differentiated by the greater severity of the symptoms of influenza. Hay fever and allied forms of allergy (q.v.) may be mistaken for coryza but differentiation usually is made with persistence of the allergic disorder.

Prognosis

Resolution of symptoms normally occurs in 4 to 7 days. In many instances, complications such as sinusitis, adenoiditis, tonsillitis, eustachitis or laryngitis, tracheitis and bronchitis (q.v.) may produce symptoms that continue beyond this period.

Prophylaxis

Many measures, including polybacterial vaccines, have been recommended for the prophylaxis or aborting of upper respiratory infection but thus far none has proved efficacious. Some believe that prophylactic vaccines tend to diminish the frequency or severity of bacterial complications. Massive doses of vitamin C taken routinely during the colder months of the year, when colds are most frequent, or at the onset of a cold, are believed by many to be beneficial. Others are of the opinion that multivitamin preparations or large doses of vitamins A and D taken regularly help to ward off colds. Some physicians recommend the use of an antihistaminic preparation such as Neo-Antergan (R 79), administered when the first symptoms appear, to combat any possible allergic component.

Treatment

Bed rest should be instituted at onset and symptomatic therapy given. Adequate rest often is the greatest single factor contributing to the patient's rapid recovery, while his temporary isolation aids in preventing the infection of other persons. Relief of most of the initial complaints is provided by various mixtures of antipyretics and analgesics (R 1 to 6). Some physicians advocate preparations (R 7, 73, 76) containing atropine (rhinitis tablets) for drying the mucosa in the early stages. Nose drops, such as 1% ephedrine (R 77), or a nasal inhaler (R 78) may be conservatively employed for relief of obstruction. Steam inhalation, alone or with tincture of benzoin (R 57) or oil of pine (R 58), often is soothing to the inflamed respiratory tract (see BEDSIDE PROC.). The diet should be light and fluids given in large quantity, especially those containing high concentrations of vitamin C. The application of counter-irritants such as mustard plasters or flaxseed poultices (*see* BEDSIDE PROC.) is useful in relieving chest discomfort. If the cough is dry and troublesome, ammonium chloride (℞ 39) alone or combined with syrup of ipecac (℞ 44), or Stokes's expectorant (℞ 47) alone, may be given. Codeine or other agents to stop a cough are often necessary, but they should not be used indiscriminately since they interfere with pulmonary drainage and may favor the development of pneumonic involvement. If used, the cough suppressive (℞ 8, 13) is best administered as a single dose at bedtime to promote sleep. Papaverine and codeine combined (℞ 14) often are beneficial in the treatment of a cold, especially in the early stages. (For treatment of complications *see* chapters devoted to these subjects.)

The patient should rest until he has been asymptomatic and afebrile for at least 2 days, after which normal activities may be resumed slowly.

ACUTE LARYNGOTRACHEOBRONCHITIS

An acute, often fulminating, respiratory infection character-ized by tracheitis, bronchitis, potential obstructive laryngitis, severe dyspnea, and high fever.

Etiology, Incidence, and Pathologic Physiology

Hemolytic streptococci, staphylococci, and *H. influenzae* are responsible for the great majority of cases; pneumococci less frequently. The syndrome is relatively rare and usually is found in infants and children, but may occur at any age. It is most often seen in late winter or early spring.

Mucous membranes of the larynx, trachea, and bronchi are acutely inflamed. Edema is severe, and this, with the copious, tenacious mucus constantly secreted, threatens to block completely the subglottic area of the larynx, or bronchi, or both. Atelectasis occurs in the lung when smaller bronchi become obstructed and, if the patient survives, pneumonia develops almost as part of the disease rather than as a complication.

Symptoms and Signs

Onset is sudden; while it may occur during the course of what appeared to be a "cold," the disease is more likely to strike individuals who are apparently well. High fever, rapidly developing toxemia, and grave dyspnea are the characteristic symptoms. At first, the patient is flushed and excited and labors violently to breathe. Cough may be almost constant but is relatively unproductive despite the heavy laryngeal secretions. There is notable retraction of the supra- and infrasternal spaces due to respiratory effort. An initial hoarseness is followed by stridor and aphonia. The latter is partly due to dyspnea, the patient not having time between breathing efforts to cry. At first, severe subglottic edema is the chief obstruction to respiration, but tenacious mucus soon fills the bronchioles and increases the dyspnea. The situation now becomes grave, the patient is pale and cyanotic, respiratory efforts are feeble, and death may follow in a few hours. Tracheotomy should be done before the obstructive stage is reached; after it has developed, the procedure is rarely lifesaving.

High fever is characteristic, but the leukocyte count is not always elevated. Prostration is severe and it is sometimes difficult to evaluate how much anoxemia contributes to it.

Diagnosis

Severe dyspnea, always the most obvious symptom, should immediately warn the physician of the possibility of laryngotracheobronchitis. The case history, elevated temperature, and absence of characteristic chest findings help to rule out a foreign body. Diphtheria also must be considered in differential diagnosis. Laryngeal diphtheria should be excluded by direct laryngoscopy and culture of secretions.

Prognosis and Treatment

The outlook in these cases is grave. Even though the acute respiratory obstruction may be relieved, there still is danger of complications, such as sepsis, failure of circulation, or pneumonia, unless adequate treatment is promptly instituted.

The principles of treatment for laryngotracheobronchitis are as follows: (1) Place patient in an atmosphere of high humidity. (2) Give sulfonamides and antibiotics in full dosage from the earliest possible moment. (3) Give oxygen. (4) Allay the patient's apprehension and restlessness by careful handling and possibly by small doses of phenobarbital (R 16). Do not use morphine or codeine. (5) Prepare early for possible tracheotomy.

Humidity can be raised sufficiently by steam from pans or steamers but these usually superheat the room. A room temperature not above 75° F., with humidity above 90%, is ideal. There are vaporizing devices that increase humidity without producing steam. Oxygen is most easily administered to infants and children by means of the open-top tent (see CLIN. PROC.) since a closed tent makes humidification difficult.

Sulfadiazine (R 31, 32) should always be given in a daily dosage of 50 to 60 mg. (gr. ¾ to i/lb. body wt.). The oral dose is divided into 6 parts and administered every 4 hours; the daily dose of sodium sulfadiazine is divided and administered I.V. every 8 hours. Penicillin (R 18, 19) also should be given,

10,000 to 60,000 u. I.M. every 3 hours, since 3 of the 4 common causative organisms are susceptible to its action.

In cases caused by *H. influenzae*, streptomycin (℞ 23) is indicated, with sulfadiazine (℞ 31, 32) and possibly with penicillin (℞ 18, 19) also, if penicillin-sensitive organisms are present. Specific antiserum (rabbit) may be administered in these cases, in a single injection of at least 100 mg. antibody nitrogen, followed by additional doses if necessary (℞ 38). Drug therapy should be continued for several days after acute symptoms have subsided.

Tracheotomy rather than laryngeal intubation is indicated when respiratory obstruction is imminent or when the dyspnea is so great as to threaten complete exhaustion of the patient. The physician unaccustomed to managing severe respiratory distress should have an otolaryngologist in consultation on cases of laryngotracheobronchitis. Tracheotomy not only permits by-passing of the subglottic edema but also allows removal of crusts and mucus from trachea and bronchi by insertion of a small bronchoscope.

The Mosher "lifesaver" is a piece of equipment with which every physician who treats children should be familiar, as it may save life by providing an airway while preparation for tracheotomy is being made, and its presence facilitates tracheotomy. It is a hollow semiflexible metal tube 12 to 15 inches long, with a ring welded to one end. The tube can be guided by hand through the epiglottis and larynx and into the trachea of a child suffering from laryngeal obstruction.

Emergency tracheotomy should be done under as aseptic conditions as possible. The child should be restrained by "mummifying," and the administration of an anesthetic where necessary. His head should be hyperextended. The midline incision must be made boldly, including the skin, superficial fascia and pretracheal muscles, bisecting the tracheotomic triangle and keeping slightly above the sternal notch and well below the thyroid cartilage. Once down to the anterior tracheal wall, one should identify the tracheal rings and incise the 3rd and 4th and, if necessary, the 5th. The cannula is inserted after the wound edges are covered with petrolatum gauze. Bleeding should be controlled only after the cannula has been inserted.

Nursing care is necessary throughout the acute stage of laryngotracheobronchitis and constant specialized nursing is required for the tracheotomized patient.

BRONCHITIS

Inflammation of the bronchial tree, which may be localized or diffuse, acute or chronic, and caused by infections, or by physical or chemical agents.

ACUTE BRONCHITIS

An acute inflammation of the tracheobronchial tree, generally self-limited, with eventual complete healing and return of normal function.

Etiology and Incidence

In the usual infectious form, acute bronchitis is part of a general acute upper respiratory infection. Onset may be due to the common cold; to a pyogenic infection of the nasopharynx, throat, or tracheobronchial tree; or to one of the influenza viruses.

Acute bronchitis is most prevalent in winter. Predisposing or contributory factors are exposure, chilling, fatigue, malnutrition, rickets. It is commonly a mild disease, but may be serious in debilitated patients and those with chronic pulmonary or cardiac disease, the special danger being the development of pneumonia.

Recurring attacks suggest a focus of infection, such as chronic sinusitis, bronchiectasis, or, in children, hypertrophied tonsils and adenoids. Allergic factors are frequently important.

Acute bronchial irritation and inflammation may be caused by such physical and chemical irritants as mineral and vegetable dusts of various kinds, strong acid fumes, ammonia, certain volatile organic solvents, chlorine, hydrogen sulfide, sulfur dioxide, or bromine. Tobacco is a bronchial irritant for some individuals. Of the war gases, the quick-acting irritants such as mustard and chlorine will cause tracheitis and bronchitis.

Pathology and Pathologic Physiology

The earliest change is hyperemia of the mucous membrane, followed by desquamation, edema, leukocytic infiltration of the submucosa, and the formation of sticky or mucopurulent exudate. With the disturbance in the self-cleansing function of the bronchial ciliated epithelium, the phagocyte cells and the lymphatics, the normally sterile bronchi become invaded with bacteria, and cellular debris and mucopurulent exudate accumulate. Cough, though distressing, is an essential mechanism in eliminating bronchial secretions.

Symptoms and Signs

Early symptoms are those of acute respiratory infection: coryza, malaise, chilliness, slight fever, pains in back and muscles, sore throat. Onset of cough usually indicates the beginning of the bronchitis itself. At first it is dry and nonproductive; after a day or two small amounts of viscid sputum are raised; later a more abundant mucoid or mucopurulent secretion appears. In uncomplicated cases, there is fever up to 101° or 102° F. for 3 to 5 days, or less, following which acute symptoms subside, though cough may continue for 2 or 3 weeks.

Physical signs in the lungs are few or absent in uncomplicated acute bronchitis. There may be scattered sibilant or sonorous rales; occasionally, crackling or moist rales at the base. Persisting localized signs suggest such a complication as bronchopneumonia or tuberculosis.

Diagnosis

Diagnosis of acute bronchitis may ordinarily be made without difficulty on the basis of the foregoing. Complications or the presence of other diseases must be ruled out, especially if symptoms are serious or prolonged. To be considered are pulmonary tuberculosis, bronchopneumonia, lobar pneumonia, influenza, sinusitis, left heart failure, aortic aneurysm, pericarditis, pleurisy, bronchiectasis, bronchial asthma, foreign body in the lung, carcinoma of the lung, mediastinal lymphoma; and, in children, measles, whooping cough, acute tonsillitis, acute otitis media.

Treatment

General: The patient should be put to bed, and remain there until fever has subsided. It is well to give a mild cathartic at the onset (*see* CONSTIPATION). Force fluids to 3,000 or 4,000 cc. daily during the febrile course. Bland diet (*see* DIETS) is indicated. An antipyretic and analgesic agent (R 1 to 6) every 4 to 8 hours relieves malaise and reduces fever during the first 2 or 3 days.

Local: For chest soreness in early stages, a mustard plaster or flaxseed poultice will give relief (*see* BEDSIDE PROC.). Mild cough may be controlled by nonopiate mixtures (R 40, 43, 45); normally, however, a codeine or opium cough mixture is most effective (R 47, 50, 51). Steam inhalations with tincture of benzoin or a similar inhalant are ordinarily helpful (*see* BEDSIDE PROC.); for constant irritative cough, a steam kettle should be kept in the room constantly to humidify the air. In later stages, an expectorant may loosen the cough (R 45, 46, 47). In asthmatic subjects, bronchodilator drugs may be indicated (R 64, 67).

Other procedures: If fever is high and persists, with the patient more than mildly ill, chemotherapy may be indicated. If the sputum shows gram-positive cocci, penicillin or a sulfonamide drug is indicated (R 18, 19, 31, 32). When the infecting organism is *H. influenzae* (Pfeiffer's bacillus) or *K. pneumoniae* (Friedländer's bacillus), streptomycin should be used (R 23). The aerosol technic of administration of the antibiotics may be employed, either alone or in conjunction with systemic therapy (R 20, 22, 24) (*see* CLIN. PROC.). After a severe attack, several days should be allowed for convalescence. For prevention, influenza vaccine may be used, especially if influenza is prevalent in the community.

CHRONIC BRONCHITIS

A long-standing disease of the tracheobronchial tree, with chronic inflammation, fibrotic and atrophic changes in mucous membranes and deeper bronchial structures, usually associated with pulmonary fibrosis, emphysema, or other chronic pulmonary disease.

Etiology

No single or specific bacteriologic agent is recognized as causing chronic bronchitis. It usually is a part of the phenomenon of chronic fibrotic pulmonary disease. Important factors, in addition to low grade chronic infection of the bronchial tree, are inadequate bronchial drainage, surrounding pulmonary fibrosis or infection, mechanical distortions, inadequate circulation, and impairment of pulmonary tissue nutrition. Thus, chronic bronchitis is a frequent accompaniment of pulmonary fibrosis, obstructive emphysema, chronic asthma, pulmonary tuberculosis, bronchiectasis, chronic sinusitis, kyphoscoliosis, congestive heart failure, or of bronchial constriction, compression, or narrowing from any cause.

Pathology and Pathologic Physiology

The bronchi are thickened and inelastic. The bronchial surface is dark red, sometimes trabeculated; it may be dry or covered with mucus or pus. Microscopically, the epithelium is deformed, with hypertrophy in some places, denudation and atrophy in others. Similar changes occur in mucous glands and muscular layers. The submucosa shows fibrous hyperplasia, and there may be peribronchial inflammation in varying degrees.

The dysfunctions associated with chronic bronchitis are those due to inflammation and chronic infection of mucous membranes, with exudate and poor bronchial drainage; tracheobronchial rigidity, with loss of pulmonary elasticity; and obstruction of the air passages.

Degenerative changes in the bronchi disturb the normal action of the ciliary apparatus and lymphatics in removing bacteria and foreign material from the bronchi. Thus, retention of mucus and pus is favored. Bronchial drainage becomes increasingly dependent upon the physiologic function of coughing.

Bronchial rigidity restricts normal ventilation, and becomes a factor in ventilatory insufficiency of the restrictive type, a prominent cause of dyspnea (*see* PULMONARY FIBROSIS).

Swollen mucous membranes, tenacious exudate and, frequently, spasm of bronchiolar muscles tend to obstruct the air passages, and produce the characteristic dyspnea of obstructive ventilatory insufficiency. This is of course much more pronounced when there is a coexistent chronic obstructive emphysema or chronic asthma (q.v.).

Disturbances of body chemistry in chronic bronchitis are those of associated chronic pulmonary disease when the latter is severe. Most important of these are lowered arterial O_2 saturation and elevated blood and plasma CO_2 levels.

Symptoms and Signs

Mild forms may exist for years with only slight cough, such as the morning "cigarette" cough, with aggravation after acute upper respiratory infection. As the condition progresses, chronic cough and sputum become worse; often an attack of bronchopneumonia marks an abrupt change for the worse. Symptoms usually are more troublesome during the winter. Sputum may be scanty or abundant, mucoid or purulent. Bloody or foul sputum ordinarily indicates some other disease: tuberculosis, bronchiectasis, or carcinoma. Cough may be loose and constant, or paroxysmal with severe spasms lasting several minutes, until sputum is raised. Asthmatic symptoms, cyanosis, or dyspnea are manifestations of other complications (see PULMONARY FIBROSIS, EMPHYSEMA, CONGESTIVE HEART FAILURE).

Chronic bronchitis is characteristically afebrile, with no change in leukocytosis or sedimentation rate. Physical signs are few. Chest expansion and vital capacity are usually diminished. Frequently, scattered rales are heard, which may be sonorous, wheezing, squeaking, or moist in character. If bronchial exudate is abundant, there may be moist or sticky rales at the bases. The physical signs of the other commonly occurring manifestations of chronic pulmonary disease—fibrosis and emphysema—may be present and of any degree of severity. Clubbing of the fingers may occur in advanced chronic bronchitis with heavy infection and purulent sputum, but this sign commonly indicates bronchiectasis, intrapulmonary suppuration, or some severe anoxic state.

Diagnosis

In the chronic form of bronchitis, as in the acute, it is essential to rule out the presence of complications, or other more serious disease. Persistent localized physical signs, with or without fever, suggest such conditions as pulmonary tuberculosis, bronchiectasis, bronchial carcinoma, or chronic pneumonitis. Other diseases with chronic cough are congestive left-sided heart failure, chronic sinusitis, lung abscess, some cases of silicosis, foreign body in a bronchus, Boeck's sarcoid, and the rarer mycotic and fungus infections.

Treatment

General: Chronic bronchitis, though rarely fatal, is an incurable disease. The patient's general health and nutrition should be cared for and his activities regulated to avoid exposure and fatigue. If tobacco is an irritant, smoking should be stopped. For children, special attention should be given to nutrition, with ample amounts of vitamins A and D (see NUTRITIONAL DEFICIENCIES). For prevention, the most important consideration is avoidance of repeated acute infections. It is desirable for the patient to live in a mild equable climate, especially during the winter months.

Local: Treatment of chronic bronchitis is essentially that for controlling cough. As indicated above, when pulmonary drainage is poor, cough is a physiologic necessity in order to clear the air passages of the accumulated exudate. The therapeutic problem is therefore threefold: to reduce or eliminate sputum when possible; to facilitate the raising of whatever sputum is formed; to reduce to a minimum the irritative and paroxysmal aspects of the cough reflex.

The most effective means of reducing sputum is to suppress infection, though this is not always possible. At times, however, especially during or after an acute febrile exacerbation, a course of 7 to 10 days of sulfonamide (℞ 31), penicillin (℞ 18, 19), or streptomycin (℞ 23) medication will be of pronounced benefit. Drugs to reduce secretion, such as belladonna (℞ 75), may be tried but, as a rule, are not of significant value.

Various measures may be used to facilitate the raising of sputum. These include expectorants (℞ 45 to 49); steam and other inhalants (*see* BEDSIDE PROC.); and, especially if there is any asthmatic tendency, bronchodilators, which often give pronounced relief (℞ 64 to 67). If a patient suffers from severe and intractable paroxysms of cough, it may be helpful, several times a day, to give an expectorant, then a bronchodilator spray, then have the patient sit in a chair or on the side of the bed and cough vigorously to raise sputum. After this, sedation may provide a long period of rest. Postural drainage (*see* BEDSIDE PROC.) is rarely helpful, unless there is coexisting bronchiectasis or lung abscess.

In addition to the above measures, cough sedatives often are needed, though these should be used as little as possible. Codeine usually is adequate (℞ 8, 50, 51). Demerol helps in many cases (℞ 10), Dionin occasionally (℞ 56). Rarely, more potent opiates may be needed in severe paroxysms, but the danger of addiction must be kept constantly in mind (℞ 9, 12). Also, if a severe degree of pulmonary failure is present, as indicated by cyanosis or dyspnea, morphine must be used cautiously, so as not to cause suppression of the cough reflex and respiratory depression. In an occasional instance, with foul sputum, a deodorant may be needed (℞ 60, 61).

SPECIAL (RARER) FORMS OF BRONCHITIS

Fibrinous Bronchitis (plastic bronchitis): Formation of fibrin casts of the smaller bronchi. Treatment is by means of expectorants and supportive measures.

Bronchiolitis Fibrosa Obliterans: Destruction and obliteration of smaller bronchioles, commonly following irritant chemical inhalation. Progressive cough, dyspnea, cyanosis. Usually fatal. Treatment, supportive: Sedation, O_2 continuously and in high concentration.

Spirochetal Bronchitis (bronchopulmonary spirochetosis, Castellani's spirochetosis): Bronchitis with abundant sputum containing spirochetes in large numbers. Treatment: Arsenic has been considered specific; arsphenamine or Mapharsen the drugs of choice (R 36, 37).

Capillary Bronchitis: Essentially a severe diffuse bronchopneumonia (q.v.) of infants or debilitated persons.

Acute Laryngotracheobronchitis (q.v.): A disease, usually of infants and young children, causing massive obstructive lesions in the subglottic region.

BRONCHIECTASIS

A chronic congenital or acquired disease characterized by cylindrical, saccular, or cystic dilatation of the bronchi, with secondary infection.

Etiology and Pathology

Congenital bronchiectasis is due to agenesis of the alveoli, with resultant cystic dilatation of the bronchial mucosa. Acquired bronchiectasis usually is secondary to bronchial obstruction or infection. Some authorities consider chronic bronchitis with necrosis of the bronchial wall to be the principal cause of bronchiectasis. The infection may be secondary to chronic sinusitis, allergy, emphysema, pertussis, pneumonia, silicosis, aspiration of foreign bodies, tuberculosis, atelectasis, and lung abscess.

Bronchiectasis may be unilateral or bilateral, and is most common in the lower lobes. The involved areas contain a secretion which may be but is not always fetid. The bronchial mucosa is inflamed, and may become ulcerated, exposing blood vessels from which small hemorrhages can originate. Adjacent pulmonary tissue may become inflamed, abscessed, or gangrenous. Compensatory emphysema is common.

Symptoms and Signs

Onset usually is insidious, with a cough that is either dry or slightly productive. As the condition progresses the cough tends to become paroxysmal and occurs particularly on arising or after changes in position. Sputum is abundant and, on standing, it may separate into 3 layers: frothy at the top, greenish and turbid in the middle, and thick with pus at the bottom. Hemoptysis is not infrequent and may be an early symptom before purulent exudate is manifest. Dyspnea on exertion may be noted in severe cases. Recurrent attacks of acute respiratory infection are usual. When drainage from the bronchiectatic cavities is obstructed, systemic manifestations appear, such as fever, malaise, loss of weight, and pallor. Drainage from the upper lobes is rarely impaired. Clubbing of the fingers and toes is evident in cases of long standing. Uncomplicated cystic bronchiectasis is asymptomatic.

Physical signs are not specific. There may be limited expansion of the chest, moist rales, diminished breath sounds, and evidence of compensatory emphysema. A significant sign is a change in the physical findings after a paroxysm of coughing, although this is more common in bronchitis than in bronchiectasis.

Diagnosis

Bronchiectasis must be suspected in all patients with the above symptoms and signs. Diagnosis is confirmed by bronchography, using contrast media, or by bronchoscopy. The sputum should be investigated in detail to determine which organisms may be involved in the infectious process. Bronchiectasis must be differentiated from tuberculosis, chronic bronchitis, and fungus infections.

Treatment

Treatment is chiefly medical. There is a small proportion of cases in which the condition is localized in one lobe or one lung, and in these the diseased area should be resected. Medical treatment is directed toward removal or alleviation of all etiologic factors such as partial obstruction of the bronchus, infection, and cough. Any existing foci of infection in the sinuses, teeth, or tonsils must be eliminated. If adequate drainage is established and infection eliminated, the anatomic changes in the bronchus do not require further treatment since they no longer represent a clinical disease. Bed rest is occasionally warranted. Bronchoscopy is essential in treatment as well as in diagnosis to rule out and correct any bronchial obstruction. Medication designed to liquefy the secretion, relieve bronchial spasm, and diminish the frequency and severity of the cough is required. These effects can be obtained by the use of expectorants (℞ 45 to 49), antispasmodics (℞ 64, 67), and cough depressants (℞ 50, 51), administered individually or in various combinations.

Because of the presence of rather large amounts of purulent secretion, it is important that the cough, although diminished, should not be suppressed completely until there is no longer any pus. For this reason morphine and its derivatives should ordinarily not be used. Codeine (℞ 8) is the best cough depressant although in severe, spasmodic cough, small amounts of morphine (0.24 Gm.), Demerol (0.75 Gm.), or Dilaudid (0.06 Gm.) may be added to 120 cc. (℥ iv) of a cough mixture, but for short periods of time only. Severe spasmodic cough also may be relieved by carbon dioxide inhalation.

Such treatment must always be accompanied by adequate postural drainage to prevent retention of bronchial secretions (*see* BEDSIDE PROC.).

Sometimes, symptoms can be relieved by medication and postural drainage alone, in which case postural drainage should be continued for about 6 weeks after symptoms have been relieved. In many cases of real chronicity, infection must be eliminated before symptoms will disappear. For this purpose, chemotherapy or antibiotics are recommended. Sulfadiazine (℞ 31) is given by mouth. Penicillin (℞ 18, 19) or streptomycin (℞ 23) can be administered parenterally, but inhalation of their aerosols (℞ 20, 24) is more successful since an adequate concentration can thus be applied directly to the affected area. Penicillin alone will eliminate many infecting organisms, but penicillin-resistant strains often remain, and for this reason a mixture of penicillin and streptomycin (℞ 22) is most effective. It is important to use a nebulizer which produces a microscopic mist, and to place the apparatus not in the mouth, but approximately 2 inches away. Oxygen or compressed air, or simply a hand bulb, may be used to produce the mist. There is no particular virtue in the use of oxygen. Since bronchial spasm is commonly associated with bronchial infection, it may be necessary to add an antispasmodic (℞ 64) to the aerosols.

In addition to aerosol therapy, medication to relieve the cough and liquefy the sputum must be given as indicated. Postural drainage should always be combined with any method of treatment and continued as long as secretion is being raised. When symptoms are relieved, further bronchography should be done to find out whether surgery is indicated. It is well to remember that the anatomic change and loss of normal defense mechanism are not altered by the treatment described. Consequently, recurrence of symptoms, frequently with entirely new organisms, may appear when a respiratory infection is incurred. Prevention of such infections is essential during the asymptomatic period in bronchiectasis.

ATELECTASIS

Collapse of the alveoli of the lung parenchyma, either massive or confined to small areas, and which may be fetal or primary, if the alveoli have never been expanded, or secondary or acquired.

Etiology

The etiologic factor in all cases of atelectasis is bronchial obstruction. In fetal atelectasis interference with the ingress of air prevents expansion of the lung when respiration begins. In secondary atelectasis, bronchial obstruction is followed by absorption of the gas contained in the alveoli with retraction of the lung to produce the airless state. The obstruction may be caused by tenacious bronchial secretion, foreign bodies, tumors within the bronchial lumen and extrinsic tumors compressing the bronchi. Massive collapse of the lung usually is seen as a postoperative complication, and most frequently when the surgical procedure involves the upper abdomen. Heavy doses of opiates and sedatives, tight dressings, abdominal distension, and immobility of the body as a whole favor its development by reason of the limitation of respiratory movement, elevation of the diaphragm, accumulation of viscid bronchial secretions, and suppression of the cough reflex.

Pathology and Pathologic Physiology

In fetal atelectasis a mucus plug obstructs the bronchus leading to the atelectatic area. The alveoli are completely collapsed, giving a cuboidal appearance under the microscope, with no spaces representing alveoli.

In secondary atelectasis, following obstruction of a bronchus by any of the mechanisms mentioned, there is cessation of ventilation of the lung area distal to that bronchus. Collapse occurs because circulation continues, gas exchange between the alveoli and the capillaries likewise continues, and the entrapped gas is steadily absorbed since it cannot be replenished.

In the average patient some bacteria always are present, resulting in inflammatory reaction. Therefore, because of filling of the alveolar spaces with secretion and some cells, the resultant atelectatic lung is not completely collapsed. The uninvolved surrounding lung becomes emphysematous, the heart and mediastinum are pushed by the greater surrounding pressure toward the atelectatic area, the diaphragm becomes elevated, and the chest wall flattened.

During this entire period of bronchial obstruction there is no replenishing of the oxygen in the alveolar space; the blood circulating in the area therefore cannot receive the additional O_2 required nor can it eliminate the necessary amount of CO_2. As a result, this blood returns via the pulmonary vein to the arterial system as the same venous blood that entered the lung. The resultant arterial blood contains less O_2 and more CO_2 than normal, producing cyanosis and dyspnea.

Absence of ventilation is followed by a diminution in blood channels until, 24 to 48 hours later, there is very little blood flowing through the airless section of the lung, and the cyanosis and dyspnea become less severe due to compensation by the uninvolved pulmonary tissue. If the obstruction is removed, air enters the affected area as expected, the inflammatory condition subsides, and the lung returns to its normal state in a variable length of time, depending upon the amount of infection that was present. If obstruction is not removed, the airlessness and lack of circulation initiate secondary changes, with the development of fibrosis. If these conditions persist, a retracted, fibrotic lung with bronchiectatic changes results.

Symptoms and Signs

The symptoms depend upon whether the obstruction is sudden, as with foreign bodies or thick postoperative secretion, or whether it develops slowly as when associated with tumor. In rapid occlusion there is pain on the affected side, sudden development of dyspnea and cyanosis, drop in blood pressure, tachycardia, elevation of temperature, and shock. On examination of the chest, dullness to flatness over the involved area is found, with diminished or absent breath sounds. The excursion of the chest in this area is reduced or absent. The trachea is deviated toward the affected side, and the heart likewise is displaced in this direction. The patient has a tendency to lie with the atelectatic area dependent. In slowly developing atelectasis there may be no symptoms other than increased dyspnea and weakness. Physical examination will reveal the same findings as in rapid occlusion.

X-ray examination shows a shadow indicating airless lung. The size and location of this will depend upon the bronchus involved. If segmental areas only are affected, the X-ray shadow will be triangular, with its apex directed toward the hilum. If lobar, the entire area occupied by the lobe is airless. The trachea, heart, and mediastinum are seen to be deviated toward the atelectatic area. The diaphragm on the affected side is elevated, and rib spaces are narrowed.

Diagnosis

Diagnosis is made from the clinical manifestations plus X-ray evidence of diminution in size of the lung (as indicated by retraction of ribs, elevation of diaphragm, and deviation of mediastinum) and of a solid, airless shadow. Further important evidence is the finding of bronchial obstruction on bronchoscopic examination. However, the number of bronchi visualized by bronchoscopy is small and unless the obstruction is in a main bronchus or in certain of the early divisions of the smaller bronchi, the examination may be reported negative.

Spontaneous pneumothorax (q.v.) will give the same clinical picture, but the percussion note is tympanitic, heart and mediastinum are pushed to the opposite side, and the X-ray establishes the diagnosis.

Massive effusion may produce dyspnea, cyanosis, and weakness, and the physical findings of flatness and absent breath sounds. However, the heart and mediastinum are deviated away from the involved area and the chest wall bulges instead of being flattened.

Pneumonic consolidation is difficult to differentiate, and there is little value in so doing, since infected atelectasis and pneumonic consolidation are very closely allied and their treatment is approximately the same.

Treatment

Fetal atelectasis is treated by aspiration of the trachea by catheter and administration of O_2 until respiratory distress ceases. Treatment of secondary atelectasis falls into two categories: special, as applied to particular etiologic factors, and general.

Postoperative massive atelectasis is best combated by prevention. Anesthetic agents with a long postanesthesia narcosis should be avoided and narcotics used sparingly after operation, since these depress the cough reflex, which is the major defense mechanism of the bronchi against obstruction by mucus. The patient must not be allowed to lie in one position more than 1 or 2 hours. Early ambulation is important. If there is beginning bronchial obstruction, as indicated by wheezing or a sharp, forced expiration, the patient should be encouraged to cough and breathe deeply. This may be aided by inhalation of a 95% O_2–5% CO_2 mixture by mask or catheter, or by a few breaths of a high concentration of CO_2 to produce a sharp cough.

Once bronchial obstruction becomes established, and the train of events leading to complete atelectasis is started, treatment must be directed toward the obstruction and the infection which is invariably present. For bronchial obstruction 95% O_2–5% CO_2 inhalation should be continued as long as necessary. The patient should be placed so that the uninvolved side is dependent, allowing for increased drainage of the affected area, and should be encouraged to cough. Prophylactic sulfathiazole (R 30), sulfadiazine (R 31), or penicillin (R 18, 19) therapy should be instituted. If there is no improvement in 1 or 2 hours, bronchoscopy should be done and as much secretion as possible aspirated. Following this, all the measures previously described should be continued until the lung returns to normal.

In all cases of atelectasis, bronchoscopy should be performed and the obstruction removed, whether it be a foreign body, tenacious mucus, or other agent. If obstruction is due to a bronchogenic tumor or to extrinsic pressure on the bronchus, the tumor must be removed and the pressure relieved by appropriate measures. Since all secondary atelectases become infected regardless of the cause of obstruction, sulfathiazole (R 30), sulfadiazine (R 31), penicillin (R 18, 19), or streptomycin (R 23) should be given, alone or in combination. The choice of drug depends upon the nature of the infecting organism. Although administration of antibiotics as aerosols may be helpful, these are less effective in atelectasis than in other infections, owing to the bronchial obstruction present. Antispasmodics (R 64, 65, 69) are of value because of the tendency of the bronchial tree to contract on expiration and produce further obstruction. Since the sputum is likely to be tenacious, liquefying agents, such as potassium iodide (R 49) and ammonium chloride (R 39) are indicated. If the obstruction is in the major bronchi, a severe hacking or spasmodic cough may result which requires treatment (R 52, 53), but too great a reduction of the cough reflex is conducive to further bronchial obstruction and should be avoided.

EMPHYSEMA

A condition, localized or diffuse, acute or chronic, characterized by loss of elasticity and overdistention of pulmonary alveoli, which become distorted and eventually rupture (alveolar or vesicular emphysema), and sometimes by the presence of air in the tissues (interstitial emphysema).

CHRONIC HYPERTROPHIC EMPHYSEMA

In this most common form, widespread partial bronchial or bronchiolar obstruction, usually due to chronic bronchitis or asthma, is the chief underlying factor.

Pathology and Pathologic Physiology

Grossly, the lungs are large, pale and dry. They fail to collapse when the thorax is opened. Distended air sacs and bullae can be seen throughout; these are more numerous at the apices and along the lung margins. Adhesions usually are present, further limiting the normal motion of the lungs. The bronchi show evidence of chronic infection, with peribronchial fibrosis. Hypertrophy of the right ventricle may be present. Loss of alveolar elastic tissue is an important histologic change. The alveolar walls are stretched and thinned. The normal architecture of atria and alveoli is destroyed; rupture of alveolar septums results in air sacs of varying sizes. There is a reduction in the number of capillaries in the remaining alveolar walls, and the pulmonary arterial vessels may show sclerotic changes.

Since the tracheobronchial airways are dilated in the inspiratory position, a state of hyperinflation is naturally assumed when there is diffuse bronchial or bronchiolar obstruction. Persistent hyperinflation leads to stretched and narrowed alveolar capillaries, and contributes to the progressive trophic changes, loss of elastic tissue, and dissolution of alveolar walls. The lungs thus slowly increase in size. The thoracic cage tends to assume the inspiratory position, and the diaphragm becomes low or flat. The normally negative intrapleural pressure approaches a mean of zero, but increased respiratory effort causes a wide swing, positive in expiration, negative in inspiration. The vital capacity is diminished and tidal air (volume of each breath) decreases, while residual air (that remaining in the lungs in extreme expiratory position) increases. The minute volume of respiration also is increased. Oxygenation of the blood often is incomplete because of decreased vascularity and changes in the alveolar walls, and also because of unequal dis tribution and poor mixing of the inspired air with the residual air in the enlarged air sacs. Oxygen saturation of the blood decreases to 80%, or even 65% (normal saturation, 95%). At the same time, the CO_2 content increases. Each of these factors should stimulate the respiratory center, but since the process develops slowly the sensitivity of the center progressively decreases, and patients complain of dyspnea while at rest only in advanced stages of emphysema. A compensatory polycythemia usually develops along with the arterial anoxia.

The reduced capillary bed may cause little strain upon the right ventricle at first, but eventually pulmonary artery hypertension develops progressively. Also, the wide swings of pressure produced by respiratory effort on inelastic lungs and the increased intrathoracic pressure due to asthma, coughing, and straining increase the strain on the right heart. In advanced cases there is right-sided congestive failure with edema.

Symptoms and Signs

There usually is a history of asthma, of exposure to silica dust, or of chronic cough and expectoration. Dyspnea of some degree is invariably present: the expiratory type with wheezing, expiratory cough is characteristic. In early cases this may be slight; in advanced cases it appears at rest or with the least exertion. General symptoms are easy fatigue, insomnia, poor appetite. Epigastric distress may occur from overstrain of the abdominal muscles. Peptic ulcer is a not infrequent concomitant. Respiration is labored. The accessory muscles of respiration are active, and expiration is a forceful straining process. The shoulder girdle is elevated; the neck appears short. The thorax may be barrel-shaped; or elongated, with lateral motion absent. Chest expansion is reduced and upper costal in type. A variable degree of cyanosis is present; orthopnea is absent except in severe asthmatic attacks. The neck veins may be distended during expiration. The cardiac impulse is faint or absent.

The percussion note is hyperresonant or even tympanitic. The area of cardiac dullness is decreased or obliterated; hepatic and splenic dullness may be difficult to demonstrate. The diaphragm is low and shows little or no movement. Breath sounds are suppressed. Inspiration is short and harsh, expiration abnormally long. Musical rales are common; moist rales occur with bronchiectasis or heart failure. Heart sounds are muffled and faint, even when no heart failure is present. Roentgen study confirms the hyperaeration, the loss of normal motion of the diaphragm, and its low position. Increased fibrosis may be found in cases associated with infection. The lateral view shows a widened air space between the sternum and the heart, and between the spine and the heart.

In its most advanced degree, obstructive emphysema is marked by three types of symptomatology which may occur in any combination: (1) extreme dyspnea, gasping and asthmatic in type, often with episodes of intractable cough or asthma; (2) anoxia, with deepening cyanosis and cerebral symptoms, insomnia, drowsiness, loss of memory, disorientation, coma; (3) cardiac failure, with cor pulmonale, sometimes also left heart enlargement, anoxia, polycythemia, and eventually right-sided congestive failure.

Laboratory studies show decreased vital capacity (*see* LAB. PROC.)—values below 60% are very significant; volume of respiration is increased despite obstructed expiratory phase, except in advanced cases with marked cyanosis, and impending right-sided heart failure; polycythemia without leukocytosis (unless there is an associated infection); decreased O_2 saturation of the arterial blood, with an increased CO_2 content; elevated plasma bicarbonate values; low chlorides.

Diagnosis

The onset is insidious. In the early stages, the diagnosis is difficult to establish, but emphysema should be suspected whenever there is a history of chronic cough or asthma, shortness of breath out of proportion to the amount of exertion, or cyanosis without signs of cardiac disease. In advanced cases the diagnosis is obvious.

Treatment

The underlying disease should be treated before irreversible changes have occurred. Any measures which decrease the bronchial obstruction will slow up or stop the progress of the disease (*see* BRONCHITIS; ASTHMA). Once the elastic tissue has been destroyed, treatment is purely symptomatic. Many patients with emphysema are obese, and reduction of weight will decrease the demands upon circulation and respiration, with symptomatic improvement. Drugs such as thyroid or amphetamine should not be used, however, since they increase the strain on the circulation.

The patient's activity should be restricted to what he can do without fatigue. Some ambulatory activity is preferable to complete bed rest. Mild sedation (℞ 16) may be helpful, but mental depression should be watched for. Anorexia with progressive weight loss should be combated by nutritious diet, appetizers (sherry with meals), and adequate vitamins. Further measures are directed against infection, obstruction of air passages, anoxia, or secondary cardiac failure.

Infection: Chronic bronchitis (q.v.), frequently present with chronic emphysema, causes cough with sputum and aggravates the bronchiolar obstruction by exudate and swollen mucous membranes. It also leads to frequent acute respiratory infections, especially in the winter. These may be mild upper respiratory and bronchial, or true bronchopneumonia (q.v.). These acute episodes are treated as required. Sometimes they clear promptly; other attacks linger for weeks. Bronchiectasis (q.v.) is a frequent complication of chronic bronchitis and emphysema; it is usually diffuse and cylindrical in type.

Bronchiolar obstruction: Much of the inability to ventilate the lungs in emphysema is due to loss of elasticity, often with fibrosis. Some, however, is caused by reversible bronchiolar obstruction due either to bronchospasm or to swollen mucous membranes. Relief of the latter often will bring marked symptomatic improvement. Control of bronchial infection is an important factor. The use of bronchodilator drugs, however, is the mainstay of therapy.

With mild symptoms ephedrine alone (℞ 67) or with a barbiturate (℞ 68) may be sufficient. If there is much cough with sputum, an expectorant (℞ 49) may give additional relief. For moderate to moderately severe obstructive dyspnea, a bronchodilator spray is most effective (℞ 64). The patient should be carefully instructed how to use this to best advantage, exhaling completely, then inhaling deeply as he vaporizes the solution with several compressions of the bulb, repeating this for 4 to 8 inhalations. With some patients, this may produce an irritating dryness of the throat; others may have mild systemic epinephrine reactions. Ambulatory patients can carry the nebulizer with them, using it at intervals through the day. If the spray is used more often than 5 or 6 times in 24 hours, however, tolerance may develop. Occasionally, a patient will receive greater benefit from epinephrine hypodermically (℞ 66). Asthmatic cough will respond to codeine (℞ 8), but large doses should be avoided.

Inhalations of aerosol penicillin (℞ 20) or streptomycin (℞ 24), or both (℞ 22), often seem to give relief, even when no definite infection can be demonstrated, but sputum should be cultured before using these agents. The specially designed steam aerosol nebulizer is an excellent method for supplying aerosols, together with warmth and moisture.

Aminophylline is a useful drug. During a chronic asthmatic state, symptoms will be alleviated by a suppository (℞ 70) at night, or night and morning. The drug may be tried by mouth (℞ 71) but usually gastrointestinal symptoms will occur if the dosage is large enough to be effective. For asthmatic seizures, aminophylline I.V. (℞ 72) usually brings relief in 5 to 10 minutes. It should be injected slowly to avoid cardiac overstimulation or arrhythmia.

A properly fitted abdominal belt often is beneficial. Primarily, this raises the diaphragm by pressure from below. As a result, there is a decrease in the residual air. The ratio of lung volume to tidal air is favorably altered and vital capacity increased. A similar result can be achieved by pneumoperitoneum although this is not yet widely accepted except for the treatment of emphysema associated with pulmonary tuberculosis.

Breathing exercises with emphasis on forceful, prolonged expiration seem to help many patients. The patient bends forward and compresses the lower part of the thorax manually during expiration. A tight elastic binder may be used instead to supply the compression. These exercises must be continued over a long period of time.

Anoxia: Oxygen inhalation will give relief in acute or chronic dyspnea. Inhalation by nasal tube or mask for $\frac{1}{2}$ to 1 hour, 2 or 3 times a day, can be carried out by the patient at home. For severe dyspnea and anoxia, continuous O_2 by mask or tent may be necessary. In cases with high blood CO_2 levels, continuous O_2 should not be given over a long period of time, as habituation may develop. With maximally severe status asthmaticus, helium-oxygen therapy may be necessary (*see* BRONCHIAL ASTHMA).

Cardiac failure: Treatment of the cardiac symptoms of advanced emphysema is that of congestive heart failure (q.v.).

BULLOUS EMPHYSEMA

Localized areas of emphysema within the lung substance. It is caused by bronchial or bronchiolar obstruction at one or more sites. It may occur with acute or chronic infections of any sort, with aspiration of a foreign body, with asthma, pneumonoconiosis, bronchogenic carcinoma, sarcoidosis, or with any other disease which involves only a part of the bronchial tree. Occasionally, a bulla attains great size; this is sometimes referred to as a pneumocyst or a balloon cyst, and may be mistaken for pneumothorax. Injudicious needling of such a pneumocyst is usually followed by pneumothorax. The same complication occurs with spontaneous rupture of a large bulla situated near the surface of the lung.

Symptoms, Signs, and Diagnosis

If bullae are small and few, symptoms may be nil. If numerous or very large, there will be dyspnea with or without cyanosis. The symptoms and laboratory findings will resemble those seen in chronic hypertrophic emphysema (q.v.).

Physical signs usually are inconclusive, but may suggest partial pneumothorax. Diagnosis is best made by X-ray, which shows one or more radiolucent areas. Infected bullae may be confused with tuberculous cavities or lung abscess.

Treatment

A solitary cyst, or a process localized to one portion of a lung, often can be removed surgically. When more widespread, and not amenable to surgery, the treatment is the same as for chronic hypertrophic emphysema (q.v.).

COMPENSATORY OR LOCALIZED EMPHYSEMA

Emphysema occurring in response to loss of functioning lung tissue due to disease, destruction, maldevelopment, or surgical removal. With the advent of thoracic surgery, preoperative determination of the status of the uninvolved lung tissue has become increasingly important. A successful operation may leave the patient with such poor function of the remaining lung tissue that he is worse off than before. Thoracoplasty, or the use of inert substances such as lucite balls, often is necessary to eliminate dead space and prevent overdistention of the remaining lung tissue. Otherwise, readjustments of various kinds occur. The thorax decreases in size; the mediastinum may shift; the diaphragm rises; the remaining lung tissue has to expand to fill any residual space. Hyperplasia of alveoli does not occur in adults, and probably not in children; the alveoli merely increase in size. There is poor mixing of gases and impaired gas exchange in the enlarged alveoli, and the total lung volume increases without a corresponding increase in vital capacity. Some loss of capillaries also occurs. These factors tend to produce a mild degree of dyspnea and some cyanosis. Restoration of the normal position of the mediastinum, and reduction of the emphysema of the remaining lung, as by a secondary thoracoplasty, often will improve pulmonary function significantly.

SENILE EMPHYSEMA

This usually represents one of the atrophic changes of old age. It is attributed to decreased mobility of the spine and ribs, with gradual elevation of the ribs and sternum, and fixation of the thorax in the inspiratory position. When it occurs in young individuals, it usually is called **postural emphysema.** The lungs are small, and collapse readily when the thorax is opened. There is no obstruction in the bronchi or bronchioles. The lung vesicles are larger than normal, and there is usually some loss of alveolar walls, but the elastic tissue is well preserved and the capillary bed shows little change. The diaphragm moves normally or shows increased excursion; respiration is abdominal. Although vital capacity is somewhat reduced there is but little impairment of respiratory function. Cyanosis is rarely seen. Treatment is seldom necessary in uncomplicated senile emphysema.

INTERSTITIAL EMPHYSEMA

A condition characterized by rupture of marginal alveoli into the subpleural space, or into the peribronchial or perivascular tissues. The air dissects along the pleura or vessel, and may reach the mediastinum. From there it may spread to the neck or to the retroperitoneal tissues. Occasionally, it ruptures through the pleura or peritoneum, causing pneumothorax or pneumoperitoneum.

Symptoms and Signs

Symptoms vary with the amount of air that escapes, and the rate at which this occurs. There may be dyspnea, cyanosis, or retrosternal pain. The disease may simulate angina, coronary thrombosis, pericarditis, pulmonary infarction, or pneumonia. Unless subcutaneous emphysema is present the diagnosis may be difficult. The lungs show little or no abnormality on physical examination. A peculiar "crunch" is sometimes heard over the mediastinum or precordium, synchronous with the heart beat. X-rays usually are necessary to establish the diagnosis in the less severe forms.

Treatment

Oxygen inhalation is given to relieve the dyspnea and cyanosis. Sometimes the use of 100% O_2 by mask, continuously, will aid in the removal of the interstitial air by denitrogenating the blood and then permitting the circulating blood to absorb this air from the tissues. This requires 24 to 48 hours of continuous O_2 inhalation.

Opiates are usually necessary to control the pain and cough until the rupture becomes sealed off and the air is absorbed (℞ 8, 11, 13). Morphine should be used with caution if there is severe respiratory embarrassment, respiratory depression, or severe cyanosis; it depresses the respiratory center. Needling of the mediastinal or subcutaneous tissues will sometimes relieve pressure and help control pain. In advanced cases, with extensive subcutaneous emphysema and vascular compression, multiple incisions are necessary to permit the air to escape. If tension pneumothorax is present, it should be controlled by intermittent or continuous suction (*see* PNEUMOTHORAX). A sulfonamide (℞ 31) or penicillin (℞ 18, 19) should be given to prevent infection of the lung and mediastinum.

PNEUMONIA

An acute infection of the alveolar spaces of the lung. Involvement of an entire lobe is called **lobar pneumonia;** of parts of the lobe only, **lobular** (or patchy) **pneumonia.** When the infection is restricted to alveoli contiguous to bronchi, it is sometimes referred to as **bronchopneumonia.**

Though many classifications have been suggested, it probably is most logical to speak of the disease as bacterial or nonbacterial pneumonia; or, when the specific etiologic agent is known, to refer to it accordingly: e.g., pneumococcal pneumonia, Friedländer's bacillus pneumonia, virus pneumonia.

The common microorganisms causing bacterial pneumonia are the various types of pneumococcus, Group A hemolytic streptococcus, *Klebsiella pneumoniae* (Friedländer's bacillus)

Types A and B, and *Pasteurella tularensis*. Pneumonia also can be caused, but rarely, by practically any other pathogenic bacterium; also by viruses, rickettsias, and fungi. Virus pneumonias are common, though it is not possible to demonstrate the virus except by special technics. Cases of virus pneumonia frequently diagnosed as "primary atypical pneumonia, cause unknown" might better be designated as "probable virus pneumonia."

Predisposing factors are chronic alcoholism, malnutrition, debility, exposure, foreign matter in the respiratory tract (such as occurs from aspiration of vomitus or other material), and hypostasis (*see* Aspiration Pneumonia; Hypostatic Pneumonia).

Bacterial pneumonia generally occurs sporadically. Healthy carriers usually are responsible for the infection of others, but there is unfortunately no way in which these carriers can be identified and eliminated.

Since the advent of chemotherapy and its successful control of upper respiratory infections, the incidence of pneumonia has been greatly reduced, and the prognosis of the disease itself has been vastly improved.

Pneumococcal pneumonia will be described in detail because it is by far the most common form of pneumonia, and many of its features are essentially similar to those of other bacterial pneumonias.

PNEUMOCOCCAL PNEUMONIA

Pneumonia caused by pneumococci and, since the infection usually involves one or more lobes, frequently called "lobar."

Pathology and Pathogenesis

Pneumococci reach the lungs via the respiratory passages, finally lodging in the alveoli. Here, they proliferate and their metabolic products set up an inflammatory process. This is first manifested by the outpouring of protein-rich edema fluid into the alveolar spaces. The fluid then serves as culture medium for the pneumococci, and as a transport vehicle from one alveolus to another, from one lobule to another, and from one lobe to another.

The early stage of pneumonia (the first 12 to 16 hours) has been called the stage of "red hepatization" because of the reddish appearance of the consolidated lung, which pathologists formerly compared with the liver. The red color is due to the widespread dilatation of pulmonary blood vessels characteristic of early pneumonia.

A few hours after the initial dilatation of lung capillaries and the outpouring of edema fluid into the alveoli, polymorphonuclear leukocytes enter the alveolar spaces. Soon they are so numerous as to form most of the bulk of the consolidated lung, though in the "zone of edema fluid," where the pneumonic lesion is advancing, they are sparse. Some of these leukocytes are

actively phagocytic, taking up pneumococci by "surface phagocytosis." This kind of phagocytosis, which does not require
the help of opsonins, occurs when leukocytes can trap bacteria
against the wall of an alveolus or against another leukocyte.
Thus, the more leukocytes in the alveolar space, the more active
will be surface phagocytosis. In tissue sections pneumococci
are hard to find in the consolidated portion of the lung but
are plentiful in the advancing margin of the lesion, where
edema fluid is more abundant than are leukocytes.

At the time of spontaneous recovery the "macrophage reaction" takes place. Large mononuclear cells enter the alveoli,
engulf any pneumococci still present, and phagocytize the polymorphonuclear leukocytes. This process continues until resolution is complete, when the lungs become clear to X-ray and
percussion.

The pathogenesis of other bacteriogenic pneumonia is essentially similar.

Symptoms and Signs

In many cases pneumonia is preceded by an upper respiratory infection. The onset of pulmonary symptoms usually is
sudden, with a shaking chill, sharp pain in the involved chest,
cough with the early production of rusty sputum, fever, and
headache. Usually, all these symptoms appear, although one
or more may be absent. Rusty sputum, when present, is practically diagnostic. Dyspnea is frequent with respiration rapid
(25 to 45/minute) and often painful because of pleuritic involvement. A peculiar expiratory grunt is characteristic. Delirium is common, especially in alcoholic patients. A convulsion may herald onset in children. In pneumococcal pneumonia, the patient sweats profusely, often is cyanotic, and
is acutely ill. The temperature rises rapidly to reach 101° to
105°F.; the pulse accelerates to 100 to 130. Signs of consolidation may be lacking during the first few hours, but soon fine
rales and suppressed breath sounds can be heard over the involved area. Frank consolidation, involving part of a lobe or
several lobes, is found later. A pleural friction rub often is
heard in the early stages.

The cough at this time is dry and hacking except when bronchitis has preceded the pneumonia, in which case it is productive, with purulent sputum. There are likely to be extremely
painful paroxysms of coughing. In the later stages, the cough
is more productive and usually painless. As the disease progresses, the appearance of the sputum changes from pinkish or
blood-flecked in the beginning to rusty at the height of the
process, and finally to yellow and mucopurulent during the
stage of resolution.

Gastrointestinal symptoms often are noted, such as abdominal
distention, jaundice, and diarrhea. Nausea and vomiting may
usher in the disease. In pneumonias involving the right mid-

dle or lower lobes, actual right upper quadrant tenderness and rigidity sometimes suggest the diagnosis of gall bladder disease, appendicitis, or peritonitis. Herpes, usually of the lips and face, is present in the majority of cases.

Diagnosis

The diagnosis of pneumococcal pneumonia should be strongly suspected in any patient with a history of acute febrile illness, associated with chill, pain in chest, and cough, especially with expectoration of viscid rusty sputum. If physical examination then reveals tachycardia, tachypnea, cyanosis, and signs of consolidation, the diagnosis of pneumonia is confirmed. X-ray may provide further confirmation, or in early cases may yield the only positive evidence of pulmonary consolidation. Ordinarily, a leukocyte count may be normal or even low. The bacterial etiology is determined by sputum cultures and, if positive, by blood cultures, also. The pneumococci may be typed by the Neufeld method.

Some cases are more gradual and insidious in onset, exhibiting an upper respiratory infection and acute bronchitis with persisting or increasing fever and leukocytosis, and physical signs consisting only of moist rales at first, with evidence of consolidation later.

Prognosis

Patients treated during the first 1 to 3 days are more likely to recover than those treated later. Also, the prognosis is generally better in persons under 50 than in older persons. Any of the following factors makes the outlook less favorable: a positive blood culture, especially if the number of colonies/cc. exceeds 100; involvement of 2 or more lobes; leukocyte count under 5,000; BUN over 70 mg./100 cc.; the presence of any chronic disease, or of meningitis or endocarditis. A complicating meningitis or endocarditis is the most adverse factor, since failure to recognize these diseases and to treat them specifically will produce a fatal outcome.

Treatment

Supportive measures must be instituted at once, with complete bed rest, administration of fluids, and of O_2 and analgesics when indicated. The initiation of specific therapy should not await demonstration of the pathogen by culture, but should be based temporarily upon the history and physical examination. After the sputum has been studied, any necessary changes in antibacterial therapy may be instituted. If pneumococcal pneumonia is suspected, penicillin is the drug of choice. One of the sulfonamides may be given in addition or as an alternative choice.

Specific therapy: Aqueous penicillin (℞ 18) in doses of 200,-000 or 300,000 u. dissolved in 2 or 3 cc. of distilled water should be administered every 12 hours for a total of 3 doses; after

that this dose should be continued at 24-hour intervals until
the temperature is normal for 48 hours: 30,000 to 50,000 u.
of aqueous penicillin every 3 hours also is effective, but this
regimen is less practical and no more efficacious than the
long-interval schedule. Repository penicillin may be given
in doses of 300,000 u. every 12 to 24 hours (R 19).

Sulfonamides available for clinical use are sulfadiazine, sulfamerazine, sulfathiazole, and sulfapyridine. Of these, sulfadiazine (R 31), sulfamerazine (R 34) and the sulfonamide
mixture (R 35), because of their lower toxicity, are preferable
(*see* SULFONAMIDE THERAPY). The initial dose for adults is 2
or 4 Gm. orally, followed by 1 Gm. every 4 or 6 hours, day
and night. Infants and children should be given 60 to 100 mg.
(gr. i to iss)/lb. body wt. every 24 hours in divided doses, following an initial dose of ½ the daily dosage. Sodium bicarbonate often is indicated to maintain an alkaline reaction
in urine (*see* SULFONAMIDE THERAPY).

Clinical improvement during sulfonamide therapy manifests
itself at about the same time as with penicillin, i.e., in 12 to 48
hours. In some cases, the response is dramatic, fever disappearing and toxicity vanishing the day after treatment is started.
In others, improvement comes by lysis.

In critically ill patients, or in patients who cannot take or
retain medicine given orally, sulfonamides should be administered I.V. as a 5% solution of the sodium salt (R 32), 3 Gm.
being given initially, followed by 2 Gm. every 8 hours. Oral
therapy should be resumed, however, as soon as it becomes
feasible.

Sodium sulfadiazine also can be given subcut. as a 1 to 3%
solution (R 33), 3 Gm. every 12 hours. Subcut. injections are
indicated in children who vomit. The dose is 50 mg. (gr. ¾)
of sulfadiazine/lb. body wt./day; ½ of the 24-hour dose is
given initially, and the remainder divided into 4-hourly doses.

Sulfonamide therapy may be hampered by poor absorption
of the drug from the gastrointestinal tract, by unrecognized
complications such as endocarditis or meningitis, by sulfonamide-resistant pneumococci or by the presence of para-aminobenzoic acid (derived from procaine). Though the optimum
therapeutic blood level has never been definitely determined,
it is generally agreed that 4 to 10 mg./100 cc. of sulfadiazine
or sulfamerazine is desirable. Endocarditis can be recognized
by the appearance of new or changing cardiac murmurs, and
particularly by the persistence of a positive blood culture.
Sulfonamide-resistant pneumococci are not common in the
general bacterial population, but may appear when treatment
is prolonged.

It has been claimed that combined penicillin and sulfonamide
therapy of pneumococcal pneumonia reduces the mortality rate.
In the average case, this is not necessary, though in seriously ill
patients it may be advisable to administer full therapeutic

doses of penicillin and sulfadiazine until improvement is manifest.

Treatment with either penicillin or sulfonamides or both should be maintained until the patient has been afebrile for 48 hours.

General supportive measures: Complete **bed rest** is essential during the acute phase of pneumonia. Patients treated during the first 2 days of illness, who have not had long febrile courses, may be allowed up after 2 or 3 days of normal temperature. Those who have survived stormy courses must remain in bed longer.

Fluids: Four to 6 liters a day will be consumed by most patients in the acute stages of bacterial pneumonia. In severely dehydrated individuals, as much as 10 liters may be required in the first 24 hours. The great majority of pneumonia patients will take water eagerly by mouth. Only in certain cases with delirium, vomiting, or meningitic complications will parenteral administration of fluid be required.

Diet: During the febrile stages the patient should remain on liquids, or at the most a soft diet (*see* DIETS). As soon as his temperature is normal he can be given a regular diet. Inasmuch as nitrogen loss always occurs, a high protein intake (100 Gm./day if possible) is advisable during convalescence (*see* DIETS, High Protein).

Oxygen: Most patients with pneumonia are cyanotic to some degree. As long as cyanosis persists, O_2 should be administered by tent, mask, or catheter (*see* CLIN. PROC.). O_2 also is helpful in ameliorating cough and restlessness and in preventing or relieving abdominal distention.

Relief of pain: Pleural pain usually can be relieved by codeine (℞ 8) 60 mg. (gr. i), repeated in 4 hours. Occasionally, morphine 10 to 15 mg. (gr. ⅙ to ¼) (℞ 9) may be required, but this drug should be avoided if possible because of its tendency to produce abdominal distention. A tight binder around the chest sometimes gives relief. Pneumothorax and intercostal block have been used when other measures have failed; the latter probably is the more effective.

Abdominal distention: Abdominal distention is less frequent since chemotherapy has shortened the course of pneumonia. However, it still occurs occasionally, and is more easily prevented than treated. A carefully given enema, repeated at appropriate intervals, during the acute stage of pneumonia may be necessary. If distention threatens, a rectal tube should be inserted. An injection of neostigmine (℞ 85) at the same time often helps. Hot stupes may give some relief (*see* CLIN. PROC.). Distention is less likely to develop in patients who receive O_2.

Shock: When shock occurs in pneumonia, it should be treated in the usual manner—by administration of whole blood or plasma, and by keeping the patient warm (*see* SHOCK).

HEMOLYTIC STREPTOCOCCAL PNEUMONIA

Etiology

Almost all hemolytic streptococcal pneumonias are caused by Group A streptococci. These pneumonias are sometimes primary infections, but more often follow tonsillitis or pharyngitis, with or without scarlatiniform rash. They may occur as a sequel to influenza.

Symptoms and Signs

These are similar to those of pneumococcal pneumonia, but in addition the pharynx is often swollen and the tonsils may be covered with exudate. If the patient has recently had scarlet fever, there may be desquamation. An important sign of streptococcal pneumonia is the presence of a large pleural effusion, frequently bloody, during the acute stage, but this does not always occur.

Diagnosis

Diagnosis of the pneumonic process is made in the same way as for pneumococcal pneumonia. Streptococcal etiology should be suspected if the pneumonia accompanies or follows scarlet fever or streptococcal tonsillitis or pharyngitis, or if empyema is present during the acute stage. The gross appearance of the sputum is not characteristic. A stained specimen may show gram-positive cocci in chains, but the diagnosis must be confirmed by cultures on a blood agar plate. Blood culture may be positive.

Prognosis and Treatment

Hemolytic streptococcal pneumonia usually is serious, particularly when complicated by bacteremia or empyema, or both. The prognosis has been immensely improved since the introduction of penicillin and sulfonamides. Mild cases are occasionally seen.

Aqueous penicillin, 50,000 u. I.M. every 3 hours (℞ 18), should be given promptly and continued in uncomplicated cases until the temperature has been normal for at least 48 hours. Because of the existence of a significant number of sulfonamide-resistant hemolytic streptococci, sulfonamides are not recommended if penicillin is available. Penicillin-resistant group A hemolytic streptococci have not yet been reported.

Proper therapy of hemolytic streptococcal pneumonia must include a careful search for empyema, and exploratory thoracentesis should be done to resolve any doubt. If free fluid is found, 1,000 cc. should be withdrawn and replaced by 50,000 to 100,000 u. of penicillin dissolved in approximately 300 cc. of sterile saline injected into the pleural cavity (℞ 21) (*see* ANTI-BIOTIC THERAPY). This procedure should be repeated daily until smears and cultures are negative. (For further details *see*

EMPYEMA.) Supportive treatment is the same as for pneumococcal pneumonia (q.v.).

STAPHYLOCOCCAL PNEUMONIA

Etiology

Most cases of staphylococcal pneumonia are caused by coagulase-positive *Staph. aureus;* a few by *Staph. albus.* Staphylococcal pneumonia may be primary, but more frequently it occurs as a complication of influenza or of staphylococcal bacteremia. Thus the infection may be either blood-borne or airborne.

Symptoms and Signs

In cases complicating influenza, the symptoms of pneumonia may appear concomitantly with the influenza, or days or weeks later. Some or all of the symptoms of pneumococcal pneumonia may be present in varying degrees of severity, i.e., pleural pain, dyspnea, cyanosis, and cough. The physical signs frequently indicate a patchy distribution, though lobar involvement sometimes occurs. Pulmonary abscesses of less than 1 cm. to several cm. in diameter are common, but may be difficult to identify by physical examination. Related signs may be a furuncular rash and evidence of abscess in liver, kidneys, brain, or elsewhere.

Diagnosis

The signs and symptoms of pneumonia, plus a blood or sputum culture positive for staphylococcus, are diagnostic. Gram stain of the sputum will show many gram-positive cocci resembling staphylococci. Roentgenographic evidence of small abscesses also is suggestive. Leukocytosis usually is present.

Prognosis and Treatment

The mortality rate is fairly high in this always serious disease. The general principles of treatment for pneumococcal pneumonia apply equally to staphylococcal pneumonia. Because of the wide variation in strain sensitivity of staphylococci to antibacterial drugs, the sensitivity of the infecting strain to penicillin and to streptomycin should be measured in each case if possible. Sulfonamide sensitivity tests are not well standardized and therefore less reliable. While the laboratory report is pending, the patient should receive both penicillin and sulfadiazine. An average dose of 50,000 u. of aqueous penicillin should be given I.M. every 3 hours (R 18). In addition, an initial dose of 4 Gm. of sulfadiazine (R 31) should be administered, followed by 1 Gm. every 4 hours. If the organism is resistant to penicillin but sensitive to streptomycin, the latter should be administered. The dosage of streptomycin in staphylococcal pneumonia has not been established, but an empirical dose of 0.5 Gm. I. M. every 6 hours may be tried

(R 23). In critically ill patients, it is justifiable to prescribe streptomycin in addition to penicillin and sulfonamide while awaiting the results of sensitivity tests. If the organism proves to be sensitive to penicillin, streptomycin should be discontinued.

Though *in vitro* sensitivity tests are useful guides in the therapy of staphylococcal infections, it must be emphasized that they can never replace sound clinical judgment.

FRIEDLÄNDER'S BACILLUS (*KLEBSIELLA*) PNEUMONIA

Etiology and Pathology

Pneumonia may be caused by type A, B, or C of Friedländer's bacillus. About 80% of such cases are due to type A.

The cut surface of the lung in *Klebsiella* pneumonia is exceedingly viscid. Necrosis and abscess formation are common in the acute stage. Chronic pulmonary abscess is a frequent sequel in patients who recover.

Symptoms and Signs

These are similar to those of pneumococcal pneumonia (q.v.). Signs of cavitation are sometimes present, especially in the chronic stage of the disease.

Diagnosis

Most patients with Friedländer's bacillus pneumonia are severely or even critically ill. The disease should be suspected in any patient who exhibits unusually rapid spread of consolidation from one lobe to another. Sometimes, 3 or 4 lobes become involved within 2 days. Sputum is viscid and may be "cherry red" in color; stained smears show gram-negative rods in varying numbers. Pneumococci are sometimes found in the sputum. Blood culture is frequently positive. In many cases, the pneumonic exudate is so thick that it produces a downward curving of the border of the upper lobe as seen by X-ray. This sign, though not pathognomonic, is more frequent in Friedländer's than in other kinds of pneumonia. In lower lobe lesions, the consolidation often is extremely dense.

Prognosis and Treatment

The mortality rate is high, particularly in bacteremic cases. Abscesses are common and may persist for many months after recovery from the acute stage of the disease.

Both streptomycin (R 23) and sulfadiazine (R 31) should be administered. The dose of streptomycin should probably be large—0.5 Gm. I.M. every 4 to 6 hours until clinical improvement appears. The dosage then can be reduced to 0.2 Gm. or 0.3 Gm. I.M. every 6 or 8 hours for 4 additional days. An initial dose of 4 Gm. of sulfadiazine followed by 1 Gm. every

4 hours should be prescribed. Supportive measures are the same as for pneumococcal pneumonia (q.v.).

TULAREMIC PNEUMONIA

Etiology

The causative organism, *Pasteurella tularensis,* is usually transmitted by rabbits (*see* TULAREMIA). Tularemic pneumonia may be associated with ulceroglandular tularemia but it sometimes occurs primarily.

Symptoms and Signs

Symptoms are those of other pneumonias. Signs of consolidation are frequently present, but in lobular tularemic pneumonia there may be only suppression of breath sounds and occasional rales. A primary ulcer on the hand or finger, as the site of initial infection, may or may not appear.

Diagnosis

A history of handling, skinning, dressing, or cooking wild rabbits or other wild animals is the most important requisite for early diagnosis. Pulmonary involvement is detected by physical signs or roentgenogram. Agglutinins against *Past. tularensis* will be found in the patient's serum, but usually do not appear until about the 10th day after infection. A rising titer of agglutinins aids in diagnosis. *Past. tularensis* can sometimes be found in the blood.

Prognosis and Treatment

The disease varies greatly in severity, from completely asymptomatic pneumonia diagnosed only by X-ray to an extensive and fatal consolidation. The prognosis is good in mild cases and has been greatly improved in severe cases by the introduction of streptomycin therapy.

Streptomycin is specific. Small doses, 0.5 to 1.5 Gm./day, I.M., have proved effective. A practical dosage is 0.5 Gm. I.M. every 12 hours (℞ 23) for 4 to 7 days. The response is frequently rapid and dramatic. Supportive treatment is the same as for pneumococcal pneumonia (q.v.). Aureomycin (℞ 28) also has been found to be effective in tularemic pneumonia.

VIRUS PNEUMONIA

Etiology

As previously stated, most cases diagnosed as "primary atypical pneumonia, cause unknown" probably are viral in origin although no etiologic agent can be recovered. Thus, this form of viral pneumonia differs from the less frequently occurring pneumonias of known viral origin, viz., influenzal pneumonia and psittacosis (q.v.).

Symptoms and Signs

The onset of "virus pneumonia," in contrast to bacterial pneumonia, usually is gradual, though acute onsets are sometimes seen. Constitutional symptoms of infection ordinarily predominate over the pulmonary symptoms. Headache, malaise, and chilliness without frank rigor are common. Cough, which is almost invariably present, with mucopurulent or more rarely rusty or frankly bloody sputum, may be severe and paroxysmal, sometimes almost incessant. Physical signs usually are sparse in comparison with the X-ray findings. Though evidence of consolidation is sometimes elicited, frequently the only physical signs are a few subcrepitant rales after cough or deep inspiration. Furthermore, the patient may not appear ill. The pulse and respiratory rate often are normal even in the presence of fever.

Diagnosis

Virus pneumonias are difficult to identify etiologically, though the history of more gradual onset of malaise, headache, and cough is generally characteristic of this group of pneumonias. The leukocyte count usually is normal, and rarely rises above 15,000. The roentgenogram reveals pulmonary involvement of varying degrees, sometimes much greater than physical signs indicate. Examination of the blood for "cold agglutinins" is positive in about 70 to 80% of the cases, but the diagnostic titers of these antibodies may not appear until the 3rd week of the disease, often after recovery has occurred.

Psittacosis should be suspected if the patient has had contact with birds, particularly parrots or lovebirds. However, pneumonia caused by the virus harbored in pigeons probably occurs in human beings more frequently than is generally realized. A definite diagnosis can be made by demonstrating an increase in titer of antibodies to the specific virus during the course of pneumonia (see PSITTACOSIS).

Prognosis and Treatment

The mortality in so-called "primary atypical" virus pneumonia is less than 1%.

In some cases of "primary atypical" virus pneumonias, aureomycin (℞ 28) has been responsible for dramatic improvement; the initial dosage is 1 Gm. every 4 hours, followed by decreasing doses as improvement is manifest. Chloromycetin (℞ 29) also has been found to be effective in this disease. Some authorities recommend the use of penicillin as a prophylactic against secondary invaders. This procedure is advisable in severe but not in mild cases. The dose is 30,000 u. I.M. (℞ 18) every 3 hours, or 300,000 u./day (℞ 19), until the temperature has been normal for 2 days.

Symptomatic treatment may include codeine (℞ 8) for headache or cough. Elixir of terpin hydrate (℞ 40) often will soothe the throat irritation in cases where cough is annoying. Expectorants (℞ 41 to 45) are sometimes helpful.

In cases where reflex bronchiolar spasm is extensive, aminophylline (℞ 71) may give relief.

ASPIRATION PNEUMONIA

Etiology

This form of pneumonia is due to foreign matter that somehow manages to enter the respiratory tract. Postoperatively, following alcoholic overindulgence, and as a result of poisoning (q.v.), the tracheobronchial reflexes are diminished and therefore, when material is regurgitated, its aspiration into the lung passages is likely to follow. Aspiration is a hazard also attending the incautious insertion or removal of a stomach tube (see CLIN. PROC.). Oily substances, especially when administered in the form of nose drops, often are aspirated into the lungs, particularly by infants, by aged and debilitated patients, or during sleep or other state of unconsciousness.

The irritation caused by foreign matter in the finer air passages is responsible for the outpouring of edema fluid, which is an ideal medium for the propagation of endogenous pathogens. When the process is extensive a typical bronchopneumonia ensues.

Diagnosis

With a minor degree of foreign body aspiration, only slight symptoms or none may be noted, but when large amounts of material have gained access to the lungs, fever, cough, dyspnea, and chest pain result. A history of foreign matter aspiration and the typical radiographic findings of bronchopneumonic inflammation are helpful in diagnosis, which may be verified by the identification of aspirated material in the sputum.

Prophylaxis and Treatment

Aspiration pneumonia can be prevented by adequate supervision of all patients postoperatively and of patients severely poisoned and those treated by stomach tube. (For methods of preventing the aspiration of foreign material, see CLIN. PROC.) The administration to children of oily substances intranasally should be avoided, and the oral administration of oily medicaments should be used with adequate precautions to prevent their aspiration.

When aspiration pneumonia does develop, and since most cases are due to a mixed infection, sulfonamides (℞ 31) and penicillin (℞ 18, 19) should be administered as described under pneumococcal pneumonia. If it is discovered that some of the pathogens are resistant to penicillin and sulfonamides, streptomycin therapy (℞ 23) should be instituted.

HYPOSTATIC PNEUMONIA

Etiology

When this condition occurs, it usually is in debilitated patients who have chronic passive congestion of the lungs. The sluggish circulation and the edema fluid present are conducive to infection by pathogens, usually endogenous, of varying degrees of virulence. Patients with long-standing heart disease and other ailments favoring pulmonary stasis are prone to develop this form of pneumonia.

Diagnosis

Since hypostatic pneumonia always is a complication of other illness, the symptoms are often indistinguishable from those of the underlying disease. Dyspnea, cyanosis, cough with expectoration of frothy pink sputum, and low grade fever are the prominent findings. On auscultation rales may be heard over both lung bases. Radiographic examination usually reveals obliteration of both costophrenic angles and a bilateral diffuse basal density.

Treatment

Control of the primary disease is essential, as is frequent change of the patient's position in bed and the earliest possible resumption of ambulation when feasible. Some physicians advocate the prophylactic administration of penicillin (℞ 18, 19) whenever passive congestion of the lungs is known to exist.

PSITTACOSIS

(Ornithosis)

An infectious, mainly intestinal, disease of birds, caused by a filtrable virus which is transmissible to man, in whom it produces an atypical form of pneumonia. The disease is found principally in psittacine birds (parrots, parakeets, lovebirds), although poultry, pigeons, and canaries may harbor a similar infection.

Etiology and Incidence

The causative virus can be filtered only through rather coarse filters and is large enough to be seen microscopically. Human infection ordinarily occurs through inhalation of dust from feathers or cage contents of infected birds; sometimes it follows a bite from a bird harboring the virus. It also may be transmitted by the cough droplets of infected patients.

Epidemics of psittacosis have occurred from time to time in various parts of the world. A pandemic in 1929-30 was traced to green Amazon parrots from South America. Since that time quarantine regulations have greatly reduced the incidence of the disease, but have not eliminated it. The infection has since been found in lovebirds in aviaries, in pigeons, and in a number of other species. Human cases are occasionally reported as occurring in laboratory workers or bird handlers.

Symptoms and Signs

Following an incubation period of 6 to 15 days, the onset may be insidious, or abrupt with fever, chills or chilly sensations, headache, backache, and anorexia. Cough, usually nonproductive, rapidly develops and may be severe. The temperature rises rapidly, reaching as high as 104° F., and ordinarily is accompanied by a relative bradycardia. As the disease progresses into the 2nd week, physical signs of pneumonitis may appear. This usually begins in the hilar areas and spreads to the periphery of the lungs. Finally, frank consolidation may occur, particularly if there is secondary invasion by pyogenic bacteria. Early in the disease, X-ray is generally necessary to demonstrate the pneumonitis. The leukocyte count usually is normal in the absence of secondary bacterial infection.

The temperature remains elevated for 2 or 3 weeks, after which it generally falls by lysis and recovery ensues. Convalescence is slow after a severe attack.

Diagnosis

The history is of prime importance, since the disease may easily be confused with influenza, other atypical forms of pneumonia, or typhoid fever. Psittacosis should always be suspected in patients with the symptoms described who have had close contact with birds, particularly those of the parrot family. The birds should be examined for psittacosis. Diagnosis can be confirmed only by actual recovery of the virus from the patient's sputum or by the complement fixation test. The latter test may be carried out by sending serial specimens of blood serum obtained early in the disease and late in convalescence to the National Institute of Health, U.S. Public Health Service, Bethesda, Maryland.

Prognosis

The prognosis depends upon the source of infection, the patient's age, and the extent of the pneumonia. Infections acquired from birds of the parrot family show a mortality rate of about 20%, which is higher than that in infections from other birds (e.g., pigeons). (There is some question as to whether the virus is the same in the different species.) In patients over 40 years of age, the mortality is extremely high. A pronounced increase in pulse and respiration rates during the illness indicates a poor prognosis.

Treatment

Psittacosis appears to be the only virus disease definitely influenced by penicillin. Excellent therapeutic results have been reported from its use in a number of clinical cases as well as in experimental animals. Large doses are required (℞ 18) for optimal results. Under this medication secondary bacterial invasion also may be prevented. Should signs of infection by bacteria insensitive to penicillin appear, sulfadiazine (℞ 31) or streptomycin (℞ 23) may be employed. Strict isolation of the patient, with appropriate precautions for protection of attendants against respiratory discharges, whether from coughing or from sputum contact, is required (see BEDSIDE PROC.). Severe cough may be controlled with codeine (℞ 8). Expectorants (℞ 43 to 45), and inhalants (℞ 57, 58), are useful to combat a dry cough or tenacious sputum. Acetylsalicylic acid (℞ 1) or analgesic mixtures (℞ 2 to 6) are useful for headache and malaise. Restlessness and insomnia should be combated with the usual sedatives (℞ 15, 16). Aureomycin (℞ 28) and Chloromycetin (℞ 29) have each been used for the treatment of psittacosis with excellent results.

LOEFFLER'S SYNDROME

A pneumonitis characterized by transient eosinophilic infiltration of the lungs and associated with a great increase of eosinophiles in the blood and sputum.

Etiology, Pathology, and Pathologic Physiology

Numerous agents are capable of inducing Loeffler's syndrome. These include *Ascaris, Ancylostoma, Trichinella, Fasciola hepatica,* and perhaps also the tubercle bacillus, privet pollen, and *Endameba histolytica.* However, in most cases, no etiologic agent is proved, nor is a possible allergic relationship certain.

Irregular patches, ranging from a few mm. to 5 cm. in diameter, are scattered throughout the lungs, and consist of a collagenous network, in the meshes of which are numerous eosinophiles, plasma cells, lymphocytes, and giant cells. Vascular lesions resembling periarteritis nodosa are present.

Symptoms and Signs

In general, symptoms are so few that the disease usually is discovered accidentally. Most patients run an afebrile course, but slight elevation of temperature sometimes occurs. Cough, with or without a "stitch" in the side, is fairly frequent. In many of the reported cases, bronchial asthma was associated with the syndrome. Physical findings usually are minimal, with but slight increased resonance and roughened breath sounds. Various types of rales are occasionally heard, including crepitant, subcrepitant, sibilant, and sonorous. Eosinophilia is common, the average level ranging from 10 to 25%.

Diagnosis

In typical cases, transient allergic pulmonary consolidation is fairly well defined, but diagnosis depends on X-ray examination. The roentgenogram reveals rapidly developing shadows in the lungs, which disappear with equal rapidity. There are points of similarity with periarteritis nodosa and tropical eosinophilia, but ordinarily these conditions should be easily excluded.

Treatment

The disease usually runs a self-limited, benign course, but cortisone or ACTH may shorten its duration. When asthma (q.v.) is present, the usual therapy is indicated. In the presence of helminth infestations, appropriate vermifuges should be used (*see* INTESTINAL PARASITES).

PULMONARY ABSCESS

A localized area of necrosis in the pulmonary parenchyma, surrounded by an inflammatory cellular tissue reaction. The term "gangrene of the lung" often is used to denote a similar process in which there is a massive area of necrosis without a surrounding inflammatory reaction. A lung abscess may be putrid or nonputrid.

Etiology

Bronchial obstruction with infection appears to be etiologic in the majority of putrid lung abscesses. The obstruction often is caused by aspirated infected blood, pus, or mucus. Aspiration is most likely to occur during operations on the nasopharynx and oral cavity under general anesthesia, particularly in patients with poor oral hygiene. Bronchial obstruction due to benign or malignant tumors or foreign bodies often leads to abscess formation resulting from infection behind the obstruction; these abscesses frequently are nonputrid.

Putrid abscesses may be caused also by septic pulmonary emboli which produce necrosis of the bronchopulmonary segment involved. Abscesses may follow penetrating wounds of the chest, particularly those with retained foreign bodies. Pneumococcal pneumonia is not likely to produce sufficient necrosis to cause abscess, but staphylococcal pneumonia is frequently followed by abscess formation. The condition may result from extension of infection from bronchiectatic or mycotic lesions, from suppuration within a pulmonary cyst, or from degeneration within a malignant tumor.

The organisms usually cultured from lung abscesses are the common pyogenic bacteria and the inhabitants of the nasopharynx. Anaerobic organisms are largely responsible for the foul odor which is characteristic of the so-called putrid lung abscess. *Bact. melaninogenicum,* an anaerobe which produces a black pigment, is sometimes found. Spirochetes and fusiform bacilli, occasionally present, increase the putrefaction. In nonputrid abscesses, only a few varieties of organisms are present, mostly aerobes. Abscess formation is also observed in the necrotizing pneumonitis that is associated with virus infection.

Pathology

Putrid lung abscesses usually are single, but may be multiple. Nonputrid lesions are generally multiple. Multiple abscesses as a rule are unilateral; they may develop simultaneously or spread from a single focus. The lower lobes, especially of the right lung, are most frequently affected. The solitary putrid lung abscess incident to bronchial obstruction or an infected embolus starts as necrosis of the major portion of the bronchopulmonary segment involved. It usually is close to the parietal pleura, and the pleural space at this point is likely to be obliterated by inflammatory adhesions. Upon occasion, however, the abscess may occupy the bronchopleural segment facing the mediastinum, diaphragm, or interlobar space ("central abscesses").

In most instances, the abscess ruptures into a bronchus and its contents are coughed out, leaving a cavity in the lung. Failing this, it may spread to adjacent portions of the lung. Following rupture through a bronchus with adequate drainage, the walls of the abscess may collapse and contract so that the cavity eventually becomes completely obliterated. If drainage is inadequate, the abscess wall becomes fibrotic and rigid, the cavity may be lined with epithelium and healing will not occur. Occasionally, the necrotizing process advances more rapidly than the obliterative pleuritis, and the abscess perforates into the free pleural cavity. Perforation of "central abscesses" may result in mediastinal, diaphragmatic, or interlobar empyema.

Bronchi or large blood vessels may be seen as ridges on the wall of a cavity. Erosion of such vessels may cause serious hemorrhage. Septic emboli may be carried through the pulmonary veins to the arterial system and set up a secondary brain abscess or meningitis.

Symptoms and Signs

Early symptoms of lung abscess are those of any acute pneumonitis—malaise, anorexia, cough, sweats, chills, and fever. Often, there is transitory chest pain, indicating pleuritic involvement. Repeated chills are suggestive of abscess. Physical signs are those of a small area of pneumonic consolidation, chiefly dullness, with breath sounds suppressed more often than bronchial. Fine or medium moist rales may be present. In fulminating gangrene of the lung there may be severe prostration and toxicity, with a temperature of 105° F. or more.

The presence of a nonputrid lung abscess is suspected when acute pneumonitis follows a persistent or unfavorable course.

The cough continues; the fever and constitutional manifestations do not abate; there is no clearing on the roentgenograms; occasionally, a small cavitation with a fluid level is seen. Abscesses of the nonputrid variety do not as a rule give rise to the foul, unforgettable odor of breath and sputum characteristic of the putrid type.

Usually, about 1 to 3 weeks after the onset of acute symptoms, putrid abscesses perforate into a bronchus, and a large amount of foul purulent sputum may be coughed out in a few hours. The sputum may be blood streaked and contain bits of gangrenous lung tissue. Chronic lung abscess is accompanied by anorexia, weight loss, anemia, weakness, dyspnea on exertion, debility, and clubbing of the fingers. With penicillin therapy these signs of pulmonary suppuration may be minimized, but this does not necessarily denote cure. A persistent cough, at times productive, perhaps with infrequent minor hemoptysis, is evidence of a persistent lung abscess.

Physical examination of the chest may be negative, but rales and rhonchi usually are present. If the cavity is large, there may be tympany and amphoric breathing. Secondary abscess, bronchiectasis, and amyloid disease may be late complications.

Diagnosis

The most important diagnostic evidence of a lung abscess is the finding of a fluid level in a cavity on X-ray examination. This, with the symptoms and signs described above, particularly the sudden appearance of purulent sputum, is highly indicative of lung abscess. Before perforation into a bronchus has occurred, the X-ray shows only an area of consolidation and diagnosis cannot be made with certainty. Bronchoscopy should be performed in cases of obscure etiology to detect a foreign body or tumor.

Lesions that simulate lung abscess are bronchiectasis, empyema with bronchopleural fistula, tuberculosis, infected pulmonary air cyst, bronchogenic carcinoma, and subphrenic or hepatic (amebic or hydatid) abscess with perforation into a bronchus. Through bacteriologic study of the sputum, serial roentgenograms, body section roentgenograms, bronchoscopy, bronchography, microscopic search of the secretions for tumor cells, and a careful evaluation of the history and physical findings, a correct diagnosis can be made in almost all instances. Sputum with a very foul odor is characteristic of putrid lung abscess and differentiates it from nonputrid abscess and other conditions.

Prognosis

The fate of nonputrid abscesses is variable: many are absorbed and disappear with few chronic changes; others rupture into the bronchi and discharge spontaneously. If drainage through a bronchus is adequate, the acute symptoms will subside within a few days and recovery will be rapid: if not, the abscess will become chronic. Sometimes the abscess points into the pleura and gives rise to an empyema. In the putrid lung abscesses, spontaneous cures sometimes result, probably through evacuation into the nearest bronchus; in other cases the lesion progresses with increasing septic manifestations to a fatal issue. Most often the general symptoms subside and the abscess enters the subacute or chronic stage. The prognosis always is best in persons otherwise healthy and under 40 years of age, and usually good in children.

Treatment

General: In acute cases this includes bed rest, a nutritious diet, vitamins and, if necessary, hematinics. The protein intake may be supplemented by highly nutritious liquids (*see* DIETS). The patient should sleep on the affected side to prevent drainage of secretions into the sound lung.

Local and chemotherapeutic: Postural drainage is an important therapeutic measure (*see* BEDSIDE PROC.).

At onset, when an abscess frequently cannot be differentiated from a nonsuppurative pneumonitis or pneumonia, it should be treated with penicillin (℞ 18). After the abscess ruptures into a bronchus, the organisms should be cultured and tested for sensitivity to penicillin and streptomycin. The agent or combination of agents most effective *in vitro* should then be used. If streptomycin is indicated, 2 Gm. daily (℞ 23) usually will be adequate. The greatest benefit may be obtained by giving these antibiotics by a combination of I.M. injections and aerosols (℞ 20, 22, 24) or by bronchoscopic instillation into the bronchus that drains the abscess. Since the patient's progress depends largely upon adequate drainage, the cough reflex should not be suppressed. Expectorants (℞ 40, 45) should be employed. However, an irritating cough that tires the patient without giving relief should be checked with codeine (℞ 8). Foul sputum may be deodorized in part with creosote carbonate (℞ 61).

Surgical: Bronchoscopic aspiration 2 or 3 times a week will promote drainage; very thick tenacious sputum can be removed and excess granulations cauterized. If the patient is not obviously improving within 3 or 4 weeks on conservative therapy, it indicates that the drainage is not adequate, and external surgical drainage should be instituted. When this is done early, the mortality is low and the chances of cure are high. Some surgical opinion favors operation promptly upon establishment of the diagnosis. When the patient does not improve and is not subjected to external drainage, the abscess passes into the stage of chronicity and, because of the rigidity and perhaps epithelization of the chronic abscess wall, the cavity will not collapse completely, so that a cure can be expected in only a certain proportion (40% or less) of cases.

Pulmonary resection offers the best chance of complete cure for the chronic lung abscess. If there is a considerable amount of purulent sputum, indicating continued infection, it may be safer for the abscess to be drained externally and pulmonary resection done at a later date. In cases of solitary chronic abscess in which sputum has been reduced to a minimum, either by conservative treatment or open surgical drainage, complete cure often may be anticipated following pulmonary resection. The average operative mortality in such cases is 5 to 10%. When adequate drainage of multiple abscesses is not possible and the patient continues to have fever and a large amount of sputum, pulmonary resection perhaps offers the only chance for cure, despite its high mortality. A chronic abscess with hemorrhage is best treated by pulmonary resection unless acute infection is present, in which case open drainage and packing may be preferable.

PULMONARY EDEMA

An edema of the lungs, usually acute, resulting from the escape of serous fluid from the capillaries into the interstitial tissue and alveolar spaces.

Etiology, Pathologic Physiology, and Pathology

Anoxia, resulting from poor circulation, or poor ventilation in the pulmonary bed, increases capillary permeability and creates alveolar edema, which in turn exacerbates the anoxia. Thus, a vicious cycle is established.

From the clinical standpoint, the most common cause of pulmonary edema is failure of the left ventricle as a result of hypertension, coronary artery sclerosis and insufficiency, aortic valvular insufficiency or, less frequently, mitral stenosis and insufficiency, myocarditis or pericarditis. The principal factors favoring anoxia and pulmonary edema in heart disease are: (1) congestion and increased pressure in the lesser (pulmonary) circulation; (2) hemodilution, especially at night when the patient is recumbent and the blood stream picks up protein-poor fluid that was forced out of dependent capillaries during the preceding day; (3) increased blood volume with nocturnal augmentation by the same mechanism. A decrease in plasma colloids from malnutrition, liver damage, or proteinuria lowers the osmotic pressure of the blood and contributes to edema formation.

Irritant gases, fumes, and vapors are capable of causing pulmonary edema by a direct effect on the pulmonary alveolar endothelium. Symptoms and signs may occur immediately or several hours after exposure to chlorine, bromine, fumes of strong acids, ammonia, sulfur dioxide, mustard gas, phosgene, and the oxides of nitrogen and phosphorus.

Intoxication with alcohol, barbiturates, iodine, morphine, or epinephrine may be followed by more or less severe attacks of pulmonary edema, as may certain pulmonary infections.

Nervous system factors in pulmonary edema are much disputed. Loss of vagus activity has been suggested as a possible causal mechanism. There is no doubt that certain C.N.S. disorders—especially brain trauma, cerebrovascular accidents, or tumor—are occasionally complicated by anoxia and pulmonary edema. The anoxia may be due to circulatory factors, alterations in capillary permeability, or to failure of the cough reflex and other mechanisms for getting rid of pulmonary secretions. The pulmonary edema of nephritis and anemia probably is in great part secondary to circulatory failure and hypoproteinemia. Edema of the lungs is frequent as a terminal event, probably due to anoxia (q.v.) which occurs as the cardiorespiratory system fails.

Edematous lungs are large, heavy, firm, and waterlogged, sometimes pale, sometimes congested with blood. They pit on pressure and the cut surface exudes a frothy blood-tinged fluid. In subacute or chronic edema, the fluid may exhibit a gelatinous consistency. Microscopically, the essential finding is albuminous fluid within the alveolar spaces. Edema of interstitial pulmonary tissues and of the alveolar walls themselves also may be present.

Symptoms and Signs

Pulmonary edema typically occurs in attacks. The onset usually is insidious, extending over several hours of progressively more alarming symptoms, but may be abrupt. Slight cough often is an initial symptom, but there also may be asthmatic wheezing due to bronchiolar spasm. Dyspnea and orthopnea occur early, and the patient has a profound sense of oppression in the chest. In a fully developed attack he is found sitting upright gasping for breath, with the nose and mouth flecked with pink, frothy sputum. The facies exhibit a terrified anguish emphasized by pallor, sweating, and cyanosis. Cough is frequent, sometimes paroxysmal. Bubbling rales, wheezing, and sonorous rhonchi and squeaks are heard in the chest. The pulse is rapid and thin, and the blood pressure falls.

In cardiac patients, attacks of pulmonary edema represent a direct extension of either paroxysmal dyspnea or cardiac asthma (q.v.). The former may be defined as an attack of acute pulmonary congestion without transudation, while the latter is the same with an added element of bronchial constriction and perhaps early transudation of fluid as well. Pulmonary edema in the moribund or comatose patient is insidious in onset, extending over hours or days. It is refractory to treatment and usually occurs as a terminal episode or indicates impending death.

Diagnosis and Prognosis

The clinical picture, plus a history of exposure to irritant gases, fumes, or vapor, drug intoxication, preexisting pulmonary or cardiac disease, or other etiologic factors, usually is sufficient to establish the diagnosis. The prognosis in mild attacks usually is good, but the condition may be progressive, and therapy should always be instituted immediately.

Treatment

As soon as it has been determined that pulmonary edema is likely to develop or is already present, appropriate measures must be taken at once to prevent or control it. Immediate therapy is indicated for all patients exposed to any irritant gas, fume or vapor when, in the opinion of the physician, the exposure has been sufficiently great to justify the fear that pulmonary edema may be an imminent possibility.

The treatment of pulmonary edema is by immediate and absolute bed rest, oxygen, and attention to the underlying cause (*see* ETIOLOGY). The patient usually will need and assume the orthopneic position during an acute attack.

Oxygen: High concentrations (75 to 100%) must be administered at once to prevent or combat anoxia. As the anoxia is controlled, the patient's restlessness, anxiety, and dyspnea will disappear. Oxygen (O_2) is inhaled under atmospheric pressure, but with expiration being made against a positive pressure of from 1 or 2 up to 6 cm. of water (*see* CLIN. PROC.). In pulmonary edema of cardiac origin, O_2 under positive pressure must be used with due caution; the resistance level selected must be the maximum that is well tolerated by the patient and the procedure should be discontinued after 1 hour if no beneficial effect is noted. (In such instances, O_2 should be continued, though not under positive pressure.)

The volume of O_2 required by patients with pulmonary edema may be initially as high as 20 to 30 liters/minute. If a favorable response occurs, positive pressure O_2 inhalation is continued until the acute symptoms subside, after which it may be tentatively discontinued. The patient must be closely observed for any evidence of subsequent cyanosis, coughing, dyspnea or increase in the respiratory rate. Should any of these manifestations appear, further periods of O_2 inhalation must be given until discontinuance no longer results in any such symptoms or signs.

Nebulized spray of 0.5 cc. of epinephrine 1:100 (℞ 64), administered before or during O_2 administration, is a useful adjunct for those patients in whom pulmonary edema is actually present and in whom bronchiolar spasm is evident. (CAUTION! Epinephrine must never be given parenterally to these patients since it may aggravate or even cause pulmonary edema.) Aminophylline 0.48 Gm. (gr. vii) I.V. (℞ 72) likewise often proves effective, but must be given slowly.

Sedation: In acute pulmonary edema due to acute left ventricular failure, morphine (℞ 9) is indicated (*see* CONGESTIVE

HEART FAILURE). However, in acute pulmonary edema due to alveolar irritation from irritant vapors, gases or fumes, or in all cases after the appearance of severe anoxia with cyanosis, or in the presence of delirium, morphine and other sedatives are contraindicated since they depress respiration and inhibit the cough reflex.

Cardiac therapy: In attacks caused by heart disease, digitalis should be administered immediately, I.V. if necessary, provided the patient has received none in the preceding 2 weeks (see CONGESTIVE HEART FAILURE). Rapid phlebotomy of 250 to 500 cc. of blood is sometimes dramatically effective in acute cardiac episodes but should not be used in acute pulmonary edema due to irritant gases, fumes, or vapors. The effect is achieved by sharply reducing the return to the right side of the heart while the left is allowed to drain some of the excess blood from the lungs. Bloodless phlebotomy with venous tourniquets placed high on the legs and arms to trap blood in the extremities is safer and sometimes equally effective. The tourniquets should be released, one at a time in rotation, for 5 minutes every ½ hour in order to avoid ischemic damage to the extremities. The effect persists after removal of the tourniquet because a protein-poor ultrafiltrate is forced out of the capillaries of the extremities and thus the total blood volume actually is reduced.

Hypertonic solutions such as 50% glucose in 20 to 100 cc. of distilled water have been used I.V. These often will "dry out" the lungs momentarily, but the effect is transitory, and the ultimate results may be harmful, as they tend to increase blood volume.

PULMONARY EMBOLISM;
PULMONARY INFARCTION

Pulmonary embolism: *Lodgment of a clot in the pulmonary vascular bed.* **Pulmonary infarction:** *Necrosis of part of the lung parenchyma due to interruption of its blood supply, most commonly by pulmonary embolism.*

Etiology

Emboli causing pulmonary infarction usually arise from thrombosis of the deep veins in the legs or pelvis, fragments of the thrombus being carried by the blood stream to the pulmonary artery (see VENOUS THROMBOSIS). They also may originate from a mural thrombus in the right auricle or ventricle, from subacute bacterial endocarditis involving the right side of the heart, or from fat droplets from the marrow of fractured long bones. Pulmonary infarction also may result from spontaneous thrombosis of a branch of the pulmonary artery or vein, especially in the presence of congestive heart failure.

Pathologic Physiology

If a small pulmonary artery is occluded, the tissue normally supplied becomes ischemic and, if the collateral (bronchial artery) circulation is not sufficient, small areas of hemorrhagic exudation develop, usually involving the alveolar walls. The affected tissue generally is roughly wedge-shaped with the base against the pleura and the apex at the site of vascular occlusion. Capillary permeability increases, and extravasation of fluid and blood cells into alveoli results. Grossly, the affected region is firm, dark red and airless. Where the overlying pleura is involved, a localized area of fibrinous pleurisy develops.

If a large branch of a pulmonary artery is occluded, widespread hemorrhagic exudation occurs in the affected area. In addition, there is sudden obstruction to the flow of blood through part of the pulmonary circuit. Reflexes are set up via the autonomic nervous system which cause spasm of the pulmonary arteries, sometimes also of the bronchi. There follows pulmonary hypertension, overloading of the right ventricle and poor filling of the left side of the heart, with both right-sided congestion and peripheral shock. Similar reflexes may affect the rate and rhythm of the heart.

Larger emboli usually cause death within a few minutes, without sufficient time for infarction to take place. Smaller emboli with infarction may eventually heal by recanalization and restoration of pulmonary tissues, but most result in brownish retracted scars.

Symptoms and Signs

The symptomatology of pulmonary infarction depends on the size and location of the infarct. The most common symptom in patients with small infarcts is a sudden onset of pleuritic pain over the involved area, associated at times with cough. Physical examination frequently is completely negative, but a small patch of crepitant rales often may be heard. There usually is a rise in temperature and in pulse and respiratory rates. Mild leukocytosis and, a few days later, elevation of the erythrocyte sedimentation rate may occur. X-rays of the chest are frequently clear, particularly in the immediate postembolic period, though a small area of increased density may be noted, which may be radiologically indistinguishable from a pneumonitis.

Moderately large infarcts may produce the same signs and symptoms with some degree of dyspnea in addition. Hemoptysis is encountered, associated with these larger infarcts. Sometimes, a friction rub can be heard. Jaundice may be seen occasionally in patients with pulmonary infarction, especially in cardiac cases with congestive heart failure. Later, evidence of pulmonary consolidation may be found. Infrequently, there are signs and X-ray evidence of pleural effusion. The fluid may be serous or serosanguineous. A chest X-ray will often show a nonspecific irregular density, and rarely a wedge-shaped shadow with its base at the periphery of the lung. An ECG made immediately may give evidence of right ventricular strain, with right bundle branch block, exaggerated S_1 and Q_3, or inverted T_3 and T_4F.

Large pulmonary infarcts cause acute dyspnea, cyanosis, and shock. At onset, there may be pleuritic pain, or a deep, nonpleuritic sort of chest pain followed within a day or two by pleuritic pain.

Infarction at different sites may give special symptoms: At the diaphragmatic surface it may cause pain in the shoulder, or abdominal pain and rigidity. In the left lower lobe the clinical picture may closely resemble myocardial infarction, with pain radiating down the left arm and sometimes a pleuropericardial friction rub. The clinical picture of acute cor pulmonale may develop with distended veins, enlarged liver, and accentuated second pulmonic sound.

Diagnosis

Pulmonary infarction can easily be confused with bronchopneumonia, pleurisy, pericarditis, myocardial infarction, spontaneous pneumothorax (q.v.), and many other conditions. It can be differentiated only by bearing its possibility constantly in mind and searching for confirmatory evidence, and especially for signs of peripheral venous thrombosis. Pulmonary infarction should always be considered when there is a sudden onset of pleuritic pain without obvious explanation; when a case of bronchopneumonia does not follow its usual course; or when there is an unexplained pleural effusion.

Prognosis

This depends upon the extent of the original infarction, the general health, cardiac status, and the number of embolic recurrences. If not treated with anticoagulants or by venous ligation, approximately 30% of patients will suffer further nonfatal emboli, and approximately 15% will die of a subsequent embolus.

In patients who are treated with anticoagulants there is an expected incidence of 2% subsequent nonfatal pulmonary emboli and less than 1% subsequent fatal emboli. Similar successful results can be obtained by deep venous ligation.

Treatment

Therapy of pulmonary embolus is aimed primarily at reducing the fatalities which result from both the original and subsequent episodes of embolism. Once a presumptive or definite diagnosis of pulmonary embolus or infarction has been made, treatment should be instituted immediately, with complete bed rest and administration of anticoagulants (*see* ANTICOAGULANT

THERAPY). In acute severe pulmonary embolism with bronchial and arterial spasm, the following medication is recommended for the first 36 hours: (a) atropine sulfate (℞ 73) 0.6 to 1 mg. I.V. or I.M. every 3 to 6 hours; (b) papaverine hydrochloride (℞ 74) 0.1 Gm. (gr. iss) I.V. or I.M. every 3 hours. For analgesia: codeine (℞ 8), Demerol (℞ 10), or morphine (℞ 9). Relief of pleuritic pain also may be obtained by poultices, chest strapping, or intercostal nerve block with 1 to 2% procaine.

Oxygen is beneficial in cases with the more severe, acute emboli, whether or not there is significant cyanosis or dyspnea.

Sudden embolization may precipitate congestive heart failure or acute cor pulmonale. Digitalization is advisable if there is evidence of congestive failure. Prophylactic antibiotic therapy is recommended to avoid secondary infection in the infarcted area of the lung. Penicillin (℞ 18, 19) is adequate for this purpose.

The patient should be kept in bed for a minimum of 6 days, or longer depending upon the severity of the lung involvement. Anticoagulant therapy (q.v.) should be instituted immediately and continued for a minimum of 1 week during ambulation. If anticoagulant measures and their control tests are not readily available, vein ligation (*see* VENOUS THROMBOSIS) is the treatment of choice, whether or not evidence of venous thrombosis is present. For recurrent embolic phenomena in the face of adequate anticoagulant management, vein ligation may be indicated in addition to the anticoagulants.

PULMONARY FIBROSIS

A pathologic increase in connective tissue in the lung, which may be localized or diffuse, and either pleural, peribronchial, interstitial, or alveolar in distribution.

Pathologic Physiology

As will be indicated below in describing the various forms of pulmonary fibrosis, the symptoms and signs depend on the type and distribution as well as the degree of fibrous infiltration or replacement. Particular diseases (q.v.) tend to produce certain types of fibrosis. Thus, local suppuration such as abscess or localized bronchiectasis will cause localized fibrosis, whereas the lesions in silicosis are diffuse and interstitial. Tuberculosis has the most protean manifestations, and can cause practically any type of pulmonary fibrosis.

LOCALIZED PULMONARY FIBROSIS

A typical example is a single apical tuberculous lesion, such as that surrounding a cavity. Other similar organizing lesions are produced by localized organizing pneumonia, localized bronchiectasis, or a healing lung abscess. The fibrous tissue in these lesions usually is rather dense, and the involved lung tissue is thus rendered immobile and functionless. Marked shrinkage of this tissue, with some degree of compensatory emphysema in the surrounding lung, is seen. Involvement of a single lobe, or of only a portion of one lobe, with the remainder of the lungs unaffected, will not significantly disturb the patient's pulmonary function, and will produce no symptoms. However, irritation or exudate in the affected region will be accompanied by coughing or occasionally the development of asthma, if the infection results in a general sensitization.

Treatment

Treatment is that of the underlying disease. For this, surgical excision (lobectomy), when feasible, is the most definitive measure. Thoracoplasty is indicated in many tuberculous cases (q.v.).

FIBROID LUNG

Long-standing fibrocaseous tuberculosis throughout one lung not infrequently results in the so-called fibroid lung, a greatly scarred, shrunken, and functionless organ, often containing multiple cavities. The lung usually is bound to the chest by adhesions, and there is considerable shrinkage of the chest wall and displacement of mediastinum and diaphragm. Mediastinal displacement may compromise heart action or distort the great veins, causing elevated venous pressure, and may induce emphysema of the opposite lung. Unilateral fibroid lung is associated with considerable limitation of physical activity because of dyspnea, since the total breathing capacity is much diminished.

Treatment

Patients with severe mediastinal displacement sometimes experience improved pulmonary function following thoracoplasty. Otherwise, treatment is that of the underlying disease, plus symptomatic treatment for dyspnea and cough.

PLEURAL FIBROSIS

Slight pleural thickening, as revealed by X-ray, gives no signs or symptoms. Moderate pleural thickening results in dullness to percussion and diminished breath sounds, but is asymptomatic. Progressing constrictive pleurisy, however, usually due to active pleural tuberculosis, causes shrinkage and diminished expansion of the chest, and if the condition continues, the fibrosis extends into the lung parenchyma, with the end result a fibroid lung. Progressing pleural fibrosis is one of the complications, fortunately not common, of tuberculous pleurisy with effusion. An interesting physical sign which may appear within a few weeks of onset, in this condition, is homolateral atrophy of the muscles of the chest wall.

Treatment

Treatment is that of the underlying tuberculosis (q.v.).

DIFFUSE INTERSTITIAL (RESTRICTIVE) FIBROSIS

The characteristic lesion is an increase in connective tissue extending through the septums and interstitial pulmonary tissues. Elastic fibers are diminished, the pulmonary vascular bed may be decreased where the fibrosis is dense, but the alveolo-capillary membranes usually are not thickened. The chief effect on pulmonary function is a loss of elasticity and expansibility; vital capacity is decreased, and maximum breathing capacity much diminished. The patient is comfortable at rest, dyspneic on effort, the dyspnea subsiding very promptly after the effort has ceased.

Restrictive pulmonary fibrosis most commonly occurs secondary to certain forms of "nonspecific" chronic bronchitis, in which the fibrosis, starting in the submucosa of bronchi and bronchioli, extends into pulmonary septums, involving eventually all pulmonary expansile tissues. The fibrosis of healing or healed disseminated (bronchogenic) pulmonary tuberculosis may produce essentially the same clinical findings. Silicosis (q.v.) also is a diffuse interstitial fibrosis. The primary lesion here is near the terminal blood vessels and lymphatics, extending to involve the entire pulmonary lymphatic system. Other forms of interstitial restrictive fibrosis are radiation (X-ray) fibrosis and sarcoidosis of Boeck (q.v.).

The chief symptom, as indicated above, is dyspnea on exertion, its severity measured by the decrease in vital capacity and in maximum breathing capacity. Other symptoms, such as cough, sputum, episodes of recurrent infection, bronchitis, or bronchopneumonia, depend on the underlying disease.

On physical examination, the chest usually is normal in resting contour but its expansion symmetrically limited. A typical sign of significant loss of pulmonary elasticity is jerking down of the trachea with each inspiration. The percussion note over the chest is not consistently altered; breath sounds may be normal, increased, or diminished. Presence or absence of rales depends on the amount of secondary infection with exudate. X-ray may show only slight diffuse change, as in 2nd stage silicosis, or there may be heavy extra densities due to fibrous tissue infiltration.

Treatment

For the exertional dyspnea, adequate limitation of activity is the chief measure. Breathing exercises accomplish little in this condition. The prevention of recurring infection (*see*

Bronchitis; Bronchopneumonia) is the best means of arresting the advance of the disease. The condition may progress rapidly, but usually is slowly progressive over many years. In advanced states of extreme dyspnea, oxygen therapy may give symptomatic relief.

PULMONARY FIBROSIS AND EMPHYSEMA

(Combined restrictive and obstructive pulmonary insufficiency)

In a great many, if not the majority, of the conditions just described, especially "nonspecific" pulmonary fibrosis, silicosis, and tuberculous fibrosis, the pulmonary pathologic changes consist of a combination of fibrosis and diffuse pulmonary emphysema. The manifestations will therefore be partly the restrictive ones due to fibrosis, and partly those due to the overdistention and air passage obstruction of emphysema.

Treatment

The management of such cases, especially as they advance in severity, becomes increasingly the treatment of pulmonary emphysema (q.v.).

DIFFUSE ALVEOLAR FIBROSIS

An uncommon but definite clinical entity may occur, in which the major lesion is fibrous or hyaline thickening in or around the pulmonary alveolocapillary membranes. The symptoms are extreme hyperventilation, dyspnea, and cyanosis, due to impaired diffusion of oxygen from the alveoli into the blood. A high degree of arterial oxygen unsaturation is present. Certain unusual types of "nonspecific" pulmonary fibrosis are in this group, as also are scleroderma of the lung and the pulmonary changes of beryllium workers (q.v.). The last may resolve and recover; the first two progress steadily over periods of years to a fatal termination.

Treatment

Treatment is that of the basic disease. Oxygen continuously and in high concentration often is needed to give symptomatic relief.

———————

THE PNEUMOCONIOSES

A group of pulmonary abnormalities resulting from the inhalation of dust particles. Following inhalation, those particles which pass the defense mechanism of the upper respiratory tract to reach the alveoli are engulfed by phagocytes and carried into the pulmonary lymphatics. They are then deposited in the many foci of lymphoid tissue scattered throughout the framework of the lung and in the regional lymph nodes.

The benign pneumoconioses resulting from the deposition of biologically inert matter (e.g., iron, carbon) are characterized by an absence of tissue reaction. The fibrogenic pneumoconioses caused by the inhalation of free silica (quartz), asbestos, talc, and diatomaceous earth result in pulmonary fibrosis with its sequelae. The character and degree of the fibrosis depend upon the size and number of the particles inhaled. As a rule relatively large particles result in a discrete, nodular, less serious type of fibrosis; small particles cause a more serious diffuse fibrosis. A third group of materials exerts harmful effects by ill-understood mechanisms. The inhalation of either bagasse (sugar-cane fiber) or cotton fiber may result in an allergic type of reaction. The syndrome of pulmonary granulomatosis in individuals exposed to beryllium compounds is placed in the miscellaneous group of pneumoconioses because its pathogenesis still is obscure.

SIDEROSIS

A benign pneumoconiosis caused by the inhalation of fumes or dust containing iron particles. From 5 to 30 years of heavy exposure in occupations involving the welding or grinding of iron or steel are necessary for the establishment of this condition. It causes no symptoms, pulmonary fibrosis, impaired lung function, abnormal physical findings, or predisposition to tuberculosis. Chest X-ray examination reveals small discrete rounded shadows disseminated throughout the lung fields. These shadows are often misdiagnosed as being due to silicotic nodulation. No treatment is necessary.

ANTHRACOSIS

A clinically unimportant benign pneumoconiosis caused by the prolonged inhalation of coal dust having no free silica content. It is characterized by the deposition of black carbonaceous particles in the interstitial tissue and lymphatics of the lungs. It is not associated with morbidity, and besides being characteristically present in coal miners and other workers with coal, it is a common postmortem finding in the lungs of city dwellers. The anthracotic material cannot be seen on chest X-ray because it is radiolucent. No treatment is necessary.

SILICOSIS

A fibrogenic pneumoconiosis caused by the inhalation of free silica (quartz) dust, characterized by discrete nodular pulmonary fibrosis and, in its more advanced stages, by impairment of respiratory function.

Etiology

The inhalation of dust containing free crystalline silica over a prolonged period, varying from 2 to 25 years or more, is necessary for the establishment of silicosis. Industrial procedures which result in the dispersion of free silica into the air include the mining of lead, hard coal, and gold; sandstone and granite cutting; sandblasting; metallurgic processes using free silica; and the manufacture and use of silica abrasives. Only dust containing small particles of free silica (less than 10 μ and especially under 5 in size) can cause silicosis. Allowable maximum concentrations of industrial dust are stated to be from 50 to 100 million particles/cu. ft. of air if the free silica content of the dust is under 10%, but down to 5 million particles/cu. ft. if the silica content is more than 50%.

Pathology

The irritative action (apparently physiochemical in nature) of free silica in the pulmonary lymphatic structures stimulates local fibroblastic proliferation with resultant collagen formation. These irritative foci become surrounded by hyaline fibrous tissue and nodules result, uniformly distributed throughout the lungs.. These nodules may coalesce as the disease progresses, especially if infection intervenes, to form massive areas of fibrosis. As a result, much of the functioning pulmonary tissue is destroyed locally. In addition, the lung immediately about such areas is disturbed further by reason of the emphysema accompanying contracture of the scar.

In the stage of discrete nodulation pulmonary function tests show little if any decrease in maximum pulmonary ventilation. With massive fibrosis and emphysema, this function is markedly reduced, with resultant decrease in vital capacity, increase in residual air, and great reduction in work endurance. In advanced stages of massive fibrosis, there may be arterial oxygen unsaturation, and right heart hypertrophy and failure.

Symptoms, Signs, and Clinical Course

Discrete nodulation does not usually result in any significant symptoms. It is the massive conglomerate fibrosis resulting from the coalescence of nodules that is responsible for the symptoms and signs. In these cases, symptoms develop very slowly over many years. Dyspnea, which becomes more severe as the disease progresses, may be the only symptom. Cough is not common in uncomplicated silicosis: when present, it is dry or only slightly productive. The sputum may contain particles of free silica if the patient still is exposed to the substance, and even after exposure has ceased. Malaise, disturbed sleep, anorexia, chest pains, hoarseness, cyanosis, and hemoptysis may occur in the advanced stages, at which time attacks of intercurrent bronchopneumonia may occur and subsequent bronchiectasis occasionally develops. When these symptoms do occur, tuberculous disease should be suspected. Fever is rarely present unless there is complicating infection or necrosis.

Physical signs usually are slight or entirely absent with discrete nodular silicosis. In advanced cases of conglomerate fibrosis, cyanosis, tachycardia, accentuated second pulmonic heart sound, decreased chest expansion and decreased excursion of the diaphragm, areas of hyporesonance and hyperresonance, diminished intensity of breath sounds, and fine to medium rales may be present.

In the terminal stage, cor pulmonale with right-sided congestive heart failure may develop. Death usually occurs either from this cause or from a secondary diffuse bronchopneumonia; less frequently, it may be due to tuberculosis.

The X-ray findings in the early prenodular stage include only increased linear and vascular markings in the hilar areas and bronchial tree. However, silicosis cannot be diagnosed without the presence of discrete nodular shadows varying in size up to 4 mm. in diameter, distributed more or less uniformly throughout the lung fields. Advanced disease is manifested by the coalescence of these nodules and the appearance of confluent fibrosis with secondary emphysema. Hilar enlargement usually is present in this stage. Occasionally, sharply demarcated annular densities appear in the hilar areas and parenchyma due to emphysematous blebs. Evidence of atelectasis, emphysema, pleural thickening and adhesions may be observed in the 3rd stage.

Silicosis may be progressive for some years after heavy exposure is stopped, but such progression usually is self-limited. Progression after mild to moderate exposures over a period of many years usually does not occur to any appreciable degree.

The incidence of tuberculosis in silicotics is above that among the general population; therefore, one should be constantly on the alert for evidence of tuberculosis in any individual who shows even a mild degree of silicotic nodulation. The tuberculosilicotic lesion usually is an exceedingly chronic one, with dense and slowly progressive fibrosis. Those cases that progress to active tuberculosis usually occur in the later decades of life but may never reach the terminal stage of the disease. These individuals more frequently die from right heart failure or pyogenic bronchopneumonia.

Diagnosis

A diagnosis of silicosis is strongly indicated by the characteristic X-ray pattern when the patient also has an adequate history of exposure to free silica dust. Diagnosis should not rest on X-ray findings alone. It is necessary to evaluate the occupational hazard present, as determined by representative air samples demonstrating the number and size of particles of free silica in the atmosphere breathed, the duration of exposure, and the past history of similar exposures. The findings of a thorough physical examination must be correlated with these other data.

Silicosis must be differentiated from the following conditions which may present a nodular pattern on chest X-ray: miliary tuberculosis, siderosis of welders and grinders, passive hyperemia, bronchiolitis, multiple pulmonary miliary abscesses, carcinomatosis, leukemic infiltration, disseminated pulmonary actinomycosis, sarcoidosis, the pulmonary granulomatosis of beryllium workers, Hodgkin's disease, lipoid pneumonitis, fusospirochetal disease, fungus infections, pulmonary vascular changes due to age and mitral stenosis, and miliary calcifications of undetermined origin.

Prophylaxis

Prevention of silicosis in exposed workers is of major importance and requires close cooperation between the physician and the industrial hygienist. The physician should ensure healthy working personnel by means of preemployment and periodic physical and other examinations including serial chest films; by prevention, control, and follow-up of respiratory infections; and by recommending the provision of adequate preventive measures, including the transfer of workers to less hazardous occupations when indicated. The hygienist should ensure healthful working conditions by employing measures designed to keep the air-concentration of dust containing free silica well below dangerous levels, and by supervising the use of personal protective equipment.

Treatment

Once fibrosis has developed in the lungs, there is no way of removing it. Symptomatic relief of disabling silicosis following the inhalation of aluminum dust has been reported, but results so far are not conclusive.

Persons with silicosis, when their general condition is good and significant impairment of lung function has not yet resulted, should be kept on the job, provided the dust exposure can be reduced to accepted safe limits. Too often silicotic workers are given well-meant but ill-considered advice to leave the only trade for which they have had training. Invalidism, malingering, and neurosis are frequently the result of such inexperienced counsel.

Bed rest is required for patients with fever, pulmonary hemorrhage, severe dyspnea, or concurrent respiratory infections, and for those in poor general condition. Restriction of activities and removal to a warm, dry climate may be necessary in certain instances of advanced disease. Symptomatic therapy is indicated for cough (℞ 40, 47), fever and malaise (℞ 1 to 6), insomnia (℞ 16, 17), hemoptysis (q.v.), anorexia (℞ 87) and chest pain (℞ 1 to 6).

ASBESTOSIS

A fibrogenic pneumoconiosis due to the inhalation of asbestos (hydrated magnesium silicate) fiber dust. The pulmonary fibrosis occurring in asbestosis is thought to be a result of mechanical irritation caused by the inhaled fibers rather than due to chemical irritation as in silicosis. The signs, symptoms, and clinical course are similar to those of severe silicosis (q.v.). The X-ray findings differ in that the fibrosis is diffuse without nodulation, and often is described as having a "ground-glass" appearance. Treatment is similar to that for silicosis (q.v.).

BYSSINOSIS

A respiratory affection resulting from inhalation of cotton dust. Exposure for 20 to 25 years is necessary for the development of severe symptoms, most of which appear allergic in nature. Pulmonary fibrosis is not characteristic of the disease. Cough, occasionally productive of an extremely tenacious sputum, dyspnea of an asthmatic type, and a chronic bronchitis are characteristic. The symptoms usually abate when the patient is not working and reappear in exaggerated form on his return to work. Emphysema and a barrel type of chest eventually develop.

Prophylaxis and Treatment

The prevention of prolonged exposure to high concentrations of cotton dust is most important. In chronic cases, measures of value in the treatment of emphysema and chronic bronchitis (q.v.) are indicated.

BAGASSOSIS

A condition resulting from the inhalation of the dust of bagasse, a residuum of sugar cane after the extraction of the sugar, used in the cellulose industry. After several months' exposure to this dust, a pneumonitis characterized by cough, foul-smelling sputum, dyspnea, and chills and fever may develop. Chest X-ray may show diffuse ground-glass mottling throughout the lung fields. The prognosis is good with recovery in 1 to 2 months the rule.

Prophylaxis and Treatment

Preventive measures to avoid excessive inhalations of the dust are most important. Supportive treatment as indicated for an acute bronchitis (q.v.) is recommended for the acute phase of the disease.

BERYLLIOSIS

("Beryllium poisoning," "Beryllium granulomatosis," "Pulmonary changes of beryllium workers")

A disease of the respiratory tract, of uncertain etiology, thought to be caused by the inhalation of fumes or dust containing beryllium compounds and products. It may occur as an acute transient inflammation of the respiratory tract, or as a chronic disseminated granulomatous lesion of the lungs.

Etiology and Incidence

The disease is predominantly an occupational hazard present in the process of extracting beryllium from its ore and in the manufacture of such products as fluorescent lamps and corrosion-resistant alloys. Workers exposed to the sulfate and halide radicals of beryllium compounds may develop an acute nasopharyngitis, bronchitis, or pneumonitis. However, cases have been reported which incriminate also beryllium oxide and metallic beryllium. The chronic form of the disease may result apparently from only very brief exposure. It has been observed in beryllium extraction plants, in the manufacture of beryllium-copper alloys, and in the preparation and use of fluorescent beryllium powders. Such exposures are not always productive of disease. Thus, a characteristic feature is the low attack rate among workers exposed—fewer than 2% of those exposed having become affected. The onset of the chronic form may at times be delayed as much as 5 years after the exposure.

A small number of instances have been reported of berylliosis involving persons not engaged in beryllium processing but living in the vicinity—the so-called "neighborhood" cases. (Skin granulomas may develop at the sites of beryllium-contaminated wounds, such as those caused by broken fluorescent bulbs.)

Pathology

The characteristic lesion in the chronic disease is the formation of granulomatous nodules in the lungs, involving also a thickening of alveolar septums.

Symptoms and Signs

In the chronic form of this disease, symptoms of respiratory insufficiency are most prominent, and out of proportion to physical or X-ray signs. They consist of dyspnea, hyperpnea, cyanosis, and cough. The chest X-ray in early cases suggests a sandstorm in appearance. In later stages, a diffuse reticular pattern appears superimposed on the granular background. Advanced chronic cases are marked by evenly distributed nodular shadows throughout the lung fields varying in size from 1 to 5 mm. in diameter. The differential diagnosis is similar to that of silicosis, with the exception that berylliosis more closely resembles pulmonary sarcoidosis.

Prognosis and Treatment

The prognosis of the acute form of the disease is good, but the chronic form often results in progressive loss of respiratory function and may cause right heart strain and death from cor pulmonale. The treatment is essentially the same as for silicosis (q.v.).

TUBERCULOSIS

(Phthisis, Consumption)

A common, acute or chronic, communicable disease, protean in its manifestations and of relatively high mortality, caused by

the Mycobacterium tuberculosis *and characterized patholog-*
ically by inflammatory infiltrations, caseation, tubercle forma-
tion, and fibrosis. It usually affects the respiratory system, but
not uncommonly involves the gastrointestinal and genitourinary
tracts, the bones and joints, the nervous system, and the skin
and lymphatics.

Etiology

Tuberculosis in man may be caused by any one of three types
of *Myco. tuberculosis,* identical in appearance—the human, the
bovine and, rarely, the avian. The bacillus is a rod-shaped acid-
fast organism, varying from 0.5 to 4.0 μ in length and often
having a beaded appearance. It has no capsule and is mainly
composed of proteins, waxes, lipids, and polysaccharides. The
high wax and lipid content of the mycobacteria may account in
part for their resistance to ordinary disinfectants, their acid-fast
staining characteristics, and certain of the tissue reactions occurring with infection due to these organisms. They are aerobic
and may live for long periods in the dark and when refrigerated. They do not survive long when exposed to daylight,
but are very resistant to drying. The bacilli are killed by pasteurization at 60° C. for 30 minutes or by boiling for 2 minutes.

Human, bovine, and avian tubercle bacilli differ from one another in their cultural characteristics and in their virulence for
different species of animals. The bovine bacilli are highly virulent for rabbits. An I.V. injection of 0.01 mg. of bovine bacilli
into a rabbit will cause its death from disseminated tuberculosis
in 6 to 8 weeks. A similar injection of human type bacilli into
a rabbit will produce only a few nonfatal lesions. The human
and bovine types are, however, extremely virulent for the
guinea pig. The human type is responsible for almost all the
tuberculosis in man in the U.S., while the bovine type plays an
insignificant role in this country because of the pasteurization of
milk and the effective eradication of tuberculosis in cattle, the
usual reservoir for bovine tuberculosis. In certain European
countries where tuberculosis in cattle still is relatively common,
the bovine type occurs in up to 50% of the extrapulmonary
varieties of tuberculosis and in up to 30% of the pulmonary
varieties. The avian form in man is so rare as to constitute a
medical curiosity when it occurs.

Epidemiology

The tubercle bacillus may enter the body by inhalation, ingestion, or direct inoculation. Inhalation of bacilli spread by
coughing, sneezing, or expectorations from tuberculous patients
with open cavities is by far the most common method of spread.
Since the tubercle bacillus can live for a considerable period in
the dry state, inhalation of contaminated dried excreta and
sputum present in dust is a serious hazard. Ingestion of bacilli,
usually bovine, accounts in part for the abdominal types of

tuberculosis. Contaminated foods and tableware are chiefly responsible for the ingestion of the human type, and milk from tuberculous cows spreads the bovine type. Children are more likely to develop gastrointestinal tuberculosis because they are more apt to mouth contaminated articles, and have a higher frequency of exposure to possible infection through milk. Direct inoculation of the skin is a rarity but does occasionally occur.

Contributing factors: Age and sex are important factors determining the type and severity of the disease. An acute form of generalized tuberculosis often is responsible for the relatively high death rate during the first 5 years of life. Between the ages of 5 and 15 years, the mortality rates are at their lowest and then gradually increase with advancing age. The peak number of deaths occur between the ages of 35 and 50, but the mortality rates are highest for the older age groups. In the 15- to 30-year age group, the death rate among females is higher than among males, in fact more females between the ages of 15 and 19 die of tuberculosis than of any other disease. The mortality rate for men increases steadily as age advances until in the older age groups the male mortality rate is considerably higher than that for females.

Population groups with little previous exposure to the disease, especially those of the nonwhite races and certain of the thin-skinned, fair-haired peoples are more susceptible to tuberculosis. In American Negroes, the tuberculosis mortality rate is 3 to 5 times that of the whites, and the individual cases usually are more severe, with more extensive caseation and greater tendency to disseminate.

Tuberculosis never is inherited. A genetically carried weakness of resistance to the infection is, however, strongly suggested, and along with substandard living conditions may help to account for the high mortality rates encountered in the colored peoples and the other groups.

Prolonged states of fatigue, chronic alcoholism, debilitating illnesses, and pregnancy may result in a diminished ability to resist tuberculous infection. Poor socio-economic conditions associated with high tuberculosis mortality rates include poor nutrition, dirty and overcrowded quarters, inadequate housing in cold climates, insufficient clothing, and the like as significant contributory causes. Occupation also is a factor. Doctors, nurses, and hospital employees are frequently exposed to open cases. Exposure to silicious dust, which predisposes to pulmonary tuberculosis, occurs in many industries.

Incidence

The incidence of tuberculous disease must be differentiated from the incidence of tuberculous infection. Sensitivity to tuberculin as evidenced by a reaction to the tuberculin test indicates that the individual has had or has a tuberculous infection, but not necessarily disease associated with morbidity. In the U.S. at this time it is estimated that between 30 and 50% of the population reacts to tuberculin; a greater percentage in the older age groups and in congested urban areas. However, the estimated morbidity rate for tuberculous disease is about 350/100,000 population, or about 0.5% of the adult population. In 1946, the mortality rate was 36.4/100,000, or approximately $\frac{1}{10}$ the morbidity rate, indicating that $\frac{1}{10}$ of the active tuberculous patients alive any one year will die of their disease during that year. The mortality rates in other parts of the world vary from a low of approximately 30 to 40/100,000 in Denmark to 500/100,000 in Warsaw in 1944. The trend in the U.S. has been extremely encouraging in that there has been over an 80% decrease in the mortality rate during the past 50 years.

Pathogenesis

The establishment of a tuberculous infection depends upon the number and virulence of the invading tubercle bacilli and the degree of immunity of the host. A large number of virulent organisms may overcome the resistance of a relatively immune individual, or a small number of a less virulent strain may be sufficient to cause disease in a nonimmune individual. Resistance to tuberculosis may be natural or acquired. The differences in race susceptibility to tuberculosis demonstrate that there probably are differences in degrees of natural resistance. A tuberculous infection results in an acquired relative immunity which develops slowly and in man may not reach its peak for a year or longer. An allergic (hypersensitive) state, in which certain of the inflammatory mechanisms of the body react with increased intensity to the tubercle bacillus, develops in from 4 to 6 weeks after the first tuberculous infection.

The Koch phenomenon demonstrates the difference of the reaction to the tubercle bacillus in a healthy animal and in one already infected and having acquired immunity and hypersensitivity (allergy). As noted in the Koch phenomenon, a healthy guinea pig inoculated with tubercle bacilli develops a local lesion which becomes necrotic; the infection spreads to the regional lymph nodes and finally the animal dies of disseminated tuberculosis. If a guinea pig already having a tuberculous infection is reinfected in a similar way, a local lesion forms more rapidly and with a greater local inflammatory reaction (result of hypersensitivity), but the regional lymph nodes are not grossly involved and the lesion remains localized for a longer time (result of acquired immunity). These principles help account for the differences between the primary phase of human tuberculosis and the later chronic progressive phases. Primary infection in man usually consists of a local lesion and a regional adenitis, the so-called primary complex. Due to a greater natural resistance in man than in the guinea pig, death from disseminated tuberculosis usually does not occur in this phase of the disease in adults. However, in children a primary infection not uncommonly results in a hematogenous disseminated tuberculosis or a tuberculous meningitis. In chronic tuberculosis, with allergy and acquired immunity exerting their influences, the lesions are less often the sources of hematogenous dissemination. However, when they become necrotic and excavated, infectious discharges often lead to surface infection of related structures. Thus, the larynx and intestine often are infected in chronic pulmonary cases; the bladder in renal cases. A reaction to the tuberculin test (q.v.) demonstrates the presence of a state of hypersensitivity to the tubercle bacillus, but is not necessarily a measure of the degree of immunity, although the two may be closely related.

Pathology

The reaction of a tissue to infection with the tubercle bacillus may vary morphologically from tubercle formation to a diffuse inflammatory exudation. The tubercle, a proliferative type of lesion, is thought to be a healing stage of a preceding focal exudation. It is characteristic in appearance and composed of a collection of giant cells, epithelioid cells and lymphocytes. The frankly exudative lesions are the result of infiltration of the tissues with mononuclear cells, leukocytes, plasma, and fibrin. The central portion of either type of lesion may undergo caseous degeneration, liquefaction, and cavitation. Progressive necrosis in the abscess cavity may result in its rupture through surrounding structures to produce a fistula through which the necrotic liquefied matter can escape. Infection may spread from the active focus by direct extension, by way of lymphatics, tubular structures (bronchi, ureters, salpinges), or via the blood stream.

In the exudative phase, as active inflammation subsides, some of the inflammatory products may be removed by resolution. Healing then proceeds by fibrous organization; caseous lesions may become encapsulated and slowly calcify.

PULMONARY TUBERCULOSIS

A form of tuberculosis—the one most frequently encountered —*which may involve the lung parenchyma, the bronchi, and the pleura, or the bronchopulmonary lymph nodes.*

Pathogenesis

Since inhalation of the tubercle bacilli is the method by which the disease is most frequently spread, the lung is the organ in which most of the organisms are deposited.

Primary phase: The disease process which develops directly following the first implantation of the tubercle bacillus in the lung is known as the primary phase of the disease. The primary tuberculous focus is usually located near the pleura in the lower lobe or in the lower part of the upper lobe. It commonly begins as a small area of tuberculous pneumonic exudation, the center of which rapidly undergoes caseation. Lymphatic spread of infection to the regional bronchopulmonary lymph nodes takes place promptly, involving them in a caseous tuberculous process. The focus of caseous pneumonia in the lung parenchyma (Ghon tubercle) together with the regional adenitis is called the primary complex. As a rule, the lesions become arrested at this stage of their development and subsequently go on to heal by fibrosis and calcification. Two remnants of the healed primary focus almost invariably remain; a calcified primary complex which may be visible on X-ray and which may contain viable bacilli, and a state of allergy manifest by a reaction to tuberculin.

At times, particularly in infants and the colored races, the primary complex does not heal but goes on to a progressive form of the disease. The hilar lymphadenitis may become very severe, or the parenchymatous lesion may go on to cavitation. Local spread from the parenchymatous lesion by direct extension or via lymphatics may cause progressive pulmonary disease. An ulcerating primary parenchymatous focus or caseous node may rupture into a bronchus and cause tubercle bacilli to be distributed throughout a large area of the lung and result in an aspiration type of tuberculous bronchopneumonia. Either component of the primary complex may rupture into a blood vessel to result in the generalized hematogenous form of miliary tuberculosis, or give rise to tubercle bacilli which by way of the lymphatics enter the venous side of the circulatory system (lymphohematogenous spread), also to result in a generalized tuberculosis.

Chronic progressive and reinfection phase: A minority of individuals successfully recovering from a usually asymptomatic primary infection subsequently develop progressive tuberculosis. Chronic pulmonary tuberculosis is the type of symptomatic tuberculosis most commonly seen in adults, and usually follows months or years after the primary infection. This may be due to uninterrupted progression of the lesions of the primary phase (particularly in adolescent youth and young adults), or to a reactivation of these after many months or years of latency. In older people (usually past 40 years), the primary lesions may have healed, and chronic progressive disease may then be due to a new infection from without; this then is defined as a reinfection phase. In either event, the process of caseous necrosis and ulceration almost always accounts for further extension of the disease—usually represented by cavity formation in the lung, seldom by rupture of a necrotic lymph node into the bronchus.

The lesion occurring first in chronic tuberculosis, whether due to exogenous reinfection or to exacerbation of previous diseases, usually appears as one or several pneumonic foci in the subapical or midlung areas. This small infiltration, microscopic or a few centimeters in diameter, is unstable and either retro-

gresses or progresses. Retrogression usually takes place by resorption and fibrous organization, at times with calcification.
In this type of tuberculosis (sometimes called the adult type of
tuberculosis), progression occurs by means of caseation, direct
spread, and cavitation with rupture of the contents of the cavity
into a bronchus. Inhalation of this infectious pus into neighboring or more distant healthy alveoli then occurs. This is
known as bronchogenic spread, which is characteristic of the
chronic type of tuberculosis as contrasted to the lymphatic type
of spread occurring in the primary phase. Hemorrhage into a
cavity followed by aspiration of the tubercle bacilli-laden blood
into healthy portions of the lungs also is a common cause of
spread. As a consequence of peripheral extension, central caseation, liquefaction, cavitation, and bronchogenic spread, the
greater portions of both lung fields may be involved with areas
of caseation and cavitation. In most cases, little hilar involvement will be present because of relatively little lymphatic
spread.

Healing may take place at any stage of chronic pulmonary
tuberculosis as a combination of resorption, fibrosis, and calcification. It often occurs in one portion of the lung while active
disease continues in other portions. The extent of pulmonary
involvement has arbitrarily been described as minimal, moderately advanced, and far advanced. Minimal lesions are those
without demonstrable cavitation and not exceeding in equivalent volume the portion of lung which lies above the 2nd
chondrocostal junction and the spine of the 4th or body of the
5th thoracic vertebra on one side. Moderately advanced lesions
may have cavities the total diameter of which should not exceed 4 cm., and the lesions may extend through not more than
the volume of one lung or its equivalent in both lungs. Far
advanced lesions are classified as those more extensive than
the moderately advanced.

Laryngeal, oropharyngeal, and intestinal tuberculosis may
result from coughing up and swallowing infectious material coming from cavities communicating with bronchi. Hematogenous
spread resulting in generalized miliary tuberculosis occurs, but
less frequently than in primary tuberculosis.

Symptoms, Signs, and X-ray Findings

Primary phase: These cases are often not recognized as
tuberculosis. Other than a short course of unexplained fever
and some failure to gain weight, most cases exhibit no symptoms
or signs. The primary complex may or may not be detectable
by X-ray during the active stage of the disease. At times it
becomes apparent only years later, following calcification. The
development of a reaction to tuberculin indicates that a tuberculous infection is present somewhere in the body.

The symptomatic type of primary tuberculosis, more commonly seen in children and adolescent youths, is characterized

by an influenza-type course with fever up to 104°F. lasting for 2 to 3 weeks. Erythema nodosum may be present. Drowsiness, fatigue, loss of weight and appetite may occur but at times the child may appear in a good state of nutrition and quite bright and lively. Cough, dyspnea, and chest pain are uncommon and physical signs are few or absent. Infrequently, massive enlargement of the mediastinal lymph nodes causes compression of main bronchi or the trachea which may result in cyanosis, labored breathing, and a bi-tonal cough. Recovery takes place by gradual defervescence and gain in weight and appetite.

The parenchymal lesion of primary infection as seen by X-ray appears as a patch of mottling or rounded homogeneous clouding varying in size from 1 cm. or less up to the area of a lobe or more, usually in the lower ⅔ of one lung. Even where there are relatively few symptoms, there may be extensive pulmonary involvement as shown by X-ray. The outstanding X-ray feature of primary tuberculosis, especially in children, is the gross enlargement of the bronchopulmonary or mediastinal lymph nodes. Occasionally, there is widening of the superior mediastinum. During follow-up X-rays the lesions may be seen to recede with striking rapidity, or gradually to become calcified over a period of a year or two. In the adult form of primary tuberculosis, the lymph node enlargement is much less often demonstrable by X-ray.

Ulceration of one of the components of the primary complex may result in a progressive type of primary tuberculosis as a result of bronchogenic spread. Anatomically, clinically, and roentgenologically, this type of primary tuberculosis does not differ significantly from progressive reinfection tuberculosis (q.v.).

Since primary tuberculosis is noted for the ease with which lymphatic, and consequently hematogenous, spread occurs, generalized hematogenous (miliary) tuberculosis (q.v.) is seen not uncommonly, especially in infants and young children.

Progressive Pulmonary Tuberculosis: The signs and symptoms of pulmonary tuberculosis usually do not become apparent until some time after the actual appearance of the lesions on X-ray. Most frequently the onset of clinical symptoms is extremely insidious and is attended by the gradual development of fatigue, unexplained loss of weight, and anorexia. At times the onset is marked by grippelike symptoms of fever, weakness, and malaise which may last for several weeks. An acute tuberculous pneumonia may cause the first clinical symptoms.

As the disease progresses, a variety of symptoms and signs appear. The constitutional symptoms caused by **toxemia** are related to the rate and degree of progression of the disease. With extension of the lesion, loss of weight becomes increasingly obvious; lassitude, fatigue and malaise may become severe; sweating, especially at night, may assume drenching proportions; and secondary anemia may become pronounced in advanced cases. Fever, although often not noticed by the patient, usually is present. An evening temperature rise of 2 to 3 degrees occurs in most cases and, during grippelike episodes or in acute tuberculous pneumonia, swings from 97° or 98°F. in the morning to 104° or 105°F. in the evening are not uncommon.

Cough, the symptom most frequently referable to the respiratory system, as well as hemoptysis and expectoration, rarely develops until the pulmonary lesion has broken down and ulcerated into a bronchus. At first, the cough occurs only in the morning as a result of material accumulated in the bronchi overnight. As the disease progresses, the cough becomes very severe and tuberculous patients may become exhausted by the almost continuous ineffective attempts to clear the respiratory passages.

The **sputum,** which with minimal ulceration is very scanty at first, may rapidly increase to 2 or 3 ounces daily as a result of progressive pulmonary excavation. With secondary infection of the cavities it is not unusual for 10 to 12 ounces of sputum to be expectorated daily. The sputum does not separate into layers. In a caseous pneumonic liquefying lesion it appears green and purulent. As the disease process becomes more chronic with less excavation, the sputum becomes yellowish and mucoid in character. Sudden increase in the amount of sputum may mean a new cavity rupturing into a bronchus or the rupture into the lung of a localized pleural collection of fluid. Very sudden decrease in the amount of sputum may be due to a bronchial obstruction.

Hemoptysis may occasionally occur as the first symptom of reinfection pulmonary tuberculosis. It may vary from slight bloody streaking of the sputum to massive hemorrhage. It occurs in more than half the cases during some portion of the course of the disease. The bleeding usually arises as a result of rupture of blood vessels in the walls of cavities or as a result of a tuberculous ulcer of a bronchus or the trachea. Fatal hemorrhages occur in only a small percentage of the cases, and then usually in cases with long-standing cavernous tuberculosis in which a vessel in the wall of the cavity ruptures after undergoing aneurysmal dilatation.

Pain in the chest aggravated by respiratory effort is not unusual when the lesion is close to the pleura and involving it. The pain may be referred to the shoulder or hypochondrium if the diaphragmatic pleura is irritated. Wheezing and stridulous breathing may be experienced as a result of partial bronchial obstruction. Dyspnea is commonly seen during the acute febrile periods and as a result of long-standing fibrogenic tuberculosis with considerable secondary fibrosis and emphysema. A sudden onset of dyspnea may result from a spontaneous pneumothorax or a rapidly developing serous pleurisy. Hoarseness may be the result of excessive coughing or laryngeal tuberculosis.

Search for the signs of pulmonary tuberculosis should include: (a) an exhaustive chest examination calculated to discover pulmonary signs by means of careful inspection, palpation, percussion, and auscultation; (b) a thorough general physical checking to evaluate the systemic effects of toxicity and to discover whether any dissemination of the tuberculous process has taken place; and (c) adequate roentgenographic studies. The chest signs frequently are minimal even though considerable pulmonary pathology is present, emphasizing the inadequacy of relying on signs alone for the diagnosis of pulmonary tuberculosis.

In limited or early pulmonary tuberculosis careful examination of the chest may reveal no abnormal signs. At times, slight dullness, bronchovesicular breathing and a few crepitant or moderately coarse rales may be discovered over an area of little more than 1 or 2 cm. in diameter. In eliciting these, it is important to have the patient exhale, then give a single short cough at the end of expiration, then inhale again. The characteristic X-ray picture of early reinfection tuberculosis consists of a small area of cloudy mottling with translucent high lights usually in the upper ⅓ of the lung. A small central rarefaction may indicate beginning liquefaction and cavitation.

Advanced pulmonary tuberculosis may present few or no physical findings or may give rise to many unmistakable signs denoting pulmonary pathology. Depression in the chest wall, with atrophy of the muscles, narrowing of the intercostal spaces, and limitation of movement of the thoracic cage on one side, along with deviation of the trachea and apex beat of the heart, may be seen by inspection, especially in long-standing fibrosing tuberculosis. Palpation may reveal changes in tactile fremitus and the presence of a pleural rub. Percussion may disclose large areas of dullness to flatness over extensive bronchopneumonic lesions and pleural effusion, and the "cracked pot" note over large cavities. The presence on auscultation of fine, medium, or coarse rales, dry, moist, or asthmatic in type, and breath sounds diminished or increased, either normal, bronchovesicular, or bronchial in character, may help to confirm the presence of fibrosis and emphysema, of consolidation, cavitation, pleural effusion, and pneumothorax.

Roentgenographic examination of a tuberculous lung is the essential diagnostic procedure, and may reveal a variety of lesions including bronchopneumonic infiltrations, nodular infiltrations, cavities, a varying amount of fibrosis and emphysema, pleural effusions, and pneumothorax.

Laboratory Findings

There are no characteristic hematologic changes in early tuberculosis. As advanced disease develops, a hypochromic anemia usually becomes evident. Rapidly advancing disease usually results in a moderate leukocytosis. In acute tuberculous pneumonia, the white blood count may rise as high as 15,000 to 20,000 with a shift to the left. The urine in febrile tuberculosis may contain some albumin, but pyuria, hematuria, heavy albuminuria, and bacilluria when present are indicative of renal tuberculosis (q.v.).

The E.S.R. is accelerated in most cases of active tuberculosis beyond the early, progressive, minimal stage. The rate usually is proportional to the severity of the lesion, being especially rapid in progressive febrile forms of the disease. It may be normal in early cases, in advanced cases at absolute bed rest, and in old fibroid cases with or without cavitation.

Tubercle bacilli should be looked for in the sputum of all patients suspected of having pulmonary tuberculosis. The sputum is most heavily laden with tubercle bacilli in cases which have actively draining cavities, but it also may contain the bacilli in cases with early or minimal lesions even when cavitation is not demonstrable. With proper collection and examination of actual sputum (not merely saliva), tubercle bacilli can be demonstrated in more than 90% of all patients with active disease and in almost 100% of patients with draining cavities. In patients (children and others) who swallow their sputum, a specimen for examination may be obtained by aspirating the fasting stomach contents early in the morning. A patient with a cavity usually expectorates sufficient sputum for examination. The sputum should be collected over a 24-hour period, its appearance noted and its volume measured. Tubercle bacilli should be looked for in Ziehl-Neelsen stained smears (*see* Lab. Proc.) made from mucopurulent particles selected from the specimen. At least 20 minutes should be spent studying the smear before discarding it as negative. If tubercle bacilli cannot be demonstrated in repeated smears, concentration by centrifugation and chemical digestion (*see* Lab. Proc.) of the pooled sputum collected over one to several days should be done. The sediment obtained by this method then is stained and examined. Approximately 25% of sputum specimens found negative for tubercle bacilli on direct smear contain undiscovered tubercle bacilli. Culture on suitable media and guinea-pig inoculation where necessary will reveal the presence of organisms in those specimens of sputums and fasting gastric contents in which there are very few tubercle bacilli. Tubercle bacilli in pus from tuberculous abscesses, urine, pleural fluid, cerebrospinal fluid, and in other body fluids also may be detected by smear, culture, and guinea pig inoculation.

Diagnosis

Tuberculin test: A reaction to the tuberculin test always indicates the presence of a tuberculous infection. It does not, however, give information as to whether the lesion is active or inactive. When there is no reaction to tuberculin the probability is that a tuberculous infection is not present. However, a tuberculous patient may not react to tuberculin if the dose is too small, if the lesions are well healed, in the presence of certain acute infectious diseases such as influenza and measles, and sometimes during pregnancy. In the first 3 to 6 weeks following infection, allergy has not yet developed, and in terminal states of tuberculosis, allergy to tuberculin may be lost (anergic state). The intracutaneous method of Mantoux is a more sensitive test than the Pirquet cutaneous scratch test or the Vollmer patch test. For routine case-finding the Mantoux test is done by injecting 0.1 cc. of tuberculin, containing either 0.1 mg. Old Tuberculin (OT) or 0.0001 mg. of the purified protein derivative (PPD) into the superficial layer of the skin to form a wheal. A reaction, reflecting the allergic state, is indicated by redness, induration, and edema of the subcutaneous tissues after 48 hours. A reaction between 5 and 10 mm. in diameter is recorded as 1+, 10 to 20 mm. as 2+, a diameter exceeding 20 mm. as 3+, and a severe reaction with necrosis is recorded as 4+. If no reaction occurs, the test may be repeated after an interval of 4 or 5 days using 10 times the original concentration. In sick patients, 0.01 mg. OT or 0.00001 mg. of PPD is used as the initial dose. The Vollmer patch test is done by applying to the skin a piece of gauze impregnated with dried tuberculin. The strip is removed after 48 hours and the area is examined after 72 to 96 hours. A reaction consists of a red papular, occasionally vesicular, eruption.

Diagnosis of pulmonary tuberculosis is made in the majority of cases by the discovery of characteristic findings on chest X-ray. The X-ray may have been taken as a routine standard-sized film or photofluorogram in a mass survey. It may have been indicated in an infant with a positive tuberculin test. Or, it may have been taken as part of the study of a patient with vague symptoms of loss of weight, easy fatigability, persistent cough, repeated or prolonged grippelike episodes, hemoptysis, pleurisy with or without effusion, persistent unexplained fever, lymphadenopathy, fistula in ano, or chronic laryngitis with hoarseness. The finding of the lesion on X-ray, together with physical signs and positive sputum, verifies the diagnosis.

An "active" case is one in which either the X-ray signs are changing (i.e., retrogressive or progressive), or in which sputum or gastric studies are positive for tubercle bacilli. A case recorded as "activity undetermined" is one in which no tubercle bacilli can be found in smears but cultures are positive and the lesions on X-ray are stable or show slight shrinkage; or a case in which a definite conclusion cannot be reached after a thorough evaluation of clinical, laboratory, and X-ray findings. An "inactive" case is one in which there are no clinical signs of illness, the sputum studies are negative for tubercle bacilli, and the lesions seen on X-ray are stable or show slight shrinkage.

Pulmonary tuberculosis must be differentiated from other diseases (q.v.) involving the lungs, especially those associated with fever, productive cough, persisting X-ray changes, hemoptysis, and chronicity. The pneumonias, especially primary atypical, bronchiectasis, lung abscess, pulmonary neoplasms, pulmonary fibrosis, and emphysema, and the fibrogenic pneumoconioses must be ruled out. Coccidioidomycosis and histoplasmosis may simulate pulmonary tuberculosis. More rarely actinomycosis, blastomycosis, and moniliosis require differentiation. Infiltrations due to sarcoidosis may very closely resemble tubercular lesions. Pulmonary lesions secondary to cardiovascular disease such as pulmonary congestion with hemoptysis, in severe mitral stenosis, must be distinguished.

Complications

The complications of pulmonary tuberculosis may result from direct spread (intracanalicular) or hematogenous spread. Direct involvement of the pleura almost invariably occurs. Acute varieties of pulmonary tuberculosis are usually associated with more intense pleural reactions than chronic cases. A small parenchymal tuberculous focus may at times be masked by its pleural reaction. A tuberculous empyema also may result from direct extension to the pleura. Spontaneous pneumothorax occasionally occurs either as the result of ulceration of a caseous focus into the pleural sac or as a result of rupture of an emphysematous bleb occurring in chronic tuberculosis with fibrosis and emphysema. Tuberculous laryngitis (q.v.) is a common complication of advanced disease and is due in most instances to the bathing of the laryngeal structures with bacilli-laden sputum from a cavity. Less frequent is tuberculous involvement of the pharynx or tongue. Tuberculous ulcers of the larger bronchi and trachea most often result from direct extension and surface contamination; uncommonly they are caused by invasion via the peribronchial lymphatics. Intestinal tuberculosis (q.v.) occurs as a frequent complication when bacilli-laden sputum is swallowed. It usually occurs in advanced pulmonary disease with cavitation. Tuberculous pericarditis may be caused by an extension of a pleural or mediastinal involvement.

Hematogenous spread accounts for a high percentage of the complications of pulmonary tuberculosis. Generalized miliary tuberculosis (q.v.) may occur in acute or chronic forms. The more important structures involved by hematogenous spread include any of the serous membranes of the body (pleura, pericardium, peritoneum, synovia, bursa, tunica vaginalis of the testes), the genitourinary tract (q.v.), the brain and meninges (q.v.), the bones and joints (q.v.), the adrenal glands, portions of the lung remote from the primary focus, and the eye.

Other possible complications of pulmonary tuberculosis include pulmonary fibrosis and emphysema (q.v.) occurring in chronic fibrosing tuberculosis, and amyloidosis (q.v.).

Tuberculosis complicating pregnancy always is a serious problem. Generally speaking, a woman with a history of tuberculosis which has been inactive for 2 years may be allowed to become pregnant. Pregnancy is contraindicated if an active lesion is present or signs of activity have been present within the preceding 2 years. Interruption of the pregnancy may be done before but not after the 12th week. If the patient is first seen after the 12th week, irrespective of the seriousness of the tuberculous process, she should be allowed to go to term. Most patients can tolerate a normal delivery.

Prognosis

The prognosis of pulmonary tuberculosis depends upon several factors. The character and extent of the lesion are perhaps the most important considerations. An early infiltration without cavitation will almost always heal under prompt and adequate treatment. In moderately advanced disease, ⅓ of the patients die within 5 years, and with far advanced disease, most patients die within 2 to 5 years. The fibroid or fibrocalcific lesions offer a better prognosis than do the exudative bronchopneumonic lesions.

The larger the size of cavities, the more severe the clinical symptoms, and the greater the quantity of sputum raised, the poorer the outlook. Tuberculosis in infancy, early childhood, and in adolescence, especially in girls, carries a high mortality rate. Men in the older age groups have a higher mortality than women. Cases occurring in families with a history of high tuberculosis mortality and in the colored races have a poorer prognosis probably because of constitutional and racial characteristics.

Prophylaxis

The prevention of the spread of tuberculosis depends upon an adequate public health program in which the general practitioner plays a key role. Finding the case, isolating it, and treating it adequately are the essential principles. A high index of suspicion for tuberculosis on the part of the physician, mass chest X-ray surveys, and the investigation of known contacts of active cases are necessary for early diagnosis and isolation of the tuberculous patient from the community. Prevention of overcrowding, with adequate ventilation of all premises used for public gatherings, slum clearance, control of tuberculosis in cattle, and pasteurization of milk are other essential public health measures. Education of the public is needed to encourage periodic chest X-rays and physical check-ups for complaints such as chronic cough and loss of weight. Adequate facilities for the treatment of tuberculous patients should be available in the community.

Contact with tuberculous patients should be kept at a minimum especially for those who are constitutionally predisposed to the disease. Individuals who cannot avoid contact with tuberculous patients should pay strict attention to isolation measures (*see* BEDSIDE PROC.). Factors responsible for the production of malnutrition and excessive fatigue should be eliminated. Loss of weight and anemia should be corrected and fatigue avoided.

Vaccination with BCG (Bacillus Calmette-Guerin) is recommended by some for groups of tuberculin nonreactors who are relatively more exposed to tuberculosis, in an attempt to produce an active immunity. These groups include doctors, medical students, nurses, technicians, and hospital employees, individuals in the home who are unavoidably exposed, and children and adults thought to have inferior resistance who live in communities having high tuberculosis morbidity rates. The method of vaccination currently recommended is similar to the multiple-pressure method used for smallpox vaccination, in which a sewing-type needle is held tangentially to the skin and 30 punctures are made through 1 drop of BCG vaccine (℞ 84) over an area of 2 × 2.5 cm. With this method, over 90% of tuberculin nonreactors become reactors within 1 month.

Treatment

The degree of activity of a tuberculous lesion will determine the type and amount of treatment needed in a given case. Patients with clinical symptoms and laboratory evidence of activity (q.v.) are obviously in need of prompt adequate therapy.

There is a group of patients who have lesions of uncertain stability and who may have vague symptoms of fatigue and loss of weight. These patients require frequent periodic checks on X-ray status, sedimentation rate, morning, afternoon, and evening temperatures and pulses, and examination of sputum, if any, for tubercle bacilli, before a decision can be reached as to whether therapy is indicated. Usually, if this type of patient is over 30 years old, he may be kept under close observation while at work; if under 25 years, he should be observed at bed rest.

Adequate treatment usually requires hospital or sanatorium care. Home treatment should be allowed only if the diagnosis is in doubt, if the patient refuses to be hospitalized, or if no hospital facilities are available. The handling of the relatively stabilized lesion in the so-called "good chronic" is a special problem calling for expert and cooperative management by institutional staffs and family physicians.

Rest: A period of complete bed rest must be required of all patients who have active pulmonary tuberculosis. The duration of the rest period depends upon a number of factors, among which are the seriousness of the lesions, the age of the patient, his mental outlook, and whether or not collapse therapy (q.v.) is employed. Strict bed rest has its greatest value in the treatment of tuberculosis of relatively recent onset in young individuals. In such cases, almost complete resolution and disappearance of the lesion as shown by X-ray may be achieved. As a general rule bed rest should be continued until all signs of activity have disappeared, plus a sufficient time for substantial healing to take place. Several months to a year or more may be necessary. When the lesions are limited to one side of the chest, the patient is advised to rest more on the affected side, or the affected side may be splinted by placing a sand bag on it. These measures may help prevent bronchogenic spread to the other lung. The use of an equalizing pressure chamber may provide more efficient "splinting," especially for the gravely ill patient with bilateral disease.

When stability of the lesion is attained gradual activity may be allowed. A period of 6 to 12 months of gradually increasing activity, starting with sitting up in bed for a short period daily, later sitting in a chair, still later bathroom privileges, and finally allowing the patient to be up and about 1 or 2 hours daily is generally recommended during convalescence. The majority of young individuals can stand prolonged periods of bed rest. In older debilitated patients, prolonged bed rest adds the hazards of thromboembolic disease. Emotional maladjustment to long inactivity is a problem in all age groups.

Climate: Climate and altitude now are considered relatively unimportant in the treatment of pulmonary tuberculosis. Elderly, poorly nourished individuals do somewhat better in a warm, dry climate. Younger patients may derive benefit from a cool, invigorating climate. Sun bathing and artificial heliotherapy are of little value and may actually be dangerous. Fresh air and air baths may be of use in stimulating appetite and for their psychotherapeutic value.

Diet: There are no virtues in many of the special diets recommended for the treatment of tuberculosis. Overfeeding is not necessary. All that is needed is a balanced diet with adequate amounts of the foodstuffs known to be necessary for the maintenance of good general health. The average patient should be given between 3,000 and 4,000 calories a day, supplemented with a glass of milk between meals. Vitamin supplementation is of value especially in advanced disease in which vitamin A and ascorbic acid deficiencies have been found.

Psychotherapy: Removal of emotional tension is necessary for the establishment of complete rest. Psychiatric counseling with the aid of the social worker may be necessary to help the patient adjust to the prospect of a long-drawn-out, confining illness, and assist him in his emotional, economic, and family problems. Recreational and occupational therapy, and helping the patient return to work when his condition improves, are further duties of the social worker.

Specific therapy: Streptomycin, dihydrostreptomycin, and para-aminosalicylic acid are chemotherapeutic agents of distinct usefulness in the treatment of tuberculosis. They favorably affect a majority of progressive or stationary exudative lesions, and are of value in the treatment of caseous pneumonia and subacute or chronic disseminated pulmonary tuberculosis. It is generally agreed that streptomycin or dihydrostreptomycin should not be used in minimal lesions which usually respond promptly to bed rest. This precaution is necessary because of the probability of the development of resistant strains of tubercle bacilli which will not respond to the antibiotic should a progressive form of tuberculosis later occur. Streptomycin and dihydrostreptomycin have little or no therapeutic effect on old fibrotic or caseating lesions or on terminal types of pulmonary tuberculosis. However, in terminal cases, even though these drugs may offer little hope of curing the disease, they often lessen the pain, cough, amount of sputum and other distressing symptoms.

Para-aminosalicylic acid is indicated chiefly as an adjuvant to streptomycin or dihydrostreptomycin therapy, since it delays the emergence of organismal resistance to these drugs. It may be used alone, however, when streptomycin and dihydrostreptomycin are contraindicated or have proved ineffective, since it possesses antituberculous activity itself.

Antibiotic substances should not be substituted for conventional measures used in the treatment of tuberculosis but should be used as adjuvants. They are useful in preparing patients for certain forms of collapse therapy or other surgical procedures. However, it is advisable not to administer the drugs as routine prophylactics, but to confine their preoperative use to cases in which ulcerative endobronchial lesions or grossly infected cavities already exist and to patients undergoing pulmonary resections. In other patients, the drugs should be held in reserve to combat possible postoperative spreads.

Certain of the complications of pulmonary tuberculosis are particularly susceptible to antimicrobial therapy. The antibiotics are definitely effective in ulcerative or granulomatous lesions of the oropharynx, larynx, and tracheobronchial tree. Draining cutaneous sinuses respond promptly and favorably. Generalized miliary tuberculosis (q.v.) often responds dramatically and tuberculous meningitis (q.v.) may be favorably affected.

The development of resistance of the tubercle bacillus to streptomycin or dihydrostreptomycin is frequent and limits the period over which these antibiotics may be effective. Toxic effects on the 8th nerve, as manifested by impairment of vestibular function in patients treated with streptomycin, may occur in perhaps 15% of patients on a dose of 1 Gm. daily for 42 days, the incidence increasing with greater dosage and prolongation of treatment. Neurotoxicity following the use of dihydrostreptomycin in doses of 1 to 2 Gm. for 42 to 60 days is significantly less and slower to appear. Involvement of the auditory portion of the 8th nerve is rare with present dosage schedules of either streptomycin or dihydrostreptomycin and deafness hardly ever occurs if the drug is stopped promptly, should tinnitus develop.

The minimal effective dose of streptomycin (℞ 23) or dihydrostreptomycin (℞ 25), and the maximum effective duration of therapy to achieve the perfect balance between the avoidance of resistance and full therapeutic effect are not yet determined. With streptomycin, between 15 and 20 mg./Kg. body wt./day is the recommended dose, which, in a 75-Kg. patient, amounts to between 1 and 1.5 Gm. daily, individual doses not to exceed 1 Gm., given for from 42 to 90 or more days. In general, the dosage of dihydrostreptomycin is the same, but, because of its lesser toxicity, this drug can be given in daily dosage up to 2 or 3 Gm. (20 to 40 mg./Kg.) when so desired. A trend to decrease the period of therapy toward the lower limit so as to reduce the hazard of developing strains of streptomycin-resistant organisms, now is giving way to the practice of concomitant use of para-aminosalicylic acid, which significantly delays the emergence of drug-resistant strains.

The recommended daily dose of para-aminosalicylic acid is 10 to 15 Gm., given orally in 4 divided doses after each meal, and with aluminum hydroxide gel at bedtime, for a period of 90 to 120 days or longer. It may be given as a tablet or capsule (℞ 26) or in solution (℞ 27).

Symptomatic treatment: Cough, hemoptysis and chest pain require symptomatic therapy. Steam inhalation (℞ 58) or oil spray (℞ 59) may lessen cough due to laryngeal irritation. Bronchodilator sprays (℞ 64) are sometimes of value for patients with asthma or asthmatic cough, to help raise sputum and ease respiration. Expectorant cough mixtures (℞ 42 to 45) may help loosen a cough productive of a thick and tenacious sputum. If large amounts of material accumulate in cavities, postural drainage 15 to 30 minutes 3 or 4 times daily, is useful in reducing the coughing (*see* BEDSIDE PROC.). The patient should not try to raise sputum until it is ready to be expectorated with little effort. Only when these measures fail to alleviate a severe exhausting cough should codeine (℞ 8) or other cough preventive (℞ 54 to 56) be used.

Chest pain may be relieved by adhesive plaster strapping, analgesics such as acetophenetidin (℞ 3), and, only if very severe, by opiates (℞ 9, 11). Infiltration of 1% procaine into the area of the affected intercostal space may be of use. Night sweats may be partially prevented by having the patient sleep in a cool and airy room and avoiding excessive bed clothes. A bedtime bath with dilute alcohol, vinegar and water (℞ 82), formaldehyde-alcohol (℞ 80), or an alum solution (℞ 81) may be helpful.

Hemoptysis, often a distressing symptom, is discussed elsewhere (q.v.). Phenobarbital (Ŗ 16) or other sedatives are often indicated to enable the patient to relax both mentally and physically. Ferrous sulfate (Ŗ 86) or other iron preparations may be of value in combating associated anemia.

Collapse therapy should be used mainly to promote cavity closure and healing and to prevent further bronchogenic dissemination or infection of other persons. Rest alone offers little or no hope for accomplishing closure if the cavity diameter exceeds 2 to 3 cm. Collapse or immobilization of all or part of a lung may be induced by artificial pneumothorax, with intrapleural pneumonolysis if adhesions prevent collapse, paralysis of the hemidiaphragm by crushing or cutting the phrenic nerve, or by pneumoperitoneum. Thoracoplasty may be necessary in those cases in which the above less drastic measures fail or when the disease process is so severe that little benefit can be expected from them. A limited thoracoplasty, 3 to 5 ribs, is sometimes the procedure of choice for selective collapse of an upper lobe lesion. Thoracotomy for the purpose of draining a cavity (cavernostomy) is occasionally of value. Lobectomy or pneumonectomy is indicated in certain cases of unilateral disease.

GENERALIZED HEMATOGENOUS TUBERCULOSIS

(Miliary tuberculosis; Lymphohematogenous tuberculosis)

A tuberculous infection involving any or all of the organs of the body, due to a "seeding" of these structures via the blood stream with tubercle bacilli, originating from an unencapsulated tuberculous focus. It may exist in acute, subacute, or chronic form.

Pathogenesis

Tubercle bacilli gain access to the blood stream by extension from a caseous focus via the lymphatics and thoracic duct into the venous circulation, or by rupture of a caseous focus directly into a blood vessel. In children, systemic dissemination usually arises from a caseating lymph node of the primary complex; in adults a secondary lesion usually is responsible. The lesions of hematogenous tuberculosis vary from purely productive (the miliary tubercle) to necrotic (a caseating focus). Pulmonary involvement may simulate a caseous pneumonia.

Depending upon the number and virulence of the invading tubercle bacilli, the site at which they gain access to the general circulation, and the relative immunity of the host, hematogenous tuberculosis takes various forms. It may be so serious as to cause death in a relatively short time or it may be so mild as to cause no symptoms. Parts of only 1 or 2 organs may be involved, or the infection may be generalized and involve almost every organ in the body.

Symptoms, Signs, and Course

Acute form: Occurs most frequently in infants and children and occasionally in highly susceptible adults. Previous to the onset of this form of the disease the patient may have appeared to be in excellent health or may have had signs of inactive or active pulmonary tuberculosis. The onset of acute generalized miliary tuberculosis usually is influenza-like in nature with muscle pain, headache, fatigue, and fever as high as 104° F. These symptoms may appear suddenly or develop over a week's time. Other symptoms depend upon which organ systems are predominantly involved. With meningeal involvement, symptoms of meningitis (q.v.) will become apparent; with serous membrane involvement, effusions may accumulate in the serous cavities; with lung involvement, dyspnea and cyanosis may be severe, but cough usually is absent or slight.

During the first week of the acute form of the disease, the signs are usually limited to those of toxemia. Then, depending upon the systems predominantly involved, other signs may develop. Rales may be heard in the lungs; fluid may be demonstrated in any of the serous cavities (pleura, peritoneum, synovia, pericardium); lymphadenopathy may be evident; the spleen occasionally becomes palpable. Miliary tubercles may be seen in the choroid upon ophthalmoscopic examination. At first, the chest X-ray shows nothing characteristic, but after 2 to 3 weeks, miliary stippling of the entire lung fields is a common finding.

Subacute form: The onset of this form of the disease is more insidious. Fatigue, loss of weight, malaise, and fever develop over several weeks. The infection is less overwhelming and fewer lesions are established in the various organs. A greater variety of manifestations develop, however, because the patient lives longer, allowing for the development of local lesions. Lymphadenopathy is more prominent, splenomegaly more frequently seen, and progressive ulcerative pulmonary tuberculosis often develops subsequent to the miliary "seeding." Symptoms and signs of genitourinary tuberculosis (q.v.), bone and joint tuberculosis (q.v.), or skin tuberculosis (q.v.) frequently develop during the illness. A majority of the patients die within 3 to 6 months but some live for many years with partially healed lesions in the organ systems involved.

Chronic and latent forms: Chronic hematogenous tuberculosis is characterized by a paucity of symptoms and signs. It is most insidious in onset and may persist for years in latent form with episodic exacerbations referable to one or another organ. Prolonged fatigability, loss of weight, and low grade fever may persist for months. Exudation or plastic inflammation of the serous membranes may appear. Physical examination of the chest may reveal few or no rales and signs of emphysema. The chest X-ray may show finely nodular densities throughout the lung fields, especially prominent in the apices. An abdominal flat film may reveal calcific areas in the region of the kidneys, spleen, or lymph nodes. Lesions in the genitourinary tract (q.v.), bones and joints (q.v.), skin (q.v.) and elsewhere may cause symptoms and signs which establish the diagnosis.

Diagnosis

Hematogenous tuberculosis must be considered in any case running an unexplained febrile course. A history of lymphadenopathy, pleurisy with effusion, osteoarticular disease, an unusually prominent primary complex on chest X-ray, or a leukopenia with an increase in monocytes, makes the diagnosis likely. The presence of a reaction to tuberculin, or, better, the change from no reaction to the appearance of a reaction during the period of observation, is confirmatory evidence. Constant observation for the development of any localizing tuberculous complication is necessary. Frequent chest X-rays may reveal the development of miliary lesions in the lungs. A pleural effusion may develop which, upon culture or guinea pig inoculation, may reveal the presence of tubercle bacilli. Tubercle bacilli may similarly be identified in the urine if the kidneys become involved, in the spinal fluid if the meninges are affected, and in the sputum if the pulmonary lesions break down.

The discovery of "typical" miliary lesions on chest X-ray is not in itself sufficient to make certain the diagnosis of miliary tuberculosis. Sarcoidosis, coccidioidomycosis, histoplasmosis, pneumoconiosis, pulmonary congestion in heart failure, diffuse bronchopneumonia, and multiple tubercular foci following a bronchogenic spread may present a similar X-ray picture. Brucellosis, typhoid fever, subacute bacterial endocarditis, malaria, Hodgkin's disease, and disseminated lupus erythematosus may clinically simulate hematogenous tuberculosis.

Treatment

The treatment of hematogenous tuberculosis varies with the acuteness of the disease and organ systems involved. The therapy of the pulmonary, meningeal, genitourinary, gastrointestinal, and osteo-articular complications of the hematogenous form of the disease is discussed in the chapters concerning these subjects. Streptomycin or dihydrostreptomycin (R 23, 25) is of considerable value in the treatment of the acute and subacute disseminated forms of the disease. An average daily total of 2 Gm. (but not exceeding 3 Gm.) is given I.M. in divided doses for 120 or more days. (For information on administration and the use of para-aminosalicylic acid, see Specific Therapy, under Pulmonary Tuberculosis.) In addition to specific antibiotic therapy, active supportive treatment is indicated for the patient with severe acute miliary tuberculosis. He may be so ill as to require I.V. hydration and alimentation (q.v.) and vitamin supplements. Blood transfusions may be helpful. In the less acute form of the disease, supportive treatment as outlined in the treatment of pulmonary tuberculosis is indicated.

HEMOPTYSIS

Coughing up of blood as a result of bleeding in any portion of the respiratory tract, most often due to tuberculosis, bronchiectasis, or mitral stenosis.

Etiology

The most frequent cause of hemoptysis is pulmonary tuberculosis. Other inflammatory lesions of the respiratory tract also responsible are: bronchiectasis; lung abscess; syphilitic ulceration of the larynx, trachea, or bronchi; fungus infection and parasitic infestation of the lung; and occasionally the hyperemia associated with catarrhal inflammation, as in pertussis. In an acute pneumonia, the sputum often contains blood, either fresh or old (rusty sputum). Vascular lesions are a common cause of respiratory tract bleeding. Diapedesis of blood into the alveoli or rupture of bronchial veins as a result of pulmonary congestion occurs frequently in congestive heart failure, especially when due to mitral stenosis. Pulmonary infarction, erosion of a bronchial wall by an aortic aneurysm, bleeding from local telangiectases of the bronchial tree, and vicarious menstruation are other causes referable to the circulatory system. Neoplasms of the trachea, bronchi, or lungs commonly cause hemoptysis. Penetrating and crushing wounds of the thorax may injure the lungs and result in bleeding. A less frequent cause is one of the hemorrhagic diseases: idiopathic thrombocytopenic purpura, the secondary purpuras, hemorrhagic disease of the newborn, leukemia, scurvy, and hemophilia. Overdosage with the anticoagulants, dicumarol and heparin, also may cause pulmonary bleeding.

Diagnosis

The bleeding may vary in amount from the small quantity causing blood-streaking of the sputum to the large amounts causing massive hemorrhage and death. Severe hemorrhage causes death by the patient's drowning in his own blood rather than as a result of blood loss, except for the almost instantaneous exitus that may occur with the sudden exsanguination of a ruptured aortic aneurysm. In hemoptysis, the blood usually is bright red and frothy, alkaline, mixed with mucus or pus, and has a salty taste. It must be differentiated from the dark red or black, acid-reacting blood of hematemesis (q.v.).

Care also must be taken to differentiate true pulmonary bleeding from blood or hemorrhagic exudate dropping down into the tracheobronchial passages from the nose, mouth, or nasopharynx.

Treatment

Proper treatment of the underlying cause is the most important factor in the control of hemoptysis. The presence of streaks of blood in the sputum requires no special symptomatic treatment. However, more severe bleeding requires symptomatic treatment, whatever the cause. The patient should be put at absolute bed rest and encouraged to lie on the affected side. He should cough with the glottis open, without straining. If the coughing is violent, codeine (℞ 8) may be given to suppress but not completely abolish the cough reflex. Sedatives (℞ 16) are indicated to relieve the patient's anxiety. If the coagulating properties of the blood are disturbed, as in the hemorrhagic diseases (q.v.), or excessive dosage with dicumarol and heparin (see ANTICOAGULANT THERAPY), then vitamin K, calcium gluconate, and blood transfusions may be indicated. For prolonged moderate or sudden severe hemoptysis, especially in cavernous tuberculosis, lung collapse by pneumothorax, pneumoperitoneum, or diaphragmatic paralysis may be indicated. Severe exsanguination may require blood transfusion and other measures of value in the treatment of shock (q.v.) due to blood loss.

PNEUMOTHORAX

Free air in the pleural cavity, between chest wall and lung.

Etiology

Induced: Pneumothorax may be used as a therapeutic measure or a diagnostic procedure (to outline masses or replace fluid for better roentgenographic visualization of structures within the chest).

Traumatic: Perforation of the chest wall (gunshot, stab, auto accidents, falls), or traumatic rupture of the lung (direct force, crushing injuries, blasts) frequently provides access of air to the pleural cavity. A fractured rib may tear both the parietal and visceral pleura, or a thoracentesis needle may puncture the visceral pleura and a small branch bronchus, thereby producing pneumothorax. Occasionally, pneumothorax follows bronchoscopy, esophagoscopy, sympathectomy, or renal operations.

Spontaneous: This term includes: (1) Pneumothorax occurring in the course of some pulmonary disease (e.g., tuberculosis, abscess, emphysema, bronchiectasis, silicosis, tumor) or occasionally from perforation of the pleura by erosion through the diaphragm (e.g., malignant tumor of the stomach or colon, or a liver abscess). Evidence of the disease process usually is present before the sudden episode of pneumothorax occurs. Roentgenographic signs of the disease usually are seen in the collapsed or contralateral lung, but sometimes in early tuberculosis the lung fields are negative to X-ray studies. Tuberculosis accounts for approximately 90% of this type of pneumothorax. (2) Idiopathic spontaneous pneumothorax (pneumothorax simplex), spontaneous pneumothorax occurring in the apparently healthy. This form occurs most frequently in the age group 20 to 40, more often in males, and more commonly in the right lung. Rupture of an emphysematous bleb on the visceral pleura is thought to be the cause. These blebs may result from a congenital defect or more likely from the effect of a valvelike obstruction of a small terminal pulmonary subdivision caused by the healed scar of a previous infection. With this mechanism established, sudden strains or violent coughs could be expected to rupture the bleb. However, some ruptures occur without cough or exertion, and have been reported during high-altitude flying. These are apparently associated with hyperventilation and atmospheric pressure change. Simultaneous bilateral spontaneous pneumothorax has occurred.

Tension pneumothorax (pressure pneumothorax, valvular pneumothorax): This includes any type of pneumothorax in which the intrapleural pressure is greater than the atmospheric. In these cases, the margins or edges of the tear in the pleura are in apposition and form a valve which permits air to enter the pleural sac, but prevents its escape so that each respiratory excursion tends to increase the pressure. This displaces the heart and mediastinum and, with the increased pressure, not only interferes with remaining ventilation, but also embarrasses the circulation.

Symptoms and Signs

The symptoms of acute pneumothorax depend largely on the speed and extent of its development. Usually, there is a sudden sharp pain in the chest, difficulty in breathing and often a dry, hacking cough. The pain may be referred to the corresponding shoulder, across the chest, or down over the abdomen and may simulate an acute coronary occlusion or an acute abdomen. Signs of shock and circulatory collapse may appear, but these are unusual. As the affected lung collapses and the intrapulmonary and intrapleural pressures become equalized, the acute distress subsides. With collapse of the lung, any opening in the parietal pleura usually closes.

On physical examination there usually is limitation of motion and hyperinflation on the affected side. Tactile fremitus is diminished or absent. The percussion note is hyperresonant. The breath sounds are diminished or absent on the affected side and exaggerated on the opposite side. When there is a positive pressure pneumothorax the coin test is positive. Displacement of the cardiac dullness and apex beat away from the affected side (more marked on expiration than on inspiration) produces the so-called shifting apex or pendulum heart, demonstrated best by fluoroscope. The chest roentgenogram usually is characteristic, showing absence of lung markings peripherally with a definite lung margin. However, in routine inspiratory roentgenograms a small pneumothorax may be easily overlooked, whereas it would be obvious in an expiratory film.

41

Treatment

Spontaneous pneumothorax ordinarily does not require any special treatment other than rest. The patient's activity should be moderately restricted until the ruptured pleura heals and the lung re-expands (usually 3 or 4 weeks). Progress should be checked by frequent fluoroscopic or roentgenographic examinations. Some consider it advisable to test the intrapleural pressure at regular intervals.

If symptoms of tension pneumothorax are present or later appear (restlessness, anxiety, increasing dyspnea), or if there is evidence of bilateral pneumothorax, immediate aspiration of air from the pleural cavity is necessary (*see* CLIN. PROC.). Sufficient air should be removed to relieve the symptoms and bring the intrapleural pressure down to zero. If symptoms recur after successive air removals, indicating a persistent tension pneumothorax, a blunt needle should be left in place in the pleural cavity connected by rubber tubing to a water trap, the end of the tubing to be not more than 1 cm. below the surface. In this way a positive pressure greater than 1 cm. of water will be relieved.

Oxygen given by mask (*see* CLIN. PROC.) is of value for dyspnea during the acute phase of tension pneumothorax. Sedatives (R 16) and codeine (R 8) for pain usually are all that will be needed. Morphine (R 9) may be used in single, small doses for severe dyspnea or anxiety, but should not be repeated within 12 hours because of its tendency to depress the respiratory center.

Recurrences develop in about 5% of pneumothoraces and usually require special treatment. There are two viewpoints as to the management of recurring spontaneous pneumothorax. The first is to maintain the pneumothorax, keeping the lung collapsed, thereby favoring healing of the ruptured area. The second method is to insert material into the pleural sac that will cause a mild pleuritis which favors the formation of adhesions between the visceral and parietal pleura, and in this way to prevent recurrences. Various substances have been used, such as sterile culture broth, 50% glucose, 1% silver nitrate, even powdered talc. The least harmful and probably the best is blood plasma with small amounts of the patient's own blood added to it. The possibility of infection is reduced by the addition of 50,000 u. of penicillin to the plasma-blood mixture. In rare instances, surgical resection of that portion of the lung that contains the fistula tract is justifiable.

PLEURISY

An inflammation of the pleura, which may be of a fibrinous ("dry") type, or a serofibrinous type accompanied by non-

purulent effusion. A third type is **empyema** (q.v.) characterized by an accumulation of purulent exudate.

FIBRINOUS PLEURISY

("Dry" pleurisy)

Etiology and Pathology

Pleurisy often is classified as primary and secondary. Most instances of so-called primary pleurisy probably represent extension of infection from an unrecognized subpleural focus. So many of these patients later develop tuberculosis that primary pleurisy should be regarded as tuberculous until proved otherwise. Epidemic pleurodynia seems to be a true primary pleuritis, presumably caused by a filtrable virus not yet isolated.

Pleurisy often accompanies inflammatory lung disease and may complicate mediastinitis, pericarditis, infections of the chest wall, and subdiaphragmatic disease. It also may accompany pulmonary infarction, malignancy, and trauma to the chest wall. Pleuritic pain may occur in uremia, rheumatic fever, disseminated lupus erythematosus, and periarteritis nodosa.

The area of pleural involvement may be small or may include almost the entire pleural surface. Grossly, the pleural membrane may show changes ranging from a slight loss of luster to those of severe inflammation with deposition of fibrin. The microscopic picture will depend on the underlying disease but will show in varying degree disruption of the pleural endothelium and fibrin deposition. The fibrin may be reabsorbed, or organized into fibrous tissue with resultant pleural adhesions.

Symptoms and Signs

Pain is the dominant symptom of pleurisy. Usually, onset is sudden. The pain may vary from vague discomfort to an intense, sharp, stabbing sensation. It is aggravated by respiration, but may be present only on deep breathing or coughing.

The pain of pleurisy is due to inflammation of the parietal pleura. The visceral pleura is insensitive. Since parietal pleura is innervated by the intercostal nerves, pain usually is felt over the site of pleuritis. The central portion of the diaphragmatic pleura is innervated by the phrenic nerve and involvement of this area causes pain referred to the neck and shoulder. The posterior and peripheral portions of the diaphragmatic pleura are supplied by the lower 6 thoracic nerves and irritation of these portions of the pleura may cause pain referred to the lower chest wall or to the abdomen. Diaphragmatic pleurisy may therefore simulate intra-abdominal disease. The patient usually prefers to lie on or press the affected side in an effort to limit respiratory excursion.

Respiration tends to be rapid and shallow, and motion of the affected side may be limited. Unless the process is long-standing and pleural thickening has developed, the percussion note and tactile fremitus will be normal. Breath sounds in acute pleuritis may be diminished because of the restriction of respiratory motion. The dominant physical sign is the pleural friction rub, which in some instances may be elicited by palpation as well as by auscultation. It varies from early fine crackles to a fully developed harsh grating, creaking, or leathery sound synchronous with respiration and usually heard in both inspiration and expiration. Friction sounds due to a pleuritis adjacent to the heart may vary with the heart beat as well as with respiration. While fever and malaise almost always accompany pleurisy, the clinical picture will vary with the underlying disease.

Diagnosis

The diagnosis of pleurisy usually is made readily, as the pleuritic pain and the friction rub are so characteristic. Diaphragmatic pleurisy may be differentiated from acute inflammatory disease of the abdomen by the presence of a respiratory infection; absence of nausea or vomiting; marked aggravation of pain by deep respirations or cough; shallow rapid breathing; tendency toward relief of pain by pressure on the abdomen.

A pleural friction rub may occasionally be heard in severely dehydrated patients. This rub disappears with hydration. The friction rub of pericarditis may be confused with that of pleurisy, but usually is heard best over the left border of the sternum in the 3rd and 4th interspaces. Unlike the pleural friction rub, the pericardial rub is not significantly influenced by respiration though there may be some variation in its intensity synchronous with respiration. Intercostal neuritis may be confused with pleurisy but the pain rarely is related to respiration and there is no friction rub. If the neuritis is herpetic, development of the characteristic herpetic eruption establishes the diagnosis; pain may be present for months after the herpetic eruption subsides.

Treatment

Therapy of the underlying disease is essential. The patient should remain in bed until the temperature has been normal for as long a period as it was elevated. Relief of pain is paramount. Regardless of the etiology of the pleurisy, pain may be lessened by the local application of heat. Strapping of the involved hemithorax with adhesive tape may relieve severe pain. Strapping should be applied with the patient holding his breath after a maximal expiratory effort. If adhesive strapping is not advisable, the involved area may be included in an elastic bandage encircling the entire thorax, snugly applied over and pinned to an undergarment. If these measures, supplemented by acetylsalicylic acid (℞ 1) or codeine (℞ 8) or both (℞ 2) do not give satisfactory relief, the intercostal nerves may be blocked by paravertebral infiltration with 1% procaine. If absolutely necessary, morphine (℞ 9) or Demerol (℞ 10) may be administered for relief of pain.

SEROFIBRINOUS PLEURISY
(Pleurisy with effusion)

Etiology and Pathology

Serofibrinous pleurisy may be regarded as a sequel to fibrinous pleurisy and of similar etiology. Many cases clinically diagnosed as fibrinous pleurisy probably have some serous exudate, which is not detected since less than 100 cc. of fluid is not apparent on routine X-ray examination. Tuberculosis is the most common cause of serofibrinous pleurisy in younger people, and malignancy in older people.

The pathology of serofibrinous pleurisy differs from that of fibrinous pleurisy described in the preceding section only by the presence of serous exudate in the pleural cavity, which may vary from a small amount to as much as 5 liters.

Symptoms and Signs

Onset of serofibrinous pleurisy depends on the underlying disease. It may be so insidious that the patient is symptom-free except for a vague feeling of malaise; or onset may be dramatic, with transient pleural pain, high fever, prostration, and rapidly developing dyspnea. Often there is a history of mild pleuritic pain lasting several months followed by a period of relative comfort presumably due to separation of pleural surfaces by the accumulation of fluid.

The effect of the effusion depends on its size and rate of accumulation. Large collections of fluid may greatly reduce the vital capacity by reducing pulmonary volume. The heart may be severely embarrassed by interference with venous return as well as by increased pressure in the pulmonary circuit. Rarely, the weight of the fluid may invert the diaphragm, further reducing respiratory capacity and hampering venous return. Large amounts of pleural fluid can be tolerated without significant dyspnea, however, if it accumulates slowly.

A friction rub may be heard early in the disease but, as the pleural surfaces become separated by the effusion, it disappears. The signs of pleural effusion depend on the amount of fluid present and the mobility of the mediastinum. A thin layer of fluid between the pleural surfaces may produce only slight dullness to percussion and slight interference with the transmission of tactile fremitus, vocal fremitus, or breath sounds. A large pleural effusion will cause diminished respiratory excursion of the affected side, bulging of the interspaces, deviation of the trachea, and a shift of the apical impulse away from the affected hemithorax. The percussion note will be dull or flat over the fluid and hyperresonant above. The area of cardiac dullness may be displaced. Tactile fremitus will be diminished or absent over the fluid, as are breath sounds and voice sounds, although there may be rather loud bronchial breathing and egophony at the upper border of the effusion. If pneumothorax is present, the upper border of fluid can be sharply defined by percussion, and succussion splashes may be heard. Small areas of atelectasis may be impossible to distinguish from small collections of fluid except by X-ray. If the physical signs are minimal, the patient may be asked to cough deeply several times, and if physical signs then change, it is safe to assume that the original findings were due to small areas of atelectasis rather than to a thin layer of fluid or to pleural thickening.

Diagnosis

Usually, the diagnosis is readily made on the basis of history and physical examination, reinforced by careful X-ray studies, and by exploratory aspiration where necessary to establish the etiology.

Because of the ready coagulability of pleural exudates it is advisable to collect fluid for study in tubes containing either sodium citrate or potassium oxalate. Pleural effusions usually are clear or only slightly turbid, and amber to straw colored. The specific gravity is 1.016 or greater and the protein content above 3 Gm./100 cc., whereas the transudates that may occur in cardiac decompensation, renal disease, hepatic disease, and nutritional deficiency have lower specific gravities and protein contents. Bloody fluid is common in carcinomatous effusions and is sometimes seen in tuberculous effusions. Chylous effusions are occasionally encountered and suggest damage to the thoracic duct, usually by tumor.

The leukocyte count of the pleural fluid may vary from a few cells to several thousand/cu. mm. An effusion due to pyogenic infection will at first show a predominance of polymorphonuclear neutrophiles and may progress to frank empyema (q.v.). In sterile postpneumonic effusions, the differential gradually shifts and monocytes become predominant. Tuberculous effusions, unless secondarily infected, will show a great predominance of lymphocytes. Malignant cells may rarely be demonstrated on a stained smear of the sediment, but cell block preparations are more often positive. In addition to Gram and Ziehl-Neelsen stained smears (*see* Lab. Proc.), cultures should be made on appropriate media. The presence of tubercle bacilli should be determined by culture on special media or by guinea-pig inoculation.

Treatment

All patients with serofibrinous pleurisy should be kept in bed. The diet should be high in protein and vitamins. Salt should be restricted until the nature of the effusion has been established: if it is an exudate rather than a transudate, salt restriction may be discontinued. Fluids need not be restricted. Specific treatment will depend on the nature of the underlying disease. If pleuritic pain is present, treatment as outlined for fibrinous pleurisy may be instituted.

Immediate aspiration of the pleural fluid is essential for diagnosis and for relief of respiratory distress, if present. Any effusion associated with pyogenic infection should be treated as an empyema (q.v.). Most nonpyogenic effusions tend to be absorbed spontaneously on bed rest, and further aspiration need be made only if there is no sign of reabsorption or if fluid reaccumulates sufficiently to cause respiratory embarrassment.

The site for thoracentesis will depend on physical and X-ray findings. In most instances, either the 6th interspace in the midaxillary line or the 8th interspace in the scapular line will be satisfactory (*see* CLIN. PROC.). To minimize the danger of acute pulmonary edema, the fluid should be withdrawn slowly and no more than 1,500 cc. removed at a time. Pneumothorax is to be avoided by careful attention to maintenance of a negative pressure.

EMPYEMA

(Purulent pleuritis)

A purulent exudate in the pleural cavity, which may be acute or chronic.

Etiology

Empyema usually results from a spread of infection from contiguous structures, most frequently the lungs. It may occur as a complication of pneumonia, bronchiectasis, pulmonary abscess, tuberculosis, or mycotic pulmonary disease, or spread from infection of the chest wall, mediastinum, pericardium, or subdiaphragmatic areas. The infection also may be introduced directly by penetrating wounds of the chest wall or during surgical procedures. Rarely, empyema may result from the trapping of infected emboli in the pleural vessels or may complicate bacteremia.

The organisms most frequent in empyema are pneumococci, hemolytic streptococci, staphylococci, tubercle bacilli, anaerobic streptococci, fusospirochetes, and coliform bacteria. Despite the fact that the incidence of empyema as a complication of pneumococcal pneumonia has been reduced by modern chemotherapy, the pneumococcus probably still is the most frequent cause. The hemolytic streptococcal empyemas common during the great pandemic of influenza now are rare; hemolytic *Staph. aureus* infections more frequently complicate influenza. Mixed infections of the pleural cavity usually are secondary to lung abscess and bronchiectasis, and generally consist of anaerobic streptococci, fusospirochetes, staphylococci, and coliform bacteria. The pus of mixed infections often is foul and this accounts for the term "putrid empyema."

Chronic empyema usually is due to inadequate treatment of

acute empyema, but it may be caused by a bronchopleural fistula, osteomyelitis of a rib, or a foreign body within the pleural space. Tuberculosis and fungus infections tend to cause chronic empyemas. Often, the chronic empyema represents repeated reinfections of the pleural cavity from persistent foci of infection in the lungs.

Pathology

The extent of the inflammation varies; only a small portion of the interlobar septum or the entire pleural cavity may be affected. Depending upon the duration of the infection and the nature of the causative organism, the appearance of the pleura also will vary from that of a fairly normal membrane with a thin fibrin layer to a tremendously thickened structure with a tough, shaggy exudate binding the lung to the chest wall and forming multiloculated cavities. The consistency of the exudate ranges from a thin fluid to a thick pus that is difficult to aspirate. Microscopically, the pleural endothelium usually is found to be destroyed and the pleural surface covered with a layer of fibrin of varying thickness containing polymorphonuclear leukocytes. If treatment is inadequate, this may later be replaced by fibrous tissue that eventually may bind the lung in an inelastic case.

Small amounts of pus in the pleural cavity do not displace the lungs sufficiently to cause respiratory embarrassment, but large accumulations may considerably reduce the vital capacity. In pneumococcal empyema, fibrin deposition is comparatively rapid and heavy, so that mediastinal stabilization and fixation of the lung to the chest wall occur early. This process, by limiting respiratory excursion, also may greatly reduce vital capacity. With neglected empyemas, the chest on the affected side may be shrunken and the lung compressed in an unyielding fibrous case so that the lung receives little ventilation.

Symptoms and Signs

Since empyema is almost invariably a secondary infection, its onset is apt to be masked by the symptoms and signs of the primary disease. Not infrequently the development of an empyema is heralded by pleural pain, but this is rarely of long duration. The patient may complain of persistent dull pain in the chest and of tenderness over the site of pleural involvement. Cough is frequently though not always present. Commonly, however, there are no specific symptoms. The disease must be suspected when pneumonia does not respond satisfactorily to treatment or a relapse occurs. In chronic pulmonary disease the development of empyema may symptomatically suggest pneumonia. A change in the amount and character of sputum produced by patients with chronic suppurative pulmonary disease may indicate the development of empyema with a pleuropulmonary fistula.

The signs of empyema are identical with those of pleural effusion. Small accumulations of fluid, particularly if interlobar, often cannot be detected by physical examination. Limitation of respiratory motion is an important physical sign and may occur even though the amount of fluid is small. Rarely, if the amount of fluid is large, a bulging of intercostal spaces may be seen. The trachea and mediastinal contents may be shifted away from the affected side if the mediastinum is not fixed. Tactile fremitus is diminished or absent. The percussion note is dull to flat, and breath sounds are diminished or absent. As with pleural effusion, there may be comparatively loud bronchial breathing and egophony over the upper border of the fluid collection.

In chronic empyema, the involved hemithorax may appear shrunken, with narrowing of the interspaces, scoliosis, elevation of the diaphragm, and retraction of the mediastinal contents to the affected side. Clubbing of the fingers is common.

Complications

Although empyema usually is secondary to pre-existing infections, such conditions as pericarditis, endocarditis, meningitis, brain abscess, and purulent arthritis often are encountered as complications. Rarely, amyloidosis with enlargement of the liver and spleen may complicate chronic empyema. Occasionally, a neglected empyema may drain spontaneously through the chest wall (empyema necessitatis).

Diagnosis

The presence of primary disease and the minimal nature of the physical signs shown by empyema often make diagnosis difficult. Therefore, it must be borne in mind that the condition may develop in any patient having infection of the contiguous structures. An unfavorable change in his condition demands careful examination of the chest. Whenever physical signs are questionable, X-ray studies of the chest must be carried out; otherwise small accumulations of fluid may be overlooked. Interlobar empyemas frequently can be detected only by X-ray examination, using the oblique and lateral as well as standard positions.

Leukocyte counts, with differentials, are of diagnostic value, since with developing empyema there may be an increase of leukocytes or in the percentage of polymorphonuclears, or both, without significant changes in the patient's temperature, pulse, or respiration. A persistent leukocytosis in a patient with pneumonia, who otherwise seems to be responding satisfactorily to treatment, necessitates careful search for empyema. The leukocyte count in empyema ranges from 15,000 to 50,000.

The diagnosis can be established only by examination of the pleural exudate. Diagnostic aspiration should be done whenever empyema is suspected. Selection of the site for thoracentesis is guided by the physical examination and roentgenograms. In early cases, the exudate usually is thin, straw or amber colored, and contains few leukocytes. Specific gravity is 1.016 or higher. As the disease progresses, the fluid becomes thicker and may contain more than 50,000 leukocytes/cu. mm. The odor of the chest fluid is significant, a foul odor indicating a mixed infection and in general a serious type of empyema, often with a bronchopleural fistula.

Wright stained smears of the exudate should be made for cytologic study, and Gram and Ziehl-Neelsen stained smears to detect the presence of bacteria. Both aerobic and anaerobic cultures should be made. If fungus disease is suspected, appropriate media should be used for culture. Cultures and guinea-pig inoculations should be carried out to determine whether tubercle bacilli are present.

Prognosis and Treatment

The prognosis of empyema has been tremendously improved with the introduction of antibiotic therapy. Now, the vast majority of patients with complicated empyema treated early may be expected to recover.

Once the diagnosis of empyema is established, treatment should be immediate. If the pleural fluid is turbid, it is best to inject 200,000 u. of penicillin (℞ 21) in 50 or 100 cc. isotonic salt solution into the pleural cavity before the needle used for diagnostic aspiration is withdrawn. If subsequent study of the fluid gives no indication for further penicillin treatment, no harm will have been done; while if penicillin is indicated, time will have been saved.

The choice of therapeutic agent is based on the bacteriologic findings. Ideally, the sensitivity of the infecting organisms to penicillin and streptomycin should be determined, but generally speaking, all empyemas due to gram-positive organisms should be treated with penicillin (℞ 18, 19), whereas those with gram-negative organisms or tubercle bacilli, or with mixed infections, should be given streptomycin (℞ 23), 0.5 Gm. I.M. every 4 hours, either alone or in combination with penicillin or a sulfonamide (℞ 31, 32). The antibiotics should be administered both systemically and by instillation into the pleural cavity. Sulfonamides may be given by mouth or, if necessary, parenterally as the sodium salt. The chest should be tapped daily, with the needle inserted into the most dependent portion of the cavity (see CLIN. PROC.). If the fluid is thick a 16-gauge needle may be needed. As much purulent material as possible should be withdrawn, shifting the position of the needle as seems necessary. An encapsulated empyema must be accurately located if aspiration is to be successful. If the fluid is thick and contains much fibrin, the cavity should be irrigated with isotonic salt solution. Finally, depending on the amount and character of the fluid withdrawn, 50,000 to 200,000 u. of penicillin (R 21) or 0.1 to 0.5 Gm. of streptomycin (R 23), or both, dissolved in 50 to 100 cc. of physiologic saline, should be instilled. In most instances, the patient's general condition will improve dramatically within the first 48 hours of treatment. Daily aspiration of the pleural fluid, together with irrigation and instillation of the appropriate antibiotic, should be continued until the exudate has become sterile. Intrapleural antibiotic therapy then may be discontinued and further aspiration done only if the fluid fails to be spontaneously reabsorbed. Parenteral antibiotic or oral sulfonamide therapy, or both, should be continued until the patient has been afebrile for 3 consecutive days.

While the treatment of empyema by repeated aspiration, together with antibiotic and sulfonamide therapy, usually will prove successful, surgicial intervention will sometimes be necessary. If the patient does not seem to be improving after a week of medical treatment, or if drainage by aspiration is unsatisfactory because of multilocular cavities or the character of the exudate, surgical drainage should be undertaken. Putrid empyema has in the past been believed to require immediate open drainage, since thoracentesis might cause an overwhelming cellulitis of the chest. However, the effectiveness of the antibiotics in combating anaerobic infections suggests that open drainage may safely be delayed and the need for surgical measures decided later, based on the patient's response to medical therapy. Chronic empyemas and those with frank bronchopleural fistulas usually require surgical treatment. Rarely, a pulmonary abscess (q.v.) will rupture suddenly into the pleural space. This constitutes an immediate surgical emergency, requiring tube drainage with drainage bottle and appropriate treatment for shock.

If the empyema is a complication of tuberculosis (q.v.) or of other infectious disease, the primary infection must of course be treated by standard methods. Tuberculous empyema is a complication of advanced pulmonary tuberculosis. It also occurs during the course of therapeutic pneumothorax in about 10% of the cases. Secondary infection with pyogenic organisms is not infrequent in this condition. In the treatment of tuberculous empyema, a trial of streptomycin therapy may be desirable, but this alone will seldom effect a cure and surgery must be resorted to. Drainage of pus, followed later by thoracoplasty to decrease the dead space, are the necessary surgical procedures.

In uncomplicated empyema, the patient should be encouraged to become ambulatory as soon as the fever has subsided. The diet should be high in proteins and vitamins. The objective of treatment is not merely to eliminate infection but also to restore normal respiratory function. Neglecting the early institution of exercises designed to promote expansion of the lung is unfortunately a common oversight which may lead to permanent impairment of respiratory function. Breathing exercises (exhaling against resistance) and careful instruction as to deep breathing are necessary as soon as the patient becomes afebrile.

NEOPLASMS

A tumor or new growth situated in the bronchial tree, or in the substance of the lungs.

Etiology and Pathology

Pulmonary tumors may be primary or secondary, malignant or benign.

The cause of primary pulmonary carcinoma is almost completely unknown. The only recognized etiology is that of certain radioactive ores, apparently responsible for a high incidence of the disease in a restricted mining population in Europe. Tobacco, oils, fumes, tarred roads, and other possible irritants have been suspected but proof of their effects is lacking.

Primary carcinoma of the lung is responsible for 5 to 10% of all deaths due to cancer. The disease is diagnosed much more frequently than it was 20 years ago: opinions differ as to whether there actually is an increased incidence or only better diagnosis. It is more common in men, 80% of cases occurring between the ages of 40 and 70.

The most important forms of pulmonary neoplasm are primary carcinoma, arising from the bronchial epithelium, and metastatic carcinoma, reaching the lungs secondarily from some other primary focus. Among the rarer tumors are benign bronchial adenoma, sarcoma, dermoid cyst, chondroma, neurofibroma, and lipoma. The pulmonary infiltrations or extensions of generalized diseases such as lymphoma (e.g., Hodgkin's disease) or leukemia (q.v.) will not be considered here.

Symptoms and Signs

Primary carcinoma of the bronchus: About 90% of patients complain of cough; it is the first symptom in more than half. It may be of various types, irritative, spasmodic, or asthmatic. In patients already subject to chronic cough, a change due to the carcinoma may be most difficult to detect. Alterations in character, severity, or persistence will sometimes be suggestive. Sputum often is scanty and mucoid; purulent only with secondary infection. Dyspnea, either an early or late symptom, is seen in almost 60% of cases. Pain in the chest is present in about half of all cases; it may be pleuritic, deep seated, or referred to the shoulder or back. Hemoptysis, usually small in amount but recurrent, is a symptom in almost 50%. Other common symptoms are loss of weight, fever, wheezing respirations, cyanosis, clubbing of fingers and toes.

A tumor at the apex (Pancoast's tumor) may cause symptoms due to pressure on the brachial plexus.

Physical signs may be absent if the tumor is in a "silent" area. If a large bronchus is occluded, there are the signs of atelectasis—shrunken chest, poor expansion, diminished breath sounds. A localized wheeze, indicating partial obstruction, is an important sign. Secondary infection may cause the moist rales of bronchiectasis, or frank pneumonia, or lung abscess. Pleural effusion usually indicates pleural invasion of the tumor, especially if the fluid is bloody. Metastatic enlargement of cervical lymph glands is common. Mediastinal gland enlargement may cause pressure symptoms.

Carcinoma of the bronchus is apt to metastasize widely to cervical and mediastinal lymph nodes, pleura, liver, brain, bones, esophagus, and adrenals. In many instances, the first observable symptoms are those caused by the metastatic tumors. Spread to the opposite lung is relatively uncommon. The primary lesion may be very small, sometimes detectable only at autopsy.

Secondary metastases in the lung: These lesions may occasionally be linear along lymphatic channels, or uniformly disseminated (the "snowstorm" appearance by X-ray), but are more commonly discrete rounded shadows in the X-ray field. The latter are usually multiple, but occasionally single, "solitary metastases."

Metastases in the lung ordinarily do not cause symptoms or signs. A metastatic nodule may press on a bronchus and produce the symptoms of bronchial obstruction; but pressure symptoms, when they occur, more frequently are due to enlargement of mediastinal lymph nodes.

Malignant neoplasms that are apt to metastasize to the lungs include sarcoma (by hematogenous dissemination), carcinoma of breast, stomach, prostate, kidney, or thyroid, and malignant tumors of the testicle.

Other tumors: The benign tumors, when they cause symptoms, usually do so by pressure on surrounding structures. Special mention should be made of endobronchial adenoma, a relatively rare tumor usually mistaken for carcinoma. A characteristic symptom of benign bronchial adenoma is repeated episodes of profuse hemoptysis.

Diagnosis

Since favorably located carcinomas of the lung now can be removed surgically, and occasionally a permanent cure effected, early diagnosis is most important. Suspicion aroused by a thorough history, or careful scrutiny of a routine X-ray or of an X-ray taken for another purpose, most often will reveal very early lesions. The diagnosis is usually established by bronchoscopy, either by direct visualization and biopsy of the tumor or by microscopic examination of bronchial secretions sucked out during the procedure. Not infrequently, the surgeon will operate directly if the X-ray evidence is sufficient, establishing the diagnosis only at operation.

In cases that have metastasized, the diagnosis may be made by biopsy of an enlarged cervical or (less often) axillary lymph node, or by examination of pleural fluid for tumor cells.

A benign tumor may at times be identified by X-ray when it has a characteristically smooth outline and sharply defined margins.

In the differential diagnosis, conditions that often are confused with lung tumors are localized tuberculous lesions, lung abscess, localized pneumonia, pulmonary infarct, abscess from Potts' disease of the spine, esophageal diverticulum, foreign body in the bronchus, and mycotic lung diseases such as the rounded lesions of coccidioidomycosis.

Prognosis and Treatment

The average survival of patients with untreated carcinoma of the bronchus, after the diagnosis has been established, is 9 months; but not infrequently a patient may live 2 years or more. With successful surgical removal of the primary tumor, the patient can be expected to live longer, though 5- and 10-year survivals still are few.

Surgical removal, when possible, is obviously the treatment of choice. Some lung tumors are radiosensitive, and a vigorous course of radiotherapy will shrink such tumors and give relief of symptoms for a few months. Therapy with the nitrogen mustard, mechlorethamine (HN_2), produces transient general improvement and alleviation of distressing symptoms in some patients with extensive inoperable primary carcinoma of the lung, particularly in cases of anaplastic or oat-cell carcinoma. Remissions usually are only 2 weeks to 2 months in duration. Improvement consists chiefly of a decrease in cough, dyspnea, amount of sputum, and hemoptysis. Some patients show an increase in appetite, weight, and strength. There may be some reduction in the amount of pleural effusion, increased aeration of atelectatic areas, and temporary control of pulmonary lesions. Treatment of relapses usually is not so successful as the first course. Mechlorethamine (R 83) is administered only I.V. in an average dosage of 0.1 mg./Kg. body wt. daily for 4 days.

In patients with inoperable or recurrent carcinoma of the bronchus, progressively increasing amounts of sedatives and narcotics usually will be required. Patients with bronchial or tracheal obstruction may need—in addition to heavy sedation —oxygen, bronchodilators, or even helium and oxygen terminally.

Solitary metastatic lesions have occasionally been removed surgically, with benefit to the patient.

Benign tumors should be removed surgically when possible. If not giving symptoms and not increasing in size, a benign tumor may in some instances be left in place but must be followed carefully by X-ray.

DYSPNEA

Breathlessness or distressed breathing. While usually a subjective symptom, it may also be an objective manifestation: labored or distressed respiration of any kind, as observed objectively in a patient, can properly be called dyspnea, whether or not the patient himself complains of it. When the patient must sit upright in order to breathe, the condition is referred to as **orthopnea.**

Pathologic Physiology

Dyspnea is primarily dependent on two factors: the amount of pulmonary ventilation required by the individual in his particular physiologic state (rest, exercise, anoxia), and the capacity of his breathing apparatus (lungs and thorax) to supply this required ventilation.

Pulmonary ventilation is a response to the total respiratory stimulus; and the rate and form, as well as the total volume, of breathing are largely determined by this stimulus, within the framework permitted by the chest wall and pulmonary structures. There are two respiratory centers: that in the medulla, responding to alterations in blood CO_2 tension and blood acidity; and that in the carotid sinus structures, responding to changes in arterial blood oxygen saturation (i.e., anoxia). In addition to these basic chemical stimuli, respiration is modified by other factors such as proprioceptive reflexes from lungs and chest, and sensory, visceral, nervous, and emotional influences of various kinds.

The breathing capacity of an individual (maximum breathing capacity or maximum minute ventilation) is the maximum volume of pulmonary ventilation that can be respired in unit time. In normal individuals, this is about 150 liters/minute in males, 100 liters/minute in females.

A useful concept is that of the breathing reserve, which is an individual's extra breathing capacity, over and above his actual ventilation or ventilatory requirement. In many of its simpler forms, dyspnea is well correlated with the breathing reserve, dyspnea being first noticed when the breathing reserve is reduced to about 65 or 70% of maximum breathing capacity.

Types

1. Physiologic: The most common form of dyspnea is that associated with physical exertion. The greatly increased ventilation is maintained chiefly through augmented respiratory stimulus provided by increased tissue and blood acidity. Dyspnea also occurs in anoxia, as at high altitude, the increased respiratory stimulus here being chiefly the effect of anoxia on the carotid sinuses.

2. Pulmonary: Dyspnea primarily from pulmonary causes is of two general forms: restrictive, due to defects in lungs or chest wall that limit and restrict lung expansion; and obstructive, due to partial obstruction of tracheobronchial air passages. In restrictive forms, such as pulmonary fibrosis, pneumothorax, or severe kyphoscoliosis, patients usually are comfortable at rest, but become intensely dyspneic on exertion sufficient to cause pulmonary ventilation to approach the greatly limited breathing capacity. In obstructive forms, such as obstructive emphysema or asthma, there may be a sense of dyspnea even at rest, with labored and retarded breathing, especially during expiration. In these cases, there is often also some anoxia, increasing the respiratory stimulus, and increasing pulmonary ventilation.

3. Cardiac: In the early stages of diminished cardiac reserve, cardiac output fails to increase sufficiently during exercise, respiratory stimulus is increased because of tissue and cerebral acidity and the patient hyperventilates. Various reflex factors also may contribute to the hyperventilation. The patient's symptoms, however, usually are not simple breathlessness, but shortness of breath combined with a sense of exhaustion, and often accompanied by a feeling of smothering or sternal oppression from relative coronary insufficiency. In the later state of true congestive failure, the lungs are turgid with blood and ventilatory capacity is much reduced, with breathing reserve thus also diminished. Here, also, reflex factors increase pulmonary ventilation. Cardiac asthma is a state of acute pulmonary congestion, with distinct hyperventilation and a considerable factor of obstruction of the air passages. Periodic or Cheyne-Stokes respiration is not fully understood, but probably is associated with a retarded cerebral and general circulation, acidity and anoxia in the respiratory centers causing hyperventilation, followed by apnea when the over-aerated blood reaches these centers.

4. Circulatory: "Air hunger" is an acute dyspnea usually seen at the terminal stages of profound exsanguinating hemorrhage. It is a grave sign calling for immediate transfusion. The dyspnea of chronic anemia is purely exertional, except when the anemia is extreme.

5. Chemical: Diabetic acidosis, with pronouncedly increased blood acidity (pH 7.20 to 6.95), induces slow deep respirations (Kussmaul breathing). There is no loss of breathing capacity, however, and only rarely does the patient complain of dyspnea. In cardiorenal acidosis, on the other hand, there sometimes is an extreme panting type of dyspnea, due to a combination of acidosis, heart failure, pulmonary edema, and anemia.

6. Central: Cerebral lesions, such as hemiplegia, often are associated with an intense hyperventilation, sometimes noisy and stertorous, occasionally irregularly periodic (Biot type). There is a rare postencephalitic condition characterized by extreme hyperventilation.

7. **Respiratory neuroses:** There are a number of forms of respiratory neurosis in which the patients complain of dyspnea. The two most common are the hysterical type, which consists in severe continuous hyperventilation, sometimes leading to acute gaseous alkalosis from "blowing off" CO_2, with positive Trousseau and Chvostek signs, and a type characterized by a series of deep sighing respirations, the patient breathing at maximal depth until he or she obtains a "satisfactory" respiration, at which time the hyperventilatory impulse subsides.

Treatment

The treatment is that of the various individual conditions (q.v.) indicated above.

ANOXIA

(Hypoxia)

A general term denoting acute or chronic oxygen deficiency in the tissues from any cause. **Anoxemia** is a deficiency in the oxygen (O_2) content of blood, usually referring to arterial blood. **Asphyxia** is a condition in which there is both anoxia and increased carbon dioxide (CO_2) tension in the blood and tissues. **Suffocation** refers to the cessation of respiration, with resultant asphyxia. **Cyanosis** is the blueness of the skin that occurs in the presence of inadequate oxygenation of the circulating blood.

Etiology, Pathologic Physiology, and Types

Normal body respiration requires the presence of an adequate supply (concentration) of O_2 in the alveoli, a sufficient amount of hemoglobin which is capable of combining with this O_2, the transportation of the oxyhemoglobin thus formed to the tissues at a rate commensurate with tissue needs, and the ability of the body cells to utilize the O_2 so supplied. Any unfavorable variation in these processes, beyond the ability of the body functionally to compensate for the change, will result in anoxia. Accordingly, 4 types of anoxia are possible:

1. **Anoxic:** The capacity of the blood to carry O_2 is normal, but there is deficient oxygenation of the arterial blood. This may be due to (*a*) insufficient O_2 in the inspired air (e.g., at high altitudes, or due to vitiation of the atmosphere by such physiologically inert gases as methane or nitrogen); (*b*) decreased vital capacity or impaired passage of O_2 through the

alveoli into the arterial blood (e.g., due to tracheal or bronchial obstruction, shallow or unduly slow breathing, pulmonary inflammation or fibrosis, asthma, pulmonary edema, emphysema, atelectasis); (*c*) congenital heart defects (q.v.) with right-to-left shunts of blood; (*d*) respiratory depression or arrest (as in electric shock, drowning, cerebral trauma, poliomyelitis, or due to respiratory depressants such as morphine, barbiturates, alcohol, or certain anesthetic agents).

2. Anemic: The O_2 carrying capacity of the blood is decreased. The hemoglobin may be reduced in quantity (as in certain types of anemia) or may be so altered by toxic agents that it cannot carry its full quota of O_2. The abnormal compounds so formed are carboxyhemoglobin (following inhalation of carbon monoxide), methemoglobin (with nitrites, nitrates, anilines, acetanilid, antipyrine, chlorates, sulfonamides, as the causative substances), and sulfhemoglobin (due to exposure to certain sulfides). It recently has been shown that infants fed a formula prepared with well water containing large amounts (above 10 parts/million) of nitrates are prone to intermittent attacks of cyanosis and anoxia due to the formation of methemoglobin.

3. Stagnant: The O_2 content and O_2 carrying capacity of the blood are normal, but the blood flow through the capillaries is slowed to such a degree that tissue demands for O_2 cannot be met. This type of anoxia may be general or localized and is associated with congestive heart failure, shock, impaired venous return, or obstruction to the arterial or venous blood flow by trauma, tourniquet, embolus, thrombosis, or peripheral vascular disease.

4. Histotoxic: The tissue cells are unable to utilize O_2 due to impairment of the oxidative-enzyme mechanism of the cell. Cyanides or alcohol are characteristic agents that may cause histotoxic anoxia.

Symptoms and Signs

The effects produced by anoxia depend on the type and degree of anoxia present, the rapidity of its development, its duration, and the relative physiologic competency of the involved cells at the onset. The brain, heart, and eye are particularly sensitive to deprivation of O_2. The physiologic lesion of anoxia consists of capillary damage with resultant minute petechial hemorrhages.

To a large extent, the clinical manifestations of anoxia will blend into or be overshadowed by those of the underlying disease (*see* Etiology). However, the manifestations of acute generalized anoxia (such as may be encountered at high altitudes) have been extensively studied. These include dyspnea, rapid pulse, cyanosis, impairment of the special senses, headache, anorexia, and mental disturbances (e.g., euphoria, delirium). In severe cases, muscular twitchings, convulsions, unconsciousness, and death may ensue. The after-effects of acute nonfatal anoxia may persist for up to 48 hours and include headache, lethargy, nausea, and vomiting.

Cyanosis is recognizable when there are abnormal blood pigments present (such as sulfhemoglobin, methemoglobin), or when the capillary blood contains an excess of reduced hemoglobin (above 5 Gm./100 cc. blood). It is most readily noted in the lips and nail beds but severe degrees of cyanosis may be evident anywhere in the skin or mucous membranes. The discoloration may vary from a pale violet to purple or even black. Major degrees of cyanosis most commonly occur in polycythemia (q.v.), congestive heart failure (q.v.), advanced emphysema, Ayerza's disease, and in certain congenital anomalies of the cardiovascular system (q.v.).

Local anoxia is characterized by symptoms and signs confined to the affected area.

Thus, there may be attacks of syncope, angina pectoris, pulmonary edema, or intermittent claudication due to anoxia of the brain, heart, alveoli, or lower extremities, respectively. The skin of a locally anoxic area may be cyanotic, often with induration which may even go on to ulceration.

Diagnosis

The diagnosis depends on a history of exposure to or evidence of action by agents or conditions known to cause anoxia. Cyanosis and dyspnea are suggestive but not pathognomonic signs. Hemoglobin determination will reveal anemia, if present. Specific laboratory tests for anoxia include determination of the O_2 saturation and content of arterial blood and spectroscopic examination of the blood for the presence of abnormal hemoglobin pigments.

Prognosis

The length of time during which extreme anoxia can persist and still be compatible with subsequent complete tissue recovery varies from a matter of seconds to several hours, depending on the tissue involved, the brain being the most sensitive. Episodes in excess of 10 minutes not infrequently result in permanent sequelae in the form of blindness, mental deficiency, or other similar defects due to damage to the more highly specialized C.N.S. centers.

Chronic experience of mild degrees of anoxia sometimes may result in compensatory physiologic changes which tend to overcome the anoxic state; such changes are well illustrated by the polycythemia and increased vital capacity which develop in persons living constantly at high altitudes.

Treatment

Because the clinical manifestations of mild or early anoxia usually are inconspicuous, it is imperative that the physician be "anoxia conscious" at all times. Only in this way can therapy be instituted promptly to combat the disorder before it is of such severity or duration as to result in tissue damage. It is hazardous and unwise to delay treatment until the appearance of cyanosis or severe dyspnea.

The treatment of anoxia is that of the underlying condition (*see* Etiology), plus O_2 inhalation for those forms of anoxia in which the O_2 saturation of the blood, though decreased, is yet capable of being elevated. Thus, O_2 inhalation is especially beneficial in the treatment of anoxic anoxia where it tends to increase the O_2 saturation of the arterial blood to or near normal (96%). In other types of anoxia, where the O_2 carrying mechanism is deficient in degree or altered in nature (as in anemic anoxia), or where the circulation flows too slowly (i.e., stagnant anoxia), O_2 alone is of only moderate or slight benefit; in histotoxic anoxia, O_2 by itself is of little therapeutic value.

For inhalation, an O_2 concentration of 75 to 100% is preferable to lesser concentrations. With such higher concentrations, the beneficial results of O_2 therapy are achieved most rapidly; they offer the greatest safeguard against increasing anoxia, and they aid in depressing the cough reflex in cases of pulmonary edema due to irritant gases, fumes, or vapors. If a patient ceases to breathe, artificial respiration (q.v.), plus the use of O_2, if available, must be started immediately. The addition of 5 to 10% CO_2 to the O_2 is not indicated in anoxia except in those cases due to carbon monoxide poisoning, where it is of definite benefit.

In conjunction with O_2 inhalation, respiratory stimulants (℞ 62, 63) are useful when respiration is depressed as a result of drugs or poisons; depressed respiration resulting from anoxia alone will not be benefited by such stimulants, O_2 being the most effective agent available. As a general rule, morphine and other sedatives which depress respiration should be avoided in the presence of anoxia, their use being limited to treatment of traumatic shock and judicious administration in cardiac cases (*see* CONGESTIVE HEART FAILURE; PULMONARY EDEMA; SHOCK).

PRESCRIPTIONS

(Wherever a prescribed "proprietary" is representative of a class of therapeutic agents, alternative proprietary preparations will be found listed in Part II.)

Analgesics, Antipyretics, Sedatives, and Antitussives

1. ℞ Acetylsalicylic acid . . . . . 0.3 Gm. (gr. v)
   2 tablets every 4 hours.

2. ℞ Acetylsalicylic acid . . . . . 0.6 Gm. (gr. x)
   Codeine sulfate. . . . . . . 0.03 Gm. (gr. ss)
   1 capsule every 4 hours.

3. ℞ Acetophenetidin . . . . .   0.12   Gm. (gr. ii)

> 1 powder or capsule every hour or two for 3 or 4 hours before expected rise in temperature.

4. ℞ Acetylsalicylic acid . . . .   0.2   Gm. (gr. iii)
    Caffeine . . . .   0.03   Gm. (gr. ss)
    Acetophenetidin . . . . . .   0.15   Gm. (gr. iiss)

> 1 or 2 tablets or capsules 1 to 3 times daily.

5. ℞ Acetylsalicylic acid . . . . .   0.3   Gm. (gr. v)
    Acetophenetidin . . . .   0.12   Gm. (gr. ii)
    Caffeine . . . .   0.03   Gm. (gr. ss)
    Codeine sulfate. . . . . . .   0.015 Gm. (gr. $\frac{1}{4}$)

> 1 capsule or powder every 4 hours if necessary.

6. ℞ Ipecac and Opium Powder N.F.
      (Dover's Powder). . . . .   0.15   Gm. (gr. iiss)
    Acetophenetidin . . . . . .   0.1   Gm. (gr. iss)
    Acetylsalicylic acid . . . .   0.12   Gm. (gr. ii)
    Camphor . . . .   0.008 Gm. (gr. $\frac{1}{8}$)
    Caffeine . . . .   0.008 Gm. (gr. $\frac{1}{8}$)

> 1 capsule every half hour for 6 doses, then 1 every 3 hours.

7. ℞ Acetophenetidin . . . .   0.2   Gm. (gr. iii)
    Acetylsalicylic acid . . . . .   0.15   Gm. (gr. iiss)
    Belladonna Extract U.S.P. . .   0.015 Gm. (gr. $\frac{1}{4}$)
    Phenobarbital . . . .   0.015 Gm. (gr. $\frac{1}{4}$)

> 1 capsule at onset of symptoms; repeat dose in 3 hours.

8. ℞ Codeine phosphate   15   mg. (gr. $\frac{1}{4}$)

> 1 to 4 tablets orally or subcut. every 4 hours for pain or cough.

9. ℞ Morphine sulfate

> 10 to 15 mg. (gr. $\frac{1}{6}$ to $\frac{1}{4}$) subcut. every 4 hours if necessary.

10. ℞ "Demerol Hydrochloride" . .   50   mg.

> $\frac{1}{2}$ to 2 tablets every 4 to 8 hours.

11. ℞ "Demerol Hydrochloride"
    (ampul)

> 50 to 100 mg. I.M. every 4 hours.

12. ℞ "Pantopon"   (ampul)

> 20 mg. (gr. $\frac{1}{3}$) subcut.

13. ℞ Methadone Hydrochloride
    N.N.R.   5   mg.

> $\frac{1}{2}$ to 1 tablet every 3 or 4 hours for pain or cough.

14. ℞ Codeine sulfate. 15   mg. (gr. ¼)
     Papaverine hydrochloride . . 15   mg. (gr. ¼)
     1 capsule every 3 or 4 hours.

15. ℞ Phenobarbital Elixir U.S.P.. . 60.0   cc. (℥ ii)
     1 teaspoon as indicated for sedation.

16. ℞ Phenobarbital 15   mg. (gr. ¼)
     1 to 4 tablets as indicated for sedation or
     insomnia.

17. ℞ Three Bromides Elixir N.F. . 120.0   cc. (℥ iv)
     1 or 2 teaspoons at bedtime.

Antimicrobial Agents

18. ℞ Penicillin   (vial)
     30,000 to 100,000 u. I.M. every 3 hours or
     300,000 u. I.M. every 12 to 24 hours.

19. ℞ Procaine penicillin   (vial)
     300,000 u. I.M. every 12 to 24 hours.

20. ℞ Penicillin   (vial)
     Dissolve 200,000 u. in 2 to 5 cc. saline and
     inhale 1 to 2 cc. by aerosol 2 or 3 times daily.

21. ℞ Penicillin   (vial)
     Dissolve 50,000 to 200,000 u. in 50 to 300 cc.
     Sterile Isotonic Sodium Chloride Solution for
     Parenteral Use U.S.P. and instill daily into
     the pleural cavity.

22. ℞ Penicillin 300,000   u.
     Streptomycin. . . . .   1.0   Gm.
     Sodium chloride, isotonic solu-
        tion. . . . . 10.0   cc.
     Nebulize and inhale 1 cc. as vapor 5 times a
     day.

23. ℞ Streptomycin   (vial)
     For nontuberculous conditions: 1 to 4 Gm.
     daily, administered I.M. in divided doses
     every 4 to 6 hours.   For intrapleural admin-
     istration: Dissolve 0.1 to 0.5 Gm. in 50
     to 100 cc. Sterile Isotonic Sodium Chloride
     Solution for Parenteral Use U.S.P. and inject
     daily.   For tuberculosis: *See* dosage described
     under TUBERCULOSIS, Pulmonary.

24. ℞ Streptomycin   (vial)
     Dissolve 1 Gm. in 10 cc. isotonic sodium
     chloride solution and inhale 1 cc. by aerosol
     every 4 to 6 hours.

25. ℞ Dihydrostreptomycin   (vial)
     15 to 20 mg./Kg. body wt. daily, adminis-
     tered I.M. in divided doses (*see* TUBERCU-
     LOSIS for dosage required).

26. ℞ Para-aminosalicylic acid . . . 0.5 Gm. (gr. viiss)

 6 capsules or tablets after each meal and (with an aluminum hydroxide gel) at bedtime.

27. ℞ Para-aminosalicylic acid . . 100.0 Gm. (ℨ iiiss)
  Sodium bicarbonate. . . . . 60.0 Gm. (ℨ ii)
  Oil of wintergreen. . . . . 0.3 cc. (♏ v)
  Distilled water. . . . q.s. ad 500.0 cc. (ℨ xvi)

 4 teaspoons after each meal and at bedtime.

28. ℞ Aureomycin (capsules) . . . 0.25 Gm.

 25 to 100 mg./Kg. body wt./day in 4 to 8 equally divided doses. With improvement, dosage may be reduced.

29. ℞ "Chloromycetin" . . . . . . 0.25 Gm.

 50 to 75 mg./Kg. body wt. initially followed by 25 to 50 mg./Kg. every 2 to 3 hours until afebrile; then every 6 hours until cured.

30. ℞ Sulfathiazole . . . . 0.5 Gm. (gr. viiss)

 4 to 8 tablets initially, then 2 tablets every 4 hours.

31. ℞ Sulfadiazine . . . . 0.5 Gm. (gr. viiss)

 4 to 8 tablets initially, then 2 tablets every 4 to 6 hours.

32. ℞ Sodium sulfadiazine (ampul)

 2 to 3 Gm. I.V. every 8 to 12 hours, administered as a 5% solution in Water for Injection U.S.P.

33. ℞ Sodium sulfadiazine (ampul)

 Dissolve 3 Gm. in 100 to 300 cc. Water for Injection U.S.P. or Sterile Isotonic Sodium Chloride Solution for Parenteral Use U.S.P. and inject subcut. every 12 hours.

34. ℞ Sulfamerazine . . . . 0.5 Gm. (gr. viiss)

 4 tablets initially, then 2 tablets every 6 to 8 hours.

35. ℞ Sulfadiazine
  Sulfathiazole
  Sulfamerazine . . . . . āā 0.17 Gm. (gr. iiss)

 8 tablets initially followed by 2 tablets every 4 hours.

36. ℞ Arsphenamine (ampul) . . . 0.6 Gm. (gr. x)

 Dissolve contents of 1 ampul in 60 cc. of Water for Injection U.S.P., neutralize with 5.1 cc. of normal sodium hydroxide, and administer slowly I.V. by the gravity method.

37. ℞ "Mapharsen" (ampul) . . . 60 mg. (gr. i)

 Dissolve contents of 1 ampul in 3 cc. Water for Injection U.S.P. and administer I.V.

38. ℞ *Hemophilus influenzae* antiserum (Rabbit) (vial)

> 100 mg. antibody nitrogen I.M.; repeated if
> necessary.

Expectorants

39. ℞ Ammonium chloride (enteric
coated) . . . .   0.5   Gm. (gr. viiss)

> 2 tablets every 4 hours.

40. ℞ Terpin Hydrate Elixir N.F.. .   120.0   cc. (℥ iv)

> 1 teaspoon every 2 or 3 hours.

41. ℞ Ammonium chloride. . . . .   15.0   Gm. (℥ ss)
Compound Opium and Glycyr-
rhiza Mixture N.F. (Brown
Mixture). . . . . .q.s. ad 120.0   cc. (℥ iv)

> 1 teaspoon every 3 hours.

42. ℞ Ammonium chloride. . . . .   6.0   Gm. (℥ iss)
Citric Acid Syrup U.S.P. . .   90.0   cc. (℥ iii)
Water. . . . . . . .q.s. ad 120.0   cc. (℥ iv)

> 1 teaspoon well diluted with water every 2
> to 4 hours.

43. ℞ Ammonium chloride. . . .   10.0   Gm. (℥ iiss)
Glycyrrhiza Syrup U.S.P.
q.s. ad 120.0   cc. (℥ iv)

> 1 teaspoon in water every 4 hours.

44. ℞ Ammonium chloride. . . . .   5.0   Gm. (gr. lxxv)
Ipecac Syrup U.S.P. . . .   15.0   cc. (℥ ss)
Glycyrrhiza Syrup U.S.P.
q.s. ad 60.0   cc. (℥ ii)

> 1 teaspoon every 2 hours.

45. ℞ Ammonium chloride. . . . .   6.0   Gm. (℥ iss)
Wild Cherry Syrup U.S.P.
q.s. ad 120.0   cc. (℥ iv)

> 1 teaspoon every 2 to 4 hours.

46. ℞ Potassium iodide . . . . . .   18.0   Gm. (℥ ivss)
Ipecac Syrup U.S.P. . . .   18.0   cc. (℥ ivss)
Tolu Balsam Syrup U.S.P. .   18.0   cc. (℥ ivss)
Water. . . . . . . .q.s. ad 120.0   cc. (℥ iv)

> 1 teaspoon as needed.

47. ℞ Expectorant Mixture N.F.
(Stokes's Expectorant). . .   120.0   cc. (℥ iv)

> 1 teaspoon every 3 or 4 hours.

48. ℞ Compound syrup of cocillana.   120.0   cc. (℥ iv)

> 1 teaspoon every 4 hours.

49. ℞ Saturated Potassium Iodide
     Solution N.F. . . . . . . 30.0   cc.   (℥ i)
     5 to 10 drops 3 times a day after meals.

Sedative Cough Mixtures

Any **one** of the following
cough depressants, in the
amounts specified, may be
added to 120 cc. (℥ iv) of ℞ 42
through ℞ 45, for short periods
of treatment only:

Codeine phosphate	0.3	Gm. (gr. v)
or "Dilaudid"	0.06	Gm. (gr. i)
or "Pantopon"	0.5	Gm. (gr. viiss)
or "Demerol"	0.75	Gm. (gr. xii)
or Morphine	0.24	Gm. (gr. iv)
or Methadone	0.06	Gm. (gr. i)

50. ℞ Codeine phosphate . . . . . 0.45 Gm. (gr. vii)
    Terpin Hydrate Elixir N.F.
            q.s. ad 120.0 cc. (℥ iv)
    1 teaspoon every 3 or 4 hours.

51. ℞ Diluted Phosphoric Acid N.F. 8.0 cc. (℥ ii)
    Codeine phosphate . . . . . 0.45 Gm. (gr. vii)
    Wild Cherry Syrup U.S.P.
            q.s. ad 120.0 cc. (℥ iv)
    1 teaspoon every 3 or 4 hours.

52. ℞ Ephedrine sulfate. . . . . . 0.8 Gm. (gr. xii)
    Codeine phosphate . . . . . 0.24 Gm. (gr. iv)
    Terpin Hydrate Elixir N.F.
            q.s. ad 120.0 cc. (℥ iv)
    1 teaspoon every 4 hours.

53. ℞ Ephedrine sulfate. . . . . . 0.8 Gm. (gr. xii)
    Codeine phosphate . . . . . 0.24 Gm. (gr. iv)
    Compound syrup of cocillana
            q.s. ad 120.0 cc. (℥ iv)
    1 teaspoon every 4 hours.

54. ℞ Codeine phosphate . . . . . 0.24 Gm. (gr. iv)
    Tolu Balsam Syrup U.S.P. . . 30.0 cc. (℥ i)
    Wild Cherry Syrup U.S.P. . . 30.0 cc. (℥ i)
    1 to 2 teaspoons every 4 hours.

55. ℞ Codeine sulfate. . . . . . . 0.2 Gm. (gr. iii)
    Diluted Hydrochloric Acid
      U.S.P.. . . . . 1.5 cc. (♏ xxiv)
    Glycerin. . . . . 15.0 cc. (℥ ss)
    Water. . . . . .q.s. ad 90.0 cc. (℥ iii)
    2 teaspoons 1 to 4 times daily.

56. ℞ "Dionin" . . . . 0.3   Gm. (gr. v)
     Ammonium chloride. . . . . 6.0   Gm. (ℨ iss)
     Tolu Balsam Syrup U.S.P.. . 30.0   cc.   (ℨ i)
     Water. . . . . . . .q.s. ad 120.0   cc.   (ℨ iv)
       1 teaspoon every 3 or 4 hours.

57. ℞ Menthol. . . . . 0.12   Gm. (gr. ii)
     Chloroform . . . . 1.0   cc.   (♏ xv)
     Compound Benzoin Tincture
       U.S.P. . . . . . q.s. ad 30.0   cc.   (ℨ i)
       Add 1 teaspoon to a quart of boiling water
       and inhale vapor 2 or 3 times a day.

58. ℞ Chloroform
     Creosote carbonate
     Eucalyptol
     Oil of pine sylvestris . . .āā   8.0   cc.   (ℨ ii)
       Add several teaspoons to 2 quarts of boiling
       water and inhale vapor.

59. ℞ Menthol. . . . . 0.2   Gm. (gr. iii)
     Eucalyptol. . . . . 0.2   cc.   (♏ iii)
     Light Liquid Petrolatum
       U.S.P. . . . . . q.s. ad 60.0   cc.   (ℨ ii)
       Spray into throat with an oil atomizer as
       necessary.

Respiratory Deodorants

60. ℞ Menthol. . . . . 3.0   Gm. (gr. xlv)
     Alcohol U.S.P. . . . .q.s. ad 30.0   cc.   (ℨ i)
       Add a few drops to ½ pint of hot water and
       inhale vapor every 1 or 2 hours.

61. ℞ Creosote carbonate . . . . 30.0   cc.   (ℨ i)
       5 drops in milk, 3 times a day after meals.

Respiratory Stimulants

62. ℞ Caffeine and Sodium Benzoate
       Injection U.S.P. (ampul) . 0.5   Gm. (gr. viiss)
       Contents of 1 ampul I.V., slowly.

63. ℞ "Metrazol" (ampul) . . . 0.1   Gm. (gr. iss)
       Contents of 1 ampul I.V., slowly.

Bronchodilators and Antispasmodics

64. ℞ Epinephrine hydrochloride,
       1:100 solution . . . . . . 30.0   cc.   (ℨ i)
       Inhale vapor from nebulizer 5 to 15 times;
       repeat 4 or more times daily.
       (Note: 0.5 to 1.0 cc. may be added to ℞ 20,
       22, or 24; or before or during O_2 administra-
       tion, when bronchodilatation is desired.)

65. ℞ Epinephrine hydrochloride,
    1:500 solution in oil   (ampul)
      1 cc. (♏ xv) I.M.

66. ℞ Epinephrine hydrochloride,
    1:1,000 solution   (ampul)
      0.3 to 1.0 cc. (♏ v to xv) subcut.

67. ℞ Ephedrine sulfate   25   mg. (gr. ⅜)
      1 or 2 capsules every 3 or 4 hours.
      (NOTE: Ephedrine sulfate, in amounts of 0.8
      Gm. [gr. xii], may be added to 4 oz. of ℞ 42
      to 45, with or without one of the cough de-
      pressants listed in the group of Sedative
      Cough Mixtures.)

68. ℞ Ephedrine sulfate   25   mg. (gr. ⅜)
    Phenobarbital   15   mg. (gr. ¼)
      1 capsule 4 times daily.

69. ℞ Ephedrine sulfate, 2% solution
      Inhale 1 cc. from a nebulizer 3 to 6 times
      daily.

70. ℞ Aminophylline (suppository) 0.5 Gm. (gr. viiss)
      1 suppository at night, or night and morning.

71. ℞ Aminophylline (enteric
    coated) . . . .   0.1 Gm. (gr. iss)
      1 or 2 tablets 3 or 4 times daily.

72. ℞ Aminophylline (ampul)
      0.24 to 0.48 Gm. (gr. iv to viii) I.V., slowly.

73. ℞ Atropine sulfate
      0.6 to 1.0 mg. (gr. 1/100 to 1/60) subcut.,
      I.M., or I.V. every 3 to 6 hours.

74. ℞ Papaverine hydrochloride
    (ampul)
      0.1 Gm. (gr. iss) I.M. or I.V. every 3 hours.

Agents Used for Rhinitis

75. ℞ Belladonna Tincture U.S.P. .   30.0   cc. (℥ i)
      5 to 10 drops in ¼ glass of water after meals.

76. ℞ Camphor   30   mg. (gr. ss)
    Belladonna Extract U.S.P. . .   8   mg. (gr. ⅛)
    Quinine sulfate   60   mg. (gr. i)
      1 capsule every 2 hours for 4 doses.

77. ℞ Ephedrine sulfate, 1% solution 15.0   cc. (℥ ss)
      3 drops in each nostril as necessary.

78. ℞ Nasal inhaler
   (Various types — vasoconstrictor, aromatic,
   or both — are commercially available.)

   Inhale vapor once through each nostril, not
   more often than every 3 hours.

79. ℞ "Neo-Antergan Maleate" . .   50   mg.
   1 or 2 tablets; repeat in 1 hour.

Anhidrotics

80. ℞ Formaldehyde . . . .   8.0   cc.   (ℨ ii)
   Ethyl alcohol 70% . . q.s. ad 180.0 cc.   (ℨ vi)
   Apply once daily to body surface avoiding
   contact with umbilical, anal and genital
   areas.

81. ℞ Alum . . . .   8.0   Gm. (ℨ ii)
   Ethyl alcohol 70% . . . . . 60.0   cc.   (ℨ ii)
   Water . . . . q.s. ad 500.0 cc.   (ℨ xvi)
   Apply to body surface once or twice daily.

82. ℞ Diluted Acetic Acid N.F. . . 120.0 cc.   (ℨ iv)
   Water . . . . q.s. ad 500.0 cc.   (ℨ xvi)
   Apply once or twice daily to body surface.

Miscellaneous

83. ℞ Mechlorethamine hydrochloride   (vial)
   0.1 mg./Kg. body wt. daily for 4 days, administered I.V.

84. ℞ BCG vaccine
   Over an area of 2 x 2.5 cm., through 1 drop
   of vaccine, make 30 skin punctures with
   needle held tangentially to the skin.

85. ℞ Neostigmine methylsulfate,
   1:2,000 solution   (ampul)
   1 cc. (0.5 mg.) subcut. for distention.

86. ℞ Ferrous sulfate . . . .   0.2   Gm. (gr. iii)
   1 tablet 3 to 4 times daily.

87. ℞ Nux Vomica Tincture N.F. .   8.0   cc.   (ℨ ii)
   Compound Gentian Tincture
   U.S.P. . . . . . . q.s. ad 90.0 cc.   (ℨ iii)
   1 teaspoon 3 times a day, before meals.

SKIN AND CONNECTIVE TISSUE

ERYTHEMA SIMPLEX

Redness of the skin, diffuse over wide areas or restricted to circumscribed patches, and due to hyperemia. The etiology is varied, with the most common causes being exposure to extremes of temperature, trauma, sensitivity to drugs, and febrile infections. There is no infiltration or elevation of the skin and the redness disappears momentarily on pressure. Pruritus and burning, alone or in combination, may be associated with this phenomenon. Since erythema simplex occurs in so many and varied disorders, it is essential to determine the cause before attempting to apply other than palliative treatment.

MILIARIA

(Heat rash, Lichen tropicus, Prickly heat, Miliaria rubra)

An acute inflammatory dermatitis due to keratin obstruction of the sweat ducts. The disease is most common in infants, in the obese, and in those exposed to excessive heat for long periods of time. Following profuse sweating, closely grouped papules and vesicopustules appear on an erythematous base, associated with itching and burning.

The sites of predilection are the chest, back, waistline, and skin folds. The inflammation subsides in a few days and may be followed by desquamation. However, recurrent attacks are common, and in prolonged cases, the sweating mechanism may become impaired (tropical anhydrotic asthenia). The condition must be distinguished from seborrheic dermatitis, contact dermatitis, secondary syphilis, drug eruption, and "id" eruptions.

Treatment

This consists in keeping the patient as cool as possible and avoiding those conditions which promote perspiration. Baths containing starch or 1:40,000 potassium permanganate (℞ 104, 105) are soothing. Calamine lotion (℞ 78) will frequently relieve itching. Desquamation may be induced by ultraviolet rays or by 5% salicylic acid (℞ 33) followed by a drying shake lotion (℞ 168, 169) or a powder (℞ 170).

INTERTRIGO

(Chafing, Erythema intertrigo)

An acute superficial inflammation of opposing skin surfaces characterized by erythema, abrasion, maceration and, in some cases, superficial fissuring. It is caused by moisture, warmth and friction incident to the mechanical factor of two opposing skin surfaces rubbing together. Bacterial or mycotic infection almost invariably ensues as a complication.

The flexures of the axillas, the groin, the anal region, the interdigital spaces of the hands and feet, and the area beneath the breasts are the sites of predilection. Obesity and hot weather are the important predisposing factors. Burning and itching are common.

Treatment

Prophylactic measures include proper cleansing and the continued use of a dusting powder (℞ 26, 171), and reduction of weight in obese individuals. Patients should be instructed to wear cool, well aerated clothing and avoid strenuous activity in hot weather if this is feasible.

The acute manifestations usually clear up promptly with therapy. However, the disease may become exceedingly chronic, especially in the obese. Potassium permanganate solution (1:12,000), as compresses or soaks, is the best single therapeutic agent (℞ 4). Tannic acid 5% (℞ 5) sprayed on every hour is often even more effective in severe cases. After the acute manifestations subside, dusting powders (℞ 124, 125, 172), or Castellani's paint (℞ 126), or both, should be used. Another useful local treatment is 1% silver nitrate (℞ 63).

PRURITUS
(Itching)

A sensation, generalized or localized, which the patient instinctively attempts to relieve by scratching the skin in the area affected.

Etiology and Manifestations

Fundamentally, itching may be produced by mildly irritant stimuli acting on the epidermal nerve endings for pain. No specific stimulus is required. Both the peripheral and central thresholds for itching may vary considerably among different individuals and in the same individual at different times. A moderate transitory pruritus is physiologic and is experienced at times by everyone; only when it is persistent and troublesome does it become pathologic. Secondary pruritus occurs in most of the skin diseases, and is especially severe in scabies, pediculosis, insect bites, urticaria, atopic dermatitis, contact dermatitis, food allergy eruptions, miliaria, and dermatitis herpetiformis. It may be the sole sign of a serious systemic disease, and as such demands careful evaluation. This must be more than "skin deep" since, specifically, the itching may be caused by diabetes mellitus, nephritis, diseases of the hepatobiliary system, carcinoma, leukemia, Hodgkin's disease, tuberculosis, gout, arteriosclerosis, and thyroid dysfunction. Pregnancy, the climacteric, focal infection, and drug or food allergy are other etiologic factors. Pruritus may also be psychogenic.

Persistent scratching may produce areas of erythema, wheals, excoriated papules, fissures, and crusts. The trauma is not always caused by the fingernails; some individuals rub the lesions with towels or against hard surfaces or apply heat in an attempt to relieve the itching. There often are signs of secondary infection. If the pruritus is of long standing, lichenification and pigmentation may be present. In patients with a high threshold for the scratch reflex, severe pruritus may be present without the concomitant scratch dermatitis.

Prognosis and Treatment

Since the prognosis of pruritus is directly related to the

underlying cause of the symptom, it is essential to find and remove that cause. To this end, all medicaments the patient may be using either internally or externally should be stopped, if feasible, since drug sensitivity often is responsible for initiating or increasing the pruritus. Many drugs in common use, such as salicylates, barbiturates, and penicillin, may produce a reaction, and innumerable pruritic dermatoses are caused by proprietary, home-concocted or prescribed topical medicaments. The patient must also avoid contact with mechanical irritants such as rough-surfaced or woolen clothing. If he cannot voluntarily refrain from excessive scratching and the condition remains unrelieved after symptomatic therapy, restraints may be necessary. Environmental temperature changes should be minimized since vasomotor responses may intensify the pruritus.

Symptomatic therapy should be instituted immediately. Antihistaminic drugs (see ALLERGY, General Treatment) afford partial relief in a moderate number of cases. Vasodilators may be of transitory benefit, but generally are disappointing: papaverine (℞ 218) is the most widely used. Procaine (℞ 81) is given I.V. in severe cases of generalized pruritus, but it must be administered slowly and with great caution since it may cause a serious reaction.

Colloid baths are advisable in extensive pruritus. The patient soaks himself for 10 to 20 minutes twice a day in a tubful of lukewarm water containing ½ to 1 lb. of cornstarch (℞ 104), and after patting himself dry applies an antipruritic preparation. There are innumerable medicaments for topical use, but the most commonly employed are those containing menthol (⅛ to 1%), camphor (⅛ to 5%), phenol (⅛ to 2%) or benzocaine (2 to 10%). Singly or in combination these antipruritic agents may be incorporated in various vehicles (℞ 82 to 85). Local antipruritic agents of all types are of only limited value, however. Many such preparations themselves tend to produce sensitivity reactions and thereby to aggravate the pruritus.

Other measures sometimes resorted to in cases of intractable localized pruritus are X-radiation, nerve section, tattooing, and nerve injection. Calcium gluconate injections I.V. (℞ 86) are sometimes helpful. Relief or arrest of any underlying disease, plus symptomatic therapy, will usually relieve the pruritus.

SEBORRHEIC DERMATITIS

An acute or subacute inflammatory disease originating on those areas most profusely supplied by sebaceous glands, especially the scalp, face, aural, presternal, axillary, and crural areas. It is characterized by superficial, irregularly sized and shaped

42

erythematous patches covered with greasy yellowish scales (e.g., dandruff).

Etiology

Seborrhea, or oiliness of the skin, generally most pronounced during puberty, is the underlying causal factor. Oily areas provide excellent sites for bacterial or fungous growth or both. Seborrhea seems definitely related to endocrine changes (disturbed androgen-estrogen balance) and yet has such varying etiologic possibilities as heredity, frank hypothyroidism, excess ingestion of fat, carbohydrate, or alcohol, gastrointestinal disturbance, fatigue, excessive perspiration, poor personal hygiene, neurogenic factors and climatic conditions.

Symptoms and Signs

The elementary lesions are perifollicular erythematous macules or papules which may become confluent. Several body areas may be involved simultaneously. On glabrous skin, the borders of the annular, circinate, acriform or serpiginous yellowish-scaled patches are papular and exhibit mild erythematous flare. The lesions may become acutely eczematous in intertriginous areas, or in other areas when modified by moisture, medicaments, or secondary invaders.

Diagnosis

This must exclude syphilids, dermatitis venenata, pityriasis rosea, atopic dermatitis, superimposed fungus infections, and psoriasis. Removing the scales and touching the lesions with a cigarette paper wrapped around a glass slide may disclose: discrete blood points which suggest psoriasis; or oily puncta, seborrheic dermatitis; or diffuse serosanguineous blotches, dermatitis venenata or neurodermatitis.

Prognosis and Treatment

The acute dermatitis ordinarily responds within a few days or weeks, while the subacute or chronic types may be extremely refractory, necessitating expert dermatologic guidance.

Medicaments are chosen according to the clinical stage of the eruption and the regions involved: hairy, intertriginous, or glabrous skin. Erythema, edema, and vesiculation generally characterize the acute stage; oozing, crusting and scaling, the subacute; pigmentary changes, thickening and fissuring, the chronic.

In the acute stage, wet compresses, soaks or baths are used, especially when impetiginous and severe inflammatory changes are present (R 2, 3, 4, 105, 106).

As the acute stage subsides, a mild sulfur ointment with or without resorcinol (R 36) is more efficacious. A paste (R 37) may be better tolerated on glabrous skin. In stubborn cases, even with mild oozing, a sulfur paste may be used (R 38).

Pragmatar (℞ 39) is excellent during the subacute stage. For subacute or chronic scalp involvement, an ointment containing oil of cade, sulfur, and salicylic acid (℞ 40) is useful; women may find a lotion (℞ 41) more convenient.

Sulfur and resorcinol preparations may cause an irritated skin, or act as sensitizing agents, requiring temporary or permanent discontinuance of therapy. Rosewater ointment (℞ 19), wet dressings, or soaks (℞ 2, 3, 4, 105, 106) then may be substituted.

The eyelids do not tolerate sulfur well, and blepharitis is treated with 2% yellow oxide of mercury (℞ 135). Painful fissures in the external ear canal or elsewhere may be treated topically once a day with 1 to 5% silver nitrate solution (℞ 63, 64), or with Castellani's paint (℞ 126). Expertly administered, superficial X-ray therapy may be helpful.

General measures: These include regular rest and sleeping periods; frequent bathing, use of soap substitutes (℞ 27, 28, 29) if soap is irritating; high protein, low carbohydrate, low fat diet; weight reduction, if indicated; prohibition of alcohol; vitamin B complex (℞ 210); twice weekly I.M. injections of 3 cc. crude liver extract (℞ 211) fortified with 100 mg. pyridoxine (℞ 212); elimination of possible contact allergens—medicaments, perfumes, deodorants, clothing, dyes, nail polish, metals (nickel in white gold); eradication of foci of infection; gradual desensitization, perhaps with *Staph. aureus* vaccine, if pyogen susceptibility exists.

––––––––––

SEBACEOUS CYST

(Wen, Seboma, Steatoma)

A slow-growing benign cystic tumor of the skin which results from occlusion of the sebaceous gland ducts, and frequently is found on the scalp, ears, face, back, or scrotum.

On palpation the cystic mass is firm, globular, movable, and nontender. It seldom causes any discomfort. Sebaceous cysts should be differentiated from lipomas, gummas, and osteomas. Fatty tumors are not so well rounded and have a characteristic "pillowy" feeling. The patient with a gumma has a positive serology and may complain of pain on palpation of the tumor. Osteomas are solid and immovable.

Treatment

Surgical excision of the intact tumor is the treatment of choice. Incision and drainage, followed by electrocoagulation applied to the inner surface of the cyst, have been successful in some cases. Recurrence is invariable if the capsule is not completely removed or destroyed.

DYSHIDROSIS

HYPERHIDROSIS

(Sudorrhea, Bromidrosis)

A condition of the skin in which the sweat glands are over-active. The resulting excessive perspiration may be general or confined to the palms, soles, axillas, inframammary regions, or groin. The exudate may be malodorous **(bromidrosis).** The skin in the affected areas often is erythematous or of a bluish white color. In severe cases, there may be maceration, fissuring and scaling of the skin, especially on the foot.

Generalized hyperhidrosis frequently accompanies certain systemic diseases such as anemia, diabetes, hyperthyroidism, and fever from any cause. Obesity and endocrine dysfunction also may cause generalized sweating. Occasionally, an abnormality or disease of the nervous system may be responsible.

The reason for **localized hyperhidrosis** is not clear, since it usually occurs in otherwise normal individuals. However, it appears at sites where normal individuals sweat when under emotional stress rather than heat stress. This fact suggests the etiologic importance of emotional factors. In **bromidrosis,** the fetid odor is caused by decomposition of the sweat and of cellular debris, brought about by the action of bacteria and yeasts.

In generalized hyperhidrosis, the prognosis is related to that of the primary disease. Localized conditions may or may not respond to therapy. The condition usually is somewhat resistant to treatment. Uncontrolled cases may lead to troublesome complications. Hyperhidrosis may be a cause or contributing factor in the production of various skin diseases, such as fungus and pyogenic infections, contact dermatitis, food allergy dermatoses, and seborrheic dermatitis.

Treatment

For **generalized hyperhidrosis,** treatment of the underlying systemic disease (including psychotherapy) is necessary. Atropine (℞ 173) may be given, rarely, to prevent excessive water loss, but as a rule local treatment with powders (℞ 174, 175), alcohol sponges, and potassium permanganate baths, 1:40,000 (℞ 105), is all that is indicated in dermatologic management.

Local hyperhidrosis may be treated with lotions (℞ 175) or dusting powders (℞ 174). Aluminum chloride solutions, 10 to 25% (℞ 176), are widely used. Formaldehyde solutions, 1 to 3% (℞ 177), often are highly effective in treating the palms and soles, but may cause sensitization. Potassium permanganate soaks (℞ 4) are useful. These and other antiperspirant solutions should be applied once a day for several days, and thereafter as indicated.

The treatment for **bromidrosis** is essentially the same as for ordinary hyperhidrosis, but the response may be more satisfactory. Cleanliness, which is essential for both forms, should be even more meticulously observed in bromidrosis. In addition, the use of fungicidal powders (℞ 124) is indicated.

If hyperhidrosis in a disabling form continues despite these remedies, local X-ray treatment or preganglionic sympathetic surgery may be required, but X-ray must be administered only by one experienced in its use, since the margin of safety is narrow.

POMPHOLYX
(Cheiropompholyx)

An acute or subacute, recurrent, vesicular, sometimes pruritic eruption of the hands, the feet, or both, of unknown cause. The diagnosis rests upon elimination of all other causative factors (e.g., dermatophytosis, food allergy, contact dermatitis or "id" eruptions). Treatment is nonspecific and consists of potassium permanganate soaks (℞ 4), salicylic acid in alcohol (℞ 33), and fractional doses of X-rays in resistant cases. Some cases respond well to psychotherapy.

HYPERTRICHOSIS
(Superfluous hair, Hirsutism)

Excessive hair growth in areas usually not hairy. There appears to be a familial tendency in a fair proportion of cases. In women and children, the endocrine system is frequently implicated. The endocrine dyscrasias most frequently associated with hirsutism are adrenal cortical tumors, basophilic adenoma of the pituitary and arrhenoblastoma of the ovary. While chronic irritation may be a causative factor, there is no positive evidence that shaving produces hypertrichosis.

Treatment

General: This should be directed against the underlying endocrine disorder if such exists. **Local:** X-ray is contraindicated in hypertrichosis. The treatment of choice is the destruction of each individual hair follicle by electrolysis. Mechanical measures include plucking, shaving, and epilating wax (℞ 114). Chemical depilatories (℞ 115, 116) are quite adequate if the directions are followed. If the hair is fine, use of a hair bleach (℞ 120) may prove satisfactory.

ALOPECIA
(Calvities, Baldness)

Loss of hair, which may be diffuse or circumscribed, and manifested as the ordinary baldness of age or as an abnormal condition resulting from a variety of causes.

DIFFUSE ALOPECIAS

Senile Alopecia: This condition occurs in elderly individuals, and may be either the end result of a previous scalp disorder (seborrhea) or a manifestation of the general atrophic processes of aging. Hair is lost slowly. There is symmetric thinning, and eventually total loss of hair on the vertex and in the temporal areas. The denuded scalp is smooth, and the hair follicles and sebaceous glands usually are atrophied. Prognosis for return of hair is poor. Occasionally, the process can be retarded.

Toxic Alopecia: This occurs following serious illnesses (e.g., typhoid fever, influenza, tuberculosis), in myxedema, in hypopituitary states and other endocrine disturbances, and sometimes during pregnancy, or postpartum. Administration of certain drugs (thallium, tin, arsenic) may be followed by alopecia. The hair loss usually is diffuse in debilitating diseases and following drug ingestion. In hypothyroidism it is marginal, while in hypopituitary states the vertex is affected. Prognosis for return of hair is fairly good in toxic alopecia after the underlying cause has been removed.

Premature Alopecia: This condition is seen in relatively youthful individuals who are otherwise normal. While no cause has been discovered, hereditary and familial tendencies seem evident. The condition is slowly progressive. The involved areas may be completely hairless or show some lanugo-like hairs. The hair follicles and sebaceous glands usually are atrophied. Prognosis for return of hair is poor.

Alopecia in Seborrheic Dermatitis (alopecia pityroides, a. furfuracea): The cause of seborrheic dermatitis (q.v.) is not known, but there seem to be familial and hereditary tendencies. There are two types: seborrhea oleosa, in which the scalp is very greasy, and seborrhea sicca in which it is dry and scaly (dandruff). Alopecia usually is much more frequent following seborrhea sicca. Hair loss begins in the frontal and temporal regions and is slowly progressive. The affected areas show only a few thin lanugo-like hairs. Prognosis is poor for return of lost hair, but good for arrest of the condition (*see* SEBORRHEIC DERMATITIS).

CIRCUMSCRIBED ALOPECIAS

Cicatricial Alopecias: These diseases usually are the direct result of some underlying disorder and therefore are not amenable to local therapy. Included in this classification are the following: lupus erythematosus, pseudopelade (Brocq), folliculitis decalvans, perifolliculitis abscedens et suffodiens, syphilitic gumma of scalp, and post-traumatic or postinfectious (kerion favus) lesions.

Noncicatricial Alopecias: Syphilitic alopecia is associated with secondary syphilis. The hair loss is patchy, but not clearly defined, producing a moth-eaten appearance. The hairs still remaining in the patches are dry and lusterless. The prognosis for regrowth of hair is very good if antisyphilitic treatment is administered. No local therapy is indicated (*see* SYPHILIS).

Tinea capitis (ringworm of the scalp) is usually caused by a microsporon. It is limited to children below the age of puberty. The lesions consist of well circumscribed patches of partial alopecia; the hairs seem clipped off, and the remaining hairs are dry and lusterless. The patches may be covered with grayish or yellowish scales, and often itch. The affected hairs fluoresce under Wood's light. While inflammatory changes usually are absent, erythema, crusting, and pustulation occasionally occur (*see* Tinea capitis in DERMATOMYCOSES chapter).

Mechanical Alopecia: The patient himself may destroy his hair by rubbing, plucking, or breaking it off, as a manifestation of neurosis or true mania. The hair loss may be regional or circumscribed. Remaining hairs in the involved areas are normal. In infants, such hair loss can occur, especially in the occipital area, as a result of lying constantly on the back and against the bed clothes. Prognosis is good in the young, but poor in the old.

Alopecia Areata (area celsi, alopecia circumscripta): In this condition there is sudden hair loss in circumscribed areas. The etiology is unknown. This type of alopecia may occur in any age group. The scalp is the site of predilection, but all hairy areas may be involved (universal alopecia). The skin of the bald spots is normal in consistency, and the hairs at the periphery are loose, easily extracted, and exhibit atrophic changes near the mouth of the follicles ("exclamation-point" hairs). Lesions are asymptomatic except for occasional burning or itching. Regrowth of hair occurs slowly. The first returning hairs are thin, lanugo-like, and usually white; they are replaced by a second sturdier crop, which may still exhibit absence of pigment. In most patients, provided involvement is not extensive with almost total loss of hair, the prognosis for eventual return of hair is excellent.

Treatment

Care of the scalp is essential, and consists of washing, brushing, and massage, frequently repeated. The hair should be washed every 5 to 7 days. Liquid soaps are recommended (℞ 30, 31, 32). The shampoo should be followed by a rinse of dilute white vinegar (teaspoon to a glass of water) then rinsed with water. Both the scalp and hair should be brushed for 2 to 3 minutes nightly to remove dirt and scales, but care should be taken not to injure the scalp. Combs and brushes should be restricted to individual use and cleansed frequently. Massage should be done for 3 to 5 minutes nightly by forcing the scalp into a ridge between the fingers, several times over the entire head.

Topical medicaments are applied to the scalp to produce local hyperemia and to correct dryness (℞ 10, 21) or seborrhea (℞ 39, 41 to 44). Erythema doses of ultraviolet rays or a single local application of pure phenol (℞ 66) may be helpful in inducing hyperemia in affected areas of alopecia areata.

Restoration of general health by such measures as rest, changes in mode of living, and elimination of foci of infection and toxic drugs, is essential to the complete treatment of all forms of alopecia.

VITILIGO

(Acquired leukoderma; Acquired achromia; Leukasmus; Piebald skin; Leukopathia)

An acquired disorder of the skin characterized by loss of pigment, resulting in variously shaped and sized milky-white patches surrounded by normal or hyperpigmented borders. Except for lack of color, the skin of the lesions is unaltered. The hairs may or may not become depigmented. The cause of true vitiligo is unknown. Consecutive achromia may be secondary to a variety of dermatoses including tinea versicolor (pseudoachromia parasitica), syphilis (leukoderma colli or syphiliticum), pityriasis rosea, postarsphenamine exfoliative dermatitis and certain other drug eruptions, psoriasis, localized and generalized neurodermatitis, lupus erythematosus, leprosy (vitiligoid leprid), lichen planus, alopecia areata, and occupational leukodermas due to antioxidants, such as agerite, used in the manufacture of rubber goods. It also may at times be associated with peritoneal tuberculosis, pernicious anemia and some endocrine disturbances. Leukoderma acquisitum centrifugum, consisting of an oval white patch with a pigmented mole in the center, is a special nevoid lesion. Vitiligo occurs most commonly in the second and third decades of life and seems to be more frequent in dark-skinned races.

Symptoms and Signs

The lesions are nonindurated, nonelevated, noninflammatory, and asymptomatic; only the pigmentation is altered. The depigmented areas show increased sensitivity to ultraviolet rays and to common cutaneous irritants. The course of vitiligo is variable, but it usually is progressive, with lesions appearing first on the hands, feet, arms, neck, and face. They may increase in size and number and spread by peripheral extension and confluence until large areas or, rarely, the entire cutaneous surface is involved (pseudo-albinism). The progress may stop at any stage, and spontaneous regression with recovery has been reported. Vitiligo is apparent when the margins of the lesions and surrounding normal skin become more pigmented or tanned.

The achromic areas may become erythematous but they do not tan.

Diagnosis

Usually, the diagnosis is simple. The patches are "dead" white, sharply demarcated, and of various sizes and shapes; often, the borders are hyperpigmented. Consecutive achromia secondary to other dermatoses as listed above should be excluded. Morphea and scleroderma are differentiated from vitiligo by their characteristic induration and atrophy.

Treatment

Although active treatment generally is useless, much can be done to alleviate the patient's apprehension and to obscure the disfigurement. He should be assured that the ailment will not affect his general health and is not particularly objectionable. Because there is frequently an associated neurocirculatory instability, general hygienic and psychotherapeutic measures are helpful.

The lesions can be made less conspicuous by staining with 0.2 to 0.5% potassium permanganate solution, 2.5% tincture of iodine, or best with a hydroalcoholic fluidextract of the green hulls of black walnuts (℞ 117). The lesions may be covered with a lotion tinted with sulfonated bitumen (ichthammol) (℞ 118). Covermark (℞ 119), regular or waterproof, or a similar preparation, is quite satisfactory.

When the lesions of vitiligo are so extensive that the most conspicuous areas are those of the intervening normally pigmented skin, or when hyperpigmentation of the borders accentuates these areas, it is better to try to bleach the normal skin than to cover the depigmented parts. Strong hydrogen peroxide in ointment form (℞ 121) or ammoniated mercury ointment (℞ 122) can be used, or the pigmented borders of the normal skin can be painted several times daily with a strong solution of mercuric chloride (℞ 45) until desquamation ensues. Since consecutive achromia results from varying primary conditions, as listed under etiology, its treatment must depend essentially on the diagnosis and correction of the original disease process. The local measures described can be used in addition.

ACNE

ACNE VULGARIS

A common chronic inflammatory disease of the sebaceous glands and the pilosebaceous follicles of the skin, characterized by comedones, papules, pustules, cysts, inflammatory plaques or nodules, and scarring, and usually associated with seborrhea.

Clinical types include acne simplex, a. seborrheicus, a. comedonicus, a. punctata, a. indurata, a. pustulosa, a. cystica, a. conglobata, a. cachecticorum.

Etiology

Although the exact cause of acne vulgaris is unknown, many contributory factors have been determined.

Predisposing causes: (1) Increased activity of the pilosebaceous apparatus, probably due directly or indirectly to endocrine factors (disturbed androgen-estrogen balance). Eunuchs and eunuchoid individuals normally have neither seborrhea nor acne vulgaris, yet both conditions can be induced in them by androgen therapy. (2) A hereditary and familial tendency toward the seborrheic habitus; i.e., thyroid-lipoid disturbances, carbohydrate metabolic alterations, psychoneurogenous backgrounds.

Exciting causes: Dietary factors, such as excess carbohydrate or fat; allergy to certain foods (e.g., chocolate, nuts, milk, cheese, tomatoes, wheat, eggs); foods with high iodine content (e.g., seafoods, spinach, cabbage) play an important role. Seborrhea of the scalp often acts as a focus of inoculation for acne. Hydration of the skin (edema) due to gastrointestinal dysfunction, excess carbohydrates and endocrine disturbances (menstrual flares) seems to promote the pustular phase of acne. Physical, mental, and emotional strain and psychoneurotic tendencies are important factors. The nervous habit of pinching and squeezing the lesions causes extensive scarring.

Infection: The part played by *B. acnes* or staphylococci still is controversial. It is generally agreed that pyogen susceptibility and allergy often are important as secondary factors.

Vitamin and other factors: Vitamin A deficiency may cause follicular hyperkeratosis with plugging of sebaceous ducts. Vitamin B deficiency may cause gastrointestinal dysfunction which tends to aggravate the disease. Pyridoxine administered parenterally has been considered by some effective in reducing excessive seborrhea. Vitamin D also has been advocated in the therapy of acne.

Ingestion of bromides or iodides may aggravate existing acne vulgaris or may be the sole exciting factor (halogen acne). Contact with tar, paraffin, and chlorinated hydrocarbons may cause acne (acne artificialis) on exposed parts or exacerbate existing lesions. "Chin fondling" and efforts to conceal acne lesions with the hands—the so-called "acne salute"—perpetuate the condition.

Symptoms and Signs

Acne vulgaris usually begins during puberty and disappears by the age of 30. The lesions are pleomorphic and are distributed chiefly over the face, sometimes extending to the presternal, scapular, and shoulder areas. The primary lesion is the comedone, or "blackhead," which is a slightly elevated papule with a black central punctum consisting of keratinous debris and chemically modified sebum (comedo acne). The elementary lesions may become more papular and erythematous (acne punctata), and the papules in turn may become pustular (acne pustulosa). Firm, deep-seated inflammatory nodules are designated acne indurata. Occasionally, the inflammatory process extends rather widely beyond the pilosebaceous system resulting in deep-seated, dusky red lenticular cystic plaques which undergo dermal abscess formation (acne conglobata). Ordinarily, a case of acne vulgaris will present several of these various lesions.

Diagnosis

The typical distribution of comedones, erythematous papules, pustules, nodules, cysts, and scarring, with history of onset during adolescence, and associated seborrhea make diagnosis easy. The differential diagnosis includes other diseases with cutaneous eruptions, such as papular and papulopustular secondary syphilis, acne rosacea, tuberculodermas, acne necrotica, variola, acneform drug eruptions, and chronic papular contact dermatitis.

Prognosis

With proper care, the vast majority of cases can be cured. In neglected cases, profound psychologic damage and personality changes may result from the disfigurement of acne vulgaris and lead to social and economic failure for the patient.

Prophylaxis

Prophylaxis may be applied to individuals with seborrheic tendencies. Scrupulous cleansing of the scalp and skin and the use of mildly antiseptic drying solutions should be recommended. The physician should evaluate and if possible correct the predisposing and exciting causes of acne in the constitution, habits and surroundings of such individuals.

Treatment

The aims of therapy are to clear existing lesions and to prevent physical disfigurement and psychologic trauma. The importance of the disease must not be minimized, and the first step should be to assure the patient that he can be cured if he will give his full cooperation. Squeezing, pinching, and picking the lesions are strictly forbidden. The entire body, especially the face, must be kept clean by frequent washing. The scalp should be washed frequently, and the face 4 times a day, using hot water and ordinary soap and allowing the lather to remain on the face for several minutes, then rinsing first with hot and next with cold water. After this, the lesions may be gently but firmly massaged between thumb and finger to express excess sebum, and the face rerinsed with warm and cold water. Steamed towels also are useful in softening tough follicular plugs.

In addition, mildly antiseptic agents such as saturated boric acid solution (℞ 1) or potassium permanganate solution (℞ 4) should be applied to the face daily. (The latter will cause slight temporary staining of the skin.) For pustular acne, 20% acetone in isopropyl alcohol (℞ 6) is preferred. If seborrhea is excessive, cleanse with cotton pledgets soaked in a solution of sodium borate (℞ 7) or triethanolamine (℞ 8), and use these solutions, tolerably hot, as wet dressings or soaks.

Each night, after washing and application of an antiseptic, an antiseborrheic lotion should be applied, beginning with a mild preparation and gradually increasing its strength. When papules and pustules predominate, a mild sulfur lotion (White Lotion N.F.) (℞ 46), resorcinol lotion (℞ 47), or sulfur-resorcinol lotion, mild (℞ 48) or strong (℞ 49), is best. These shake lotions are applied with cotton pledgets. Use resorcinol only at night, as light discolors it. (CAUTION: *Mercury and sulfur are incompatible, forming black mercury sulfide.*) Sulfurated lime solution (Vleminckx's solution) (℞ 50) is effective but has an objectionable odor. In severe cases of acne pustulosa, acne indurata, or acne conglobata a sulfur-resorcinol paste (℞ 51) or Quinolor (℞ 52), an ointment of chlorhydroxyquinolines and benzoyl peroxide, is indicated. If the skin becomes excessively erythematous and scaling, these drying agents should be stopped temporarily and soothing preparations such as calamine lotion (℞ 78) or unscented cold cream substituted. After washing the face in the morning, an astringent lotion of 2.5% salicylic acid in alcohol may be applied (℞ 33).

Cosmetics: Greasy preparations should be avoided. The face powder should contain 2 to 4% finely powdered precipitated sulfur. If it is necessary to continue specific therapy during the day, neutracolor may be added to the white lotion (℞ 46) to match the patient's skin. Lipstick and small amounts of rouge are permissible. If the face is considerably disfigured, Covermark or similar preparations give good cosmetic effects, but require meticulous skin cleansing between applications. Stains of the skin resulting from therapy or superficial pigmentations may be bleached with an ointment containing hydrogen peroxide solution (℞ 121) or with 5% ammoniated mercury ointment (℞ 138).

Acne surgery: The physician should evacuate the comedones with a comedone extractor at regular intervals to prevent the development of numerous papular, pustular, cystic, and nodular lesions which would result in extensive scarring. If there is difficulty in removing the plugs, the patient should use strong free-alkali soap several times a day, or soap containing pumice, or a sulfur-salicylic acid ointment (℞ 53). Application of steamed towels for 5 to 10 minutes prior to surgery is helpful. Deep cysts and abscesses should be opened by a thin scalpel, iridectomy knife, or electrodesiccation needle.

Diet: In order to evaluate the factor of food allergy in acne, the common allergens—milk, eggs, wheat, nuts, chocolate, pork, cheese, bananas, tomatoes, onions, and citrus fruit—should be eliminated for a trial period of 3 to 4 weeks. Foods containing bromides and iodides should be avoided. Although opinions vary as to dietary management, the consensus is that the diet should be sparing in fats. (For further general measures, *see* Exciting Causes.)

Specialized therapy: The measures outlined above will control the average case of acne vulgaris. Cases that fail to respond within 2 to 3 months and those with extensive and severe lesions should be referred to a dermatologist for specialized therapy. X-ray: Superficial X-ray therapy by a competent expert is required in a high percentage of cases, and, given early, will prevent extensive scarring and disfigurement. It cannot be overemphasized, however, that a course of X-ray treatments alone does not constitute the successful management of acne. Cold quartz local irradiation is useful for its peeling action. Cryotherapy probably is of little value but, if used, should be carried out by experienced specialists. Dermato-allergic food and contact dermatitis factors should be evaluated and controlled. Bacterial vaccines are of questionable value for routine use but are indicated in cases showing pyogen susceptibility or allergy. Vaccines containing lysed *Staph. aureus* and its toxoid and bacteriophage components seem most suitable for desensitization procedures. Foci of infection should be located and eliminated. Endocrine therapy is logical and has shown some promise, but no general recommendations can yet be made. Desiccated thyroid gland is indicated in patients of the obese and Fröhlich types and in those with basal metabolism rates below normal. Foreign protein therapy (e.g., I.M. or intradermal injection of whole sterile milk) and autohemotherapy have proved helpful in certain cases of acne conglobata. Vitamin therapy, even in the absence of definite hypovitaminosis, is helpful. One or two multivitamin capsules daily (℞ 213) are recommended. These often are supplemented by weekly I.M. injections of crude liver extract (℞ 211) with 50 to 200 mg. of pyridoxine (B₆) added (℞ 212). Vitamin A (50,-000 to 100,000 u. daily) has been recommended but its usefulness is not fully established. Anemia, if present, should be treated with iron (℞ 214) or crude liver extract injections (℞ 211), or both.

ACNE ROSACEA
(Rosacea, Acne erythematosa, Telangiectasis faciei)

A chronic disease of the skin, involving the flush areas of the face (nose, cheeks, chin, and lower central forehead), occurring

*in either sex, usually in middle life, and characterized by vary-
ing degrees of erythema, telangiectasis, comedones, erythematous papules, and pustules, and in a few instances terminating
with moderate to marked hypertrophy of the tissues, particularly of the nose (rhinophyma).*

It is a disease of multiple etiologic components chief among
which are neurovascular instability, endocrine disorders, gastrointestinal disturbances, food idiosyncrasies, focal infections,
alcoholism, external irritants, and dysvitaminosis. Any of these
factors and possibly others, alone or in combination, are productive of a vasomotor neurosis which is considered to be the
basic mechanism responsible for this condition.

In diagnosis, the following must be ruled out: acne vulgaris,
rosacea-like tuberculid of Lewandowsky, lupus vulgaris and
other facial tuberculids, lupus erythematosus, syphilids, acneform drug eruptions (iodides and bromides), and seborrheic
dermatitis.

Prognosis is fairly good if the many etiologic factors of the
rosacea complex are evaluated and corrected, otherwise recurrences and relapses are common. At times, especially if there
is a deep-seated emotional conflict or complex, the affection is
most difficult to relieve.

Treatment

General: The diet should be bland and low in calories.
Obesity should be corrected. All very hot foods or drinks,
especially caffeine-containing beverages, should be strictly forbidden, as should alcoholic beverages and all highly seasoned
foods or drinks. In some cases, certain foods seem to act as
food allergens, as for example chocolate, tea, coffee, milk, nuts,
or pork, and these and any other suspected foods should be
given a period of trial elimination. The ingestion of bromides
(sedative medicaments) and iodides (iodized salt) should be
avoided. The face should be protected against exposure to
wind, sand, sun, extremes in temperature, and any other external irritants. Any existent dysvitaminosis should be corrected.

Local: The face should be kept clean and as free as possible
of oiliness, but it is unwise to use very hot water. The skin
should be cleansed with lukewarm water and ordinary white
soap, and after being rinsed, should be blotted dry rather than
vigorously rubbed. If there is an obvious seborrheic factor a
sulfur-resorcinol-calamine lotion (℞ 36) should be applied several times daily. If the lotion proves too drying, a sulfur-
resorcinol paste (℞ 37) is generally effective and well tolerated.
The scalp should be kept clean and free from oiliness and dandruff. Shampoo once or twice weekly. If the seborrhea persists,
one may use a resorcinol-mercury lotion (℞ 41) or Pragmatar, a
sulfur-salicylic acid-cetyl alcohol-coal tar distillate in a hydrophilic base (℞ 39). Strong antiseborrheic measures are gener-

ally not advisable, but at times, such modalities are necessary
and Vleminckx's solution (℞ 50) is effective.

Cases severe and resistant to therapy should be referred for
dermatologic consultation. Superficial roentgen therapy in the
hands of a fully qualified expert gives excellent results in selected cases. Telangiectases may be made to disappear by
electrolysis, electrodesiccation and by use of solid carbon dioxide (dry ice). The removal of these permanently dilated vessels brings about marked improvement in the condition. The
nodular and lobulated hypertrophy of the nose (rhinophyma)
can be helped greatly by multiple scarification, electrolysis,
electrodesiccation, surgical excision, or decortication. Good
results in the treatment of acne rosacea have been reported from
the use of a mixture of crushed solid carbon dioxide, 10% finely
powdered sulfur and acetone (cryotherapy, slush method). This
procedure requires specialized training and technic. All cases
of acne rosacea complicated by rosaceal keratitis or other ocular signs should have ophthalmologic consultation.

ACNE NECROTICA

(Acne varioliformis, Acne frontalis, Acne rodens, Impetigo
rodens, Folliculitis varioliformis, Necrotic granuloma)

*A comparatively rare skin affection occurring in both sexes,
usually in middle life, and characterized by development on
the scalp, hairline, forehead, nuchal and frontal areas, the nose,
lateral aspects of the cheeks, very occasionally the anterior and
posterior chest, of pinhead to lentil-sized reddish brown papules
or papulopustules which undergo central necrosis, with formation of brownish crusts which eventually slough, leaving vario-
liform depressed scars.* The lesions are discrete, indolent, slow
to develop, tend to be follicular, appear in crops and are very
apt to recur over periods of months or years. In their incipi-
ency, the lesions may sting, itch or have a warm burning sensation. If they become deep-seated, destruction of hair follicles
of the scalp results in cicatricial alopecia. Marked disfigurement from scarring may occur.

The exact cause of the disease is unknown, but some evidence
indicates that the condition may be due to necrotizing staphylococci acting through an allergic mechanism. Seborrhea usually
is coincident.

Acne necrotica is a distinct disease entity and must be distinguished from other acnes, i.e., a. vulgaris, a. rosacea, and
from acneform syphilids, tuberculids, simple folliculitis, neurotic excoriations and drug eruptions. Serologic tests for syphilis, and tuberculin intradermal tests (starting with a high dilution, 1:1,000,000 Old Tuberculin), are necessary diagnostic procedures.

The prognosis should be guarded insofar as complete cure is concerned, since acne necrotica often is resistant to therapy and tends to recur.

Treatment

Local: The scalp should be kept scrupulously clean by frequent shampoos (2 or 3 times weekly). Facial cleanliness is essential. If there is seborrhea, a mercury and resorcinol lotion (R 41) should be applied to the scalp each night by means of a medicine dropper and rubbed in with a toothbrush. An antiseptic ointment, 5% ammoniated mercury ointment (R 138), should be rubbed into each lesion and surrounding areas for 3 minutes twice daily, and application should be continued for several weeks after the lesions have subsided. Quinolor, an ointment containing chlorohydroxyquinolines and benzoyl peroxide in a hydrophilic base (R 52), often is very effective. At times, use of ointments is not advised for hairy areas since coccic follicular disease often travels under an ointment. In such instances, a lotion (R 41) should be used 2 or 3 times daily.

General: Picking, scratching, or squeezing the lesions must be strictly avoided. The diet should be reduced in caloric value, chiefly by reduction of fats, but should be high in vitamins. The vitamin intake may be supplemented by taking 2 multivitamin capsules (R 213) daily. The elimination of chocolate, nuts, and the like, as described under acne vulgaris (q.v.) should be tried.

Specialized therapy: If the patient does not respond to the above listed local and general modalities after 3 or 4 weeks, referral for dermatologic consultation and further specialized forms of therapy is indicated. Superficial X-ray therapy, given only by those fully qualified in this technic, often will cause rapid resolution of lesions and aid in preventing recurrences. In severe cases, it is sometimes necessary to treat lesions with caustics, electrodesiccation, or galvanopuncture. Staphylococcus ambotoxoid (toxoid and bacterial antigens) often is effective as supplemental therapy in clearing the lesions and preventing recurrences. It should be administered according to directions contained in the package insert. An autogenous vaccine also should be tried in resistant cases.

IMPETIGO

IMPETIGO CONTAGIOSA

(Impetigo vulgaris, Impetigo simplex, Streptococcic impetigo, Phlyctenular impetigo)

A common, contagious, autoinoculable, acute, pyogenic skin infection, whose lesions are characterized by thin-walled vesi-

cles, bullae, pustules, and thick superficial crusts, with hemolytic streptococcus and coagulase-positive staphylococcus as the causative organisms. Predisposing factors are poor hygiene, overcrowding, and faulty diet. The disease is most prevalent in hot moist climates. It usually occurs in infants and children and readily becomes epidemic in institutions such as hospitals and orphanages. The newborn are especially susceptible.

Symptoms and Signs

The early lesion is a flat erythematous macule or a superficial vesicle or vesicopustule which rapidly ruptures, leaving a denuded exudative epidermis. The exudate is thin and straw colored and dries to form yellowish, superficial crusts that have a "stuck on" appearance. If the initial lesions do not rupture, there may develop in rapid succession within 12 to 24 hours vesiculopapules, vesicopustules, or bullae which may rupture at any stage, leaving a similar oozing erythematous base. Sometimes the lesions tend to clear centrally and spread peripherally (impetigo gyrata). In infants they usually are bullous (impetigo neonatorum); occasionally they appear as a superficial perifolliculitis (impetigo of Bockhart). The sites most commonly affected are the face, scalp, and extremities—particularly hands and arms. Lesions may appear around the fingernails or on the conjunctival, oral and nasal mucous membranes. Sometimes there is a rather general distribution. Constitutional symptoms are rare but do occur with extensive eruptions in debilitated or very young patients, in whom a febrile reaction may be pronounced.

Diagnosis and Prognosis

Impetigo is to be distinguished from tinea corporis, contact dermatitis, secondary syphilis, herpes simplex, and drug eruptions (q.v.). Unless complicated by constitutional symptoms, impetigo can be relieved in 3 to 10 days by effective treatment; without treatment the course is unpredictable. Acute glomerulonephritis is a possible, but infrequent, sequel.

Treatment

Removal of crusts and tops of vesicles, vesicopustules, and bullae before attempting local treatment is the first and most important step. In mild cases, crusts can be removed by thorough cleansing of the lesions and surrounding skin with soap and water. If this is ineffective, removal can be facilitated by softening the crusts with compresses wet with a mildly antiseptic solution such as boric acid (℞ 1), 1:11,000 potassium permanganate (℞ 4), or a 1:20 dilution of Burow's solution (℞ 2), applied at least 4 times a day. The crusts then are easily removed by mild débridement. The tops of vesicles and bullae should be cut off with sterile scissors after the application of alcohol or other antiseptic. An antiseptic bath (e.g., of potassium permanganate) can be used for extensive eruptions (℞

105). If the lesions are on the beard area, shaving should be done only every other day, using a sharp blade each time and a brushless cream. Extension of infection is unlikely if appropriate hygienic precautions are carried out, and autoinoculation may be prevented by maintaining rigid cleanliness of the hands and nails, towels, and bed linen. If scabies, pediculosis, or other disease is present on the skin, it must be controlled before antipyogenic measures can be effective (q.v.).

For subsequent local treatment, ammoniated mercury ointment 2.5% (℞ 137) is beneficial, but is contraindicated if the patient has a history of sensitivity to mercury or if tincture of iodine has previously been applied to the lesions. For infants, a 1% mercury ointment (℞ 136) is recommended, but should not be used over large areas because of possible skin absorption. For hairy parts (beard, scalp), Quinolor ointment (℞ 52), full strength or diluted with a suitable base, or tyrothricin (℞ 155) is recommended. To patients with extensive lesions and those who fail to respond to local measures, penicillin (℞ 147) or a sulfonamide (℞ 150, 151) should be given. Early reports are encouraging concerning bacitracin (℞ 153), and aureomycin (℞ 139), antibiotic agents suitable for topical use in the treatment of pyogenic infections.

IMPETIGINIZED DERMATITIS

A form of pyogenic skin infection, characterized by serous or serosanguineous exudation, vesicles and vesicopustules, pyogenic crusts and peripheral erythema, that frequently is a complication of pruritic dermatoses (seborrheic dermatitis, scabies, pediculosis, fungus infections and contact dermatitis) when secondary infection with staphylococci or streptococci occurs. Local discomfort in the form of itching, burning, and tenseness is commonly present. Fever, malaise, headache, and local lymphadenopathy also are frequently noted. Impetiginization often becomes such a prominent feature of the skin eruption that it may be difficult to diagnose the underlying condition.

Treatment

In order to effect cure, control of the primary disease is essential. For details regarding specific dermatoses, *see* the respective chapters. Therapy for relief of impetiginized dermatitis is the same as that for impetigo contagiosa (q.v.).

ECTHYMA
(Ulcerative impetigo)

A pyogenic infection involving the entire epidermis and extending deep enough into the dermis so that a superficial or deeper ulceration covered by a crust is formed. Healing results in scar formation. The condition is closely related to impetigo contagiosa (q.v.) in that it is similar in its etiology, predisposing factors, and onset. Many believe that it differs from impetigo only in being more severe and in spreading more slowly.

Diagnosis

The disease occurs most frequently on the lower extremities, below the knees. Usually, the initial lesion begins as a vesicle or a vesicopustule, which ruptures and becomes excavated to form an ulcer. This is covered by a pyogenic crust consisting of dried seropurulent exudate. Pus can frequently be expressed from beneath the crust which, when removed, reveals a superficial saucer-shaped ulcer with an irregular, granulating, purulent base. An inflammatory halo or areola usually is present. Often, scattered inflammatory papules and pustules are seen on the surrounding skin. In the simple type of ecthyma, the lesions rarely exceed 1 to 2 cm. in diameter. Ecthyma is to be differentiated from secondary syphilis, tertiary nodulo-ulcerative syphilis, erythema induratum (Bazin's disease), sickle cell ulcer, furuncle, and ulcers due to such causes as cancer, cutaneous diphtheria, tuberculosis, and drug eruptions.

Prognosis and Treatment

With effective therapy healing occurs in 2 to 3 weeks. The treatment of ecthyma is similar to that of impetigo (q.v.).

SYCOSIS VULGARIS

(Barber's itch; Folliculitis barbae)

A chronic follicular skin infection due to invasion of the pilosebaceous follicles by coagulase-positive staphylococci. Allergy may play a part. The disease is characterized by inflammatory papules and pustules which are usually pierced by a hair. It occurs in males after puberty and is almost always limited to the bearded region, although it may sometimes be seen on other hairy parts of the body.

Symptoms and Signs

The initial lesions are irregularly distributed, superficial follicular pustules. As the disease progresses, the skin of the involved region becomes erythematous and somewhat edematous, and additional pustules appear. Exudation may be abundant, with serous crusts suggesting impetigo, but this can be easily ruled out by the presence in sycosis vulgaris of glassy sheaths on the epilated hairs. Involution of several lesions may be followed by fresh crops and sooner or later distinct patches are

formed. Early in the process the hairs are usually fixed firmly
in their follicles, but when suppuration becomes pronounced
they are loose and easily removed. In cases of long standing,
the hairs are thinned and poorly nourished. Subjective symptoms of burning, itching, and pain may be associated with the
individual lesions. Furuncles, abscesses, cicatrices, vegetations,
and impetiginized dermatitis may complicate the process.

Diagnosis

Sycosis vulgaris must be differentiated from impetigo contagiosa and Bockhart's impetigo, tinea sycosis, seborrheic dermatitis, lupus erythematosus, and secondary syphilis (q.v.).

Prognosis and Treatment

The disease is occasionally acute, but more often chronic and
resistant to treatment. The prognosis must be guarded, but
usually it is good if general therapeutic measures are carried
out along with local treatment.

Local: This necessarily varies according to the condition,
but in all cases epilation of all infected hairs is obligatory to
achieve satisfactory therapeutic results. When there is much
tenderness, pain, swelling, pustulation, and crusting, warm compresses of potassium permanganate solution 1:9,000 (℞ 4) are
indicated. In the acute types, penicillin (℞ 146, 147) or sulfonamides (℞ 150, 151) systemically are of benefit if the organism is sensitive to these agents. Other forms of local treatment include Quinolor ointment (℞ 52), or ammoniated mercury ointment (℞ 138), Burow's solution ointment (℞ 18), or
tyrothricin solution (℞ 155).

General: Often, local therapy alone will not effect satisfactory therapeutic results. It then becomes necessary to evaluate
possible contributory etiologic factors, such as diet and foci
of infection elsewhere. In many cases, specific allergens such
as chocolate, nuts, milk and milk products, or other foods, must
be eliminated to obtain relief. Not infrequently, bacterial
sensitivity is an important factor, and desensitization can be
obtained by the use of autogenous or stock vaccines. Superficial X-ray therapy, supervised by an experienced physician, is
an important therapeutic adjunct.

PYODERMA

*Those acute inflammatory skin diseases which are caused by
pyogenic bacteria, usually Staph. aureus or Str. hemolyticus.
(See also* IMPETIGO CONTAGIOSA; ECTHYMA; SYCOSIS VULGARIS.)
Pyodermas differ only in severity and in the skin structures involved. Among the predisposing factors one should be on the
alert for are general debility, hyperglycemia (diabetes mellitus),

avitaminosis, scabies, pediculosis, contact dermatitis, seborrheic dermatitis, and local trauma.

The inflammatory process is usually accompanied by erythema, tenderness and edema in the adjacent area. Commonly, in severe forms, there is burning pain at the site of the lesion. Constitutional symptoms of malaise, chills and fever may be present; some degree of leukocytosis is usual. The various pyodermas often must be differentiated from cellulitis, anthrax, syphilis, the bubo of lymphogranuloma venereum and chancroidal bubo, and secondarily infected sebaceous cyst.

FURUNCLE AND CARBUNCLE

Furuncle (Boil): *A tender, acute, perifollicular, inflammatory nodule which becomes a pustule with central necrosis discharging, either spontaneously or as a result of incision, a central core of necrotic tissue and a variable amount of sanguineous, purulent exudate.* It is autoinoculable, and the lesions are apt to be multiple (furunculosis). They may occur anywhere on the skin, but the sites of predilection are the neck, axillas, breast, extremities, face, and ear. Lesions within the external auditory canal and the nose, and on the central part of the face often are painful and a cause for great concern. Nasal lesions may be complicated by the development of sinus thrombosis.

Carbuncle: *A multiple perifollicular abscess characterized by sloughing at numerous points on the surface.* The lesion resembles a furuncle except for being larger, flatter, denser, less rapidly developed, and more painful. It may be accompanied by severe constitutional symptoms (prostration, somnolence, stupor). It is most frequently seen in men, often occurring on the nape of the neck, and may be either superficial or deep. It is followed by extensive sloughs, ulcers, and large scars.

Treatment

Furuncles and small carbuncles are best treated conservatively. They should be protected from irritation, and moist heat should be applied intermittently. The skin must be kept scrupulously clean by frequent washing with soap and water. Superficial X-ray treatment by a qualified physician may shorten the clinical course. Locally, ointments containing ammoniated mercury 5% (℞ 138), tyrothricin (℞ 154), or Furacin (℞ 140) may be applied. Bed rest is necessary in severe cases.

When the lesions are large or situated on the central portion of the face (nose, upper lip, or near the eyes), penicillin (℞ 146, 147) or a sulfonamide (℞ 150, 151), or both combined, should be given to prevent possible complications of meningitis or sinus thrombosis. Penicillin also is effective when injected locally into the lesion, using a concentration of 50,000 u./cc. in water or normal saline. When the lesion is seen late and is about to point, incision and drainage should be done.

This is followed by application of warm compresses of 1:9,000 potassium permanganate solution (℞ 4) or tyrothricin solution (℞ 155) for half an hour, 3 or 4 times daily, to prevent reinfection.

HYDRADENITIS AXILLARIS
(Abscess of the apocrine sweat glands, Hidradenitis suppurativa acquisitum)

A pyogenic disease of the axillary sweat glands. It is characterized by the development of tender, erythematous nodules, which are at first firm, but later become fluctuant and tend to suppurate and produce sinus tracts. New nodules may appear and coalesce to form cordlike bands. Lesions occur occasionally in the labia majora, scrotum, anal region, and nipples. Women are more often affected than men.

Treatment
Substantial improvement may be obtained by use of a medical regimen similar to that described for furunculosis (q.v.). In addition, administration of thyroid, 30 to 60 mg. (gr. ss to i) daily (℞ 216), plus a low fat diet, has been recommended. Local irritation, as from clothing, should be eliminated.

PYOGENIC PARONYCHIA
(Panaritium, Whitlow)

An inflammation of the periungual tissues, which may be acute, subacute or chronic. It usually is most prominent in the lunula area. The condition generally occurs in persons who keep their hands in water excessively (e.g., housewives, bartenders). In the acute form there is severe inflammation and suppuration, and the nail may be lost. It is necessary, but often difficult, to differentiate subacute bacterial paronychia from monilial paronychia.

Treatment
Acute paronychia often requires incision and drainage. Local applications and X-ray, as described for furuncle (q.v.), are effective. It is important to keep the hands clean, but they must be protected from excessive exposure to water.

GRANULOMA PYOGENICUM
(Botryomycosis hominis, Granuloma telangiectaticum, Septic granuloma)

A benign, pedunculated or sessile, vascular granulomatous tumor characterized by relatively rapid growth, intense bleeding upon slight trauma, and persistence unless properly treated. It frequently develops at the site of trauma. The areas of predilection are the hand, foot, lip, cheek, chin, shoulder, back, and umbilical region. The lesions frequently are moist and fleshy, and at times are covered by purulent exudate. They must be differentiated from angioma, papilloma, simple granuloma or "proud flesh," bromoderma, dermatitis vegetans, Kaposi's idiopathic hemorrhagic sarcoma, epithelioma, and amelanotic melanoma.

Treatment

Any destructive sterilizing procedure, such as electrodesiccation, is a favored method of treatment. Other modes of therapy are superficial X-radiation (by a qualified physician) or penicillin solution (50,000 u./cc.) injected into the lesion. The removal site should be dressed with one of the bactericidal ointments or solutions (℞ 4, 138, 139, 154, 155).

ERYSIPELAS

An acute infection of the skin caused by the hemolytic streptococcus, and characterized by a sharply demarcated, red, swollen area, with accompanying fever and malaise.

Etiology, Epidemiology, and Pathology

Erysipelas may be due to any one of several different types of group A hemolytic streptococci. It is no longer believed that the disease is caused by strains capable of producing a specific toxin. The same type of hemolytic streptococcus may cause acute pharyngitis, scarlet fever, and erysipelas among a group of contacts. The organisms may enter through a gross skin lesion but ordinarily the site of entry is not apparent.

The disease appears sporadically even during epidemics of other diseases caused by group A hemolytic streptococci. The incidence of erysipelas, as of other streptococcal diseases, is highest during the winter and early spring. While it may be noted at any age it is most often encountered among older people. It is particularly common among persons suffering from chronic debilitating disease. It may be superimposed upon other streptococcal diseases such as scarlet fever, otitis media, sinusitis, tonsillitis, pharyngitis, empyema, wound infection, and puerperal sepsis.

The characteristic red, shining skin lesion is caused by dilatation of and damage to the minute vessels with consequent accumulation of fluid of high protein content in the tissue spaces. Numerous polymorphonuclear leukocytes gather in the inflamed area. Streptococci may be readily cultured from the lesions.

Symptoms and Signs

Ordinarily the onset of erysipelas is relatively acute, with chills, fever, nausea and vomiting a day or so before the skin lesions appear. However, the lesions may develop without significant systemic manifestations. They appear as well demarcated, elevated, pink to red areas with a shiny surface on which vesicles or bullae occasionally develop. The margins are sharply defined and the lesions spread by direct extension. In facial erysipelas, a characteristic "butterfly" appearance is frequent, due to symmetrical distribution of the process, beginning at the bridge of the nose and extending over the cheeks. Simultaneous involvement of more than one area is unusual. The patient may complain of burning or itching, but local discomfort is rarely severe. The area of inflammation may remain small but in the more serious cases it may involve the entire face and extend onto the scalp or occupy an equivalent area on the trunk or extremities. Temperatures as high as 105°F. may accompany the spread of the lesion. In the untreated patient the skin becomes reddish purple on the 4th or 5th day and the swelling begins to subside. Desquamation begins in about a week. There is no scarring, but repeated attacks involving the same area may damage the lymphatics and result in a chronic edema. The severity of the systemic manifestations parallels the course of the cutaneous inflammation.

The most frequently encountered complications are (1) streptococcal bacteremia and (2) pneumonia, usually streptococcal, but occasionally of other etiology. Orbital cellulitis and meningitis are rare complications. Occasionally, secondary invasion by *Staph. aureus* occurs with resulting tissue destruction. Glomerulonephritis or rheumatic fever may, in rare instances, follow erysipelas.

The disease does not confer immunity: repeated attacks of erysipelas in the same individual are not uncommon. The involved area may become sensitized to streptococcal toxins and the site may become inflamed in the presence of streptococcal disease elsewhere in the body.

Diagnosis

The facial type of the disease usually is readily recognized because the red, shining, elevated and sharply demarcated lesion is so characteristic. Lesions on the trunk and extremities show the same characteristics and the difficulty in diagnosis lies in failure to think of the disease as occurring elsewhere than on the face. In doubtful cases the diagnosis may be established by recovering streptococci from a small amount of tissue fluid aspirated from the margin of the lesion or from blebs if present. The temperature may be very high. Except in cachectic patients and chronic alcoholics there is a leukocytosis. Regardless of the total leukocyte count, all patients will show a relative increase in polymorphonuclear leukocytes.

Erysipelas is to be differentiated from erysipeloid, caused by *Erysipelothrix rhusiopathiae*, which is most common in food handlers. Erysipeloid affects the skin of the hands, is slowly progressive, and rarely accompanied by fever. The lesions are of a purple hue instead of red. Eczematous dermatitis may be differentiated by absence of the elevated, sharply defined margins so characteristic of erysipelas, and the patient usually is afebrile. A deep-seated cellulitis, or a thrombophlebitis with tissue swelling and cutaneous erythema may be difficult at times to differentiate from true erysipelas.

Treatment

Reasonable precautions should be taken to isolate the patient. Disposable materials contaminated by the patient should be destroyed. Bed and body clothing should be disinfected.

The patient should be kept in bed and given a high protein, high vitamin, bland diet with liberal amounts of fluids (3,000-4,000 cc. a day). Local discomfort may be relieved by the application of packs soaked in a cold saturated solution of magnesium sulfate. Acetylsalicylic acid may be used for analgesia, and occasionally codeine may be needed (℞ 194, 195, 196). Rarely, the discomfort may be sufficiently severe to require Demerol or morphine (℞ 197, 198, 199). Sedation with a barbiturate or paraldehyde may be indicated (℞ 200, 201, 202). The introduction of the sulfonamides and more recently of penicillin has tremendously improved the prognosis of erysipelas. Penicillin (℞ 146, 147) is the drug of choice, but sulfonamides (℞ 150, 151) may be used. Sulfonamide therapy should not be instituted until the patient is properly hydrated because of the hazard of renal damage. Furthermore, a daily urinary output of at least 1,200 cc. should be maintained during the course of sulfonamide therapy. Penicillin or sulfonamide therapy generally should be continued until the patient has been afebrile for 3 days.

HERPES SIMPLEX

(Fever blister, Herpes labialis, Cold sore, Herpetic keratitis, Herpes progenitalis, Herpes menstrualis, Herpes gestationis)

An acute virus infection characterized by the formation of groups of vesicles, individual or multiple, filled with clear fluid, on slightly raised inflammatory bases. These occur on the skin, mucous membranes, or conjunctiva. Primary infection may be accompanied by constitutional symptoms, but the typical recurrent form is a localized eruption.

Etiology

The infecting agent is a medium-sized virus. An initial systemic or severe local infection is believed to occur in most persons during infancy or childhood. This produces sufficient antibodies to prevent further generalized attacks, but not local eruptions. Local irritation or trauma, mechanical or thermal, may initiate the eruption. Lowered resistance from acute febrile diseases (e.g., pneumonia, meningitis) or the common cold, is the usual precipitating factor. Trigger mechanisms such as exposure to sunlight, menstruation, sexual intercourse, pregnancy, emotional disturbances, and ingestion of certain foods, may produce recurrent outbreaks of herpes simplex. Frequently, there is no apparent cause.

Symptoms and Signs

The manifestations vary with the site of eruption. Typical lesions (small vesicles on an erythematous base) develop rapidly, with burning, itching and tingling, persist for 5 to 10 days, then gradually subside and disappear without scarring. Vesicles do not rupture spontaneously but, when broken, a thin yellowish crust forms which tends to fall off easily. As drying occurs, superficial painful fissures or cracks may form, which heal slowly. Secondary infection occurs readily and exacerbates the process.

Skin lesions are most common on the face, about the mouth or on the lips (h. labialis). Lesions may also occur on the trunk or extremities. As a primary infection, herpes may complicate infantile or atopic eczema (Kaposi's varicelliform eruption, eczema herpeticum), producing severe systemic reactions, occasionally fatal.

Mucous membrane eruptions occur most frequently as small, whitish plaques or aphthous ulcers (canker sores); vesicles are uncommon. A gingivostomatitis in young children may develop, with symptoms of irritability, anorexia, fever, oral fetor, whitish plaques and ulcers of the mouth, red swollen gums, and regional adenopathy. Herpes of the vagina also appears as plaques or ulcers.

Eye lesions may involve the lids, conjunctiva, or cornea. The common corneal lesions consist of recurrent herpetic keratitis, which appears as an irregular dendritic ulcer on the superficial layers. A more severe but infrequent type, disciform keratitis, produces a permanent disk-shaped opacity in the deep layers.

Other varieties occur on or about the genitalia (h. progenitalis, h. praeputialis). Lesions may reappear regularly at the same site—labia majora, buttock, nose, cheek, elbow, palm—at the menstrual period (h. menstrualis). Herpes gestationis frequently begins on the abdomen, around the umbilicus, during the 2nd half of pregnancy. Rarely the disease may invade the C.N.S., producing severe and usually fatal encephalitis.

Diagnosis

Genital herpes must be distinguished from moniliasis, syphilis, and primary lymphogranuloma venereum. Eczema herpeticum often is indistinguishable clinically from eczema vaccinatum (both of which may be called Kaposi's varicelliform eruption). History of recent vaccination or exposure to a recently vaccinated person may help distinguish the two. Biopsy of a vesicle may reveal the characteristic eosinophilic intranuclear inclusion bodies of herpes as distinguished from the basophilic cytoplasmic inclusion bodies of vaccinia. Herpes zoster (q.v.) may be identified by its distribution along the course of a nerve.

Treatment

There is no specific treatment. Symptomatic relief and prevention of secondary infection should be attempted.

Skin lesions may be mopped with cotton soaked in 95% alcohol, spirits of camphor, or benzalkonium chloride (R 141), followed by a dusting powder (R 179) or a drying lotion (R 46, 78). Tincture of benzoin (R 112) or collodion (R 222) may be applied and renewed once or twice daily, especially when fissures or cracks are present. Hard, dry crusts may be softened by a soothing ointment (R 113). Extensive skin lesions may be treated with wet dressings of Burow's solution (R 2) or applications of calamine lotion (R 78).

Mouth and other mucous membrane lesions may be benefited by a detergent and bactericidal solution such as benzalkonium chloride (R 141) or cetylpyridinium chloride (R 142) as mouthwash or application.

Ulcers (canker sores), when persistent and painful, may be touched with a silver nitrate stick or a swab dipped in 10% silver nitrate solution (R 65), followed by thorough rinsing with water. The opposed surfaces of mucous membrane lesions (kissing ulcers) should be kept apart by a liberal application of dusting powder (R 179) and a layer of gauze.

Eye lesions should be treated by a competent ophthalmologist.

Systemic symptoms when severe may require general supportive treatment such as parenteral fluids, amino acids mixtures, and blood transfusions.

Chronic recurrent cases may be benefited by X-ray therapy administered by one experienced in its use. Repeated smallpox vaccinations (8 to 10) performed at intervals of 1 or 2 weeks have been reported as helpful. (If the vaccination "takes," it is not repeated until the reaction subsides.) Trigger mechanisms must be sought and eliminated when possible. Proprietary sunburn lotions containing an ultraviolet filter may prevent eruptions due to exposure to sunlight.

WARTS

(Verrucae)

Circumscribed benign epithelial proliferations induced by a filtrable virus. The disease is readily transmitted among per-

sons in close association, although the factors that predispose
to infection are not well known. The incubation period varies
from 3 weeks to several months.

Warts may appear anywhere on the cutaneous surface, the
lips, or the genital mucous membrane. They occur most commonly on the dorsum of the hand, less frequently on the sole
of the foot, the face, and the genitalia. They have a characteristic pebbly, cauliflower-like surface, on which thrombosed blood
vessels appear as black dots. Paring the outer keratinous layer
will reveal numerous tiny papillae and large superficial bleeding points. On exposed surfaces such as the face or the dorsum
of the hand, they may be of the common exuberant type (v.
vulgaris), the barely elevated type (v. plana), or the finger-like
type (v. filiformis or digitata). On pressure-bearing areas, such
as the foot, they become depressed below the surface, often are
exquisitely painful and cause formation of a thick surrounding
callus (v. plantaris or plantar wart). On mucous surfaces they
grow luxuriantly, have a whitish macerated surface, and are
known as **condylomata acuminata** (venereal warts).

Diagnosis

Careful inspection of the lesion with the aid of a magnifying
glass after removal of the outermost horny layers usually is adequate to differentiate verrucae from other circumscribed
lesions. Not infrequently plantar warts may be obscured by
surrounding callosities. Biopsy may occasionally be required.
Genital and perianal lesions call for special attention, including darkfield examinations and a serologic test for syphilis, in
order to rule out the smooth-topped condylomata lata of secondary syphilis.

Prognosis

Some warts disappear spontaneously, but others persist for
many years. Response to treatment varies from cure with the
simplest measures to persistence despite intensive therapy.
Plantar warts seem to have the least tendency to spontaneous
regression.

Treatment

Since warts have a tendency to spontaneous disappearance,
the theory of psychotherapeutic suggestion is difficult to establish but is worth bearing in mind in evaluating other forms of
therapy. Systemic treatment, such as bismuth injections,
probably is of little or no value apart from its problematical
psychologic effect.

Specific treatment is available only for condylomata acuminata, and consists of podophyllin (℞ 70, 71) carefully applied
to each lesion with an applicator stick. Normal mucous membrane should be avoided and the patient instructed to wash
the medicament off with soap and water after 4 to 8 hours.

Within a few days, the condylomata usually turn white and fall off. Retreatment is occasionally necessary. Prophylactic measures to prevent recurrences include circumcision, treatment of lesions of marital partner, careful daily soap and water hygiene and daily application of a drying dusting powder (℞ 171, 172).

All other warts are treated locally with destructive agents. No treatment should be used so vigorously as to leave a scar. Fractional applications repeated at intervals produce the best cosmetic results and cure a higher percentage of patients. Concomitant hyperhidrosis, mycotic infections, or orthopedic deformities should be treated before other measures are started. Electrodesiccation under procaine anesthesia, if lightly and expertly done, often is the simplest way of treating the common, filiform, and digitate warts. X-ray therapy, in the hands of an expert, is frequently effective. Freezing with solid carbon dioxide is often successful. Warts also may be destroyed by repeated application of strong acids such as trichloroacetic (℞ 69). Flat warts frequently extend over large areas and are best treated by the daily application of a keratolytic such as Vleminckx's solution (℞ 50) or Castellani's paint (℞ 126).

Plantar warts are the most painful and often the most difficult to treat. Electrodesiccation is effective in some cases. X-ray therapy, by qualified experts, in cancericidal doses, will cure about 50 to 75%. However, the following plan of treatment is preferred:

(1) Pare down callus and wart, stopping before bleeding occurs. (2) Touch the wart carefully with "liquefied crystals" of phenol (℞ 66), using a bare applicator stick to keep excess acid from normal skin. (3) Follow this with "fuming" nitric acid (℞ 67), again using only a bare applicator. (4) Fashion a ring pad from heavy felt and apply it so that the hole just fits over the wart (multiple holes for multiple warts). (5) Apply a speck of 60% salicylic acid in petrolatum (℞ 68) to the wart but do not fill the hole with it. (6) Tape the pad to the foot securely, using multiple strips of 1-inch adhesive tape, covering the hole and the entire pad. When the patient walks on this the wart will be extruded and thus become accessible for further treatment. Vigorous exercise, or wetting the tape during bathing or swimming, should be avoided. After 5 days repeat steps 1 through 6. If meticulously carried out, the wart will be gone in about 3 to 7 treatments. See the patient at 2-week intervals thereafter, to watch for recurrences. These, or new warts should be retreated as many times as necessary. If properly and persistently treated, the most resistant plantar warts can be cured on an ambulatory basis without painful scars or residuals. This treatment may be used when other modalities, such as X-ray therapy, have failed.

Excision of warts is undesirable since it may produce a painful scar. Curettage of the abnormal tissue with a small, sharp spoon curet is frequently effective and will not cause scarring if normal tissue is not injured. This procedure may be carried out under local anesthesia.

CUTANEOUS TUBERCULOSIS

Any skin lesion due to Myco. tuberculosis, *either directly by local infection, or indirectly from infection elsewhere in the body* (*tuberculids*). About 85% of cases are caused by the human type of tubercle bacillus, the remainder by the bovine type. The disease is relatively rare in the United States. While it may be seen in tuberculous children or adolescents, it occurs most frequently in persons in the lower income groups living under unhygienic conditions.

General Characteristics

The skin lesions frequently are associated with tuberculous lesions elsewhere, and the basic pathology is similar to that of tuberculosis generally. The great variation in clinical appearance of the cutaneous lesions is due to the varied response of the human body to tubercle bacilli. Once established on the skin, the tuberculous process can spread by contiguity or through the vascular system. Allergy to tubercle bacilli is best measured by skin tests with tuberculin. There are various technics, of which the Mantoux test and the Vollmer patch test (q.v.) are the most frequently employed. Reactions to the tuberculin test vary in strength or may be absent (*see* below). A reaction is seldom obtained in primary tuberculous processes of less than 6 to 8 weeks' duration.

Clinical Types

A. Localized lesions: (1) **Tuberculous chancre:** This primary tuberculous complex consists of a nondescript ulcer at the site of inoculation, accompanied by lymphangitis and satellite lymphadenitis in an individual previously free of tuberculous infection. Usually, the lesion tends to heal spontaneously. At first there is no reaction to the tuberculin test, but in 6 to 8 weeks a reaction may be obtained. (2) **Tuberculosis verrucosa cutis** (Verruca necrogenica) results from reinfection of an individual already partly immune owing to a previous tuberculous process. It is caused by direct inoculation with tuberculous material from cadavers, tuberculous cattle or a patient's sputum. Men are most often affected, and the usual sites are the exposed surfaces of arms and legs. The lesions consist of brownish verrucose patches, which may show some suppuration and peripheral extension, with lymphatic involvement. A tuberculin reaction can be obtained. (3) **Tu-**

berculosis cutis orificialis is tuberculosis of the mucous membranes, secondary to tuberculosis of the internal organs. It consists of chronic indolent ulcers of the oral, genital, and anal regions. The lesions are not indurated, and may or may not be painful. These ulcers usually are teeming with tubercle bacilli. The tuberculin reaction is present except in the terminal stages of tuberculosis. The prognosis is generally poor. (4) **Scrofuloderma** (tuberculosis colliquativa) is a cold abscess of the skin, secondary to a subcutaneous tuberculous focus, usually of bone or of lymph nodes. It is most common on the neck or chest and appears as an indolent bluish ulcer. It usually occurs in young persons. The tuberculin reaction is present. Prognosis is fairly good. (5) **Lupus vulgaris** can occur anywhere, but the face is the usual site. The primary lesion is a soft brownish tubercle resembling apple butter, which persists under diascopic examination ("apple-butter nodule"). Later, the eruption can assume various forms. There may be psoriasis-like plaques, hypertrophic verrucose masses, or shallow crusted ulcers. The lesions heal by scar formation which may be disfiguring. The tuberculin reaction is present. Untreated, the disease slowly progresses, but it rarely is a direct cause of death.

B. **Hematogenous types** originating from some internal tuberculous focus: (1) **Acute miliary tuberculosis** produces a generalized, often hemorrhagic, papular eruption. It occurs most frequently in children. The tuberculin reaction usually is lacking and the prognosis is poor. (2) **Lupus miliaris disseminatus** consists of a brownish folliculopapular eruption which can occur anywhere but is most common on the flush areas of the face. Diascopic inspection discloses typical lupus nodules. The eruption is essentially benign and heals with scarring. A reaction to tuberculin is present. (3) **Rosacea-like tuberculid** is most common in women. Small brown papules are symmetrically distributed over the cheeks and forehead, exempting the chin and nose. The course is chronic and without serious complications. The tuberculin test is strongly positive. (4) **Papulonecrotic tuberculid** consists of symmetrically distributed bluish papules, usually on the extremities, which develop central necrosis and on healing leave punched-out scars. Spontaneous healing is the rule. A strong reaction to tuberculin is present. (5) **Tuberculosis indurativa** (erythema induratum) usually occurs in women. It consists of large indurated cutaneous nodules which may terminate in absorption or necrosis and ulceration. The lesions may appear anywhere but are most frequent on the lower extremities, especially the calf. The eruption runs a chronic course. The tuberculin reaction is present. (6) **Follicular tuberculid** appears as patches of grouped follicular lesions, particularly on the trunk, which have to be differentiated from the grouped follicular syphilid and from trichophytid lesions.

Treatment

All the therapeutic measures for tuberculosis (q.v.) apply equally well in cutaneous tuberculosis and only a few special procedures are necessary. For ulcerative lesions a local antiseptic ointment (℞ 138) is useful. In lupus vulgaris and tuberculosis verrucosa cutis, excision, electrocoagulation or various escharotic agents (℞ 61, 69) may be employed. Bed rest is essential in tuberculosis indurativa. Vitamin D_2 (℞ 209) is highly beneficial, especially in lupus vulgaris, but not specific for all types of cutaneous tuberculosis. Streptomycin or dihydrostreptomycin therapy holds considerable promise in many types of cutaneous tuberculosis, but it should be used with due caution (*see* ANTIBIOTIC THERAPY).

DERMATOMYCOSES

Superficial fungus infections of the skin or its appendages. They include tinea capitis, t. favosa, t. barbae, t. corporis, t. versicolor, t. cruris, t. pedis, t. unguium, erythrasma, and trichomycosis axillaris. These diseases are produced by various *Hyphomycetes,* of which the most important clinically are *Microsporon, Trichophyton, Epidermophyton,* and *Achorion.*

The causal organisms usually can be identified by direct microscopic examination of potassium hydroxide-mounted hairs, skin scrapings or other specimens from suspected areas, or by culture (*see* LAB. PROC.). The trichophytin test for cutaneous sensitivity is of limited diagnostic value, since a reaction may indicate either a previous or an existing infection. Failure to react, however, tends to rule out a fungus origin for the lesions. Wood's light provides confirmation of a diagnosis of t. capitis and also is a guide during treatment. These ultraviolet emanations of the order of 3,500 angstroms produce brilliant fluorescence of the fungus-infected hairy areas.

Dermatophytid, or "id" eruptions are easily confused with primary fungus infections. They occur secondarily in another, often distant, part of the body. The usual sequence is a primary fungus infection of the feet (e.g., athlete's foot) followed by a secondary vesicular "id" eruption on the hands. Dermatophytids are caused by antigenic substances produced by fungi at the primary site and disseminated through the body to remote areas of sensitized skin, where they cause various types of eruptions—erythematous, eczematous, vesicular, or bullous—not necessarily resembling the original eruption. Microscopic and culture examinations of material from such secondary lesions are negative for fungi, and the primary focus must be sought for diagnosis. Dermatophytids usually disappear without treatment once the primary infection is curbed or eradicated.

Tinea capitis (ringworm of scalp, t. tonsurans): Usually caused by *Microsporon audouini*, but *Trichophyton* and fungi of animal origin are occasionally responsible. The disease occurs in children, is highly contagious, and often becomes epidemic in schools. It begins as one or more small, rounded, elevated scaly grayish patches upon any portion of the hairy scalp. Follicles become prominent, and affected hairs are dry, brittle, lusterless, and usually broken. Eventually the hair is lost, leaving "rubbed off" bald patches. As the patches increase in size and number, they coalesce and slowly spread over the entire scalp. Some cases exhibit a highly inflammatory exudative reaction (kerion) in the infected areas. Except for slight itching, the disease usually is asymptomatic. It may persist for years despite local therapy and resolve of itself with the onset of puberty.

Tinea favosa (favus, crusted ringworm, honeycomb ringworm, porrigo scutula): This disease, now rare in the United States, is caused by *Trichophyton schoenleinii, gypseum,* or *violaceum.* The scalp is primarily affected, but the nails and glabrous skin also may be involved. The disease begins as a superficial circumscribed inflammation, with scaling and thick diffuse crusts which later become elevated, tenacious yellowish scutula (shield-shaped crusts). The crust usually is friable and on removal leaves a red, shiny, sometimes suppurating, cup. A "mousy" or "damp straw" odor is characteristic. The course is slow and chronic. After healing there is scar formation and some degree of permanent alopecia. When the nails are involved they become brittle, discolored, and irregularly thickened, with crust formation under the free edges. Patches occurring on glabrous skin appear as thickly crusted yellowish disks which through fusion and extension eventually cover large areas.

Tinea barbae (t. sycosis, barber's itch, ringworm of beard): Caused by *Microsporon lanosum* or *Trichophyton gypseum, violaceum,* or *purpureum.* The disease is not common. It is incurred by contact with animals or by exposure to infected material, often in barber shops. Lesions are confined to the beard region. The inflammatory process begins as small, slightly scaly, hyperemic patches, which spread peripherally and clear at the center. The borders are raised and are pustular or scaling. Contiguous patches may increase to form a large irregular lesion. With invasion of hair and follicles, induration and lumpy swellings develop. Deep-seated nodules, which tend to ulcerate (kerion), may be found. Hairs become dry and brittle, then break off and fall out or are easily extracted. Tinea barbae must be differentiated from anthrax, actinomycosis, syphiloderma, contact dermatitis, and bromide or iodine eruptions. Culture and microscopic examination are indicated for diagnosis.

Tinea corporis (t. trichophytina, glabrosa, or circinata;

43

trichophytosis corporis; ringworm): Either *Trichophyton* or *Microsporon* may be causative. Lesions appear on any part of the glabrous skin, as single or multiple papulosquamous erythematous plaques which spread peripherally. A raised vesiculopapular or crusted border of several millimeters' width appears, and as the lesion expands the center tends to clear, producing characteristic annular lesions. In the chronic form there is less central clearing and the lesions are dull red or brownish, erythematous, scaling plaques, slightly elevated above the surrounding skin. The patient may complain of slight burning and varying degrees of pruritus.

Tinea versicolor (pityriasis versicolor, dermatomycosis furfuracea, chromophytosis): This benign fungus process, confined to the most superficial layers of the skin—usually that of the upper trunk and lower neck—is caused by *Microsporon furfur*. The lesions appear as gyrate, circumscribed or diffuse, furfuraceous, brownish red, scaling plaques, which may be macular or almost imperceptibly elevated. When they are stroked, superficial scaling is revealed. The disease usually is asymptomatic, but may cause slight pruritus. Treatment usually results in remission rather than permanent cure.

Erythrasma: This chronic infection of the stratum corneum with *Microsporon minutissimum* (*Nocardia minutissima*) is characterized by well circumscribed maculopapular, brown to reddish brown plaques. These are fairly extensive (palmsized) and usually occur in the axillary, crurogenital, and intertriginous regions. Obese adults are most frequently affected. The plaques show evidence of gradual spread from serpiginous, slightly erythematous borders, with no tendency to central clearing. Differentiation must be made from intertrigo, t. cruris, and seborrheic dermatitis. The causative organism can be seen microscopically in potassium hydroxide mounts stained with methylene blue. The prognosis is good, but recurrences are frequent.

Trichomycosis axillaris (trichomycosis nodosa): Causative organism, *Nocardia tenuis*. An asymptomatic affection of the axillary, and sometimes the pubic, hairs, which become covered with reddish, yellowish, or blackish concretions or sheaths of a sandpaper appearance. It is unimportant clinically and often goes unnoticed.

Tinea cruris (eczema marginatum, ringworm of groin, jock itch, dhobie itch): Infection can be caused by various Trichophyton fungi, but *Epidermophyton inguinale* is the most common etiologic agent. Contact surfaces of the scrotal and crural regions or anogenital and gluteal areas are the sites of predilection. In the acute phase, erythema is prominent, with superficial oozing and crusting which may be accompanied by intense burning and pruritus. Subacute and chronic lesions are dry, scaling, and moderately erythematous or hyperpigmented. Lichenification occasionally occurs. Asymmetrical involvement is the rule and this feature aids in differentiating t. cruris from intertrigo, seborrheic dermatitis, and other cutaneous disease in this area.

Tinea pedis (ringworm of the foot, athlete's foot, dermatophytosis, trichophytosis pedis): This probably is the most common of fungus diseases. The majority of cases are caused by *Trichophyton purpureum* (which frequently produces the more chronic and refractory lesions) and *T. gypseum.* Distribution of these fungi is widespread and apparently persons acquire this infection because of predisposing factors, such as excessive sweating, friction, uncleanliness, and a skin *p*H conducive to fungus growth. The incidence is greatest in warm weather. Onset usually is insidious, and in its milder state, the infection may be practically asymptomatic. There may be excessive scaliness and maceration of the skin between the toes. As the disease progresses, multilocular vesicles appear singly or in patches along the sides and undersurfaces of the digits and the sole of the foot. In severe cases the lesions may coalesce to form bullae. The skin becomes raw and eroded, and the entire area edematous. Secondary pyogenic infection is frequent. Subjective symptoms of burning, pruritus, and pain often are severe.

A squamous hyperkeratotic type of t. pedis sometimes occurs, which is characterized by thickened hyperkeratotic plaques with scaling and eczematous changes, with or without superficial fissuring, and occasionally shows small vesicles at the periphery of the plaques.

Rarely, a similar infection may occur primarily on the hands (t. manis). Involvement of the hands usually is in the form of a dermatophytid, with the original focus in the feet. When an acute vesicular dermatitis appears on the hands it is infrequently due to a primary fungus infection. The final diagnosis of tinea of either the hands or the feet rests upon direct potassium hydroxide examination and cultures from the tops of vesicles or scrapings. Under appropriate treatment, the condition may be completely cured, but its tendency is to become subacute and chronic, and reinfections are numerous.

Tinea unguium (onychomycosis, fungus infection of the nails): In most cases the causative fungus is *Trichophyton purpureum,* although the condition also can be due to other fungi including *Epidermophyton inguinale* and *Trichophyton gypseum.* These are the same fungi that cause infections of the feet and hands.

The toenails are more commonly affected than the fingernails. Ungual involvement always begins peripherally and is characterized by loss of luster at the free edge or at the lateral border. This is followed by varying degrees of thickening, friability, separation from the nail bed, and the accumulation of grumous material under the free edge of the nail. This condition usually progresses until the entire nail is involved.

It often is difficult to differentiate from psoriasis. In psoriasis, more nails and more of each nail are affected and there is a characteristic shallow pitting of the nail; also psoriatic lesions usually are found elsewhere. In monilial infection, the nail may appear darkened, ridged, pitted, or even somewhat fragmented at its peripheral border.

Treatment

Incorrect treatment of superficial dermatomycoses probably causes more disability than the disease itself. Irritating forms of therapy for an acute dermatomycosis, such as full-strength Whitfield's ointment, tincture of iodine, or X-radiation, may precipitate a dermatophytid reaction in another part of the body.

General: The application of fungicides should be preceded by control of any complicating "treatment dermatitis" (dermatitis venenata, q.v.) or secondary infection, the removal of involved hair, nails, and crusts, and frequent scrupulous cleansing of the part. Systemic administration of sulfonamides (℞ 150, 151) or penicillin (℞ 146, 147) may be indicated to combat secondary bacterial infections. However, penicillin should be given with caution since it is similar antigenically to pathogenic fungi and may exacerbate primary foci, or of itself cause dermophytid reaction. During the acute phases of any fungus infections, mild antiseptic ointments (℞ 12, 137, 138), or applications, 3 to 5 times daily, of potassium permanganate (℞ 4), coal tar (℞ 107), boric acid (℞ 1), acriflavine (℞ 143), or Burow's solution (℞ 2) may be employed to dry exudative surfaces and reduce inflammation.

A wide variety of fungicidal preparations are available (℞ 39, 72, 124 to 134). It may be necessary to try several before the most beneficial agent for a specific case is found. Ointments are best applied at bedtime and removed in the morning, to be replaced by a light coating of drying powder (℞ 181). Contiguous skin surfaces should be kept dry of sweat by placing absorbent cotton or lamb's wool between them. In chronic eczematous infections, especially chronic t. cruris, crude coal tar paint (℞ 9) or ointment (℞ 16) is beneficial.

Tinea capitis: The scalp should be shampooed at least every 3 or 4 days. Infected hairs, identified by their fluorescence under Wood's light, should be plucked out, and loose hairs, crusts and debris removed frequently. It is advisable to clip the hair closely about every 10 days. Oral ingestion of thallium salts for epilation is to be condemned because of their high toxicity. Of the many fungicides that may be tried, the use of salicylanilid ointment or Salundek (℞ 127, 128) is particularly valuable in this condition. These fungicides should be rubbed into the scalp twice daily for several months. When this therapy is conscientiously followed, although less than half the cases will clear up after 3 to 4 months of treatment, virtually all will be cured if therapy is continued for 6 months or, as is occasionally necessary, for up to 1 year. If adequate local therapy of t. capitis has proved ineffective, X-ray epilation of the scalp may then be advised. It should be done only by one experienced in this procedure since even the slightest overdosage may cause permanent loss of hair in some patients.

Tinea favosa: Crusts (scutula), debris, and infected hairs should be removed after softening with salicylic acid ointment (℞ 35) or oil application (℞ 24). Fungicidal preparations (℞ 39, 72, 124, 125, 127 to 134) may be tried in this infection. It often is necessary to resort to X-ray epilation of the entire scalp by a qualified physician.

Tinea barbae: The inflammatory type is best treated with applications of solutions of potassium permanganate (℞ 4), Burow's solution (℞ 2) or acriflavine (℞ 143) several times daily. Infected hairs should be plucked. Fungicidal ointments (℞ 39, 124, 125, 127 to 130) applied between wet applications, or alone in mild infections, usually are beneficial.

Tinea corporis: Soap and water cleansing of lesions plus use of ammoniated mercury (℞ 137, 138) or a fungicide (℞ 124 to 134) usually effects rapid improvement and cure. Fungicidal powders (℞ 124, 125) are recommended for daytime use on intertriginous surfaces, rather than ointment vehicles.

Tinea versicolor and Erythrasma: Vigorous cleansing of the skin plus the application of a fungicide (℞ 39, 124, 125, 131, 133, 134) several times daily usually is curative. Mild erythema doses of ultraviolet rays will accelerate improvement. Wood's light is useful in revealing areas requiring treatment.

Trichomycosis axillaris: Involved hair should be shaved off and a fungicide (℞ 39, 124, 125, 131) applied daily for several weeks.

Tinea cruris: For the acute manifestations sitz baths (℞ 105, 107) are effective for drying exudative surfaces. Half-strength Castellani's paint (℞ 126) may be used cautiously after bathing. In the chronic cases, fungicidal ointments (℞ 39, 124, 125, 127 to 132, 137, 138) may be applied at night, and Castellani's paint (℞ 126) or a fungicidal powder (℞ 124, 125) during the day. Crude coal tar paint (℞ 9) or coal tar ointment (℞ 16) may be helpful in eczematized chronic t. cruris.

Tinea pedis: In the acute stage, ambulation should be restricted and the feet soaked 2 to 3 times daily for 30 minutes in potassium permanganate (℞ 4), acriflavine (℞ 143) or Burow's solution (℞ 2). Water-soluble fungicidal ointments (℞ 124, 125) or ammoniated mercury (℞ 137, 138) should be applied between soaks. Daily débridement is essential and, in the acute stage, consists of clipping off the tops of vesicles or, in the chronic stage, a foot bath followed by vigorous wiping, thus removing keratinous debris. In mild or chronic fungus infections any of the fungicides (℞ 39, 124 to 134) may be effective if combined with a daily foot bath, scrupulous wiping, use of boiled socks and control of hyperhidrosis. Excessive sweating may be eliminated with daily application of powders (℞ 124, 125, 181) or a foot bath (℞ 178, 180).

Tinea unguium: In mild cases, scraping the involved nail surface and area around and beneath the cuticle, plus the application of a fungicide (℞ 39, 72, 125, 129 to 134), may control the infection. Favorable results have been reported with weekly applications of ammoniacal silver nitrate (℞ 74). In more resistant cases it may be necessary to excise the nail. This should be attempted only after the nail has been softened by application of a 40% salicylic acid plaster (℞ 73) cut to its exact size.

SCABIES

(The itch)

A highly contagious parasitic skin disease, characterized by burrows in the skin, multiform eruptions, and intense itching that occurs chiefly at night.

Etiology and Incidence

Scabies is caused by the itch mite (*Sarcoptes* or *Acarus scabiei*). The impregnated female burrows into the horny layer (stratum corneum) of the skin and deposits her eggs along the tunnel. Within 4 to 8 days the larvae are hatched. These later emerge from the burrow, travel across the skin and enter the hair follicles. Sensitization of the host to the parasite is responsible for the itching. True sensitization occurs approximately one month after infestation.

Scabies is acquired through intimate contact with an infested individual or infested clothing, and is most prevalent among persons living under crowded, unhygienic conditions. Infestation often involves an entire household.

Symptoms and Diagnosis

Pruritus, most intense at night because of the nocturnal activity of the parasites, is the most common complaint. The characteristic lesion is the burrow, which appears as a fine, wavy, dark line varying in length from a few millimeters to several centimeters. In fair-skinned individuals, burrows usually are well marked and are accompanied by vesicles. After development of the burrows, the eruption may become multiform with papules, pustules, crusts, excoriations, and hyperpigmentation. The areas most frequently involved are the interdigital surfaces and web spaces of the hands, the volar aspects of the wrists and forearms, the anterior axillary folds, the waist, the breasts of women, the buttocks in children, and the genital region. The lesions may appear anywhere on the body; however, they rarely are noted above the neckline. In doubtful cases, microscopic demonstration of the parasite or ova should be attempted by removing the burrow and its contents with a Hagedorn needle and placing the specimen in 10% potassium hydroxide on a slide beneath a cover glass.

When the disease has been of long duration and neglected, eczematization, lichenification, furunculosis, impetigo, paronychia, and other manifestations of pyoderma frequently develop. Pediculosis often may be coexistent. Not infrequently the appearance of the scabies eruption has become modified by previous treatment. The most common complication is a sulfur dermatitis characterized by a dry, erythematous, pruritic, scaly skin.

Scabies must be differentiated from papular urticaria, secondary syphilis, Paget's disease, exudative neurodermatitis, pediculosis corporis, lichen planus, tinea versicolor, pityriasis rosea, drug eruptions, and food allergy dermatoses.

Treatment

Treatment is entirely external. If there is the slightest suspicion that other members of the household are infected, they must be treated simultaneously to prevent reinfestation. If the disorder is associated with any pyogenic infection, appropriate therapeutic measures should be carried out.

The standard antiscabetic course is as follows: (1) First night: hot bath, soak thoroughly, scrub with soap and water, using a wash cloth or soft brush to open the burrows, with special attention to the sites of predilection (hands, arms, axillas, perianal and genital regions). (2) Apply sulfur ointment over the entire body, except for the scalp and face. In infants, even the face and scalp must be treated. (3) Next morning: rub in ointment, but omit bath. If hands are washed during day, ointment should be reapplied. (4) Second night: repeat application of sulfur ointment, but no bath. (5) Second morning: bathe with soap and water, dry by gentle rubbing, and cover the body with talcum powder. Change and send all underwear and night clothing to the laundry. If possible, air the rest of the bed clothing. Also, air outer clothing (coats, suits, dresses).

Sulfur ointment (℞ 191) is the time-honored antiscabetic medicament. The strength of the sulfur prescribed is dependent upon the presumed toleration of the patient's skin. In infants and small children, 2 to 5% sulfur is used; in older children and in women with delicate fair skin, 5% sulfur; in all other adults, 10% sulfur. Perhaps a more effective antiscabetic is a preparation incorporating balsam of Peru in the above formulas, using the same concentration as the sulfur (℞ 192). Any resulting sulfur dermatitis may be treated with an antipruritic lotion (℞ 78), colloidal baths (℞ 104), and the avoidance of soap.

Benzyl benzoate lotion or emulsion (℞ 193) has a more rapid effect and is cleaner to use. The incidence of some degree of contact dermatitis following this form of treatment is from 2 to 8%. After a preliminary soap and water bath, the emulsion is applied with a stiff brush to all parts of the body except the head and neck, and repeated after 5 minutes. The 2nd application is allowed to dry before the patient dresses. This procedure (except for the bath) is repeated after 12 hours. After 24 hours the patient bathes and puts on clean clothing. All possibly contaminated clothes or bedding are then washed or aired. Many other preparations are useful, but the success of therapy depends far more on the thoroughness with which it is carried out than on the particular antiscabetic agent. To avoid sequelae of overtreatment, it is important to warn the patient not to treat himself any oftener than a single course without seeking medical advice. Reassurance often is necessary after adequate treatment, to discourage acarophobia. A second course, if necessary, should not be given in less than 7 to 10 days.

PEDICULOSIS

(Lousiness, Phthiriasis)

Infestation of man by lice. Three varieties may occur, involving respectively the head, the body, and the pubic areas.

PEDICULOSIS CAPITIS

Due to Pediculus capitis *(head louse), and limited to the scalp (rarely the beard and eyebrows).* Transmission occurs through intimate contact (hats, brushes, personal contact). This infestation is more common in people with longer hair (women and children). No known diseases are transmitted by *P. capitis.*

Diagnosis is made by finding pediculi and nits (ova). These oval nits are fixed to the hair shaft, and can be moved up or down on the shaft. The nits mature in 3 to 14 days. The pediculi are of a grayish color, and are most frequently found around the occiput and behind the ears. Usually, there are numerous infected excoriation marks on the scalp, and a moderate, discrete, posterior cervical adenopathy. Occasionally, a generalized pruritus can be traced to *P. capitis.* All patients with itching and infected eczematous dermatitis of the scalp and neck should be examined for pediculi. In cases of prolonged infestation, the eyebrows may be involved.

Treatment

All possible sources of infestation should be examined and treated as necessary. All personal headgear, combs, and hairbrushes should be disinfected. Locally, DDT is the treatment of choice, either as a powder (℞ 182) or as a lotion (℞ 183).

Cuprex (℞ 184), 50% kerosene (℞ 185), tincture of larkspur (℞ 186), bichloride of mercury lotion (℞ 187) or lauryl thiocyanate (℞ 190) also may be used. Application should be followed by a vinegar rinse (℞ 188) to remove nits. Clipping of hair is a good measure when feasible. Where secondary infection is present, this should be controlled with an antiseptic ointment (℞ 138) before parasiticidal measures are started.

PEDICULOSIS CORPORIS OR VESTIMENTI

Due to Pediculus corporis (*body louse*), *which inhabits the seams of clothing worn next to the skin and feeds on the skin covered by such clothing.* Except in abnormal situations (crowding, during wars), this is a disease of unhygienic environment and is common in dirty or neglected individuals. *P. corporis* is the vector of typhus fever, trench fever, and recurrent febrile spirochetosis (relapsing fever).

Intense itching is the most evident symptom. In heavy infestations, occasionally there are headache, fever, and malaise. The skin reveals small red punctae (bites), urticarial eruptions, pyodermas, and scratch marks. These scratch marks often are very suggestive of *P. corporis,* especially when there are parallel linear marks on shoulders, buttocks, and abdomen. The hands are not involved in *P. corporis* infestation. The parasites and nits are found in the seams of clothing and underclothes, though ova may be present on body hairs. Protracted severe cases may develop generalized hyperpigmentation (including mucous membranes), weakness and debility.

Treatment

Sources of infestation should be investigated and cleared up. Parasiticidal measures (dry heat at 140° F. for 5 minutes, hot water at 150° F. for 5 minutes or immersion in gasoline followed by dry cleaning) should be used on all clothing and bedding. In addition, dusting of clothes with DDT powder (℞ 182) is practical and effective. If dusting alone is used, it should be continued daily for 2 to 3 weeks. A thorough bath and scrubbing with soap followed by application of bichloride of mercury lotion (℞ 187) to hairy areas suspected of harboring nits will ensure complete removal of all parasites. For treatment of the skin, soothing baths (℞ 104), lotions (℞ 78), antihistaminic drugs such as Neo-Antergan (℞ 219), and a mild antiseptic ointment (℞ 138) if a pyogenic element is present, are recommended.

PEDICULOSIS PUBIS

Due to Phthirus pubis (*crab louse*) *which usually infests hairs of the genital region but is occasionally found in hairs of the axillas, eyebrows, eyelashes, beard, and body surface (in hairy individuals).* The infestation can be acquired through sexual intercourse, toilet seats, and bed clothing. No known diseases are transmitted by *P. pubis.*

All cases of itching of the genital and crural regions should be examined for *P. pubis*. The parasite often is hard to find. Its ova are attached to the bases of hairs. Excoriations and dermatitis in the genitocrural area are common and usually secondary to self-medication. Bluish spots (taches bleues), pea to fingernail size, may occur on the skin and are caused by the toxin of the parasite.

Treatment

All sources of infestation should be sought and eliminated. Underwear should be boiled. Patients should wash toilet seats with an antiseptic after use. Any secondary dermatitis should be treated before the parasiticidal remedies are applied, since the parasiticides often will aggravate any coexisting dermatitis. Therapy should consist of potassium permanganate soaks (℞ 4), if oozing and crusting are present, and a soothing lotion (℞ 78), if the eruption is less acute.

DDT is the remedy of choice either as a powder (℞ 182), or as a lotion (℞ 183). Cuprex (℞ 184), tincture of larkspur (℞ 186), bichloride of mercury lotion (℞ 187), ammoniated mercury ointment (℞ 138), or xylol (℞ 189) in instances of intolerance to mercury, are the other effective measures. Shaving of hair in the affected area may be necessary in stubborn cases. In case the eyelids and eyelashes are affected, the parasites are carefully removed with forceps and 2% yellow oxide of mercury ointment (℞ 135) is rubbed into the hairy areas. Any dermatitis developing secondary to the use of parasiticides should be treated like any other dermatitis of the same stage (℞ 4, 78, 104).

ATOPIC DERMATITIS

(Disseminated neurodermatitis, Prurigo hebra)

A chronic superficial inflammation of the skin characterized by thickening, excoriation, and lichenification, with associated pruritus. It often begins in infancy and usually occurs in individuals with a high familial incidence of allergic diseases.

Etiology

Basically, atopic dermatitis is allergic in origin, with a strong hereditary factor. Neurocirculatory and emotional instability are frequent predisposing and exacerbating conditions. Numerous allergens have been responsible for precipitating the dermatitis, the most important being foods (e.g., chocolate, oranges, strawberries, tomatoes) and contactants (e.g., wool, cotton, paint, cosmetics, oils). Inhalants (e.g., dander, pollen, dust) also frequently responsible. In infants, the role of food allergy is more important than in adults. Thus, the older the child, the less likely is food allergy to prove of etiologic significance. Finally, bacterial foci of infection occasionally act as causative or exacerbating factors.

Symptoms, Signs, and Diagnosis

Atopic dermatitis is commonly seen in asthenic, dry-skinned individuals. Asthma or hay fever sometimes coexists or alternates with the dermatitis. There is generally a significant family history of allergy.

Pruritus, usually worse at night, is the outstanding subjective symptom, and papules with excoriated and crusted tops are the primary cutaneous lesions. Poorly defined plaques are formed when the papules become confluent. The sites of predilection are the face, neck, and flexural aspects of the elbows and knees. Other areas often involved are the dorsal surfaces of the hands and feet, the buttocks, and the inguinal and axillary folds. In cases of long duration the lesions often coalesce over the face and form a hard mask composed of dried exudate, colored brownish to purplish with blood from scratching. Secondary infection may supervene, resulting in a predominantly pyogenic dermatitis.

Scratch, intradermal and patch tests, plus elimination diets (see ALLERGY), may be helpful in determining the single or multiple allergens which precipitate the eruption.

Course and Prognosis

Atopic dermatitis frequently begins in early infancy and continues with remissions and exacerbations (usually during the spring and autumn) until about the age of 2 years, when it may disappear or improve significantly. A period of freedom may then ensue, but only to be followed by the appearance of another allergic disease (e.g., asthma), which in turn often disappears after several years. Atopic dermatitis may thereafter recur during puberty or early adulthood. Thus, a history of alternating allergic diseases frequently is obtained. Occasionally the initial onset may occur in adults with no history of earlier allergic episodes. Because recurrences and exacerbations are common, the prognosis must be guarded. The dermatitis often disappears spontaneously after the 4th decade of life, but complete elimination of the exciting allergens may bring about earlier recovery. Often, however, after a variable period of regression, new sensitivities develop and the dermatitis recurs.

Treatment

Patients should be taught to avoid emotional upsets as much as possible. Foci of infection, if present, should be eliminated. In order to avoid irritation of the skin, soap substitutes (℞ 27, 28, 29) should be used for routine cleansing. Ocean bathing may be beneficial but too frequent baths and showers are not advised since they may further dry an already dry skin. Undue exposure to the sun also is contraindicated.

When sensitivity to a contactant, inhalant, or ingestant has been demonstrated, further exposure should be avoided or appropriate desensitization procedures tried (*see* ALLERGY). To allay pruritus, a starch bath (℞ 104) may be necessary, or lotions (℞ 87, 88), an ointment (℞ 89, 90), or compresses (℞ 2, 4) applied locally. Preparations containing phenol are contraindicated since sensitization to phenol not infrequently develops. A tar ointment (℞ 15) or paint (℞ 9) is helpful in the dry lichenified stage but should not be applied in the acute stage. Antihistaminic drugs, such as Neo-Antergan (℞ 219), often are beneficial. If complicating pyogenic infection occurs, it should be treated as described *under* Impetiginized Dermatitis (q.v.).

———————

ECZEMATOUS DERMATITIS

An acute, subacute, or chronic skin disease characterized by erythema, papules, and vesicles, with varying degrees of infiltration, oozing, crusting, scaling, and lichenification. (The term "eczema" is best avoided, since it means different things to different people.)

Etiology and Incidence

The etiology is protean, and single or multiple factors may be involved. In some patients, the eruption persists even after removal of all seemingly possible causes. Although eczematous dermatitis may occur in apparently healthy individuals, predisposing and exacerbating factors are debility, an abnormally dry or extremely oily skin, a fair complexion, maceration of the skin due to excessive sweating or immersion in water, exposure to extremes of heat or cold, emotional instability, focal infections, and, to a limited extent, heredity. Exciting factors which, alone or in combination, may precipitate the eruption include the following: (1) Contact, frequently occupational, with irritating and sensitizing agents such as strong acids or alkalis, mercury, sulfur, formalin, alcohol, streptomycin, cosmetics, medicaments used locally, cleansing agents, and a wide variety of other substances. Thus, confectioners, barbers, printers, chemists, and workers in almost every modern industry may be exposed daily to potential irritants that may cause the development of eczematous dermatitis. Also included here are patients overtreated with local medication. (2) Exposure to thermal or actinic rays from the sun, or other sources such as furnaces and artificial lights. (3) Trauma, from friction or pressure (e.g., garters, corsets, trusses). (4) Pyogenic infection, beginning as a pyogenic dermatitis and becoming eczematous through the development of sensitivity to the bacteria or their products. A secondary variety is exemplified by the invasion of a preexisting dermatitis with pyogenic bacteria. (5) Peripheral vascular disorders such as varicose veins. (6) Allergy to either food or inhalants (*see* ATOPIC DERMATITIS). (7) Fungus infection, which may be responsible (rarely) for chronic eczematous dermatitis.

This form of dermatitis is the one most commonly encountered, and individuals of both sexes and all ages are equally subject to it.

Symptoms, Signs, and Diagnosis

Itching is almost always present and usually becomes worse at night. Burning or smarting may occasionally be the chief complaint. The lesions appear anywhere on the body, but the sites of predilection are the hands, feet, ears, and legs. The acute form is characterized by edema, erythema, papules, vesicles, pustules (if secondary infection occurs), oozing, and crusting. In the subacute type, erythema, vesicles, and papules likewise occur, but there is more infiltration and scaling. The chronic form is characterized by less erythema, fewer papules or vesicles, occasional pustules, and a greater degree of lichenification, fissuring, and infiltration.

Eczematous dermatitis must be differentiated from psoriasis, seborrheic dermatitis, dermatomycosis and the dermatophytids, impetigo and scabies.

Prognosis

The prognosis usually is favorable if the causative agents or predisposing conditions can be determined and eliminated. This may be difficult to achieve, however, because of the multitudinous factors that can be contributory. Thus, despite thorough investigation and attempts at correction, the dermatitis may change from acute to chronic and persist for years. There may be intervals of resolution or diminution of lesions, alternating with reappearance or exacerbation when deleterious influences become operative.

Treatment

Obviously, the first step is to eliminate the exciting factor, if this can be determined. If not, therapy is largely a matter of trial and error. The skin should be protected against further contact with irritants, if these have been indicted, by the wearing of protective clothing and the application of a suitable ointment (R 111) to exposed areas. Nonirritating preparations (R 27, 28, 29) rather than soap should be used for cleansing the skin. To prevent scratching and subsequent secondary infection the patient's fingernails should be cut short, or the hands covered with mittens. In cases due to allergy to foods or inhalants (e.g., pollens, dusts), avoidance or specific desensitization should

be tried (*see* ALLERGY). Emotional upsets should be avoided as
far as possible; a mild sedative (℞ 200) may be palliative.

   Because of the intense pruritus, care of the lesions is of immediate importance. They should not be washed with soap and
water, but cleansed with a bland oil. Medicated compresses
(℞ 2, 4) are useful to control infection, oozing, crusting and
pruritus. When the lesions are widespread, potassium permanganate or cornstarch baths may be helpful (℞ 104, 105).
For more localized lesions, soothing lotions (℞ 87, 91, 92)
should be applied to control itching. In many cases, especially
those of the dry lichenified type, ointments are preferable.
Burow's solution ointment (℞ 93) is helpful in allaying pruritus. Preparations containing phenol are best avoided, since
they cause sensitivity reactions in a small percentage of patients. For chronic and subacute eruptions, a bland ointment
(℞ 12, 13) or one which is mildly stimulating (℞ 111) is indicated. Since there is no drug which all patients can tolerate,
any of these preparations should first be tried on a small area
of affected skin. If the lesions show no sign of aggravation
after 24 hours, general application may be made. Antihistaminic drugs, such as Neo-Antergan (℞ 219), have been used
with benefit in some cases to allay the pruritus and resolve the
eruptions. If the lesions are pustular, due to secondary infection, ammoniated mercury (℞ 137, 138) may be applied provided the patient is not sensitive to it, but bacitracin ointment
(℞ 153) or medicated compresses (℞ 2, 4) often are preferable.
In the presence of extensive pyogenic lesions, penicillin (℞
147) may be given I.M., or sulfonamides (℞ 150, 151) orally.
Complicating fungus infections should be treated as described
in the chapter on Dermatomycoses (q.v.). It is highly important to avoid overtreatment; a long list of therapeutic agents
including penicillin ointment, sulfonamide ointment, local anesthetic agents, and many other ointments cause sensitivity reactions in a varying percentage of cases and their use should be
avoided. Eczematous dermatitis presents a difficult therapeutic problem and in many cases dermatologic consultation is
essential.

CONTACT DERMATITIS

(Dermatitis venenata, including Rhus
[e.g., poison ivy] dermatitis)

*An acute or chronic, superficial inflammation of the skin
caused by contact with sensitizing or irritating agents, including
vegetable, animal and mineral substances.*

Etiology

Normally, there is a balance between the resistance of the

skin and the contactants to which it is exposed. This balance can be upset by excessive exposure to an allergen or by predisposing factors which decrease skin resistance, such as trauma, excessive sweating with maceration, prolonged exposure to water and soap, ichthyosis, age (skin of young and old is less resistant), complexion (light more susceptible than dark), area of the body (eyelids and genitalia most susceptible), and overexposure to sunlight.

The causative factors may be encountered in the patient's occupational or home environment. Following are listed some of the most common sensitizers: (1) **Plants:** poison ivy, oak, and sumac; primrose, chrysanthemum, timothy, marsh elder, ragweed, bitterwood, cocklebur, feverfew, sneezeweed. (2) **Trees,** especially tropical varieties: mahogany, teakwood, ebony, balsa, kapok, European oak, Canadian spruce, elm, pear, poplar, Brazilian walnut, white pine. (3) **Fruits and vegetables:** tomatoes, onions, citrus fruits, celery. (4) **Chemicals:** paraphenylenediamine, mercury, chromic acid, pyrethrum, paradichlorobenzene, DDT. (5) **Therapeutic agents,** externally applied or encountered, constitute an important group of irritants. Persons who handle such products in the course of their manufacture, sale, or administration may develop contact dermatitis from occasional or constant exposure. Many patients are injudiciously treated with local preparations through the well intended but often harmful advice of friends, druggists, newspaper writers, and even some physicians. Such preparations often contain arsenic, mercury, iodine, salicylic acid, resorcinol, quinine, penicillin, the sulfonamides, streptomycin, or local anesthetics, and are a common cause of chronic dermatitis, especially on the hands. (6) **Cosmetics:** hair dyes, bleaches, and tonics; deodorants, depilatories, nail polishes, face creams, and powders. (7) **Clothing materials** such as nylon, wool, silk, linen, leather, fur. (8) **Miscellaneous substances:** tobacco, soaps, lacquers, metals (particularly gold, silver, nickel), vegetable gums (acacia, tragacanth), animal danders (dog, cat, cow, horse), feathers (chicken, duck, goose, turkey, as used in pillows), and an almost limitless number of household contactants including polishes and waxes.

Hypersensitivity depends upon previous contact with the causative substance. Usually, 6 to 10 days must elapse between the first contact and the appearance of sensitization dermatitis. Such a period apparently is required for the development of true specific allergy or hypersensitivity.

Symptoms and Signs

Usually, only the exposed portions of the skin are affected, specifically the dorsal surface of the hands and feet, forearms, face, and neck. Frequently, the so-called "friction areas" such as axilla, groin, and interdigital surfaces of the hands are involved. The dermatitis may be sharply limited to the site of actual contact or may advance beyond this area and even become widespread, depending upon the degree of cutaneous sensitivity present and the concentration of the offending allergen.

All degrees of inflammation ranging from simple erythema to gangrene may be present. Most patients first present erythema limited to the area of contact. Later, edema, papules, vesicles, and pustules may appear. Three types, or stages, of dermatitis venenata are recognized: (1) The **acute** type consists of edema, erythema, vesicles, and bullous primary lesions; if severe, the vesicles and bullae rupture, thereby producing denudation, oozing, and crusting. Usually, pruritus and burning, alone or in combination, are pronounced. (2) The **subacute** stage is characterized by papules, scaling, thickening, excoriations, crusting, and some itching or burning, or both. (3) In the **chronic** phase there is lichenification, dryness, hyperpigmentation, fissuring, scaling, and varying degrees of pruritus or burning. During the acute stage the causative agent may be absorbed (from necrotic cells) by the blood stream and transported to other cutaneous sites or spread via direct contact. At any of the 3 stages the lesions may become secondarily infected and thereby complicated by fever, chills, malaise, lymphangitis, lymphadenitis, or even bacteremia.

Diagnosis

The first step is to consider the distribution of the dermatitis and to ascertain whether the affected sites are those which readily come in direct contact with a sensitizing agent. If so, it is necessary to take a detailed history including the patient's occupation, home surroundings, trips to woods or country, cosmetics used, hobbies, animal pets, previous eruptions, and treatment if any. In this way, a number of potential contactant allergens may come under suspicion. Specific diagnosis can then be made by means of the patch test (*see* ALLERGY). Careful differentiation should be made between an allergic response and one due to a primary irritant (i.e., a chemical substance that will cause dermatitis in the majority of individuals). Primary irritants will produce severe bullous eruptions similar to those of a 2nd degree burn, whereas the specific allergic reaction will vary from a simple erythema to edema, vesiculation, and oozing, depending upon the sensitivity of the patient. The patient should be instructed to remove the patch earlier if the test site begins to itch; otherwise, in highly sensitive individuals, generalized reactions may result. Patch testing is a specialized procedure, and in general it should be done by one experienced in its use. It should never be attempted during the acute stage of the eruption.

Prognosis

Once the sensitizing agent has been determined, simple avoidance of it usually results in clearing of the lesions in a few days or weeks, with no residual scarring. Some individuals after one mild attack apparently acquire an immunity to the allergen under continued exposure (as in industry). In other cases, further contacts cause severe exacerbations.

Treatment

Avoidance of contact with the specific allergen usually is curative. Exposed individuals known to be sensitive, or others unavoidably in contact with a substance known to be highly sensitizing to the skin (e.g., in occupation), should wear protective clothing. Absolute cleanliness should be observed, and any of the contactant deposited on the skin or clothing promptly washed away with soap and water. It may be necessary for the patient to change his job or to make changes in his habits and environment. If such measures cannot be carried out, desensitization is helpful in preventing recurrences. Thus, in patients with Rhus (poison ivy) dermatitis, weekly injections of an extract are initiated in January, February, or March and continued throughout the summer. The initial dose is 0.02 cc. subcut.; subsequent doses are progressively doubled unless a reaction occurs. Then the previous dose may be readministered. Possible untoward reactions include local inflammation, malaise, fever, muscle pain, nausea, vomiting, urticaria, and angioneurotic edema. Occasionally, toxic nephrosis may occur.

Local treatment of infected contact dermatitis may be accomplished by use of potassium permanganate, as compresses (℞ 4) or baths (℞ 105). Ammoniated mercury (℞ 137) and boric acid (℞ 12) are alternative local medications. Severe secondary infections may necessitate the use of penicillin (℞ 146, 147) or sulfonamides (℞ 150, 151) systemically; local application of these drugs is contraindicated. Itching and burning may be relieved by compresses of Burow's solution (℞ 2), starch baths (℞ 104), or lotions (℞ 94, 96, 97). Menthol-phenol (℞ 98) or ichthammol-zinc oxide ointment (℞ 13) may be used as a dressing once the vesicles have broken and are drying up.

The oral administration of antihistaminic drugs (see ALLERGY, General Treatment) will relieve many patients with dermatitis venenata. Barbiturates (℞ 200) often are helpful for sedation if pruritus is severe, or ephedrine combined with a barbiturate (℞ 99) may be used.

DRUG ERUPTIONS

(Dermatitis medicamentosa, Toxicoderma)

An eruption on the skin and mucous membranes in which a drug previously administered is definitely implicated as the causative agent. Any drug may cause such a reaction and, while the mechanism by which the eruption is produced has not been clearly established, individual idiosyncrasy or hypersensitivity in the patient appears to be involved.

Symptoms and Diagnosis

The cutaneous manifestations vary from slight itching or faint erythema to severe, persistent and occasionally fatal eruptions. Thus, drug eruptions can resemble many different dermatologic entities. Also, one drug does not always cause the same type of eruption in different individuals, or in the same individual at different times. Thus, in some patients, cutaneous sensitivity to penicillin may result in an urticarial eruption, while in others the manifestation may be an oozing vesicular dermatitis of the groin, feet, and hands. A partial list of more commonly used drugs and the skin lesions they may cause is as follows: (1) **Sulfonamides:** toxic erythema-like eruptions, erythema nodosum, and erythema multiforme. (2) **Penicillin:** Urticaria, angioneurotic edema, and eczematous eruptions, particularly of groin, hands, and feet. (3) **Phenolphthalein:** fixed hyperpigmented plaques, sometimes bullous with involvement of mucous membranes and genitalia. (4) **Barbiturates:** toxic erythema and erythema multiforme. (5) **Bromides and iodides:** acneform eruptions, pustular folliculitis, fungating ulcerative granulomas. (6) **Arsenic; gold:** exfoliative dermatitis. (7) **Atabrine:** lichenoid and eczematous eruptions.

Many of the eruptions are accompanied by constitutional symptoms such as malaise, fever up to 105° F., jaundice, granulocytopenia, and signs of kidney and heart damage. Complete blood and urine examinations are therefore necessary.

Diagnosis often is difficult and usually is made tentatively from the circumstantial evidence available. The physician should always suspect drug eruptions when confronted with atypical or unusual dermatoses. The usual allergies should be ruled out. Skin tests with suspected drugs are useless and may aggravate the existing eruption. A history of previous drug intake is significant but often difficult to elicit. Repeated inquiries concerning daily habits, drug ingestion, self-medication, and the use of patent medicines must be made. Improvement after withdrawal of a suspected drug is strong evidence for drug eruption. Recurrence of the eruption on its readministration is also important evidence, but this is not a measure to be used frequently, as the resulting eruption may be severe and possibly dangerous to the patient. If such a test is done, a very small dose of the drug should be used initially (e.g., 20 to 30 mg. of sulfathiazole).

Prognosis

Almost all drug eruptions will clear up on discontinuation of the causative agent, but those due to iodides and bromides may persist for several years. Sometimes, sensitivity to a single drug may develop into multiple drug sensitivities, with a poorer prognosis.

Treatment

Prophylactic: All drugs administered in any condition should be as few as possible and discontinued as soon as feasible. The drugs that are frequent offenders should not be prescribed indiscriminately, as their therapeutic effects may be outweighed by the development of sensitivity. This is especially true of the bromides, sulfonamides and penicillin, which often are administered for trivial conditions.

General: All drugs being taken by the patient should be stopped. If this is not feasible, the drug most likely to be the cause of the eruption should be discontinued and replaced, if necessary, by a chemically unrelated drug with similar physiologic action. Elimination of the drug from the body can be hastened by forcing fluids, and by administration of "safe" cathartics (℞ 220, 221). In arsenical or gold salt eruptions, BAL should be used (℞ 166). For iodine and bromide eruptions, give sodium chloride 12 to 15 Gm. daily, to increase elimination. For purpuric and hemorrhagic eruptions, vitamins C (℞ 207) and K (℞ 208) should be administered. Sodium thiosulfate (℞ 161) can be used in many drug eruptions, as a "detoxifying or neutralizing agent," though its efficacy is doubtful. Antihistaminic drugs such as Neo-Antergan (℞ 219), or ephedrine and phenobarbital (℞ 99) are effective in urticarial eruptions. Use of cortisone or ACTH often is highly effective.

All patients deserve a complete physical examination. Hospitalization is indicated for extensive eczematous or exfoliative dermatitis (especially that due to arsenicals) and in cases with purpuric, hemorrhagic, or bullous manifestations. Patients with constitutional symptoms, such as jaundice, granulocytopenia, and cardiac or kidney damage, also should be hospitalized and given treatment appropriate to these disorders (q.v.).

Local: This depends upon the clinical manifestations irrespective of etiology. Thus, eczematous or other lesions due to drugs are treated in the same way as those due to other agents. Such therapy is discussed in detail in the appropriate chapters (q.v.). Nevertheless, a few additional prescriptions are listed for acute eczematous lesions (℞ 4, 93, 94) and those with secondary infection (℞ 137) or pruritus (℞ 95), and for exfoliative eruptions (℞ 11, 104).

ERYTHEMA NODOSUM

An inflammatory disease of the skin characterized by tender, red nodes appearing usually upon the legs over the tibias. It is most common in females under 30 years of age. The condition is so frequently associated with sore throat, arthritis, and endocarditis, which are characteristic of rheumatic fever (q.v.), that a similar causation must be postulated for many cases. It also has been observed in tuberculosis; in children, it signifies activity of the infection. In adults, erythema nodosum may be associated with a variety of diseases and drugs. A condition resembling erythema nodosum may occur in secondary syphilis.

The disease begins abruptly with headache, muscular and joint pains, and fever. Within 48 hours, ill-defined plaques appear symmetrically upon the legs, usually over the tibias, and less commonly over the outer side of the forearm. Initially, they are deep-seated and sensitive, but they rapidly approach the surface and become elevated as firm, nut-sized nodules. The color of the lesions gradually changes from red to bluish to brown, like a bruise. Suppuration is rare. Individual lesions may disappear in 7 to 14 days but the disease runs a course of 3 to 4 weeks. Recurrence is unusual and the prognosis is excellent.

Treatment

Therapy is entirely symptomatic. Bed rest, elevation of the affected parts, supportive dressing on the legs, and salicylates (℞ 194) are most useful. Soothing lotions (℞ 78, 79) may be applied locally. Associated disease should be sought for and appropriately treated.

ERYTHEMA MULTIFORME

(Herpes iris, Erythema multiforme bullosum, Erythema multiforme exudativum)

An acute or subacute skin disease characterized by well defined reddish or multicolored patches of erythema, macules, papules, vesicles, or nodules. It may be caused by a variety of toxic, infectious, or allergenic agents such as drugs, serums, or foods. It may be a complication of various types of infection. Frequently, the basic cause cannot be determined. The disease is most frequently encountered in young females, particularly in the spring and fall.

Malaise and arthralgia often may precede the skin changes. The dermatitis appears suddenly. The lesions are bilaterally symmetrical, spread peripherally, and fuse into polycyclic plaques. Lesions are seen on any part of the body but are found especially on the dorsa of the hands and feet, the mouth, and the genital regions.

The prognosis usually is excellent. A single attack passes off in 2 to 3 weeks. Rarely, the lesions may recur over a period of many years. The bullous form of the disease must be differentiated from dermatitis herpetiformis, lupus erythematosus, and pemphigus.

Treatment

Possible causative factors must be determined and corrected in order to avoid recurrence. Symptomatic therapy depends on the stage of the dermatitis. Compresses (℞ 4), colloid baths (℞ 104, 108), liniments (℞ 80) and ointments (℞ 12), each may be useful. An antihistaminic drug, such as Neo-Antergan (℞ 219), may hasten involution of the process.

PITYRIASIS ROSEA

(Pityriasis circinata, Pityriasis rubra, Herpes tonsurans
maculosus, Pityriasis maculata et circinata)

A self-limited, acute, mildly inflammatory disease of the skin, of unknown origin, and characterized by papulosquamous lesions. Some consider it a mildly infectious exanthem due to a viral agent. It occurs in both sexes, generally between the 2nd and 4th decades of life, but may appear at any age. The incidence is highest during spring and autumn.

Symptoms and Signs

Prodromal symptoms of malaise, low grade fever, headache, and generalized adenopathy are not usual but can occur. A "herald patch" often appears about 7 to 10 days before the generalized eruption. This is a rose or fawn colored, well demarcated, oval or circinate patch covered by a dry scale. By the time it has increased 1 to 4 cm. in diameter and perhaps begun to fade, similar lesions appear on the trunk, buttocks, or extremities. Lesions are rare on the face but occasionally have been noted on the buccal mucosa and, in children, on the scalp. In a typical case, the eruption develops rapidly and often is accompanied by a moderate pruritus in the early stages. The individual lesions and their distributions are characteristic. Lesions usually are oval, 0.5 to 2.0 cm. in diameter, and arranged with their long axes along the folds of the skin. They are slightly elevated, very slightly infiltrated, papular or maculopapular, covered with a fine adherent dry scale, and similar in color to the original eruption. If compressed longitudinally, fine "cigarette-paper" crinkling is seen. When present on the palms and soles (exceedingly rare), the eruptions usually are vesicular. On the buccal mucosa, they appear as annular, erythematous plaques. In the Negro they often are papular.

Diagnosis

Pityriasis rosea must be differentiated from seborrheic dermatitis, tinea corporis, secondary syphilis, psoriasis, lichen planus, parapsoriasis (rare), drug eruptions, and "id" eruptions. The characteristic arrangement of the eruptions, and particularly the "herald patch," are diagnostic. However, a serologic test for syphilis should always be made.

Prognosis and Treatment

The disease is self-limited. Without treatment, it may persist for 6 to 8 weeks—occasionally much longer. Under appropriate treatment, recovery without permanent residua is the rule. Recurrences are rare.

Because the course of pityriasis rosea is self-limited, treatment is difficult to evaluate. If constitutional symptoms are present, acetylsalicylic acid (℞ 194) may be given. Local treatment should be mild. If pruritus is distressing, a mild colloidal or starch bath (℞ 104) should be used, together with an antipruritic shake lotion (℞ 100). A sedative (℞ 200) may be necessary to ensure sleep. When the eruption persists after acute symptoms have subsided, mild exfoliation can be attained with repeated, generalized exposures to ultraviolet rays in suberythema to slight erythema doses. This actinotherapy can be expedited by the use of a mild keratolytic agent such as Pragmatar (℞ 39). Caution should be observed, however, in using ultraviolet rays when the eruption is in the acute phase. Local application of 30% sulfur ointment (℞ 75) is of value in resistant cases, when cautiously employed.

LICHEN PLANUS

(Lichen ruber planus, Lichen psoriasis)

An inflammatory dermatosis, manifested by multiple, small, flat-topped, angular, or polygonal papules exhibiting a reddish or violaceous color, and covered by a horny, glistening film. The etiology is unknown. The disease is more common after the 2nd decade of life, is rare in children and affects both sexes equally. Anxiety, overwork, and nervous instability are contributory factors.

Symptoms and Signs

Usually, the condition has a gradual onset and a chronic course, but an acute, explosive, generalized form is observed in some patients.

The individual primary lesion is an angular or polygonal, flat-topped, sharply defined papule covered with a firmly attached, thin, transparent, horny film which gives the lesion a waxy or varnished appearance. Close examination with magnification often reveals a network of bluish white lines over the surface, which are known as Wickham's striae. The early lesions are erythematous with a violaceous tinge. Older lesions usually are dull purple or darker in color. Rarely, vesicles and bullae may be found if the inflammation is intense.

The lesions may be discrete and isolated or grouped irregularly, but may become confluent to form large plaques with sharp outlines. The lesions may extend peripherally and heal centrally, producing an annular or circinate form (annular lichen planus). Very rarely the center of the lesion may show atrophy (atrophic lichen planus). If the eruption is of long standing, large hypertrophic plaques may be formed, particularly on the anterior surface of the legs (hypertrophic lichen planus). Patches may form in response to trauma (Koebner phenomenon).

The lesions are generally symmetrical in distribution and the characteristic locations are the flexor surfaces of the forearms and wrist, the buccal mucosa, and the genital mucocutaneous junctions. Involution of the papules often leaves residual pigmentation.

The subjective symptoms are those of intense pruritus, often interfering with sleep and nutrition. In the acute, generalized forms there may be coincident febrile symptoms with mild systemic disturbances.

Diagnosis

Secondary syphilis, psoriasis and lichen planus-like drug eruptions, especially those due to gold, arsenic, and atabrine, often are confused with this disease. Hypertrophic lichen planus is to be differentiated from lichen simplex chronicus (neurodermatitis). Lichen planus of the oral mucous membranes is sometimes extremely difficult to differentiate from leukoplakia.

Prognosis and Treatment

The prognosis is generally favorable. However, hypertrophic lichen planus usually is most resistant to therapy and may persist for years, despite the use of all forms of therapy. Recurrences are common. Malignant changes have not been reported.

The following nonspecific measures are used in the treatment of this disease, which is benign and tends to be self-limited:

The patient should be examined from an over-all point of view. Many of these patients need psychotherapy and mild sedation for a brief time. Traditionally, mercury (R 163), arsenic (R 164), or bismuth (R 159), has been used on empirical grounds. In some patients such therapy does seem to affect the course of the disease favorably; however, considerable judgment should be exercised in the use of the various therapeutic agents mentioned above, inasmuch as reactions from such drugs can sometimes be more troublesome than the disease itself. In any event, they should not be continued for more than a few weeks.

Local treatment is essentially symptomatic (R 14, 40, 101); R 14 and R 40 should be used only in the more chronic cases, particularly the hypertrophic variety. Ultraviolet ray treatment is not contraindicated, but it is of doubtful value. Superficial X-ray therapy probably is the most useful single modality, but should always be given under the supervision of a qualified roentgenologist.

LICHEN SIMPLEX CHRONICUS

(Lichen Vidal; Chronic circumscribed neurodermatitis)

A chronic superficial inflammation of the skin, characterized by thickened, dry, desquamating, well demarcated, excoriated plaques, of oval, irregular, or angular shape, associated with severe pruritus. A fully developed plaque has an external zone of brownish, discrete papules and a central zone of confluent papules covered with scales. Hyperpigmentation often is seen. These occur on parts of the body accessible to scratching. The cause is unknown, but various predisposing factors have been suggested, such as emotional instability, avitaminosis, debility, and exhaustion from strenuous mental or physical activity. Allergy, as judged by skin tests, appears to play no part. Onset usually is in the 3rd, 4th, and 5th decades of life, and females are affected more frequently than males. The lesions often disappear spontaneously during the summer and recur in the fall and winter. Prognosis for complete cure is poor, but with adequate treatment improvement usually can be obtained.

Treatment

Control of pruritus (q.v.) is the chief aim of therapy. This may be accomplished by the use of a sedative (℞ 200) and antipruritic lotions (℞ 102, 103). Keratolytic ointments (℞ 39) are useful when lichenification is pronounced. Since ordinary soaps tend to dry the skin and increase the pruritus, soap substitutes should be employed (℞ 27, 28, 29). Patients should be advised to avoid emotional strain, if possible. In resistant cases, X-radiation administered by a physician experienced in its use often is effective.

PSORIASIS

(Alphos, Psora)

A chronic, occasionally acute, recurrent, papulosquamous, inflammatory skin disease.

Etiology and Incidence

The cause is unknown. Among the many etiologic concepts that have been advanced, most support has been given to its being a constitutional disturbance of fat and fat-soluble vitamin metabolism. Some investigators contend that the eruption is an allergic manifestation of a fungus infection. Trauma may influence psoriasis, as indicated by the Koebner phenomenon in acute psoriasis, which consists of the development of typical lesions at the site of chemical or mechanical irritation. Additional factors such as climate and psychic maladjustment definitely can play important parts in influencing the course of the disease. Psoriasis characteristically occurs between the ages of 15 and 35 and is uncommon in children and Negroes. It afflicts males and females with equal frequency, apparently with some familial tendency.

Symptoms and Signs

The initial lesions may be acute or insidious in onset, appearing as small papules which increase in size by peripheral extension and coalesce to form sharply demarcated, erythematous plaques. The plaques are covered with imbricated, glistening "mother of pearl" scales. Peeling off the scales leaves a smooth shiny hyperemic surface studded with tiny bleeding points. The lesions may occur anywhere on the body but have a predilection for extensor surfaces of extremities (elbows and knees) and for the scalp and sacral region. The eruption varies from a single lesion to one sparing little of the body surface. Hair growth is not altered by the disease. As a result of peripheral extension of the lesions and central healing, circinate, gyrate, and serpiginous lesions are commonly noted on the trunk. In acute cases marked pruritus may be associated with the eruption, although in the majority truly constitutional symptoms are absent. As the eruption disappears, scales fall off, leaving the underlying skin discolored, pigmented or paler than the surrounding skin. Irritation by chemical or physical agents often causes old lesions to spread and the wide appearance of new ones.

The nails are frequently involved, as evidenced by stippling, pitting, thickening, brownish discoloration, cracking, and elevation of the distal portion of the nail. In many instances of nail involvement, fungus infection must be ruled out. Rarely there is an accompanying psoriatic arthritis (q.v.) clinically similar to rheumatoid arthritis. Joint involvement clears with the regression of the skin lesions.

Diagnosis

The more common psoriasiform eruptions from which psoriasis must be differentiated are seborrheic dermatitis, psoriasiform syphilis, pityriasis rosea, tinea circinata, acute lupus erythematosus, eczema and lichen planus, and localized neurodermatitis.

Prognosis and Treatment

The disorder does not materially interfere with the health of the affected individual. It runs an inconstant course and characteristically tends to recur. No method of therapy ensures a cure; however, with persistent treatment a remission may be obtained. The frequency of recurrence varies with individuals, the outlook being better if the patient can move to a warm climate.

One of the most important aspects of treatment is education of the patient regarding his disease so that he can live a normal existence, avoiding tension, and with a high morale. He should be cautioned against self-medication, since overtreatment causes exacerbations. Exposure to natural sunlight in gradually increasing doses is especially recommended.

In the **acute stage** of the disease bland local therapy should be prescribed. Daily colloid baths (starch, oatmeal) (R 104, 108) followed by a soothing ointment containing boric acid (R 12) or Vioform (R 17)— or a mild sulfur-salicylic acid preparation (R 60)—may be used. Injection of 10 cc. of the patient's blood I.M. once weekly for 6 to 8 weeks has been recommended by some therapists.

In the treatment of the **chronic stage**, caution should be exercised to avoid overtreatment irritation. Daily exposure to ultraviolet rays in suberythema to very mild erythema doses is helpful. In cases of widespread involvement the Goeckerman regimen, consisting of the application of crude coal tar ointment (R 15) which is removed with mineral oil (R 24) prior to ultraviolet ray exposure the next day, is very effective. This procedure may be carried on from one to several weeks depending on the results obtained.

Preliminary studies indicate that refined undecylenic acid, 2 to 5 Gm. orally in capsules, 3 times daily between meals, may be helpful.

The patient should bathe daily and remove all scales by applying a mild soap and gently scrubbing the lesions with a soft skin brush. Many local applications are available including ammoniated mercury-salicylic acid ointment (R 54) and coal tar paint (R 9). Chrysarobin ointment 0.1 to 5% (R 55) has been recommended. It should be used cautiously, and never on the face or scalp, since it stains the skin and clothing. Isolated chronic lesions may be treated with anthralin (R 56) starting with the weaker concentrations. All applications should be limited to the areas of skin involved. Scalp lesions are particularly resistant to therapy and may require trial of various local medications as with Pragmatar (R 39), ammoniated mercury (R 57), sulphur and salicylic acid (R 58), and compound oil of cade ointment (R 59). The scalp should be shampooed 3 times weekly.

Resistant cases may be benefited by a course of arsenic therapy, as Fowler's solution (R 165). Superficial X-ray therapy is contraindicated in the treatment of this disease.

Therapy with cortisone or ACTH is proving helpful.

PEMPHIGUS

A rather rare but grave skin disease characterized by the development of bullae on apparently normal skin and mucous membranes. The cause of pemphigus is unknown. Of the many theories advanced, those based on an infectious or toxic origin have the greatest support. This disease frequently is seen in butchers and others who handle meat and meat products.

Signs and Symptoms

Three variants of pemphigus are seen: pemphigus vulgaris, pemphigus foliaceus and pemphigus vegetans.

Constitutional symptoms generally are absent at the onset of **pemphigus vulgaris.** The bullae vary greatly in size and are filled with clear exudate which later becomes turbid or purulent. Concomitantly the skin surrounding the bullae may become erythematous. The bullae either rupture, leaving a raw surface, or desiccate, leaving crusts. The sites of predilection for the eruption are the face, scalp, flexural areas, and the mucous membranes. The membranes of the mouth, eye, nose, and vagina may all be affected. In the mouth, the bullae promptly rupture, leaving a whitish film-coated erosion. The severity of the process varies greatly, but almost invariably the course is downhill. Lesions continue to appear, with constitutional symptoms and debility ensuing. The skin may become covered with oozing, crusted malodorous eruptions. Painful lesions in the mouth and on the larynx may make speech and ingestion of food almost impossible.

Pemphigus foliaceus is a form of chronic pemphigus, in which the entire cutaneous surface is involved. In this type, the skin presents no elevated bullous lesions, but collections of fluid can be found in the epidermis. These lacunas result in a flaky, scaly exfoliation. Large areas of denuded skin are intermingled with exfoliating plaques.

Pemphigus vegetans is a rare type of chronic pemphigus, in which warty excrescences develop at the site of the bullae.

Diagnosis

The diagnosis of pemphigus is based on the history, type, and topography of the lesions. Nikolsky's sign often is helpful as a diagnostic aid. It consists of the demonstration of a lack of cohesion between the layers of the skin. The outer layer is easily rubbed off by slight trauma. A phytopharmacologic test (Macht-Pels) also has been described. Histopathologic study of biopsy material is valuable, but the changes found are not entirely diagnostic.

The differentiation of pemphigus vulgaris from other bullous dermatoses is important because the disease is so grave. Six other diseases may be distinguished by the following criteria:

dermatitis herpetiformis (grouped pruritic vesicles and papules, mucous membrane lesions exceedingly rare); erythema multiforme bullosum (localization and collateral lesions); bullous drug eruptions (history of drug intake); bullous dermatitis factitia (artificial bizarre patterning); bullous syphilid (occurs in infants with congenital syphilis); bullous impetigo (course and response to antibiotic therapy).

Pemphigus foliaceus resembles generalized exfoliative dermatitis, but shows distinctive features in its flaccid bullae, raw eroded areas, and fetid odor. Pemphigus vegetans may resemble the fungating iodide or bromide eruptions or condyloma latum. In many cases, the final diagnosis in all types of pemphigus depends on the course of the disease and experienced evaluation of all its aspects.

Prognosis and Treatment

Pemphigus vulgaris usually is fatal after a course of months to years, during which partial or complete remissions may occur at any time. Death results from toxemia or from some intercurrent infection, commonly pneumonia, to which these patients become increasingly susceptible. Prognosis must be guarded in view of the grave nature of this disease with its tendency to relapses.

Pemphigus foliaceus and pemphigus vegetans are variants of pemphigus vulgaris with the same treatment.

No cure for pemphigus is known. The disease has been controlled in some cases with cortisone or ACTH. Some good results have followed the administration of suramin sodium (℞ 162), but this drug often has caused toxic reactions including renal damage, erythema, purpura, and gastrointestinal disorders, and must be used with caution.

Hospitalization is indicated for treatment of all but the most benign cases. Supportive measures as employed in the treatment of grave systemic diseases are indicated. A high caloric, high protein diet plus vitamin supplements is essential. Parenteral feeding and fluids must be given to patients unable to eat because of intractable pain in the oropharyngeal lesions. Repeated small blood transfusions, especially those from a pemphigus patient in remission are thought to be valuable. Adrenal cortex extract (℞ 217) and crude liver extract (℞ 211) also may be given. Ultraviolet ray therapy produces beneficial results. Other treatment that has been used includes various forms of arsenic such as Fowler's solution (℞ 165) and Stovarsol (℞ 167), vitamin D_2 (℞ 209), and injections of foreign protein such as boiled milk. Some of the agents that have been tried are toxic in large doses and must be given with caution to avoid possible complications.

External treatment must not be neglected. Bullae should be opened daily and the bases painted with a 1% solution of gentian violet (℞ 144). Pressure dressings with vaseline gauze

do much to promote healing and prevent new bullae from
forming. The use of benzocaine in lotions (℞ 204) is necessary
at times to alleviate pain. Occasionally, soothing ointments
(℞ 13, 93) are desirable. Mouth lesions demand special attention. An aqueous solution of potassium permanganate (℞ 4) can
serve as a mouthwash, and erosions should be treated with 5%
silver nitrate solution (℞ 64).

For bedridden patients, liberal sprinkling of the sheets with
talcum (℞ 25), containing 5% benzocaine (℞ 203) if necessary,
affords relief. If the involvement is extensive, the patient may
derive the greatest benefit from immersion in a continuous
water bath, or baths containing 1:40,000 potassium permanganate (℞ 105) for about 20 to 30 minutes several times daily.

LUPUS ERYTHEMATOSUS

(Lupus erythematodes, Lupus sebaceus, Seborrhea
congestiva)

*A relatively rare systemic disease characterized by cutaneous
lesions consisting of erythematous scaling patches of various
sizes and configurations which result in superficial atrophy of
the skin and scar formation.* **Lupus erythematosus disseminatus** (q.v.), an acute fulminating form, is discussed separately.

Etiology and Incidence

The cause is unknown. The disease is more common in
women than in men (3:1) and appears most often during the
3rd decade of life. The first attack frequently follows overexposure to the sun. Tuberculosis, streptococcal and virus
infections, abnormality of the reticulo-endothelial system, and
bacterial allergy have been suggested as etiologic factors.

Symptoms and Signs

Clinically, the disease may be either chronic or subacute.

1. Chronic (Discoid) **Lupus Erythematosus:** This begins
as one or several erythematous macular lesions on the exposed
parts, varying in diameter from 0.5 cm. to 6 cm., which become covered with grayish brown adherent scales. On close
examination, dilated follicular openings can be seen, into which
the scales extend as keratotic plugs. Often the eruption is
symmetrical, appearing on the cheeks and across the nose in a
butterfly pattern. The face, neck, ears, and scalp are the chief
sites, but other exposed areas may be involved and (rarely)
the lips and oral mucosa. Subjective symptoms usually are
absent or slight. The lesions increase by peripheral extension
and soon present an erythematous border with a slightly depressed and paler center. In several months or years the

typical triad of erythema, scaling, and atrophy becomes established. Healed lesions leave depressed, atrophic, noncontractile scars and may show peripheral telangiectasis. On the scalp, the atrophy is more severe and permanent alopecia results. Itching may be troublesome. In the mouth, the lesions, usually on the buccal mucosa, appear as elevated, circumscribed plaques with sharply defined bluish red borders, and tend to ulcerate superficially. The vermilion border of the lips may become bluish red, slightly swollen and covered with scales (silvering of the lips). Occasionally, the regional lymph nodes are slightly enlarged but not tender.

2. **Subacute Lupus Erythematosus:** This may occur alone or be superimposed upon a chronic discoid lupus erythematosus. It is characterized by sudden onset with occasional fever, headache, and indefinite pains. The eruption differs from that of the chronic form in the sudden appearance of extensive lesions symmetrically arranged on the thorax, arms, and legs in addition to the sites involved in the chronic type (q.v.). The lesions are more diffuse, covering large areas, and erythematous with a livid hue; scaling is slight. All degrees of severity are seen.

Diagnosis

The mild and chronic forms of lupus erythematosus are to be distinguished from seborrheic dermatitis, psoriasis of the face and scalp, acne rosacea, dry forms of neurodermatitis, alopecia areata, tinea capitis, pseudopelade, folliculitis decalvans, lupus vulgaris, sarcoid, and late syphilis. Leukoplakia and lichen planus lesions of the mucous membrane occasionally present considerable diagnostic difficulty. Careful inspection usually will reveal the triad of erythema, scaling, and atrophy, occasionally combined with telangiectasis, silvering of the lips, and lesions of the buccal mucosa. However, biopsy is essential in all questionable cases.

Prognosis

In the chronic discoid form the course is capricious. Atrophy and scarring may or may not occur. The lesions may disappear spontaneously or remain stationary for months or years. Carcinomatous changes may develop in lesions of long standing, or subacute or acute forms suddenly appear.

In the subacute form the eruption may undergo involution without leaving any trace, or slight atrophy may result. Some lesions remain stationary and present the picture of chronic lupus erythematosus, or develop into the acute form (see LUPUS ERYTHEMATOSUS DISSEMINATUS).

Treatment

Early treatment often prevents progression and may cause existing lesions to heal without sequelae, but once atrophy has appeared, treatment cannot reverse the process. A thorough physical examination with a search for foci of infection is indicated in all cases. However, it is extremely important to choose the correct time for eradication of these foci. In chronic lupus erythematosus this may be done immediately, but in the acute and subacute forms tampering with a focus of infection is absolutely contraindicated. A period of remission must be awaited before any focus can be attacked with reasonable safety. The practical importance of rest, avoidance of overwork, and supportive care cannot be overemphasized in the treatment of all forms of the disease. It is imperative to avoid exposure to sunlight, either direct or reflected, and ultra-violet ray treatments are contraindicated. Protective lotions and creams (℞ 109, 110) should be used more or less constantly, and especially when the patient is exposed to sunlight. Gold therapy (℞ 157) has given gratifying results in selected cases, but it must be used with caution because of its high toxicity (*see* RHEUMATOID ARTHRITIS). Bismuth (℞ 159, 160) is beneficial in many cases, though probably less so than gold. Quinine orally (℞ 158) may be useful in early cases. Because of the possibility that infection may play a role in etiology, penicillin (℞ 146, 147) merits a trial, particularly in the acute and subacute forms. Liver extract (℞ 211) and vitamin B complex (℞ 210), especially the nicotinic acid component (℞ 206), are valuable as adjuvants. Mapharsen (℞ 156) may be useful in cases refractory to other treatment.

Carbon dioxide snow is the best agent now known for topical application to chronic lesions (but not to others). Freezing the lesions with moderate pressure for 5 to 15 seconds at intervals of 2 to 3 weeks may cause their rapid disappearance, leaving white scars. An ointment (℞ 62) may be of some benefit.

LUPUS ERYTHEMATOSUS DISSEMINATUS

(Disseminated lupus erythematosus; Atypical verrucose endocarditis, "Libman-Sacks syndrome")

A degenerative process of unknown etiology, involving primarily the collagen system and ground substance of a wide variety of tissues, with characteristic, acellular lesions in the skin, serous surfaces, heart valves, kidneys, lymph nodes, and smaller blood vessels. It is most common in young adult females.

Symptoms and Signs

The clinical picture of disseminated lupus varies with the acuteness of the process and the anatomic distribution of the lesions. Some, or all, of the following manifestations are encountered in a typical illness: fever with leukopenia, progressive cachexia with periods of remission, cutaneous erythema, polyarthritis, nephritis, polyserositis, and verrucose endocarditis. Symptoms and signs referable to almost every system of the body may be noted in special instances. The disease may begin abruptly with high fever simulating an acute infection, or so gradually that the date of onset is indeterminable. An important finding in most cases is the rash, which first appears as discrete, erythematous, scaly, nonitching patches on exposed surfaces such as the cheeks, chin, forehead, and neck. Across the bridge of the nose the lesions often coalesce to form a butterfly pattern. The rash is unfavorably affected by sunlight. The fingertips, mucous membranes, and other skin surfaces also may become involved.

The arthritic manifestations consist of swelling and stiffness of the larger joints, with little tenderness or redness and few permanent deformities. The typical renal lesion, found in about half the cases, is a hyaline thickening of some of the glomerular capillaries, giving a "wire loop" appearance. These lesions cause albuminuria, cylindruria, and slight hematuria, but seldom azotemia, oliguria or hypertension. Cardiac lesions are due to fibrinoid degeneration of the subepicardial and subendocardial connective tissue and are marked by swelling and coalescence of collagenous fibrils into matted amorphous masses of eosinophilic material. Pericardial adhesions develop and vegetations composed essentially of elevated masses of denatured collagen appear on the valves and walls of the heart. The endocardial verrucae seldom give rise to murmurs or lead to cardiac insufficiency. Similar lesions of fibrinoid degeneration are commonly found in the tissues of the mediastinum, pleura, and peritoneum, and give symptoms of intermittent friction rubs and local discomfort. Other occasional findings are nonsuppurative lymphadenopathies, transitory perivascular exudations in the retina, and inconstant C.N.S. derangements. The lesions in the blood vessels consist of fibrinoid changes in the walls of the terminal arterioles and groups of capillaries, which lead to nutritive and functional disturbances in nearby tissues. In contrast to periarteritis nodosa, however, they seldom cause gross infarction.

Laboratory Findings

Common observations are moderate hypochromic anemia, leukopenia, and thrombopenia. The E.S.R. is greatly accelerated. The serum albumin usually is diminished and gamma globulins are increased. False positive Wassermann reactions and misleading cephalin flocculation tests indicate qualitative abnormalities in the globulin complex.

Diagnosis

Disseminated lupus erythematosus is easily recognized when a febrile wasting disease occurs in a young woman, in combination with a patchy erythematous skin eruption, vague joint pains, and intermittent pleuritic and abdominal pain, accompanied by leukopenia, albuminuria, and hyperglobulinemia. The condition is not to be confused with discoid lupus, which is generally regarded as an unrelated local disorder of the skin. Differential diagnosis must exclude chronic wasting infections and toxic erythemas, but most confusing are the other so-called "collagen diseases," e.g., rheumatic fever, periarteritis nodosa, rheumatoid arthritis, dermatomyositis, and scleroderma (q.v.). Cutaneous, arthritic, and vascular disturbances are common in all such conditions and, while each has its typical manifestations, in some instances sharp differentiation is impossible.

Prognosis and Treatment

The prognosis in well defined cases is grave. The acute disease may terminate fatally within a few weeks, with acute toxemia. The cause of death often is obscure, and lesions are surprisingly few at autopsy. On the other hand, the disease may run a chronic remittent course, causing semi-invalidism for years. Apparent spontaneous recovery has been noted in a few cases.

Because the highest incidence is in young women, androgens, estrogens, and even castration, have been tried, but with no benefit. Administration of quinine, salicylates, urea, ichthammol, tincture of iodine, arsenicals, liver extract, and sulfapyridine has given indifferent results. Gold salts, such as Myochrysine (R 157), are useful in chronic, but contraindicated in acute disseminated, lupus. Direct sunlight is to be avoided. A well balanced, high caloric diet should be supplied. Transfusions temporarily diminish the anemia and improve the patient's general well-being. Antibiotics are useful only for secondary infection. Rest is important in chronic cases, since relapses often follow overexertion.

Encouraging results are being reported in the treatment of disseminated lupus, scleroderma, and dermatomyositis with cortisone or ACTH, although final evaluation must await further studies.

SCLERODERMA

(Dermatosclerosis, Sclererema adultorum, Hidebound skin)

A chronic localized or diffuse skin disease, of unknown etiology, characterized by fibrosis, rigidity, and atrophy of the skin and subcutaneous tissues. It is most common in females and during middle life.

Symptoms and Signs

The onset usually is gradual. Initially, there is painless edema of the skin, followed successively over a period of months or years by hardening, atrophy, and finally immobility. The distribution usually is symmetrical and may be localized (circumscribed scleroderma, morphea) or diffuse. The skin becomes smooth and shiny and the face assumes a masklike appearance. Immobility of the skin may interfere with breathing, chewing, and joint movements. Trophic ulcers are common and vascular changes of the Raynaud type may develop. Constitutional symptoms usually are minimal or absent. The disease usually is slowly progressive, with periods of remission. Spontaneous recovery has been observed, particularly among children.

Treatment

(For mention of recent investigative therapy, *see* the preceding chapter.) A balanced diet, preferably with general vitamin supplementation, should be maintained, although there is no evidence that the disorder is due to nutritional deficiency. Methyl testosterone (℞ 215) has caused regression of lesions and increased muscular strength in some cases. Thyroid extract, various extracts of pancreas, foreign protein I.V., neostigmine, ammonium chloride, parathyroidectomy, and surgical correction of obvious endocrinopathies have each proved beneficial in isolated instances. Measures to soften the skin and improve blood supply to the tissues may be useful. These include massage, warm baths, and bland ointments containing 1% pilocarpine (℞ 20) or 1% salicylic acid (℞ 34). Niacin (℞ 206), or acetylcholine by iontophoresis (*see* CLIN. PROC.) may promote vasodilation.

DERMATOMYOSITIS

A grave but rare systemic disorder of the collagenous tissues, characterized by inflammatory and degenerative changes in the skin and voluntary muscles.

Etiology and Incidence

The cause of dermatomyositis is unknown. Preceding infections are regarded as precipitating factors in some cases. The syndrome occurs predominantly between the ages of 10 and 50 years, and may appear during the course of neoplastic disease.

Symptoms and Signs

Onset may be abrupt, with fever, prostration, bright erythema of the skin, and painful swollen muscles; or insidious, with vague fatigability and gradual weakness in a single muscle group with inconspicuous scaling and pigmentation of the skin. Early symptoms may predominate in the skin or the muscles.

Muscular involvement may be widespread or localized. The shoulders, pelvic girdle, and proximal muscles are most commonly affected, but any group of muscles may be affected. The myocardium and unstriated muscles usually escape serious damage. The initial muscular signs usually are brawny swelling with pain, tenderness, stiffness, and weakness, followed eventually by atrophy and fibrous contractures.

Skin manifestations are variable. Erythema and brawny edema particularly about the eyes, on the face, and over affected muscles are common. The eruption may be patchy and localized or widespread, involving the mucous membranes as well as the skin. The dermatitis may be transient or may be followed by excessive brownish pigmentation or by scarring indistinguishable from that of scleroderma (q.v.).

Visceral lesions also are occasionally present, giving rise to dysphagia, pleural pain, effusions into serous cavities, retinal exudates, splenomegaly, lymphadenopathies, and joint pain and stiffness. Vasomotor disturbances in the hands, resembling Raynaud's disease, have been described. Fever usually is high in acute forms of the disease, and slight or absent in chronic cases. In most cases the course is marked by repeated acute exacerbations. Laboratory findings are not diagnostic. The blood may show a moderate secondary anemia and a definite eosinophilia in some cases. The erythrocytic sedimentation is accelerated. Hyperglobulinemia is a common finding. Urinary excretion of creatine is increased, and the output of creatinine proportionately reduced.

Diagnosis

The similarities of some forms of dermatomyositis to disseminated lupus (q.v.) and to diffuse scleroderma are striking, and it is widely held that these disorders are fundamentally related, differing primarily in the distribution of the lesions, the extent of vascular thickening, and the degree of residual scarring. Scarring is less prominent than in scleroderma, and the visceral involvement is less striking than in disseminated lupus, but biopsies are often necessary for a final differentiation. Clinically, the muscular involvement characterizes dermatomyositis. Other conditions, such as trichinosis, toxic erythemas, acute fibrositis, and primary myopathies, also must be considered.

Prognosis

The course of the disease varies. Remissions are frequent and complete recovery may occasionally occur. Death often occurs within 2 years due to cardiorespiratory disease. Usually, however, the disease progresses to a certain indefinite point and then remains stationary.

Treatment

(For mention of recent investigative therapy, *see* the chapter on Disseminated Lupus.) Oral administration of alpha tocopherol (vitamin E), 40 to 120 mg. daily, once widely advocated, has proved disappointing. Androgens, estrogens, ephedrine, antihistaminics, and many other agents have been tried without benefit. Splinting to immobilize painful muscles, local heat, and gentle passive motion to prevent contractures are important palliative measures. Codeine (℞ 196) and acetylsalicylic acid (℞ 194) may be given every 4 hours to control pain. Habit-forming analgesics cannot be withheld during the agonizing episodes of dermatomyositis, but drug addictions often are acquired, which complicate the subsequent management of the disease.

PERIARTERITIS NODOSA

(Kussmaul-Maier disease, Polyarteritis,
Diffuse necrotizing arteritis)

A grave disease characterized by focal degenerative and inflammatory lesions of the smaller arteries, leading to functional impairment of tissues supplied by the affected vessels.

Etiology and Incidence

The cause of periarteritis nodosa is not known. Until recently the disorder was generally regarded as a rare type of infection, but accumulating evidence indicates that allergy may be of prime significance in some cases. The patients frequently give a history of allergy or antecedent infection. The disease is predominantly one of middle life, but may occur from infancy to old age. The incidence is about 3 times greater in males than in females.

Pathology

The distinguishing feature is focalized swelling of collagen fibers limited to the media and adventitia of the smaller arteries. An intense cellular accumulation of polymorphonuclear leukocytes, eosinophiles, lymphocytes, and plasma cells develops at the point of injury, with narrowing of the vessel lumen and weakening of the wall. Local aneurysms form and may rupture. After a few weeks or months the lesion heals with resolution of the exudate, proliferation of endothelium, and replacement of the original structures by fibroblasts.

Symptoms and Signs

Onset may be abrupt, with fever as the initial symptom, and the course may be that of an acute febrile disease, with fatal termination after several months, or it may be insidious and give the clinical picture of a chronic wasting disease. The symptoms vary widely and are determined largely by the location and severity of the arteritis and the extent of secondary circulatory impairment. They may be referable to the heart, kidneys, lungs, gastrointestinal tract, nervous system, and eyes. Fever is the most common systemic symptom. Skin manifestations include purpura, urticaria, edema, and erythema. Subcutaneous nodules may sometimes be palpated. There usually is a severe leukocytosis (40,000 to 60,000) with moderate eosinophilia. Secondary anemia is frequent.

Diagnosis

Diagnosis often is difficult since the acute form of periarteritis may simulate trichinosis, rheumatic disease, bacterial endocarditis, typhoid fever, miliary tuberculosis, polymyositis, acute hemorrhagic nephritis, pyonephrosis, multiple neuritis, gastroenteritis, sepsis, serous tuberculosis, influenza, and purpura hemorrhagica. The chronic form frequently is mistaken for chronic nephritis, generalized arteriosclerosis, chronic myocarditis, tuberculosis, syphilis, neoplasm, or C.N.S. degeneration. The diagnosis often rests on the exclusion of these conditions, which at times is impossible. Microscopic examination of sections of indurated skin and tender muscles or of material removed at exploratory operations furnishes the only certain means of diagnosis. The condition often can be recognized clinically if it is considered in the differential diagnosis of all obscure febrile illnesses, or when a case simulating nephritis or a cardiac disorder is accompanied by eosinophilia or by unexplained derangements in other systems, such as joint pains, muscle tenderness or weakness, subcutaneous nodules, purpuric skin rashes, or pain in the abdomen or extremities. A rapidly developing hypertension with wide excursions of blood pressure also should suggest the possibility of periarteritis nodosa.

Prognosis and Treatment

Periarteritis nodosa, whether acute or chronic, is almost universally fatal, due to vascular insufficiency of one or more vital organs such as the heart, kidneys, or lungs, caused by occlusion of the affected vessels. Acute ischemia of the intestines may lead to perforations with secondary peritonitis. Fatal hemorrhage from a ruptured viscus also is common.

Treatment has been entirely symptomatic. Recently, encouraging results have been reported following the administration of cortisone or ACTH to a few patients; further study, however, must precede final evaluation of this or related therapeutic innovations. Allergens must be avoided and any chronic infections eliminated by appropriate therapy. Antihistaminic drugs are not effective. Supportive and palliative measures, such as repeated transfusions, high caloric diet, and adequate sedation, are indicated. Supplements of a standard vitamin complex are usually added, but there is no evidence of a deficiency state in this disease. Prompt repair of perforations of the gastrointestinal tract may circumvent fatal peritonitis.

ICHTHYOSIS

(Fish skin disease, Alligator skin disease,
Ichthyosis simplex, Xeroderma)

A congenital heredofamilial disease of the skin characterized by dryness and scaliness, and due to an abnormality of the cornification process.

Symptoms and Signs

Ichthyosis presents all degrees of change. In the mild form, the skin is dry and presents fine scaling, chiefly on the extensor surface of the extremities. Small keratotic papules also may be seen. The skin has a grayish hue. In the more severe forms, the process is generalized but the extensor surfaces continue to present the greatest changes. The scales are quadrangular and attached centrally. The skin may become extremely thick and inelastic. The nails become coarse and are easily broken; the hair becomes dry and the function of both the sebaceous and sweat glands is greatly reduced. The severity of the process is greater in the winter than in the summer.

Diagnosis and Prognosis

The diagnosis rests upon clinical appearances and history. Ichthyosis is differentiated from other scaling dermatoses by the fact that it is noninflammatory and comparatively asymptomatic. It progresses to a given stage, remaining stationary except for seasonal fluctuations. Complete recovery is not seen, yet persistent proper therapy can do much to reduce the severity of ichthyosis.

Treatment

There is no specific cure for this disease. Efforts must be directed toward conservation of sebum and artificial replacement therapy. The patients should be advised to avoid all factors which lead to the removal of the sebum of the skin. Soap, hot water, and fat solvents, such as gasoline, alcohol, and carbon tetrachloride must be avoided as much as possible. Cleansing should be accomplished by the use of colloid baths (℞ 104, 108) and soap substitutes (℞ 27, 28, 29). Frequent inunctions of oils or ointments (℞ 22, 23) will do much to relieve this disease. For many, living in a warm environment is of benefit. Ultraviolet rays also may aid when given in small stimulating doses.

In certain patients, thyroid (℞ 216) and vitamin A (℞ 205) administration have effected improvement.

CALLOSITY; CORN

(Callositas, Tyloma, Keratoma, Clavus)

Callosity: *An acquired superficial, circumscribed, horny patch of epidermis which occurs at the site of repeated trauma.*
Corn: *A circumscribed, cone-shaped hypertrophy of the epidermis, the apex of which presses on the corium.*

Callosities result from long-continued, intermittent pressure or friction on the skin as occurs from wearing tight shoes, grasping tools or athletic equipment, plucking stringed musical instruments, and kneeling or going barefoot. Corns result from persistent trauma to the skin. Ill-fitting footwear is a common cause of corns and callosities of the feet.

Symptoms and Signs

Callosities are smooth, dirty yellowish white hyperkeratoses, usually insensitive to pain, which develop chiefly on the hands and feet, but may occur over bony prominences such as the knees or ischial tuberosities. Their position at certain characteristic sites on fingers or hands often is a reliable stigma of the patient's occupation, such as bricklayer, drummer, harpist. Because of their protective action, callosities often are essential to the prosecution of the work.

Corns are pea-sized or larger lesions which occur on the feet at the site of greatest trauma. Their whitish center or core consists of condensed keratin. They are spontaneously painful, especially with change of weather, and tender when compressed. "Hard" corns occur on the prominent protuberances of the foot and especially the toes. "Soft" corns occur between the toes and, because of the moisture and maceration, are whiter and softer.

Diagnosis

Plantar warts must be differentiated from simple callosities because callus forms around the protuberance of the wart and simulates the former entity. By paring away this callus, its verrucous structure will be revealed. Bunions (the inflamed bursa over the metatarsophalangeal joint of the big toe) may resemble a corn or callosity in appearance. Hyperkeratotic mycotic infections are more diffuse and often are accompanied by such lesions as vesicles and scaling, which aid in differentiation. Microscopic and cultural examinations of these lesions for fungi may be of further help. Arsenical keratoses are symmetrically distributed, sometimes pigmented, on palms and soles with many discrete individual lesions. A history of arsenic ingestion (Fowler's solution), 10 or more years before, often can be obtained. Psoriasis, eczema, congenital keratoderma palmaris et plantaris, keratoderma blennorrhagica, and angiokeratoma also are to be considered.

Treatment

Prophylaxis is of the greatest importance. Avoidance of the offending trauma will cure most cases. This may be done by changing the patient's activity or the manner in which he performs it. If the lesions are on the feet, footwear designed to redistribute the pressure more evenly is essential for a lasting cure.

Local treatment with various softening and destructive agents will give temporary relief or hasten cure with other measures. To soften the lesions they may be soaked in hot water to which soap or washing soda has been added. The excess keratin then can be removed by paring or with emery paper. Care must be taken especially in diabetics not to cause bleeding or infection. Keratolytics such as 20% salicylic acid in collodion (R 76) or 40% salicylic acid plasters (R 73) may be applied so as to cover just the lesions. After several days these may be pared with ease and the material reapplied if necessary. Caustics such as a silver nitrate stick (R 77) or trichloroacetic acid (R 69) touched to the center of the lesions twice a week also are used, especially for painful soft corns or after softening and trimming hard corns. A ringed felt pad with salicylic acid plaster (corn plaster) often will give temporary relief. Recent observations indicate that massive doses of vitamin A (R 205) given for a month or more will sometimes reduce callosities and diffuse plantar hyperkeratosis. This therapy is recommended in severe or resistant cases, but its effect will not be evident for several weeks.

DECUBITUS

(Bed sore, Pressure sore, Trophic ulcer)

Local necrosis of the skin and subcutaneous tissues overlying a bony prominence which has been subjected to prolonged pressure against an external object (e.g., bed, cast, splint). It is most frequently seen in patients long bedridden. The lesions may develop over the pelvis, the sacrum, greater tuberosities, crest of the ilium, condyles of the femur, and prominences about the ankle.

Etiology

The essential cause is local pressure upon the tissues. The partial or complete occlusion of blood supply leads to necrosis and gangrene. First the more sensitive subcutaneous and deeper tissues are damaged, and later the skin becomes necrotic. Predisposing factors are trauma, maceration of the skin, and malnutrition (hypoproteinemia). Pressure combined with injury to the skin from ill-adjusted supports or wrinkled bed covers or clothing may cause small breaks in the skin through which infection is introduced. Maceration of the skin often follows soaking of the bed and clothing by perspiration or by incontinence of urine or feces. Malnutrition reduces the ability of the tissues to resist breakdown under pressure or to repair the damage when pressure is reduced.

Symptoms and Signs

Three stages of decubitus are recognized: threatened, inevitable, and ulcer. Threatened decubitus is indicated by a redness of the skin which disappears on pressure. At this stage the skin and tissues are still soft. An inevitable decubitus is diagnosed by the presence of redness, or local cyanosis, unaffected by digital pressure. The tissues are indurated and occasionally a vesicle may be present. Ulcer is characterized by tissue necrosis. It may involve not only the skin and subcutaneous tissues, but fascia, muscle, and bone as well. It is at this stage that infection is most common.

Prophylaxis

Prophylaxis should be vigorously employed to combat the causative factors of pressure, injury or maceration of the skin, and malnutrition.

Frequent change of posture and redistribution of points of contact will minimize excessive pressure over vulnerable areas. Frequent changing of the patient alternately from the supine to the prone position, and to the side, if permissible, is one means of preventing long periods of pressure over the same site. The Operative Turning (Stryker) Frame facilitates turning paraplegic patients and should be used if available. Air mattresses, rubber-foam mattresses, and rubber rings will protect sensitive areas. Fluffed pillows or rolled blankets under the knees allow pressure to be borne on the plantar surfaces of the heels rather than the more vulnerable posterior portion.

Care should be observed in the operating room to protect the bony prominences of debilitated patients against prolonged pressure with resultant shutting off of the blood supply. Nasal and oral suction tubes should be shifted frequently whenever possible to prevent pressure ulceration in the nose and throat.

Injury to the skin is avoided by seeing that bed linens and clothing are taut and clean, and free from wrinkles or small, hard particles. Crumbs of food, tobacco, and other foreign bodies must be removed.

Maceration is prevented by keeping the patient's skin dry and clean at all times. Essential measures are the frequent changing of bed clothes, sponging the skin in hot weather, thoroughly drying it after baths, and hardening it by gentle massage with alcohol. After the skin has become completely dry, a dusting powder such as zinc stearate (℞ 179), talc (℞ 25), or boric acid (℞ 26) is applied. Urinary incontinence must be controlled. This may be done by an indwelling catheter, in which case sulfonamides (℞ 150, 151) should be given prophylactically against infection. Control of fecal incontinence is especially important. For this purpose enemas should be used. Dressings should be changed frequently.

Malnutrition as manifested by anemia and hypoproteinemia is an important causative factor in decubitus. Active measures for restoring the nitrogen balance from negative to positive include a high protein, high caloric diet; supplementary between-meal feedings; administration of amino acids or of protein hydrolysate; and plasma and whole blood transfusions as indicated by hemoglobin, hematocrit, and total blood protein levels. Vitamins parenterally are indicated if avitaminosis is demonstrated or suspected.

Treatment

Threatened decubitus requires forceful employment of all the prophylactic measures just outlined in order to prevent necrosis of the tissues. Stimulation of the circulation by gentle massage and infrared radiation and protection of the skin by coating it with tincture of benzoin may be helpful.

Inevitable decubitus and ulcer may be treated conservatively or surgically. Surgical intervention greatly reduces healing time.

Ulcer will require treatment as follows:

General: Improvement of nutritional status and maintenance of positive nitrogen balance are necessary, through high protein, high caloric, high vitamin diet (*see* Diets), with supplementary repeated I.V. injections of amino acids mixtures or whole blood transfusions, or both. Pressure must be kept off the involved area as much as possible by adjustment of patient's position or of casts or other appliances.

Local: Conservative débridement of necrotic tissue should be done. Topical application of the common antiseptics is condemned, since they do not penetrate or sterilize the sloughing tissue. However, irrigations with medicinal zinc peroxide (℞ 145) sometimes are useful against anaerobic or microaerophilic bacteria. If there is discharge from the ulcer, sterile dressings are recommended. Antibiotics are helpful in controlling infection. *Staph. aureus* and hemolytic streptococcus are the most serious invaders, and since these usually are sensitive to penicillin, wet dressings containing 1,000 u./cc. (℞ 148) may be applied. In the presence of fecal incontinence, streptomycin-sensitive organisms may contaminate the lesion, and streptomycin in a concentration of 5 mg./cc. (℞ 149) may be applied as a wet dressing for a short time. Streptomycin

(℞ 149) or penicillin (℞ 148), or both, may be applied as a dusting powder in dehydrated plasma or in sterile lactose. Streptomycin-fastness develops rapidly, however, since the organisms are meshed in the sloughing tissues and thus protected from the full antibacterial action of the drug. Tyrothricin is less effective than either penicillin or streptomycin and therefore is not recommended.

Systemic: In the presence of spreading cellulitis, I.M. penicillin (℞ 146, 147) is a necessary adjuvant to local therapy.

Surgical: When positive nitrogen balance and freedom from active infection are established and healthy granulation tissue appears, complete excision of the necrotic tissue, with immediate plastic closure of the ulcer by sliding full-thickness skin flaps, is the treatment of choice. Split-thickness and pinch grafts are not recommended over bony prominences except to make the patient a good operative risk. The same considerations and precautions as for threatened decubitus apply to the management of the operative site.

NEVI

(Moles, Beauty spots, Birthmarks)

Circumscribed, benign new growths of the skin that occur as the result of congenital maldevelopment or as later hyperplasia of "embryonal rests." Although many cutaneous entities can be included under the term "nevus," only the common ones are discussed below.

Diagnosis and Treatment

Pigmented nevi include the following types:

Freckles (ephelides) and **chloasma** (liver spots) are abnormal collections of pigment, which are small and circumscribed in freckles, and larger and more diffuse in chloasma. The color may be various shades of brown, occasionally even blackish. In predisposed individuals, freckles usually develop during childhood over areas exposed to sunlight, though some may be present over the covered parts of the body. Chloasma may occur as a result of the action of such agents as friction, heat or light, application of various irritant substances to the skin, or in association with pregnancy and systemic diseases such as tuberculosis, cancer, liver diseases. Chloasma may occur anywhere on the body, but is more common on the face and trunk. In both chloasma and freckles the only physical findings are areas of pigmentation of the skin. Freckles and some types of chloasma are worse in the summer but become lighter in the winter. Chloasma associated with systemic disease may disappear after cure of the disease, but freckles, once developed, will not disappear entirely. Patients predisposed to freckling should avoid overexposure to sunlight. Patients with chloasma should be checked for any evidence of systemic disease. Local therapy, which often is unsatisfactory, consists of application of "bleaching cream" (R 123) regularly, or a masking cream (R 119).

Hyperkeratotic and **verrucose nevi** occasionally are present at birth or in early childhood. They occur anywhere on the body and may be various shades of brown. They may be of a linear distribution or may assume a variety of patterns. Prognosis for the disappearance of lesions is poor, and rarely they become malignant. Therapy of choice, when feasible, is surgical excision.

Pigmented nevi proper may occur anywhere on the body and the color may vary from light brown to slate blue. They may be hairy or hairless, flat or elevated, and vary in size. In general, the flat, smooth, hairless, deeply pigmented nevus has more tendency to become malignant. This is especially true on the lower extremities. All nevi can become malignant, and constant trauma, irritation, and inadequate removal predispose to such malignant changes. Nevi containing hairs, especially soft nevi, rarely undergo malignant transformation. Indications for removal are cosmetic, the presence of a nevus at a site exposed to frequent irritation, and recent growth or inflammatory changes in the nevus. Pigmented nevi disappear only rarely without therapy. When properly removed, recurrences are unusual. If there is anything unusual about a nevus, expert opinion should be sought. The nevus should be removed by wide and deep excision and a pathologic examination of the specimen made. Hairy nevi can be treated by application of trichloroacetic acid at 14-day intervals, after the hairs have been removed by electrolysis.

Hemangiomas, localized hyperplasias of the blood vascular tissue of the skin, are classed among the nevi. They include:

Flat Angioma (Nevus flammeus, Port-wine mark): A macular, superficial hemangioma which can occur on any part of the body. It does not become malignant and is not affected by radiotherapy or any local treatment. It can be disguised to some extent by covering with a cosmetic cream (R 119).

Cavernous Angioma (Strawberry mark): A nodular, soft angiomatous mass, fairly deep-seated, which blanches on pressure. It may occur anywhere, but is common on the face and neck. Such angiomas are present at birth or soon thereafter. Usually, they disappear without active therapy in a few years. They do not become malignant. The various types of therapy include repeated applications of solid carbon dioxide, X-ray therapy, radium, and injection of sclerosing solution. Treatment should be started early in infancy. Some of these lesions tend to disappear spontaneously.

Stellate Angioma (Spider nevus): An angioma consisting of a central point from which numerous telangiectatic vessels radiate in a star fashion. The lesions may occur anywhere on the body, but are most frequent on the face. They may be associated with hepatic disease, hypertension, and pregnancy, but can occur in normal persons. Disappearance occurs spontaneously only in pregnancy. These angiomas do not become malignant. Therapy consists of destruction of the central point by electrolysis.

Senile Angioma (Ruby spot): A small compressible mass of blood vessels which can develop anywhere on the body of elderly individuals. It is of no significance and requires no therapy.

EPITHELIOMA

A skin cancer. Malignant skin tumors may be primary or secondary. Primary varieties originate from the skin itself, whereas secondary growths may occur as a result of direct extension of neoplasms from adjacent structures, or from lymphatic or hematogenous spread of metastases. The types of skin cancer most commonly encountered are basal cell epithelioma, squamous cell epithelioma, and basal squamous cell epithelioma, which are here described.

Basal Cell Epithelioma (Rodent ulcer): This lesion usually occurs in older individuals with fair, dry skin, who have been exposed to strong sunlight for long periods of time. The tumor is asymptomatic, superficial, and may occur anywhere on the body but is most common on exposed areas. It begins as a small shiny translucent nodule, grows slowly and develops a hard pearly border. Frequently, small telangiectatic vessels are present over the lesion. Central crusting and ulceration or papillary growths may develop.

Untreated basal cell epitheliomas do not metastasize but do spread by extension and cause deformities. Inadequate treatment may alter such a lesion to the more malignant type of squamous cell epithelioma and therefore it is essential that suspicious growths should be biopsied and treated by one very familiar with these tumors. These lesions may be removed by irradiation, surgical excision, or by chemical or electric cautery.

Squamous Cell Epithelioma (Prickle cell epithelioma): This type of tumor commonly involves the lips, tongue, and mucosa of the nose, eyelids, penis, or vulva, although it may appear on any part of the body. The growth originates from the squamous cells of the epidermis and in the early stages it is a small nodule or flat papule which grows slowly. A fungoid growth may develop or the surface may break down to form an ulcer with an indurated base, hard, undermined edges, and covered with a crust. Growth proceeds inward, as well as peripherally, with involvement of the underlying tissues and development of metastases. The tumor must be differentiated from lesions of syphilis, tuberculosis, and various precancerous conditions. Examination of a suspected growth should always include a biopsy examination. Untreated squamous cell epithelioma may progress to a fatal outcome quite rapidly. Lesions of the mucous membranes and mucocutaneous junctions always have a grave prognosis; even with adequate therapy the prognosis is not very good in extensive lesions, lesions of long duration, and those in which metastases are suspected. However, adequately treated small early lesions are usually cured. Treatment should be only by a specially trained physician. Destructive measures employed to treat the tumor and its metastases include surgical excision, X-ray, and radium.

Basal Squamous Cell Epithelioma (Mixed or transitional cell epithelioma): A small proportion of the typical basal cell epitheliomas contain areas of squamous cell epithelioma. The cause of this is unknown, and the diagnosis can be made only after pathologic examination. Such lesions behave like a squamous cell epithelioma, eventually invade other tissues and metastasize. Therapy should be that of squamous cell epithelioma, as the prognosis is the same.

PRESCRIPTIONS

(Wherever a prescribed "proprietary" is representative of a class of therapeutic agents, alternative proprietary preparations will be found in Part II.)

Emollients and Protectives

1. ℞ Boric acid, saturated solution . 120.0 cc. (℥ iv)

> Apply to face with cotton pledgets several times daily.

2. ℞ Aluminum Acetate Solution
    N.F. (Burow's Solution) . 240.0 cc. (℥ viii)

> Dilute with water 1:10, or 1:20, and use as wet compresses or soaks.

3. ℞ Resorcinol . . . . 5.0 Gm. (gr. lxxv)
    Boric acid . . . . 15.0 Gm. (℥ ss)
    Glycerin . . . . 15.0 cc. (℥ ss)
    Warm water . . . q.s. ad 1,000.0 cc. (℥ xxxii)

> Store in refrigerator. Use as cold compresses. (Do not use on blond or white hair.)

4. ℞ Potassium permanganate . . 0.12 Gm. (gr. ii)

> Dissolve 1 tablet in 2 to 3 pints of water (1:9,000–1:12,000). Use as a compress, wash, or soak for 15 to 20 minutes 4 times daily. (Solution must be freshly prepared each day.)

5. ℞ Tannic acid . . . . 6.0 Gm. (ʒ iss)
   Distilled water. . . . q.s. ad 120.0 cc. (ʒ iv)
   Use in a fly sprayer, treating affected areas
   every hour when patient is awake.

6. ℞ Acetone . . . . 20.0 cc. (ʒ v)
   Isopropyl alcohol . . . . . 80.0 cc. (ʒ iiss)
   Apply to face daily. (For pustular acne)

7. ℞ Sodium borate . . . . . . 16.0 Gm. (ʒ iv)
   Water. . . . . . q.s. ad 2,000.0 cc. (ʒ lxiv)
   Apply to face as wet dressing. (For sebor-
   rheic acne)

8. ℞ Triethanolamine . . . . . 6.0 Gm. (ʒ iss)
   Boric acid . . . . 2.0 Gm. (ʒ ss)
   Glycerin. . . . . 4.0 cc. (ʒ i)
   Ethyl alcohol 50% . . . . 30.0 cc. (ʒ i)
   Rose Water U.S.P. . . q.s. ad 120.0 cc. (ʒ iv)
   Apply as wet dressing. (Seborrheic and
   comedo cleansing lotion)

9. ℞ Acetone . . . . 4.0 cc. (ʒ i)
   Collodion . . . . 4.0 cc. (ʒ i)
   Crude coal tar. . . . q.s. ad 30.0 cc. (ʒ i)
   Apply to affected area and allow to dry.
   Cover with plain talc.

10. ℞ Castor Oil U.S.P. . . . . . 4.0 cc. (ʒ i)
    Expressed Almond Oil U.S.P. 24.0 cc. (ʒ vi)
    Glycerin. . . . . 10.0 cc. (ʒ iiss)
    Ethyl alcohol 70% . . . q.s. ad 100.0 cc. (ʒ iiiss)
    Apply nightly to scalp.

11. ℞ Hydrophilic Ointment U.S.P.. 72.0 Gm. (ʒ iiss)
    Water. . . . . 48.0 cc. (ʒ xii)
    Apply to skin during interval between
    starch baths.

12. ℞ Boric acid, 10% ointment . . 60.0 Gm. (ʒ ii)
    Apply locally once or twice daily.

13. ℞ Ichthammol N.F. . . . . . 2.0 Gm. (ʒ ss)
    Zinc Oxide Paste N.F. q.s. ad 60.0 Gm. (ʒ ii)
    Apply locally 2 or 3 times daily.

14. ℞ Coal Tar Solution N.F. . . . 6.0 cc. (ʒ iss)
    Zinc oxide . . . . 24.0 Gm. (ʒ vi)
    Starch. . . . . 24.0 Gm. (ʒ vi)
    Glycerin. . . . . 36.0 cc. (ʒ ix)
    Water. . . . . q.s. ad 120.0 cc. (ʒ iv)
    Apply locally 4 times daily.

15. ℞ Crude coal tar . . . . 4.0 cc. (ʒ i)
Zinc oxide . . . . 4.0 Gm. (ʒ i)
Castor Oil U.S.P. . . . . . . 4.0 cc. (ʒ i)
Starch . . . . 30.0 Gm. (ʒ i)
Hydrophilic Ointment U.S.P. 26.0 Gm. (ʒ viss)

> Apply locally twice daily, or after ultra-violet ray therapy.

16. ℞ Crude coal tar . . . . 3.0 cc. (♏ xlv)
Lanolin U.S.P. q.s.
Zinc oxide . . . . 3.0 Gm. (gr. xlv)
White Petrolatum U.S.P.
q.s. ad 60.0 Gm. (ʒ ii)

> Apply once or twice daily.

17. ℞ "Vioform" . . . . 2.0 Gm. (ʒ ss)
White Petrolatum U.S.P.
q.s. ad 60.0 Gm. (ʒ ii)

> Apply to lesions, following a colloid bath.

18. ℞ Burow's solution ointment
Aluminum acetate . . . . 1.5 Gm. (gr. xxiiss)
Lanolin or Hydrophilic Oint-
ment U.S.P. . . . q.s. ad 30.0 Gm. (ʒ i)

> Apply twice daily.

19. ℞ Rose Water Ointment U.S.P. 60.0 cc. (ʒ ii)

> Apply to sensitized areas, as required.

20. ℞ Pilocarpine, 1% ointment . . 120.0 Gm. (ʒ iv)

> Apply to affected area daily.

21. ℞ Rosin . . . . 16.0 Gm. (ʒ iv)
Lanolin U.S.P. . . . . 16.0 Gm. (ʒ iv)
White Petrolatum U.S.P.
q.s. ad 100.0 Gm. (ʒ iiiss)

> Apply nightly to scalp.

22. ℞ Lanolin U.S.P. . . . . 240.0 Gm. (ʒ viii)

> To be rubbed into affected areas twice daily.

23. ℞ Olive oil . . . . 240.0 cc. (ʒ viii)

> To be rubbed into skin twice daily.

24. ℞ Liquid Petrolatum U.S.P.

> To be kept on the affected area continuously until softening has been accomplished.

25. ℞ Talc

> Dust on patient's sheets liberally.

26. ℞ Boric acid

> Dust as a powder on affected areas.

Soap Substitutes and Shampoos

27. ℞ "pHisoderm"
      Use instead of soap.

28. ℞ Dermolate
      Use instead of soap.

29. ℞ "Lowila"
      Use instead of soap.

30. ℞ Medicinal Soft Soap U.S.P. .   64.0 Gm. (ʒ ii)
      Water. . . . .   24.0 cc. (ʒ vi)
      Ethyl alcohol, 70%. . q.s. ad 100.0 cc. (ʒ iiiss)
      Use as a shampoo.

31. ℞ Castile soap shavings . . . .   40.0 Gm. (ʒ x)
      Olive oil . . . .   4.0 cc. (ʒ i)
      Medicinal Soft Soap U.S.P. .   4.0 Gm. (ʒ i)
      Potassium carbonate, 5% solu-
        tion. . . . .   4.0 cc. (ʒ i)
      Ethyl alcohol 50%. . q.s. ad   100.0 cc. (ʒ iiiss)
      Perfume as desired.
      Use as a shampoo.

32. ℞ Coal Tar Solution N.F. . . .   4.0 cc. (ʒ i)
      Medicinal Soft Soap U.S.P. .   32.0 Gm. (ʒ i)
      Ethyl alcohol 50% . . . . .   50.0 cc. (ʒ xiiss)
      Water. . . . . q.s. ad 100.0 cc. (ʒ iiiss)
      Use as a shampoo.

Keratolytics

33. ℞ Salicylic acid. . . . .   6.0 Gm. (ʒ iss)
      Ethyl alcohol 70%. . q.s. ad   120.0 cc. (ʒ iv)
      Paint affected areas several successive days,
      until desquamation. Acne vulgaris: Use
      half strength, each morning.

34. ℞ Salicylic acid, 1% ointment .   60.0 Gm. (ʒ ii)
      Apply to affected area daily.

35. ℞ Salicylic acid, 10% ointment . 60.0 Gm. (ʒ ii)
      Employ until lesions are softened.

36. ℞ Precipitated sulfur . . . . .   5.0 Gm. (gr. lxxv)
      Resorcinol . . . .   2.4 Gm. (gr. xxxvi)
      Prepared calamine . . . . .   9.6 Gm. (ʒ iiss)
      Zinc oxide . . . .   9.6 Gm. (ʒ iiss)
      Glycerin. . . . .   2.4 cc. (♏. xxxvi)
      Bentonite Magma U.S.P. . .   48.0 cc. (ʒ xii)
      Calcium Hydroxide Solution
        U.S.P. . . . . . . q.s. ad   120.0 cc. (ʒ iv)
      Apply twice daily to affected area.   (NOTE!)

The amount of sulfur and resorcinol may be
doubled if necessary. Substitute resorcinol
monoacetate for resorcinol when intended
for patients with blond or white hair.)

37. ℞ Precipitated sulfur . . . . .   6.0 Gm. (℈ iss)
     Resorcinol . . . .   2.0 Gm. (℈ ss)
     Zinc oxide . . . .   16.0 Gm. (℈ iv)
     Starch . . . .   16.0 Gm. (℈ iv)
     White Petrolatum U.S.P. . .   30.0 Gm. (℈ i)
     Lanolin U.S.P. . . . .   30.0 Gm. (℈ i)

     Apply twice daily. (May be used on the
     face. Reduce content of sulfur and resor-
     cinol by half if indicated. Substitute
     resorcinol monoacetate for resorcinol when
     intended for patients with blond or white
     hair.)

38. ℞ Precipitated sulfur . . . . .   24.0 Gm. (℈ vi)
     Lanolin U.S.P. . . . .   20.0 Gm. (℈ v)
     White Petrolatum U.S.P.
                        q.s. ad 60.0 Gm. (℈ ii)

     Apply twice daily. (Particularly useful for
     resistant dermatitis behind the ears.)

39. ℞ "Pragmatar"

     Apply ointment to lesions at night. (NOTE!
     May become irritating to intertriginous or
     genital sites. Wash such areas free of oint-
     ment in the morning, and dust with powder
     containing equal parts talc, boric acid, and
     zinc oxide, to which may be added 2 to 4%
     finely powdered precipitated sulfur.)

40. ℞ Cade Oil U.S.P. . . . . . .   6.0 cc. (℈ iss)
     Precipitated sulfur . . . . .   3.0 Gm. (gr. xlv)
     Salicylic acid . . . .   1.5 Gm. (gr. xxiiss)
     White Petrolatum U.S.P.
                        q.s. ad 30.0 Gm. (℈ i)

     Rub thoroughly into scalp daily for 1
     month, then 3 times weekly for 3 to 6
     months. Shampoo twice weekly.

41. ℞ Resorcinol . . . .   4.0 Gm. (℈ i)
     Salicylic acid . . . .   4.0 Gm. (℈ i)
     Mercury bichloride . . . . .   0.12 Gm. (gr. ii)
     Glycerin . . . .   4.0 cc. (℈ i)
     Ethyl alcohol 70% . . q.s. ad 240.0 cc. (℈ viii)

     Apply to affected areas 1 to 3 times daily
     and shampoo the scalp twice weekly. (For
     patients with blond or white hair substitute
     resorcinol monoacetate for resorcinol. See
     also note following ℞ 42.)

42. ℞ Chloral hydrate . . . . . .   4.0 Gm. (℈ i)
     Salicylic acid . . . .   4.0 Gm. (℈ i)
     Glycerin . . . .   2.0 cc. (℈ ss)

(Continued on next page)

Mercury bichloride . . . . . .   0.2   Gm. (gr. iii)
Alcohol U.S.P.
Water. . . . . . . .āā q.s. ad 240.0   cc.   (℥ viii)

> Use as scalp lotion daily for 1 week, then reapply after a short rest period. (For people with blond or gray hair. NOTE! If hair is dry, replace glycerin of ℞ 41 or 42 with castor oil 1 to 4%.)

43. ℞ Sulfur. . . . .   2.0   Gm. (℥ ss)
     Salicylic acid. . . . .   2.0   Gm. (℥ ss)
     Coal Tar Solution N.F. . . .   8.0   cc.   (℥ ii)
     Hydrophilic Petrolatum U.S.P.
     Lanolin U.S.P. . . āā q.s. ad   60.0   Gm. (℥ ii)

> Apply nightly to scalp for 1 week, then reapply after short rest period. Shampoo every 3 to 5 days. (For mild or moderate seborrhea)

44. ℞ Precipitated sulfur . . . . .   3.0   Gm. (gr. xlv)
     Salicylic acid. . . . .   1.8   Gm. (gr. xxvii)
     Resorcinol . . . .   1.9   Gm. (gr. xxviii)
     Castor Oil U.S.P. . . . . . .   6.0   cc.   (℥ iss)
     Hydrophilic Petrolatum U.S.P.
                  q.s. ad   60.0   Gm. (℥ ii)

> Massage well into scalp once or twice a day for 1 week. Shampoo every 2 or 3 days. (For severe seborrhea)

45. ℞ Mercury bichloride . . . . .   1.0   Gm. (gr. xv)
     Alcohol U.S.P. . . . .   24.0   cc.   (℥ vi)
     Distilled water . . . .   75.0   cc.   (℥ iiss)

> Paint on hyperpigmented areas frequently, until skin peels.

46. ℞ White Lotion N.F.
     Zinc sulfate . . . .   4.0   Gm. (℥ i)
     Sulfurated potash. . . . .   4.0   Gm. (℥ i)
     Distilled water. . . q.s. ad 100.0   cc.   (℥ iiiss)

> Apply at bedtime. Antiseborrheic and comedo shake lotion. If to be used during daytime, neutracolor may be added to match patient's skin color. For very oily skin 20% acetone may be added to white lotion formula. (The sulfur content of this formula may be varied as desired.)

47. ℞ Resorcinol . . . .   4.0   Gm. (℥ i)
     Glycerin. . . . .   16.0   cc.   (℥ iv)
     Ethyl alcohol 70% . . . . .   90.0   cc.   (℥ iii)
     Rose Water U.S.P. . . q.s. ad 120.0   cc.   (℥ iv)

> Apply at night and remove by thorough cleansing the following morning. (For comedo and seborrheic forms of acne.)
> CAUTION! When this preparation may possibly come in contact with blond or white hair, substitute resorcinol monoacetate for resorcinol.

48. ℞ Sulfur and resorcinol lotion
(weak)

Resorcinol	2.0 Gm.	(℥ ss)
Precipitated sulfur	5.0 Gm.	(gr. lxxv)
Zinc oxide	20.0 Gm.	(℥ v)
Talc.	20.0 Gm.	(℥ v)
Glycerin.	10.0 cc.	(℥ iiss)
Distilled water	35.0 cc.	(℥ ix)
Alcohol U.S.P.	35.0 cc.	(℥ ix)

Apply in same manner as ℞ 47. (*See* CAUTION, ℞ 47.)

49. ℞ Sulfur and resorcinol lotion
(strong)

Same as ℞ 48 (weak lotion) except that resorcinol is increased to 4% (5.5 Gm.) and sulfur to 10% (14.0 Gm.). Apply in same manner as ℞ 47.

50. ℞ Sulfurated Lime Solution N.F.
(Vleminckx's Solution)

Calcium oxide	20.0 Gm.	(℥ v)
Sublimed sulfur.	30.0 Gm.	(℥ i)
Water. . . . . . . .q.s. ad	120.0 cc.	(℥ iv)

Dilute 1:10 to 1:20 and apply to face with cotton pledget each night.

51. ℞ Sulfur-resorcinol paste (strong)

Precipitated sulfur	6.0 Gm.	(℥ iss)
Resorcinol	2.0 Gm.	(℥ ss)
Zinc oxide	16.0 Gm.	(℥ iv)
Starch.	16.0 Gm.	(℥ iv)
White Petrolatum U.S.P. . .	20.0 Gm.	(℥ v)
Lanolin U.S.P.	20.0 Gm.	(℥ v)

Rub small amount on face each night. (NOTE! It is often advisable to commence treatment with the sulfur and resorcinol reduced to as low as half the above content. *See* CAUTION, ℞ 47.)

52. ℞ "Quinolor" (ointment)

Rub into affected areas 1 to 3 times daily.

53. ℞ Precipitated sulfur . . . . . 3.0 Gm. (gr. xlv)

Salicylic acid.	3.0 Gm.	(gr. xlv)
Anhydrous Lanolin U.S.P. . .	60.0 Gm.	(℥ ii)
White Petrolatum U.S.P. . .	60.0 Gm.	(℥ ii)

Rub into affected areas each night.

54. ℞ Salicylic acid. . . . . 2.0 Gm. (℥ ss)

Ammoniated mercury	2.0 Gm.	(℥ ss)
Hydrophilic Ointment U.S.P.		
	q.s. ad 100.0 Gm.	(℥ iiiss)

Apply to lesion, being careful to treat only

the involved skin. (Note! The concentration of the above compounds may be increased to as high as 5% salicylic acid and 10% ammoniated mercury.)

55. ℞ Chrysarobin, 0.1 to 5% ointment . . . . 60.0 Gm. (℥ ii)

> Apply daily to lesions on body. (Caution! Never use on face or scalp.)

56. ℞ Anthralin, 0.1 to 1.0% ointment . . . . 60.0 Gm. (℥ ii)

> Apply daily to lesions, starting with 0.1% and gradually increasing to 1%.

57. ℞ Ammoniated mercury, 10 to 20% ointment . . . . . 60.0 Gm. (℥ ii)

> Use locally on scalp. Shampoo every 2 to 3 days.

58. ℞ Precipitated sulfur . . . . .   2.0 Gm. (℥ ss)
     Salicylic acid. . . . .   2.0 Gm. (℥ ss)
     Coal Tar Solution N.F. . . .   8.0 cc. (℥ ii)
     Lanolin U.S.P. . . . .   8.0 Gm. (℥ ii)
     Hydrophilic Petrolatum U.S.P.
                               q.s. ad 60.0 Gm. (℥ ii)

> Use locally on scalp as directed before retiring. Shampoo every 2 to 3 days.

59. ℞ Cade Oil U.S.P. . . . . . .   6.0 cc. (℥ iss)
     Precipitated sulfur . . . . .   3.0 Gm. (gr. xlv)
     Salicylic acid. . . . .   1.5 Gm. (gr. xxiiss)
     Hydrophilic Petrolatum U.S.P.
                               q.s. ad 30.0 Gm. (℥ iv)

> Use locally; shampoo every 2 or 3 days.

60. ℞ Precipitated sulfur . . . . .   1.8 Gm. (gr. xxvii)
     Salicylic acid. . . . .   1.8 Gm. (gr. xxvii)
     Hydrophilic Petrolatum U.S.P.
                               q.s. ad 60.0 Gm. (℥ ii)

> Apply to affected parts after use of ℞ 1.

61. ℞ Pyrogallol . . . .   20.0 Gm. (℥ v)
     White Petrolatum U.S.P.
                               q.s. ad 100.0 Gm. (℥ iiiss)

> Apply only to lesions twice a day for 1 week.

62. ℞ Pyrogallol . . . .   1.5 Gm. (gr. xxiiss)
     Ichthammol N.F. . . . .   1.5 Gm. (gr. xxiiss)
     Zinc Oxide Ointment U.S.P.
                               q.s. ad 30.0 Gm. (℥ i)

> Massage into affected parts morning and night. (May prove to be irritating.)

Caustics and Corrosives

63. ℞ Silver nitrate, 1% solution . . 30.0 cc. (℥ i)

  Paint affected areas once daily.

64. ℞ Silver nitrate, 5% solution . . 15.0 cc. (℥ ss)

  Apply topically to fissures once daily.

65. ℞ Silver nitrate, 10% solution. . 15.0 cc. (℥ ss)

  Apply with cotton swab to sides and base of
  ulcer. Rinse with water after application.

66. ℞ Liquefied Phenol U.S.P.

  Paint affected areas, allow to remain briefly
  until blanching occurs, then wipe off with
  cotton moistened with alcohol.

67. ℞ Nitric acid (fuming)

  Apply to lesions only. (Dispense in glass-
  stoppered bottle.)

68. ℞ Salicylic acid . . . . 36.0 Gm. (℥ ix)
    White Petrolatum U.S.P.
                q.s. ad 60.0 Gm. (℥ ii)

  Apply to lesions only.

69. ℞ Trichloroacetic acid
    Water   q.s. to liquefy

  Apply to lesions with a swab once daily,
  being careful to avoid injury to adjacent
  normal skin.

70. ℞ Podophyllin . . . . 7.5 Gm. (gr. cxii)
    Compound Benzoin Tincture
      U.S.P. . . . . . . q.s. ad 30.0 cc. (℥ i)

  Shake well before using. (For condylomata acuminata)

71. ℞ Podophyllin . . . . 6.0 Gm. (℥ iss)
    Liquid Petrolatum U.S.P.
                q.s. ad 30.0 Gm. (℥ i)

  Shake well before using. (For condylomata acuminata)

72. ℞ Chrysarobin . . . . 0.6 Gm. (gr. x)
    Chloroform . . . . . q.s. ad 30.0 cc. (℥ i)

  Apply once or twice daily.

73. ℞ Salicylic acid, 40% plaster

  Cut to exact size of nail and keep applied
  until nail is softened.

74. ℞ Ammoniacal Silver Nitrate
      Solution N.F. . . . . . . 60.0 cc. (℥ ii)

  Apply weekly, covering area of nail involved
  with the aid of a capillary tube dropper.

75. ℞ Sulfur, 30% ointment
>Apply to individual lesions twice daily.

76. ℞ Salicylic acid . . . .   6.0 Gm. (ʒ iss)
Collodion U.S.P. . . . q.s. ad   30.0 cc. (℥ i)
>Apply nightly until callus becomes soft.

77. ℞ Silver nitrate, fused sticks
>Apply to corn twice a week. (CAUTION!
>Do not touch to fingers or normal skin.)

Antipruritics

78. ℞ Calamine Lotion U.S.P. . . . 180.0 cc. (℥ vi)
>Apply to affected areas as required.

79. ℞ Phenolated Calamine Lotion
>   N.F. . . . . 180.0 cc. (℥ vi)
>Apply to affected areas as required.

80. ℞ Calamine Liniment N.F. . . 120.0 cc. (℥ iv)
>Apply 4 times daily to affected areas.

81. ℞ Procaine hydrochloride . . .   1.0 Gm.
>Sterile Isotonic Sodium Chlo-
>ride Solution for Parenteral
>Use U.S.P. . . . . . . 1,000.0 cc.
>Calculate procaine dosage as 3 mg./Kg. of
>body wt.   Administer I.V. at a rate of 30
>to 50 drops/minute.

82. ℞ Menthol . . . .   0.6 Gm. (gr. x)
Camphor . . . .   1.2 Gm. (gr. xviii)
Calamine Lotion U.S.P. q.s. ad 120.0 cc. (℥ iv)
>Apply to affected areas as needed.

83. ℞ Menthol . . . . 0.15 Gm. (gr. iiss)
Phenol . . . .   0.6 Gm. (gr. x)
Ichthammol N.F. . . . . .   3.0 Gm. (gr. xlv)
Zinc Oxide Ointment U.S.P.
>   q.s. ad   60.0 Gm. (℥ ii)
>Apply in thin layer to areas involved.   Re-
>move later with mineral oil.

84. ℞ Benzocaine . . . .   6.0 Gm. (ʒ iss)
Calamine Lotion U.S.P. q.s. ad 120.0 cc. (℥ iv)
>Apply to affected areas.

85. ℞ Benzocaine . . . .   3.0 Gm. (gr. xlv)
Hydrophylic Ointment U.S.P.
>   q.s. ad   60.0 Gm. (℥ ii)
>Apply to affected areas.

86. ℞ Calcium gluconate, 10% solu-
>tion (ampul)
>10 cc. (1 Gm.) I.V., slowly.

87. ℞ Zinc oxide . . . . 20.0 Gm. (ʒ v)
   Glycerin. . . . . 2.4 cc. (♏ xxxvi)
   Bentonite U.S.P. . . . . . . 48.0 Gm. (ʒ xii)
   Calcium Hydroxide Solution
   U.S.P. . . . . . q.s. ad 180.0 cc. (℥ vi)
   Apply locally as necessary.

88. ℞ Menthol. . . . . 0.8 Gm. (gr. xii)
   Camphor . . . . 0.8 Gm. (gr. xii)
   Zinc oxide . . . . 20.0 Gm. (ʒ v)
   Glycerin. . . . . 2.4 cc. (♏ xxxvi)
   Bentonite U.S.P. . . . . . . 48.0 Gm. (ʒ xii)
   Calcium Hydroxide Solution
   U.S.P. . . . . . q.s. ad 180.0 cc. (℥ vi)
   Apply locally as necessary.

89. ℞ Phenol . . . . 0.15 Gm. (gr. iiss)
   Calomel . . . . 1.0 Gm. (gr. xv)
   Zinc Oxide Ointment U.S.P.
   q.s. ad 30.0 Gm. (℥ i)
   Apply locally as necessary.

90. ℞ Menthol. . . . . 0.15 Gm. (gr. iiss)
   Camphor . . . . 0.15 Gm. (gr. iiss)
   Rose Water Ointment U.S.P.
   q.s. ad 30.0 Gm. (℥ i)
   Apply locally as necessary.

91. ℞ Menthol. . . . . 0.25 Gm. (gr. iv)
   Coal Tar Solution N.F. . . . 10.0 cc. (ʒ iiss)
   Resorcinol . . . . 4.0 Gm. (ʒ i)
   Benzocaine. . . . . 12.0 Gm. (ʒ iii)
   Calamine Liniment N.F.
   q.s. ad 240.0 cc. (℥ viii)
   Apply 3 times daily.

92. ℞ Zinc oxide . . . . 20.0 Gm. (ʒ v)
   Talc. . . . . 20.0 Gm. (ʒ v)
   Glycerin. . . . . 15.0 cc. (℥ ss)
   Water. . . . . q.s. ad 120.0 cc. (℥ iv)
   Apply locally.

93. ℞ Aluminum Acetate Solution
   N.F. (Burow's Solution) . 10.0 cc. (ʒ iiss)
   Lanolin U.S.P. . . . . . . 20.0 Gm. (ʒ v)
   Zinc Oxide Paste N.F.. . . . 30.0 Gm. (℥ i)
   Apply locally 3 times daily.

94. ℞ Zinc oxide . . . . 20.0 Gm. (ʒ v)
   Talc. . . . . 20.0 Gm. (ʒ v)
   Glycerin. . . . . 15.0 cc. (℥ ss)
   Water. . . . . 35.0 cc. (℥ ix)
   Alcohol U.S.P. . . . . . . 35.0 cc. (℥ ix)
   Apply during interval between soaks.

95. ℞ Menthol. . . . .   0.25 Gm. (gr. iv)
       Phenol . . . .   0.75 Gm. (gr. xii)
       Zinc oxide . . . .   20.0 Gm.   (℥ v)
       Talc. . . . .   20.0 Gm.   (℥ v)
       Glycerin. . . . .   15.0 cc.   (℥ ss)
       Water. . . . .   35.0 cc.   (℥ ix)
       Alchohol U.S.P. . . . .   35.0 cc.   (℥ ix)
       Apply to affected areas 2 or 3 times a day.

96. ℞ Liquefied Phenol U.S.P. . . .   1.0 cc.   (♏ xv)
       Boric acid . . . .   4.0 Gm.   (℥ i)
       Glycerin. . . . .   8.0 cc.   (℥ ii)
       Water. . . . . . .q.s. ad   180.0 cc.   (℥ vi)
       Apply locally as necessary.

97. ℞ Menthol. . . . .   0.25 Gm. (gr. iv)
       Phenol . . . .   0.5 Gm.   (gr. viiss)
       Coal Tar Solution N.F. . . . 10.0 cc. (℥ iiss)
       Zinc oxide . . . .   20.0 Gm. (℥ v)
       Talc. . . . .   20.0 Gm. (℥ v)
       Glycerin. . . . .   15.0 cc. (℥ ss)
       Bentonite U.S.P. . . . .   4.0 Gm. (℥ i)
       Water. . . . . . .q.s. ad   100.0 cc. (℥ iiiss)
       Apply locally as necessary.

98. ℞ Menthol. . . . .   0.15 Gm. (gr. iiss)
       Phenol . . . .   0.15 Gm. (gr. iiss)
       Zinc Oxide Paste N.F. .q.s. ad 30.0 Gm. (℥ i)
       Apply locally twice daily and cover with a
       bandage. (Note! Camphor 0.6 Gm. (gr. x)
       may be added for greater antipruritic
       effect.)

99. ℞ Ephedrine sulfate. . . . .   25.0 mg. (gr. ⅜)
       Phenobarbital . . . . . .   15.0 mg. (gr. ¼)
       1 capsule 3 or 4 times a day.

100. ℞ Menthol. . . . .   0.6 Gm. (gr. x)
        Camphor . . . .   2.4 Gm. (gr. xxxvi)
        Prepared calamine . . . .   9.6 Gm. (℥ iiss)
        Zinc oxide . . . .   9.6 Gm. (℥ iiss)
        Glycerin. . . . .   2.4 cc. (♏ xxxvi)
        Bentonite Magma U.S.P. . .   48.0 cc. (℥ xii)
        Calcium Hydroxide Solution
           U.S.P. . . . . . q.s. ad 120.0 cc. (℥ iv)
        Apply as necessary.

101. ℞ Phenol . . . .   1.0 Gm. (gr. xv)
        Prepared calamine . . . .   8.0 Gm. (℥ ii)
        Zinc oxide . . . .   8.0 Gm. (℥ ii)
        Olive oil. . . . .   50.0 cc. (℥ xiiss)
        Calcium Hydroxide Solution
           U.S.P. . . . . . q.s. ad 100.0 cc. (℥ iiiss)
        Apply locally as needed.

102. ℞ Coal Tar Solution N.F. . . . 2.0 cc. (℥ ss)
     Phenol . . . . 2.0 Gm. (℥ ss)
     Glycerin . . . . 8.0 cc. (℥ ii)
     Menthol . . . . 0.6 Gm. (gr. x)
     Alcohol U.S.P. . . . . . . 60.0 cc. (℥ ii)
     Camphor Water U.S.P.
                    q.s. ad 120.0 cc. (℥ iv)
          Apply locally 3 or 4 times daily.

103. ℞ Coal Tar Solution N.F. . . . 10.0 cc. (℥ iiss)
     Zinc oxide . . . . 20.0 Gm. (℥ v)
     Talc . . . . 20.0 Gm. (℥ v)
     Glycerin . . . . 15.0 cc. (℥ ss)
     Bentonite U.S.P. . . . . . . 4.0 Gm. (℥ i)
     Water . . . . q.s. ad 100.0 cc. (℥ iiiss)
          Apply locally 3 or 4 times daily.

Medicated Baths

104. ℞ Starch
          Add 8 to 16 oz. of cornstarch to an average
          tub bath.

105. ℞ Potassium permanganate,
          1:40,000 solution (approx.)
          Prepare by dissolving 1 to 4 tsp. of potas-
          sium permanganate crystals in an adult-size
          bath (40 to 60 gallons). Soak body for 20
          to 30 minutes.

106. ℞ Potassium sulfide
          One handful to an adult-size bath (40 to 60
          gal.). Soak body for 20 to 30 minutes twice
          daily.

107. ℞ Coal Tar Solution N.F. . . . 120.0 cc. (℥ iv)
          Add 1½ ounces (45 cc.) of coal tar solution
          to one-half tub (20 to 30 gallons) of warm
          water or water to which 8 oz. of starch has
          been added.

108. ℞ Oatmeal
          Place 4 to 8 ounces of oatmeal in a cloth
          bag and use the bag as a washcloth.

Protective Applications

109. ℞ Tannic acid . . . . 6.0 Gm. (℥ iss)
     Salol . . . . 2.4 Gm. (gr. xxxvi)
     Glycerin . . . . 12.0 cc. (℥ iii)
     Ethyl Alcohol 70% . . q.s. ad 120.0 cc. (℥ iv)
          Apply liberally to exposed parts before going
          outdoors.

110. ℞ Methyl anthranilate. . . . . . 7.0 Gm. (gr. cv)
     Stearyl alcohol . . . . 25.0 Gm. (ℨ vi)
     White Petrolatum U.S.P. . . 25.0 Gm. (ℨ vi)
     Glycerin . . . . 12.0 cc. (ℨ iii)
     Sodium laurylsulfate . . . . 1.0 Gm. (gr. xv)
     Methyl parahydroxy benzoate 0.025 Gm. (gr. ⅜)
     Distilled water . . . . 38.0 cc. (ℨ iss)

> Apply to all exposed surfaces before going outdoors.

111. ℞ Zinc oxide . . . . 5.0 Gm. (gr. lxxv)
     Talc. . . . . 5.0 Gm. (gr. lxxv)
     Iron oxide . . . . 1.0 Gm. (gr. xv)
     Irish moss . . . . 2.0 Gm. (ℨ ss)
     Benzoin . . . . 2.0 Gm. (ℨ ss)
     Water. . . . . 10.0 cc. (ℨ iiss)
     Alcohol U.S.P. . . . . . . 15.0 cc. (ℨ ss)
     Hydrophylic Ointment U.S.P. 60.0 Gm. (ℨ ii)

> Apply locally as protective ointment.

112. ℞ Compound Benzoin Tincture
     U.S.P. . . . . 15.0 cc. (ℨ ss)

> Paint on lesions and allow to dry. For fissures at angles of mouth, apply and allow to dry while mouth is wide open.

113. ℞ Compound Benzoin Tincture
     U.S.P. . . . . 4.0 cc. (ℨ i)
     Rose Water Ointment U.S.P.
     q.s. ad 30.0 Gm. (ℨ i)

> Apply to crusts and, after crusts are removed, directly to lesions.

Epilators and Depilators

114. ℞ Epilating wax
     Rosin . . . . 50.0 Gm. (ℨ xiiss)
     Beeswax. . . . . 25.0 Gm. (ℨ vi)
     Paraffin . . . . 15.0 Gm. (ℨ ss)
     White Petrolatum U.S.P. . 10.0 Gm. (ℨ iiss)

> Melt and apply to hairy areas over a strip of gauze. Allow to cool, then strip off the gauze.

115. ℞ Liquid depilatory
     Sodium sulfide . . . . . . 10.0 Gm. (ℨ iiss)
     Glycerin. . . . . 10.0 cc. (ℨ iiss)
     Alcohol U.S.P. . . . . . . 5.0 cc. (♏ lxxv)
     Water. . . . . 74.0 cc. (ℨ iiss)
     Perfume. . . . . 1.0 cc. (♏ xv)

> Apply to area and allow to remain for about 10 minutes; then wipe off. Cleanse with water, then apply cold cream or Rose Water Ointment U.S.P.

116. ℞ Paste depilatory

Strontium sulfide	15.0 Gm.	(ℨ ss)
Barium sulfide	15.0 Gm.	(ℨ ss)
Talc	10.0 Gm.	(ℨ iiss)
Starch	20.0 Gm.	(ℨ v)
Glycerin	15.0 Gm.	(ℨ ss)
Water	25.0 cc.	(ℨ vi)

Apply in same manner as ℞ 115.

Masking Agents and Bleaches

117. ℞ Carmine

Carmine	6.0 Gm.	(ℨ iss)
Fluid extract of walnut	12.0 cc.	(ℨ iii)
Aromatic Ammonia Spirit U.S.P.	15.0 cc.	(ℨ ss)
Alcohol U.S.P. q.s. ad	60.0 cc.	(ℨ ii)

Bismarck brown } q.s. to match complexion
Henna

Apply lightly, coat upon coat, until desired color is obtained.

118. ℞ Tragacanth

Tragacanth	2.0 Gm.	(ℨ ss)
Glycerin	10.0 cc.	(ℨ iiss)
Zinc oxide	20.0 Gm.	(ℨ v)
Prepared calamine	20.0 Gm.	(ℨ v)
Distilled water q.s. ad	240.0 cc.	(ℨ viii)

Ichthammol N.F. q.s. to match skin tint

Add 5 to 30 drops as required for cosmetic tinting of patches.

119. ℞ "Covermark" (or similar type of masking agent)

Proper tint to be selected and method of use demonstrated by representative of the manufacturer.

120. ℞ Hair bleach

Hydrogen peroxide, 17% solution	5.0 cc.	(♏ lxxv)
Ammonia Water U.S.P.	4.0 cc.	(ℨ i)
Water	91.0 cc.	(ℨ iii)

Wash area thoroughly with soap and water, and apply bleach for 3 to 5 minutes. Rinse with cool water following application.

121. ℞ Hydrogen peroxide, 17% solution

	6.0 cc.	(ℨ iss)
Anhydrous Lanolin U.S.P.	18.0 Gm.	(ℨ ivss)
White Petrolatum U.S.P. q.s. ad	30.0 Gm.	(ℨ i)

Rub into hyperpigmented borders or patches several times daily. (For bleaching of pigmented areas)

122. ℞ Ammoniated mercury . . . .   6.0   Gm. (ʒ iss)
      Bismuth oxychloride . . . . .   2.0   Gm. (gr. xxx)
      Lemon Oil U.S.P. . . . . . .   0.13 cc.   (ℳ ii)
      Rose Water Ointment U.S.P.
               q.s. ad   30.0   Gm. (ʒ i)

> Rub into hyperpigmented borders or pigmented patches. (Same purpose as ℞ 121)

123. ℞ Ammoniated mercury . . . .   0.75 Gm. (gr. xii)
      Bismuth subnitrate . . . . .   2.0   Gm. (ʒ ss)
      Lanolin U.S.P. . . . .   8.0   Gm. (ʒ ii)
      White Petrolatum U.S.P.
               q.s. ad   15.0   Gm. (ʒ ss)

> Apply at bedtime. (It is advisable to begin with 5% concentration of ammoniated mercury, then increase to 10%. Protect eyes and eyelids by first applying petrolatum.)

Fungicides

124. ℞ "Desenex"   (ointment or powder)

> Apply to affected areas frequently each day.

125. ℞ "Sopronol" (powder or ointment)

> Apply to affected areas once or twice daily.

126. ℞ Castellani's paint:
      Basic fuchsin, saturated
         alcoholic solution . . . .   10.0   cc.   (ʒ iiss)
      Phenol, 5% solution. . . . 100.0   cc.   (ʒ iiiss)
      Filter and add:
      Boric acid . . . .   1.0   Gm. (gr. xv)

      After 2 hours add:
      Acetone . . . .   5.0   cc.   (ℳ lxxv)

      After 2 more hours add:
      Resorcinol . . . .   10.0   Gm. (ʒ iiss)

> Paint affected areas once or twice daily using full strength or half strength. (CAUTION! Sensitization possible. Keep in dark stoppered bottle and discard after 1 month.)

127. ℞ Salicylanilid . . . .   5.0   Gm. (gr. lxxv)
      Hyamine 1622, 25% . . . .   5.0   Gm. (gr. lxxv)
      Hydrophylic Ointment U.S.P.
               q.s. ad 100.0   Gm. (ʒ iiiss)

> Apply ointment 2 or 3 times daily with vigorous rubbing.

128. ℞ "Salundek"

> Apply ointment 2 or 3 times daily with vigorous rubbing.

129. ℞ Zinc undecylenate . . . . . 20.0 Gm. (℥ v)
      Undecylenic acid . . . . . . 5.0 Gm. (gr. lxxv)
      Hydrophylic Ointment U.S.P.
        or Talc. . . . . . . .q.s. ad 100.0 Gm. (℥ iiiss)
         Apply once or twice daily.

130. ℞ "T-CAP"
         Apply ointment once or twice daily.

131. ℞ Precipitated sulfur . . . . . 3.0 Gm. (gr. xlv)
      Salicylic acid. . . . . 3.0 Gm. (gr. xlv)
      White Petrolatum U.S.P. or
      Hydrophilic Ointment
        U.S.P. . . . . . q.s. ad 60.0 Gm. (℥ ii)
         Apply once or twice daily.

132. ℞ Whitfield's Solution
      Benzoic acid . . . . 7.2 Gm. (gr. cviii)
      Salicylic acid . . . . 3.6 Gm. (gr. liv)
      Ethyl alcohol 70% .q.s. ad 120.0 cc. (℥ iv)
         Apply once or twice daily.

133. ℞ Whitfield's Ointment N.F.
      White Petrolatum U.S.P.
      (or Hydrophilic Ointment
        U.S.P.) . . . . āā 30.0 Gm. (℥ i)
         Apply once or twice daily.

134. ℞ Sodium thiosulfate . . . . . 10.0 Gm. (℥ iiss)
      Ethyl alcohol 70%
      Distilled water . . āā q.s. ad 120.0 cc. (℥ iv)
         Apply once or twice daily.

Antimicrobial Agents

135. ℞ Yellow mercuric oxide, 2%
      ointment. . . . . 15.0 Gm. (℥ ss)
         Apply to eyelids 3 times daily.

136. ℞ Ammoniated mercury, 1%
      ointment. . . . . 30.0 Gm. (℥ i)
         Apply 3 times daily after removal of crusts.

137. ℞ Ammoniated mercury, 2.5%
      ointment. . . . . 30.0 Gm. (℥ i)
         Apply 3 times daily after removal of crusts.

138. ℞ Ammoniated mercury, 5%
      ointment. . . . . 60.0 Gm. (℥ ii)
         Rub into affected areas 1 to 3 times daily.

139. ℞ Aureomycin, 3% ointment   .   30.0 Gm. (ℨ i)

   Apply to affected areas once or twice daily.

140. ℞ "Furacin" . . . . 15.0 Gm. (ℨ ss)

   Apply ointment externally twice daily.
   (CAUTION! Sensitization may develop.)

141. ℞ Benzalkonium chloride,
   1:1,000 solution . . . . . 500.0 cc.   (ℨ xvi)

   Apply freely to affected skin or mucous
   membrane and use as mouthwash after each
   meal and at bedtime.

142. ℞ Cetyl Pyridinium Chloride
   N.N.R., 1:3,000 solution. . 240.0 cc.   (ℨ viii)

   Use as mouthwash after each meal and at
   bedtime.

143. ℞ Acriflavine. . . . . 0.1 Gm. (gr. iss)

   Dissolve 1 tablet in 2 quarts (2,000 cc.) of
   water, and use as a wet dressing (1:20,000
   solution).

144. ℞ Gentian violet, 1% solution. . 30.0 cc.   (ℨ i)

   Apply to denuded areas and to base of bullae
   3 times daily.

145. ℞ Medicinal Zinc Peroxide, U.S.P.

   Prepare and apply to wound according to
   the manufacturer's directions contained in
   the package.

146. ℞ Penicillin   (vial)

   30,000 to 50,000 u. I.M. every 3 hours, or
   300,000 u. every 12 hours.

147. ℞ Procaine penicillin   (vial)

   300,000 u. I.M. every 12 to 24 hours.

148. ℞ Penicillin   (vial)

   Add 100,000 u. to 1 Gm. of dehydrated
   plasma or sterile lactose and dust on lesion,
   or dissolve in 100 cc. of sterile water and
   apply as wet dressing. For local infiltration
   of a lesion, a concentration of 50,000 u./cc.
   is recommended. (CAUTION! Sensitization
   may develop.)

149. ℞ Streptomycin   (vial)

   Mix 1 Gm. of streptomycin in 4 Gm. of dehydrated plasma or sterile lactose and dust
   on lesion, or dissolve in 200 cc. of sterile
   water and apply as a wet dressing. (CAU-
   TION! Sensitization may develop.)

150. ℞ Sulfadiazine
    Sulfamerazine
    Sulfathiazole . . . . . . āā   0.17 Gm. (gr. iiss)
    8 tablets initially, then 2 tablets every 4
    hours.

151. ℞ Sulfadiazine . . . .   0.5 Gm. (gr. viiss)
    8 tablets initially, then 2 tablets every 4
    hours.

152. ℞ Sulfadiazine, 5% ointment . .   60.0 Gm. (℥ ii)
    Apply 3 times daily after removal of crusts.
    (CAUTION! Sensitization.)

153. ℞ Bacitracin ointment (500
    u./Gm.) . . . .   30.0 Gm. (℥ i)
    Apply to affected parts 3 or 4 times daily
    after removal of crusts.

154. ℞ Tyrothricin cream (500
    micrograms/Gm.)
    Apply locally twice daily.

155. ℞ Tyrothricin solution (500
    micrograms/cc.)
    Use as wet compress 4 times daily.

Other Chemotherapeutic Agents

156. ℞ "Mapharsen" (ampul)
    20 to 40 mg. I.V. weekly, up to a total of
    1.2 Gm. (Course may be repeated after an
    interval of several months or may be alter-
    nated with a course of bismuth.)

157. ℞ "Myochrysine" (ampul)
    5 mg. I.V. (slowly) weekly; increase by 5
    mg./week until a weekly dose of 25 mg. is
    reached. (A course includes 8 to 12 injec-
    tions.)

158. ℞ Quinine sulfate 60   mg. (gr. i)
    1 capsule 3 times a day before meals for 1
    week; then 2 capsules 3 times a day for 1
    week; then 3 capsules 3 times a day for 1
    week. (CAUTION! Intolerance may de-
    velop.)

159. ℞ Bismuth Subsalicylate Injec-
    tion U.S.P. . . . .   0.2 Gm. (gr. iii)
    0.2 Gm. I.M. (gluteal) weekly for total of
    8 to 10 weeks. (CAUTION! Intolerance
    may develop.)

160. ℞ Sobisminol mass . . . . . .   0.75 Gm. (gr. xii)
    2 capsules 3 times a day before meals.
    (CAUTION! Intolerance may develop.)

161. ℞ Sodium thiosulfate (ampul) .   1.0   Gm. (gr. xv)
> Contents of 1 ampul I.V. daily.

162. ℞ Suramin Sodium U.S.P.
>   (ampul)
> Use a freshly prepared 10% solution for
> I.M. injection every 5 days.   The first dose
> is 0.25 Gm. and each dose thereafter is in-
> creased by 0.25 Gm. until a dose of 1 Gm.
> is reached.   Continue until a total of 6 in-
> jections have been given.

163. ℞ Yellow mercurous iodide. . .   8   mg. (gr. ⅛)
> 1 tablet 3 times daily after meals.   (If well
> tolerated, the dose can be doubled.)

164. ℞ Arsenic trioxide.   4   mg. (gr. 1/15)
> To be taken after meals: 1 capsule 1st day;
> 2 capsules 2nd day; and so on, until 9 to 12
> capsules are taken daily.

165. ℞ Potassium Arsenite Solution
>   U.S.P. (Fowler's Solution). 120.0 cc.   (℥ iv)
> Gradually increase the dose from 1 to 10
> drops 3 times daily.   (Do not give more
> than 30 cc. in a single course.   Course may
> be repeated twice after intervening 2-week
> rest periods.)

166. ℞ BAL (2,3-dimercaptopropanol),
>   10% solution in peanut oil
>   (ampul)
> Give deeply I.M., after carefully cleansing
> skin, as per procedure outlined under toxic
> manifestations of gold compounds (see
> RHEUMATOID ARTHRITIS).

167. ℞ "Stovarsol" (acetarsone). . .   0.25 Gm. (gr. iv)
> 1 tablet by mouth 3 or 4 times a day, after
> meals and on retiring.   (Rest periods of 4
> days after every 4 days of treatment.)

Drying Agents

168. ℞ Camphor . . . .   0.5   Gm. (gr. viiss)
>   Menthol. . . . .   1.0   Gm. (gr. xv)
>   Zinc oxide . . . .   20.0   Gm. (℥ v)
>   Talc. . . . .   20.0   Gm. (℥ v)
>   Glycerin. . . . .   15.0   cc. (℥ ss)
>   Water. . . . .   35.0   cc. (℥ ix)
>   Alcohol U.S.P. . . . . . .   35.0   cc. (℥ ix)
> Apply to affected areas several times daily.

169. ℞ Resorcinol . . . .   2.0   Gm. (℥ ss)
>   Sulfur. . . . .   5.0   Gm. (gr. lxxv)
>   Zinc oxide . . . .   20.0   Gm. (℥ v)

(Cont'd on next page)

Talc.	20.0	Gm.	(℥ v)
Glycerin.	10.0	cc.	(℥ iiss)
Water.	35.0	cc.	(℥ ix)
Alcohol U.S.P.	35.0	cc.	(℥ ix)

Apply to affected areas twice daily.
CAUTION! When this preparation may possibly come in contact with blond or white hair, substitute resorcinol monoacetate for the resorcinol.

170. ℞ Menthol. . . . . 1.0 Gm. (gr. xv)
       Boric acid . . . . 40.0 Gm. (℥ x)
       Talc. . . . . 40.0 Gm. (℥ x)
       Zinc oxide. . . . . q.s. ad 120.0 Gm. (℥ iv)

Dust on affected areas several times daily.

171. ℞ Tannic acid
       Boric acid
       Talc. . . . . . . āā q.s. ad 30.0 Gm. (℥ i)

Use daily as dusting powder.

172. ℞ Boric acid
       Talc
       Zinc oxide. . . . . āā q.s. ad 120.0 Gm. (℥ iv)

Dust on affected areas frequently during the day.

173. ℞ Atropine sulfate . . . . . . 0.6 mg. (gr. 1/100)

1 tablet by mouth every 6 hours.

174. ℞ Tannic acid
       Talc
       Zinc oxide. . . . . āā q.s. ad 120.0 Gm. (℥ iv)

Use locally as dusting powder as needed.

175. ℞ Zinc oxide . . . . 25.0 Gm. (℥ vi)
       Talc. . . . . 25.0 Gm. (℥ vi)
       Glycerin. . . . . 10.0 cc. (℥ iiss)
       Water. . . . . . . q.s. ad 120.0 cc. (℥ iv)

Apply to affected areas frequently as required.

176. ℞ Aluminum chloride, 10 to 25%
       solution . . . . 240.0 cc. (℥ viii)

Apply to affected site on alternate nights.
Do not use soap prior to application.

177. ℞ Formaldehyde, 40% solution . 0.8 cc. (♏ xii)
       Water. . . . . q.s. ad 30.0 cc. (℥ i)

Paint on soles on each of several successive nights.

178. ℞ Formaldehyde, 40% solution

Add 6 ounces (180 cc.) to 2 quarts of water and use as a foot bath for 5 minutes.

179. ℞ Zinc stearate . . . .   30.0 Gm. (ℨ i)
    > Dust freely on affected area. (CAUTION!
    > Keep lid tightly closed when not in use.
    > Keep out of hands of small children.)

180. ℞ Tannic acid, 1% solution
    > Bathe feet for 20 minutes once daily for sev-
    > eral days, as necessary.

181. ℞ Astringent foot powder
    Bentonite (or Kaolin) . . .   8.0 Gm. (ℨ ii)
    Tannic acid . . . .   8.0 Gm. (ℨ ii)
    Boric acid . . . .   8.0 Gm. (ℨ ii)
    Zinc oxide . . . .   15.0 Gm. (ℨ ss)
    Talc . . . . .q.s. ad 180.0 Gm. (ℨ vi)
    > Apply to feet each morning as necessary.

Pediculicides

182. ℞ DDT . . . .   3.0 Gm. (gr. xlv)
    Talc . . . . 60.0 Gm. (ℨ ii)
    > Apply to scalp and hair daily for 2 weeks.
    > Shampoo hair every 5 days.

183. ℞ Benzyl benzoate . . . . . 10.0 Gm. (ℨ iiss)
    Benzocaine . . . .   2.0 Gm. (ℨ ss)
    DDT . . . .   1.0 Gm. (gr. xv)
    Alcohol U.S.P. . . . .q.s. ad 100.0 cc. (ℨ iiiss)
    > Rub into affected areas at night and the next
    > morning. Protect the eyes. Do not wash
    > areas involved for 7 to 10 days. Reapply in
    > 10 days.

184. ℞ "Cuprex"
    > Rub Cuprex thoroughly into scalp and hair
    > with care to avoid eyes and wounds. Allow
    > to remain on head for 15 minutes, then wash
    > hair thoroughly with soap and water.
    > After rinsing, comb hair carefully with a fine
    > comb to remove dead pediculi and ova. Do
    > not apply more than twice in 48 hours. In
    > pediculosis pubis, apply Cuprex to affected
    > areas, then after 15 minutes wash body thor-
    > oughly with soap and water.

185. ℞ Kerosene
    Any vegetable oil (cotton-
    seed, olive oil) . . . . āā 120.0 cc. (ℨ iv)
    > Apply to head in evening, turban the head
    > overnight. In morning, use vinegar rinse
    > (℞ 188) followed by thorough combing.

186. ℞ Acetic Tincture of Larkspur
    N.F. . . . . 180.0 cc. (ℨ vi)
    > Apply in same manner as ℞ 185.

187. ℞ Mercury bichloride . . . . . . 0.24 Gm. (gr. iv)
    Diluted Acetic Acid N.F. . . 8.0 cc. (ℨ ii)
    Ethyl Alcohol 70%. . q.s. ad 120.0 cc. (ℨ iv)

> Apply to areas involved twice a day, being careful to protect the eyes. Follow by combing with fine comb.

188. ℞ White vinegar, undiluted

> Rinse scalp and hair thoroughly, then turban for 2 hours. Follow by combing with fine comb while still wet.

189. ℞ Xylol . . . . 15.0 cc. (ℨ ss)
    White Petrolatum U.S.P.
              q.s. ad 30.0 Gm. (ℨ i)

> Apply to involved areas daily.

190. ℞ Lauryl thiocyanate . . . . . 25.0 Gm. (ℨ vi)
    Liquid Petrolatum, Light,
      U.S.P. . . . . 75.0 cc. (ℨ iiss)

> Apply 2 teaspoons to scalp and allow to remain for 10 days before shampooing. (A single treatment usually suffices.)

Antiscabetics

191. ℞ Sulfur, 2 to 10% ointment . . 240.0 Gm. (ℨ viii)

> Indications for various strengths and details of how to apply may be found in the text (see SCABIES).

192. ℞ Sulfur. . . . . 5.0 Gm. (gr. lxxv)
    Peruvian Balsam U.S.P. . . . 5.0 Gm. (gr. lxxv)
    White Petrolatum U.S.P.
           q.s. ad 240.0 Gm. (ℨ viii)

> Indications for alternative strengths and instructions about method of application may be found in the text (see SCABIES). (The content of sulfur and Peruvian Balsam may be adjusted as required between 2 and 10%.)

193. ℞ Benzyl benzoate, 25% lotion
    Benzyl benzoate . . . . . 30.0 Gm. (ℨ i)
    Distilled water
    Tincture Green
      Soap U.S.P. . .āā q.s. ad 120.0 cc. (ℨ iv)

> Shake thoroughly and apply 2 times as directed.

Analgesics and Sedatives

194. ℞ Acetylsalicylic acid . . . . . 0.3 Gm. (gr. v)

> 1 to 2 tablets every 4 hours as required.

195. ℞ Acetylsalicylic acid . . . . . 0.3 Gm. (gr. v)
    Codeine sulfate. . . . . . . 0.03 Gm. (gr. ss)

> 1 tablet or capsule every 4 hours as required.

196. ℞ Codeine sulfate. . . . . 30 mg. (gr. ss)
    1 tablet every 4 hours as required.

197. ℞ Morphine sulfate
    15 mg. (gr. ¼) subcut., every 4 hours for
    severe pain.

198. ℞ "Demerol Hydrochloride" . . 50 mg.
    1 or 2 tablets every 4 hours for severe pain.

199. ℞ "Demerol Hydrochloride"
    (ampul)
    25 to 100 mg. I.M. every 4 hours for severe
    pain.

200. ℞ Phenobarbital . . . . 0.1 Gm. (gr. iss)
    1 tablet at bedtime.

201. ℞ Phenobarbital sodium
    (ampul)
    0.1 to 0.2 Gm. (gr. iss to iii) subcut.

202. ℞ Paraldehyde . . . . 60.0 cc. (ℨ ii)
    1 to 2 teaspoons at bedtime; repeat in 2
    hours if necessary.

203. ℞ Benzocaine. . . . . 25.0 Gm. (ℨ vi)
    Boric acid . . . . 25.0 Gm. (ℨ vi)
    Talc. . . . . .q.s. ad 500.0 Gm. (ℨ xvi)
    Dust patient's sheets liberally as needed.

204. ℞ Benzocaine. . . . . 5.0 Gm. (gr. lxxv)
    Zinc oxide . . . . 20.0 Gm. (ℨ v)
    Talc. . . . . 20.0 Gm. (ℨ v)
    Glycerin. . . . . 15.0 cc. (ℨ ss)
    Water. . . . . .q.s. ad 120.0 cc. (ℨ iv)
    Apply locally as required.

Vitamins and Hematinics

205. ℞ Vitamin A . . . . 100,000 u.
    1 capsule daily.

206. ℞ Nicotinic acid . . . . 50 mg.
    1 tablet twice a day.

207. ℞ Ascorbic acid . . . . 50 mg.
    2 to 6 tablets daily.

208. ℞ Menadione . . . . 2 mg.
    1 to 3 tablets daily.

209. ℞ Calciferol (Vitamin D₂)
    100,000 to 200,000 I.U. daily, with addition
    of a quart of milk daily to the customary
    diet. This therapy should be terminated in
    4 to 6 months. (CAUTION! Hypervita-
    minosis D may occur.)

210. ℞ Vitamin B complex
> 1 to 3 capsules (of any potent preparation)
> daily.

211. ℞ Liver Injection (Crude) U.S.P.
> (vial)
> 3 cc. I.M., twice weekly, in combination
> with ℞ 212.

212. ℞ Pyridoxine hydrochloride
> (Vit. B$_6$)   (ampul)
> 50 to 200 mg. I.M. twice weekly with ℞ 211.

213. ℞ Hexavitamin Capsules U.S.P.
> 1 to 2 capsules daily.

214. ℞ Ferrous sulfate . . . .   0.3   Gm. (gr. v)
> 2 tablets 3 times daily.

Hormones

215. ℞ Methyl testosterone.   10   mg.
> 6 tablets daily.

216. ℞ Thyroid U.S.P..   60   mg. (gr. i)
> 1 tablet daily.

217. ℞ Adrenal cortex extract   (vial)
> 250 to 500 u. daily subcut.

Miscellaneous

218. ℞ Papaverine hydrochloride
> (ampul)
> 30 mg. (gr. ss) I.V., repeated in 6 hours if
> necessary.

219. ℞ "Neo-Antergan Maleate" . .   50   mg.
> 1 tablet 4 times a day.

220. ℞ Magnesium sulfate
> 1 tablespoon, dissolved in a glass of warm
> water.

221. ℞ Cascara Sagrada Fluid extract
> U.S.P.. . . . .   30.0   cc.   (℥ i)
> ¼ to ½ teaspoon at night.

222. ℞ Collodion . . . .   15.0   cc.   (℥ ss)
> Apply to cracks or fissures once or twice
> daily.

VENEREAL

GONORRHEA

An infectious disease caused by the gonococcus (Neisseria gonorrheae), *involving chiefly the mucous membranes of the genitourinary tract, occasionally of the eye, and with hematogenous spread possible to serous and synovial membranes in other parts of the body.*

Etiology

The causative organism is a gram-negative diplococcus with its flattened concave surfaces in apposition. The organisms never form chains. In the acute stage of the disease the gonococci are chiefly intracellular but they may occur extracellularly in subacute or chronic infections. The gonococcus loses its viability promptly on drying or at temperatures above 106° F. In moist exudates, it may live for many hours, and at refrigerator temperatures, for several days.

Sexual intercourse is the principal mode of transmission, but direct inoculation may result from contact with contaminated hands, instruments, clothing, or bath water, especially in persons extremely susceptible, e.g., female infants and children under puberty. The incubation period varies from 2 to 8 days, but in the majority of patients, there is clinical evidence of infection between the 4th and 5th days after exposure. When the incubation period is reported as longer than 8 days, the infection usually is mild and early symptoms have been overlooked by the patient.

Symptoms and Signs

In the male, an acute anterior urethritis usually is the first manifestation of the disease. Initially, there is a scant serous or milky urethral discharge, accompanied by a varying degree of burning at the meatus, more severe during micturition. The lips of the meatus become red and swollen and, as the disease progresses, the urethral discharge increases, often becomes thick and greenish yellow, and is blood-tinged. Burning and pain are accentuated. The entire anterior urethra soon becomes inflamed and swollen, with edema of the meatus. Chordee (bent painful erection) may occur as a result of submucosal inflammation of the urethra. If therapy is not instituted promptly, phimosis and paraphimosis may result. In boys under puberty the onset and course usually are stormier than in the adult male.

In the adult female, signs of urethritis, vaginitis, cervicitis, and inflammation of Skene's and Bartholin's glands are often associated with the onset of infection. The symptoms may be so slight, however, that a woman may have a gonorrheal infection without realizing it. As a rule, the urinary symptoms of frequency, nocturia, dysuria, and at times terminal hematuria, are more pronounced in patients with first infections. A purulent yellow urethral discharge usually can be seen at the meatus or can be expressed by "milking" the urethra with digital pressure. There generally is some redness and swelling of the lips of the meatus. Also some degree of inflammation of the vulva may be seen, accompanied by itching and burning of this area and increased vaginal discharge. The cervix frequently shows evidence of inflammation. The character of the cervical discharge is variable but in highly active infections it often is tenacious and blood-tinged.

In female infants and children, typical infections are associated with marked redness and edema of the vulva and a profuse purulent vaginal discharge. However, a vaginal discharge, without other signs, should be considered gonococcal until proved otherwise.

Diagnosis

In the male: The diagnosis of gonorrhea is established by the microscopic demonstration of typical gonococci in a gram-stained smear of the urethral discharge (*see* LAB. PROC.). A thin spread of this exudate should be made to avoid confusion with other bacteria which, by superimposition, might give a false impression of being intracellular. A gram-stained smear is not reliable if the spread is too thick. A doubtful or negative result should not be construed as proving the absence of gonococci, but rather should be rechecked on one or two further occasions before it is definitely concluded that the infection is not gonorrhea. When a definite diagnosis cannot be established by the above technic, an attempt to culture the organism should be made (*see* LAB. PROC.). This applies especially to cases refractory to treatment. The two-glass urine test is suggestive of early gonorrhea since in other infections it is seldom that the 1st glass is grossly cloudy and the 2nd glass entirely clear. It is, of course, important that sufficient urine be voided into the 1st glass to thoroughly cleanse the anterior urethra. A cloudiness due to urates will clear on heating and if due to phosphates will clear on addition of acetic acid. If neither test clears the urine, the cloudiness is almost certainly due to pus or blood, or occasionally spermatozoa. A drop of uncentrifuged urine examined microscopically aids in identifying the cause of the cloudiness.

With the more effective methods of treatment of gonorrhea, a differential diagnosis is exceedingly important since other infections as a rule are distinctly less amenable to treatment with the sulfonamides and penicillin. Some of the common conditions in males that must be differentiated from gonococcal infection are: nonspecific urethritis or prostatitis, urethral stricture, chemical and traumatic urethritis, subpreputial lesions, trichomonad infestations, intraurethral chancres and chancroids, and pyuria from sources within the bladder or upper urinary tract. In the most common of these, nonspecific urethritis, the first voiding in the two-glass test seldom is grossly cloudy but contains shreds, while the prostatic exudate usually contains pus. However, prostatic massage is contraindicated until at least 3 consecutive examinations for gonococci have proved negative. Any of the above conditions can exist, unrecognized, concomitant with gonorrhea.

In the adult female: A gram-stained smear should be made of exudates from the urethra and cervix as well as from Bartholin's gland if it is exuding. Skene's gland should be expressed prior to making the urethral smear. Because of the large number of associated bacteria the microscopic examination is not so clear-cut as in the male. Gram-negative bacteria of similar morphology may be confusing and even if not actually intracellular, they may appear at times to be so. Cultures often are needed to establish the diagnosis.

The differential diagnosis in women is concerned with other causes of vaginal and cervical discharges, chief of which are trichomonad and monilial infections and nonspecific endocervicitis of various origins. The acute disturbance of urination is like that of acute cystitis due to other organisms.

In female infants and children, particularly in the older age group, the diagnosis is made chiefly by smear, but here, too, cultures are required frequently, as in the adult female, since there is a rather high incidence of nongonococcal infections. Culture may be taken through the vaginoscope, a method which also serves to rule out foreign bodies and other rare causes of vaginitis. Trichomonad and monilial infections also may occur as in the adult. Chronic infections may result, with intermittent acute exacerbations, although less frequently than before the era of the sulfonamides and penicillin. Gonococcal proctitis may occur, as it may in adults of either sex.

Complications

Local and regional: (1) In the male: The most common local complication is direct extension of the infection into the posterior urethra and the prostatic adnexae. Involvement of the seminal vesicles, Cowper's glands, and the urethral follicles is less frequent. There generally is some inflammation of the trigone, but a true gonococcal cystitis is uncommon and extension to the upper urinary tract extremely rare. Vasitis and epididymitis may occur, but since the advent of penicillin therapy, extension beyond the anterior urethra occurs mostly in neglected infections or those infections in which inadequate therapy is used. Nonspecific urethritis and prostatitis may follow gonococcal infections due to the greater resistance to therapy of the associated mixed flora. Here, suitable follow-up treatment is indicated. Strictures also may result, but usually are of the larger-caliber type. (2) In the female: Local complications include acute Bartholin abscess formation and persistent infection of Skene's glands. Regional complications result from direct extension of the infection up the female generative tract. Chronic gonococcal endocervicitis, endometritis, and salpingitis occur as a result of ascending infection. Sterility frequently results from closure of infected tubes. Gonococcal parametritis, pelvic peritonitis, and proctitis are results of further extension of infection. Pelvic inflammatory disease may so closely simulate appendicitis that differentiation is difficult. Fever, nausea, vomiting, and low abdominal pain are usually encountered. Peritoneal involvement is manifested by abdominal splinting and rebound tenderness. Bimanual or rectal examination frequently will cause pain and tenderness on palpation of the portion of the genital tract involved.

Systemic: Various remote complications may occur in either sex and at any age and are more likely to occur in individuals who had complications with prior infections. Arthritis is the most common result of metastatic infection by the gonococcus in both sexes. More than one joint is most often involved. Iritis or iridocyclitis formerly was not uncommon and often associated with arthritis, as was, occasionally, keratodermia blennorrhagicum. There are many other, rarer, complications, notably gonococcal myositis, serosynovitis, pleuritis, meningitis and endocarditis. There has been a considerable reduction in the incidence of systemic complications since the advent of more effective therapy. Overly aggressive local therapy unquestionably contributed to the high incidence in former years of both local and systemic complications.

Prophylaxis

It is highly important that all possible precautions be taken to prevent accidental infection of female children in homes where adult members are known to be infected. Likewise, in schools or institutions, caution should be used to prevent transmission of the disease. The use of condoms to avoid contamination of the urethra with infected exudates is undoubtedly the most effective measure for preventing the spread of infection by sexual intercourse, although it is not fully reliable. Local chemical prophylaxis in the male has been proved to lower the incidence of infection, but it must be used promptly after exposure and with the following fairly precise technic: The patient should urinate immediately after intercourse, and wash the genitalia with soap and water. Six cc. of a strong silver protein solution (R 17), or 10% mild silver protein solution (R 18), then is injected into the anterior urethra with an aseptic syringe and retained for 5 minutes. The genitalia then are anointed with 30% calomel ointment (R 19), to be left on for 3 hours.

Although not strictly prophylactic, the oral administration of 250,000 u. of penicillin (R 3b) shortly after intercourse has been useful in lowering the incidence of gonorrhea in military personnel, apparently by aborting gonococcal infection in its earliest stages.

Treatment

Penicillin is used almost universally as the preferred treatment of gonorrhea in both sexes. Two methods of administration are commonly employed for the acute uncomplicated gonococcal infection. Both are applicable to ambulatory patients. An aqueous solution of 50,000 u. (R 1a), given at hourly intervals for 4 injections, will cure about 95% of such infections. A single injection of 300,000 u. as procaine penicillin (R 2a), is effective in about 90% of the cases. Occasional treatment-resistant cases may require as much as 500,000 to 1,000,000 u. of penicillin given in doses of 30,000 to 50,000 u. every 3 hours. As an alternative, single daily doses of 300,000 u. of procaine penicillin in oil, supplemented by the administration of 100,000 u. orally in tablet form (R 3a) 12 and 18 hours after the injections, for several days, may be effective. The use of oral administration alone is unwise because of the danger of inadequate therapy inherent in penicillin ingestion without proper supervision. In cooperative patients, however, good results have been reported with the administration of 100,000 u. orally (R 3c) every 3 hours for 1 or 2 days.

Patients sensitive or refractory to penicillin therapy should be given sulfathiazole or sulfadiazine in a dose of 1 Gm. every 6 hours for 5 days (R 7). If an inadequate response is obtained, a second course of therapy is given in a somewhat larger dose of 1 Gm. every 4 hours for 5 days.

Streptomycin is used in patients refractory to both penicillin and the sulfonamides. A single injection of 0.3 Gm. to 0.5 Gm. (R 4), repeated once if necessary, usually is sufficient dosage to result in a cure. Aureomycin and Chloromycetin have been used in the treatment of gonorrhea with reported success.

Since syphilis is frequently acquired along with gonorrhea, the penicillin treatment of gonorrhea may mask an early syphilitic infection. Therefore, serologic tests for syphilis should be done monthly for at least the first 4 months following exposure.

Gonorrheal vulvovaginitis in children is amenable to penicillin therapy. A dose of 200 u./lb. body wt. by I.M. injections every 3 hours for at least 6 to 8 doses usually results in recovery. In resistant cases, estrogen suppositories (℞ 26) will aid in recovery by inducing proliferation of an adult type vaginal epithelium more resistant to gonococci.

Determination of Cure

Following satisfactory response to therapy, a further observation period of at least 21 days is necessary, during which favorable clinical results or laboratory findings can be sought and evaluated as criteria of cure in patients of either sex. In the male, complete absence of urethral discharge and symptoms, repeatedly negative two-glass urine examinations, and repeatedly negative smears and cultures for gonococci (at least 3 in succession) are required as evidence for cure. However, persistence of other bacteria resistant to therapy may result in the continuation of a nongonococcal discharge. If no urethral discharge is present, smears and cultures should be made of prostatic secretion expressed by prostatic massage. For the female, the determination of cure is somewhat more difficult. The criteria of cure are, as in the male, 3 successive negative smears and cultures, obtained during the standard observation period. However, infection may persist in the fallopian tubes after treatment without being detected, and at a later date may cause an acute exacerbation.

SYPHILIS

(Lues venerea, Morbus gallicus, Pox)

A chronic contagious venereal disease capable of involving any organ or tissue of the body, and characterized by florid manifestations, frequent relapses, and years of asymptomatic latency.

Etiology and Incidence

Syphilis is caused by infection with *Treponema pallidum* (*Spirocheta pallida*), a spirochete 4 to 10 μ in length (average 7) with 3 to 26 spirals or windings, and seldom more than 0.25 μ in thickness. The organism grows readily and apparently naturally in human tissues. Certain animals can be experimentally infected, but culture on artificial media or infection of common laboratory animals is unsatisfactory or impossible. The organism is transmitted by direct contact (usually sexual) between human beings, or contact with freshly contaminated material, by transfer of infected blood or plasma, and by passage through the placenta from mother to fetus. Some authorities believe that an active spirochete can penetrate the intact skin; in any case, the many minute abrasions ordinarily present offer the organism fairly easy access to the body.

It is estimated that 500,000 or more new infections occur each year in the U.S.A. More than 4% of draftees examined during World War II were found to be syphilitic, and estimates as high as 10% in some sections of the country have been made. The incidence is highest among persons of promiscuous sexual habits and poor personal hygiene. Syphilis is world-wide in distribution, and was definitely described in Europe as early as the 16th century, where it existed in epidemic form for many years. The original source of the disease remains debatable.

Pathology

Spirochetes from the initial lesion (chancre) are disseminated throughout the body via the blood and lymphatics. They lodge in and about the smaller vessels and, under favorable conditions, proliferate. *T. pallidum* can exist in human tissue without causing a pronounced reaction. Chemotaxis for neutrophiles is absent and, unless secondarily infected, the lesions are not acutely inflammatory. Plasma cells and lymphocytes infiltrate the area inhabited by active organisms, producing characteristic painless induration, and in the skin the "raw ham" or copper coloration. Eventually, immunologic balance is reached, spirochetes disappear or become difficult to find, and the chronic inflammatory mass resorbs with minimal scarring. From this time on, the remaining spirochetes apparently exist without producing any local reaction until such time as trauma, concurrent infection, or debility lowers the local or general body resistance and the ever-present spirochetes again find conditions favorable for resuming activity. At this time, the tissue reaction is more violent, since the products of spirochetal activity have sensitized the cells, and characteristic late lesions result (*see* Tertiary Syphilis). Another basic type of activity produces a slowly progressive fibrosis, with minimal cellular infiltration and much less immunologic response. This probably results from a different strain of *T. pallidum*. Certain tissues exhibit a natural resistance to continued spirochetal activity (lung, liver, kidney, skeletal muscle) and, while capable of being infected, rarely develop lesions, except in congenital syphilis.

Symptoms, Signs, and Diagnosis

Syphilis has been called the "Great Imitator" because its clinical manifestations are legion and can simulate those of almost any other disease. In general, based on strain differences in the causative organism, 2 patterns exist: in the one, skin manifestations predominate in the early stages, and gummatous lesions in the late stages; the other type, with minimal and often missed skin reactions, has a tendency toward latency and a predilection for the nervous and cardiovascular systems, being responsible for late manifestations such as paresis and tabes, or aneurysm and aortic insufficiency.

The protean nature of syphilis necessitates consideration of its several phases or stages, and highly elaborate classifications are available. For the purposes of this MANUAL, however, a simple and workable grouping has been attempted (*see* below). Specific details concerning various forms will be found in the respective parts of this chapter.

ACQUIRED SYPHILIS	CONGENITAL SYPHILIS (Heredosyphilis)
Early (primary and secondary)	Syphilis in the fetus
Latent (early and late)	Early (infantile)
Late	Late (tardive)
Cardiovascular syphilis	
Neurosyphilis	
Syphilis in pregnancy	

The diagnosis in each case is established on combined findings from the history, physical examination and laboratory tests. Many cases (some estimate 30%) provide no history or physical findings directly pathognomonic of syphilis, no primary or secondary lesions or scars, and no constitutional symptoms definitely pointing to syphilis. Many cases of latent or slightly active syphilis are discovered purely by accident during routine serologic tests performed in insurance, pre-employment or other periodic examinations, such as school or military health surveys, or in premarital or prenatal tests.

Vague complaints of fatigue, "run-down feeling," multiple aches and pains, signs of slight anemia, if unexplainable clinically, all warrant a meticulous history. This should include questions designed to uncover previous manifestations of primary or secondary lesions (atypical attacks of so-called smallpox, measles, or transient skin disorders), results of blood tests, cerebrospinal fluid examinations, I.V. or I.M. therapy (arm or hip "shots"), miscarriages, or a history of syphilis in the marital or sex partner and children. Occipital or basilar headaches, recurrent, throbbing, often worse at night or on relaxing, frequently accompany syphilitic invasion of the meninges or arteries of the brain. The differential diagnosis of migraine should include a serologic test for syphilis (preferably of the spinal fluid). Visual and auditory disturbances warrant consideration of syphilis.

Physical examination must be especially complete whenever the possibility of syphilis exists. In addition to the usual search for a chancre scar or other skin manifestation, a careful neurologic check of the cranial nerves and tests of all reflexes must be included. Unexplained findings require diagnosis. Widening of the aorta seen on fluoroscopic examination is a definite clue demanding a search for syphilis.

Laboratory Findings

Laboratory tests are an essential part of any diagnostic routine for syphilis. A mild, transient, hypochromic anemia may accompany early syphilis; or a severe anemia, late syphilis. Urinary findings generally are negative except for an occasional transient albuminuria during the invasive stage; more pronounced abnormalities may be associated with a rare gumma of the kidney. Blood chemistry changes are not pathognomonic and occur only as a result of syphilitic damage to an organ or system.

None of the serologic tests for syphilis is absolutely specific. Nevertheless, although a response may occur in nonsyphilitic conditions, such as vaccinia, exanthems, and other acute infectious diseases, these procedures, properly used and interpreted, are highly reliable. Since variable results may occasionally be obtained on the same specimen in the same laboratory by the same technician, repeated tests perhaps by another laboratory are indicated when findings are doubtful or incompatible. In general, the reactions to blood serologic tests are negative for several days or weeks after appearance of the chancre. In secondary syphilis they are almost invariably positive. In late syphilis (especially neurosyphilis), the blood reaction may be positive or negative; spinal fluid examination may provide the only clue. For latent syphilis, serologic tests give the only indication of infection.

The Wassermann test depends upon a complement fixation reaction. The Kolmer modification is more widely used. Quantitative (titer) determinations are of value in determining prognosis as well as diagnosis. The Kahn and Kline tests depend upon the precipitation of a protein fraction rather than complement fixation and are valuable checks on the Wassermann reaction. The Eagle test depends upon flocculation. The highly sensitive Hinton test is based upon agglutination, becomes positive earlier and remains positive longer, especially in neurosyphilis. A highly specific, yet relatively simple microflocculation test employing cardiolipin antigens has been recently developed.

Spinal fluid examination is essential in the recognition of early neurosyphilis and should be made at some time in every case of syphilis. It should be carried out immediately upon recognition of the disease and regardless of the treatment status, except in primary and secondary syphilis, when it is done usually about 6 months after completion of treatment. Examination of the spinal fluid should include the following procedures, aimed at the positive findings mentioned: immediate cell count (lymphocytic pleocytosis), qualitative globulin (present), quantitative albumin (increased), Wassermann test (positive), and colloidal gold tests (characteristic types of curve).

Darkfield examination is necessary to demonstrate T. *pallidum* in fresh material obtained from chancres and other syphilitic lesions, since ordinary staining methods do not color the organism. Certain characteristics help to identify the spirochete of syphilis: 3 types of movement are typical; leisurely to-and-fro motion, slower rotation on a longitudinal axis, and flexion of angulation (it can achieve "L", "C", or "U" shape like a stiff spring, without losing its coils). No other spirochete shows such a variety of changes in form. The distance between 2 consecutive spirals is shorter than the total width. The spiral forms of fusiform bacilli offer little difficulty in differentiation, but the inexperienced examiner may be confused by *Spirocheta microdentium* or *refringens*. (CAUTION! When obtaining a specimen for darkfield examination, always wear gloves.) Remove crusts or scabs; wash lesion with normal saline and dry with a sponge; abrade sufficiently to provoke the exudation of serum; carefully wipe off the first few drops, especially if blood is present, and wait for clear serum to appear; take sample from the depth of the lesion. If surface chancres are not available or are repeatedly negative, a deep lesion or lymphatic node may be aspirated. The overlying skin is painted with iodine or alcohol, the gland or indurated base of the lesion steadied, and a drop or two of sterile normal saline solution in a small syringe with a 20 gauge needle injected well into the tissues. The needle is manipulated so as to macerate the surrounding tissues, and the injected solution and tissue juice are then aspirated and examined. If laboratory facilities are not at hand, a few drops of the liquid may be aspirated into a capillary tube, the tube's ends sealed with beeswax (not heat), and the specimen sent by the fastest possible means to the nearest laboratory.

When the only evidence of syphilis is the history, a single blood test, whether positive or negative, is not sufficient to establish or rule out the diagnosis. If the infection is more than 6 months old, diagnosis cannot be considered complete without a spinal fluid examination. Unless the physician is familiar with diagnosing neurosyphilis, cardiovascular syphilis, bone syphilis, late congenital syphilis, or latent syphilis, he should enlist the aid of a specialist.

Course and Prognosis

Untreated primary and secondary lesions tend to heal spontaneously after varying periods of time. Tertiary or late lesions may appear early, within the first few months or any time thereafter, but they usually follow a latent period of 5 to 25 years without evidence of disease other than positive spinal fluid or blood serum findings. Spontaneous "cure" (i.e., extension of the latent period till death takes place from other causes) has been estimated to occur in 20 to 30% of all cases. Another 15 to 30% develop one of the forms of late neurosyphilis, and the remainder show cardiovascular manifestations, disfiguring gummatous lesions, or involvement of one or more of the other systems or tissues (e.g., eye, bones, gastro-intestinal tract). Syphilis is not often recorded as the primary cause of death, but because of numerous confirmatory postmortem findings, some pathologists believe that the disease is fundamentally responsible in many more cases than are recognized or reported clinically. Syphilis in pregnancy causes a large proportion of miscarriages and stillbirths. More than 50% of viable infants born of syphilitic mothers show evidence of early or late syphilis, or already are in an unsuspected latent phase which may not produce clinical manifestations for many years (tardive congenital syphilis).

Insufficient treatment of syphilis, or treatment with penicillin for another disease (e.g., gonorrhea) where the dosage is too small for syphilis, may mask or eliminate the primary lesion, lessen or delay secondary manifestations, or produce a state of latency. Secondary relapses and late or recurrent appearance of lesions characteristic of early syphilis, occur with inadequate treatment programs, and occasionally after what are considered adequate courses.

Syphilis, recognized early, treated vigorously and adequately, and followed carefully, can be controlled in close to 100% of cases. Congenital syphilis is preventable even when the mother's disease is recognized as late as the 7th month of gestation.

Prophylaxis

As a **mechanical prophylactic,** the condom is not particularly reliable, since infection may take place through the base of the penis, scrotum, pubes, thighs, fingers, or in kissing.

For **chemical prophylaxis** (also none too reliable), medical supervision is necessary in either sex to ensure efficient application. In the case of the female, a physician must actually administer the proper care. Chemical prophylaxis has its greatest value in the first hour after exposure and may have some value after 8 or 12 hours. Accepted procedures include:

For the male: The patient is required to urinate, after which the genitalia, thighs, and lower abdomen are washed with soap and water (with special attention to folds of frenum and foreskin), and dried thoroughly. Then, 4 cc. of fresh 2% solution of strong protein silver (℞ 17) or 10% of mild (℞ 18) is injected into the urethra. The patient holds the end of the penis firmly to retain the solution for 5 minutes, relaxing his hold from time to time sufficiently to allow a drop or two to escape. At the end of 5 minutes, the solution is permitted to drain out without stripping the penis; for the next 5 minutes the patient rubs 2 to 4 Gm. of 30% calomel ointment (℞ 19) into all parts of the penis, scrotum, thighs, and pubic area, especially the retracted prepuce, frenum, and glans. Finally, the genitalia are wrapped in paper, preferably waxed to protect the clothing, and the patient is instructed not to wash the parts or urinate for 5 hours. Even though correctly applied, this method does not give absolute protection.

For the female: Before applying prophylaxis to the female, have the patient urinate; then place her in the lithotomy position; wash genitalia and adjacent parts with soap and water, with special attention to labial folds and clitoris; douche with 2 quarts sterile water, temperature 100° F., followed by 2 quarts of 1:2,000 mercury bichloride solution; wash external genitalia with the latter solution; sponge the vulva and vagina dry; swab the entire vagina through a speculum with 2% strong (℞ 17), or 10% mild (℞ 18), protein silver solution, reaching every fold (especially the posterior vault and external os); swab the vulva in the same fashion, paying special attention to the openings of Bartholin's glands and Skene's ducts; instill enough of the same solution into the urethra to distend it moderately; have the patient retain the solution by holding her rubber-gloved finger against the meatus for 5 minutes; douche the vagina and vulva with sterile water and sponge dry; apply 30% calomel ointment (℞ 19) to cervix, vagina, vulva, and adjacent parts, rubbing thoroughly into every fold and recess of the skin and mucous membrane for at least 10 minutes. (CAUTION! Never use more than 4 Gm. of the 30% calomel ointment in the vagina.) Cover external parts with wax paper, and instruct the patient not to wash or urinate for 5 hours or more.

The use of penicillin injections, ointment or suppositories has been proposed, but has not yet been approved.

Treatment

In most respects, penicillin has become the drug of choice for specific therapy. Its effect upon late cardiovascular syphilis and late neurosyphilis has not been entirely evaluated.

Some physicians still prefer to treat syphilis with a combined course of heavy metals (arsenicals and bismuth) and penicillin. It is generally recommended, however, that this combination be reserved for cases representing treatment failure by penicillin. (For details, *see* the respective treatment portions of this chapter.)

ACQUIRED SYPHILIS

EARLY SYPHILIS: PRIMARY

The stage of invasion and dissemination of T. pallidum *throughout the body.* This stage begins with the entrance of the spirochete into the body, where it usually produces a primary chancre, and exists up to the time when clinically detectable secondary lesions appear or, if secondary manifestations are delayed, until the activity of the primary focus subsides, and early latent syphilis ensues. Except when the organism is transmitted by I.V. inoculation, a chancre of some degree probably always forms, but may not be observed or suspected. Primary syphilis frequently goes unrecognized.

Etiology and Incidence

Primary syphilis, of which there are an estimated 500,000 cases each year in the U.S.A., is acquired by contact with active *T. pallidum*. Since these organisms do not survive drying or minimal temperature changes, and are very susceptible to soap or mild antiseptics, transmission is only possible from sexual intercourse, kissing, other direct physical contact between human beings, and occasionally from accidental contact with fresh, moist, warm, infectious material on contaminated objects (syphilis innocentum). A spirochetemia of some degree probably is present in all syphilitic individuals; therefore, the disease may be acquired by blood transfusion or transfer. The chancres, the accessible lesions of secondary and early congenital syphilis and the lesions of secondary relapse, are all highly infectious. External lesions of late syphilis are relatively noninfectious even when of a wet or exudative character. Acquired syphilis is not limited to adolescents and adults; chancres in children and newborn infants have been observed (*see* Congenital Syphilis).

Pathology

The lesion of primary syphilis is the chancre, essentially similar pathologically to other syphilitic lesions. It differs in gross appearance, however, because the source of infection was external and the direction of development, in a sense, inward, while later lesions must spring from embolic foci within the tissues. Microscopically, the typical vascular and perivascular infiltration of plasma cells, lymphocytes, and large mononuclear macrophages, with surrounding fibroblastic proliferation and occasional development of multinucleated giant cells, may be observed. The infecting spirochete gains access to the subcuticular lymph space, temporarily pauses to become adapted to its new surroundings, and then begins vigorous proliferation. The local tissue reaction varies with the inherent virulence of the organism, the host's resistance, and probably the number of spirochetes inoculated. Section of the initial lesion often reveals spirochetes in unbelievably large numbers, lying in the lymph spaces adjacent to the arterioles and venules, with minimal evidence of tissue reaction. General dissemination occurs when clumps or masses of spirochetes, floating with the lymph from the original focus to and past regional lymph nodes, get into the general circulation. This spirochetemia, responsible for the widespread seeding of the infectious organisms, may develop more rapidly when a venule is entered directly. Dissemination may take place within the first 24 hours.

Symptoms and Signs

The chancre usually develops at the site of inoculation within

12 to 40 days, but the incubation period may be prolonged to 3 or more months (penicillin given for gonorrhea or other diseases is becoming a common cause of prolonging or masking primary syphilis). The primary lesion tends to be single, but repeated exposures during the incubation period, autoinoculation from contact of opposing body surfaces, or the presence of other skin lesions (e.g., herpes, scabies) during exposure may result in multiple chancres. Extragenital chancres are common and are found most frequently on the thigh, lower abdomen, lip, tongue, buccal mucosa, and pharynx. Other sites include the female breast and, in physicians, dentists, nurses, and laboratory technicians, the fingers. Hidden chancres may develop within the urethra, in the posterior vault of the vagina (most frequent site in the female), or in the cervix.

The characteristic uncomplicated lesion (Hunterian chancre) is 0.5 to 2 cm. in diameter and is eroded rather than ulcerated, with a sharply defined border. The base is indurated and usually clean, with a faint gray or raw-muscle color and a serous exudate. The chancre is relatively painless and, untreated, heals slowly (3 to 8 weeks), leaving a thin atrophic scar. Other forms occur, including the eroded type—small, smooth, superficial, with slight thin induration, and dark red or grayish in color; the indurated papule, a small, flat, dark red papule with slight indurated base and some scaling at the apex; the herpetiform; the "silvery spot"; and a diffuse painless syphilitic edema (chiefly on long prepuces or the vulva).

Painless, discrete, noninflammatory, regional adenopathy occurs in about 75% of cases—bilateral with genital lesions and, as a rule, unilateral with extragenital lesions. Fever, malaise, anorexia, and generalized aches and pains of mild degree are frequently remembered by the patient on questioning, but are rarely severe enough to attract attention during the primary stage.

Diagnosis

The minimal septic manifestations and lack of pain often lead the patient to miss the significance of the solitary lesion and to regard it as a mere pimple, insect bite, or slight abrasion. The relatively indolent nature of the syphilitic lesion, the long period of incubation, the induration, and the lack of response to local medication are typical, and when these characteristics are observed, measures to prove or disprove the presence of syphilis are required.

Tonsillar and pharyngeal involvement is grossly indistinguishable from diphtheritic and other infections. Lesions of granuloma inguinale, tuberculosis, or malignancy may resemble the hard chancre of syphilis, but ordinarily can be readily identified. Mixed chancres (chancroidal and syphilitic) may confuse the diagnosis by a tendency to extensive and multiple ulceration, characterized by early development after exposure (3 to

10 days), a markedly inflammatory aspect with foul discharge, and early painful, often suppurating (chancroidal) involvement of the inguinal nodes. Diagnosis of syphilis in these cases is often delayed until the appearance of secondary eruptions or a positive reaction to serologic tests, but could be made early by careful darkfield examination. Since the clinical characteristics of the primary lesion are not pathognomonic, and although within 2 weeks of infection 35% of cases develop positive serology, identification of *T. pallidum* by the darkfield is necessary to establish the diagnosis. Repeated examinations may be required before the spirochete is found, yet syphilis cannot be ruled out by failure to find the organism.

Treatment

Therapy of early syphilis, primary, and of early syphilis, secondary, has been combined at the end of the sub-chapter on the latter condition (*see* below).

EARLY SYPHILIS: SECONDARY

The stage of the disease when the spirochetes, disseminated through all tissues of the body during the primary invasion, produce lesions: a stage which can be identified clinically when such secondary lesions or their effects are observed. Lesions show a predilection for tissues of ectodermal origin.

Pathology

All secondary lesions reveal the characteristic syphilitic change: low grade localized tissue reaction, cellular infiltration, moderate fibrosis, and eventual healing with little or no scar formation. The sites depend upon both chance and predilection, but the nature of the lesion is determined by the tissue characteristics and the virulence of the spirochete. Strain differences are responsible for variations, from cases with skin lesions predominating to those with extensive nervous or cardiovascular system involvement but with little or no cutaneous reaction.

Symptoms and Signs

The symptoms of secondary syphilis usually are mild and attract the patient's attention in only 25 to 50% of cases. Malaise occurs in about 50%, and persistent headache in about 30%. Numerous other complaints, such as nausea, vomiting, vertigo, tinnitus, deafness, and hoarseness, may sometimes be present. Infrequently, pruritus may occur.

Skin lesions may simulate other dermatologic conditions. Some textbooks give the false impression that lesions are definite and obvious; the description of "raw ham" or "copper color" may be misleading. Skin eruptions are less frequent in white patients than in Negroes, while mucosal lesions (other than condylomas) are more so. There are 5 types of skin lesions: (1) **Macular,** usually seen on shoulders, upper arms, back, and flanks. (2) **Papular,** which may appear in the same areas, but more often on the face, palms, and soles, often in ring formation. These lesions are indurated and seem, on palpation, to be in the skin. (3) **Pustular,** uncommon, but when present usually associated with papular lesions about the nose and forehead of Negro patients. (4) **Follicular,** usually seen in groups on the back and extensor surfaces of the extremities. (5) **Cicatricial**—rare. Combinations of the different types and different stages of development may be seen at the same time, in the same area or on separated areas. Secondary skin lesions tend to be mild and chronic; they appear slowly, persist for several weeks and then gradually fade. Alopecia may occur with a follicular eruption of the scalp and appear as moth-eaten patches. It also may involve the eyebrows. This is a temporary condition and normally regrowth of hair occurs later.

Mucosal and mucocutaneous lesions appear in 50% or more of patients. They usually are painless and last for several weeks, but may disappear in a few days. The following forms are seen: (1) Syphilitic sore throat, a diffuse involvement of the pharynx and tonsils (sometimes extending into the larynx and producing impairment of function, and hoarseness), with marked edema and erosion of the mucous membrane, which becomes covered with a grayish exudate. (2) Mucous patches of the mouth, which are homologues of the macules and papules of the skin, altered by moisture, friction, trauma, and local irritation. They usually are raised, faintly inflammatory, have an eroded surface covered by a delicate grayish membrane, and are comparatively painless unless secondarily infected. (3) Genital mucous membrane lesions, similar to the mouth lesions and more common in women. (4) Condylomata lata, which are elevated lesions beginning as smooth papules that mushroom out over a short, thick base. They are most common in the vulvar region, and in the anal region of both sexes.

Lymphadenopathy usually occurs, and commonly involves the suboccipital, postauricular, inguinal, and submaxillary nodes. The nodes are discrete, visibly enlarged, painless, and nonsuppurative. The extent of involvement has no relation to the severity of the infection. Epitrochlear enlargement, when present bilaterally, suggests the diagnosis.

Osseous lesions are most frequent in the long bones, especially the tibia; they consist of a sharply localized periostitis on the anterior surface of the bone and give rise to a tender palpable mass. Periosteal changes also may occur in the sternum, clavicles, scapulas, and skull. Osteomyelitis may develop. Arthritis, tenosynovitis, and bursitis are rare. Ostealgia and myalgia are common complaints without distinctive features.

Visceral syphilis: Hepatitis occasionally occurs and may precede a florid eruption. A slight painless enlargement of the liver and varying degrees of icterus may be present. Differentiation from arsenical hepatitis and infectious hepatitis is necessary. Splenic enlargement occurs in about ⅓ of the cases. Acute syphilitic nephritis is rare, but evidence of mild early kidney involvement is seen in transient albuminuria, with occasional casts and pus cells.

Eye lesions: Asymptomatic neuroretinitis appears in a small percentage of cases, and disappears rapidly under treatment. Iritis is one of the most common eye complications of secondary syphilis, but is a delayed manifestation seldom appearing before the 6th month. Pain and circumcorneal injection are the first changes.

Ear: Syphilitic auditory neuritis and acute syphilitic labyrinthitis are uncommon manifestations of C.N.S. involvement. The presence of partial deafness or of tinnitus should be a special warning to avoid the Herxheimer reaction (q.v.), since prompt, total, and permanent deafness may result from this reaction in a patient apparently in good condition.

Blood: The average patient seldom develops secondary anemia unless the infection is severe. Women become anemic more often than men.

Cardiovascular: ECG changes may take place before treatment in secondary syphilis, but clinical evidence of cardiovascular involvement is unusual at this stage.

Central nervous system: One-third or more of the cases have spinal fluid changes, but only a few show concomitant clinical signs. The earliest, most conspicuous, and most trustworthy sign of meningeal irritation is an increase in the spinal fluid cell count. There is no necessary correlation between the severity of the syphilitic involvement and the cell count. Counts as high as 300 to 400/cu. mm. may be found in asymptomatic patients. Later, there is an increase in the globulin content of the spinal fluid. The complement fixation reaction is negative at first. Clinical symptoms when present indicate meningeal or meningovascular infection. Acute syphilitic meningitis may be diffuse with headache, nausea, vomiting, and stiff neck, or localized with inflammation at the base of the brain and involvement of the cranial nerves, usually the 6th, 7th, and 8th. Symptoms vary with the nerve affected. The process also may be localized over one convexity of the brain, producing mental confusion and convulsive seizures. Vascular lesions with thrombosis or occlusions may be associated with meningeal involvement with resultant hemiplegia, aphasia, or hemianopsia, depending upon the location. Spinal lesions, ranging from a mild myelitis to complete transverse myelitis, also may occur.

Relapse: Symptoms of the disease may recur after the lesions of secondary syphilis have disappeared with or without treatment, but more commonly after inadequate treatment. There may be a series of recurrent lesions, often insignificant in appearance, sometimes on the skin, but usually on the mucocutaneous tissues of the mouth, anus, and genitalia. These lesions contain large numbers of spirochetes and are infectious. Relapse also may involve the C.N.S. Serologic relapse without signs or symptoms also may occur. Over 90% of the relapses will appear within the first 2 years.

Diagnosis

In 50 to 70% of cases of secondary syphilis, the diagnosis is plainly indicated. The remainder can be diagnosed only through constant suspicion and alertness. Many cases are discovered only by chance, because of failure to recognize the primary lesion, plus the frequent evanescence and mildness of secondary manifestations. Positive diagnosis can be established by laboratory findings only (serologic, darkfield, or both), but the following clinical patterns are highly suggestive and when present indicate the necessity of laboratory studies to prove or disprove the presence of syphilis: (1) macular or papular eruption, sore throat, flat papules on the palms or soles; (2) macular or papular eruption, with erosions of mouth or genital papules; (3) macular or papular eruption with marked general adenopathy; (4) macular or papular eruption with sore throat persisting over a week; (5) rapidly falling hair and severe headache; (6) papular eruption of palms and soles without lesions on scalp, elbows, or knees, and without fissuring or patches of dermatitis elsewhere on the body; (7) grouped follicular lesions with hyperpigmentation; (8) persistent sore throat or aphonia; (9) persistent headache with sore throat and eruption.

Laboratory findings: The serologic test for syphilis will have a positive reaction in about 99% of secondary cases, but previous treatment may render it weakly positive or temporarily negative. False positive serologic findings may occur in the presence of pityriasis rosea, tuberculids, atypical cases of acute exanthems (especially measles and scarlet fever), and vaccinia following vaccination against smallpox. Darkfield examination of superficial scrapings of papular, genital, anal, or lip lesions will reveal *T. pallidum* in a high percentage of cases, and the diagnosis can thus be established, even when a history of chancre or exposure is lacking.

Prognosis

When early syphilis is left untreated, the probable outcome after 5 years will be a division of cases into four groups of approximately 25% each: spontaneous "cure," latent syphilis, gummatous lesions, and cardiovascular or neurosyphilis. With early and adequate treatment, the response will be satisfactory in most cases.

Treatment

General: It is necessary to maintain the patient's nutrition, to reassure him as to prospects of recovery, and to explain the plan of treatment sufficiently to ensure his cooperation. He must be instructed to sleep alone, avoid coitus or kissing, use separate eating and drinking utensils and toilet articles, destroy used surgical dressings, and air all clothing; keep away from barber shops, undergo no dental treatment without warning the dentist of his condition, and temporarily discontinue any such employment as that of domestic, cook, waiter, barber, manicurist, teacher, dentist, nurse, or physician, in which he might infect others.

Specific: Penicillin is considered the drug of choice in the treatment of early syphilis, owing to ease of administration, decreased cost, short period of treatment required, and high percentage of favorable responses. Procaine penicillin (℞ 2b) is given in doses of 600,000 u. a day for a period of 10 days in treatment of the ambulatory patient. For the hospitalized patient, a dosage schedule of 50,000 u. of crystalline penicillin in aqueous solution may be administered every 2 hours, day and night, by I.M. injection for 8 days for a total of 4,800,000 u. (℞ 1b). Treatment failures should be given a 2nd course of penicillin therapy combined with injections of 60 mg. Mapharsen (℞ 11) I.V. twice a week and 200 mg. bismuth subsalicylate (℞ 13) in oil I.M. once a week for a total of 20 injections of Mapharsen and 10 injections of bismuth. For the small percentage of cases that experience an additional treatment failure, the 26-week course of combined arsenical and bismuth therapy is recommended as follows:

Weeks:	*Treatment:*
1 to 5	Mapharsen (℞ 11) twice weekly, bismuth (℞ 13) once a week.
6 to 10	Mapharsen twice weekly
11 to 16	Bismuth once a week
17 to 21	Mapharsen twice weekly
22 to 26	Mapharsen twice weekly, bismuth once a week. (To be completed within a 9-month period or less)

For patients who fail to continue this type of treatment or are lax in keeping their appointments, a change to one of the older, less intensive schedules, is advised: e.g., 18 months of treatment without a rest interval, giving approximately 30 injections of an arsenical and 40 to 60 of bismuth.

Aureomycin has been used in the treatment of early syphilis with encouraging results. Many years of experience will be necessary before its efficacy can be fully established.

Assistance from specialists may be required for advanced or unusual cases and especially for patients showing ocular, neurologic, or cardiovascular complications.

Post-treatment observation consists of a monthly physical examination for evidence of relapse, with special attention to the common sites of mucocutaneous relapse (mouth, anus, genitalia), plus quantitative serologic tests for syphilis for the first year. Thereafter, semiannual examinations, including serologic tests for syphilis will suffice in favorably progressing cases.

Post-treatment spinal fluid examination should be made during the 6th month of follow-up observation, but if clinical or serologic relapse occurs, it should be made immediately, regardless of the treatment status.

Resistance: *T. pallidum* has not been shown to develop resistance to penicillin during treatment of syphilis. The slow response of some large chancres and other early syphilitic lesions should not be regarded as instances of treatment resistance unless darkfield examination reveals the continued presence of living *T. pallidum*. The possibility that the residual lesion is nonsyphilitic must be considered: e.g., the penile ulcer may have a chancroidal component; the generalized eruption may not be a secondary syphiloderm; the condyloma may be acuminate verruca.

Response: The rate of healing of primary and secondary lesions varies, but chancres of small size, mucous patches and macular eruptions are ordinarily healed by the time the penicillin course is completed. Large ulcerated chancres, deeply infiltrated papular eruptions, and large condylomata lata may not heal completely for 1 to 3 weeks after the course.

The serologic test for syphilis does not result in a negative reaction immediately after completion of penicillin treatment. Seronegative primary cases often become seropositive, and seropositive cases often show a higher titer of the quantitative test following penicillin therapy. However, the titer of the serologic test declines gradually in the post-treatment period, the negative phase being attained in a variable period of time. The majority of cases become negative between the 2nd and 4th months, although earlier and later reversals occur. In general, the higher the initial titer of the quantitative serologic test, the longer the reactions will take to become negative. Since lesions almost always heal following penicillin therapy, even in eventually unfavorable cases, the serologic test must be regarded as the most sensitive index of the progress of the case.

Relapse: Relapses occur and the critical period (clinical and serologic) appears to lie between the 3rd and 9th post-treatment months, although relapses have been observed occasionally at earlier or later periods.

Failure: Great care should be exercised in the determination of treatment failure, since patients may experience intercurrent infections, smallpox vaccination, and other conditions which may cause temporary swings of the serologic tests from negative to weakly positive, or elevation of the titer of the quantitative serologic test for syphilis (biologic false positive reactions). All forms of clinical relapse are generally preceded or accompanied by serologic relapse, or by persistently high serologic titers.

1. **Infectious relapse:** Mucous or cutaneous syphilitic lesions, sometimes both, appear, particularly in the oropharynx

and anogenital regions. If darkfield examinations are negative, quantitative serologic tests for syphilis should be repeated, and these will reveal a progressively rising titer in the relapsing case, or a persistently high titer without tendency to decline.

2. Serologic relapse: This is manifested by a rising titer of the quantitative serologic test for syphilis after a previously falling trend, or by a reversal of the reactions from a negative state to a persistently positive state. The rise in titer or the change from negative to positive that often occurs during or soon after completion of penicillin treatment is not considered evidence of serologic relapse. When a serologic relapse is suspected, the patient should be thoroughly and frequently examined for clinical symptoms, since these usually accompany or follow serologic relapse. Serologic relapse should be diagnosed only when a series of consecutive tests show persistently increasing titers over a period of 3 or 4 weeks. If the titer test is not available, a change from a doubtful or negative reaction to a persistently positive reaction will serve for diagnosis.

3. Serum-fastness: This is manifested in primary and secondary syphilis by a failure of the quantitative serologic test to show a marked decline within an arbitrary period of 6 months after completion of therapy. Minor fluctuations in the titer may be observed, and also a drop to a lower sustained level, but there is no consistent gradual and maintained fall to a negative reaction. This condition is uncommon in primary and secondary syphilis, but not in latent syphilis. In latent syphilis, it will not, without clinical evidences of relapse, be considered adequate reason for re-treatment.

4. Neurologic relapse (neurorecurrence) may occur as acute syphilitic meningitis, with headache, dizzy spells, fever, and neck rigidity. In fulminating cases, coma may rapidly supervene. Less commonly, relapse in the nervous system may appear as an isolated cranial nerve palsy or partial paralysis of one or more extremities. Diagnosis should be confirmed by spinal fluid examination.

5. Asymptomatic neurosyphilis may be revealed only by an abnormal spinal fluid.

6. Ocular relapse may occur as iritis (usually unilateral), optic neuritis or neuroretinitis (unilateral or bilateral). The latter conditions may be accompanied by headache with blurring and progressive failure of vision.

7. Osseous relapse is manifested by severe pain, often nocturnal, in the long bones, most often the tibias, or by severe headache when the cranial bones are involved. Local tenderness over the affected bones often is severe. Roentgenograms may assist in the diagnosis.

8. Visceral relapse, including hepatitis with jaundice, or other forms of visceral relapse, has thus far not been reported following penicillin therapy, but is possible.

Reactions: All precautions should be taken to make sure

that the drugs used are fresh and properly prepared, and are
injected properly. Prior to each injection it should be determined if there was any reaction from the previous injection.
If any uncertainty as to reaction exists, it is best to discontinue
treatment, especially with arsenicals, and obtain expert advice
before resuming therapy. Penicillin reactions are rare and
seldom severe. Therefore, treatment with penicillin hardly
ever need be interrupted because of reactions.

1. Arsenical reactions: If there are minor toxic symptoms
(nausea, vomiting, diarrhea, headache), the dose should be reduced by half for the next injection. With severe symptoms,
such as erythema on the 9th day (Milian's syndrome), drug fever,
drug eruption, jaundice, blood dyscrasias (thrombocytopenic
purpura, agranulocytosis, aplastic anemia), neurologic reactions
(hemorrhagic encephalopathy, peripheral neuritis), treatment
should be discontinued immediately. The following prompt,
energetic measures are of value: 5% dextrose solution I.V.;
high vitamin, high carbohydrate, low fat diet; supplementary
vitamins, especially B_1 and B complex; blood transfusions; a
course of penicillin in agranulocytosis and aplastic anemia to
assist in preventing bacterial infections. The prompt use of
BAL (*see* ARSENIC POISONING) (℞ 16) is indicated in the
severest conditions (encephalopathy, jaundice, exfoliative dermatitis, and blood dyscrasias), which may be fatal.

2. Bismuth reactions: This drug must be administered only
by I.M. injection in the upper outer quadrant of the buttock.
Great care should be taken to make certain that it is not injected into a blood vessel. Side effects are exceedingly rare,
except for stomatitis, which can be reduced by oral hygiene.
For rare serious reactions, such as dermatitis, BAL (℞ 16) and
other measures used for arsenical dermatitis are indicated.
When stomatitis occurs, bismuth should be discontinued and
appropriate local treatment instituted (*see* BISMUTH POISON-
ING).

3. Penicillin reactions: The most common is the Herxheimer reaction (therapeutic shock) which also can occur with
any other type of specific therapy. It is usually manifested
by fever during the first 24 hours of treatment, often with
aggravation of the syphilitic lesions and such symptoms as
headache, malaise, chilly sensation, and weakness. This reaction apparently signalizes the effectiveness of treatment, since
it is ascribed to the abrupt, massive destruction of *T. pallidum*
in the lesions and blood stream. It is observed most frequently
in primary and secondary syphilis. N.B.: Ordinarily, the
Herxheimer reaction is not an indication for interruption or
discontinuance of penicillin therapy, except when the reaction
is acutely severe or threatens to be fatal, or in the presence of
laryngitis (evidenced by hoarseness), acute syphilitic auditory
neuritis, or acute syphilitic labyrinthitis (tinnitus, beginning
or partial deafness). A Herxheimer reaction in these tissues

may lead to complete laryngeal obstruction or total and permanent deafness. Moderate Herxheimer reactions usually subside spontaneously within the first 24 to 36 hours despite continued penicillin treatment and require only symptomatic therapy, such as the codeine or aspirin. Specifically toxic or allergic penicillin reactions, less frequently observed, include mild or moderate secondary fever, beginning toward the end of the course and terminating shortly thereafter; urticaria and other minor skin eruptions; generalized pruritus without eruption; herpes labialis and progenitalis; and mild gastrointestinal symptoms. None of these manifestations calls for interruption of treatment, except in the case of moderate to severe urticaria, or of angioneurotic edema involving the upper respiratory tract. Injections of epinephrine or oral administration of an antihistaminic (*see* ALLERGY) usually will control the eruption until penicillin treatment has been completed. At times, substitution of another brand of penicillin obviates these reactions.

LATENT SYPHILIS: EARLY AND LATE

The phase of syphilitic progression that is not recognizable clinically (i.e., "hidden" syphilis) and when the diagnosis can be made only by serologic tests. Latency begins with the healing of early lesions (spontaneously or after treatment insufficient to eliminate the spirochetes from the system) and may extend from a few months to a lifetime.

By considering the first 4 years of an infection of known duration as the over-all period of potential infectiousness, latency may be divided into potentially infectious (early latent) and noninfectious (late latent) stages. In the absence of history of any primary or secondary manifestation, it may be assumed that most syphilis is acquired before the age of 25, and therefore latent syphilis in patients under 26 may be assumed to be early. (This arbitrary division is convenient for public health and treatment purposes.)

Diagnosis

Latent syphilis is usually discovered during routine blood examinations. To establish the diagnosis, positive serologic tests must be confirmed by repetition, preferably with a different standard technic. Spinal fluid findings must be negative. Since this is diagnosis by exclusion, a careful history and a complete painstaking examination, with special attention to the eyes, nervous system, heart, and great vessels, are essential. Investigation of the family and sexual contacts is necessary. A prenatally infected child is presumptive proof of its mother's latent infection even in the presence of her seronegativity. Children of suspected mothers also should be examined. The possibility of false positive reactions must be remembered and excluded by repeating the tests and searching for possible causes for such reactions. In doubtful cases, consultation with a qualified syphilologist is advisable.

Prognosis and Treatment

Latent syphilis, previously untreated, is given the same course of therapy as early syphilis (q.v.). In untreated cases, the prognosis is essentially the same. The patient has a 25 to 30% chance of developing serious lesions, about half of which will be incapacitating. Cardiovascular syphilis is the chief risk, since the danger of neurosyphilis is largely past by the time true latency is reached. With early latent syphilis, since there are no discoverable lesions, no observations as to healing can be made. Under appropriate treatment, the serologic curve may take the same course as in primary or secondary syphilis, especially in very early latent cases. Later, cases often exhibit serologic refractiveness with little or no tendency to decline, and may eventually become serum-fast. Such cases are not ordinarily re-treated after having received an adequate therapeutic course unless there is evidence of clinical progression on follow-up.

LATE SYPHILIS
(Tertiary syphilis)

Any clinical manifestation of syphilitic infection that follows the primary and secondary phases. Late syphilis is characterized by the development of typical tertiary lesions, or the ultimate destruction of a vital center or part of an organ from the continual slow progression of a hidden (latent) syphilitic process. Tertiary syphilis usually appears many years after an infection, but characteristic lesions may occur early in the disease (precocious gumma). The skin and mucous membranes, cardiovascular system, skeletal system, and C.N.S. are most commonly involved, but almost any organ or tissue may be affected. For public health and treatment purposes, syphilis existing 4 years or longer is considered late syphilis.

Etiology and Incidence

T. pallidum, constantly present in all untreated or inadequately treated cases of syphilis, may remain inactive or in a state of immunologic balance with the tissues for many years (*see* Latent Syphilis). Then, when local or general resistance becomes lowered, e.g., through trauma, concurrent infection, or debility, the spirochetes are able to invade a distant injured site or begin activity in their own immediate surroundings. Bursas, and especially the so-called "housemaids' knee" and "weavers' bottom," are frequent sites of syphilitic activity. The tissues, exposed for a considerable period to the chemical by-products of syphilitic infection, have been altered or sensitized and thus react differently from tissues initially invaded.

In another type of syphilitic infection, the spirochetes remain continually active for years, deep within the tissues. There may have been no clinical and frequently no serologic evidence of this activity. Eventually, the organ or tissue is damaged sufficiently to produce detectable effects. Both types of late manifestations may occur in the same patient at the same or at different times.

Lesions may appear a few months after secondary symptoms have subsided or as long as 50 years or more later, but the usual time is 3 to 5 years after the chancre. Prior to modern methods of treatment, about 30% of syphilitic patients developed some form of tertiary syphilis. At present, no valid statistical estimates of late syphilis are possible. Disfiguring, destructive lesions now are uncommon wherever modern care is available, but reliable pathologists have reported, from autopsy findings, an increased incidence of late syphilis, thereby suggesting the true etiology of numerous "idiopathic" disorders.

Pathology

The lesions of late syphilis are similar to those of the other stages, but with modifications suggesting tissue sensitivity. A granulomatous aspect is apparent for the individual tertiary syphilid as well as for the gumma, the difference being basically one of degree. There is increased but more undifferentiated cellular infiltration, with giant cell formation. A tendency is noted toward peripheral extension, plus central fibrosis or necrosis, with tissue destruction and scarring. The gumma, characteristic of late syphilis, is a slowly growing, destructive granulomatous mass of undifferentiated tissue with central softening or necrosis and containing relatively few spirochetes in the inflammatory border. Ulceration occurs when the necrotic center extends to the skin or mucous membrane. Serpiginous or circinate lesions result from extension along a blood vessel, or from peripheral spread along the line of least resistance, with the earlier central portion healing or fibrosing rather than ulcerating.

Continually active, hidden syphilis involves a low grade process of fibrosis with minimal inflammatory change. Detectable manifestations result when the fibrosis reaches a vital part or when sufficient tissue has been destroyed to weaken an important structure (e.g., aortitis, aneurysm).

Symptoms and Signs

Cutaneous: Skin lesions of late syphilis tend to be chronic, localized, asymmetric, infiltrated, and destructive, and to leave scars after healing. The individual lesions often are grouped in arciform or serpiginous configurations. There are 2 principal forms: (1) **Nodular and nodulo-ulcerative syphilids:** These are multiple, flat, circumscribed, roundish, indurated, copper-colored nodules, often beginning as macules. The individual lesions vary in diameter from about 0.5 to 3 cm. They are usually covered with scales or crusts and grouped in a circinate distribution which is characteristic of late syphiloderms in general. The evolution of these lesions is very gradual, and they eventually break down and ulcerate (nodulo-ulcerative) or resolve by absorption and commonly leave characteristic pigmented atrophic scars upon healing. Ulcerated lesions sometimes become secondarily infected. (2) **Gummatous syphilids:** These commonly start as one or more painless subcutaneous tumors, movable on palpation. They slowly enlarge and become attached to the overlying skin. Eventually, ulceration results with the formation of deep "punched-out" craters. These have an arciform contour with rather well defined borders and a gummy-appearing base. Healing is by granulation from the ulcer base and contraction of the edges. Although scarring often results, it usually is less extensive than might be expected from the appearance of the gumma at its height. The most common sites are the extremities, forehead, face, and scalp.

Mucous membranes: Late syphilids may occur on mucous membranes or tongue as nodular, gummatous, or leukoplakial lesions. Early recognition and adequate treatment are important, since they may become highly destructive.

Skeletal system: Frequently, there is a periostitis, gummatous osteitis (simulating osteomyelitis), perichondritis, or arthritis. Usually, no swelling or redness occurs, but myalgia and myositis are present, with pain generally worse at night.

Eye: Late syphilis may cause an iritis (gummatous), chorioretinitis (gummatous infiltration of the choroid), optic atrophy (*see* Tabes Dorsalis), or paralysis of the ocular muscles (*see* Neurosyphilis).

Ear: Involvement is rare, but there may be a gumma of the auricle, or deafness (frequently unilateral).

Respiratory system: Laryngeal involvement usually is in the form of gummatous infiltration of the laryngeal mucosa with tissue destruction; occasionally, laryngeal cartilages are destroyed. Tracheobronchial involvement is rarely encountered, although gummatous lesions of mucosa with some destruction and scarring may occur occasionally. The lung is rarely affected. Gummas, suggesting tumor formation on X-ray, may occur but are rare. A syphilitic stenosing tracheobronchitis has been described.

Gastrointestinal system: The liver is most frequently affected. Multiple gummas of varying size occur and upon resolution leave extensive scarring which gives the picture referred to as hepar lobatum. Gastric syphilis is manifested by single or multiple ulcers (gummas). Linitis plastica (leather-bottle stomach) has occurred. Tertiary lesions of the intestines and rectum are relatively rare. Esophageal involvement is seldom seen, but gummatous lesions have been recorded.

Genitourinary system: Involvement is rare, but gummas

of the kidney, bladder wall, testicle, ovary, tubes, or uterus may occur. Orchitis and epididymitis, chronic and relatively painless, are possible.

Cardiovascular and neurosyphilis: These are described separately (q.v.).

Diagnosis

Lesions of late syphilis may be confused with those of tuberculosis, malignancy, leprosy, psoriasis, and other multiform disorders, specific or nonspecific. Spirochetes are relatively few in number and difficult to demonstrate. Diagnosis must be established by positive serology and not infrequently, when serologic tests for syphilis are negative, by elimination. The indolence, induration, asymmetry, arciform configuration, and sharp margination of the lesions, together with their solitary occurrence and the tendency toward central or one-sided healing, serve as guides in distinguishing tertiary syphilis.

Visceral syphilis is one of the possibilities that should be considered in any adult with vague symptoms (especially cardiovascular, gastrointestinal, or nervous) that do not point to a clear-cut diagnosis. Such complaints may be too readily misdiagnosed as psychogenic or nutritional and treated accordingly, when the actual cause is tertiary syphilis. This possibility should be investigated through repeated serologic tests. The presence of pigmented scars, the history of a cutaneous eruption or an unusually persistent furuncle or carbuncle also should arouse suspicion of late syphilis.

Prognosis

The prognosis varies in accord with the site of involvement. If untreated, skin lesions and gummas in most cases eventually heal, and with less scarring than might be expected. With treatment, healing is greatly accelerated, but tissues destroyed or weakened cannot be restored.

Treatment

It is essential that the treatment of late syphilis be carefully individualized. The Herxheimer reaction (q.v.), which may occur with penicillin therapy, is extremely dangerous in late syphilis and must be guarded against. A combination of carefully planned specific and symptomatic therapy is required. Nutrition of the patient should be maintained and exposure to cold and wet avoided. Analgesics or sedatives (℞ 20, 21, 22) may be given as necessary.

Tertiary mucocutaneous, osseous, and visceral syphilis (except cardiovascular) should be treated by the administration of a total dosage of 6,000,000 u. of crystalline Penicillin (℞1f) given in 120 consecutive I.M. injections of 50,000 u. each at 3-hour intervals, day and night, for 15 days. If this treatment fails, the same schedule of penicillin should be repeated along

46

with Mapharsen and bismuth as outlined under the treatment of early syphilis (q.v.). Consultation with a syphilologist to obtain a suitable plan of treatment usually is advisable.

CARDIOVASCULAR SYPHILIS

A form of syphilis involving invasion of the heart and great vessels.

This is one of the most dangerous manifestations of late syphilis, and many investigators believe its incidence to be as high as 75% for untreated or inadequately treated syphilitic infections. A coexisting neurosyphilis is frequently observed. Invasion of the cardiovascular system probably occurs with the initial spirochetemia, but clinical symptoms do not usually appear for many years. Whether because of strain difference or the nature of the tissue, the organisms lodging in the great vessels of the heart or brain do not ordinarily provoke a significant tissue reaction. The process is one of slow, continued fibrosis, with little or no evidence of the typical pathologic changes of syphilis. Gummatous lesions may occur in the myocardium with symptoms similar to those of myocardial disease from other causes (e.g., bundle branch block).

The most common form of syphilitic cardiovascular disease is aortitis, which may be detected, years before actual symptoms appear, by the tambour quality of the aortic 2nd sound. Fluoroscopic and X-ray examinations often will confirm the presence of aortic dilatation. Aortitis (q.v.) may progress to insufficiency of the aortic valve with the characteristic symptoms and findings of aortic regurgitation: the water-hammer (Corrigan) pulse, the "to-and-fro" aortic murmur (heard best at the 3rd left interspace near the sternum), the femoral "pistol shot" sound and double murmur (Duroziez's sign), cor bovinum, and eventually heart failure. The process may involve the coronary ostia, producing typical angina and other signs of coronary artery disease (q.v.). Aneurysm (q.v.) of the aorta and the larger arteries is another frequent manifestation. This is due to spirochetal invasion of the aortic wall via the vasa vasorum, resulting in destruction of the elastic fibers with weakening and dilatation. Such a process may progress for years without causing symptoms. The first signs (dysphagia, hoarseness, pain, pupillary inequality) often arise from pressure of the aneurysm upon the surrounding mediastinal structures. The Wassermann and flocculation tests show positive reactions in the vast majority of cases, but negative results do not rule out syphilis. Spinal fluid tests should be made in every case to detect possible C.N.S. involvement, and these may give positive reactions when the blood is negative. Cardiac insufficiency or failure (q.v.) is treated in the manner indicated.

Little can be expected of treatment once the aortic ring has been widened, the myocardium fibrosed, the coronary ostia blocked, or the aorta weakened and stretched. In some cases, however, effective therapy may delay the ultimate outcome.

Treatment

Treatment of the syphilitic factor in this form of cardiovascular disease must be highly individualized and carefully undertaken in all cases. Any untoward reaction (therapeutic paradox) is dangerous and may cost the patient's life. Reports on the use of penicillin are encouraging but its use has not yet been completely evaluated for cardiovascular syphilis. If it is employed, a conservative course of potassium iodide (℞ 14) or bismuth (℞ 13) should be given first (for details of treatment, *see* ANEURYSM; AORTITIS). With evidence of a favorable response and absence of reaction, therapy may be increased cautiously. Penicillin, when used, should be given in doses of 50,000 u. I.M. every 3 hours over a period of 15 days or more to a total of at least 6,000,000 u. (℞ 1f). Cardiac insufficiency or failure (q.v.) should be treated as indicated.

NEUROSYPHILIS

Any involvement of the meninges, brain, or spinal cord by T. pallidum, *and which can coexist with other forms of syphilis.* It may be asymptomatic (latent), meningovascular, or parenchymal (i.e., tabes, paresis, taboparesis). The manifestations overlap, yet predominant findings suggest additional distinctions such as syphilitic encephalitis, meningomyelitis, transverse myelitis, neuritis, spastic paraplegia (Erb's), or gummatous involvement.

T. pallidum is undoubtedly distributed as widely in the nervous system as elsewhere in the body within the first hours after infection. Present-day spinal fluid findings suggest a higher incidence of C.N.S. infection than former clinical estimates of 30%. Spirochetal strain variation probably is responsible for the frequency of treacherous periods of asymptomatic latency in neurosyphilis. With few exceptions (notably, acute meningovascular syphilis), the tissue reaction is minimal and unsuspected, and cutaneous manifestations (chancre and secondaries) may be insignificant, transient, or absent. On the other hand, the spinal fluid findings are almost always positive in the early stages, and these constitute the most valuable clues to neurosyphilis.

The several clinical forms of neurosyphilis will be discussed individually.

1. ASYMPTOMATIC NEUROSYPHILIS

A form of neurosyphilis evidenced only by abnormal spinal fluid findings, occurring in a large number of persons who have syphilis, and which may represent the stage of slow but continuous tissue destruction which often precedes symptomatic neurosyphilis. Laboratory spinal fluid examination almost invariably reveals its presence. A diagnosis of C.N.S. syphilis should be made when patients with a history of syphilis have increased protein (globulin fraction) in the spinal fluid and a pleocytosis, without other possible causes (e.g., acute infectious disease, trauma).

Treatment

Early treatment will halt the progress of the disease in most patients. Penicillin (℞ 1d or 1e), 9,600,000 to 20,000,000 u., administered in divided doses over a period of 12 to 24 days, or a combined course of bismuth (℞ 13) and an arsenical (℞ 11) is generally effective (see Early Syphilis, Secondary). Success in treatment is indicated by a gradual decline in the titer of the quantitative Wassermann of both blood and spinal fluid.

2. MENINGOVASCULAR NEUROSYPHILIS

A form of neurosyphilis, localized or general, involving the meninges or the vascular structures of the brain and cord, or both.

Symptoms and Signs

When **meningeal infection** predominates, this form occurring in secondary syphilis or in relapsing early syphilis (neuro-recurrence) may appear as acute syphilitic meningitis (q.v.); in late syphilis, as chronic meningitis. Symptoms vary, from slight recurrent headaches (usually at the base of the skull and becoming worse at night) to typical meningitic signs, such as stiff neck and coma, depending upon the extent and location of the meningeal inflammation. Basilar syphilitic meningitis occasionally is seen in late syphilis, with resulting paralysis of one or more of the cranial nerves. The 3rd nerve is affected in about 30% of cases, producing ptosis, strabismus, and mydriasis. Optic neuritis is frequent and may be followed by atrophy of the optic nerve. Involvement of the 5th nerve causes neuralgic pain and disturbed sensation in the face. Lesions of the 7th nerve may cause facial paralysis, and those of the 8th nerve unilateral deafness.

When **vascular involvement** predominates (vascular syphilis; endarteritis of vessels supplying the C.N.S.), convulsions and paralyses (mono- or hemiplegias) occur. Differentiation from arteriosclerotic or cardiovascular hypertensive disease (q.v.) is relatively simple.

Spinal syphilis may appear between the 3rd and 6th months after initial infection. The meninges, blood vessels, or nerve roots are affected. Ataxic paraplegia may appear early or late. It develops insidiously with a sensation of heaviness, burning, prickling, and formication in the legs. The patient has difficulty in emptying his bladder. He walks with a characteristic gait due to rigidity and spasticity of the legs.

Treatment

Therapy of meningovascular syphilis is governed by the stage at which the condition appears (early or late). Penicillin (℞ 1d or 1e) alone or combined with an arsenical (℞ 11) and bismuth (℞ 13) is indicated (*see* Early Syphilis, Secondary).

3. TABES DORSALIS
(Locomotor ataxia)

A parenchymatous form of neurosyphilis marked by a chronic and usually progressive degeneration of the ascending sensory neurons, and which affects the posterior columns of the spinal cord, posterior nerve roots, and frequently certain cranial nerves, especially the optic nerve. Sensory disturbances, muscular incoordination, and disorders of gait and station result. Preataxic and ataxic stages are described, but these overlap, with no sharp demarcation. Tabes dorsalis develops in 2 to 5% of syphilitic patients, usually in the 4th decade of life. As a rule, it appears 15 to 20 years after the infection, but sometimes earlier or later. Children and young persons with congenital syphilis (q.v.) may be affected (juvenile tabes), most often between the ages of 5 and 20. Occasionally, the disease occurs in infants.

Symptoms and Signs

Onset is insidious and gradual. Lancinating pains may antedate other manifestations by years. These occur in 90% of cases and are the initial symptom in 60%. The pains are sharp, stabbing, and paroxysmal, lasting for 1 or 2 seconds, and darting from place to place (lightning pains). While not usually localized (tending to follow dorsal root areas), they may occur in a definite location (spot pains) such as legs, arms, and groin. The joints are seldom affected, and the pain is not increased by motion. It usually is worse at night. In the head, the pains simulate neuralgia. The overlying skin may be tender. (Alopecia, herpes, petechiae, or erythema may occur, though rarely.) Patients also complain of tingling, numbness, formication, disturbances of temperature sensation, and a girdle-like feeling of constriction about the waist or chest. The pains are apt to occur when general health is impaired or following excesses. Cold, damp weather seems to aggravate them, and the patients seek eagerly to warm themselves. They often burn themselves accidentally because of the disturbances in sensation.

These **disturbances of sensation** are an early sign. The vibration sense is lost or diminished. Hypesthesia and especially hypalgesia may occur over the nipple, ulnar border of the arm, perianal area, outer leg, and sole of foot. The testicles become insensitive to pain and there is delayed sensation on pricking the sole of the foot or the ulnar surface of the arm.

Hyperesthesia often precedes anesthesia or analgesia, although trunk anesthesia to light tactile impressions frequently is one of the earliest signs. Loss of tendon reflexes usually occurs years before the onset of ataxia. The patellar reflex (Westphal's sign) and the ankle jerk are constantly absent in tabes. Initially, the knee jerk and the tendo achilles reflex are diminished and may be elicited only by reinforcement (Jendrassik's maneuver, i.e., having the patient link his fingers tightly together then forcibly pull his hands apart during the test).

Eye findings include the following: Argyll Robertson pupil in about 75% of cases (loss of reaction to light with accommodation retained; sometimes unilateral); pupillary dilation in response to pain is absent or diminished, but paradoxically pupillary reaction may be present; pupils often are contracted, and may be irregular or unequal. Optic atrophy occurs in about 10% of cases and may be the first symptom. Gradual loss of vision terminating in blindness frequently follows. The fundus has a pale or grayish appearance but vessels appear normal. Paralysis (frequently transitory) of one or all of the extrinsic ocular muscles may cause strabismus and diplopia. A single nerve (3rd most frequently, 4th rarely) may be permanently affected. Ptosis, unilateral or bilateral, often is an early ocular sign.

Auditory, olfactory, or facial nerves may be affected. Bladder symptoms—difficulty in starting micturition, emptying the bladder, or retaining urine—may occur early. Incontinence develops later. Satyriasis frequently is an early sexual change, but impotence is a constant late finding. Constipation is common.

Crises may occur at any period. Gastric crises, the most frequent, are characterized by recurrent abdominal distress, vomiting, pallor, sweating, cold extremities, and weak pulse. The paroxysmal pain may be severe, or consist only of nausea and vomiting, with mild distress. Attacks may develop suddenly, persist for hours or days, and then cease abruptly. Laryngeal crises (paroxysmal cough, stertor, dyspnea, with cyanosis and sometimes temporary unconsciousness) occasionally occur. Intestinal (diarrhea), rectal (tenesmus), vesical, clitoridean, renal, and ocular crises also have been observed.

Ataxia is evidenced by muscular incoordination. Inability to move in the dark or to maintain equilibrium with the eyes shut (Romberg's sign) is noticed; walking becomes unsteady, and the characteristic staggering gait appears. The patient walks with legs far apart, head bent forward, eyes fixed on the ground. Leg movements are excessive, the foot being thrown out high and the heel coming down sharply (slapping gait). Sudden stopping or quick turning causes staggering and sometimes a fall. Canes are necessary until all locomotion becomes impossible. Incoordination is manifested also by inability to touch the tip of the nose with the fingers, or to bring together the finger tips of opposing hands with the eyes closed. Muscular power is retained, but muscle tone is diminished (hypotonia). The legs become flexed and flaccid and the joints can be placed in extreme hyperextension or hyperflexion (genu recurvatum). Trophic disturbances, such as perforating painless ulcer on the plantar surface of the big toe or ball of foot and ulceration of the nasal septum or hard palate, may occur (trophic, to be distinguished from gummatous). Charcot's joints (q.v.), most common in knee or ankle, are possible also in the vertebrae or elsewhere. They are characterized by painless swelling, accumulation of fluid, hypermobility, eventual destruction of epiphyses, and weakening of the capsule and ligaments. Deformity and often dislocation result. Spontaneous fracture of bones is uncommon but, when it occurs, should arouse suspicion of a syphilitic etiology.

Laboratory Findings

Cerebrospinal fluid examination usually reveals lymphocytosis, a positive Wassermann reaction, and increase of globulin, and a typical colloidal gold reaction. Blood serologic findings are frequently negative.

Diagnosis

The characteristic history and symptoms should be sufficient to establish the diagnosis of tabes, even when positive serologic findings have not been obtained.

Prognosis

In about 50% of cases the disease becomes stationary; in the remainder, it progresses. The "paralytic" patient confined to bed or chair because of severe ataxia may live 15 to 20 years, but is prone to succumb to intercurrent disorders such as pneumonia, tuberculosis, or pyelonephritis. Tabes itself rarely causes death. Early, vigorous treatment improves the prognosis.

Treatment

Encouragement, full explanation, and maintenance of the patient's morale are vital. Rest in bed for 12 hours per day is essential and all overexertion, fatigue, and mental stress are to be avoided; yet absolute confinement to bed must be delayed as long as possible. Unless there are mental changes, patients should continue with their occupation as long as they are able to perform ordinary duties. However, because of the doubtful prognosis, patients even in the preataxic stage who contemplate marriage should be warned against it. Good nutrition should be maintained, alcohol avoided, and constipation corrected. Occupational therapy, reeducation in use of the extremities, passive and active exercise, and hydrotherapy are of definite value. Many bedridden patients have been taught to walk and work again by these methods. Rest, protection from wet and cold, and the application of heat or counter-irritants are helpful in alleviating pain. Sedatives and analgesics (℞ 20, 21, 22) may be required. Morphine is best avoided because of the increased likelihood of addiction in these patients, but may be necessary on occasion. For gastric crises, withholding food, application of counterirritants (e.g., mustard plaster) over the epigastrium, gastric lavage, and administration of cerium oxalate (℞ 24) may be helpful. Extreme measures such as spinal puncture and X-radiation have been used successfully. Prolonged administration of the nitrites (℞ 25) in tabetic patients with hypertension (with caution in cases of aortic insufficiency) has been recommended for relieving pain and diminishing the frequency of crises. Patients with bladder symptoms should be trained to urinate frequently in order to avoid overdistention. Routine catheterization should be delayed as long as possible. For incontinence, belladonna (℞ 27) may be beneficial, and for urinary discomfort, agents such as Pyridium (℞ 15) are helpful. A snugly-fitting binder may relieve girdle pains. Perforating ulcers require surgical dressings. Decubitus ulcers (q.v.) must be scrupulously guarded against. Good nursing care is lifesaving for the bedridden.

Treatment of syphilis must be on an individualized basis. Penicillin (℞ 1e), 9,600,000 to 20,000,000 u. administered over a period of 12 to 24 days, has been recommended. Fever therapy by means of hypertherm, typhoid-paratyphoid I.V. injections, or malaria (*see* General Paresis), although not so effective as in paresis, should be tried (unless specifically contraindicated), if other measures fail to halt progression.

4. GENERAL PARESIS
(Dementia paralytica)

Parenchymatous neurosyphilis of the cerebral cortex and overlying meninges. The inflammatory process, meningoencephalitis, may appear on any brain area, but tends to localize at the basal and frontal aspects. In adults, it results from untreated or inadequately treated syphilitic infection, develops in 5 to 20 years (average 12), and is seen most frequently in males between the ages of 35 and 55. A juvenile form (juvenile paresis) may occur in congenital syphilis (q.v.).

Symptoms and Signs

Onset usually is insidious, but may be sudden or explosive following trauma to the head, prolonged mental or physical stress, or an alcoholic debauch. Manifestations are protean, often changing from month to month, or even day to day. Several types, distinct or overlapping, may develop: depressive, with hypochondriasis; manic, with megalomania, exalted and euphoric; agitative, with motor activity; and schizophrenic, perhaps with delusions of persecution. When spinal cord and nerve root involvement develops concurrently with paresis, the symptoms of tabes dorsalis are added, and the complex is known as taboparesis.

Frequently, the initial mental symptoms consist of insidious changes in personality, such as deterioration in table manners and in cleanliness of clothing and body. Irritability, inattentiveness, apathy, slight memory loss, and impoverishment of ideas, may indicate intellectual impairment. Contradictory behavior and foolish monetary speculations often bespeak an accompanying impairment of judgment. Previously conscientious and morally upright, the patient may now indulge in indecencies of speech and action and in alcoholic and sexual debauches. Delusions concerning his property, position, family, or personal attainments may appear. With boastfulness and grandiosity he may believe himself a potentate or deity, the possessor of priceless jewelry, beautiful women, and fabulous wealth. Such a patient's mood usually is one of euphoria. In another patient, nihilistic ideas which accompany severe depression may be paramount, and consist of ideas that his body is changed, or that he has no heart, lungs, or stomach. Because of these beliefs, the patient may refuse to eat.

At the onset, either the physical signs or mental symptoms of general paresis may predominate; generally, it is the former which first calls attention to the disease. If dysarthria develops, it usually is early. The lips are tremulous, and the speech may be slow and drawling. In particular, the consonants "l" and "r" are difficult for the paretic to enunciate. Hence, he cannot readily articulate such test phrases as "truly rural," "thirty-third artillery brigade," "around the rough and rugged rocks the ragged rascal ran," and "Methodist Episcopal." The handwriting may undergo significant changes: the lines waver, the letters are unequal in size, and both letters and syllables may be elided or repeated. Eye changes occur early and often are one of the first neurologic signs of paresis noted. Argyll Robertson pupils (loss of reaction to light with preservation of that to accommodation) usually occur. In other patients, the reaction both to light and accommodation may be sluggish or absent. Ordinarily, the consensual light reflex is lost early. Pupillary irregularity and inequality are frequent. Mydriasis, miosis, ptosis, or transient diplopia may develop. Although optic atrophy is frequent in paresis, it occurs less often than in tabes. The paretic's facies may become relatively immobile and present a vacuous expression, and intention tremors of the hands, lips, tongue, and facial muscles generally are present. Skeletal muscle disturbances occur, and consist of transient but recurrent weakness or rigidity in the arms, legs, or back. Disturbances of the deep tendon reflexes are the rule. More frequently these are exaggerated, but if a tabetic process coexists, the knee jerks are absent. Epileptiform convulsions are frequent and may be fatal. Apoplectiform episodes may result in monoplegia or hemiplegia, either permanent or transient. Attacks of focal (jacksonian) epilepsy or petit mal may occur. Sharp pains, itching or numbness, or changes in cutaneous sensibility vary with the predominant location of the lesions in the brain. Vesical and rectal symptoms may appear. The paretic's gait usually is impaired.

Diagnosis

Early diagnosis is relatively easy once suspicion is directed at the presence of this disease. Personality changes, neurasthenia-like symptoms, or the development of migrainous headaches or of convulsions in an individual past 40 should alert the physician. In such situations, serologic tests on the blood and spinal fluid are obligatory. Confusion with a neurotic or other psychotic reaction, cerebral neoplasm, arteriosclerotic degenerative disease, epilepsy, or encephalitis is possible, but from careful analysis of history, physical findings, and laboratory data, early differentiation is possible in most cases. Trauma to the head not infrequently precipitates the symptoms. General paresis, as well as tabes dorsalis and other forms of neurosyphilis, must always be kept high on the list when a diagnosis of C.N.S. disease is attempted.

Laboratory Findings

Tests for syphilis usually give positive reactions in paresis. The spinal fluid shows a slightly increased cell count (average 25 to 50 cells, 98 to 100% lymphocytes), increased protein, positive Wassermann reaction in most cases, and a positive colloidal gold reaction (95 to 100% of cases), generally with a typical paretic curve (high in the first tubes, low in the last—e.g., 5555542100). Spinal fluid findings may be positive during a long, clinically asymptomatic period (paresis sine paresi). The blood Wassermann reaction is positive in 95 to 100% of cases.

Prognosis

The course generally is one of slow progression with fatal termination in a few years from exhaustion or intercurrent infection, but it may be prolonged for 10 to 15 years. Infrequently, remissions may occur to the extent of the patient being able to resume his occupation. Early, adequate treatment ordinarily halts the progression (any existing cerebral changes being irreversible). It must be kept in mind that the rapidly developing type with subtle psychic changes, not diagnosed early, may within a few weeks of onset destroy the patient's previous good reputation and financial standing.

Treatment

The aim is to halt the progress of the disease. Penicillin alone (℞ 1e) or combined with fever therapy (see below), is useful. An arsenical (℞ 11) and bismuth (℞ 13) may occasionally be of value (*see* Early Syphilis, Secondary). Symptomatic treatment is required for delirium and apoplectiform and epileptiform attacks. Phenobarbital (℞ 22) is useful against convulsions. Opium (℞ 23) still is valuable in the melancholic and hypochondriacal states. Tube or parenteral feeding may be necessary when a patient refuses to eat. Institutional care is indicated in order to protect the patient and his associates against acts of indiscretion and violence. In any event, the patient's affairs should be placed in responsible hands as soon as the diagnosis is made. An attitude of friendliness and optimism will aid in securing cooperation and is an important adjunct to successful treatment.

Fever therapy: Fever may be induced by means of malaria or the hypertherm. Malaria is transmitted to the patient by injecting I.V. or I.M. 2 to 5 cc. of blood from a patient known to have malaria (tertian in the older method, quartan in the modern). After 10 to 15 chills (40 to 50 hours of fever) antimalarial therapy (q.v.) is instituted. If electrically induced, fever must be administered by a physician or technician experienced in the procedure; the patient is treated with a fever of 104° F. or above for 40 to 50 hours. Fever is very occasionally induced by means of typhoid vaccine, rat-bite fever, or colloidal sulfur. Any type of fever therapy is contraindicated in the presence of debility, severe anemia, or advanced cardiovascular disease.

SYPHILIS IN PREGNANCY

Syphilis in pregnancy, when untreated, causes 8 times as many stillbirths as occur in all other pregnancies. The mortality rate for infants born of untreated syphilitic mothers is excessively high, and 50% of the survivors have syphilis. Clinical evidence of early syphilis often is masked by pregnancy, but positive serologic findings are present and valid.

Routine serologic tests, performed during the first half of pregnancy, are the only reliable means of detecting the disease and, since syphilis can be acquired during pregnancy, repeat tests during the 7th month also are indicated. In general, the more recent the mother's infection, the greater the chance of fetal infection, and Kassowitz's "law" (abortions occurring later in successive pregnancies; a stillbirth or two; finally viable infants, syphilitic or healthy) must be kept in mind.

Treatment

Syphilis in the fetus can be prevented in most cases by its early recognition in the mother, followed by adequate treatment of the mother. Penicillin is preferred to the metals for treating syphilis in pregnancy, regardless of the stage of the disease. Penicillin G in aqueous solution (℞ 1b), 50,000 u. I.M. every 2 hours for 8 days (total 4,800,000 u.), is advised

for those in whom the disease is discovered after the 5th
month of pregnancy. Procaine penicillin (℞ 2b), 600,000 u.
I.M. every day for 10 days, may be used for other cases. If
seronegativity is not obtained or the titer of the quantitative
test falls too slowly, a repeat course may be given in the 3rd
trimester.

CONGENITAL SYPHILIS
(Prenatal syphilis, Heredosyphilis, Syphilis innata)

Syphilis acquired prior to passage through the birth canal.
Manifestations are altered by the duration of the infection in
utero, the efficacy of maternal or fetal defense mechanisms, and
the characteristics of the spirochetal strain. Any of the following conditions may result: (1) **Syphilis of the fetus,** producing early or late abortion, stillbirth, or birth of a live infant with
late syphilis already manifest. (2) **Early, or infantile, syphilis;** a live infant with evidence of infection delayed several
days or weeks. (3) **Late, or tardive, congenital syphilis,**
wherein the infant appears normal and frequently is seronegative, the infection remaining latent for months or years.

Syphilis incurred during the birth process or soon thereafter
is acquired syphilis, and quite frequently a primary lesion
(chancre) occurs, but the effects may be otherwise indistinguishable from early (infantile) or late (tardive) congenital syphilis.

Etiology

It has been possible to demonstrate *T. pallidum* in spermatozoa, but it is generally believed that the infection is transmitted
from mother to fetus through the placenta (diaplacental passage). Syphilis, although an important cause of miscarriages
and stillbirths, seldom if ever produces abortion before the 4th
month of gestation. Spirochetes may be found in the syphilitic
mother's milk and in lesions along the birth canal or on the
skin, but infection from these is actually acquired syphilis
(q.v.).

Pathology

Evidence of syphilis may at times be demonstrated in any
of the products of conception. An unusually large placenta,
more than ¼ the body weight of the fetus, is common. An infected fetus may be literally overwhelmed with *T. pallidum,*
including organs and tissues not ordinarily involved in adults
(e.g., liver, lung, kidney, myocardium, and skeletal muscle).
Although cord Wassermanns and placental examinations may
give negative results, spirochetes are readily demonstrable in
specimens of liver or other tissues. Microscopic examination
reveals characteristic syphilitic changes, perivascular and vascular infiltration with plasma cells and lymphocytes, and fibrotic
processes. Vesicular, bullous, or pemphigoid lesions are seen

more frequently in congenital syphilis than in the acquired adult form.

Clinical Manifestations

1. **Syphilis in the fetus** often is characterized by skin lesions, especially bullae containing serous or hemorrhagic fluid. A macerated fetus is suggestive. Syphilitic pneumonia or pneumonia alba frequently is found on autopsy.

2. **Early congenital** (prenatal) **syphilis** may not be apparent in the live infected infant until several weeks after birth. "Snuffles," the aphonic "cry," skin and mucous membrane lesions, increasing irritability, fever, failure to gain weight, and a senile facies ("little old man") are the common presenting symptoms. Enlarged spleen, generalized lymphadenopathy, hepatomegaly, and bone lesions may be observed. Cutaneous lesions resemble those of secondary syphilis. Maculopapular eruptions are most common, but annular lesions often are seen in affected Negro infants. They may be generalized, or localized in the circumoral and anogenital regions, palms, soles, or extremities. The pemphigoid syphilid, with vesicles on palms and soles, may be seen. Mucous membrane lesions in the form of mucous patches, condylomas, fissuring of the lips, and erosions at the angles of the mouth are characteristic. Bone involvement usually takes the form of osteochondritis, chondroepiphysitis, or periostitis. Parrot's pseudoparalysis (limitation due to bone involvement) may be the first clinical indication of osseous syphilis, but X-ray examination of the long bones will provide the earliest evidence. Early C.N.S. involvement, such as a chronic meningitis, and hydrocephalus, may be a resultant complication. The majority of cases, however, are latent and evidenced only by positive spinal fluid findings. Other manifestations of neurosyphilis include paralysis, epileptiform seizures, optic atrophy, and eventual mental retardation from meningovascular involvement.

3. **Late congenital syphilis** (tardive) may not become apparent for years (occasionally, 25 to 30), but most patients exhibit symptoms during childhood or adolescence. A very small percentage may show no more than positive serology throughout life. Interstitial keratitis, the most common lesion of late congenital syphilis, usually develops between the ages of 5 and 16. This is an inflammation of all the layers of the cornea with vascular infiltration and exudation. Beginning in one eye it eventually becomes bilateral and, unless arrested, results in clouding of the cornea and visual impairment. Neurosyphilis is the next most frequent manifestation of late congenital syphilis. Lesions are similar to those of adult neurosyphilis: meningeal, meningovascular, or parenchymal involvement manifested as syphilitic meningitis, meningoencephalitis, epilepsy, paralysis of cranial nerves or extremities, juvenile tabes, paresis, or taboparesis. Mental retardation may become evident, vary-

ing from mild "backwardness" to imbecility. Certain stigmas, believed to be the result of spirochetal infection of the anlage of affected structures and perhaps of the endocrine glands, are characteristic. These include Hutchinson's teeth (deformity and notching of central incisors), "moon" or "mulberry" molars (malformed 6-year molars), saber tibias, 8th nerve deafness, scaphoid scapula, high-arched palate, "open bite," Higoumenakis' sign (thickened medial ends of clavicles), ulnar deviation of the middle fingers, hypertrichosis, enlarged spleen, and typical facies (flat, high, prominent forehead, saddle nose, rhagades or scars about the mouth or nose). Other manifestations may be periostitis of the long bones or skull, gummas in long bones or skull with erosion of bone and later ulceration through the skin, or Clutton's joints (painless arthritis, most often of the knees, with effusion into the joints.

Diagnosis

Each offspring of a syphilitic mother requires diagnostic procedures, regardless of the amount of prenatal treatment that may have been given the mother. Fetal death also requires diagnosis, and serologic tests or tissue examinations will ordinarily reveal syphilis when present. Routine early and late serologic tests of pregnant women and the testing of cord blood will disclose syphilis, when the disease is present, in the great majority of cases. Occasionally, however, in infants with latent congenital syphilis, positive spinal fluid findings (increased cell count, increased lymphocytes, protein, and positive Wassermann and colloidal gold reactions) are the only indication. Blood serology may not become positive for 6 months or more. Therefore, when there is the slightest suspicion of syphilis, blood and spinal fluid serologic tests must be repeated at 6 months and 1 year. The possibility of a positive Wassermann from the infant's blood as a result of syphilis in the mother but without infection in the infant, must be considered. Here, the titer of the test serves as a guide. Repeated tests and careful interpretation are necessary to rule out syphilis in these cases.

Course and Prognosis

The earlier the appearance of symptoms, the more serious the prognosis. Response to treatment is generally satisfactory, but structural damage cannot be repaired, especially after the paralytic and mental changes of neurosyphilis. Interstitial keratitis is notoriously resistant and undependable in response to treatment. Even though response is satisfactory and clinical and laboratory evidences of infection disappear, reexamination and retesting at yearly intervals should be required.

Treatment

Congenital syphilis should be considered as practically always preventable. However, prevention depends upon early diagnosis and adequate treatment of the infected mother.

Penicillin is the drug of choice for treatment of congenital syphilis. For the first 48 to 72 hours, dosage should be small in order to avoid severe therapeutic shock, i.e., Herxheimer reaction (q.v.). For early congenital syphilis, penicillin in aqueous solution (℞ 1c) should be given I.M. every 2 hours for 10 days (120 injections). The total dosage is 220,000 u./Kg. body wt. (100,000 u./lb.); dividing this total amount by 120 gives the amount of each injection to be administered I.M. every 2 hours. For late congenital syphilis, 50,000 u. I.M. every 2 hours for 8 days (℞ 1b) or 600,000 u. of procaine penicillin I.M. every 24 hours for 10 days (℞ 2b) is recommended.

Arsenicals may occasionally be necessary, especially for interstitial keratitis and possibly some forms of neurosyphilis. Intravenous drugs can be injected into jugular, antecubital, or scalp veins. Mapharsen (℞ 11) is preferable, but sulfarsphenamine (℞ 12) is favored by some for congenital syphilis, since it can be given I.M.

Bismuth may be used in combination with other drugs or to begin therapy, in order to avoid reactions. Bismuth subsalicylate suspended in peanut oil (℞ 13) and always given I.M., in a dose of 2 to 3 mg. (in terms of bismuth metal)/Kg. of body weight, is administered once a week for 8 to 12 injections, followed by a rest period of 4 to 8 weeks.

A suggested routine scheme of treatment is outlined below:

Week	Treatment	Week	Treatment
1	Arsenical in one-third to one-half full dose	29–40	Bismuth—note overlap
2–10	Arsenical in full dose	41–48	Arsenical
10–19	Bismuth—note overlap	48–59	Bismuth—note overlap
		60–65	Arsenical
20–29	Arsenical	65–72	Bismuth—note overlap

Fever therapy (*see* General Paresis) is valuable in certain cases of interstitial keratitis and symptomatic neurosyphilis.

Response to penicillin usually is satisfactory in early congenital syphilis. The serologic test for syphilis decreases gradually in quantitative titer over a period of months; the majority of cases become negative within a year. Abnormal spinal fluid findings also tend to reverse, and the incidence of clinical or serologic relapses has been low. In late (tardive) congenital syphilis, clinical response is good, but a greater number tend to remain seropositive (latent).

Reactions to treatment apparently are infrequent; mild febrile Herxheimer reactions (q.v.) are encountered, and sometimes transient urticaria, vomiting, and diarrhea. In general, infants and small children tolerate antisyphilitic treatment well, but when therapeutic shock (Herxheimer) does occur, it may be more serious than in adults.

CHANCROID
(Ulcus molle, Soft chancre)

An acute, localized, autoinoculable, venereal disease charac-terized clinically by necrotizing ulcerations at the site of in-oculation. The primary lesion usually occurs on the genitals and is frequently accompanied by inflammatory swelling and suppuration of the regional lymph nodes.

Etiology and Epidemiology

The infectious agent, *Hemophilus ducreyi*, is a fine, short, gram-negative bacillus with rounded ends. It often is referred to as a streptobacillus because of its tendency toward chain formation.

The mode of infection is predominantly venereal, although chancroid of the fingers may be acquired accidentally by doc-tors, nurses and orderlies. The disease is spread mainly by sexual intercourse with active cases or carriers.

Pathology

The pathologic changes are not specific. Chancroidal lesions are characterized by superficial necrosis, with infiltration by poly-morphonuclear leukocytes. Plasma cells, lymphocytes, and endothelial leukocytes are present in the surrounding area. There is acute peri- and endovasculitis with pronounced swell-ing of the endothelium, frequently blocking the lumen of the capillaries and leading to necrosis. The vascular changes are characteristic and produce superficial necrosis and unhealthy granulation.

Symptoms and Signs

The incubation period generally is 3 to 5 days. If an abrasion is present at the time of contact, a lesion may appear within 24 hours. However, a low virulence of the infectious agent may delay its appearance.

The disease begins as a vesicopustule, which breaks down rapidly and soon ruptures, leaving a sharply circumscribed, saucer-like ulceration, which is tender and painful. The edges of the ulcer may become ragged and undermined. The base is moist and covered with grayish necrotic exudate, removal of which reveals uneven purulent granulation tissue. The ulcer is surrounded by an erythematous halo. Multiple lesions may develop rapidly by autoinoculation. Systemic reactions are rare in all varieties of the disease.

A rare type of **transient** chancroid occurs which may be con-fused with lymphogranuloma venereum. It is characterized by a small superficial ulceration which, in 4 to 6 days, undergoes spontaneous involution without scar formation.

Often, 10 to 20 days after the disappearance of the primary lesion, there may be an acute regional lymphadenopathy followed by suppuration. The **phagedenic** type (ulcus molle gangrenosum) is a rapidly destructive form. The **giant** chancroid, another variety, originates as a simple lesion which extends peripherally and is characterized by extensive ulceration. The **serpiginous** type (ulcus molle serpiginosum) spreads by extension and autoinoculation to the groin or thigh. The lesions may spread rapidly. The ulcerations usually are shallow, but show no tendency to heal and may persist for months or years.

Bubo: Inguinal adenitis develops in over 50% of cases. The typical chancroidal bubo is unilateral, moderately large in size, erythematous, and painful. It consists of inguinal nodes which have become fused by an acute inflammatory process. The mass gradually softens, becomes fluctuant, and unilocular suppuration results. Spontaneous rupture of the bubo may occur.

Complications

Of so-called typical lesions, 12 to 15% are mixed syphilis and chancroid (mixed chancre). In its initial stage, the mixed chancre has all the characteristics of a chancroid, but after 15 to 20 days some of the characteristics of a syphilitic chancre may be manifest. The possibility of concurrent lymphogranuloma venereum or granuloma inguinale and chancroid must be borne in mind. Balanitis, phimosis, and paraphimosis are frequent and annoying complications. Superimposed fusospirochetal infection (fusospirochetosis) often leads to rapid and extensive destruction of tissue.

Diagnosis

The diagnosis of chancroidal infection may be substantiated by the recovery of *H. ducreyi* from lesions in smears or cultures, by intradermal tests, by autoinoculation, and by biopsy of suspected lesions. Smears, prepared of the exudate from the undermined edges of the lesion, are stained with Gram, Unna-Pappenheim, Wright, or Giemsa stain. Identification of the organism in smears from the open lesion usually is difficult because of contamination or superimposed infection. The demonstration of *H. ducreyi* is greatly enhanced if the Pappenheim stain is used. Pus cells stain bluish green; bacteria, a brilliant red. *H. ducreyi* may frequently be grown from the bubo pus, aspirated under sterile conditions, by culturing on agar slants to which 1 cc. of defibrinated human or rabbit blood has been added. Culture of the primary lesion yields a mixed infection, but occasionally *H. ducreyi* is readily demonstrated.

Either of two intradermal tests may be used. In one, bubo pus antigen is employed and in the other, a bacillary vaccine (Ducrey vaccine). The latter is better standardized and gives earlier and more clear-cut reactions. The test is performed on the forearm by injecting 0.1 cc. of the vaccine intradermally. A reaction is positive if a 7 mm. area of induration appears by 48 hours afterward. The reaction usually becomes positive from 8 to 25 days after the appearance of the primary lesion, the average being about 12 to 14 days. Since the reactions probably remain positive for life, a positive reaction permits a diagnosis of past or present chancroid. A negative reaction is often obtained when the lesion is superficial, without lymphatic involvement.

In autoinoculated lesions the Ducrey bacillus is more readily demonstrable than in the original ulcers. Material from the lesion is rubbed into a scarified area on the thigh. In 2 or 3 days tiny vesicopustules usually appear and these break down to become the site of a typical chancroidal ulceration.

A biopsy of the lesion may reveal the findings described *under* Pathology, above. They are suggestive of the diagnosis but not pathognomonic.

Chancroid is frequently complicated by syphilis and, to rule out the coexistence of this complication, darkfield examination of all genital lesions should be performed. In addition, every patient should have a serologic test (Wassermann, Mazzini, Kahn, Kline, or others) at the initial examination and again 1 month after all lesions have healed.

Prognosis

Usually, the disease is self-limited and causes only minor discomfort. Systemic reactions are rare or mild. Pain is the most frequent complaint. The primary ulceration may heal gradually or ulcerations may spread by autoinoculation, and there may be much pain and inflammation of the affected parts.

Prophylaxis

Where abstinence is rejected, the proper use of a condom during intercourse is the most reliable method of preventing venereal infection. Thorough washing of the genital regions with soap and water after intercourse also is essential. In addition, several chemical prophylactics are commercially available; these should be used carefully according to the instructions accompanying the kit.

Treatment

Good results have been obtained in the treatment of chancroid lesions with either sulfadiazine 1 Gm. every 4 hours for 5 days (℞ 7), or streptomycin 0.5 Gm. I.M. every 4 hours for 8 doses (℞ 4). Sulfathiazole and urea (℞ 8) applied to the lesion will reduce the foul odor and stimulate healing. Aureomycin and Chloromycetin also have shown promising results in the treatment of chancroid.

The bubo should never be incised. If fluctuation is present it should be aspirated aseptically, repeatedly if necessary. The aspiration point should be dusted with sulfathiazole-urea powder (℞ 8), or a dressing of 5% sulfathiazole cream (℞ 6) may be applied.

Severe phimosis or paraphimosis may be treated by immersion in hot magnesium sulfate or saline solution. Circumcision or a dorsal slit rarely is necessary.

GRANULOMA INGUINALE

(Granuloma pudendi, Granuloma venereum)

A mildly contagious, chronic, progressive, autoinoculable disease involving the skin and occasionally the lymphatics, and usually occurring in the inguinal region.

Etiology and Epidemiology

The etiologic agent is *Donovania granulomatis,* a pleomorphic rod 1 to 2 microns in length, occurring intracellularly, singly or in clusters. It has been grown in the yolk sac of chick embryos. The disease has been reproduced in man by inoculation with aspirated pus from pseudobuboes of granuloma inguinale that contained no microorganism other than *Donovania granulomatis.*

Granuloma inguinale is generally regarded as a venereal disease. Although this has not been proved, the consensus is that it is acquired through coitus. The frequency of a history of sexual exposure, and the antecedent appearance of a primary penile lesion in the vast majority of males suffering from the disease, points to a venereal origin. In this country, granuloma inguinale occurs predominantly in Negroes.

Pathology

Granuloma inguinale, in the pure or unmixed form, reveals a uniform histologic picture. The pathognomonic cell is of relatively large size (25 to 90 microns) and contains many intracytoplasmic cysts filled with deeply stained bodies (*Donovania granulomatis,* or Donovan bodies).

Symptoms and Signs

Little is known about the incubation period of granuloma inguinale, although case reports in the literature suggest that it varies between 8 and 12 weeks. The onset of the disease is insidious, without premonitory constitutional symptoms. The first evidence of infection is the appearance of a vesicle, papule, or nodule, usually on the genitalia. The surface epithelium may become excoriated or eroded, leaving an ulcer with a beefy-red granular base. The early lesions may appear as small button-like elevations or as a fine granular film covering the glans, with occasional nodules gently bulging the surface. An early form frequently observed is a clean, raised, velvety tuft of granulation tissue, with a sharply defined margin, situated at the mucocutaneous border of the vaginal or preputial orifice, on the glans, or on the inner surface of the prepuce. In the female, the primary lesion usually is found on the vulva or vagina—occasionally on the cervix or in the perigenital zone. The granulation tissue bleeds easily when traumatized. Since the early lesions are not painful, the patient rarely seeks medical care until the disease is well advanced.

The inguinal manifestations are secondary to the genital. When they appear alone, a history of a previous genital lesion which healed spontaneously is frequently obtained. However, the lesions usually show very little tendency to heal; on the contrary, they tend to spread, by continuity or contiguity. As a rule, extension is very slow, but occasionally it is rather rapid and there is a predilection for moist contact surfaces, particularly in the crurosacral folds. The advancing border of the lesion has characteristic rolled edges, the granulation tissue piling over onto the bordering epithelial surface. The ulcerative process may reach a stage at which it remains more or less stationary for many years. The lesions may show a tendency to scar formation at one margin and chronic progression at another. After several months or years, they develop a characteristic sour and peculiarly pungent odor.

In about 6% of all cases of granuloma inguinale, extragenital lesions have been found. These usually are secondary, but in a few instances purely extragenital lesions have been described.

Complications

Fusospirochetosis is the most common complication of granuloma inguinale. The infected lesions become ulcerative, progressive, foul-smelling, and painful, and often are refractory to specific therapy. Syphilis, chancroid, and lymphogranuloma venereum may be coexistent. Occasionally, superimposed malignancy may complicate the picture. Secondary elephantoid enlargement of the penis, scrotum, or vulva and clitoris may occur.

Diagnosis

Granuloma inguinale should be diagnosed only when Donovan bodies are demonstrated in spreads or when biopsy reveals the pathognomonic cell.

Spreads are made by obtaining a minute piece of granulation tissue from the surface of the lesion if it appears to be clean, or from the deeper part if it appears infected. The exudate covering infected lesions should first be removed. The small piece of granulation tissue is best obtained with a sharp instrument, such as a small bone curet. It is smeared along several glass slides or crushed between two slides and then spread along the slides. The slides then are dried and stained with Wright or Giemsa stain. The demonstration of Donovan bodies is possible, by some means, in every case of granuloma inguinale. When spreads fail to corroborate the clinical diagnosis, histologic methods may be resorted to in order to demon-

strate the pathognomonic cell and the characteristic inclusion
bodies.

Prognosis

With the availability of streptomycin and aureomycin therapy, hope of cure now may be offered to almost every patient
suffering from granuloma inguinale. Cases resistant to streptomycin may be encountered, but they are few. Reactivation of
lesions frequently occurred with older forms of therapy in
debilitated patients. In such persons and in neglected and
treatment-resistant cases, the ulcerations may become extensive, occupying the whole pudendal region, lower abdomen,
buttocks, and thighs, with the patients becoming anemic, bedridden and cachectic, and finally succumbing.

Treatment

Streptomycin 1 Gm. I.M. every 6 hours for 5 days (R 4), and
aureomycin 0.25 to 0.5 Gm. every 6 hours for 15 to 30 days
(R 5), have proved to be effective therapeutic agents for
cure of this disease. Streptomycin-resistant cases may respond
satisfactorily to aureomycin or Chloromycetin, with ultimate
cure. Prior to the advent of streptomycin, antimonial therapy
with anthiomaline, tartar emetic 1%, or Fuadin was used with
some success for control of granuloma inguinale.

LYMPHOGRANULOMA VENEREUM

(Poradenitis, Lymphopathia venereum)

*A contagious disease caused by a filtrable virus and usually
incurred as a result of sexual intercourse.* The characteristic
initial symptom is a small papular or ulcerative lesion on the
genitalia. This is evanescent and is frequently followed by a
subacute regional lymphadenitis or a chronic inflammatory reaction in the subjacent connective tissue, or both. Cytoplasmic
inclusions (gamma bodies) varying in size have been seen in
cells from infected lymph nodes. As long as contaminating
exudate is present, whether it originates from a proctitis,
urethritis, discharging sinus, or an open ulcerative lesion, the
disease is contagious.

Clinical Course

The primary lesion usually appears from 5 to 21 days after
the infective contact and often is so transitory or hidden as to
escape notice. The inguinal bubo, which appears 10 to 30 days
after exposure, is frequently the first visible manifestation of
the disease.

The lymphotropism of the virus leads to the development of an adenitis in the lymph nodes nearest the primary lesion. Involvement of the inguinal lymphatic drainage area usually is followed by the characteristic inguinal bubo. When the perirectal glands are involved by either direct or retrograde extension of the infection, anorectal complications are inevitable. These occur far more commonly in the female, because the lymphatic drainage from the vagina is toward the perirectal glands.

Constitutional symptoms often are present during the stage of lymphatic progression of the infection, particularly during lymph node involvement. Fever, chills, headache, vague abdominal aches, joint pains, and anorexia are common complaints. Occasionally, such severe manifestations as meningism or a typhoidal state supervene. Splenomegaly is sometimes present.

The clinical course varies from person to person. Symptoms may be so slight that the patient never is aware of the disease, or chronic residual lesions may be so debilitating as to cause lifelong invalidism. Any combination of the following syndromes may be present.

Inguinal syndrome: Involvement of the inguinal lymphatics may be unilateral or bilateral, accompanied by pain and stiffness, followed by local swelling and tenderness. With progression of the adenitis, areas of softening develop. Eventually, the nodes tend to become matted together and adherent to the overlying skin, which has a purplish hue. Suppuration through multiple fistulous tracts may occur and occasionally a unilocular abscess is formed. Healing often ensues with extensive scarring.

Genital syndrome: In the male, secondary ulceration and occasionally massive elephantiasis of the penis may occur. In the female, elephantiasis of the vulva or clitoris is very common, particularly in Negroes. This syndrome is frequently referred to as esthiomene. The surface of the enlarged and swollen parts may be smooth or verrucose, polypoid, or ulcerated. Pedunculated tumors of the labium or clitoris are frequent. Vaginal stricture or rectovaginal fistula sometimes develops.

Anal syndrome: Polypoidal and lobulated growths, lympheroids, about the anal orifice occur either alone or with a genital or rectal syndrome. In the early stages, indurated rubbery anal tabs are present and may be mistaken for hemorrhoidal tags.

Rectal syndrome: Rectal stricture frequently is found without other manifestations of lymphogranuloma venereum and often with no history of a primary lesion or bubo. The stricture usually is of the cylindric "rubber hose" variety, but may be of the simple ring type. Intestinal obstruction may result. Conditions such as a swollen, redundant, indurated rectal mucosa, proctitis, rectal granuloma, polypoid and verrucous hypertrophy of the mucosa occasionally are present. Involvement of the perirectal tissue causes perirectal abscesses which result in ischiorectal abscesses or chronic anal fistulas.

Urethral syndrome: Stained spreads of urethral discharge which do not reveal pathogenic bacteria but show an abundance of leukocytes suggest a diagnosis of lymphogranuloma venereum. Urethral strictures and fistulas may occur. In the female, swelling and ulcerations of the urethra, or papillary elevations of mucosa about the urethral meatus have been observed.

Extragenital lymphogranuloma venereum: Axillary buboes have occurred in physicians through accidental infection of the upper extremity. Laboratory workers who are constantly exposed to high concentrations of the virus have developed generalized systemic infections with symptoms which are fairly characteristic, i.e., fever, chills, sweats, articular rheumatism, and headache. Cases of conjunctivitis and keratitis due to the virus of lymphogranuloma venereum have been reported.

Diagnosis

In the presence of a genital lesion, darkfield examination should be performed to rule out syphilitic infection. Frequently, positive low-titer Wassermann reactions may be obtained in the course of the infection. Such a positive reaction will become negative over a period of time with repeated serologic examinations, after the infection has been cured. This false positive serologic reaction is due to the increased globulin content of the serum, which also may cause a positive formol gel test.

Frei test: This is the most important confirmatory test in routine diagnosis: 0.1 cc. of the antigen obtained from infected chick embryo is injected intradermally in the forearm so that a wheal is raised. In positive cases, an inflammatory infiltration or nodule, measuring at least 5 or 6 mm. in diameter, with a surrounding zone of erythema, is present at the end of 48 to 72 hours. The control test reaction, when uninfected chick embryo material is used, should measure not more than 3 mm.

Biopsy: Histopathologic study frequently proves useful. In the bubo form, there are inflammatory and suppurative changes in the lymph nodes as well as the perilymphoid tissue. There is a polymorphogranulomatous reaction; tiny foci of necrosis or micro-abscesses surrounded by macrophages with occasional giant cells are seen. **Autoinoculation:** Autoinoculation of aspirated pus from a bubo of lymphogranuloma venereum does not produce local ulceration, while in chancroid autoinoculation of aspirated pus frequently produces a typical chancroidal ulcer. **Complement fixation test:** A serologic complement fixation test using antigen from lymphogranuloma venereum virus of chick embryo origin is commercially available. It is very sensitive and of much value in early diagnosis as well as in gauging the efficacy of treatment or progress of the disease. **Inverted Frei test:** Sometimes a negative Frei test is obtained even in the presence of a suppurative bubo. Pus aspirated from such a bubo may be made into an antigen that, on injection into patients known to have lymphogranuloma venereum, will produce a positive reaction.

Treatment

Chemotherapy: Sulfonamides (R 7) are of value, particularly in the acute phase of lymphogranuloma venereum. They are especially useful in ulcerative processes, draining sinuses, proctitis and colitis, and may be applied locally in combination with urea (R 8). However, little benefit is noted for purely strictural rectal lesions or for elephantiasic vulva. In selected cases of ulcerative colitis and rectitis due to the virus of lymphogranuloma venereum, sulfaguanidine (R 9) or succinylsulfathiazole (R 10) orally has proved of some value. Recently, it has been shown that aureomycin (R 5) is effective in the therapy of this disease. Excellent results have followed its use in the acute bubo, in proctitis and in ulcerations. Rectal strictures and elephantiasic lesions are not benefited. **Aspiration:** Fluctuant buboes should be aspirated, repeatedly if necessary, but never incised. **Vaccinotherapy:** Satisfactory therapeutic results have been obtained by subcutaneous and intradermal administration of Frei antigen (R 28). Biweekly or weekly injections of ascending doses of antigen from 0.05 to 1 cc., or repeated injections of 0.1 or 0.2 cc. over a period of months, have occasionally given striking results. Ascending doses of Frei antigen (0.05 to 0.5 cc.) of mouse brain or pus origin, may be administered I.V. at 4- to 7-day intervals to produce fever as well as focal reactions. To assure beneficial results, chemotherapy (R 7) should follow this treatment. It appears to be of some value for chronic recalcitrant lesions. **Surgery:** Polypoid excrescences, pedunculated tumors, and elephantiasic vulvas may be excised. The wounds usually heal readily. In some cases, recurrences of the ulceration have been observed after several years. Excision of the matted glands is permissible and is indicated when the inguinal mass remains chronically indurated for months without signs of suppuration or regression. However, as a general practice, excision is not advisable because it may be followed by severe elephantiasis of the genitals.

Management of rectal stricture: Pain, rectal leukorrhea, and most other complaints incident to rectal stricture are greatly lessened by sulfonamide therapy. The stricture should be gently dilated manually at weekly intervals, or not less often than every 2 weeks, to prevent recurrence of stenosis. Long-wave and short-wave diathermy benefit the inflammatory process and aid in softening the stenotic lumen. When the rectum will not admit the index finger, digital dilation under anesthesia or caudal block is necessary. Hegar dilators then may be used to obtain adequate dilatation. When strictures are beyond reach of the examining finger, colostomy is justifiable.

PRESCRIPTIONS

(Wherever a prescribed "proprietary" is representative of a class of therapeutic agents, alternative proprietary preparations will be found listed in Part II.)

Antibiotics

1. ℞ Penicillin   (vial)

   a. Gonorrhea: 50,000 u. I.M. every hour for 4 doses; for treatment-resistant cases, give 30,000 to 50,000 u. I.M. every 3 hours for 10 to 20 doses.

   b. Primary, Secondary, Latent, Late, Late Congenital, and Syphilis in Pregnancy: 50,000 u. I.M. every 2 hours day and night for 8 days (96 injections, 4.8 million u.).

   c. Early Congenital Syphilis: Inject I.M. every 2 hours for 10 days (120 doses). Total dose is 220,000 u./Kg. body wt. (100,000 u./lb.); each injection contains total dose divided by 120.

   d. Meningovascular Neurosyphilis—Asymptomatic, Acute Syphilitic Meningitis (*see also* MENINGITIS), Diffuse Meningovascular, Vascular, or Gumma: Give a total of 9.6 to 20 million u. I.M. in 12 to 20 days.

   e. Parenchymal Neurosyphilis (paresis, tabes) and Optic Atrophy: Give a total of 9.6 to 20 million u. I.M. in 12 to 24 days as adjunct to other indicated treatment.

   f. Mucocutaneous, Osseous, and Visceral Syphilis: Give 6 million u. or more I.M. in divided doses every 3 hours over a period of 15 or more days. In the case of cardiovascular syphilis, this regimen is not to be started until after several weeks' preparation with bismuth (℞ 13) therapy (*see also* ANEURYSM; AORTITIS).

2. ℞ Procaine penicillin   (vial)

   a. Gonorrhea: 300,000 u. I.M. daily—for 1 day in acute cases, longer in chronic cases.

   b. Primary, Secondary, Latent, Late, Late Congenital, and Syphilis in Pregnancy: 600,000 u. I.M. once every 24 hours for 10 days.

3. ℞ Penicillin sodium   (oral tablets)

   a. 100,000 u. orally 12 and 18 hours after ℞ 1a or 2a.

b. For early gonorrheal prophylaxis, give 250,000 u. as soon as possible after exposure.

c. For acute gonorrhea, 100,000 u. every 3 hours for 1 or 2 days.

4. ℞ Streptomycin (vial)

Gonorrhea: 0.3 to 0.5 Gm. I.M., repeated once if necessary.

Chancroid: 0.5 Gm. I.M. every 4 hours for 8 doses.

Granuloma Inguinale: 1 Gm. I.M. every 6 hours for 5 days.

5. ℞ Aureomycin . . . . 0.25 Gm.

1 or 2 capsules every 6 hours for 15 to 30 days. Continue treatment for at least 1 week after healing is complete.

Sulfonamides

6. ℞ Sulfathiazole, 5% cream

Apply to bubo at point of aspiration.

7. ℞ Sulfadiazine . . . . 0.5 Gm. (gr. viiss)

Gonorrhea or Chancroid: 2 tablets every 4 to 6 hours for 5 days; repeat course if necessary.

Lymphogranuloma Venereum: 1 tablet 4 times a day for 2 to 4 weeks.

8. ℞ Sulfathiazole (powdered)
Urea (powdered) . . . . . āā 10.0 Gm. (℥ iiss)

Apply locally to lesions or during each dressing.

9. ℞ Sulfaguanidine . . . . 0.5 Gm. (gr. viiss)

50 mg./Kg. every 4 to 8 hours for 7 to 14 days.

10. ℞ Succinylsulfathiazole

0.25 Gm./Kg. daily in divided doses for 1 or 2 weeks.

Other Chemotherapeutic Agents

11. ℞ "Mapharsen"

Administer I.V. according to schedule given in treatment sections.

Men: 40 mg. initially followed by doses up to 60 mg.

Women: 30 mg. initially, followed by doses up to 40 mg.

Children: initial dose not to exceed 0.5 mg./Kg. body wt.; later doses not to exceed 1.0 mg./Kg.

12. ℞ Sulfarsphenamine U.S.P. (ampul)

    For infants: 10 to 15 mg./Kg.

    For I.M. or subcut. injection, dissolve in ratio of 0.1 Gm./0.3 cc. Water for Injection U.S.P. (maximum volume of 2 cc.).

    For I.V. injection, 0.1 Gm./1 to 4 cc. diluent (4 cc. preferred): Total volume 5 to 20 cc.

13. ℞ Bismuth Subsalicylate Injection
      U.S.P. (vial)

    Average dose, 0.1 Gm.; administered I.M. weekly usually in a series of 6 to 10 injections. The bismuth series is generally combined with an arsenical series in a typical schedule of treatment.

14. ℞ Potassium iodide . . . . 30.0   Gm. (℥ i)
      Glycyrrhiza Syrup U.S.P. . . . 90.0   cc.   (℥ iii)
      Water . . . . q.s. ad 120.0   cc.   (℥ iv)

    1 teaspoon in milk 3 times daily after meals.

15. ℞ "Pyridium" . . . . 0.1   Gm. (gr. iss)

    1 or 2 tablets 3 times daily for relief of bladder symptoms (warn patient of coloring of urine).

16. ℞ BAL (2,3-dimercaptopropanol)
      (ampul)

    To be given deeply I.M. in accordance with procedure outlined in text under toxic manifestations of gold (*see* RHEUMATOID ARTHRITIS, *also* ARSENIC POISONING).

Venereal Prophylactics

17. ℞ Strong silver protein, 2% solution 30.0   cc.   (℥ i)

    Instill 4 to 6 cc. into urethra and retain for 5 minutes; in females, also apply by swab to entire vaginal mucosa and external os.

18. ℞ Mild silver protein, 10% solution . 30.0   cc.   (℥ i)

    Instill 4 to 6 cc. into urethra and retain for 5 minutes; in females, also apply by swab to entire vaginal mucosa and external os.

19. ℞ Calomel, 30% ointment . . . . . 60.0   Gm. (℥ ii)

    Anoint genitalia immediately after exposure. Wash off with soap and water after 3 hours.

Sedatives and Analgesics

20. ℞ Acetylsalicylic acid . . . . 0.2   Gm. (gr. iii)
      Acetophenetidin . . . . 0.12 Gm. (gr. ii)
      Caffeine . . . . 0.09 Gm. (gr. iss)

    1 or 2 capsules or tablets every 4 hours as necessary.

21. ℞ Codeine phosphate
> 30 mg. orally or subcut. every 4 hours as necessary.

22. ℞ Phenobarbital. . . . . 0.1 Gm. (gr. iss)
> 1 tablet every 4 hours as necessary.

23. ℞ Powdered Opium U.S.P. 60   mg.   (gr. i)
> 1 capsule 3 times daily after meals for melancholia and hypochondriasis.

24. ℞ Cerium oxalate . . . . 0.15 Gm. (gr. iiss)
> 1 or more powders every 2 hours for relief of vomiting in gastric crisis.

25. ℞ Sodium nitrite. . . . . 0.1 Gm. (gr. iss)
>   Potassium nitrate . . . . 0.3 Gm. (gr. v)
>   Sodium bicarbonate . . . . . . 1.0 Gm. (gr. xv)
> 1 powder in water 3 times daily for visceral crisis.

Miscellaneous

26. ℞ Estrone   (suppository). . . . . 2,000 u.
> Insert one suppository into vagina nightly until infection is controlled.

27. ℞ Belladonna Tincture U.S.P. . . . 30.0 cc.   (℥ i)
> 5 to 10 drops in water as necessary for incontinence of urine.

28. ℞ Frei antigen   (vial)
> *See* LYMPHOGRANULOMA VENEREUM for details of administration.

PART II

———

ROUTINE IMMUNIZATION PROCEDURES

Optional pediatric immunization schedules and timetables for the administration of booster or re-immunization doses are presented. A table outlining the use of human serum immune (gamma) globulin also is included. Although many pertinent details are given, actual dosage must be regulated according to individual circumstances and to the instructions accompanying packages of the various immunizing agents. (For special immunization procedures against such diseases as typhoid fever, yellow fever, cholera, plague, and other conditions not ordinarily included in pediatric practice, *see* the respective chapters.)

BASIC IMMUNIZATION

OPTIONAL SCHEDULE No. 1

Age	Agent
3 months	Pertussis Vaccine (Alum Precipitated)
4 "	" " " "
5 "	" " " "
6 "	Diphtheria-Tetanus Toxoid (Alum Precipitated)
6 "	Smallpox Vaccine
7 "	Diphtheria-Tetanus Toxoid (Alum Precipitated)
11 "	Schick Test
11 "	Pertussis Vaccine (Alum Precipitated)

OPTIONAL SCHEDULE No. 2

Age	Agent
As soon as umbilicus is healed and baby is thriving	Smallpox Vaccine
3 months	Diphtheria-Tetanus-Pertussis (Alum Precipitated or Aluminum Hydroxide Adsorbed)
4 "	Diphtheria-Tetanus-Pertussis (Alum Precipitated or Aluminum Hydroxide Adsorbed)
5 "	Pertussis Vaccine (Alum Precipitated)
7 "	Diphtheria-Tetanus-Pertussis (Alum Precipitated or Aluminum Hydroxide Adsorbed)
11 "	Schick Test

BOOSTER DOSES AND RE-IMMUNIZATION

(This schedule applies only when basic immunization
has been previously accomplished.)

Age and Indication	Agent
2 years	Diphtheria-Tetanus-Pertussis (Alum Precipitated or Aluminum Hydroxide Adsorbed)
5 "	Diphtheria-Tetanus-Pertussis (Alum Precipitated or Aluminum Hydroxide Adsorbed)
	Schick Test
5 "	Smallpox Vaccine
Every 2 years	Tetanus Toxoid (Alum Precipitated)
Every 5 years or upon exposure to smallpox, or during threatened smallpox epidemic	Smallpox Vaccine
Any age, upon possible exposure to tetanus	Fluid Tetanus Toxoid
Any age, upon exposure to diphtheria	Fluid Diphtheria Toxoid
Any age, upon exposure to pertussis	Pertussis Vaccine (N.B., in Isotonic Saline)

HUMAN SERUM IMMUNE GLOBULIN
(GAMMA GLOBULIN)

Age and Indication	Dose
0–3 years, upon exposure to measles*	0.1 cc./lb. body wt. (for complete protection)
Over 3 years, upon exposure to measles*	0.025 cc./lb. body wt. (for modification of measles)
Any age, upon exposure to infectious hepatitis*	0.1 cc./lb. body wt.; repeat in 3 wks.

* For best results, gamma globulin should be given within 6 days following exposure. (*See* WHOOPING COUGH, GERMAN MEASLES, CHICKENPOX, for other suggested prophylactic and therapeutic uses.)

GENERAL CONSIDERATIONS

1. Alum precipitated preparations are best given I.M. to avoid nodule or cold abscess formation. (CAUTION! I.V. injection is contraindicated.)

2. After 6 to 10 years of age, sensitivity to diphtheria protein may have developed. If protection is imperative when the Moloney test (0.1 cc. of 1:100 dilution of Fluid Diphtheria Toxoid intradermally) is positive, very small doses, repeated at weekly intervals, should be employed.

3. Smallpox vaccination is preferably done on the arm since there is a tendency toward a less violent reaction, less temporary interference with limb function, and smaller likelihood of secondary infection than when the thigh is used. Eczema, open skin lesions, diabetes mellitus (uncontrolled), and active tuberculosis are generally considered contraindications to routine smallpox vaccination.

4. Optimum protection against pertussis is not obtained unless 70 to 100 billion organisms are used in the basic immunizing course. For booster doses on exposure, a pertussis vaccine in normal saline is recommended, since the alum precipitated preparation is too slow-acting for this purpose.

5. With the exception of such combinations as Diphtheria-Tetanus Toxoid with Pertussis Vaccine, the simultaneous use of 2 or more immunizing agents capable of producing coincident febrile or other generalized reactions is ordinarily to be avoided.

6. *Immunization for Foreign Travel:* Under this title, information concerning immunization requirements applying in various parts of the world is published by and available from the Federal Security Agency, U.S. Public Health Service, Washington 25, D.C.

CLINICAL PROCEDURES

Under this heading are described several important procedures commonly carried out by the physician or under his direct supervision. In a separate chapter, BEDSIDE PROCEDURES, technics that fall more frequently into the field of nursing will be found. Likewise, the details of office laboratory tests are treated separately, in the chapter entitled OFFICE LABORATORY PROCEDURES.

ROUTES FOR MEDICATION

Oral

This is the easiest, most common, and generally most economical method of drug administration. Absorption of ingested medicaments into the blood stream takes place almost entirely at the level of the small intestine, within 30 to 90 minutes. A relatively empty gastrointestinal tract, or the concomitant drinking of hot liquids, favors rapid absorption. Medicines already in solution are more readily absorbed than those in tablet or capsule form. Pills having an "enteric" coating pass through the stomach unchanged, and their medicinal content is absorbed from the bowel at a later period, once the protective coating has been dissolved by the intestinal juices. Gastric irritants, e.g., salicylates and bromides, are best administered with large quantities of water or at a time when the stomach is full of food. This also is the ideal time to give drugs for prolonged systemic action. However, some nauseous drugs or very large doses of drugs are preferably given, with ample fluid, on an empty stomach, so as to avoid causing the vomiting of meals. Stomachics are most effective when taken shortly before a meal. Hypnotics and cathartics give best results when their action coincides with the natural times of sleep and defecation, respectively. Incorporating drugs in pleasant-tasting vehicles makes them more acceptable to the patient. Solid medicines of unpleasant taste can be given in gelatin capsules. Pills, tablets, or capsules are swallowed easily by most persons if placed on the tongue as far back as possible and washed down with one or more generous gulps of fluid. Some individuals are helped by being instructed to place the pill or other object loosely under the tip of the tongue, then drink copiously, whereupon the fluid automatically flushes the medication down with it.

Sublingual

Many drugs are readily absorbed into the systemic circulation when placed in contact with the sublingual mucosa. This is a convenient, effective, and fast method of administering substances that may be destroyed by the digestive juices, altered in passage through the portal circulation, or urgently needed for self-administration. Tablets that dissolve rapidly,

47

such as the hypodermic variety, are the most satisfactory for this purpose. The steroid sex hormones, nitroglycerin, and other freely soluble medicaments are commonly administered by this route.

Intranasal

Drugs may be administered intranasally for either local or systemic action. Nose drops and jellies are usually applied to the nasal mucosa for their vasoconstrictive effect (e.g., ephedrine) or antiseptic effect (e.g., penicillin, tyrothricin, silver proteinate). Preparations containing oil should not be given indiscriminately by this route since they may be aspirated and cause lipoid pneumonia. Vapors are commonly inhaled for their local effect, especially vasoconstrictive. Inhalations for such purposes should not be performed by the patient more frequently than once every 2 or 3 hours.

Nose drops should be instilled by placing the patient in the supine position with his head tilted far back and turned slightly to the side being treated. Or the patient may lie on his side, with no pillow, allowing the solution to stay in contact with the mucosa of the lower nostril for several minutes before he turns onto the opposite side for similar treatment.

Drugs may occasionally be insufflated into the nose, to be absorbed directly into the systemic circulation. Posterior pituitary extract is commonly given in this manner, as in cases of diabetes insipidus.

Inhalation

Various masks, nebulizers, vaporizers, friable ampuls, and other devices are used for administering medicaments (e.g., epinephrine 1:100 solution, penicillin, streptomycin, ether, nitrous oxide, amyl nitrite, and ammonia) in relatively high concentrations to the nose, sinuses, pharynx, bronchial tree, and lung alveoli. Drugs for this purpose may be in the form of vapor or fine particles. They generally exert their greatest effect locally on the air passages. The technic of administration depends on the kind of drug given, the type of device used, and the vehicle carrying the drug. Air, oxygen, and steam are the vehicles most commonly employed for medication by inhalation.

The mechanism containing the drug should be applied to the nose or mouth at the beginning of inspiration so that the medicated gas can be carried as far as possible into the respiratory tract. Drug solutions should not exceed 2 cc. in quantity per treatment, since it takes approximately 30 minutes to vaporize and inhale this amount of liquid.

Oxygen may be administered by means of nasal catheter, mask, funnel, or some form of tent. The amount of O_2 given therapeutically should be sufficient to provide a concentration of 50% or more in the inhaled air. Care must be exercised not to permit a spark or open flame in the vicinity of the apparatus. It is advisable to humidify the gas by bubbling it through water. This also permits estimation of the rate of flow. A filled, large-sized, standard cylinder, at 2,200 lbs. pressure, when delivering O_2 at a rate of 6 liters/minute, will last approximately 19 hours.

For intranasal administration, curved metal tubes are available which fit into the nostrils and are then strapped to the forehead. However, almost any small-gauge rubber catheter (usually No. 10 Fr.) may be used. It is advisable to lubricate the rubber catheter with petrolatum before inserting it, and to spray the nostril with a local anesthetic such as 2% butacaine or metycaine. The catheter should be passed gently along the nasal passage into the nasopharynx until the tip is visible slightly below the soft palate. Care should be taken not to insert the catheter so deeply that the tip will cause the patient to gag, and its eye should be turned away from the posterior pharyngeal surface so that the stream of O_2 will not dry out the membrane and produce irritation. A fresh catheter should be inserted at least once, preferably twice, daily, and the nostrils used alternately. Giving 5 liters/minute will provide approximately 37% concentration in the alveolar air, and 8 liters/minute approximately 40%; somewhat less is utilized if the patient breathes through his mouth.

Some patients are unusually sensitive to the presence of a nasal catheter. In such patients, a mask may be used, unless contraindicated by the need for frequent coughing, expectoration, or oral feedings. Oxygen masks are available in two general types, nasal and oronasal. The nasal mask is more comfortable but the oronasal is more efficient. Masks should fit snugly and the flow should be so regulated that the breathing bag is not completely collapsed during inspiration. With a flow of 5 liters/minute, concentrations of 50 to 60% may be obtained in the alveolar air, and 12 liters/minute will produce concentrations approaching 100%. The inhalation of 75 to 100% O_2 should be interrupted for a few minutes at least every 12 hours. In infants and young children, where a catheter or mask may not be practicable, a funnel can be attached to the tube supplying O_2 and the large end held over the patient's nose and mouth, but this is a wasteful and not very effective mode of administration.

The administration of O_2 under positive pressure may be necessary, as in pulmonary edema. Positive pressure is achieved by using a special face mask with a valve which, by governing the caliber of the exit airway, permits expiration against a controlled calibrated resistance ranging up to 6 cm. of water. The optimum pressure is the maximum tolerated by the patient.

An oxygen tent may be employed whenever other technics are not feasible. It often is the method of choice with very sick, restless, or uncooperative patients. When using a tent, it is necessary to check it constantly for possible leaks, and to open the tent for nursing procedures as briefly and seldom as possible. A type of open-top tent has been designed for giving O_2, especially to children or in cases where extra humidification is desirable. (Oxygen chambers would, of course, be the ideal way to administer O_2, but they are costly to build and operate, and seldom available.) The air in the tent should be cooled (to 65° or 70° F.) and humidified for the patient's comfort. Under ordinary circumstances, a flow of 8 to 12 liters/minute will provide a concentration of 50% O_2 within the tent.

Percutaneous

Administration of medicaments (e.g., mercury salts) for systemic effect by application to the intact skin is no longer widely practiced because of its inconvenience and relative inefficiency.

Drugs given in this manner are usually applied in the form of a water-soluble ointment to the thinner (e.g., flexor) areas of the skin.

Iontophoresis (Ion transfer)

The introduction of drugs into the deeper layers of the skin by means of an uninterrupted and unidirectional flow of electric current (galvanic) often is very useful for local effect. For example, Mecholyl Chloride, 1:500 to 1:200 aqueous solution, may be administered in this manner, though never to a patient with a history of asthma, nor over an area of broken skin or a papule.

Prior to treatment, the patient should, if possible, empty his bladder and rectum. The area to be treated should be cleansed of all grease, then wetted with the Mecholyl Chloride solution. A solution-soaked fabric (reinforced asbestos paper, cotton gauze, or stockinette) is applied, care being taken that it lies smoothly, without any wrinkles, against the skin. The positive electrode, usually a thin sheet of soft malleable block tin measuring not less than 325 sq. cm. (50 sq. in.), should be shaped to fit the area and applied snugly and evenly against the fabric. Caution should be exercised to keep the electrode from direct contact with the skin. It is best held firmly in place by an elastic bandage. The negative electrode pad, soaked with water or physiologic saline, should be placed under the patient's back or some other area distant from the positive electrode.

The current is turned on and gradually increased, 2 to 3 minutes being taken to reach a reading of 25 or 30 milliamperes. The current should be advanced only to the point of comfortable tolerance. If, during the procedure, the patient experiences a burning sensation or pain, it is necessary to shut off the current and investigate the cause. A decrease in the meter reading usually is a sign that the pads are becoming dry and need remoistening. At the conclusion of the treatment, which usually is given for 20 minutes, the patient should remain quiet, and be kept warm for at least 30 minutes before he resumes his ordinary activities.

Intracutaneous (Intradermal, Endermic)

The injection of small amounts of material between the skin layers is a procedure commonly used in diagnosis, treatment, and local anesthetization. By using a very fine needle (25 or 26 gauge) and injecting only a small quantity of fluid, usually not more than 0.1 cc., the discomfort of the injection can be minimized. Small quantities of fluid are most accurately administered with a tuberculin syringe. Using a suitable antiseptic, such as alcohol, the area to be treated is cleansed. Then, the needle, kept almost parallel to the skin, is inserted as superficially as possible. If the point of the needle is in the corium, the injection of fluid will raise a small wheal. Examples of substances frequently introduced in this manner include allergenic extracts, tuberculin, diphtheria toxoid, epinephrine, and procaine.

Hypodermic Injection

Small quantities of fluid medicament can easily be injected subcut. by pinching up the skin, previously cleansed with an antiseptic (e.g., alcohol), between thumb and forefinger and then firmly and quickly inserting the needle through all layers of the skin. The solution is injected with ease if the point of the needle (22 gauge or smaller) has penetrated into the subcut. tissues and is not lodged in skin or muscle. In order to avoid injection into a vein, which may have dangerous consequences, gentle aspiration should be attempted prior to injection. If blood appears, another site must be chosen. The favorite sites of administration are the extensor surfaces of the upper arms, the back, and the lateral aspects of the thighs.

Occasionally, solid materials such as steroid hormones are administered subcut. for a prolonged effect. Subcutaneous implantation may be accomplished by making a small incision into the anesthetized skin, under aseptic precautions, and inserting the pellet. A skin suture and a pressure dressing usually will suffice to control the bleeding and keep the pellet in place. Implanting devices are available which automatically insert such pellets.

Hypodermoclysis

Large volumes of fluid (3 or 4 liters/day) can easily be given by this means. The most practical sites of administration are the anterior and lateral aspects of the thighs, the flanks, and the loose tissues at the sides of the chest below the axillas. The needles (2 inch, 22 gauge or less) are inserted hypodermically (*see* above) after the skin has been well cleansed (over an area of 10 cm. in diameter) with alcohol or a similar antiseptic. Usually, two needles are used, one for each side, and are introduced about 2 inches subcut. at an acute angle to the skin surface. The needles should be covered with sterile gauze and fastened to the skin with adhesive tape, in order to avoid their being pulled out or contaminated. The flow of fluid should not be too rapid, since overdistention of the tissues is painful. It is desirable to shut off the flow temporarily from time to time in order to permit the fluid to be absorbed and the distention decreased. Gentle massage of the area and local heat facilitate absorption and provide some relief of pain. To diminish the patient's discomfort, 30 cc. of 1% procaine may be added to each liter of solution administered after it has been made sure that the patient is not procaine-sensitive.

Hypodermoclysis usually is not successful in a patient who is in shock, or whose serum protein level is low, or whose heart is so damaged that local tissue edema is present. Only isotonic or approximately isotonic fluids should be administered in this manner.

Intramuscular Injections

Because of the relatively great vascularity of the muscles, drugs injected I.M. are absorbed more quickly than those given subcut. The favorite sites for I.M. injection are the deltoid or triceps muscles of the upper arm and the upper lateral quadrants of the buttocks. The skin should be cleansed with alcohol or similar antiseptic and the needle ($1\frac{1}{2}$ inch, 19 or 20 gauge) then inserted with a quick thrust at right angles to and through the skin and into the muscle. It is essential to aspirate before finally injecting, to make sure that the needle is not in a blood vessel. If blood is aspirated, withdraw needle and inject at a different site. Preparations with an oily base, e.g., procaine penicillin, estrogens, testosterone, and ephedrine, usually are given I.M.

Intravenous Administration (Venoclysis)

Injection of fluids by vein is indicated under the following circumstances: when rapid absorption is desired; when fluid cannot be taken by mouth; when it is too irritating to be given by hypodermic injection; and when the volume is so great that it could not be efficiently absorbed if given by hypodermoclysis. Fluids given by vein may, under certain circumstances, induce a febrile reaction and therefore should be administered with great care (see INFUSION REACTIONS). In patients with active cardiovascular disease, fluids should either not be given I.V. at all or else they should be administered slowly and in small amounts. A convenient way to ensure slow I.V. administration is to use a small-gauge needle (26 gauge). Certain medications should never be given by vein since they may cause dangerous reactions.

The veins most frequently utilized for medication are the

basilic and median cubital veins of the forearm. Others that may occasionally be employed are those on the dorsum of the hand, the anterior malleolar veins of the foot, veins of the leg, the external jugular vein, the femoral vein, and the superior sagittal sinus. The thin-walled, movable cutaneous veins often are more difficult to use than certain less conspicuous but fixed palpable deeper veins. In infants, the superior sagittal sinus, and the external jugular are frequently chosen.

The site of injection should be prepared by cleansing with a suitable antiseptic, following which the portion of the body involved should be placed in a comfortable position so that movement during the procedure is minimized. The veins are distended by applying a tourniquet. Gently slapping the area or milking the limb toward the tourniquet also is helpful in filling the veins. Before inserting the needle, all air must be removed from the syringe or tubing, in order to avoid air embolism. The point of the needle, with the bevel upward, is quickly inserted through the skin.

During insertion, the needle should be kept parallel and lateral to the vein so that the momentum, after the needle has traversed the skin, does not carry it on clear through the vein. Once through the skin, the needle is introduced into the vein at an oblique angle. When the vein is entered, blood escapes into the needle and can be seen in the glass adapter of the syringe or in that of the rubber tubing. At this point, the tourniquet is promptly released and the injection, or gravity flow, is begun.

For continuous I.V. administration of fluids, it is advisable to immobilize the needle. This is best accomplished by placing a piece of cotton or gauze beneath the hub of the needle to hold it at an angle of about 30 degrees, and anchoring it in this position with strips of adhesive tape. The rubber tubing also should be fixed in place with adhesive strapping.

The rate of flow should be regulated so that no more than 1 liter is given in 2 hours, or 120 drops/minute.

The causes of failure in starting or maintaining I.V. fluid administration are: (1) neglecting to release the tourniquet; (2) not having the needle in the lumen of the vein; (3) an obstruction in the needle; (4) allowing the bevel of the needle to rest too firmly against the inside of the vein wall; (5) a thrombosed vein.

Extravasation of fluid or blood into the tissues is a common complication of I.V. therapy. It usually is responsible for swelling and pain at the site of injection. The pain may be severe if the solution administered is hypertonic or acid or alkaline. Occasionally, extravasation is followed by a slough; therefore it is important to remove the needle immediately when extravasation is noted, and to massage the area so as to disperse the fluid more rapidly. The area may be infiltrated with physiologic saline or Water for Injection U.S.P. to dilute the irritant. The application of local heat also will help to relieve pain and promote the removal of the irritant substance.

In rare instances it is found necessary to cannulate a vein, because it is impossible to locate one large enough to be entered by a needle. This situation may be encountered when a patient is in shock and all normally accessible veins are collapsed, or in the obese, or the very young. Cannulation of a vein also is indicated when large amounts of fluid must be given within a short period of time. The anterior malleolar vein is usually best adapted for this purpose. Under local anesthesia and with aseptic precautions, the vein is exposed by incising the skin of the ankle directly over it. The vein then is tied off with a catgut ligature and a second ligature is passed proximal to the first, under the vein, but left untied. The vein is then cut partially through between the two ligatures. A cannula or a large bore needle (15 gauge) is inserted into the vein and the second ligature is tied around it. Sterile dressings should be applied and the rubber tubing securely fixed to the foot. Once the administration of fluid has been completed, the cannula can easily be removed by withdrawing it gently. The application of a pressure dressing will effectively complete the procedure.

Intramedullary

Although other sites occasionally are used for intramedullary injection (anterior superior spine of ilium and the tibia), the most frequent site is the sternomanubrial junction. After surgical preparation of the skin over the sternomanubrial junction, the area is anesthetized by injection of procaine 1%, subcut. and into the periosteum. The needle of the sternal puncture instrument is thrust through the skin at the angle of Louis, perpendicular to the surface of the sternum. Once it is through the skin, a boring motion is used to pass it through the external lamina of the bone. After penetration, the direction of the needle is changed so that it points upward. With the point of the needle in the marrow, the obturator is removed, the syringe attached, and suction applied to verify that the marrow space has been reached (and to obtain a specimen of bone marrow if such is the purpose of the procedure).

Fluids may be administered into the bone marrow when I.V. administration is not feasible. In such instances the sternal needle is merely attached to the infusion apparatus and fluids are given just as in I.V. administration.

Intracardiac

In certain emergencies, such as cardiac standstill, it may be necessary to inject a drug (e.g., epinephrine 1:1,000) directly into one of the cardiac chambers or the musculature, so that it may rapidly enter the circulation or stimulate the heart itself. In such extreme instances, the injection is accomplished by first surgically cleansing the skin in the precordial area and then quickly inserting the needle (usually 3- or 4-inch, 20 gauge) into the 4th intercostal space, just to the left of the sternum. Once the needle point has entered the cardiac chamber, blood can easily be aspirated into the syringe. In cardiac standstill, it is preferable to make the injection into the ventricular wall. This is done by first entering the cardiac chamber, as above, then withdrawing the needle point slightly until blood no longer can be aspirated. Whether into the chamber or the muscle of the heart, the injection is made rapidly and the needle immediately thereafter completely withdrawn.

Intrathecal

In order most satisfactorily and safely to introduce a needle into the subdural space of the spinal cord, the patient should be made to lie on his side at the edge of the bed or table with his spine in hyperflexion. Extreme flexion is best obtained by having the patient draw his knees upward and force his head downward. Placing him with his spine in hyperflexion often is effective also as a means of restraint during the procedure. However, some physicians prefer a method of lumbar puncture, which they use successfully with the patient sitting bent forward on a stool, or even when he is kept lying comfortably stretched out on his side.

The site usually selected for lumbar puncture is in the midline between the 3rd and 4th lumbar vertebrae. The skin in this area should be surgically prepared with a suitable antiseptic and the area anesthetized with procaine 1% by first using a hypodermic injection, followed by one employing a 2-inch, small (21) gauge needle inserted deeply.

It often is helpful to mark the site of puncture before administering the local anesthetic. The intervertebral space between the 3rd and 4th lumbar vertebrae is easily identified by drawing an imaginary line from the top of one iliac crest to the other. Careful palpation will reveal the depression between the spines of the vertebrae. The lumbar puncture needle then is inserted through the skin in the midline between the spines. Once through the skin, the needle is directed slightly upward while being passed inward. If it impinges upon the bone it should be withdrawn and reinserted in a different direction. The bevel of the needle should be kept facing laterally so as to separate the fibers of the ligaments and the dura without breaking or tearing through them. When the needle penetrates the dura a slight "give," or sensation of released resistance, may be felt. The stylet of the needle then is withdrawn and drops of spinal fluid will at once appear. Spinal fluid should be removed cautiously since, in some cases of skull fracture or brain tumor, rapid removal may have serious consequences. An amount of fluid should be withdrawn equal to the volume of medicament to be introduced or sufficient for the laboratory investigation planned. In some instances, the removed fluid is used as a diluent for the medicament to be injected. Intrathecal injections should be made slowly. Drugs commonly injected intrathecally include streptomycin, penicillin, and procaine.

Rectal

Drugs may be given per rectum either in the form of liquids (e.g., Avertin, paraldehyde) or suppositories (e.g., aminophylline, benzocaine) for local or systemic effect. In such instances, absorption from the rectum and colon often may prove to be faster and of greater degree than from the small intestine after oral administration. Enemas used for medication should be as small as possible, yet not so concentrated as to produce local irritation. The usual volume is 25 to 75 cc. (For details of administration of nutrients per rectum, see BEDSIDE PROC.)

Vaginal

Most medication via this route is for local effect and the drug used may be either in the form of suppository (e.g., penicillin), powder (e.g., silver picrate), or paint (e.g., gentian violet). Occasionally, a medicament, such as penicillin, may be given in this manner for systemic effect because absorption occurs so readily through the vaginal mucosa. (See BEDSIDE PROC. for details on vaginal douching.)

LOCAL ANESTHESIA

Procaine hydrochloride is the drug most frequently used as a local anesthetic. The 1% solution containing epinephrine is preferred by most physicians, since the concentration is low yet effective, and the epinephrine serves to sustain the anesthesia.

The patient to be operated upon should be reclining if possible and, when the procedure is to be extensive, he should receive a preoperative hypodermic injection of morphine 10 or 15 mg. (gr. ⅙ or ¼) and occasionally scopolamine 0.4 mg. (gr. ¹⁄₁₅₀). Preoperative administration of a quick-acting barbiturate alone, such as pentobarbital 0.1 Gm. (gr. iss) often provides sufficient sedation for the performance of minor operations (see PREOPERATIVE AND POSTOPERATIVE CARE).

Regional anesthesia is achieved by blocking off the sensory nerves at some distance from the region (nerve blocking) or by blocking nerve endings in the region itself (infiltration). The procedure is begun by sterilizing with an antiseptic the area of skin to be operated on, then producing a small wheal in the skin with a short, fine caliber needle (½ inch, 26 gauge). The needle then is slowly advanced deeply into the tissues while injection of the anesthetic solution is made ahead of it. This principle of advancing the needle with the anesthetic preceding it should always be followed. From 2 to 4 cc. of solution should be injected for each 6 sq. cm. (1 square inch) infiltrated.

If long flexible needles are properly used a large area can be covered without raising additional wheals. Subcutaneous wheals may be made around the original intradermal wheal when only a superficial anesthesia is desired.

Should a reaction to procaine occur following accidental penetration of a vein or because of drug sensitivity, caffeine 0.5 Gm. or Sodium Amytal 0.5 Gm. (gr. viiss) should be given I.V. Patients experiencing mild reactions need be treated only with a few inhalations of ether, after which they should be placed temporarily in the head-down position.

ASPIRATION OF FLUIDS

Venipuncture

This often is performed to obtain blood for laboratory examination. Apply a tourniquet to the extremity and then insert the needle into the vein (as described above under Intravenous Injection) and aspirate with the tourniquet kept in place until just before withdrawing the needle. Occasionally, an emergency arises in which it is necessary to remove a large volume of blood and quickly reduce the circulatory volume, e.g., in the course of acute cardiac failure. The usual technic is to insert a large-bore needle into an accessible vein (median cephalic or basilic) under sterile precautions, after injecting a local anesthetic and applying a tourniquet. The needle should be inserted in a direction opposite to the flow of blood. The blood may be allowed to run through sterile tubing into a flask or basin. In some instances, the vein is simply incised (phlebotomy) instead of punctured with a needle. This should be done under strictly sterile conditions and with the aid of a local anesthetic. If the flow of blood is great at first and then diminishes, loosen the tourniquet somewhat, since it may have been so tight as to stop the arterial flow.

Arterial Puncture

The brachial or the femoral artery is most frequently selected for this procedure. The site is easily marked after palpation of the pulse. The skin over the artery is prepared with a suitable antiseptic, the area is anesthetized with 1% procaine and the procedure carried out under sterile conditions. The needle (1½ inch, 20 gauge) usually is easily inserted into the artery and, upon its entry, blood surges into the syringe. Arterial puncture usually is performed to obtain a sample of arterial blood for determination of its O_2 content. In such instances, about 2 cc. of sterile oil is first placed into the syringe. The blood is evacuated into tubes containing oil, with care not to expose it to the air. Medicaments may be injected intra-arterially once the needle point is within the arterial lumen. This procedure has been used for injection of penicillin solution into patients suffering from peripheral vascular disease. By this means a high concentration of penicillin is obtained in the blood reaching the peripheral vascular lesion.

Sternal, Iliac Crest, or Tibial Puncture (*see* Intramedullary Puncture, above)

Paracentesis Abdominis

Puncture of the abdominal cavity in order to remove fluids or inject various therapeutic agents is best performed with the patient on a stool. The bladder should be empty and the skin below the umbilicus and overlying the rectus muscles prepared with iodine or other suitable antiseptic. The skin and underlying tissues are anesthetized with procaine 1%. The trochar should be inserted in the midline below the umbilicus and approximately ⅓ of the distance to the pubis. This site should be high enough to avoid the bladder. Since the trochar is of rather large caliber, it usually is best to make a small skin incision (0.25 to 0.5 cm.). The trochar should not be inserted any farther through the abdominal wall than is necessary to penetrate to the peritoneum. If omentum or intestine is swept up against the trochar opening, the flow will be stopped. A slight, cautious change in position usually remedies this situation. It is advisable not to withdraw fluid too rapidly nor to remove too much at one time due to the danger of circulatory collapse as the abdominal veins become refilled.

Thoracentesis

Before attempting to aspirate fluid from the pleural cavity, the site of fluid accumulation should be determined by physical and radiographic examination. Aspiration is best performed, whenever feasible, with the patient in the sitting position, otherwise, he should lie on his side, with the affected hemithorax uppermost. The site of thoracentesis depends on the findings, but the one most frequently used is the 7th interspace, just below the angle of the scapula in the posterior axillary line. The needle is inserted close to the superior edge of the lower rib so as to avoid the intercostal nerve and vessels which lie at the lower edge of the upper rib. After the skin has been cleansed with an appropriate antiseptic, the area is anesthetized, infiltration extending down to the pleura. The aspirating needle is introduced through the skin and then cautiously through the chest wall until it has just penetrated the pleura. Upon puncturing the pleura there may be felt a slight snap or a noticeable "give." Care must be taken not to injure the lung parenchyma or to permit entrance of air into the pleural cavity. In administering pneumothorax, air is deliberately placed in the pleural cavity in controlled amounts and therefore the entrance of unmeasured quantities is to be avoided as is the case in aspiration of pleural fluid. The needle having been successfully inserted into the chest wall so that the point is just within the intrapleural space, aspiration of pleural fluid is performed by keeping a negative pressure in the syringe. When the procedure has been completed, the wound should be sealed with collodion to prevent leakage.

Pericardial Paracentesis

Aspiration of pericardial fluid is indicated when an excessive accumulation produces compression or tamponade of the heart. The area most satisfactory for pericardial paracentesis is the 5th left intercostal space, 1 to 2 cm. mesial to the left outer border of cardiac dullness. Using a fine needle, 25 or 26 gauge, the skin is infiltrated with procaine 1% after having been surgically cleansed with a suitable antiseptic. The aspirating needle (2½ inch, 18 gauge) is cautiously inserted at a right angle to the skin, while a negative pressure in the syringe is maintained by pulling on the plunger. When the pericardial space is entered, fluid will be aspirated. The needle should not be inserted any deeper than necessary since it may puncture the heart.

Paracentesis of the Tympanum (*see* Myringotomy, *under* OTITIS MEDIA)

Lumbar Puncture

(For details of spinal needle insertion, *see* Intrathecal Administration, above.) Once the needle is in place, it is advisable to note the spinal fluid pressure before and after taking a specimen.

The presence or absence of hydrostatic block may be determined by means of the Queckenstedt test. This is performed by putting pressure upon the jugular veins bilaterally, with the result that egress of blood from the cranium is interfered with and the intracranial pressure increased. This causes increase of pressure within the spinal canal, provided no obstruction exists. This test should not be performed on a patient who may have a tumor of the medulla, since the increased intracranial pressure may force the cerebellum and medulla into the foramen magnum with unfortunate, perhaps fatal, results. This may occur if too much fluid is removed rapidly, especially when the intracranial pressure is elevated.

Cisternal Puncture

This more heroic procedure is indicated when the conditions described above are suspected, or when intracranial administration of therapeutic materials or aspiration of fluid or blood is essential. This procedure should be undertaken only by a well qualified physician. The scalp over the base of the skull should be shaved and the area prepared surgically with antiseptic. Procaine 1% is injected for local anesthesia. Under aseptic conditions, a large spinal needle (18 gauge) is inserted, with the bevel directed caudally, in the exact midline just at the

upper border of the 1st cervical spinous process. The needle
must at all times be kept in the midline and directed at a
point in the exact midline at the usual level of the brow hair
line. When the needle has passed through the skin and outer
ligaments, the stylet is removed. A steady and gradual advancement of the needle can be obtained by holding it with
both forefingers and thumbs, keeping the remaining fingers
against the neck and head. As soon as the needle penetrates
the dura (less than 3 cm. deep), spinal fluid usually appears.
Once the needle point is in the cisternal space, fluid may be
removed or medicaments introduced.

Gastric and Intestinal Aspirations

Lavage of the stomach may be called for when poisonous
substances have been ingested. Solutions used are sodium bicarbonate (5%), tap water, physiologic saline, and antidotes
(*see* POISONING). This procedure also is useful to relieve nausea
and vomiting and gastric dilatation. It should not be carried
out within 3 to 5 hours after a meal except in an absolute
emergency. The tube is passed with the patient sitting up.
Placing the tube in ice prior to insertion may be helpful, since
this stiffens the rubber. By passing the moist tube along the
roof of the mouth and then having the patient swallow continuously and breathe deeply once the tube enters the pharynx,
passage to the stomach can easily be accomplished. Before administering fluids, care should be taken to see that the tube is
not in the trachea. A simple test consists of placing the end of
the tube under water; if the trachea has been entered, bubbling
will occur; also, entrance into the trachea usually causes violent
coughing. For lavage, approximately 1 pint of the desired
solution is administered through the funnel; then aspiration is
begun and the stomach contents siphoned off. The process
should be repeated until the return is clear. The tube should
be pinched tightly during withdrawal to avoid spillage into
the trachea. Fluid nourishment can be administered through
the tube, but should be given at a slower rate and, of course,
left in the stomach.

Since the standard stomach tube is of large caliber (usually
14 mm. diameter) it often is difficult to pass it by mouth and
it can be kept in place for only a short time. A smaller caliber
tube therefore may sometimes be preferable: The Rehfuss tube
is 4 mm. in diameter and is equipped at the end with a metal
"bucket," or "olive," which the patient swallows. The danger
of getting the tube into the trachea is thus obviated. The
Levin tube is of the same diameter and has several openings at
the tip. It can be passed via the mouth or nose. Another tube
frequently passed into and through the stomach is the Miller-
Abbott tube. This is much longer than the others and has a
balloon at its end which can be blown up after the tube has
been passed. The inflated balloon fills the lumen of the gut and

the tube then may be moved along by peristaltic action. These smaller diameter tubes are usually employed for the administration of fluids, aspiration of intestinal contents, or relief of dilatation, especially when these procedures are to be of long duration. Graduated markings on the tubes, when opposite the level of the incisor teeth, indicate the penetration already achieved. The average length of tube passed for gastric aspiration in adults is 55 cm., and for duodenal (biliary) aspiration 75 cm. A tube may kink up within the lumen of the tract, and checking by fluoroscope or X-ray film is a wise safeguard. No tube should be left too long in place since the irritation may cause esophageal ulceration.

Continuous aspiration may be provided by attaching the tube, once it has been passed, to a Wangensteen apparatus. This consists of 3 bottles so arranged that water dripping from 1 bottle into a 2nd causes negative pressure in the 3rd. The empty 3rd bottle becomes the receptacle for fluid and gases aspirated from the intestinal tract. This apparatus and the indwelling tube should be checked frequently to make sure that no obstructions or kinks develop, and to change the positions of the bottles so that the negative pressure is continuously maintained.

CIRCULATION TIME DETERMINATION

The following procedures may be of diagnostic and prognostic value in disorders such as congestive heart failure, congenital heart disease, and hyperthyroidism. Right circuit (arm-to-lung) time is measured by rapidly injecting Ether U.S.P. (0.3 cc.), plus sterile physiologic saline (0.7 cc.), into the antecubital vein and then having the patient report the moment he detects the odor of ether in his exhaled breath. The normal value for the right circuit is between 3.5 and 9 seconds.

Right and left circuit time is approximated by quickly injecting calcium gluconate, sodium dehydrocholate or saccharin into the antecubital vein and recording the instant the patient feels a sensation of warmth, or a bitter or a sweet taste, respectively. The normal time for the left and right circuit for calcium gluconate is 10 to 16 seconds; for sodium dehydrocholate, 8 to 14 seconds; and for saccharin, 9 to 16 seconds.

BEDSIDE PROCEDURES

Here are described briefly a number of important nursing procedures. Many of these require the services of an experienced nurse; others are simple enough to be carried out by untrained attendants in the patient's home. In either case, it is essential that the physician, who is primarily responsible for

the welfare and treatment of his patient, should have a knowledge of routine nursing technics so that he may supervise or
instruct as the situation demands.

Advice on how to feed patients will be given here, while
the appropriate foods are discussed in the Diets chapter. Many
procedures in which the nurse is called upon to assist the physician are detailed in the chapter on Clinical Procedures. A
separate chapter has been devoted to Preoperative and Postoperative Care.

ROUTINE NURSING CARE

The attention given to a patient's comfort, environment,
personal hygiene, and feeding will do much to lessen complications, promote recovery, and hasten convalescence.

Nurses and all other attendants must maintain absolute
cleanliness of their persons and clothing and be free from colds
or other infections. The sickroom should be clean and well ventilated at all times, and free from drafts and glare, but with
sufficient light, properly placed, for the patient's needs. Unnecessary noises or other interruptions to the patient's rest
must be avoided. Unpleasant odors in the room may be
masked by a spray containing ½ tsp. each of oil of clove and
oil of lavender in 1 pt. of water.

Unless specifically contraindicated, the position in which the
patient will be most comfortable should be sought. In the
home, a satisfactory sloping back rest may be provided by
using the back of a small chair, turned on its face with its legs
braced against the headboard of the bed. A pillow under the
knees will add materially to the patient's comfort, and one
placed between the sheets at the foot of the bed will relieve
pressure of the bedclothes on the patient's feet. When the
patient sits up in bed, a pillow under the forearms is restful.

A reasonable amount of movement in bed and directed leg
exercises are to be encouraged as prophylaxis against hypostatic
pneumonia (q.v.) or venous thrombosis (q.v.). These exercises
may consist of rolling from side to side, flexing the hips and
knees, and pressing the feet against the foot of the bed.

The temperature, pulse, and respiration should be taken and
recorded every 4 hours during an acute illness, but only 2 or 3
times daily during convalescence or a chronic illness. In infants and children, the normals for these determinations tend
to be higher than in adults; the temperature range is 99° to
99.6° F.; the pulse rate is about 140/minute at birth and 110
to 120 at 1 year; thereafter it gradually slows to an average of
72 for males and 80 for females beyond 14 years; the respiration
rate is about 40/minute at birth and 30 at 1 year; the adult
rate of 17 to 20 becoming gradually established by the 16th
year. Depending on the patient's illness and the physician's
orders, it may sometimes be desirable to note and record such
additional data as fluid intake and output, bowel movements,

appearance of stools, urinary frequency, production of sputum, and the like.

Care of the Bed

The bedstead should be dusted daily and washed as necessary. When indicated, rubber sheeting is placed under the lower sheet and pillow case. To change the sheets while the patient is in bed, proceed as follows: Loosen all the bedclothes at the edges; place the patient (safely) near one edge of the bed; go to the opposite side of the bed and roll the soiled undersheet lengthwise toward the patient (if there is a rubber sheet to be replaced, roll this also; or leave it in place, wash with soap and water and dry thoroughly); place clean sheet on mattress in the position it is to occupy and push the farther edge up to the patient's body, tucking the sheet in at head and foot on the unoccupied side; then go to the opposite side of the bed and turn the patient over onto the clean sheet; remove the soiled sheet; pull the remaining half of the clean sheet over and tuck it in tightly and smoothly on all sides. The upper bedclothes and pillow case are easily replaced in the usual manner.

Care of the Skin, Nails, and Hair

A daily bath in a warm room is both cleansing and refreshing to most patients. If a bed bath is necessary, a foot tub half full of water at a temperature of 110° F. is placed near the bed together with soap, toothbrush, dentifrice, talcum powder, washcloth, and towels. (It is desirable to have the patient first use the bedpan.) The patient's teeth should then be brushed, with the bedding protected by a towel. Pillow and all bedclothes except the sheets then are removed. Next, a bath blanket should replace the upper sheet, and another bath blanket or rubber sheet may be placed beneath the patient (using the technic outlined above for changing sheets). The eyes are bathed with washcloth and clear water. Face, neck, and ears then are washed with soap and water. The foot tub is brought to the bed, and the patient's hands are immersed and washed; the nails are cleaned, and trimmed if necessary. The tub then is removed from the bed, and small areas of the body are uncovered at a time, each being washed, dried, sprinkled with talcum powder, and covered before proceeding to another area. Special care should be given to cleansing the armpits, umbilicus, genitals, and buttocks, placing the patient in a suitable position to make these sites accessible. Set the basin on the bed and allow the patient to place one or both feet in the water to soak a few minutes; this helps to keep the skin and nails soft.

The hair should be thoroughly combed every morning and evening. Obstinate tangles usually can be loosened with 50% alcohol solution. Sometimes the hair becomes so matted as to require cutting. In a hospital, this should be done only after securing a signed consent from the patient or his guardian. Evidence of pediculosis, excessive dandruff, or scalp eruptions should be noted and suitably treated (*see* appropriate chapters in section on Skin and Connective Tissues). The hair should be washed at least once a month. If the patient cannot be taken to the sink, he should be moved to the edge of the bed, and his head elevated by a hard pillow under the neck and shoulders. The bedclothes and the upper part of his body are protected with bath towels and rubber sheeting beneath the head and shoulders. The edges of the overhanging rubber sheeting may be rolled to form a trough which will carry off the water to a pail at the side of the bed. Liquid castile soap is rubbed into the hair and scalp, and water is poured on from a small pitcher. After the shampoo, the hair is dried and, in the case of women, it may be braided.

Alcohol back rubs, followed by talcum powder, are refreshing and may be given several times daily. Bed sores are prone to develop, particularly over the bony prominences, in debilitated or chronically ill patients; if impending or evident, such lesions should be treated intensively (*see* Decubitus). The frequent cleansing, alcohol rubs, and changes of position described above are prophylactic.

Feeding the Patient

A bed patient should be offered a bedpan and a wash basin before receiving the tray. He should be placed in a comfortable position for eating; the food should be attractively served and the tray put within convenient reach. It may be necessary to give assistance, such as cutting meat or spreading butter. It may be necessary to feed patients whose physical activity is sharply restricted, even though they may be elevated to a sitting position in bed. After the meal the patient should be made clean and comfortable. Attention to these details and the creation of a cheerful atmosphere, if possible, help to maintain the patient's nutrition. If the patient is unable to sit up, solid foods must be given him slowly and in small amounts. For drinking, his head should be raised slightly, supported, and liquids given from a cup (regular or equipped with a spout) or, preferably, through a drinking tube.

With delirious, psychotic, or unconscious patients any removable denture must be removed. Such persons must never be fed with a drinking tube or sharp utensils. Liquids are given very slowly, using a spoon, a rubber syringe, or a medicine dropper with a long rubber tip. If the patient cannot swallow, tube feedings are indicated (*see* Clin. Proc.). Restraints (q.v.) may be needed for a restless patient.

Dental and Oral Hygiene

To promote cleanliness and prevent oral infection, the teeth should be brushed for 3 to 5 minutes at least twice daily, using any preferred dentifrice, salt, or baking soda. During this brushing, frequent rinsings are required to wash out loose particles of food. Dentures should be washed with cold water after each meal. Any evidence of oral infection should be noted and intensive treatment instituted (*see* STOMATITIS). Dry or chapped lips should be treated with a glycerin preparation or petrolatum salve.

In helpless, but conscious, individuals, the teeth must be cleaned by the nurse, care being taken to avoid gagging the patient lest vomiting result. For this reason, it is wise to postpone toothbrushing for ½ hour after a meal.

In unconscious or semiconscious patients, the jaw is held open by a tongue blade wrapped heavily with gauze. The teeth and mouth are cleansed with cotton applicators, or cotton balls or gauze (held firmly in an artery clamp), which have been moistened with Tincture of Myrrh U.S.P. or a 1:4 solution of hydrogen peroxide. The lips and tongue may be kept moist with a mixture of equal parts of glycerin and lemon juice. Mouthwashes may be required for a dyspneic patient whose mouth is dry and parched.

ENEMAS

Cleansing enemas are used to promote bowel evacuation by softening the feces and stimulating peristalsis. Carminative enemas serve to relieve distention. Retention enemas act to soothe or lubricate the rectal mucosa, to apply absorbable or local medicaments, and to soften feces. Other types are nutrient enemas (*see* Proctoclysis) and colonic irrigations (q.v.).

The patient should lie, on his side preferably, with the upper thigh flexed (Sims' position). The solution should always be administered at or just above body temperature. With the irrigating can held or suspended 12 to 18 in. above the anus, the air and any cooled solution in the tubing are expelled and the lubricated catheter or rectal tip then is gently inserted into the rectum for about 2 to 4 inches. The solution is administered slowly, over a period of 5 to 10 minutes if necessary, to prevent acute discomfort. Should cramps occur due to overstimulation of the bowel, the flow must be temporarily stopped by pinching the tube. Gentle pressure against the anus with a folded towel may prevent the expulsion of solution and tube. The enema tube should be clamped during its withdrawal to prevent spillage. A toilet stool or warmed bedpan must be readily accessible.

Cleansing Enemas: The principal solutions used are tap water, weak soapsuds (with any mild soap), and saline (1 tsp. salt to 1 pt. water). Quantities are 1 pt. for children, 1 qt. for adults. If possible, cleansing enemas should be retained for 5 to 10 minutes.

For colostomy irrigation, the procedure is the same as for a cleansing enema except that a lubricated catheter is inserted through the colostomy opening. The proximal loop of the colostomy is irrigated first and then the distal portion.

Carminative Enemas: (NOTE: Abdominal distention often may be relieved by the insertion of a rectal tube, or by the application of a flaxseed poultice or hot stupes containing water or 1:3 turpentine in oil, to the abdomen.) Where carminative enemas are necessary, they are administered in the same manner as the cleansing variety. The preparations used include:

1. **Milk and molasses:** Add 8 oz. of molasses slowly to an equal amount of warm (115° F.) milk.
2. **Turpentine and oil:** Add ½ oz. oil of turpentine to 6 oz. of warm (110° F.) olive oil. Follow in ½ to 1 hour with a cleansing enema of weak soap solution (q.v.).
3. **Turpentine and soap suds:** Add ½ oz. oil of turpentine to 8 oz. of warm (110° F.) weak soap solution (½ oz. soap to 1 pt. water). (CAUTION! Not to be retained.)
4. **Sugar and soda:** Use 8 oz. each of sugar, soda, and water.

Retention Enemas: The patient must first be told that the solution is not to be expelled but retained within the rectum until the next bowel movement takes place. Administration should be extremely slow to avoid stimulating peristalsis. The principal types of retention enema are:

1. **Emollient:** Mix 1 to 2 tsp. starch with sufficient cold water to make a thin paste; add 5 oz. boiling water, and boil for 5 minutes.
2. **Lubricant:** 3 to 6 oz. of olive, cottonseed, or mineral oil.
3. **Medicated:** 6 to 8 oz. coffee, or 1 oz. whisky added to 6 oz. isotonic saline, may be given for their stimulating effect. Other medicines should be diluted with 2 to 4 oz. of water or olive oil.

CATHETERIZATION

Catheterization of the bladder is indicated to combat urinary retention or to ensure an empty bladder. Sterile technic is absolutely essential. The meatus is first cleansed with green soap and water. A soft rubber catheter, lubricated with a sterile water-soluble jelly or boiled mineral oil is then slowly inserted (from a sterile basin) through the meatus and into the bladder. In males, while the gloved hand manipulates the catheter, light traction should be put on the penis by the ungloved hand in order to straighten out the urethra during passage. Should the progress of the catheter be obstructed, a smaller catheter may be tried, but force must never be applied. In the presence of pronounced urethral obstruction, as from stricture or an enlarged prostate, catheterization should be performed only by a qualified urologist.

IRRIGATIONS

Irrigations are given at low pressure to cleanse, soothe, deodorize, or medicate wounds, body orifices, or body cavities. Irrigations also are employed to promote healing and to hasten suppuration. Sterile solutions are indicated for use in wounds and in the normally sterile body cavities. The solution should be at or somewhat above body temperature (100° to 120° F.), and the temperature may be kept constant by means of hot water bottles around the irrigating can. Air and any cooled solution must be expelled from the tube before the irrigation is started; after which the flow of fluid should be even and uninterrupted; force should not be used under any circumstances. The patient's position should be such that gravity will aid in draining off the irrigating fluid conveniently and comfortably.

Eye: Solutions used include sterile boric acid (2%), normal saline, or bichloride of mercury (1:10,000). If only one eye is infected, the other should be protected with an eye shield. After separation of the lids, avoiding pressure on the eyeball, the flow is directed from the inner to the outer canthus. The rubber tip of the irrigating bulb must be close to the eye but not touching it. A kidney basin is held to catch the overflow. Anywhere from 1 oz. to 1 qt. may be necessary to accomplish a thorough irrigation, after which the eye is dried with sterile gauze. The attendant's hands must be thoroughly washed before touching the opposite eye.

Ear: Solutions for irrigation of the external auditory canal include soda bicarbonate (1 to 2%), isotonic saline (0.9%), and tap water. Impacted cerumen may be softened with hydrogen peroxide solution, glycerin, or olive oil prior to attempted removal by irrigation. Ear irrigations must always be applied at low pressure; if the drum is perforated irrigations must be done with extreme caution, *if at all.*

Nose: Solutions include physiologic saline, boric acid (2%), and soda bicarbonate (1 to 2%). After the patient has blown his nose, his head is placed with the unaffected nostril uppermost so that the flow will be from the normal to the affected naris. A minim medicine dropper is used as an irrigating nozzle. The irrigating can is held 2 in. above the upper nostril. The patient breathes through his mouth during the irrigation and is instructed to pinch the tube whenever he feels it necessary to stop the flow. Each nostril is irrigated with 2 to 3 oz. of solution at a time. After the treatment, the nose should not be blown for at least 3 minutes.

Throat: Solutions up to 1 qt. of warm (120° F.) physiologic saline (0.9%), tap water, boric acid (2%), or soda bicarbonate (1 to 2%) are employed. With the patient's head dropped so that his chin touches his chest, place the irrigating can 1 to 2 ft. above. A glass irrigating tip is inserted into his mouth as far as the 2nd or 3rd molar, and the solution is directed over all parts of the affected area. The patient is instructed to avoid swallowing, and the flow is stopped by compressing the tube whenever necessary to allow easier breathing.

Bladder: Solutions for intermittent irrigation include 1 pt. or more of sterile distilled water, boric acid (2%), potassium permanganate (1:3,000 to 1:5,000), protargol (1:1,000), silver nitrate (1:1,000), or argyrol (1 to 3%). Other solutions are often used for specific purposes. The patient is catheterized and a funnel is attached to the air-free catheter (or suprapubic tube, if present). From 3 to 4 oz. of solution is allowed to flow slowly into the bladder from a height of 6 to 12 in. and then made to run out into a basin by lowering and inverting the funnel. After this procedure has been carried out twice, the catheter is removed (but not a suprapubic tube, if in use). A special method of irrigating and emptying the bladder at regular intervals in cases of neurogenic bladder is known as Munro-Tidal drainage. For details of the apparatus and the technic, the reader is referred to textbooks on nursing or urology.

Vagina: From 1 to 2 qts. of warm (105° to 115° F.) tap water, isotonic saline (0.9%), boric acid (2%), lysol (0.2 to 0.5%), soda bicarbonate (1 to 2%), green soap (1%), potassium permanganate (0.1 to 1%), bichloride of mercury (1:3,000 to 1:10,000), or vinegar (1 oz./qt.) may be used. Sterile solutions are required if the douche follows any operative procedure on the vagina or cervix. The douche pan should be warmed and the irrigating can held 12 to 18 in. above the vagina. The douche nozzle is inserted up to the cervix with a gentle rotating motion and the solution allowed to run in by gravity; pressure must never be used, although it is permissible to balloon out the vagina by closing the labia intermittently during the douche.

Colon: (Enteroclysis): Suitable solutions include 2 to 3 gallons, at a temperature of 105° to 110° F., of tap water, isotonic saline (0.9%), or soda bicarbonate (1 to 5%). Colonic irrigations are given to provide fluid, cleanse the colon, relieve intestinal colic, and supply warmth. The objective is to inject a steady stream of fluid under low pressure into the colon, with provision for immediate escape of all fluid not absorbed. A cleansing enema (q.v.) should be given at least ½ hour before the treatment. The lubricated inflow catheter (Fr. 14) is inserted 6 in. into the rectum, whereas the larger, outflow, lubricated catheter (Fr. 32) is inserted only 4 in. Both tubes are then fastened to the buttocks with adhesive tape. After all air has been expelled from the tubing attached to the irrigating can, the tubing is connected with the inflow catheter; the outflow catheter is attached to a tube whose free end rests in a bedpan. The outflow tube should be clamped shut until 1 qt. of solution has been given, after which it is unclamped and the remainder of the solution administered slowly and evenly at the rate of 1 gal./15 minutes. If cramps occur, the inflow must be temporarily discontinued until they cease, and the irrigation then is resumed at a slower rate. The outflow tube should be observed for signs of clogging, in which case the inflow is stopped while the outflow catheter is removed, cleansed, and reinserted. During withdrawal the tubes are pinched to avoid spillage.

PROCTOCLYSIS

Murphy Drip: Fluids, nutrients, and medicaments, at body temperature, may be administered through a lubricated rectal catheter inserted into the rectum to a depth of 4 in. A preliminary cleansing enema should be given. Hypotonic solutions are absorbed best; these include tap water, physiologic saline (0.9%), glucose (2 to 5%, never stronger), soda bicarbonate (2 to 5%), or the desired medicine dissolved in distilled water. A single proctoclysis should not exceed 6 oz. It is administered slowly, at a rate of 40 to 60 drops/minute to avoid stimulating peristalsis. The solution in the clysis bottle is kept at the desired temperature by means of hot water bottles, and about 18 to 24 in. above the patient's buttocks. The patient's position should be changed frequently during the clysis. Should gaseous cramps occur, the gas is allowed to escape by clamping the tube and disconnecting the catheter for a few moments. The patient should urinate frequently to reduce the sensation of pressure in the abdomen. If nausea, abdominal pain, or severe distention develops, the clysis must be discontinued.

Harris Drip: Abdominal distention may be prevented or relieved by repeatedly siphoning warm tap water (maintained at 105° F. by means of hot water bottles around the irrigating can) into and out of the rectum through a lubricated rectal tip or catheter inserted 4 in. into the rectum. In addition, some absorption of fluid can occur. With the irrigating tube free of air and attached to the rectal tip or catheter, the inflow is started by raising the irrigating can 1 ft. above the buttocks; the return is secured by lowering the can 1 ft. below the buttocks. When siphonage has become established by repeating this procedure 3 or 4 times, the can is placed on a level with the rectum; as flatus escapes, the solution flows back and forth. At intervals of at least every 45 minutes, more frequently if distention and discomfort occur, the can is raised and lowered to maintain siphonage and the soiled solution is replaced with a fresh supply, the amount absorbed being measured in the process. The can must never be allowed to empty completely lest air be drawn into the bowel.

STEAM INHALATIONS

Steam inhalations promote expectoration, moisten the inspired air, and help to relieve inflammation and spasm in the respiratory tract. Steam may be derived from any kitchen utensil containing boiling water (CAUTION! Avoid danger of spilling) or from an electric steam vaporizer. The steam is administered to the patient through a paper cone, under a large towel or other canopy, in a croup tent, or freely within the room. The last named method is preferable in most instances. Compound tincture of benzoin, oil of turpentine, menthol, creosote, oil of eucalyptol, and other drugs may be added to the water (1 tsp./qt.) each time the vaporiums are used. The inhalations should continue for 20 to 30 minutes or continuously, when used freely in the room, care being taken between and during treatments to avoid either chilling or burning the patient. An electric steam generator must never be allowed to run dry, lest it become a fire hazard. (Benzoin stains may be removed from utensils with benzine and from linen with ether or denatured alcohol.)

POSTURAL DRAINAGE

Postural drainage prevents the accumulation of pulmonary secretions in the presence of such conditions as chronic bronchitis, bronchiectasis, and pulmonary abscess. The patient's head and shoulders are placed lower than his waist, i.e., by having him lean face down over the edge of the bed, or by raising the foot of the bed. Thus drainage, especially from the lower lobes, is aided by gravity. Egress of material from the right or left lung can be favored by placing that side uppermost. At first the procedure should be carried out for only 1 minute twice a day, so as to avoid the production of nausea and dizziness; this period may be gradually increased, as tolerated, to 15 to 20 minutes twice daily.

EXTERNAL APPLICATIONS

Applications are used to supply heat, cold, or a medication to part or all of the body, and may be carried out in a variety of ways.

Local Applications

Moist heat: The object of applying moist heat to the body is to ease pain, supply moisture, and promote circulation, muscle relaxation, or wound drainage. It may be given in the form of soaks or compresses, which also serve to wash away any discharge that may be present. The principal solutions employed are water, isotonic salt solution (0.9%), magnesium sulfate (3 to 6%), and boric acid (3%), but many other medicinal substances sometimes are applied as dressings. Hypertonic solutions are useful in drawing water out of the tissues at the site of application, when this is desirable. Sterile solutions and compresses are required for use on open wounds. All solutions should be at a temperature of about 120° F. when applied, and may be kept warm by repeatedly adding small amounts of reasonably hot solution. Moist compresses, using cotton, gauze, flannel, or towels, may be kept at the desired temperature by overlaying with one or more hot water bottles and enclosing the whole area in oilskin or cellophane; this also will prevent rapid drying out of the compress. Electric pads must not be used in this manner because of the danger of electric shock (q.v.) in the presence of moisture. Moist heat may be applied intermittently, or almost continuously with brief interruptions to permit some drying of the skin and thereby avoid maceration or waterlogging.

Dry heat: Hot bricks, salt bags, hot water bottles, heat lamps, electric pads, or diathermy are all safe means of applying local heat, if judiciously used. The degree of heat should be such as to produce a comfortable and soothing sensation of warmth. Towels are placed next to the skin to absorb perspiration and also to prevent overheating, especially of the bony prominences. Hot objects must never be applied to patients who are asleep or unconscious.

The heat produced by short-wave diathermy is the most penetrating and also the most dangerous; the patient must always be told beforehand that he need not endure intense heat in order to obtain relief, and instructed to mention any discomfort immediately. All metal objects must be removed from the field during treatment, and collection on the skin of pools of perspiration must be combated by the use of absorbent towels or other wrappings. A patient receiving heat from a radiant lamp or diathermy should never be left alone without having easy access to the switch so that he may stop the flow of current in case of overheating. Automatic timers are useful for keeping the treatments within safe limits.

Plasters (poultices): Various materials are used as plasters for the relief of local pain. Flaxseed and mustard are perhaps the most common. Flaxseed when made into a hot poultice retains heat for a considerable period of time and thus simply affords another means of local heat application. Mustard, on the other hand, acts as a counterirritant. It produces a high degree of erythema in the skin over the affected area, and probably by a reflex mechanism reduces pain in the underlying tissues or viscera. The irritant effect of mustard is due to a volatile oil, which is released in the presence of moisture.

Either of these substances, made into a warm paste or dough, is spread between 2 pieces of muslin somewhat larger than the area to be treated. While the poultice is being prepared, the underpiece of muslin may be laid over a hot water bottle to prevent cooling. The open edges of both pieces are folded in to prevent leakage. The plaster then is laid on the patient's lightly oiled skin and held firmly in place with a cloth binder. Constant observation is necessary to prevent burning or undue irritation. When the plaster is removed, the skin should be washed with soap and warm water, dried, greased with petrolatum, and covered with a piece of warm flannel. The method of preparation is as follows:

Mustard plaster: Mustard, 1 part, is mixed with from 4 to 6 parts of flour, for adults—12 parts of flour, for children—and enough tepid (not hot) water to make a smooth paste. (The release of the irritant volatile oil is prevented by exposure to heat over 140° F.) The paste then is spread over the muslin about ¼ in. thick and applied to the skin in the manner de-

scribed above. The skin should be examined every 5 minutes
for erythema and the plaster removed as soon as definite pink-
ness appears—usually after 5 to 20 minutes. (CAUTION! Severe blistering will result if the plaster is left on too long.)

Flaxseed poultice: Flaxseed, 1 cup in 1½ cups water, is
boiled to a doughy consistency. The heat is then turned off
and ½ tsp. soda bicarbonate added to the mixture, which then
is thoroughly beaten for a few minutes to incorporate air. With
the same technic as for a mustard plaster (q.v.), the mixture
is spread ½ to 1 inch thick on muslin, applied to the skin, and
left in place for 30 to 45 minutes, or as long as heat is retained.
(NOTE: The empty pot should immediately be filled with cold
water to facilitate cleansing later.)

Various prepared **medicinal plasters** can be bought in drug-
stores.

Cold: Cold applications are used for decreasing the local
blood supply and metabolism, relieving congestion and swelling, controlling hemorrhage and lessening ecchymosis, and for
producing partial or complete anesthesia. Ice or ice water is
most often employed, being applied directly to the affected area
in the form of an ice cap, collar, soak, compress, or pack
(crushed ice). An ice coil may be used but requires more
elaborate equipment. A compress may be kept cold by incorporating ice cubes or an ice bag within it and wrapping the
whole in oilskin. Medicated compresses may be kept cold in
the same way. The application is continued for 30 minutes
or longer, depending on the therapeutic response. Ethyl
chloride spray is a practical means for anesthetizing very small
areas by freezing, such as a furuncle requiring incision and
drainage. Ice water enemas have been used to combat extreme hyperpyrexia (*see also* General Applications, below).

General Applications

Heat or cold may be applied to the entire body in the form
of baths or packs. The tepid sponge and alcohol sponge bath
are described elsewhere (*see* Baths). The purpose of a hot bath
or pack is to induce perspiration. Cold packs reduce the body
temperature and promote the patient's comfort.

Hot packs: A dry, hot pack may be given by a well warmed
blanket wrapped around the patient; a moist one, by a blanket
first soaked in very hot water and then wrung as dry as possible. In either case, several dry blankets are wrapped over
the original one and the treatment is continued for 20 to 40
minutes. During the application of the hot pack, apply an ice
cap to the head and give fluids unless contraindicated.

Cold sheet pack: Generalized cooling may be accomplished
by wrapping the patient's body and arms in a sheet soaked in
cool water (75° F.). The sheet should be well tucked in at the
neck and axillas, and between the thighs. A hot water bottle
is placed at the feet. The bed is protected by a rubber sheet.

The cooling effect may be enhanced by an ice cap at the head or by allowing an electric fan to blow across the sheet. Additional water may be sprinkled on as needed, but care must be taken not to chill the patient. The skin should be briskly chafed through the sheet. Treatment is continued for 20 to 30 minutes. After the wet covers have been removed, the patient's back should be rubbed with alcohol and his body covered with a blanket. Half an hour later the ice cap and hot water bottle are removed.

Cold sponging: With rubber sheeting on mattress and pillow, cold wet compresses are applied to the body, which should first be warm in order to secure the proper reaction. The room should be warm, and brief friction should be applied to the skin before treatment is started. A hot water bottle is placed at the feet, an ice cap to the head, and cold compresses to the axillas and groins. The body is sponged with tepid water followed by cool water (40° to 75° F.). The patient then is turned on his side and the posterior surfaces similarly sponged. If the patient is in poor condition, sponging should be confined to a small area at a time, which is dried and covered immediately; if in good condition, he may be transferred without drying to fresh bedclothing or wrapped in cool wet towels.

After the application of cold water, an alcohol rub should be given. Simultaneously, the skin is chafed to stimulate circulation. This procedure is repeated 2 or 3 times. The importance of vigorous stimulation of the skin cannot be overemphasized; without it, the cool water may simply induce cutaneous vasoconstriction and thus impede the desired loss of heat.

SPECIAL BATHS

Tepid sponge: This serves to promote relaxation, relieve discomfort, stimulate circulation, and temporarily reduce a high fever. One part of the body at a time should be sponged with water at a temperature of about 80° F., and lightly dried. It is imperative to avoid chilling the patient: the room should be warm and free from drafts, and covers are to be used judiciously. The water bath should be followed by sponging with a 25% alcohol solution warmed to 105° F.

Sitz: This bath is aimed at relieving urinary retention, tenesmus, and local (pelvic) pain, congestion, and muscle spasm. The patient sits, preferably on a folded bath towel, for 5 to 30 minutes in a tub containing at least 6 inches of water at a temperature of 110° to 120° F. A blanket draped around his shoulders will prevent chilling. If any evidence of exhaustion appears, the bath should be terminated at once, and the patient dried and returned to bed.

Emollient: Emollient baths are given to relieve skin irritation. The patient remains for 10 to 30 minutes or longer in ⅔ tub of water heated to about 100° F., and containing an emollient such as starch, bran, or oatmeal. Immediately following the bath, the skin is patted dry in such a way as to leave on it a thin film of the agent used. No friction should be applied when alkaline, sulfur, or emollient baths are given. These baths are prepared as follows:

1. Starch: Mix 1 lb. of cornstarch with enough cold water to make a smooth paste. To this, add hot water, boil until thick, and add to water in tub.

2. Bran: Place 2 lb. of bran in a closed muslin bag and soak in a pot of hot water for 10 to 15 minutes. Then, the water and muslin bag are added to the bath water, and the bag is used as a washing sponge by repeatedly squeezing it against the skin.

3. Oatmeal: Use 3 cups of cooked oatmeal (porridge), tied in a cheesecloth bag, as a washing sponge. Soda bicarbonate (8 oz.) may be added to the oatmeal bath.

4. Sodium bicarbonate (alkaline): Dissolve sodium bicarbonate, 8 oz./30 gallons of water.

5. Potassium permanganate: This acts to dry exuding surfaces and to deodorize foul-smelling superficial lesions. Completely dissolve 1 to 4 tsp. of the crystals in water and add to ⅔ tubful of water. The patient should remain in the bath about 30 minutes. (NOTE: This bath will stain the tub.)

6. Sulfur: A mild fungistatic and keratolytic effect is produced by a sulfur bath. It is prepared by adding one of the following compounds to a tub ⅔ filled with water: potassium sulfide, 3 oz.; or zinc sulfate, 5 to 10 tsp.; or Sulfurated Lime Solution N.F., 5 to 7 oz. The patient must not be left in a sulfur bath for more than 20 minutes.

7. Tar (antipruritic): Prepared by dissolving 3 oz. of Solution of Coal Tar N.F. in an adult bath. The patient is immersed for 20 to 30 minutes.

8. Mustard: To produce counterirritation and cutaneous congestion over a large area. The adult bath should contain 1 to 2 tbsp. of mustard/gallon of warm water (80° to 90° F.). The period of exposure is for 15 to 20 minutes and must never exceed 30 minutes. Children's baths are of half strength or less. (Mustard must not be exposed to a temperature above 140° F. as the volatile oil which produces its effect is destroyed at this level.)

9. Saline: These baths, given at or somewhat above body temperature, are useful in cases of extensive burns, sepsis, or dermatitis. Slight hypertonicity of the bath is desirable and this is secured by adding 5 to 8 lb. of ordinary table salt to 30 gallons of water (70° F.). For burns, immersion should be almost continuous; for other conditions, 10 to 30 minutes.

ISOLATION TECHNICS

One or more of the following procedures should be carried out when a patient is being treated for an infectious disease. The necessary measures are selected with regard to the character of the infection, whether respiratory (e.g., tuberculosis, pneumonia, streptococcal throat), gastrointestinal (e.g., typhoid, amebic dysentery, Shigella dysentery), or other, in which sputum, nasal discharges, feces, vomitus, blood, or other material may be a vehicle for spreading the infection.

The patient should be placed in a private room, or his bed surrounded by screens. A scrub basin, with brush, containing 0.5% creosol solution should be kept near the patient's cubicle if running water is too far distant. Visiting by other persons must be rigidly restricted. Anyone entering the isolation area must wear a gown, cap, and mask. If the nasopharyngeal discharges are likely to be infectious, the patient also should wear a mask. Gauze alone does not make an effective mask. Several layers of tissue placed directly over the patient's nose and mouth, and held in place by a gauze or muslin mask, are satisfactory, since the tissues may be disposed of following use. Caps and masks should be worn by an attendant only once and for not longer than 2 hours without sterilization, but the gown may be worn longer, provided isolation technic is observed. The preferred method is to hang the gown on a hook near the door, inside the patient's room, with the opening away from the patient, neckband upright, and edges together in the back, so that the neckband and inside of gown are kept "clean." The collar string of the gown must never be touched without thoroughly washing the hands with soap, water, and brush before and after. Such articles as the stethoscope and sphygmomanometer may be kept "clean" during use by covering the skin site with a towel, and should be lightly sponged with alcohol following use.

Care must be taken to avoid contaminating a "clean" area with anything that has been in the vicinity of the infected patient. Articles possibly contaminated should be carefully handled during their disposal or preparation for re-use; rubber gloves are worn where indicated. Soiled linens are kept in closed, labeled containers, and later sterilized by completely covering with water and boiling for 20 minutes. Paper towels and napkins should be used when possible, stored in a bedside bag, and finally burned. As indicated for each disease, body discharges, soiled dressings, waste food, vomitus, excreta, bedpan rinsings, or irrigation wastes should be burned if possible, or, if not, thoroughly mixed with an equal volume of either 10% chloride of lime for 1 hour, or of 4% lysol or 10% cresol for 5 minutes. Eating utensils and bedpans should be emptied and sterilized by boiling 10 minutes immediately after use. Contaminated rubber articles that cannot be boiled must be washed with green soap and water, dried, and aired for several hours.

When the isolation period is terminated, the bed, chairs, table, and other washable furnishings should be cleansed with hot soapy water and the entire room aired for several hours. Articles that can be, should be boiled. The mattress and pillows should be aired in the sun for at least 6 hours.

RESTRAINTS

Restraints are employed to prevent a patient from injuring himself or his attendants. Padded sideboards should be used in all cases where there is danger of falling out of bed (as in the case of children, the aged, and the delirious or unconscious patient). Wrist and ankle restraints may be applied when needed, but they often tend to make the patient more restless. A strap or a clove-hitch knot is used. Before such restraints are placed, the skin should be powdered and covered with cotton wadding. The color and temperature of the restrained extremity must be watched closely for signs of impaired circulation, and the patent's position should be changed frequently. A strap around the waistline is useful, since it will permit the patient to sit up and turn on his side. A tucked-in sheet often suffices to restrain infants. Psychiatric patients should never be given sharp or pointed eating utensils, neckties, shoestrings, glassware, razor blades, or any other article with which they might injure themselves or others. They also must be carefully observed to make sure they swallow their medicines, lest these be hoarded and then be taken in a dangerous amount.

CARE AND STERILIZATION OF EQUIPMENT

Syringes: Syringes and other glassware should be rinsed with cold water immediately after use, and later washed with warm, soapy water, thoroughly rinsed, then sterilized by boiling for 10 minutes in alkali-free water. Alkali will attack glass and cause defects. This danger can be avoided in a hospital by drying and autoclaving, instead of boiling, with the syringe and plunger wrapped first in gauze, then in paper. Glass must never be heated or cooled too rapidly or it is liable to crack.

Metal instruments: These also should be rinsed with cold water after use; later, washed with warm, soapy water, rinsed again, and sterilized. Sharp-edged instruments are injured by heat and should be sterilized by placing in 70% alcohol for 10 to 20 minutes. If this is impossible, gently place in water which already is boiling and boil for 10 minutes only. Instruments (including needles) must never be left in the sterilizer after boiling, as a film of rust will form. They should be removed at once with sterile forceps (while still hot), shaken free of excess water, and stored in sterile containers.

Rubber articles: Unboilable rubber articles may be washed with soap and water, rinsed and dried, then sterilized by immersion in 70% alcohol for 20 minutes or in 1:40 phenol solution for 2 to 6 hours. They are then dried and stored. Paper placed between the folds will prevent sticking and creasing of the rubber.

Rubber gloves should be washed inside and out with warm soapy water, rinsed, and tested for holes by inflating with air and submerging under water. If indicated, they may be sterilized, before or after washing, by boiling for 5 minutes. To put on wet sterile gloves the scrubbed hands also must be wet. In the hospital, the gloves are dried and powdered on both sides, paired, wrapped, and autoclaved for 15 minutes.

Rubber catheters should be rinsed in cold water at once and later washed with soapy water and rinsed again. The lumen can be cleaned with a cotton applicator or by running through it a strip of gauze guided by a flexible wire. The catheter then is sterilized by boiling for 10 minutes or autoclaving for 30 minutes. (Silk or filiform catheters are sterilized by placing them in 1:1,000 bichloride of mercury for 2 hours and then rinsing with sterile water.)

Enamelware: Exposure to sudden changes of temperature should be avoided as this may produce chipping. The utensils should be cleaned by washing with soapy water and rinsing, and sterilized by boiling for 10 minutes. Most stains can be removed with weak chlorine solution. Steel wool should never be used, as it will scratch the surface.

PREOPERATIVE AND POSTOPERATIVE ROUTINES

Optimum surgical results require adequate preparation of the patient prior to operation, experienced and competent handling during it, and careful observation and management thereafter to avoid postoperative complications. Whether or not a physician himself is engaged in surgical practice, it frequently will be his responsibility to cooperate with the surgeon in supervising the patient's preoperative and postoperative care.

This chapter outlines briefly a workable preoperative and postoperative routine. It also mentions the more common postsurgical complications to be avoided where possible or combated if necessary. However, no elaboration of the principles will be attempted in those instances where the subjects are discussed in detail in other chapters of the MANUAL.

For example, fluid and electrolyte relationships are explained in the chapter on Acid-Base and Allied Disorders. Likewise, the appropriate chapters should be consulted for the management of such possible complicating factors as diabetes mellitus, anemia, nutritional deficiencies, hemorrhagic diseases, venous thrombosis, pain, shock, atelectasis and massive collapse of the lung, hiccup, anuria, infusion reactions, and decubitus. In chapters on Antibiotic Therapy and Sulfonamide Therapy are summarized the latest facts concerning the prophylactic and therapeutic use of drugs that have almost revolutionized certain phases of surgical practice. A wide choice of diets is presented in the Diets chapter, while much information relevant to the care of persons undergoing surgical treatment appears in the chapters on Bedside and Clinical Procedures.

PREOPERATIVE ROUTINE

Patients scheduled for elective operation should enter the hospital as far in advance as necessary for adequate baseline determinations and preparation for the intended surgical procedure. Routine blood and serologic tests and urinalyses in all patients, with chest X-ray and cardiovascular clearance in the middle and advanced age groups, are of primary importance. Every effort should be made to prepare patients psychologically and to ensure a good night's sleep by the use of a suitable hypnotic or analgesic or both. Cathartics are to be avoided, but a cleansing enema the night before, or the morning of the operation is advisable. Water and food are forbidden after midnight for all who are to have general anesthetics or major operations under spinal anesthesia. Where time permits, any existing anemia, dehydration, or malnutrition should be corrected prior to operation.

Nutrition: If a patient who is to have a purely elective operation gives a history of faulty diet or shows evidence of malnutrition, he should be built up preoperatively by an appropriate diet. Otherwise no dietary change is necessary. Deficiency in protein, ascorbic acid, or vitamin K is particularly hazardous to the surgical patient (*see* VITAMIN DEFICIENCIES; PROTEIN DEFICIENCY). Where prompt surgery is necessary the risk involved in operating on a malnourished individual must be carefully weighed against the danger of postponement. Parenteral alimentation sometimes is necessary for patients who cannot take or retain food. In any surgical patient it should be remembered that carbohydrates are quick, economical sources of energy, and that their metabolism spares proteins, helps prevent formation of ketone acids, and reduces the quantity of urinary solutes.

Fluid and electrolyte balance: Ordinarily, the kidneys are the principal regulator conserving or excreting water and salts as required to maintain fluid and electrolyte balance. They excrete 35 to 40 Gm. of solids a day, requiring, at maximum renal concentration, 500 cc. of urine. To allow for any diminution in renal function, 1,500 cc. is regarded as the optimum amount for a 24-hour period and indicates that the fluid intake is adequate. Even though the urinary volume is satisfactory, the patient still may suffer from an electrolyte imbalance. This should be treated appropriately (*see* ACID-BASE AND ALLIED DISORDERS).

In uncomplicated preoperative water depletion, correction by orally-given fluid, when feasible, is preferable. Too much fluid by vein can produce heart failure, especially if given with too much sodium, too rapidly, or in the form of blood or plasma. However, if the fluid imbalance cannot be corrected quickly or conveniently by the oral route, enough 5 to 10% glucose should be given I.V. to bring the daily urinary output to 1,500 cc. Intake and output records are essential in these cases. If the cardiac and urinary functions are not impaired, normal saline solution may be alternated with the glucose solution in equal amounts.

Blood and plasma requirements: Transfusions of blood can frequently convert a chronically ill, debilitated patient into a good surgical risk. Their proper use will correct anemia, facilitate wound healing, and aid in preventing infections and other complications. Blood is given preoperatively in the presence of (1) anemia, (2) decreased blood volume, (3) significant weight loss, (4) hypoproteinemia, or (5) chronic infection. The hematocrit is the best single guide to blood needs, but the red cell count and hemoglobin also are useful in estimating transfusion requirements. Unless severe hemorrhage has occurred, it is better not to exceed 1 liter of blood/day; 500 cc./day usually is preferable. Blood should be given daily until the hematocrit reaches the desired level, at which it should be maintained by subsequent transfusions, given as needed. In patients with cardiac damage this level should be 40 to 42; in chronic debilitating disease, 45 to 47 usually is safe. In cases of acute hemorrhage, large amounts of blood may be given rapidly, the speed depending mainly on the patient's blood pressure. If a major operation is planned, or if the patient is a poor surgical risk, matched blood should be constantly available, up to 1,500 cc. being kept ready for use.

Preoperative medication: Preceding general anesthesia, morphine, 10 to 15 mg. (gr. ⅙ to ¼) subcut. is given together with 0.4 mg. (gr. ¹⁄₁₅₀) of atropine or scopolamine for sedation and to lessen bronchial secretions. Debilitated patients require smaller doses, calculated on weight. Since infants tolerate morphine poorly, they usually are given atropine only, in small doses. In older patients who are to receive morphine, a quick-acting barbiturate, such as pentobarbital sodium 0.1 to 0.2 Gm. (gr. iss to iii), given subcut. 1 hour before operation helps to allay apprehension. Spinal anesthesia requires the same premedication because this method may fail during the operation and have to be supplemented by inhalation anesthesia. However, in these patients only morphine and a barbiturate, or a barbiturate alone, will be required. With local anesthesia, the cooperation of the patient often is needed; hence, morphine alone is administered, although a barbiturate also may be used if indicated.

Upper gastrointestinal preparation: It usually is desirable to have the gastrointestinal tract empty or nearly so before operation. If it is emptying itself normally, little more than routine care will be needed. To obtain an empty stomach is relatively easy, but if an empty ileum is required, it will be necessary to begin the preoperative fast at noon of the preceding day. In cases of intestinal obstruction, mechanical or paralytic, the stomach and proximal intestine are emptied by means of a tube, usually with continuous suction. For pyloric obstruction a Levin tube suffices, but for lower intestinal obstruction the Miller-Abbott tube (or one of its modifications) is more efficient (see CLIN. PROC.). When the end of the tube lies in the ileum, it still is possible to feed the patient orally because he will obtain some absorption through the proximal gut, while material reaching the more distal ileum will be removed. However, if the end of the suction tube lies at more proximal levels, fluids by mouth will tend to wash out electrolytes and increase their loss; small amounts of water may be allowed intermittently, with due caution. Indwelling tubes are utilized for varying periods, depending on the circumstances. They frequently are left in place during operation for use later. Indwelling tubes must be irrigated at intervals to ensure freedom of function and to clear out mucus or food particles which may obstruct the tube.

Large bowel preparation: Preoperative attention to the colon and rectum is aimed at obtaining an empty bowel and a reduction in the bacterial flora. The first may be accomplished by diet, enemas, colonic irrigations, Miller-Abbott tube, or colostomy. A low residue diet is helpful, and a completely liquid diet for a few days preoperatively may sometimes be necessary (see DIETS). It always is advisable to keep the patient on liquids alone after luncheon of the day preceding operation. Reduction of the bacterial flora, prior to colonic surgical operation, can be effected by the oral use of streptomycin, or the nonabsorbable sulfonamides, or both (see ANTIBIOTIC THERAPY; SULFONAMIDE THERAPY). During use of nonabsorbable sulfonamides, vitamin K in adequate doses must be given to compensate for the lack of bacterial action in production of this vitamin.

In cases of bowel obstruction with distention, continuous suction with a Miller-Abbott tube for decompression, together with a colostomy, often is indicated; suction can be discontinued as soon as the colostomy begins to function. These procedures are subject to variation; thus, it is often necessary to establish a colostomy without resorting to suction by tube, while sometimes a nonresidue diet and enemas will suffice. Enemas, though helpful, must not be relied upon exclusively.

Bladder preparation: An indwelling catheter is inserted, shortly before major operations on the pelvic colon or rectum, to assure an empty bladder. In many other pelvic operations, catheterization is done shortly before or at the start of the operative procedure, but the catheter need not be left in place unless there is some special indication for so doing.

Prophylactic chemotherapy: Antimicrobial therapy is indicated prophylactically before and after surgical procedures in which there exists a hazard of postoperative complications such as wound infections, bronchopneumonia, or spread of infection from operative areas. Penicillin in aqueous or repository forms (*see* ANTIBIOTIC THERAPY), 300,000 to 600,000 u. daily I.M., begun 24 hours before operation, and maintained for 2 or 3 days postoperatively, or until all likelihood of complications is past, is almost a routine procedure in major surgery. Streptomycin, 0.5 to 2 Gm. I.M. daily, also should be given if the development of a mixed infection with both streptomycin and penicillin sensitive organisms is likely (e.g., in intestinal surgery following contamination with intestinal contents containing both gram-negative and gram-positive organisms). A sulfonamide, such as sulfadiazine, also may be given in the usual dosage (*see* SULFONAMIDE THERAPY) to reinforce the antimicrobial action of the antibiotics.

POSTOPERATIVE ROUTINE

Fluid administration: Glucose solution 5% usually is given I.V. during and after all major operations. The amount will depend on the patient's anticipated needs based on the degree of dehydration, the length of the operation, and the continuing loss of fluids. Ordinarily, 2 or 3 liters are given during the first 24 hours; often, more is required. Thirst, when present, is a significant symptom. Glucose solution alone is given on the day of operation, and thereafter as needed. (Cardiac patients must always be closely observed for evidence of impending decompensation, and should never be given fluids too rapidly or in unduly large amounts.) Saline solution, 1 liter, may be given the day after operation and thereafter every 2nd or 3rd day if indicated. During continuous gastric suction the patient will require about 3,000 cc. of saline every 24 hours. A useful rule of thumb, particularly with the aid of intake-output charts, is to add 1,000 cc. of fluid (insensible loss) to the amount of output from all orifices (e.g., suction, drainage, urine). If at any time it is necessary to administer 3 or more liters of fluid I.V./day, it is well to give 2 liters in the morning, remove the needle, and give the remainder in the late afternoon or the evening. This spares the patient the tedium of unduly long administration. As the patient succeeds in taking increasing amounts of liquids by mouth, I.V. fluids are gradually reduced and finally stopped. In the very young or extremely old patient, mild dehydration is the safest state.

Blood and plasma requirements: Postoperative blood transfusions now are almost routine, but the possibility of precipitating cardiac failure must be borne in mind. The amount necessary will vary greatly with the circumstances. Immediately after operation the blood pressure and the estimated amount of blood lost are the best guides. Afterward, the patient's appearance, the hematocrit reading, the blood count and the hemoglobin are the indices. Late in convalescence, blood transfusion is sometimes needed. Too often this fact is overlooked. Preferably, the hematocrit should be maintained at the desired level by giving transfusions before it has fallen significantly; in this manner wide fluctuations in the hematocrit findings are prevented.

Oxygen administration: Inhalation of O_2 (*see* CLIN. PROC.) is advisable postoperatively for all patients following thoracic surgical procedures or during thyroid crises. It also is essential for the prevention of imminent anoxia or the correction of actual anoxia (q.v.) due to any cause.

Sedation: Morphine, 10 to 15 mg. (gr. 1/6 to 1/4) subcut., or a suitable substitute such as Demerol (50 to 100 mg.) or methadone (5 to 10 mg.) I.M., is usually indicated, although morphine depresses respiration, reduces the cough reflex, and may cause the patient to lie too motionless. These disadvantages should always be kept in mind, since they predispose to such postoperative complications as venous thrombosis, atelectasis and hypostatic pneumonia (q.v.). As little sedation should be employed as is consistent with the comfort, individual tolerance, and general medical condition of the patient. Phenobarbital, 60 to 100 mg. (gr. i to iss), is useful as a long-lasting sedative, but has little effect on pain.

Nutrition: For the postoperative surgical patient, the amount and form of his diet (liquid, solid) usually is more important than its chemical composition (*see* DIETS). Milk has a constipating effect and fruit juices often are poorly tolerated. Intake by mouth should be forbidden for the unconscious or stuporous patient. Even after he recovers from the anesthetic, he should not receive liquids orally until there is auscultatory evidence of peristalsis, or free passage of gas from the anus. The diet then is increased as tolerated, except after intra-abdominal operations, where it is best to limit the intake to certain liquids, omitting milk and fruit juices, until the patient begins to expel gas per rectum, after which the diet can be cautiously increased.

Following gastric or intestinal surgery, the food intake is increased more slowly, an unrestricted liquid diet being reached by the 6th postoperative day, a soft diet by the 9th day, and a normal diet by the 13th day. Where evidence suggests that fat is not being properly absorbed by the intestine, in particular following subtotal gastrectomy or short-circuiting anastomotic operations, absorption of fat may be aided by the use of a wetting agent, such as the polyoxyethylene derivative of sorbitan monooleate, given in doses of 1.5 Gm. with each meal.

After colonic surgery the diet will depend largely on the

degree of ileus present and on the ability of the bowel to propel gas and feces past the operative site. It is well routinely to institute continuous suction with a Levin tube in the stomach and to discontinue it when the patient begins to pass gas per rectum. Thereafter, unlimited fluids by mouth and a soft diet usually are well tolerated. A full nonresidue diet is withheld until at least the 7th day. To reduce the frequency of movements through a colostomy, a low residue diet is of value.

Position and activity in bed: Following a general or spinal anesthetic the patient should be kept flat in bed, without pillows, until the effects have worn off and the blood pressure becomes stabilized. Then, with rare exceptions, he should be encouraged to move and turn himself freely; herniorrhaphies or abdominal operations are not exceptions. Strict attention to active or passive leg exercise of the bedridden patient is of utmost importance. If the patient does not or cannot move himself, his legs should be elevated and flexed by the nurse several times every ½ hour. He should also be turned from side to side.

Ambulation: Early ambulation contributes to the welfare of the patient by hastening convalescence and lessening the incidence of certain postoperative complications (*see* below). The contraindications to getting the patient up early are congestive heart failure, hemorrhage or threatened hemorrhage, thrombophlebitis with its attendant danger of pulmonary infarction, spinal and head injuries, and certain fractures. Some surgeons feel that, following abdominal operations (including herniorrhaphies), ambulation by the 2nd or 3rd day is advisable; others, although permitting free movement in bed, do not allow these patients up for 6 to 7 days. Some patients with repair of extremely large hernias or abdominal wounds closed under tension are best kept bedfast for 12 days, but with passive and active exercise in bed within safe limits.

Care of the bowel: Ordinarily, constipation (q.v.) is treated in the usual way but, following operations on the intestinal tract or operations that produce ileus (q.v.), special treatment is required: prophylaxis, by keeping the intestine undistended, is most important. While the bowel is not functioning, little benefit will be derived from cathartics, parasympathetic stimulants, or enemas; indeed, these measures may be harmful. They are helpful only when the bowel is regaining its function, as shown by the patient's ability to pass gas or feces and the resumption of auscultatory intestinal sounds. Cathartics (*see* Constipation) should generally not be given until 4 days after any operation, 6 days after an appendectomy, and 9 days after a colon resection. They should never be given in the presence of peritonitis. Enemas are contraindicated for 9 days after colon resection and 6 days after appendectomy, unless limited to 200 cc., in which case they can be begun about the 4th day. Fecal impaction is detected by digital examina-

tion. If soft, it may be broken up by flushing the rectum with
half-strength hydrogen peroxide, a rectal tube being inserted
and kept in place for a few minutes afterward. Retention
enemas of mineral oil are helpful (see BEDSIDE PROC.). If these
measures fail, the impaction should be broken up with the
gloved finger.

Care of the bladder: In some operations on the bladder
and in the pelvis, particularly in elderly men, an indwelling
catheter is left in place. In the female especially, catheterization every 8 hours, if necessary (see BEDSIDE PROC.), usually suffices, but if function does not return after 2 to 3 catheterizations,
an indwelling catheter should be inserted. Efforts always should
be made to avoid catheterization. It often is better to let the
patient stand or sit up to urinate, if this will facilitate spontaneous bladder emptying. Urecholine, 10 mg. orally, or 2.5
mg. subcut., is useful in preventing and correcting postoperative
urinary retention; when given subcut., its effect is more rapidly
achieved. Frequent small voidings should arouse suspicion of
overflow dribbling, incontinence, or cystitis. Such patients
should be catheterized to determine the amount of retained
urine and to examine the specimen thus obtained.

Application and care of dressings and binders: Tight,
constrictive dressings are to be avoided, particularly over the
upper abdomen and the chest. Binders should never be used
unless applied loosely, and then only to hold a dressing in
place. Care of the skin adds greatly to the patient's comfort.
At each dressing, the skin should be cleaned with ether and
protected from any discharges present (see Fistula, below).

Fistula: Intestinal fistulas present problems in maintaining
fluid and electrolyte balance as well as in the care of the
surrounding skin. A duodenal fistula causes the greatest disturbance because of the extensive loss of fluids and electrolytes,
the loss of food before it can be absorbed, and the digestive
and extremely irritating effect of the secretions on the skin.
The lower the intestinal origin of the fistula, the less the
metabolic disturbance produced. Thus, a sigmoid colostomy
produces little disturbance, whereas high fistulas bring about
rapid deterioration of the patient's condition. With high
fistulas, fluid and electrolyte replacement becomes a major
problem (see ACID-BASE AND ALLIED DISORDERS).

There are many methods of protecting the skin, either by
coating it or by attempting to remove secretions before they
reach it. As a coating, aluminum paste (50% finely powdered
aluminum metal in Zinc Oxide Ointment U.S.P.) has proved
most effective, although 25% zinc oxide ointment, vaseline
gauze, and kaolin paste (prepared by adding enough water
to kaolin powder to form a thick paste) have been used successfully. All of these are more effective when applied to dry
intact skin before maceration or ulceration takes place. In
order to remove the wound secretions, particularly those con-

taining proteolytic enzymes, continuous suction is necessary. This is best accomplished by first inserting a wide, perforated glass tube in the wound, then placing in it a rubber catheter which is attached to the source of suction. A combination of this maneuver and protective skin coatings often proves effective.

Care of colostomies: Management of a colostomy should begin as soon as function commences. If the opening is to be permanent, the patient should be assured that convenient management is possible, provided he cooperates. Use of a colostomy bag should be prohibited. Relative constipation is achieved by limiting the amount of fruits and vegetables in the diet, after which early colostomy irrigations are begun (see BED-SIDE PROC.). Often, several months are required for complete training. When this has been accomplished, the diet can be liberalized and the patient will require only a small dressing over the opening, with assurance that there will be no bowel movement until the next irrigation. Fecal odors emanating from a colostomy may be controlled by a drop or two of half-strength phenol on the gauze overlying the colostomy opening.

Care of ileostomies: Immediately after establishment of an ileostomy, a salt deficiency often occurs. Continuous efforts must be made to prevent or correct any fluid or electrolyte imbalance or nutritional deficiency. Special appliances are available to take care of the copious discharge always present. Some surgeons prefer to leave a projecting loop of ileum, which is covered with grafted skin, for the application of the special fittings that are necessary.

POSTOPERATIVE COMPLICATIONS

Much of the routine already described is directed at the prevention of complications, which may result from dehydration, anemia, oversedation, venous thrombosis, restricted bodily movement, hypoproteinemia, avitaminosis, or constant pressure on parts. The aim, therefore, is to correct by appropriate measures any of these conditions that may be present before operation. When complications do occur, they require specific measures to minimize their effects on the patient and to eliminate them as soon as possible.

Ileus: Adynamic ileus is a normal sequel to any intra-abdominal operation but, if treated properly, will be short-lived unless some complicating factor is present, such as peritonitis; sympathetic irritation following sympathectomy, nephrectomy, retroperitoneal hemorrhage or infection; carcinomatosis; or intraperitoneal hemorrhage. The only constant clinical sign is a diminution of auscultatory intestinal sounds, although these may not be entirely absent if the paralysis is regional. In full-blown paralytic ileus, the abdomen is silent. When fluid accumulates in the intestine it causes distention, abdominal discomfort, and sometimes vomiting. X-rays reveal gas in the small bowel, usually with several fluid levels. Prophylaxis should begin at operation by reducing operative trauma and the handling or exposure of tissues to a minimum and by avoiding or combating the complications listed above.

Active treatment must begin immediately after the operation by attempting to render the intestine relatively empty and undistended through restriction of oral intake, continuous suction by stomach tube, and decompression of the intestine. Distention seldom is present immediately after operation; hence, it can be held to a reasonable degree by prohibiting everything by mouth. Swallowed air accounts for about 70% of the intestinal gases (mainly nitrogen); larger quantities of air are swallowed with sips of water than are realized. With all oral intake suspended, if vomiting does not occur, swallowed air, gastric juice, bile and pancreatic fluid pass into the intestine. Continuous gastric suction with a Levin tube (*see* CLIN. PROC.) effectively removes air, gastric juice, and some of the bile and pancreatic juice. Once the small intestine becomes distended, the Miller-Abbott tube provides the most efficient method of artificial decompression (*see* CLIN. PROC.).

Lesser degrees of distention may respond to the use of a lubricated rectal tube, small (200 cc.) carminative enemas, or the application of warm turpentine (1:3 in oil) stupes (*see* BEDSIDE PROC.). In the absence of any obstruction, peristaltic stimulants such as Urecholine 2.5 mg. subcut., Pitressin 0.5 cc. (♏ viii) I.M., or neostigmine methylsulfate, 0.5 mg. subcut., may sometimes prove beneficial, particularly when used in conjunction with a rectal tube; if necessary, these stimulants may be repeated, once only, after 2 hours. Their value in preventing the postoperative development of ileus is debatable, however.

From a practical standpoint, continuous suction by stomach tube is advisable after all but the simplest gastrointestinal operations. Auscultation of the abdomen should be done daily at least. If the operation has not been too extensive, the tube may be removed as soon as satisfactory intestinal sounds return; however, repeated passage of gas or feces is the best evidence that normal bowel function has been resumed. The diet then can be increased rapidly, provided there are no other contraindications. The most common mistakes are giving enemas too frequently and the overenthusiastic use of such agents as neostigmine or Pitressin.

Respiratory diseases: Pulmonary complications are common after major operations of all types, and prophylaxis should be begun at the operating table. The air passages should be cleared of excess secretion by means of suction; constrictive dressings should be avoided and sedation kept at a minimum. Aspiration of vomitus into the lungs during the recovery period can be avoided by placing the patient in the head-down position, turning his head to the side, or removing the vomitus with a gauze sponge or by suction. With the return of consciousness the patient should be made to turn himself in bed as soon as possible, to breathe deeply, and to cough as necessary. All possible measures should be directed toward ensuring complete aeration of the lungs (*see* ATELECTASIS) and preventing pulmonary infections.

Wound rupture: This complication usually occurs, if at all, by the 10th day. Predisposing factors include faulty closure, hypoproteinemia, excessive tension or strain, vitamin C deficiency, edema from any cause, and anemia. Treatment consists of surgical repair of the wound and the correction of the primary cause (q.v.).

Decubitus ulcers: Pressure ulcers (bedsores) are likely to develop in debilitated, emaciated, and chronically ill patients who must undergo prolonged bed rest. In such cases, the patient should be frequently turned in bed and pressure points protected by pneumatic rings or other suitable devices. The skin should be kept dry and scrupulously clean, and special attention be given to building up the patient's nutritional status. (For details of prophylaxis and treatment, *see* chapter on DECUBITUS.)

Thromboembolic phenomena: Venous thrombosis and embolism occur more frequently in bed patients than is commonly suspected. The most frequent sites are the veins of the foot, calf, and pelvis. Many times a fatal embolism is preceded by one of a nonfatal type; hence, the physician should be alert to detect early signs of embolization. The anticoagulants, dicumarol and heparin, are effective in combating embolic and thromboembolic phenomena, when used in suitable cases and with the proper precautions. (*See* VENOUS THROMBOSIS; ANTICOAGULANT THERAPY.)

DIETS

Foods are composed of varying proportions of protein (P), carbohydrate (C), fat (F), minerals, salts, vitamins, and water. These are all essential to vital processes, but only protein, carbohydrate, and fat are sources of energy. One Gm. of C or P yields approximately 4 calories, whereas 1 Gm. of F produces 9 calories.

Dietary requirements depend on the age, sex, height, weight, and activity (metabolic and physical) of the patient. The objective is to achieve and maintain the "ideal" weight of the patient (TABLE 1). Before the age of 25, an individual's weight is variable and characterized by progressive increase. It is extremely doubtful if progressive weight gain is normal or desirable after the age of 25 years. Recommended dietary allowances are given in TABLE 2.

A normal intake of all essential nutrients requires the daily ingestion of several basic foods whose nutritional value is analyzed in TABLE 3. Further nutritional needs may be supplied by increasing the daily intake of these basic foods or by

TABLE 1

A. IDEAL WEIGHTS FOR MEN*
(Ages twenty-five and over)

Height (in shoes with average heels)		Weight in Pounds (as ordinarily dressed)		
Feet	Inches	Small Frame	Medium Frame	Large Frame
5	2	116–25	124–33	131–42
5	3	119–28	127–36	133–44
5	4	122–32	130–40	137–49
5	5	126–36	134–44	141–53
5	6	129–39	137–47	145–57
5	7	133–43	141–51	149–62
5	8	136–47	145–56	153–66
5	9	140–51	149–60	157–70
5	10	144–55	153–64	161–75
5	11	148–59	157–68	165–80
6	0	152–64	161–73	169–85
6	1	157–69	166–78	174–90
6	2	163–75	171–84	179–96
6	3	168–80	176–89	184–202

B. IDEAL WEIGHTS FOR WOMEN*
(Ages twenty-five and over)

Height (in shoes with average heels)		Weight in Pounds (as ordinarily dressed)		
Feet	Inches	Small Frame	Medium Frame	Large Frame
4	11	104–11	110–18	117–27
5	0	105–13	112–20	119–29
5	1	107–15	114–22	121–31
5	2	110–18	117–25	124–35
5	3	113–21	120–28	127–38
5	4	116–25	124–32	131–42
5	5	119–28	127–35	133–45
5	6	123–32	130–40	138–50
5	7	126–36	134–44	142–54
5	8	129–39	137–47	145–58
5	9	133–43	141–51	149–62
5	10	136–47	145–55	152–66
5	11	139–50	148–58	155–69

* Figures from Metropolitan Life Insurance Company, Statistical Bureau, 1943.

the addition of other appropriate foods rich in the desired nutrient (*see* Food Tables, later in this chapter). For example, the increased need for calcium during pregnancy and lactation may be met by giving larger amounts of milk daily.

The following pages contain a reasonably complete outline of dietotherapy. For more detailed information, the reader is referred to standard textbooks of nutrition.

Normal Diet

A normal diet is one which requires no modification and which will supply necessary nutrients. It should be served in 3 meals, as follows:

Breakfast		Lunch		Dinner	
Fruit	1 orange	Meat		Meat, fish	
	or ½ grapefruit	(or equiv.)	2 oz.	or fowl	3 oz.
Cereals*	½ cup	2 Vegetables	200 Gm.	Vegetables	100 Gm.
Egg	1 or 2	Bread*	1 slice	Salad	100 Gm.
Bread*	1 slice	Butter**	1 pat	Bread*	1 slice
Butter**	1 pat	Fruit		Butter**	1 pat
Beverage with		Whole milk	8 oz.	Fruit or	
cream and				dessert	
sugar				Whole milk	8 oz.

* Whole wheat or enriched.   ** Or enriched oleomargarine.

The total fluid intake should be at least 2,500 cc. daily. Additional foods may be added to the diet to supply needed calories, but no food should be taken between meals.

Prenatal Diet

Principle: To meet the increased nutrient requirements of pregnancy (TABLE 2) by supplementing the normal diet (q.v.).

Content: Increase the daily intake of the components of the normal diet (TABLE 3): viz.—milk (1 qt.), lean meat or equivalent (6 oz.), liver once or twice weekly.

Avoid: Excess salt.

The nausea and vomiting of early pregnancy may be alleviated by small frequent feedings of foods rich in carbohydrate (noodles, potato, rice, banana, fruit juice). After the 1st trimester, such foods should be kept at the minimum necessary to meet caloric requirements, in order to avoid excessive weight gain. If necessary, the daily diet may be served in 4 to 6 feedings. Supplementary polyvitamins are advisable because of increased requirements during pregnancy (TABLE 2).

During lactation, the mother should continue on the diet of late pregnancy except that the daily milk consumption should be increased to 3 pts.

TABLE 2. RECOMMENDED DAILY DIETARY

	CALO-RIES[a] PER DAY	PRO-TEIN Gm.	CAL-CIUM Gm.	IRON mg.
Men (154 lb.)				
Sedentary	2400	70	1.0	12[d]
Active	3000	70	1.0	12[d]
Laborer	4500	70	1.0	12[d]
Women (123 lb.)				
Sedentary	2000	60	1.0	12
Active	2400	60	1.0	12
Very active	3000	60	1.0	12
Pregnancy (last half)	2400[f]	85	1.5	15
Lactation	3000	100	2.0	15
Children up to 12 yrs.[g]				
Under 1 yr.[h]	110/Kg.	3.5/Kg.	1.0	6
1– 3 yrs. (29 lb.)	1200	40	1.0	7
4– 6 yrs. (42 lb.)	1600	50	1.0	8
7– 9 yrs. (55 lb.)	2000	60	1.0	10
10–12 yrs. (75 lb.)	2500	70	1.2	12
Children over 12 yrs.[g]				
Girls				
13–15 (108 lb.)	2600	80	1.3	15
16–20 (119 lb.)	2400	75	1.0	15
Boys				
13–15 (103 lb.)	3200	85	1.4	15
16–20 (141 lb.)	3800	100	1.4	15

* Revised 1948, Food and Nutrition Board, National Research Council.

[a] Calorie allowances must be adjusted up or down to meet specific needs. The calorie values in the table are therefore not applicable to all individuals but rather represent group averages.   The proper calorie allowance is that which over an extended period will maintain body weight or rate of growth at the level most conducive to well-being.

[b] The allowance depends on the relative amounts of vitamin A and carotene. The allowances of the table are based on the premise that approximately two-thirds of the vitamin A value of the average diet in this country is contributed by carotene and that carotene has half or less than half the value of vitamin A.

[c] For adults (except pregnant and lactating women) receiving diets supplying 2000 calories or less, such as reducing diets, the allowances of thiamine, riboflavin and niacin may be 1 mg., 1.5 mg. and 10 mg. respectively.   The fact that figures are given for different calorie levels for thiamine, riboflavin and niacin does not imply that we can estimate the requirement of these factors within 500 calories, but they are added merely for simplicity of calculation.   Other members of the B complex also are required, though no values

ALLOWANCES FOR MEN, WOMEN AND CHILDREN*

VITAMIN A[b] I.U.	THI-AMINE[c] mg.	RIBO-FLAVIN[c] mg.	NIACIN[c] mg.	ASCOR-BIC ACID mg.	VITAMIN D I.U.
					[e]
5000	1.2	1.8	12	75	
5000	1.5	1.8	15	75	
5000	1.8	1.8	18	75	
					[e]
5000	1.0	1.5	10	70	
5000	1.2	1.5	12	70	
5000	1.5	1.5	15	70	
6000	1.5	2.5	15	100	400
8000	1.5	3.0	15	150	400
1500	0.4	0.6	4	30	400
2000	0.6	0.9	6	35	400
2500	0.8	1.2	8	50	400
3500	1.0	1.5	10	60	400
4500	1.2	1.8	12	75	400
5000	1.3	2.0	13	80	400
5000	1.2	1.8	12	80	400
5000	1.5	2.0	15	90	400
6000	1.7	2.5	17	100	400

can be given. Foods supplying adequate thiamine, riboflavin and niacin will tend to supply sufficient of the remaining B vitamins.

[d] There is evidence that the male adult needs relatively little iron. The need will usually be provided for if the diet is satisfactory in other respects.

[e] For persons who have no opportunity for exposure to clear sunshine, and for elderly persons, the ingestion of small amounts of supplementary vitamin D may be desirable. Other adults probably have little need for such supplements.

[f] During the latter part of pregnancy the calorie allowance should increase approximately 20% above the preceding level. The value of 2400 calories represents the allowance for pregnant, sedentary women.

[g] Allowances for children are based on the needs for the middle year in each group (as 2, 5, 8, etc.) and are for moderate activity and for average weight at the middle year of the age group.

[h] Needs for infants increase from month to month with size and activity. The amounts given are for approximately 6 to 8 months. The dietary requirements for some of the nutrients such as protein and calcium are less if derived largely from human milk.

TABLE 3. MINIMUM DAILY REQUIREMENTS OF BASIC NUTRIENTS

FOOD	MEASURE	WEIGHT Gm.	CALORIES	C Gm.	P Gm.	F Gm.	CALCIUM Gm.	IRON mg.	VIT. A I.U.	THIAMINE mg.	RIBOFLAVIN mg.	NIACIN mg.	ASCORBIC ACID mg.
Milk	1 pt.	480	330	24	18	18	0.56	0.4	760–940	0.2	0.8	0.6	2–6
Meat (including liver at least once each 10 days)	3 oz.	90	220	1	23	13	0.01	3.5	2,700	0.3	0.4	5	0
Egg	1 (med.)	50	80	0	6	6	0.03	1.4	500	0.06	0.18	0	0
Butter (or enriched oleomargarine)	½ oz.	15	115	0	0	12.5	0	0	500	0	0	0	0
Bread (whole wheat or enriched)	3 slices	90	240	43	8	2.5	0.04	2.4	0	0.24	0.12	1.8	0
Cereal (whole wheat or enriched)	½ cup	20	80	15	2	0.5	0.01	0.7	0	0.08	0.03	0.6	0
Fruit, Citrus: 1 medium orange or ½ grapefruit	—	100	55	10	0	0	0.02	0.6	200	0.06	0.03	0.2	30–40
Fruit, Noncitrus	2 servings	200	70–130	10–40	2	0–1	0.04	1.0	300	0.1	0.1	0.7	0–10
Vegetables: 3 green or yellow, cooked, and 1 raw	4 servings	400	150	30	7	0	0.2	1.5	5,500	0.15	0.25	0.15	30–40
Protein (additional): 1 egg, 8 oz. milk, or 1 oz. meat or cheese	—	—	100	0–8	6–7	4–9	0.1	0.1–1.0	500–900	0.1	0.1–0.4	0–1	0–1
Total	—	—	1,440–1,500	133–171	72–73	56.5–62.5	1.01	11.6–12.5	10,960–11,540	1.29	2.01–2.31	9.05–10.05	62–97

High Caloric Diet

Indications: Protracted fever, hyperthyroidism, under-weight, malnutrition.

Principle: The normal diet (q.v.) is supplemented with high caloric foods such as sugars, jams, honey, butter, cream, gravy, eggnog with cream, and rich desserts. Bulky or low caloric foods, such as additional vegetables or fruit, should be avoided. Febrile patients may require liquid or semisolid foods of high caloric value (*see* High Caloric Semifluid Diet). These foods may be given with the regular meals, as interval feedings, or both. When indicated, the appetite may be stimulated by the injection of regular insulin (5 u.) before meals, or by a cocktail or glass of dry sherry.

Sample Menu

Breakfast		Lunch		Dinner	
Fruit juice with added sugar	8 oz.	Cream soup with butter**		Meat, fish or fowl	3 oz.
Cereal* with cream and sugar		Meat (or equiv.)	2 oz.	Vegetable with butter**	100 Gm.
Egg	1 or 2	Vegetable with butter**	100 Gm.	Potato with butter**	100 Gm.
Bread* with butter** and jam	2 slices	Potato, spaghetti, or rice	100 Gm.	Salad with dressing	
Beverage with cream and sugar		Bread* with butter** and jam	2 slices	Bread* with butter** and jam	
		Fruit		Dessert (rich)	
		Cream 10 to 20%	8 oz.	Cream (10 to 20%)	8 oz.

Midafternoon and bedtime (when desired or necessary): Eggnog with cream and sugar, sandwiches, or cake with 8 oz. cream (10 to 20%).

* Whole wheat or enriched.   ** Or enriched oleomargarine.

Low Caloric Diet

Indication: Obesity.

Principle: To produce weight reduction by a diet which is deficient in caloric but adequate in essential nutrients. This is achieved by eliminating cereal, sugar, and cream from the normal diet (q.v.) and the liberal use of boiled vegetables which are low in carbohydrate content (*see* Food Tables). Unnecessary fats may be eliminated by the use of broiled lean meat. Saccharin is used in place of sugar for sweetening.

Avoid: Fried foods, fats or oils, sugar, cream, cereal, fat meat, high carbohydrate vegetables and fruits (*see* Food Tables), gravy, sweets, nuts, sweetened beverages.

Sample Reducing Diet
(1,200 calories)

Breakfast	Lunch	Dinner

Fruit   1 orange
  or ½ grapefruit
Egg   1
Bread*   1 slice
Butter**   1 pat
Beverage with
  milk and
  saccharin
	Broiled lean meat
	  (or equiv.) 2 oz.
	Boiled 5%
	  vegetable 100 Gm.
	Salad with lemon,
	  spices and
	  vinegar*** 100 Gm.
	Bread* ½ slice
	Butter** 1 pat
	Fruit
	  (5 to 20%) 100 Gm.
	Skimmed milk 8 oz.
		Broiled lean
		  meat, fish
		  or fowl 3 oz.
		Boiled potato 1 small
		Boiled
		  vegetables 200 Gm.
		Bread* ½ slice
		Butter** 1 pat
		Fruit
		  (5 to 20%) 100 Gm.
		Skimmed milk 8 oz.

* Whole wheat or enriched.   ** Or enriched oleomargarine.   *** Celery, lettuce, endive, and cucumber, prepared with lemon, spices, and vinegar (but without oil or dressing), may be taken freely between meals to allay hunger.

Sample Reducing Diet
(1,000 calories)

Eliminate the potato and one slice of bread (or equiv.—*see* Food Tables) from the 1,200 calorie diet.

Sample Reducing Diet
(800 calories)

Eliminate the potato, 2 pats of butter, and 1½ slices of bread from the 1,200 calorie diet. This diet now is deficient in vitamins A, B₁, and B₂, so that supplementary polyvitamins should be given daily.

Sample Reducing Diet
(700 to 800 calories)

A simple but very effective reducing diet, containing 700 to 800 calories, consists of 2 qt. of skimmed milk (or its equivalent in powdered skimmed milk plus water), 1 medium apple, and 1 multivitamin capsule. The milk and apple are divided and consumed as desired through the day.

Sample Reducing Diet
(600 Calories)

Eliminate the potato, all the butter, all the bread, and one serving of fruit from the 1,200 calorie diet. Polyvitamin supplementation is required.

High Protein Diet (With some restriction of fat)

Indication: Cirrhosis of the liver, nephrosis, hypoproteinemia, malnutrition.

Principle: To provide needed protein, the normal diet (q.v.) is supplemented with protein-rich foods such as meat, fish, fowl, egg white, cheese, and milk.

Sample Menu

Breakfast		Lunch		Dinner	
Fruit	1 orange	Meat		Meat, fish	
or	½ grapefruit	(or equiv.)	4 oz.	or fowl	4 oz.
Cereal*	½ cup	Potato, rice,		Potato	100 Gm.
with milk		dry beans or		Vegetable	100 Gm.
and sugar		spaghetti	100 Gm.	Bread*	1 slice
Eggs	2	Salad	100 Gm.	Butter**	1 pat
Bread*	1 slice	Bread*	1 slice	Dessert	
Butter**	1 pat	Butter**	1 pat	Milk	8 oz.
Beverage with		Fruit			
cream and		Milk	8 oz.		
sugar					

Midmorning		Bedtime
Milk	8 oz.	Eggnog with milk.

* Whole wheat or enriched.   ** Or enriched oleomargarine.

The above diet supplies approximately 130 to 140 Gm. of protein. If additional protein intake is desired, cottage cheese, other nonfatty cheeses, high protein drinks, or protein hydrolysates are indicated. The drinks are prepared by adding casein, powdered milk, or egg whites to skimmed milk or an eggnog and flavoring the mixture with cocoa and glucose or maltose.

Low Protein Diet

Indications: Nephritis, nitrogen retention.

Principle: To give only sufficient protein to maintain nitrogen balance.

Content: The following foods may be included but not in excess of the amount specified: egg (1), milk (1 pt.), meat or equivalent (1 to 2 oz.), butter (15 Gm.), cereal (1 or 2 serv-

Sample Menu

Breakfast		Lunch		Dinner	
Citrus fruit or		Vegetable	100 Gm.	Meat, fish	
fruit juice		Potato or		or fowl	1 or 2 oz.
Cereal* with		rice	100 Gm.	Potato or	
milk 4 oz.		Salad	100 Gm.	rice	100 Gm.
and sugar		(without		Vegetable	100 Gm.
Egg	1	dressing)		Bread*	1 slice
Bread*	1 slice	Bread*	1 slice	Butter**	1 pat
Butter**	1 pat	Butter**	1 pat	Milk	6 oz.
Beverage with		Fruit			
cream and		Milk	6 oz.		
sugar					

* Whole wheat or enriched.   ** Or enriched oleomargarine.

ings), fruit (2 servings), bread (3 slices), vegetables (3 servings), 1 potato, or corn (1 or 2 servings).

Avoid: Cheese, gelatin, peas, lentils, beans, nuts, and desserts containing milk or egg in excess of the maximum daily allowance.

If restriction of salt and fluid is desired, along with that of protein, the principles of the low salt diet (q.v.) should be incorporated into the low protein regimen.

High Residue Diet

Indication: Atonic constipation.

Principle: The atonic intestinal musculature is stimulated by supplementing the normal diet (q.v.) with foods which are bulky and high in cellulose content (fruits and vegetables). In addition, at least 6 to 8 glasses of water must be taken daily.

Sample Menu		
Breakfast	*Lunch*	*Dinner*

Fruit 1 orange
  or ½ grapefruit,
  with pulp
Stewed fruit
Cereal* ½ cup
  with milk
  and sugar
Egg 1 or 2
Bread* 1 slice
Butter** 1 pat
Beverage with
  cream and
  sugar
	Meat 2 oz.
	  (or equiv.)
	Potato, rice
	  or spaghetti 100 Gm.
	2 Vegetables 200 Gm.
	Salad 100 Gm.
	Bread* 1 slice
	Butter** 1 pat
	Fruit
	Milk or
	  buttermilk 8 oz.
		Meat, fish
		  or fowl 3 oz.
		Potato 100 Gm.
		2 Vegetables 200 Gm.
		Bread* 1 slice
		Butter** 1 pat
		Fruit
		Milk or
		  buttermilk 8 oz.

Bedtime		
Fruit or fruit juice		

* Whole wheat or enriched.   ** Or enriched oleomargarine.

Low Residue Diet

Indications: Gastrointestinal irritability or inflammation, and both before and after gastrointestinal surgery.

Principle: To spare the gastrointestinal tract by furnishing, in frequent small feedings, necessary nutrients that are easily digested and low in residue content.

Content: Sugars, milk, egg, ground lean meat (beef, lamb, or chicken), gelatin, fine white cereal (cooked), enriched white bread, crackers, butter, cottage or cream cheese, strained fruit or vegetable (cooked), potato, soup, spaghetti, beverages, dessert (custard, ice cream, cookies, tapioca, gelatin, rice pudding, plain cake).

Avoid: Raw fruit and vegetables, whole wheat cereal or bread, pork, veal, spices, fried food, excessive fat, rich desserts, nuts.

Sample Menu

Breakfast	Lunch	Dinner
Fruit juice	Lean meat 2 oz.	Lean meat 3 oz.
White (fine, cooked)	(or equiv.)	Potato
cereal with milk	Potato, rice,	Strained
and sugar	or spaghetti	vegetable
Egg	Bread* with	Bread* with
Bread* with	butter**	butter**
butter**	and jam	and jam
and jam	Dessert	Dessert
Beverage with	Milk 8 oz.	Milk 8 oz.
milk and sugar		

Midmorning	Midafternoon	Bedtime
Milk 6 oz.	Milk 6 oz.	Eggnog with milk
Soda crackers	Soda crackers	and sugar

    * Enriched white.   ** Or enriched oleomargarine.

Low Fat Diet (Containing 60 Gm. fat)***

Indications: Certain diseases of the liver and gallbladder.

Principle: The diseased organ is spared from the demands made upon it by fatty foods. The diet should consist largely of easily digested foods (carbohydrates). Egg yolk and meat should be restricted but egg white and cottage cheese are permitted freely. Vegetables are allowed to the limits of tolerance.

Sample Menu

Breakfast		Lunch	Dinner	
Fruit	citrus	Cottage cheese 2 oz.	Lean meat,	
Cereal*	½ cup	Potato, spa-	fish or	
with milk		ghetti or rice 100 Gm.	fowl 3 oz.	
and sugar		Salad (without	only	
Egg	1 only	oil or dressing)	Potato	
Bread*	1 slice	Vegetable 100 Gm.	(no butter)	
Butter**	1 pat	Bread* 1 slice	Vegetable 100 Gm.	
Beverage with		Butter** 1 pat	Bread* 1 slice	
milk and sugar		Fruit	Butter** 1 pat	
		Milk 8 oz.	Fruit or	
			cake	
			(no cream)	
			Milk 8 oz.	

    * Whole wheat or enriched.   ** Or enriched oleomargarine.   *** If further reduction in fat intake is desirable, omit all butter, use skimmed milk for whole milk, and prescribe a vitamin A supplement since the diet then will be deficient in vitamin A.

Low Purine Diet

Indication: Gout.

Principle: To supply foods which are low in purine content, high in carbohydrate (to promote urate excretion), and low in fat (fats decrease urate excretion). The proteins are derived from food which contain little or no purine.

Content: Milk, egg, fruit, most vegetables (*see* restricted and forbidden foods, below), cheese, enriched bread or cereal, butter, and all nonprohibited foods.

Restrict: Certain foods may be eaten sparingly, such as beans, peas, spinach, mushrooms, oatmeal, whole wheat bread or cereal, coffee, tea, or cocoa. Some patients may be allowed 2 oz. twice weekly of beef, veal, mutton, lamb, pork, fish, or fowl, if tolerated.

Avoid: Sweetbreads, sardines, anchovies, kidney, liver, brain, meat, meat extracts, gravies, fish, game, fowl, lentils, wine. Distilled liquors or beer may be taken in moderation.

Sample Menu

Breakfast	Lunch	Dinner
Fruit or fruit juice	Cream soup (without meat extracts)	Egg or cheese
Cereal* with milk and sugar	Cheese or egg	Potato
Egg	Potato, rice or spaghetti	Vegetables (2)
Bread* with butter**	Salad (without dressing)	Bread* with butter**
Beverage with milk and sugar	Bread* with butter**	Dessert
	Fruit	Milk
	Milk	

* Enriched white.　　** Or enriched oleomargarine.

Low Salt Diet

Indication: Cardiovascular or renal edema.

Principle: To inhibit and eliminate edema and reduce blood and interstitial fluid volumes by avoiding foods rich in sodium and preparing the meals without adding salt.

Content: The following foods are allowed within the maximal specified limits: fresh meat (3 oz.), milk (1 pt.), egg (2), sweet butter, unsalted cottage cheese (2 to 3 oz.), whole wheat cereal (1 serving), vegetables (2 servings), potato, fresh fruit (2 servings), unsalted bread (matzoth or specially prepared salt-free bread), and all other nonprohibited foods which can be prepared and served without salt. Pure, salt-free spices (clove, mustard, pepper, onion, vinegar, horseradish) and commercially available, safe, salt substitutes may be used for seasoning. (CAUTION! Avoid lithium salt preparations.)

Avoid: Salted or canned fish or meat, all cheese not listed above, canned vegetables or soups, salad dressings, nuts, prepared biscuits or bread, desserts containing milk in excess of the amount permitted daily, salt butter, salted spices, relish, pickle, bouillon cubes, catsup, olives, and salt substitutes which contain sodium. (NOTE: Since the sodium ion is the important one to rule out, care must be taken that the patient does not use laxatives, dentifrices or other substances with a sodium content.)

Sample Menu

Breakfast	Lunch	Dinner

Fruit—   citrus
Cereal*   ½ cup
  with milk (4 oz.),
  and sugar
Egg
Bread* **
Butter** ***
	Egg or cottage
	  cheese**
	Potato, rice or
	  spaghetti
	Vegetable (1)
	Salad (without
	  dressing)
	Bread* **
	Butter** ***
	Fruit
	Milk 6 oz.
		Fresh meat, fish
		  or fowl**
		Potato
		Vegetable (1)
		Bread* **
		Butter** ***
		Dessert**
		Milk 6 oz.

* Whole wheat or enriched.   ** Unsalted.   *** Or enriched oleomargarine.

If a soft, low salt diet is required, the above foods may be ground or strained and the raw salad eliminated entirely.

Rice Diet (Kempner)

Indications: Essential hypertension, renal disease.

Content (daily): 200 to 350 Gm. (dry) rice, 100 to 500 Gm. sugar, all nonprohibited fruit and fruit juices, 1,000 cc. fluid (including fruit juices).

Avoid: Nuts, more than one banana daily, tomato or vegetable juices, dates, salt, avocados, dried fruits to which any substance other than sugar has been added.

This daily diet contains 2,000 calories, 1,000 cc. fluid, 20 Gm. protein, 5 Gm. fat, 0.2 Gm. chloride, and 0.15 Gm. sodium. About half the calories should come from rice (100 Gm. dry rice = 350 calories) which has been boiled or steamed in unsalted water or fruit juice. The remaining calories are furnished by fruit juices, fruit, and sugar. Additional chloride or calories may be needed to combat hypochloremia or undesirable weight loss, respectively. Maintenance doses of all the vitamins should be given daily in the form of a multivitamin preparation.

For best results, the diet should be continued for at least 2 to 5 months. Thereafter, if tolerated, the diet may be gradually expanded to include nonleguminous vegetables, potato, lean meat, fish, and fowl.

Elimination Diets

Indication: Suspected food allergy.

Principle: To eliminate or incriminate certain foods as allergens by their individual and gradual addition to a basic diet composed of relatively nonallergenic foods. Common food allergens are milk, egg, wheat, citrus fruits, tomato, potato, chocolate, and oatmeal, and all products containing one or more of these ingredients. However, any food occasionally may be responsible.

TABLE 4

ELIMINATION DIETS

FOODSTUFF	DIET No. 1* (No beef, pork, fowl, milk, rye, corn)	DIET No. 2* (No beef, lamb, milk, rice)	DIET No. 3* (No lamb, fowl, rye, rice, corn, milk)
Cereal	Rice products	Corn products	
Vegetable	Lettuce, spinach, carrots, beets, artichokes	Corn, tomatoes, peas, asparagus, squash, string beans	Lima beans, beets, potato (white and sweet), string beans, tomatoes
Meat	Lamb	Chicken, bacon	Beef, bacon
Flour (Bread or biscuits)	Rice	Corn, 100% rye (ordinarily, rye bread contains wheat)	Lima bean, soy bean, potato
Fruit	Lemon, pear, grapefruit	Peaches, apricots, prunes, pineapple	Grapefruit, lemon, peaches, apricots
Fat	Cottonseed oil, olive oil	Corn oil, cottonseed oil	Cottonseed oil, olive oil
Beverage	Tea, coffee (black), lemonade		Tea, coffee (black), lemonade
Miscellaneous	Tapioca, gelatin, cane sugar, maple sugar, salt, peanut butter, olives, synthetic vinegar	Cane sugar, gelatin, corn syrup, salt, synthetic vinegar	Tapioca, gelatin, cane sugar, maple syrup, salt, olives, synthetic vinegar

* DIET No. 4: Should symptoms persist on the above 3 elimination diets, the daily diet may be restricted to 2,000–3,000 cc. of whole milk.

The choice of the diet to be used will depend on the patient's history and skin tests. Most of the common allergens and all suspected foods must be eliminated from any starting diet. No foods or fluids must be consumed other than those specified within the starting diet. The patient (and physician) must know the exact composition of all meals, so that eating in restaurants is not advisable. Furthermore, one always must be certain of the purity of products used—for example, ordinary rye bread contains some wheat flour.

Several such diets, modified after Rowe, are offered above. The physician should start with the one which best meets the patient's needs. If no improvement occurs after 2 weeks on any one diet, another should be tried. When definite improvement is noted, one new food may be added every 3 days. Aggravation of symptoms following the addition of a new food is the best evidence of allergy to that item. Such evidence should be verified by noting the effect of removing that food from the diet for several days and then restoring it.

Vitamin supplements daily are necessary until a normal vitamin intake is otherwise assured.

Soft Diets

Indications: Inability to tolerate a normal solid diet, due to poor teeth, general physical weakness, or gastrointestinal disturbances.

Principle: To provide essential nutrients in a form which is low in residue, well tolerated, and easily digested.

Content: Strained soups and vegetables, fine wheat cereals, bread, cooked fruit (without skin or seeds), ripe banana, potato, rice, ground beef, fowl, fish, egg, cheese, milk, custard, gelatin, tapioca, puddings, cake, cookies.

Avoid: Raw fruits and vegetables, coarse cereal, rich desserts, strong spices, veal, pork, all fried foods.

Sample Menu

Breakfast		Lunch		Dinner	
Fine cereal* with milk and sugar	½ cup	Strained soup		Ground meat, fish or fowl	3 oz.
		Ground beef (or equiv.)	2 oz.	Potato	
Egg—not fried		Potato, rice or spaghetti	100 Gm.	Strained vegetable	100 Gm.
Bread*	1 slice	Strained vegetables (2)	200 Gm.	Bread*	1 slice
Butter**	1 pat	Bread*	1 slice	Butter**	1 pat
Cooked fruit or dilute fruit juice***		Butter**	1 pat	Dilute fruit juice***	
Beverage with cream and sugar		Cooked fruit*** or ripe banana		Dessert	
		Milk	8 oz.	Milk	8 oz.

* Whole wheat or enriched.   ** Or enriched oleomargarine.   *** Taken at the end of the meal.

Bland (Ulcer) Diet

Indications: Gastritis, peptic ulcer.

Principle: To dilute the gastric juices frequently by providing several feedings daily of easily digested, palatable, non-irritating foods. Milk is the basis of any bland diet, with other foods being gradually added as tolerated.

Ulcer Diet for Ambulatory Patients

Breakfast	Lunch	Dinner
Cereal with milk and sugar Egg Bread* with butter** Beverage with milk and sugar Strained fruit or fruit juice***	Cream soup Lean meat 2 oz. (or equiv.) Potato, rice or spaghetti Bread* with butter** Milk 8 oz. Strained fruit juice***	Lean meat, fish or fowl Potato Strained cooked vegetables (2) Bread* with butter** Dessert Milk 8 oz. Strained fruit juice***

Between Meals and at Bedtime

Milk   6 oz.
White crackers
NOTE: Milk may be taken at any time.

* Enriched white.   ** Or enriched oleomargarine.   *** Taken at meal's end.

Sample Menu (4-Week Sippy Regimen)

1st to 3rd days: Give hourly from 7 A.M. to 7 P.M., 3 oz. of a mixture containing equal parts of milk and 20% cream; serve cold or chilled.

4th to 10th days: Continue the hourly feeding of the milk—20% cream mixture, and gradually add egg and fine cereal to the diet so that the patient is receiving (in place of the milk-cream feeding scheduled for that hour) an egg twice daily (7 A.M. and 7 P.M.) and 3 oz. of cooked cereal 3 times daily (10 A.M., 1 P.M., 4 P.M.) by the 10th day.

11th to 28th days: As tolerated, other permitted foods are added to replace the hourly milk-cream mixture until the patient's diet is gradually converted to one of modified low residue (q.v.) and then to an ambulatory ulcer diet. Supplementary iron and polyvitamins are indicated during the Sippy regimen.

Modified Sippy Regimen

Several modifications of the original Sippy regimen have been devised to eliminate its monotony, its deficiency in iron and vitamins, and the absence of food intake from 7 P.M. to 7 A.M. These consist of giving 2 to 4 oz. of the milk-cream mixture every 1 to 2 hours up to 11 P.M. and (if the patient is awake) during the night, plus the more rapid addition to the diet of permitted cereal, egg, toast, crackers, and strained fruits and vegetables. Thus, a soft diet (q.v.) is soon being taken and this in turn is supplanted by the ambulatory.

Content: Milk, cream, fine white, or prepared cereals (farina, cream of wheat, strained oatmeal, corn flakes, puffed rice, cornmeal), gelatin, soup, potato (without skin), rice, butter or oleomargarine, enriched white bread, white crackers, sugars, egg, strained cooked fruit and vegetable, ripe banana, fruit juice, lean fresh meat (beef, lamb, veal), fresh fish, cream or cottage cheese, dessert (custard, tapioca, rice or cornstarch pudding, gelatin, cookies, plain cake).

Avoid: Fried food, spices, carbonated beverages, coffee, pastry, alcohol, tobacco, meat broths, coarse cereal or bread, raw fruit or vegetable, pork, strong cheese, rich desserts.

High Caloric Semifluid Diet

Indications: Fever or illness wherein the patient cannot tolerate a normal or a soft diet.

Principle: To supply needed nutrients in a form that the patient can tolerate. Frequent small feedings permit more complete ingestion of the diet and are tolerated better than 3 large meals.

Sample Menu

Breakfast	Lunch	Dinner
Fruit juice with added sugar	Cream soup with butter**	Broth
White or prepared (fine) cereal with cream and sugar	Cheese 2 oz.	Egg or cheese 2 oz.
	Potato with butter**	Potato with butter**
Egg	Bread* 1 slice	Bread* 1 slice
Bread* 1 slice	Butter** and jam	Butter** and jam
Butter** and jam	10% cream 8 oz.	Dessert
Beverage with cream and sugar		10% cream 8 oz.

Midmorning	Midafternoon	Bedtime
10% cream 6 oz.	Fruit juice with added sugar	Eggnog with cream and sugar
Soda crackers		

Salt: 4 Gm. or more daily (total)
Fluids: 3,000 cc. daily (total)

* Enriched white.   ** Or enriched oleomargarine.

Content: Beverages, fruit juices, enriched white bread, fine white or prepared cereal, cream, butter, ripe banana, dessert (plain), strained vegetables containing 10 to 20% carbohydrate (*see* Food Tables), potato, cream soups, eggs, cream or cottage cheese, gelatin, milk, sugars, jams.

Avoid: Coarse cereals, raw fruits and vegetables, strong cheese, fried food, rich desserts, meat, fish, and fowl.

Liquid Diet

Indication: Inability to consume soft or solid foods.

Principle: To supply essential nutrients in fluid form.

Content: Any food which can be served in strained or liquid form plus custard, ice cream, plain pudding, tapioca, gelatin, and soft-boiled eggs.

Avoid: All food in solid form.

Sample Menu

Breakfast	Lunch	Dinner
Fruit juice 6 oz.	Fruit juice 6 oz.	Fruit juice 6 oz.
Strained cereal with milk and sugar	Cream soup with butter*	Cream soup with butter*
Soft-boiled egg with butter*	Strained vegetables (2)	Strained vegetables (2)
Beverage with cream and sugar	Strained fruit	Dessert
	Milk 8 oz.	Milk 8 oz.

Between Meals and at Bedtime

Eggnog, milk, malted milk, or fruit juice.

* Or enriched oleomargarine.

Additional protein may be administered by the addition of gelatin, whole egg, egg white, casein, powdered milk, or protein hydrolysates, to the above foods.

When tube feedings are required, nutrition may be maintained by the administration of a suitable formula at frequent intervals. A 1-day supply of such a formula should contain strained cereal (100 Gm.), milk (1,000 cc.), 10% cream (300

TABLE 5. INFANT FEEDING

Age (months)	¼	¾	1	2	3	4	5	6	7	8	9	10	11	12
Weight (pounds)	7	8	9	11	12	13	14	15	16	17	18	19	20	21
Feedings per Day	7	6-7	6	5-6	5	5	5	5	5	5	4-5	4	4	3-4
Orange Juice* (oz.)	—	1/8	½	1-2	2-3	3	3	3	3	3	3	3	3	3
Cereal** (tbsp.)	—	—	—	1	2	2	3-4	4	4-5	5	5	5	5-6	6
Vegetable, strained (tbsp.)	—	—	—	1	2	2	2	3	4	4	4	4	4	4
Fruit, strained (tbsp.)	—	—	—	1	2	2	3	3	4	4	4	4	4	4
Egg Yolk	—	—	—	—	—	½	1	1	1	—	—	—	—	—
Meat, finely ground (oz.)	—	—	—	—	—	—	—	½	1	1½	2	2	3	3
Dessert (tbsp.) Gelatin Custard	—	—	—	—	—	—	—	—	1	2	2	2	2	2
Whole Egg	—	—	—	—	—	—	—	—	—	1	1	1	1	1-2
Additional**** Food	—	—	—	—	—	****	—	****	—	****	****	—	—	—

Required Daily Calorie Intake: 45 to 50 calories/lb. body wt.

Vitamins A and D: Sufficient supplementary vitamins to supply 1,500 I.U. Vitamin A and 800 I.U. Vitamin D.

Formula:
1. Boiled milk (whole): 1.5 to 2 oz./lb. body wt./day; maximum, 35 oz. (Whole milk, 20 calories/oz.)

2. Boiled water: Sufficient to furnish total fluid intake of 3 oz./lb. body wt./day; maximum, 35 oz.

3. Sugar: Add sufficient to furnish the number of calories required in the formula in addition to the calorie value of the milk. (Sugar = 4 calories/Gm.)

* Allergy to orange juice requires the substitution of twice the volume of tomato juice or the use of ascorbic acid tablets (30-50 mg. daily). ** Servings, 1 or 2, as required and tolerated. *** Current trends favor even earlier addition of these foods to the infant diet. **** Ripe banana (4 mo.); dry toast, potato (6 mo.); chopped vegetables (8-9 mo.).

cc.), orange juice (100 cc.), maltose (25 Gm.), glucose (75 Gm.), eggs (3), butter or oleomargarine (25 Gm.), and salt (3 Gm.). Additional vitamins, calories, and protein may be assured by the addition to the formula of a polyvitamin liquid, olive oil, or protein hydrolysate powder respectively. The eggs should be thoroughly beaten and the entire mixture warmed, strained, divided, and bottled into the desired number of feedings, and then stored in the refrigerator. Each bottle should be warmed to body temperature before administration.

Infant Diets

Infant nutrition is based on the use of a formula containing milk, water, and a sugar. Whole milk may be replaced in equal volume by evaporated milk or one of the dried milks, the concentration of which can be adjusted to correspond to that of whole milk. The sugar component may consist of maltose, honey, cane sugar, lactose, or other suitable saccharide. Cereal includes any prepared infant cereal, or farina. Each new food added to the infant diet must be given in small amounts initially, and not within 1 week of any other new food, in order to reveal any allergy to it. The foregoing table gives the basic pattern of infant feeding and is self-explanatory.

Diabetic Diet

Principles: To supply necessary nutrients in a manner compatible with the patient's impaired carbohydrate metabolism. Any food may be consumed, and substitution of food equivalents always is permissible, as long as the total intake (both per meal and per day) of carbohydrate, protein, and fat does not differ significantly from that which is prescribed for each individual diabetic. Fruits and vegetables are grouped according to their approximate percentage of carbohydrate content. Saccharin is used for sweetening.

Slight undernutrition is desirable. The optimum daily caloric intake is that which is 5 to 10% below that of a normal individual of the same "ideal weight," sex and activity (TABLES 1 and 2). The protein requirement is 1 to 1.5 Gm./Kg. daily. Of the remaining nonprotein calories which are allowed, 50 to 65% should be supplied by carbohydrates (1 Gm. = 4 calories) and the remainder by fats (1 Gm. = 9 calories).

Individual tastes and the economic status of the patient must be considered in computing a diabetic diet. The basic nutrients of a normal diet (TABLE 3), but with less cereal and bread, are the foundation of any diabetic menu. Other foods are then added to supply the daily requirements of carbohydrate, protein, and fat. These foods should be divided appropriately into 3 meals as shown below, with the nutritional

content, weight, and household measure for each carefully specified. Protein balance may be achieved by controlling the intake
of egg white, meat, cheese, and milk. Fat intake may be controlled by regulating the butter or oleomargarine allowance.
A set of household scales is essential to assure the degree of
accuracy required in weighing out and preparing diabetic diets.

If no insulin, or if regular insulin, is being taken, the daily
carbohydrate allowance may be administered in 3 approximately equal parts, ⅓ at each meal. With protamine insulin,
the carbohydrate intake is divided as follows: breakfast, 20%;
lunch, 40%; dinner, 40%. Globin insulin requires the largest
carbohydrate meal at noon so that the division is: breakfast,
25%; lunch, 50%; dinner, 25%. Occasionally, in patients receiving globin or protamine insulin, a small carbohydrate feeding (milk and soda crackers) may be indicated in midafternoon, or at bedtime, respectively.

Sample Menu in Diabetes

Diet prescription—C: 165; P: 75; F: 65; Calories: 1,545

Food	Gm.	Household Measure	C	P	F
BREAKFAST					
Fruit 10%*	150	1 orange	15	0	0
Cereal**	20	½ cup	15	2	1
Milk for cereal, etc.	120	½ cup	6	4	4.5
Egg*	50	1 medium	0	7	6
Bread* **	30	1 slice ½″ thick	15	3	1
Butter* ***	5	Square 1″ x 1″ x ¼″	0	0	4
Beverage with saccharin	0		0	0	0
		Total	51	16	16.5
LUNCH					
Meat*	60	3″ x 5″ x ⅓″	0	15	8
Vegetable 5%	100		5	1	0
Vegetable 10%	100		10	2	0
Bread* **	15	½ slice, ½″ thick	7.5	1.5	0.5
Butter* ***	5	1″ x 1″ x ¼″	0	0	4
Fruit 20%	100		20	2	0
Milk—whole	240	1 glass	0.2	8.5	9
		Total	55.5	30.0	21.5
DINNER					
Meat*	90	3″ x 5″ x ½″	1	23	13
Vegetable 5%	100		5	1	0
Vegetable 15%	100		15	3	0
Bread* **	30	1 slice, ½″ thick	15	3	1
Butter* ***	5	1″ x 1″ x ¼″	0	0	4
Fruit* 10%	100		10	0	0
Milk—whole	240	1 glass	12	8.5	9
		Total	58	28.5	27
		Daily Total	164.5	74.5	65

* Or equivalent. ** Whole wheat or enriched. *** Or enriched oleomargarine.

FOOD TABLES

Showing Percentage of Carbohydrate, Protein and Fat
Present in 100 Gm. Portions of Common Foods

I. Vegetables

Group 1 (Approx. 5% C)

Vegetable	100 Gm. Portion Household Measure	Percentage (1 Gm. C or P = 4 cal.) (1 Gm. F = 9 cal.) C	P	F
Artichokes (French)	1 medium	3	1	0
Asparagus	½ cup (tips), 10 stalks	3	1	0
Beans, string	¾ cup	3	1	0
Beet greens	½ cup	4	2	0
Broccoli	⅔ cup	4	3	0
Brussels sprouts	10 sprouts	5	1	0
Cabbage	⅔ to 1 cup	4	1	0
Cauliflower	⅔ cup	2	1	0
Celery	2 hearts or 4 stalks	3	1	0
Chard leaves	2 to 3 cups	4	3	0
Cucumber	½ cup	2	1	0
Eggplant	¾ cup	4	1	0
Endive	2 small	2	1	0
Escarole	⅔ small head	2	1	0
Kale	⅔ cup	5	2	0
Leeks	¾ cup	5	2	0
Lettuce	⅓ small head	2	1	0
Mushrooms	½ cup	1	1	0
Okra	½ cup	4	1	0
Peppers, green	1 medium (3″ to 4″ long)	4	1	0
Pumpkin	½ cup	6	1	0
Radishes	10 medium	3	1	0
Rhubarb	⅔ cup	3	1	0
Sauerkraut	⅔ cup	3	1	0
Spinach	½ cup	2	1	0
Squash, summer	⅔ cup	3	1	0
Tomatoes	1 medium or ½ cup	4	1	0
Turnip (beet or greens)	½ cup	5	1	0
Watercress	1 medium bunch	2	1	0

Group 2 (Approx. 10% C)

Beans, dry soy	½ cup	7	35	18
Beetroot	½ cup	9	2	0
Carrots	⅔ cup	8	1	0
Dandelion greens	½ cup (cooked)	7	3	1
Onion, white	½ cup (5 or 6 small)	9	2	0
Peas, green (fresh or canned)	½ cup	9	4	0
Peppers, red	1 medium (3″ to 4″ long)	7	1	1
Rutabaga	⅔ cup	7	1	0
Squash, winter	¾ cup	7	1	0

Group 3 (Approx. 15% C)

Beans, lima	½ cup	15	4	0
Parsnips	½ cup	16	2	1

I. Vegetables (*Continued*)

Group 4 (Approx. 20% C)

Vegetable	100 Gm. Portion Household Measure	Percentage (1 Gm. C or P = 4 cal.) (1 Gm. F = 9 cal.)		
		C	P	F
Beans, baked, canned	½ cup	19	6	2
Beans, kidney, canned	½ cup	17	7	0
Chili sauce	⅓ cup	20	0	0
Corn	⅓ cup	19	3	1
Potato	1 medium (2½″ dia.)	19	2	1
Succotash, canned	⅔ cup	18	4	1

Group 5 (Above 20% C)

		C	P	F
Beans, dry	⅖ cup	62	22	2
Lentils	½ cup	57	25	1
Potato chips	4 cups	49	7	37
Potato, sweet	1 small or ½ medium	26	3	0

II. Fruits

Group 1 (Approx. 5 % C)

Fruit	100 Gm. Portion Household Measure	Percentage (1 Gm. C or P = 4 cal.) (1 Gm. F = 9 cal.)		
		C	P	F
Avocado	½ (4″ long)	3	2	26
Muskmelon (cantaloupe or honeydew)	¼ melon (5″ dia.)	5	1	0
Watermelon (edible portion)	1 slice (2″ x 2″ x 2″)	6	0	0

Group 2 (Approx. 10% C)

		C	P	F
Blackberries	½ cup	8	1	1
Cranberries	¼ cup (cooked)	10	1	1
Currants	½ cup	10	2	0
Gooseberries	⅔ cup	8	1	0
Grapefruit	½ (4″ dia.) or ⅖ cup juice	10	0	0
Lemon	1 (2½″ long) or ½ cup juice	8	1	0
Papaya	¼ (5″ dia.)	9	1	0
Tangerine	2 small or ½ cup juice	9	1	0

Group 3 (Approx. 15% C)

		C	P	F
Apple	1 small (¾ medium)	14	0	0
Apple juice	½ cup	13	0	0
Apple sauce	½ cup	13	0	0
Apricots (fresh)	1½ average	13	1	0
Blueberries	⅔ cup or ⅖ cup juice	15	1	1
Grapes	⅖ cup	15	1	1
Huckleberries	⅔ cup or ⅖ cup juice	14	0	0
Limes	1 (2½″ long)	13	0	0
Loganberries	⅔ cup	14	1	1
Mulberries	⅔ cup	13	0	0

II. **Fruits** (*Continued*) Group 3 (Approx. 15% C) (*Continued*)

Fruit	100 Gm. Portion Household Measure	Percentage (1 Gm. C or P = 4 cal.) (1 Gm. F = 9 cal.)		
		C	P	F
Nectarines	2 medium	14	0	0
Orange	1 medium or ⅖ cup juice	13	0	0
Peaches	1 medium (2½″)	12	1	0
Pears	1 medium	14	1	0
Pineapple, fresh or canned	⅔ cup or 1 slice (3″ thick)	14	0	0
Pineapple juice	½ cup	14	0	0
Plums, fresh	3 (1½″ dia.)	12	1	0
Quinces, fresh	⅓ (2½″ x 3″)	12	0	0
Raspberries	⅔ cup or ½ cup juice	12	1	1
	Group 4 (Approx. 20% C)			
Banana	1 medium, ½ large	22	1	0
Cherries	⅔ cup	17	1	1
Figs, fresh	2 medium (1½″)	18	1	0
Grape juice	½ cup	19	0	0
Persimmons, Japanese	1 large	18	1	0
Prune juice (canned)	½ glass	18	0	0
Prunes, fresh	3 to 4	19	1	0
	Group 5 (Above 20% C)			
Cherries, maraschino	½ cup	50	0	0
Currants, dried	½ cup	70	2	0
Dates, fresh	18 medium	65	2	0
Dates, dry	14 medium	78	2	3
Figs, dry	8 to 10	68	4	0
Persimmons, native, fresh	2 small	28	1	0
Prunes, dried	10 medium	65	2	0
Raisins, dried	⅔ cup	75	3	3

III. **Meats** (raw, unless otherwise specified)

Type of Meat	100 Gm. Household Portion	Percentage (1 Gm. C or P = 4 cal.) (1 Gm. F = 9 cal.)		
		C	P	F
Bacon	10 slices (2″ x 4″ x ⅛″)	0	9	65
Bacon, crisp	20 slices (2″ x 3″ x ⅛″)	0	30	50
Beef, medium fat, medium roasted	2 slices (2″ x 3″ x 1″)	0	20	11
Beef, lean, broiled	2 slices (2″ x 3″ x 1″)	0	28	5
Beef, fat, medium done	2 slices (2″ x 3″ x 1″)	0	13	18
Chicken or duck		0	21	5
Frankfurter (all meat)	2 average size	1	19	18
Ham, fresh, lean	2 slices (2″ x 2″ x ½″)	0	25	14
Ham, fresh, fat	2 slices (4″ x 3″ x ½″)	0	12	40
Heart, beef	2 slices (2″ x 3″ x ½″)	0	16	20
Heart, pork	1 slice (2″ x 3″ x 1″)	0	17	6
Kidney	½ cup	0	16	6
Lamb (or mutton)	2 slices (1″ x 4″ x 1″)	0	19	15
Lamb (or mutton) chops	2 chops	0	20	22

III. Meats (*Continued*)

Type of Meat	100 Gm. Household Portion	Percentage (1 Gm. C or P = 4 cal.) (1 Gm. F = 9 cal.)		
		C	P	F
Liver	2 slices (3″ x 2″ x ½″)	0	20	5
Pork, lean	1 slice (2″ x 3″ x 3″)	0	16	24
Sausage (all meat)	6 (3″ x ¾″)	0	18	38
Tongue	5 slices (¼″ thick)	0	16	15
Turkey	2 slices (4″ x 3″ x ½″)	0	22	18
Veal, medium fat	2 slices (2″ x 3″ x ½″)	0	20	8

IV. Fish (raw, unless otherwise specified)

Type of Fish	100 Gm. Household Portion	Percentage (1 Gm. C or P = 4 cal.) (1 Gm. F = 9 cal.)		
		C	P	F
Bass	2 slices (4″ x 2″ x ½″)	0	20	2
Clams, meat only	½ cup	5	11	1
Cod	2 slices (4″ x 2″ x ½″)	0	20	1
Crabmeat, canned	⅔ cup	1	17	3
Fish, other	⅔ cup	0	19	8
Halibut	2 slices (4″ x 2″ x ½″)	0	18	6
Herring	½ medium fish	0	20	7
Herring, smoked	½ medium fish	0	37	16
Lobster, fresh or canned	¾ cup	0	18	1
Oysters, meat only	4 or 5 large	5	8	1
Salmon, fresh or canned	¾ cup	0	21	12
Sardines, canned	4 large or 10 small	0	23	20
Scallops	½ cup	3	15	0
Shrimp	½ cup	1	18	1

V. Bread, Cereals and Flour Products

Type of Product	100 Gm. Household Portion	Percentage (1 Gm. C or P = 4 cal.) (1 Gm. F = 9 cal.)		
		C	P	F
Bread: white, rye or whole wheat	3½ slices (½″ thick)	50	9	3
Cake or cookies (without fruit or icing)	1 slice (3″ x 3″ x 1½″)	65	6	9
Cereal: whole wheat, rice, rye or oat		77	11	1
Crackers, graham	10 to 12 large	72	9	9
Crackers, matzoth		70	15	0
Crackers, soda	25 (2″ x 2″)	73	10	9
Doughnuts	2	52	7	22
Hominy, cooked	½ cup	15	2	0
Macaroni, cooked	⅔ cup	18	3	0
Macaroni, raw	¾ cup	74	13	1
Noodles, cooked	½ cup	20	4	0
Rice	½ cup	24	3	0
Spaghetti, cooked	½ cup	20	4	0

VI. Dairy Products

Type of Product	100 Gm. Household Portion	Percentage (1 Gm. C or P = 4 cal.) (1 Gm. F = 9 cal.)		
		C	P	F
Milk, whole	⅖ cup	5	4	4
Milk, skimmed	⅖ cup	5	4	0
Milk, evaporated	⅖ cup	10	7	8
Milk, powdered, skimmed	¾ cup	52	36	1
Milk, malted, dry	¾ cup	72	15	9
Buttermilk	½ cup	5	4	1
Cream, 10% (light)	⅖ cup	5	4	12
Cream, 20% (average)	⅖ cup	5	3	19
Cream, 40% (heavy)	⅖ cup	3	2	41
Ice Cream (without fruit or nuts)	½ cup	20	4	13
Butter (or oleomargarine)	10 squares (1″ x 1″ x ½″)	0	1	81
Cheese, American	1 slice (4″ x 2″ x 1″)	2	27	32
Cheese, cottage	6 level tbsp.	4	20	1
Cheese, cream	5 squares (1″ x 1″ x ¾″)	2	7	34
Cheese, other	⅖ cup	2	20	32
Egg, whole	1 medium (60 Gm.)	0	6	6
Egg white	1 white only	0	3	0
Egg yolk	1 yolk only	0	3	6

VII. Miscellaneous Foods

Type of Product	100 Gm. Household Portion	Percentage (1 Gm. C or P = 4 cal.) (1 Gm. F = 9 cal.)		
		C	P	F
Beer	⅖ glass	4	0	0
Broth, clear	½ cup	0	0	0
Carbonated drinks	⅖ glass	8 to 16	0	0
Catsup	⅖ cup	24	2	0
Chocolate, sweet, dry	⅖ cup	60	2	25
Chocolate, unsweetened, dry	⅖ cup	25	12	52
Cocoa, dry, unsweetened	¾ cup	38	18	20
Coconut, prepared	1 cup	52	4	39
Cod liver oil	⅖ cup	0	0	100
Custard	½ cup	5	6	7
Dextrose	⅖ cup	100	0	0
Fat, cooking	⅖ cup	0	0	100
Flour	1½ cup	76	11	1
Gelatin, dry	⅔ cup	0	85	0
Honey	⅓ cup	81	0	0
Jelly	⅓ cup	70	0	0
Lard (or other shortening)	⅖ cup	0	0	100
Marmalade	⅓ cup	65	1	0
Mayonnaise	⅖ cup	0	2	75
Molasses	½ cup	60	0	0
Nuts, miscellaneous (meats)		20	20	60
Oils, salad and cooking	⅖ cup	0	0	100
Olives, ripe or green	18	3	2	15
Pickles, sour	⅓ cup	2	0.5	0

VII. **Miscellaneous Foods** (*Continued*)

Type of Product	100 Gm. Household Portion	Percentage (1 Gm. C or P = 4 cal.) (1 Gm. F = 9 cal.)		
		C	P	F
Pickles, sweet, mixed	1 cup	25	1	0
Popcorn, popped	6 cups	80	12	5
Salad dressing	⅓ cup	15	5	10
Soup, commercial, undiluted (see labels)	⅖ cup	10	3	2
Soup, creamed	½ cup	4	2	13
Soy bean, dry	½ cup	12	34	18
Soy bean, fresh	⅔ cup	6	13	7
Starch, corn	¾ cup	87	1	0
Sugar, granulated	⅖ cup	100	0	0
Tapioca pudding	⅔ cup	28	3	3
Vinegar	⅖ cup	4	0	0
Yeast	100 Gm.	8	8	0

The exact content of manufactured foods may vary, due to such factors as added sugar, and always should be determined from the label or from the manufacturer.

Food Equivalents

To permit wide variety in the menu and to avoid those foods which are disliked or not tolerated, alternative foods may be substituted in amounts which are approximately equivalent in their content of C, P, and F. Every item in any one list of foods is mutually equivalent. For example, since 100 Gm. of a Group 1 (5%) vegetable is equivalent to 50 Gm. of a Group 2 (10%) vegetable or 25 Gm. of a Group 4 (20%) fruit, then also 25% of a Group 4 fruit is equivalent to 50 Gm. of a Group 2 vegetable. However, the mineral and vitamin content may not be equivalent, so that the possibility of creating deficiencies in these nutrients must not be overlooked.

When the fat value of desired equivalents differs significantly,

Approximate Equivalent Values (in Gm.) of Fruit and Vegetable Groups (100 Gm. Portions)

100 Gm. Portion	Group 1 (5%)	Group 2 (10%)	Group 3 (15%)	Group 4 (20%)
Group 1 (5%)	100 Gm.	50 Gm.	33 Gm.	25 Gm.
Group 2 (10%)	200 Gm.	100 Gm.	66 Gm.	50 Gm.
Group 3 (15%)	300 Gm.	150 Gm.	100 Gm.	75 Gm.
Group 4 (20%)	400 Gm.	200 Gm.	133 Gm.	100 Gm.

the situation may be corrected by adding to, or removing from, the meal an appropriate amount of butter. Furthermore, a single food may be replaced by two items—for example, 1 egg is equivalent to 8 Gm. of liver plus 11 Gm. of bacon.

Approximate Equivalents of 1 Slice (30 Gm.) Bread:
C: 16; P: 3; F: 1

	Gm.	Household Measures
Group 1 (5%) fruit or vegetable	320	
Group 2 (10%) fruit or vegetable	160	
Group 3 (15%) fruit or vegetable	106	
Group 4 (20%) fruit or vegetable	78	
Corn flakes	20	1 cup
Crackers	23	3 squares
Macaroni (cooked)	80	⅓ cup
Peas, fresh, shelled	106	⅔ cup
Potato, white	89	1 small
Potato chips	34	1¼ cup
Potato, sweet	61	½ medium
Rice (cooked)	67	½ cup

Approximate Equivalents of 1 Egg (60 Gm.):
C: 0; P: 6; F: 6

	Gm.	Household Measures
Cheese, American	20	1 slice (3″ x 2″ x ½″)
Cheese, cream (deduct 10 Gm. butter)	60	4 tbsp.—minus
Cheese, cottage (add 5 Gm. butter)	30	
Fish (add 3 Gm. butter)	30	⅙ cup
Fowl	30	1 slice (4″ x 1″ x ½″)
Liver	8	1 slice (1″ x 1″ x ½″)
Bacon	11	3 slices (3″ x 2″ x ⅛″)
Meat, medium fat	30	1 slice (2″ x 3″ x 1″)

Approximate Equivalent of 100 Gm. Meat (Medium Fat):
C: 0; P: 20; F: 20

Give 3⅓ times the equivalent allowed for 1 egg (60 Gm.) above.

Approximate Equivalent of 20 Gm. Butter:
C: 0; P: 0.5; F: 17

	Gm.	Household Measure
Cooking fats	17	1 tbsp.
Cream (40%)	40	2½ tbsp.
Lard	17	1 tbsp.
Mayonnaise	23	1½ tbsp.
Salad oil	17	1 tbsp.

OFFICE LABORATORY PROCEDURES

Diagnostic laboratory procedures ordinarily of value in a general office practice are described in this chapter. Those outlined in detail are, with few exceptions, the ones that can be performed with a limited amount of equipment and technical assistance. In the case of certain more complex laboratory procedures, however, instructions are given as to how specimens should be collected and handled prior to examination in hospitals, health departments or private laboratories.

URINE

Physiologic Normals

Average amount in 24 hours	1,200 to 1,500 cc.
Reaction to litmus	faintly acid
Specific gravity	1.005 to 1.022
Color	amber
Constituents (in 24-hour specimen):	
Urea	20.0–30.0 Gm.
Uric acid	0.6– 0.75 Gm.
Total nitrogen	10.0–16.0 Gm.
Ammonia	0.5–15.0 Gm.
Chlorides	10.0–15.0 Gm.
Phosphate	2.0– 4.0 Gm.
Total sulfur	1.0– 3.5 Gm.
Creatinine	0.3– 0.45 Gm.
Total solids	50.0–70.0 Gm.
Total acidity	equiv. to 400–600 cc. of N/10 NaOH

Collection of Specimen

A specimen voided at random is usually satisfactory for routine qualitative tests. Urine voided about 3 hours after meals is most likely to contain abnormal constituents. For quantitative tests a sample of pooled urine collected over 24 hours should be used. If the urine is to be kept for an appreciable time before examination, and especially in warm weather, a preservative should be added. Toluol, 2 cc./100 cc. urine, is satisfactory for this purpose.

Specific Gravity

The specific gravity is read off the graduated stem of a urinometer floated in a specimen of urine. Care should be taken to make the reading at the bottom of the meniscus and to be sure that the urinometer is not in contact with the side of the tube. Urinometers are standardized to give accurate readings only at specific temperatures. If the urine is brought to the optimum temperature for the instrument used, no correction is necessary; otherwise it is necessary to add 0.001 to the urinometer reading for every 3 degrees C. above the temperature for which the urinometer is standardized, and to subtract a like amount for every 3 degrees C. below that point.

Reaction

Test acidity with litmus paper (acid—red; alkaline—blue). Normal urine usually is slightly acid, but may be alkaline for several hours after meals.

Albumin (Purdy's Heat Test)

Filter or centrifuge the urine if it is not clear. Take a test tube ⅔ full of the urine and boil upper portion for 2 minutes. If a precipitate forms it may be due to albumin, phosphates or carbonates. Add several drops of 10% acetic acid; if the precipitate persists, it is due to albumin. The amount of albumin present is directly proportional to the density of the precipitate.

Bence-Jones Protein

Slightly acidify the urine with 10% acetic acid. Heat half a test-tubeful slowly in a water bath. If Bence-Jones protein is present the urine becomes turbid at about 40° C., a definite precipitate appears at about 60° C. and redissolves as the boiling point is reached. On cooling, the precipitate reappears. The presence of albumin may mask the Bence-Jones protein. Albumin may be removed by filtering the specimen while near the boiling point.

Glucose (Benedict's Qualitative Test)

To 8 drops of urine in a test tube add 5 cc. of Benedict's qualitative reagent. Boil in water bath for 5 minutes. If no glucose is present the solution will remain blue. A yellow-green precipitate (1+) will appear if less than 0.5% glucose is present (this may appear only after cooling). A greenish yellow precipitate (2+) indicates 0.5 to 1%; a yellow precipitate (3+), 1 to 2%; and an orange or red precipitate (4+), more than 2%. Other reducing sugars (levulose, lactose, and pentoses) give positive reactions. Salicylates excreted in the urine may produce an opaque green precipitate, which can be confusing. Streptomycin in concentrations above 200 micrograms/cc. in the urine also reduces Benedict's solution.

Acetone (Lange's Test)

To a small quantity of urine add glacial acetic acid to about ¹⁄₂₀ of its volume (1 drop for each cc. of urine) and sufficient fresh concentrated aqueous solution of sodium nitroprusside to slightly tint the solution. Carefully lay a few cc. of ammonia upon its surface. If acetone is present, a reddish purple ring will appear within a few minutes at the plane of contact between the two fluids.

Bilirubin (Bile)

Dip the lower ¼ inch of a strip of barium paper into the urine for 5 or 10 seconds. Remove the strip and lay it on white absorbent paper. Place a drop of Fouchet's reagent (25%

trichloroacetic acid containing 0.9% ferric chloride) at the brown line which marks the level of immersion. A green color denotes the presence of bilirubin. The intensity of the color is proportional to the amount of bilirubin present.

Urobilinogen

To 10 cc. of freshly voided urine add 1 cc. of Ehrlich's reagent; mix, and let stand for 5 minutes. The presence of pathologic amounts of urobilinogen causes a cherry red color to appear.

Blood (Benzidine Test)

To a mixture of equal parts of hydrogen peroxide and a saturated solution of benzidine in glacial acetic acid, add an equivalent amount of urine. A greenish blue color indicates the presence of hemoglobin.

Calcium (Sulkowitch Test)

Place patient on a neutral, low calcium diet for 3 days. Then collect a 24-hour urine specimen. To 5 cc. of this urine add an equal quantity of Sulkowitch reagent (oxalic acid 2.5 Gm., ammonium oxalate 2.5 Gm., glacial acetic acid 5 cc., and distilled water to 150 cc.). Let stand for 3 to 5 minutes and read: no precipitate—no calcium present, serum calcium level probably 5 to 7.5 mg./100 cc.; fine white cloud—moderate amount of calcium, serum level probably normal; definite precipitate—increased calcium; heavy precipitate (like milk)—likelihood of hypercalcemia.

Microscopic Examination of Urine

Centrifuge slowly for several minutes a fresh sample of urine. Place a portion of the sediment thus obtained on a microscope slide, with or without a cover slip, and examine first with a 16 mm. objective, then with a 4 mm. objective. Red blood cells, leukocytes, epithelial cells, casts, mucus threads, and bacteria (in a catheterized specimen only) should be looked for. A quantitative estimate may be arrived at by counting the numbers of these formed elements/low or high power field. In an acid urine, uric acid or calcium oxalate crystals and amorphous urates may be seen; in an alkaline urine, ammonium biurate or phosphate crystals and amorphous phosphates may be present.

Concentration and Dilution Tests

Concentration test: After the patient has had a high protein supper with only 200 cc. of fluid allowed, all fluids and foods are withheld until the following noon. Urine specimens are collected at 8 A.M. and 11 A.M. Normally, the specific gravity should be 1.025 or higher in one of the specimens. If not, allow a dry lunch and supper and test the specific gravity of each specimen voided up to 8 A.M. the following morning. If no specimen approximates a specific gravity of 1.027 or more, an impairment of the renal ability to concentrate is present.

Dilution test: Allow nothing by mouth after 8 P.M. on the day preceding the test. At 8 A.M. on the day of the test have the patient first empty his bladder and then drink 1,500 cc. of water as soon as possible. Have him void every ½ hour until noon and collect the specimens in separate containers. The specific gravity of at least 1 specimen should be 1.003 or lower. The total volume of the pooled specimens should exceed 80% of the water ingested.

BLOOD

Physiologic Normals (for Blood Chemistry, *see* page 1542)

Volume	7 to 9% body wt.
	(4,000–6,000 cc.)
pH	7.35 to 7.45
Erythrocytes	4,500,000–5,000,000/cu. mm.
Leukocytes	5,000–9,000/cu. mm.
Polymorphonuclear neutrophils	60–70%
Lymphocytes	25–33%
Monocytes	2–6%
Eosinophils	1–4%
Basophils	0.25– 0.5%
Reticulocytes	0.5 – 1.5%
Platelets	200,000–600,000/cu. mm.
Hemoglobin (average for both sexes)	14–15 Gm./100 cc.
Hematocrit (men)	38–48%
Hematocrit (women)	36–47%
Color index	0.9–1.1
Volume index	0.9–1.1
Mean corpuscular volume	80–94 cu. μ
Mean corpuscular hemoglobin	27–32 micromicrograms
Mean corp. hemo. concentration	32–38%
Bleeding time	1–3 min.
Coagulation time	2–8 min.
Clot retraction time	begins in 1 hr.; complete in 24
Sedimentation rate, in 1st hr. (men)	0–10 mm.
(women)	0–20 mm.
Prothrombin time (Quick)	10–15 sec.

Collection of Specimen

Blood may be obtained by venipuncture, or by skin puncture with a blood lancet. The technic of venipuncture has been described under Clinical Procedures (q.v.). The usual sites for skin puncture are the edge of the earlobe, the palmar edge of the tip of the middle or ring finger or, in infants, the plantar surface of the big toe or heel. Rub the skin vigorously with alcohol-soaked gauze to cleanse it and also to stimulate circulation. Make a quick stab with a sterile sharp blood lancet. The first drop of blood should be wiped off with sterile gauze and specimens for testing obtained from the blood which follows. Gentle pressure will reopen the puncture each time an additional drop of blood is necessary for a period sufficient to allow for several tests; at no time should the site be squeezed or milked to obtain more blood; instead, when necessary, repeat the puncture. When the tests are completed, cover the wound and maintain firm pressure with alcohol-soaked cotton or gauze until bleeding stops.

Blood obtained by venipuncture may be oxalated and used for certain tests including red blood cell count, white blood cell count and differential, and hemoglobin determination, provided these procedures are done within a reasonably short time (30 minutes) after the blood is obtained. This permits the performance of most of the tests on a single specimen and avoids the annoyance of an additional finger puncture. The oxalated blood should be shaken thoroughly to ensure even distribution of the cells before specimens for counts are taken from the container.

Red Blood Cell Count (R. B. C.)

Draw blood to the 0.5 mark of a clean, dry, red-cell pipet (identified by the 101 mark above the bulb). Quickly and carefully wipe excess blood from the tip with gauze and then plunge the pipet into a wide-mouthed bottle containing Hayem's fluid (mercuric chloride 0.5 Gm., sodium sulfate 5 Gm., sodium chloride 1 Gm., distilled water 200 cc.) and fill to the 101 mark, meanwhile rotating the pipet and avoiding bubbles. Encircle the pipet with a broad, heavy rubber band to prevent spilling and drying, and shake to mix contents thoroughly. The count should be made the same day the specimen is obtained.

To make the count, close both ends of the pipet and shake it well for at least 3 minutes. Discard half the contents. Allow a small drop to form at the tip, and with this, charge the counting chamber. If the drop is too large it will overflow the ruled platform. The counting chamber and the cover slip then will have to be cleaned and dried, and the chamber recharged. On the other hand, make sure the chamber is completely charged, with no bubbles present.

Examine under low power of the microscope to see that the cells are evenly distributed, center the ruled red-cell counting area (Neubauer), and under high power count the number of red cells in 80 of the smallest squares (5 of the larger squares containing 16 small squares each). To the sum thus obtained add 4 zeros, which will give the number of red blood cells/cu. mm. of blood.

Hemoglobin Determination (Hb.)

Several methods are available and confusion may occur since with each method 100% hemoglobin is based on a different value. The instrument used should be standardized to give readings in grams/100 cc. against blood from normal healthy adults with a red cell count of 5,000,000. The average for normal adults is approximately 16 Gm./100 cc. blood. For purposes of simplification an arbitrary standard of 16.6 Gm./100 cc.

blood has been suggested to represent 100% hemoglobin, since any figure obtained as grams per 100 cc. in a hemoglobin determination, when multiplied by the factor 6, is thereby converted to the percentage of normal of the hemoglobin present.

Blood is drawn into a hemoglobin pipet to the 20 mm. mark. It then is expelled into a graduated tube containing about 1 cc. of dilute (0.1 normal) hydrochloric acid (the amount varies with the type of apparatus). On mixing, the hemoglobin is converted into acid hematin. Water is added drop by drop and mixed until the color of the preparation matches a prepared standard. The amount of hemoglobin present is read from the graduation on the tube reached by the surface of the fluid. Other methods include the addition of standard amounts of diluting fluid and then determination of the amount of hemoglobin present by matching the specimen against graded color standards or by matching it in a colorimeter.

White Blood Cell Count (W. B. C.)

Use a clean dry white-cell pipet (11 mark above the bulb). Draw blood to the 0.5 mark and 1% acetic acid solution to the 11 mark. (The acetic acid solution should be filtered frequently, and prepared fresh every 2 weeks.) The technic is the same as for the red cell count except that additional care must be taken in filling, measuring, mixing, and handling the pipet, since the bore is considerably larger than that of the red-cell pipet. The counting chamber is charged and under low power the white blood cells in the 4 largest corner squares (1 sq. mm. each) are counted. Their sum multiplied by 50 gives the number of white cells in 1 cu. mm. of blood. For accuracy, the determination should be done several times and the average taken.

White Blood Cell Differential Count

Touch the surface of a clean glass slide to the drop of blood on the fingertip or earlobe. Spread the blood thinly and evenly by sliding the edge of another slide held at an angle of about 30 degrees to the surface of the first. Wave the smear in the air to obtain rapid drying; in cases of severe anemia where the amount of plasma is relatively increased, the slide should be gently heated to hasten drying, since the cells will deteriorate with slow drying. Stain the smear with Wright's or Giemsa's stain (see below). With stains containing methyl alcohol, such as Wright's, no special fixation procedure is required. Examine the smear under oil immersion. Since an even distribution of leukocytes is difficult to obtain, a total of at least 200 cells should be counted in areas of the slide, which should include both edges of the smear as well as the central portion. Count is kept on each type of leukocyte identified and the differential is figured on a percentage basis. Highly experienced individuals are able to obtain a rough estimate of the percentage of mononucleated and multinucleated white cells by means of the "chamber count," performed during the total white cell count, but this method is subject to gross inaccuracies.

Reticulocyte Count

Place a drop of filtered 1% brilliant cresyl blue stain in 0.9% saline, near one end of a glass slide. Add a drop of blood of equal size from earlobe or fingertip puncture and stir with a pin or toothpick. In 1 minute, make thin smear and stain with Wright's (leave water on for 1 minute only). Examine under oil immersion. A piece of paper with a small rectangular hole, placed inside the ocular, helps to limit the microscope field and prevent confusion in counting the cells. At least 1,000 cells should be counted and the percentage of reticulocytes determined. These appear as red cells either stippled, wreathed, or covered with blue pigment; they normally represent about 0.5 to 1.5% of the total red cells.

Platelet Count

Platelets may be counted on the slide prepared for the reticulocyte count. Count all the platelets seen among 1,000 red cells, and determine their ratio. Then, by calculating from the red cell count, the number of platelets present in 1 cu. mm. of blood also can be determined. The normal platelet count by the indirect method is 250,000 to 500,000/cu. mm. A direct method of counting is to draw platelet solution (sodium citrate 3 Gm., neutral formalin 5 cc. in 100 cc. water) to the 0.5 mark in a red-cell pipet, then draw blood to the 0.5 mark and, after wiping the tip of the pipet, draw platelet solution to the 101 mark. Mix and count in the hemocytometer and calculate in the same manner as for the red cell count (q.v.). This method is more accurate.

Hematocrit

Centrifuge oxalated blood (6 mg. ammonium oxalate and 4 mg. potassium oxalate/5 cc. blood) in a hematocrit tube for 30 to 40 minutes. Use low speed for the first half of the time, and high speed for the remainder. The red cells become packed in the bottom of the tube and the plasma remains on top, with a thin yellowish layer of leukocytes intervening. The reading is made at the top of the column of packed red cells, and the hematocrit calculated according to the type of tube used. The hematocrit represents the percentage of red cells by volume. The average normal is 46 to 48% of whole blood.

Erythrocyte Sedimentation Rate (E.S.R.)

The rate at which red blood cells settle in a standing tube is measured. Ammonium oxalate and potassium oxalate (6 and 4 mg., respectively), preferably dry, should be placed in the tube before the blood (5 cc.) is added. In most types of hematocrit tubes this test can be performed before centrifuging. Care must be taken to ensure a vertical position of the tube during the test, since tilting alters the rate of settling. Findings vary according to the tube and method used. With normal or near normal hematocrits, no correction is necessary; however, when the hematocrit varies from normal, corrections in the sedimentation rate must be made. Prepared tables for calculating the correction are available in standard manuals on laboratory procedure. Normal rates of sedimentation vary with the method of determination used. With the Wintrobe-Landsberg method (hematocrit tube, column of blood 100 mm. high), they are 0 to 9 mm./hr. for men, and 0 to 20 mm./hr. for women; with the Modified Westergren (1 cc. of blood, column 200 mm. high), 0 to 10 mm./hr. for men, and 0 to 20 mm./hr. for women. Modified Cutler method (2 cc. blood, column 50 mm. high), 2 to 8 mm./hr. for men, and 2 to 10 mm. for women.

Color Index (C.I.)

The color index represents the relative quantity of hemoglobin in each red cell as compared with the standard of 100% hemoglobin in an erythrocyte count of 5,000,000/cu. mm. of blood. The percentage of hemoglobin (relative to the standard) found in a given sample, divided by the percentage of red cells (relative to the standard count), gives the color index. Hence, a color index of 1 indicates that each red cell contains the normal amount of hemoglobin, and an index of 0.5 indicates that each has only half of the normal value.

Volume Index (V.I.)

Divide the hematocrit (percent by volume of red blood cells/100 cc. of blood) by 45 (as normal hematocrit) to obtain the percentage of normal volume of red blood cells present. Divide this figure by the percent of normal of the number of red cells/cu. mm. blood to obtain the volume index.

Mean Corpuscular Volume (M.C.V.)

Divide the volume of packed cells in 1,000 cc. of blood (hematocrit multiplied by 10) by the number of red blood cells in millions/cu. mm. Normal, 80 to 94 cu. μ.

Mean Corpuscular Hemoglobin (M.C.H.)

The average weight of hemoglobin in each red cell is determined by dividing the amount of hemoglobin in Gm./1,000 cc. of blood by the red cell count in millions/cu. mm. of blood. Normal: 27 to 32 micromicrograms.

Mean Corpuscular Hemoglobin Concentration (M.C.H.C.)

Divide the hemoglobin in Gm./100 cc. by the hematocrit. Multiply the result by 100 to obtain the concentration of hemoglobin as a percentage of the volume of a corpuscle (normal: 33 to 38%).

Coagulation (Clotting) Time

Place 1 cc. of venous blood in a standard serologic test tube. Tilt the tube at 1-minute intervals. Clotting is evident when the blood gels. The clotting time from the withdrawal of blood to clot formation normally varies from 5 to 10 minutes.

Clot Retraction Time

Place 1 cc. of venous blood in a standard serologic test tube; incubate at 37° C. Inspect at hourly intervals until retraction begins, and then again at 18 or 24 hours. Normally, retraction begins within a few minutes to 2 hours after the clot is formed, and is complete within 18 to 24 hours.

Bleeding Time

Make stab wound in earlobe or fingertip (stab used for determining the coagulation time may be used). Record time from the moment of the stab, and at ½-minute intervals blot wound with a piece of absorbent paper until bleeding stops. Normally, bleeding stops after 2 to 6 blots (1 to 3 minutes).

Red Blood Cell Fragility Test

In each of 18 small, clean test tubes place 1 cc. of NaCl solution varying in concentration in steps of 0.02% NaCl, the 1st tube to contain 0.26%, and the last tube 0.6%. Add 1 drop of venous blood to each test tube and let the tubes stand at room temperature for 2 hours. Read the percentage of NaCl at which hemolysis begins and at which it is complete. Normal red blood cells begin to hemolyze at a concentration of about 0.44% NaCl or less, and the process usually is complete at a concentration of 0.3%. A control test, using normal blood, should always be performed at the same time with identical solutions.

Blood Typing and Cross Matching

Blood is obtained from both donor and recipient. Each specimen is divided into two portions, one of which is converted into a cell suspension by adding 1 drop to a test tube containing 1 cc. of a 1% solution of sodium citrate in 0.85% saline solution, and the other into a serum portion made by placing several cc. of the blood in a test tube and allowing the clot to form, thereby separating the cells and serum. (CAUTION! Accuracy in labeling is imperative.)

For typing, a drop of the unknown cell suspension is mixed with a known type A serum and another drop mixed with a known type B serum on opposite ends of a glass slide. A china-marking pencil can be used to encircle and identify each area. (All precautions must be taken to ensure the potency of the test serums.) Mix with a toothpick and observe fre-

BLOOD CHEMISTRY FINDINGS: NORMAL AND ABNORMAL

	Minimal Quantity Necessary for Determination	Normal Range, Values/100 cc.	Conditions in which Variations from Normal May Occur (See appropriate chapters)	
			Increase	Decrease
Glucose	5 cc. serum, oxalated whole blood or plasma. 0.1 cc. (micro method)	80–120 mg.	Diabetes mellitus; hyperthyroidism; acromegaly; hemochromatosis; adrenal tumors, cortical or medullary	Hyperinsulinism, Addison's disease, adenoma or carcinoma of islands of Langerhans
Total Serum Protein	5 cc. serum	6.0–7.5 Gm.	Dehydration (See Globulin, below)	Cachectic illnesses, renal disease, severe burns, malnutrition, liver disease
Albumin	5 cc. serum	3.5–5.5 Gm.	Dehydration	Renal disease, malnutrition, liver disease
Globulin	5 cc. serum	2.5–3.0 Gm.	Chronic infectious diseases such as tuberculosis, syphilis, malaria, rheumatoid arthritis, lupus erythematosus, periarteritis nodosa, kala-azar, lymphogranuloma venereum. Sarcoidosis, cirrhosis, myeloma, carcinomatosis	
Albumin-Globulin (A/G) Ratio		1.3:1 to 3:1	See Albumin and Globulin, above	
Fibrinogen	5 cc. oxalated serum	0.25–0.5 Gm.	Most infectious diseases, conditions producing inflammation or destruction, traumatic injuries	Liver disease, cachexias
Nonprotein Nitrogen	5 cc. serum, oxalated whole blood or plasma	25–38 mg.	Renal disease, urinary obstruction; cardiac failure; intestinal obstruction; gastrointestinal hemorrhage; metallic poisoning; dehydration and shock	
Urea Nitrogen	5 cc. serum, oxalated whole blood or plasma	8–20 mg.	Same as Nonprotein Nitrogen	Severe liver damage

			Increased	Decreased
Creatinine	5 cc. serum, oxalated whole blood or plasma	1–2 mg.	Renal disease, urinary obstruction, metallic poisoning	
Uric Acid	5 cc. serum, oxalated whole blood or plasma	1.5–4.0 mg.	Gout, nephritis, eclampsia	
Calcium	5 cc. serum	9.5–11.5 mg.	Hyperparathyroidism, parathyroid administration, vitamin D overdosage	Hypoparathyroidism, severe nephritis, uremia, rickets
Phosphorus (Inorganic)	5 cc. serum	2.5–3.5 mg. (adults) 3–5 mg. (children)	Tetany, nephritis, uremia, rickets	Hyperparathyroidism
Sodium	5 cc. serum	0.315–0.340 Gm.		Addison's disease, severe diarrhea, high fevers, diabetic acidosis
Potassium	5 cc. serum	16–22 mg.	Addison's disease	
Chlorides as NaCl	5 cc. serum	0.57–0.62 Gm.	Nephritis, eclampsia, cardiac failure	Gastrointestinal disturbances, febrile conditions, acidosis, vomiting, shock
Cholesterol	5 cc. serum	150–250 mg.	Lipoid nephrosis, amyloidosis, biliary cirrhosis, myxedema, obstructive jaundice, diabetes	
Cholesterol Esters	5 cc. serum	50–75% of total cholesterol (above)	Obstructive jaundice	Severe liver disease
Total Lipids	5 cc. serum	0.57–0.82 Gm.	Nephrosis, diabetes, arthritis, hypothyroidism	
Serum Acid Phosphatase	5 cc. serum	1–3 King-Armstrong u. 0–1 Bodansky u.	Metastasizing prostatic carcinoma	
Serum Alkaline Phosphatase	5 cc. serum	1–13 King-Armstrong u. 1–4 Bodansky u.	Increased osteoblastic activity (Paget's disease, osteogenic sarcoma, osteoplastic bone metastases, rickets, hyperparathyroidism), obstructive jaundice	
CO₂ Combining Power	5 cc. serum taken under liquid petrolatum	50–70 volumes/100 cc.	Emphysema, chronic; vomiting, alkalosis	Acidosis, ketosis; intestinal obstruction, diarrhea; traumatic shock

quently for a period of 20 minutes for signs of agglutination. The type is determined as follows:

Type O —No agglutination in either mixture
Type A —Agglutination with type B serum
Type B —Agglutination with type A serum
Type AB—Agglutination in both mixtures

Cross matching should be performed before each transfusion. Mix a drop of the donor's cells with a drop of the recipient's serum (major cross match) and, on the other end of the same slide, mix a drop of the donor's serum with a drop of the recipient's cells (minor cross match). Observe for at least 20 minutes. Agglutination can be seen with the unaided eye, but all mixtures should always be checked under the low power of the microscope. Agglutination will occur either within 20 minutes or not at all. The appearance of agglutination, especially in the mixture of donor's cells and recipient's serum, contraindicates the use of the donor's blood for that recipient.

In addition, Rh typing generally is advisable but a description of this procedure is beyond the scope of this chapter. For a discussion of the significance of the Rh groups *see* Erythroblastosis Fetalis.

Blood Culture

Obtain blood by venous puncture (*see* CLIN. PROC.), during a chill or at the height of a fever when possible. Use extra sterile precautions, prepare site for needle puncture with iodine and alcohol, flame mouths and stoppers of test tubes and containers used. Have agar melted just sufficiently to liquefy, pour into 2 plates and mix each with 1 cc. of the blood. If anaerobic culture is indicated, pour an additional plate to be cultured under anaerobic conditions. Next, inject 5 cc. of the blood into each of 2 flasks containing 50 cc. of blood infusion broth. If other tests are to be made, 5 cc. of blood may be placed in a sterile citrated test tube, mixed and capped, and sent to the laboratory as a source for further cultures. If the patient has received sulfonamide medication, 5 mg. para-aminobenzoic acid should be added to each 100 cc. of culture medium. Likewise, the addition of 10 u. of penicillinase to 15 cc. of culture media is thought by some authorities to inhibit the effect of penicillin or streptomycin, when present in the blood. (Penicillinase must be handled aseptically.)

Blood Smears

The 2-slide method of blood smear preparation has been described under White Blood Cell Differential (q.v.). The cover glass method consists of collecting a single drop of blood on a clean dry cover glass. A second cover glass is placed on top of the drop and the blood permitted to spread between the two. As soon as it has spread, separate the cover glasses by sliding them apart. Stain both and examine. By this method all the white blood cells in 1 drop of blood may be studied.

Thick smears may be made by the 2-slide method by using a larger drop of blood and holding the spreading slide at a less acute angle. Another method is to collect on a clean slide a drop of blood sufficiently large to spread by itself the size of a dime. Let this dry evenly, protected from heat and dust, then stain and examine.

Blood Sugar

Carefully measure 2 cc. citrated blood with a pipet and add to 16 cc. of $\frac{1}{12}$ normal sulfuric acid. When the mixture has become dark in color, add 2 cc. of 10% sodium tungstate solution. Filter until the filtrate is crystal clear. (This protein-free filtrate represents a blood dilution of 1:10 and may be used for other determinations requiring a protein-free filtrate.) Next, place 2 cc. of the filtrate in a Folin-Wu blood sugar tube. Into a similar tube, introduce 2 cc. of a solution containing 0.2 mg. of glucose, and into a third, 2 cc. of a solution containing 0.4 mg. glucose (last 2 standard tubes not required when prepared standards are available). To each of these tubes add 2 cc. of alkaline copper tartrate and boil in a water bath for 6 minutes. When cool, add 2 cc. molybdate-acid solution to each tube and dilute with distilled water to the 25 cc. mark. Match in the colorimeter against the standard whose color is most like the unknown. Set the known standard at 20 and calculate as follows:

$$\frac{20}{\text{Unknown reading}} \times 100 = \text{mg. glucose/100 cc. whole blood}$$

When using 0.4 mg. glucose/2 cc. standard solution, multiply by 200.

CEREBROSPINAL FLUID

Physiologic Normals

Volume	approx. 130 cc.
Color	colorless and clear
Specific gravity	1.003–1.008
Reaction	alkaline
Protein	16 – 38 mg./100 cc.
Glucose	45 – 80 mg./100 cc.
Chloride (NaCl)	720 – 750 mg./100 cc.
Phosphate (inorganic)	1 – 2 mg./100 cc.
Calcium	4.5 – 5.5 mg./100 cc.
Cells	0 – 10/cu. mm.
Pressure	5 – 7.5 mm. of mercury
	60 – 100 mm. of water

Collection of Specimen

The technics of performing a spinal tap and determining the spinal fluid pressure are described under Clinical Procedures (q.v.). For routine testing purposes 5 to 8 cc. of spinal fluid is required. Discard the first few drops, especially if the puncture technic has been faulty or unusually difficult. Collect the remainder in 2 or 3 sterile test tubes. Microscopic examination must be done at once; specimens for chemical determinations should be refrigerated, or dispatched immediately to a nearby laboratory; spinal fluid to be cultured may, if necessary, be incubated overnight in the original sterile test tube.

Gross Examination

Normal spinal fluid is clear and colorless, and does not coagulate. Haziness appears when 200 to 500 cells/cu. mm. are present. More than 500 cells/cu. mm. produce a turbid or purulent fluid. Bloody fluid which does not coagulate on standing and has a uniform appearance in all test tubes is obtained in cases of bleeding into the subarachnoid space. Fluid that is at first bloody but clears on continued collection, is the result of trauma due to faulty technic. Xanthochromic (yellow or amber tinged) spinal fluid is obtained whenever blood has been present for more than 4 hours or when bile pigment is present. The fluid may appear faintly yellow, when the protein content is greater than 100 mg./100 cc. Clots, either coarse or in the form of delicate webs, indicate the presence of fibrinogen and fibrin ferment. Coarse clots commonly form in fluids with high leukocyte counts. Web formation is common in cases of tuberculous meningitis. (For differential diagnosis of abnormal spinal fluid findings *see* table, p. 986.)

Protein

Globulin: Qualitative determination requires a clear spinal fluid and is valueless when blood is present. The Pandy qualitative test consists of adding 1 cc. of spinal fluid to 1 cc. of a saturated solution of phenol in distilled water. A faint turbidity appears with normal fluid. A definite white cloud indicates increased globulin; the intensity of the precipitate is roughly proportional to the amount of globulin present.

Total protein: Quantitative determination can be performed rapidly by adding 3 cc. of 3% sulfosalicylic acid to 1 cc. of spinal fluid. Mix and let stand for 5 minutes. Compare degree of turbidity with prepared tubes of known concentrations. Protein content above 38 to 40 mg./100 cc. is abnormal. Average normal is 25 mg./100 cc.

Sugar

Normally, spinal fluid sugar varies between 50 and 80 mg./100 cc., or about half the blood sugar level. Benedict's qualitative test (q.v.), as performed with urine (q.v.), can be done and will provide a rough estimate of major alterations in sugar content. Accurate determination of the content may be obtained by diluting 1 part of spinal fluid with 4 parts of distilled water and substituting this for the protein-free filtrate in the blood sugar determination (q.v.). (NOTE: Since the specimen is diluted 1:4, the result of the calculations must be multiplied by 5.) For use in diagnostic interpretation the spinal fluid sugar value is not significant unless it is compared with a blood sugar level simultaneously determined.

Microscopic Examination

This must be performed as soon as possible after the specimen is collected. For the cell count the fluid may be unstained, or Unna's polychrome methylene blue may be used. Draw the Unna's fluid to the 1 mark in a white blood-cell pipet and then fill to the 11 mark with spinal fluid. Fill a hemacytometer counting chamber and count the number of cells in the ruled area. Calculate the number/cu. mm. and multiply this figure by 1.1 to correct for dilution by the staining fluid. With unstained counts this correction is unnecessary. Unna's fluid colors white blood cells blue, and red blood cells yellow.

A differential count also should be made. Centrifuge the specimen and smear the sediment on a slide by means of a wire loop. Dry and stain with Wright's stain. Report the types of cells found by per cent.

Two additional slides should be smeared in the same manner, the first stained with Gram's stain and the second with methylene blue for morphologic studies of bacteria. (Remember to examine for Torula, which are gram-positive.) If tuberculosis is suspected, an additional slide should be prepared for acid-fast staining; centrifuge at least 10 cc. of spinal fluid at high speed for 1 hour; pour off supernatant fluid; to the sediment add about 3 cc. of 95% alcohol and a drop of dilute egg albumen solution; recentrifuge at high speed for 30 minutes; smear slide and stain. If a pellicle or web is present, transfer it to a slide for staining, since the organisms often are retained in this.

Spinal Fluid Culture

It is preferable to culture spinal fluid as soon as possible, but the specimen may be incubated overnight in the original sterile test tube when necessary. Cultures should be planted on chocolate slants and on blood agar for routine cultures, but special media or animal inoculation may be required.

GASTRIC CONTENTS

Physiologic Normals

Total acidity	50–100 degrees*
Free HCl	25– 50 degrees
Combined HCl	10– 15 degrees
Organic acids and acid salts	3– 5 degrees

* Degrees are equivalent to the number of cc. of decinormal NaOH required to neutralize 100 cc. of gastric contents.

Collection of Specimen

The examination is conducted after a 12-hour fast. The patient is seated with the head forward, chin tilted up, and lap covered with towels or a rubber apron. To obtain cooperation, the whole procedure should be explained to him in detail. He should be urged not to swallow saliva during the test, since it will alter the findings. The tube (Sawyer, Rehfuss, or Levin) is inserted until the first marking-ring reaches the front teeth (40 cm.), at which time the tip of the tube is in the stomach (for technic and precautions, see CLIN. PROC.).

The fasting content is withdrawn with an asepto-type syringe, the amount measured, and the specimen set aside for testing, in a labeled test tube or beaker. Secretions then are collected 3 times at 10 to 15 minute intervals, measured, and set aside for testing.

Next, gastric secretion is stimulated by administration of a test meal, alcohol, or histamine. The Ewald-type test meal consists of 300 to 400 cc. of water, or weak tea without cream or sugar, and 2 slices of bread or toast or a shredded wheat biscuit served plain. Ethyl alcohol (50 cc. of a 7% solution) or water alone (200 to 300 cc.) often is preferred, since either may be administered through the tube, thereby eliminating the withdrawal and reinsertion of the tube, necessary with the test meal to permit mastication. Histamine, 0.01 mg./Kg. body wt. injected subcut., also stimulates gastric secretion. (CAUTION! Patients must be carefully selected for histamine stimulation, since physical discomfort, flushing, and increased pulse rate frequently ensue. Severe and even dangerous reactions may occur in histamine-sensitive patients.) After gastric stimulation by any of these methods, a 5 cc. specimen is withdrawn every 15 minutes. The peak of acidity usually is reached within 1 hour. Since specimens from different parts of the stomach may vary in acidity, a portion of the gastric contents may be drawn into the syringe and forcibly reinjected (provided there is no contraindication) just before withdrawing the sample to be tested. The rate of secretion and the rate at which the stomach empties cannot be ascertained by the fractional method described but can be estimated by withdrawing and measuring the total contents obtainable at 15 and 30 minutes after the test meal. Samples are taken and the remainder of the specimen then may be reinjected into the stomach. This procedure is useful in postvagotomy tests to demonstrate gastric motility.

Gross Examination

The amount of fasting specimen varies from 20 to 100 cc., averages 40 cc., and should not exceed 100 cc. Following an Ewald-type test meal, 50 to 100 cc. usually can be obtained in 1 hour, and the secretory volume following histamine stimulation (no test meal) averages 20 to 50 cc.

Normally, the fasting specimen is colorless, slightly opalescent, and contains varying amounts of mucus which can be removed, if desired, by centrifuging. Food particles should not be present after a 12-hour fast. Fresh blood has its normal appearance but blood from chronic bleeding, as in ulcer or carcinoma, is partially digested and appears as dark brown particles in the fluid, which also is stained a dark, greenish brown (coffee-grounds appearance). Bile, freshly regurgitated, imparts a lemon yellow color, while bile that has been in the stomach for a considerable time produces a green and turbid appearance.

Total Acidity (Töpfer's method)

Place 10 cc. of filtered stomach contents in a white evaporating dish (5 cc. may be used, but this amount provides less accurate data); add 4 drops of 1% alcoholic solution of phenolphthalein. Titrate with decinormal sodium hydroxide solution. A rose red color indicates the end point. Saturation of the specimen with sodium chloride produces a sharper end reaction. Each degree of acidity is equivalent to 0.00365 Gm. of HCl. To determine the number of degrees in 100 cc. of gastric juice (normally 50 to 100 degrees) multiply the number of cc. of decinormal NaOH used in titrating by 10 for a 10 cc. specimen, or by 20 for a 5 cc. specimen.

Free Hydrochloric Acid (Töpfer's method)

The procedure is the same as for total acidity determination, except that 4 drops of 0.5% alcoholic solution of dimethylamino-azobenzol is used instead of phenolphthalein. On adding the indicator, a red color denotes the presence of free HCl. The decinormal NaOH is added until the last trace of red disappears. The number of cc. of decinormal NaOH so required is used as above in calculating the degrees of acidity present (normally 25 to 50 degrees). When the quantity of test material is limited, the same specimen may be used for both the free HCl and the total acidity determinations. Find the amount of free HCl first, then add the phenolphthalein and continue the titration.

Combined Hydrochloric Acid (Töpfer's method)

If no free HCl is found, it is necessary to determine whether or not any is present in combined form. This test is performed in the same manner as the preceding test, except that 4 drops of a 1% aqueous solution of sodium alizarin sulfonate is used as an indicator. Titrate until a violet color appears and the shade does not deepen. The number of cc. of decinormal NaOH used multiplied by 10 (for a 10 cc. specimen) gives the number of degrees of all the acidity (lactic acid, other organic acids and acid salts) except that of the combined HCl. Then subtract this figure from that obtained in the test for total acidity (q.v.); the difference, if any, represents the degrees of combined HCl present (normally 10 to 15 degrees).

Lactic Acid (Kelling's Test, Simon's Modification)

Add ferric chloride solution to a test tube of distilled water until a faint yellow color is obtained. Place half of this in another (control) tube. Add several drops of the specimen to the first tube: if lactic acid is present, the solution will assume a much stronger yellow color than that of the control. Lactic acid is not present in gastric contents under normal conditions.

Blood

Mix equal parts of hydrogen peroxide and a saturated solution of benzidine in glacial acetic acid. To several cc. of this mixture add an equal portion of gastric juice. The appearance of a blue color indicates the presence of hemoglobin.

Microscopic Examination

Place a drop of unfiltered gastric juice on a slide, cover with a cover slip and examine under the 16 mm. and 4 mm. objectives. By lowering the condenser and closing the diaphragm of the microscope, structures in the gastric contents may be seen more readily. A drop of diluted Lugol's solution run under the cover slip also aids visualization. Starch granules, occasional epithelial cells, yeast cells and bacteria are ordinarily found. Any red blood corpuscles and pus cells that may be present can be identified.

DUODENAL CONTENTS
(Gallbladder Drainage)

Collection of Specimen

After the patient has fasted for 12 hours, an Einhorn, Rehfuss, or Ågren-Lagerhöf tube is inserted into the stomach and the gastric contents removed, as described above. The patient then lies on his right side, with hips slightly elevated; in 30 to 45 minutes, the tip of the tube will usually pass into the duodenum, excepting the Ågren-Lagerhöf tube, which takes an hour or more. Specimens of 5 to 10 cc. each are collected in series. To obtain fresh bile, introduce 50 to 100 cc. of sterile 25% saturated magnesium sulfate solution into the duodenum through the tube (Lyon's method). This relaxes the sphincter of Oddi and promotes gallbladder drainage. The tube is left in place, and after 5 minutes the duodenal contents are aspirated.

Gross Examination

Duodenal fluid is normally clear and colorless, but may be yellowish. It is viscid in consistency and alkaline in reaction. Cloudiness is due to mixture with gastric juice or to the presence of pus cells from duodenal or biliary inflammation. Following the introduction of magnesium sulfate or other biliary tract stimulant, light yellow bile from the common duct is obtained (A bile). Soon thereafter a darker, more viscid type of bile from the gallbladder appears in amounts of 25 to 75 cc. (B bile). Finally, a less viscid, clear yellow bile, which presumably has been freshly secreted, can be collected.

Microscopic Examination

This must be done immediately after collection, since digestive ferments rapidly destroy the cellular elements. Very few leukocytes and tissue cells are found in normal duodenal contents. Numerous pus cells suggest inflammation. *Giardia lamblia* and *Strongyloides stercoralis* can be identified when present. *Endameba histolytica* (vegetative or cystic forms) indicate liver or bile duct involvement. In centrifuged bile specimens, obtained by stimulation, the finding of cholesterol crystals, dark yellow-brown calcium bilirubinate crystals, amorphous yellow bilirubin, and characteristic bile-stained epithelial cells or leukocytes is strongly suggestive of cholelithiasis. Bacteriologic examination, with present methods, is incapable of providing information of definite clinical value in most cases.

FECES

Collection of the Specimen

The patient should first urinate, so that the stool does not become contaminated with urine. The stool then is passed into a clean receptacle and examined as soon as possible, since decomposition occurs within a few hours. The stool should be obtained without the aid of enemas or cathartics, if possible, except in examinations to determine a suspected typhoid carrier state when a saline cathartic may be of use in collecting a suitable specimen. Special technics often are necessary for collecting stool specimens in suspected cases of amebiasis (q.v.).

Gross Examination

The frequency of the bowel movements and the quantity, color, consistency, and odor of the stools should be noted. Blood, mucus, pus, concretions (gallstones), and macroscopic parasites should be looked for.

Chemical Test for Blood

Whenever feasible, keep the patient on a meat-free diet for 3 days preceding this test. Then emulsify a portion of the stool in about 15 cc. of water. Add an equal amount of ether, shake to extract the fat, and discard the supernatant ether. Add about 3 cc. of glacial acetic acid to 10 cc. of the remaining material, and again extract with 10 cc. of ether. Blood, if present, can be detected in this ether extract by the benzidine test, as described under examination of the urine (q.v., above).

Bilirubin

Filter 10 cc. of fecal emulsion through a small filter paper. Add a drop of concentrated nitric acid to the partially dried filter paper. A play of colors on the filter paper indicates the presence of bile.

Urobilin

Shake a small quantity of stool in a test tube of water. Filter. Test the filtrate for urobilin as described in the test for urine urobilinogen (q.v., above).

Microscopic Examination

Several portions of the specimen should be examined, especially those containing blood or pus. The material is placed on a glass slide, thinned with water or physiologic saline, and covered with a cover slip. It then is examined for the character of food remnants, and the presence of fat, red blood cells, pus cells, epithelial cells, parasites, and ova.

Stool Culture

Insert a rectal swab into a piece of soft rubber tubing 7″ long and ¼″ in diameter. Sterilize. Lubricate the outside of the tube and insert it into rectum, then withdraw the tubing an inch or two, leaving the swab at its original level. Remove swab and tube and send swab to laboratory in infusion broth.

SPUTUM

Collection of Specimen

The specimen should be as free of saliva as possible, and preferably should be the product of a deep explosive cough. For routine examination, other than culture, it may be collected in a clean wide-mouthed bottle or paper cup. The entire amount produced in 24 hours should be saved and examined.

Gross Examination

The quantity, color, odor, and presence or absence of blood and pus should be noted. The sputum may be classified as serous, mucoid, bloody, blood-streaked, purulent, seropurulent, or mucopurulent, according to its consistency. A tendency toward layering should be looked for. Bronchial casts and pneumoliths may be present.

Microscopic Examination

Unstained sputum: The portions to be examined should be selected carefully. Those containing blood or pus are the ones most likely to contain pathologic materials. Small amounts of this suspected material may be picked up with a wire loop or cotton applicator and spread on a slide. Cover, and examine first with a 16 mm. objective and then with a 4 mm. objective. The important pathologic constituents that may be seen in the unstained smear include pus cells, pigmented cells (heart-failure cells, carbon-laden cells), Charcot-Leyden crystals, Curschmann's spirals, the ray fungus of actinomycosis, molds and yeasts, elastic fibers, and myelin globules.

Stained sputum: Several thin smears of material from suspicious areas of the sputum, selected and prepared as described above, are allowed to dry. The smear is heat-fixed by passing the slide, face up, 10 or 12 times through the flame of a Bunsen burner or alcohol lamp, with care not to scorch the preparation. A Gram stain should be made to identify gram-negative or gram-positive organisms and spirochetes; a Ziehl-Neelsen stain for acid-fast organisms; and a Wright stain for eosinophiles and other cells (see Staining Methods, below).

Sputum Concentration

Chemical digestion of the sputum and examination of the centrifuged sediment help to identify tubercle bacilli in a sputum specimen containing relatively few acid-fast bacilli. Collect all sputum for 24, 48, or 72 hours. Mix equal amounts of sputum and sodium hydroxide-alum digester with a few drops of bromthymol blue as an indicator. Incubate at 37° C. until a homogeneous mass forms. Add 2.5 normal HCl in drops until a light bluish green color appears. Centrifuge at high speed for 5 minutes; remove supernatant fluid. Examine acid-fast stained smears for tubercle bacilli.

Sputum Culture

Have patient rinse mouth with hot water before attempting to cough up sputum. Avoid contamination of specimen with saliva. Collect and send material to a laboratory in a well stoppered, sterile container.

SEMEN

Collection of Specimen

The specimen should be collected by appropriate means in a clean sterile glass receptacle. Condoms are not suitable, since they contain chemicals which inhibit spermatozoa, and semen taken from the vagina may be altered by secretions and other vaginal contents. Collection should be made during the hours when the laboratory is open, and the specimen should be kept as close as possible to body temperature until it can be examined. If transportation requiring considerable time is necessary, the specimen container may be placed in a vacuum bottle. The time of the last previous ejaculation should be noted.

Gross Examination

Normally, semen is viscid, opaque or opalescent, yellowish white or cream colored. The usual volume of a specimen is 2.5

to 7 cc., with an average of 4 cc. The volume, opacity and viscosity are diminished following frequent ejaculations. Examine for evidence of pus or blood.

Microscopic Examination

For **direct examination** place a small amount of semen on a warmed slide and cover with a cover slip. Normally, the majority of the spermatozoa are actively motile.

For **sperm count** use a white blood cell pipet and draw semen to the 0.5 mark. Fill to the 11 mark with 0.5% chlorazene. Shake for 2 to 3 minutes. Fill counting chamber of hemacytometer and count the number of spermatozoa in 2 of the large squares (2 sq. mm.). The addition of 5 zeroes gives the number of sperm/cc. semen: normal, 80 to 200 million.

A **smear** is made in the same manner as a thin blood smear. Air dry for several hours and fix over a flame. To stain, immerse in 0.5% chlorazene for 3 minutes, wash in water; dehydrate in 95% alcohol, air dry, stain with 0.25% crystal violet for 2 minutes, wash in water; decolorize in 95% alcohol for not more than 20 seconds, wash in water; stain with 1% rose bengal for 8 to 10 seconds, wash with water, and dry. Make a count of 300 to 500 spermatozoa and differentiate between the normal and abnormal heads. More than 20% abnormal heads is pathologic. (*See* also p. 601.)

Identification of Semen

Soak and occasionally agitate the stained portion of clothing or other material in normal saline or dilute alcohol for 1 hour or longer. Centrifuge, discard supernatant fluid and examine the sediment. The presence of spermatozoa is positive proof, accepted legally, that the stain was sperm. However, animal sperm cannot always be distinguished from human sperm by this method.

Florence's reaction: Place a few drops of the reagent (iodine 2.54 Gm., potassium iodide 1.65 Gm., distilled water 30 cc.) on the suspected material on a glass slide. By low-power examination with the microscope, dark brown rhombic shaped crystals can be seen if semen, crushed insects, and certain tissue extracts are present. Failure of the crystals to appear is proof that semen is absent.

MISCELLANEOUS

Cultures, Smears, and Biopsy Material

Collect specimens whenever possible from a portion of the lesion or area where the pathogenic organisms are most likely to be present, such as the spreading edge of an ulcer, the base of a vesicle or pustule, beneath a crust, or from an exudate. Do not use the same swab for both smear and culture. For smears, roll swab on surface of slide, or, when specimen is liquid, spread in the same manner as a thin blood smear. It usually is advisable to prepare at least 2 slides, one for the Gram stain, the other for special staining. For broth cultures, dip the swab in the medium and twirl; use sterile pipet for liquid specimens. For plate or slant cultures, place material on the surface with a swab but spread with a sterile wire loop. Specimens are ordinarily cultured in infusion broth or on blood agar, but other media often are necessary. Special technics and media are usually required for anaerobic cultures. Most health department and private laboratories supply slides and culture material in packages suitable for mailing or messenger delivery. These packages generally contain any necessary special instructions.

Eye: Use sterile cotton swab or wire loop, avoid contact with eyelashes and lids. Prepare 2 slides, 1 for Gram's stain and 1 for morphologic study; send swab sealed in a sterile tube, or immersed in culture broth, to a laboratory for culture.

Nose and Throat: Use a sterile cotton swab; avoid contact with skin in taking specimen from the nose, and with tongue and teeth in taking them from the throat. Make 3 smears, 1 for Gram's stain, 1 for gentian violet stain to detect Vincent's organisms, and 1 for Loeffler's alkaline methylene blue for diphtheria organisms. (CAUTION! Only a tentative diagnosis of diphtheria can be made from a smear, and the absence of suggestive organisms does not rule out diphtheria.) Cultures also should be made on Loeffler's serum and chocolate tellurite plates for diphtheria; other organisms may be cultured in infusion broth or on blood agar and chocolate tellurite plates, and thioglycollate media may be used when indicated.

Urethra: When discharges are profuse, material can be obtained with a wire loop or swab. In the male, prostatic massage and stripping of the penis may be required to produce a specimen. In the female, the orifice of the urethra may be spread and slightly evaginated to obtain the specimen or to visualize the duct openings of Skene's glands. Massage of the urethra, with the gloved index finger in the anterior vagina, also may be necessary. Prepare 2 smears, 1 for Gram's stain and 1 for methylene blue. Culture on chocolate agar.

Vagina and Cervix: Use a sterile dry vaginal speculum. In most cases this can be inserted without the aid of a lubricating jelly. With cotton swab, touch area selected, or for routine smears, touch swab to cervical os. Avoid contact with other areas of cervix and the vaginal walls. Prepare smears and cultures and make as for urethral specimens or other special examinations as required.

Exudates and Transudates: Exudates are pathologic fluids of inflammatory origin. They contain varying amounts of cells, are rich in albumin and tend to coagulate on standing; specific gravity usually is above 1.016 to 1.018. Seromucin, a mucus-like substance, is present and can be detected by the development of a cloudy white precipitate on adding several drops of 5% acetic acid to a specimen of the fluid. This aids in distinguishing an exudate from a transudate.

Transudates are noninflammatory in origin, and usually are clear or opalescent, contain but few cells, do not coagulate on standing, and have a specific gravity below 1.016 to 1.018.

For microscopic study, a tube of fresh fluid is obtained, mixed with several cc. of citrated saline solution, and centrifuged for 5 to 10 minutes. The supernatant liquid is carefully poured off and the sediment is smeared on a slide. Apply Wright's stain diluted with 1 part pure methyl alcohol to 3 parts of stain; then examine slide under the oil immersion lens. If there is reason for making a cell count, the procedure is that described under Cerebrospinal Fluid (q.v.).

Cultures and other bacteriologic studies are made by inoculating the fluid or the centrifuged sediment on suitable media.

Fungi: To obtain specimen, remove material from moist surfaces, vesicles, pustules, ulcers, or abscesses, using a scalpel or syringe, as necessary. When the lesions are superficial, as on the nails, hair, or skin, pluck a few hairs or shave a thin slice from the suspected area. In collecting sputum or aspirating the bronchi, avoid contact with saliva and food particles. To examine, place specimen in a drop of 20% NaOH on a slide and cover with a cover glass; wait 30 minutes before examining. Culture on Sabouraud's medium and blood agar plates; make 2 of each, one set for incubation at 37° C., the other to be left at room temperature. In some instances, growth does not appear for 1 to 3 weeks.

Tumor Cells in Body Fluids: The identification of tumor cells in body fluids requires special staining technics and considerable experience in the cytologic method of cancer diagnosis. Bronchial, uterine, cervical, urethral, and rectal secretions may contain tumor cells if the regions producing or bathed by the secretions are neoplastic. Likewise, urine, ascitic fluid or pleural fluid may contain tumor cells if urinary tract, abdominal or pleural neoplastic disease is present. A portion of the secretion or exudate should be smeared on a glass slide in the usual manner, fixed in a solution of equal parts of 95% alcohol and ether, and examined with the special stains required for cytologic diagnosis (Papanicolaou stains). If the specimen is a large quantity of dilute fluid such as urine or ascitic or pleural fluid, a concentrated centrifuged sediment should be fixed in 10% formalin and imbedded by the usual histologic method before being examined with special stains.

Biopsy Material: Specimens are usually placed in small, wide-mouthed, corked specimen jars containing 10% formaldehyde solution or formol-alcohol solution, for preservation until they can be fixed, sectioned, and studied. It is best to consult the pathologist who will examine the material as to the preservative he prefers.

STAINING METHODS

Gram Stain

1. Fix smear by heat.
2. Apply 2% crystal violet in pure methyl alcohol for 30 seconds.
3. Wash with water.
4. Apply Gram's iodine solution for 90 seconds.
5. Wash in 95% alcohol and acetone, equal parts, until the purple color stops coming off (about 30 seconds).
6. Counterstain with Bismarck brown, weak fuchsin or safranin. For safranin, use a 2.5% solution in 95% alcohol for 1 minute, then wash with water, and dry. Gram-positive organisms appear dark blue or purple, gram-negative organisms are colored by the counterstain.

Methylene Blue Stain

1. Apply Loeffler's alkaline methylene blue (saturated alcoholic solution of methylene blue, 30 parts; potassium hydroxide, 1:10,000 aqueous solution, 100 parts). For average smears, leave on 30 seconds; for diphtheria or Vincent's organisms leave on 3 to 5 minutes.
2. Wash with water.

Wright Stain

1. Flood slide with Wright's stain for 5 minutes.
2. Add an equal amount of distilled water (10 to 15 drops) and gently agitate the slide for 3 minutes.
3. Wash with water until the stain no longer comes off.
4. Dry in air and examine with oil immersion objective.

Acid-Fast Stain (Ziehl-Neelsen)

1. Cover fixed smear with carbofuchsin, steam over water bath for 5 minutes or over direct flame for 5 minutes.
2. Wash with water.
3. Apply acid alcohol, decolorize until a faint pink remains.
4. Wash with water.
5. Stain with methylene blue (q.v.).

Giemsa Stain

For blood smears: 1. Immerse slide with fixed smear in stain diluted 1:10 for 20 minutes, or 1:50 for 45 minutes.
2. Rinse with distilled water for at least 3 minutes.
3. Dry and examine. (Do not blot.)
For spirochetes: 1. Fix smear in absolute alcohol for 15 minutes.
2. Add 10 drops of stain to 10 cc. of distilled water containing 1 drop of 1% potassium carbonate solution; immerse slide in this solution for 2 to 3 hours.
3. Wash with distilled water, air-dry, and examine.

THE PHYSICIAN'S BAG

Obviously, for reasons of portability, the contents of the physician's bag will be restricted to those therapeutic agents and mechanical devices required for immediate use in medical emergencies and for dealing with the more commonly encountered types of illness. However, it is important that the physician shall have readily available certain other materials necessary for meeting relatively unusual situations; these items may be carried conveniently in an auxiliary bag or other suitable container kept ready in the physician's automobile. Unused drugs which tend to deteriorate must be replaced periodically, always in advance of their expiration dates.

The following list of relatively essential items to be carried in the physician's bag is representative of the needs and preferences of most physicians. Drugs and instruments of supplemental value are listed as "elective." A physician specializing in a given field may find it necessary to alter or expand these lists to satisfy the requirements of his practice.

I. ESSENTIAL CONTENTS

Therapeutic Agents

Morphine sulfate (hypo. tab. or sterile solution)
Codeine phosphate (hypo. tab.): 30 mg. (gr. ss)
Acetylsalicylic acid: 0.3 Gm. (gr. v)
Analgesic ear drops
Phenobarbital: 30 mg. (gr. ss)
Sodium phenobarbital (ampul): 0.3 Gm.
Paraldehyde: 30 cc. (℥ i)
Procaine penicillin (vial): 300,000 u./cc.
Streptomycin (vial): 1 Gm.
Sulfonamide preparation: 0.5 Gm. (gr. viiss)
Water for Injection U.S.P.
Antihistaminic (e.g., "Neo-Antergan"): 25 mg.
Nitroglycerin (hypo. tab. for sublingual use): 0.6 mg. (gr. 1/100)
Amyl nitrite (perl)
A synthetic antispasmodic
Quinidine sulfate: 0.3 Gm. (gr. v)
Digitalis preparation (oral and parenteral)
"Mecholyl" (ampul): 25 mg.
Mercurial diuretic (ampul): 2 cc.
Caffeine and sodium benzoate (ampul): 0.5 Gm. (gr. viiss)
Aromatic spirits of ammonia (perl)
Analeptic (Picrotoxin, Amphetamine, or "Metrazol")
Atropine sulfate (hypo. tab.): 0.4 mg. (gr. 1/150)
Epinephrine, 1:1,000 (ampul): 1 cc.
Epinephrine, 1:500 in oil (ampul), 1 cc.
Aminophylline (ampul): 0.24 Gm. (gr. iv)
Dihydroergotamine (ampul): 1 mg.
Apomorphine (hypo. tab.): 6 mg. (gr. 1/10)
Pituitrin, obstetrical (ampul) 1 cc.
Alcohol, 70%

Instruments and Materials

Stethoscope
Sphygmomanometer
Otoscope-Ophthalmoscope

Percussion hammer
Tourniquet
Measuring tape

Clinical thermometers (oral and rectal)
Syringes (2 cc. and 10 cc.)
Needles (19 and 27 gauge)
Tongue depressors
Cotton applicators
Skin antiseptic solution
Scissors (bandage)

Adhesive tape (½″, 1″ & 3″)
Sterile gauze pads
Gauze (roller) bandage (1″, 2″ & 3″)
Elastic bandage (2″ or 3″)
Rubber glove; finger cot
Flashlight
Prescription pad

II. "ELECTIVE" MATERIALS

Glucose, 50% (ampul): 50 cc.
Syringe: 50 cc.
Calcium gluconate (ampul): 1 Gm.
Procaine hydrochloride, 2% (ampul)
Anesthetic ointment
Ophthalmic anesthetic (topical)
Ophthalmic ointment (of choice)
Neostigmine (ampul): 1.5 mg.
Surgical kit (sterile): gloves, scissors, hemostats, forceps, splinter forceps, probe, scalpel, needle holder, rubber drain, sutures, suture needle
Sterile dressings: cotton, gauze, towels, vaseline gauze, packing
Sterile needles for phlebotomy, thoracentesis, or lumbar puncture
Tetanus antitoxin (vials): 3,000 u.
"Vinethene" (inhalation anesthetic)
Catheter (Fr. 12)
Urinalysis kit for sugar and acetone
Safety razor and blades
Glass slides
Specimen bottle (wide-mouthed)
Stomach tube
Sterile swab in sterile test tube
Splints (1 or 2 light weight, adjustable)

ALTERNATIVE PROPRIETARY PREPARATIONS

In many chapters throughout THE MERCK MANUAL, it has been necessary, in accordance with authors' prescriptions and for reasons of clarity, to refer to medicaments by their proprietary names. The mention in the text of any single proprietary agent, however, in nowise implies the unavailability of other proprietary preparations which, according to manufacturers' claims, have equivalent action and are equally efficacious. In such instances, therefore, so as to provide the physician with a wide choice of such commercially available drugs, the following groups of alternative proprietary preparations of similar therapeutic action are listed. Every effort has been made to include, so far as known, all available proprietaries in the groups represented.

The metric or apothecary dose given for any proprietary refers to the average, single, adult dose recommended for that drug. Whenever applicable, the dose of a compound substance is given (in the metric column) as the number of capsules, tablets, or suppositories to be employed. When a medicament is to be administered parenterally, this fact is indicated by an asterisk (*) placed beside the dose.

DOSE TABLE OF ALTERNATIVE PROPRIETARY PREPARATIONS

Medicament	Gm. or cc. (* = parenteral dose)	gr. or ℳ	Medicament	Gm. or cc. (* = parenteral dose)	gr. or ℳ
Analeptics			Allisatin	2 tab.	
			Alutropin	8.0	120
Benzedrine	0.005–0.015	$1/12$–$1/4$	Alzinox	1–2 tab.	
Coramine	1.5–5*	22–75*	Amesac	1 cap.	
Desoxyn	0.0025–		Aminet	1 suppos.	
	0.005	$1/25$–$1/12$	Amodrine	1–2 tab.	
	0.015*	$1/4$*	Antrocol	1 tab.	
Dexedrine	0.005–0.010	$1/12$–$1/6$	Arlcaps	1 cap.	
D-O-E	0.0025	$1/25$	Asminyl	1 tab.	
Drinalfa	0.005–0.010	$1/12$–$1/6$	Asthmolysin	0.5–1.0*	8–15*
Metrazol	0.1–0.3*	$1\frac{1}{2}$–5*	Atrocholin	1–3 tab.	
Soduxin	3–5*	45–75*	Aubromid Elixir	4.0–8.0 cc.	60–120
			Auri-Tussin	0.25–0.6	4–10
Antihistaminics†			Barbephine	1–2 tab.	
			Barbedonna	1–2 tab.	
Antistine	0.1	$1\frac{1}{2}$	Barbonate	1–2 tab.	
Benadryl	0.05	$3/4$	Belbarb	1 tab.	
Chlorothen	0.025	$3/8$	Belbarb Solution	4.0	60
Chlor-Trimeton	0.004	$1/15$	Bellabulgara	1 tab.	
Decapryn	0.05	$3/4$	Belladenal	1–2 tab.	
Diatrin	0.05	$3/4$	Bellafoline	1–2 tab.	
Di-Paralene	0.05	$3/4$	Bellafoline Solution	0.6–1.3	10–20
Histadyl	0.05	$3/4$	Bellal	1–2 tab.	
Hydryllin	2 tab.		Bellergal	1 tab.	
Neo-Antergan	0.05	$3/4$	Belnesium	2–3 tab.	
Neohetramine	0.05	$3/4$	Belphedribarb	1–2 tab.	
Pentryl	1 or 2 tab.		Benzylet	0.3–0.6	5–10
Pyribenzamine	0.05	$3/4$	Bi-Oxalate		
Pyrrolazote	0.05	$3/4$	Compound	1–2 tab.	
Tagathen	0.05	$3/4$	Bromaurate Elixir	4.0	60
Thenylene	0.05	$3/4$	Bromsalizol	1–3 tab.	
Thephorin	0.05	$3/4$	Butisol-Ephedrine		
Trimeton	0.025	$3/8$	Compound	1–2 cap.	
			Camatropine	1–2 tab.	
Anticonvulsants			Chovanol	1–2 tab.	
			Copavin	1 tab.	
(*see also* Hypnotics			Copavin Solution	4.0	60
and Sedatives)			Delkadon	1–2 tab.	
			Depropanex	2.0–3.0*	30–45*
Dilantin Sodium	0.1–0.2	$1\frac{1}{2}$–3	Disco	1–2 tab.	
Mebaral	0.1	$1\frac{1}{2}$	Donnatal	1 tab.	
Mesantoin	0.1	$1\frac{1}{2}$	Dorsamin	1–2 tab.	
Tridione	0.3–0.6	5–10	Ephcaben	1–2 tab.	
			Ephedrate	1–2 tab.	
Antispasmodics			Ephedrital	1–2 tab.	
			Ephedromal	1 cap.	
Adnephrin	1–2 cap.		Ephenate Elixir	8.0–16.0	120–240
Adrenalin	0.0005*	$1/120$*	Ephetal	1–2 tab.	
Adrephine	0.5–1.0*	8–15*	Ephetonin	$\frac{1}{2}$–1 tab.	
Adrin Solution	0.6–1.0*	10–15*	Epinephrine-Gel	1.0*	15*
Al-Si-Cal	4 tab.		Epinine	0.3–0.6	5–10
Alephed	1 cap.		Epiphedrine		
			Compound	1.0*	15*

† NOTE: Some of the above antihistaminic agents are available also as elixirs, ointments, creams, or ophthalmic solutions, or in combination with other agents.

Medicament	Gm. or cc. (* = parenteral dose)	gr. or ♏	Medicament	Gm. or cc. (* = parenteral dose)	gr. or ♏
Epragen	1–2 cap.		Pseudoephedrine	0.06	1
Eprinal	0.5 cc.*	8*	Rabellon	¼–1 tab.	
Eumydrin	0.0001	1/600	Racedal	1–2 tab.	
Eu-Phed-Ital	1–2 tab.		Racephedrine	0.024–0.05	⅜–¾
Felsol	1 powd.		Riona	1 cap.	
Fepetal	1 cap.		Sedatal	1 cap.	
Franol	1–2 tab.		Sethyl	1–2 tab.	
Gelatin-			Solanital	1 tab.	
Epinephrine	1.0*	15*	Spasmalgin	1–2 tab.	
Glucophylline	0.15–0.3	2½–5		1.0–2.0*	15–30*
Glytheonate (with			Spasmolysin	1.0*	15*
Racephedrine)	1–2 tab.		Spastosed	2–3 tab.	
Homabitol	1–2 tab.		Syntronal	1–2 tab.	
H.V.C.	8–12	120–180	Syntropan	0.05	¾
Hybephen	1 tab.			0.01*	⅙*
Injectable			Taladonna	1–3 tab.	
DeHeckel	2.0*	30*	Taludon	1–2 tab.	
Iocapral	1–2 tab.		T-Bardrin	1 suppos.	
Isuprel	0.01–0.015	⅙–¼	Tedral	1–2 tab.	
Kiophyllin	1–2 tab.		Teprin	1–2 tab.	
Lascodonna	2.0–3.0	15–45	Thalfed	1 tab.	
Lobiodrin	1 tab.		Theocin	1–2 tab.	
Luasmin	1 tab.		Theoprofedrine	1–2 tab.	
Lubismin	8.0	120	Theopropanol	1 tab.	
Lumodrin	1–2 tab.		Thephyldine	0.1–0.2	1½–3
Lusyn	1–2 tab.		Trasentine	0.075–0.15	1¼–2½
Matrobarb	1–2 tab.			0.05*	¾*
Meditab	1 tab.		Tresan	1 tab.	
Mesopin	1–2 tab.		Triatal	1–4 tab.	
Methatropin	1–2 tab.		Tribromauro	4.0–8.0	60–120
Metropine	1–2 tab.		Triophen (with		
Nebulin A	By inhalation		atropine)	1 tab.	
			Trisidonna	2–4 tab.	
Nergestic	1–3 tab.		Triz	4.0–16.0	60–240
Nervinal	1–2 tab.		Trocinate	1–2 tab.	
Nespamal	4.0–8.0	60–120	Urised	2 tab.	
Nethacetin	1–2 tab.		Viburnum		
Nethacol	4.0–8.0	60–120	Compound	1–2 tab.	
Nethamine	1 tab.		Vinobel	0.0025–	
Neurosine	4.0–8.0	60–120		0.004	1/25–1/15
Novalene	2 tab.		Vinotal	1–2 cap.	
Novatropine	1–2 tab.		W-T Powder	4.0	60
Octin	0.13	2			
Odi-Late	1–2 tab.		**Barbiturates**		
Padrophyll	1 tab.		(see Sedatives)		
Pama No. 1001	1–2 tab.				
Passiflora-Lupulus			**Coal Tar Preparations**		
Compound	1–2 tab.				
Pavatrine	0.12–0.25	2–4	Co-Tar-Ox		
Paxonin	1 tab.		Cot-Tar		
Pentaphedrine	4.0–8.0	60–120	Creo-Derma		
Perparin	0.02–0.05	⅜–¾	Creolin-Pearson		Apply according to
Phedretal	1 tab.		Daxalan		the manufac-
Phenocyamus	1–2 tab.		Dermatole		turer's instruc-
Phyatromine	1.0*	15*	Nu-Kol-Tar		tions.
Phycillin	1 tab.		Pixalbol		
Phyllophed	1 tab.		Pix-Gel		
Profenil	0.12	2	Pragmatar		
Propadrine	0.024–0.05	⅜–¾			

Medicament	Gm. or cc. (* = parenteral dose)	gr. or ℳ	Medicament	Gm. or cc. (* = parenteral dose)	gr. or ℳ
Starzin			Theodigital	1–2 cap.	
Sul-Tarbonis			Theomine	1 tab.	
Supertah			Theontrate	1–2 tab.	
Syntaclo			Theopropanol	1 tab.	
Tar Dermament			Theorate	1–2 tab.	
Tar Distillate	Apply according to the manufacturer's instructions.		Thephyldine	0.1–0.2	1½–3
Taralba			Thesodate	0.5	7½
Tarbonis			Thiomerin	1–2*	15–30*
Taroxide			Thol	1–2 tab.	
Tarpaste			Uroxyl Compound	4.0–8.0	60–120
Tarzole			Uvatalis	12–20	180–300
Ultarzole			Xan-Ca-Cyl	1–2 tab.	
Vantar			Xancylate	1–2 tab.	
			Xaniomine	1–2 tab.	
			Xaniophen	1–2 tab.	

Detergents

Acidolate		
Almay		
Asapo		
Lamo	Use according to manufacturer's instructions.	
Lowila		
pHisoderm		
Prozemoil		
Tersus		

Ear Drops

Auralgan		
Aural-Ol		
Aurazine		
Myrinol	Instill several drops or more as necessary into the external auditory canal of the affected ear.	
Oltogesic Liquid		
Otomide		
Otosmosan		
Otozole		
Pyricain		
Typanide		

Diuretics

Amchlor	4 tab.	
Cactina Pillets	1–4 pillets	
Calpurate	0.5–1.0	7½–15
Cardinate	1 cap.	
Diuretin	0.5–1.0	7½–15
Diurodan	1 tab.	
Diurol	8.0–16.0	120–240
Glucophylline	0.15–0.3	2½–5
Glytheonate	1–3 tab.	
Kavacaps	2 tab.	
Kiophylline	1–2 tab.	
Lithiated Sorghum Compound	4.0–8.0	60–120
Magnephylline	1–2 tab.	
Mercuhydrin	0.5–2.0*	8–30*
Mercurin	1 suppos.	
Mercuzanthin	0.5–2.0*	8–30*
Phyllicin	1 tab.	
Predaten	4–8	60–120
Salyrgan-Theophylline	0.5–2.0*	8–30*
Synophyllate	1–3 tab.	
Tachidrol	1–2*	15–30*
TCS Tablets	1 tab.	
Teotine	1 tab.	
Theacetin	2 tab.	
Theamin	0.06–0.2	1–3
Theobarb	1 tab.	
Theobutin	1–3 tab.	
Theocalcin	1–2 tab.	
Theocin	1–2 tab.	

Fungicides

Anthralin		
Benoxal		
Ben-Sal-Caine		
Benzo-Sal		
Benzo-Salicylic Compound		
Benzox		
B.F.I.		
Ceepryn		
Cerosal		
Chlormercrol		
Cignolin		
Colebenz	Apply according to manufacturer's instructions.	
Collo-Sul		
Cresatin		
Croleum-Suspensoid Copper Sulfate		
Cute-Asepto		
Danusol		
Desenex		
Di-Spor		
Fliktena		
Glycerite of Hydrogen Peroxide		

Medicament	Gm. or cc. (* = parenteral dose)	gr. or ℳ	Medicament	Gm. or cc. (* = parenteral dose)	gr. or ℳ
Hetoxin..........			**Hypnotics and Sedatives**		
Hydrophen.......					
I-C-Z...........					
Iocamphen.......			Abasin...........	0.25–0.5	4–7½
Iodolate........			Adalin...........	0.06–0.13	1–2
Iso-Par..........			Allonal..........	0.3–0.6	5–10
Kasal...........			Alurate..........	0.06–0.13	1–2
Korium..........			Amytal..........	0.1–0.3	1½–5
Lenigallol.......			Aphcotabs.......	1 tab.	
Mazon..........			Barbromid.......	1 tab.	
Medicone........			Bral............	1–3 tab.	
Mercarbolide.....			Bromidia........	4.0–8.0	60–120
Mercresin.......			Bromionyl.......	4.0–6.0	60–90
Merseptal.......			Bromiphen.......	1–2 tab.	
Merthiolate......			Bromobarb......	4.0–8.0	60–120
Monarden.......			Bromocol.......	0.15–0.3	2½–5
Myalete.........			Bromo-Valerianate.	8.0–16.0	120–240
Mycocide........			Bromo-Vess......	1–2 tab.	
Mycofan........			Bromural........	0.3–0.6	5–10
Mycozol........			Brosedan........	4.0–12.0	60–180
Naprylene.......	Apply according to manufacturer's instructions.		Brothane........	8.0	120
Octophen........			Butisol..........	0.15–0.3	2½–5
Oilzo			Calcibronat.....	1 tab.	
PMN			Cal-Sed.........	1–2 cap.	
Peroguent.......			Carbrital........	1 cap.	
Phe-Mer-Nite ...			Chloretone......	0.6–1.0	10–15
Phenitol.........			Chlorobutanol....	0.6–1.0	10–15
Phenmerzyl......			Cyclopal	0.05–0.15	¾–2½
Podosan........			Cyclopen........	0.1–0.2	1½–3
Quinolor.........			Delvinal.........	0.1–0.2	1½–3
Riazol..........			Dial............	0.03–0.3	½–5
Salicresin.......			Dormelix........	4.0–16.0	60–240
Salundek........			Elixsed.........	4.0	60
S.D.O.			Ethalyl.........	0.13	2½
Sopronol........			Eudital.........	1–2 tab.	
Sulfo-Merthiolate..			Evidorn.........	1 tab.	
Sulfur Diasporal...			Evipal..........	0.25–0.4	4–6
T-Cap..........			Fello-Sed	2.0–8.0	30–120
Tenicide........			Genoscopolamine..	0.001–	
Thio-Boric Powder.				0.003	1/60–1/20
Thi-Oxiquin			Glyco-Bromides		
Thisal..........			Compound.....	4.0–12.0	60–180
Tineasol.........			Ipral............	0.05–0.4	¾–6
Tricocide........			Luminal.........	0.03–0.1	½–1½
Trydecyl........			Mebaral.........	0.03–0.3	½–5
			Medinal.........	0.06–0.3	1–5
Gold Salts			Menthyval.......	0.25–0.5	4–8
(antiarthritics)			Nalgised	1 tab.	
			Nembutal.......	0.05–0.2	¾–3
Aurocein........			Neonal..........	0.05–0.4	¾–6
Aurolake........			Neo-Sedaphen...	4–8	60–120
Aurol-Sulfide.....			Nervival........	1–2 tab.	
Collosol Aurum ...	Administer according to the manufacturer's package insert.		Neuralin........	1–2 tab.	
Myochrysine.....			Neurinase.......	1 tab.	
Rexaurum.......			Neuronidia......	2.0–8.0	30–120
Solganol-B			Neurosine.......	4.0–8.0	60–120
Oleosum........			Nevrotose.......	1–2 cap.	
Triphal..........			Nostal..........	1–4 tab.	
			Nurobromyds.....	4.0–8.0	60–120

Medicament	Gm. or cc. (* = parenteral dose)	gr. or ℳ	Medicament	Gm. or cc. (* = parenteral dose)	gr. or ℳ
Nurodol	4.0–8.0	60–120	Glysulfed		
Ortal	0.3–1.0	5–15	I-Sedrin		
Passiphen Compound	1–2 tab.		Isofedrol		
			Isohalant		
Palapent	8.0–16.0	120–240	Iso-Phedrizem		
Pembules	0.06–0.1	1–1½	Liqua-Phedra		
Pentabromides	4.0–8.0	60–120	Manadrin		
Pental	0.05–0.3	¾–5	Metaphedren		
Pernoston	0.2	3	Nafedrose		
Phanodorn	0.2–0.4	3–6	Narakon		
Phenaphen	1–2 cap.		Nasafedrin		
Sandoptal	0.2–0.4	3–6	Neo-Synephrine		
Seconal	0.1	1½	Normardrine		
Sedabrome	1–2 tab.		Paredrine	To be used in ac-	
Sedobarb	1 tab.		Par-Pen	cordance with	
Sedobrol	2–4 cubes		Pharynol	the manufac-	
Sedormid	0.5–0.8	7½–12	Pineoleum	turer's instruc-	
Sigmodal Sodium	8–12	120–180	Privine	tions.	
Slowten	1 tab.		Prohexinol		
Sodium Alurate	0.12	2	Propadrine		
Sodium Amytal	0.06–0.2	1–3	Prothricin		
	0.2–0.5*	3–7½*	Racephedrine		
Solfoton	1 tab.		Rhinazine		
Solmides	1 tab.		Sinorol		
Somnifene	1.3–2.6	20–40	Sulfadrine		
Somnos	8.0–16.0	120–240	Sulfadex		
Sulfonal	0.75–1.0	12–15	Sulmefrin		
Sulfomethane	0.75–1.0	12–15	Symedral		
Trional	0.6–1.0	10–15	Thizodrin		
Tuinal	0.1–0.2	1½–3	Tuamine		
Valerianets	1–3 dragees		Vasodrine		
Veronal	0.3	5	Vonedrine		

Mydriatics

Eumydrin	Instill according
Euphthalmine	to the manufac-
Methatropin	turer's instruc-
Paredrine	tions.

Nasal Decongestants

Adrenalin Inhalant with Chloretone	
Adrephine	
Albomist	
Anesthone	
Aqua Drin	To be used in ac-
Benzedrex	cordance with
Camolus	the manufac-
Efedron	turer's instruc-
Efemist	tions.
Ephedazole	
Epinine	
Eprinal	
Gluco-Fedrin	

Ophthalmic Antiseptics

(excluding antibiotics and sulfonamides)

Argentis	
Argolaval	
Argyn	
Argyrol	
Butesin Picrate	
Ceepryn	
Colsargen	
Hyzin	
Ichthargan	
Lunargen	
Lunosol	To be used in ac-
Merbromin	cordance with
Mercarbolide	the manufac-
Mercurochrome	turer's instruc-
Mercurophen	tions.
Metaphen	
Merthiolate	
Novoxil	
Phemerol	
Protargol	

Medicament	Gm. or cc. (* = parenteral dose)	gr. or ♏	Medicament	Gm. or cc. (* = parenteral dose)	gr. or ♏
Sarcol	To be used in accordance with the manufacturer's instructions.		Suprarenalin Solution	0.2–1.0*	3–15*
Silloid			Suprarenin Solution	0.06–1.0*	1–15*
Silvol			Sympatol	0.1–0.3	1½–3
Solargentum			Vasodrine	0.06–1.0*	1–15*
Targesin					
Zephiran					

Parasiticides
(Systemic)

Anayodin	0.25–1.0	4–15			
Atabrine	0.1	1½			
Crystoids	1.0	15			
Diodoquin	0.5	7½			
Fuadin	1.5–5.0*	22½–75*			
Neostibosan	0.2	3			
Quinoxyl	0.25–1.0	4–15			
Stovarsol	0.25	4			
Vioform	0.25	4			

Pediculicides

B.B.S.	Apply according to the manufacturer's instructions.	
Bornate		
Cuprex		
Kwell		
Lorthio		
Pyreb		

Sympathomimetic Agents

Adrenalin	0.0005*	$^1/_{120}$*
Adrephine	0.5–1.0*	8–15*
Adrin	0.06–1.0*	1–15*
Benzedrine	0.005–0.015	$^1/_{12}$–¼
Desoxyn	0.0025–0.005	$^1/_{25}$–$^1/_{12}$
	0.01–0.02*	$^1/_6$–$^1/_3$*
D-O-E	0.0025	$^1/_{25}$
Drinalfa	0.005–0.010	$^1/_{12}$–$^1/_6$
Ephedrate	1–2 tab.	
Ephetonin	0.05	¾
Epinine	0.003–0.010*	$^1/_{20}$–$^1/_6$*
Eprinal	0.06–1.0	1–15
Neo-Synephrine	0.01–0.025	$^1/_6$–$^3/_8$
	0.001–0.01*	$^1/_{60}$–$^1/_6$*
Nethamine	0.05	¾
Oenethyl	0.05–0.10*	¾–1½*
Pit-Ren	1–2 cap.	
Propadrine	0.025–0.050	$^3/_8$–¾
Racephedrine	0.025–0.050	$^3/_8$–¾
Supranephrin Solution	0.06–1.0*	1–15*

Urinary Antiseptics
(excluding sulfonamides and antibiotics)

Amdelate	8.0–12.0	120–180
Ammoform Compound	4.0–8.0	60–120
Amphomate	20.0–60.0	300–600
Arheol	0.6	10
Benzochrome	1–3 cap.	
Buchuform	1 tab.	
Camdelate	6 tab.	
Caprokol	2–4 cap.	
Cystodyne	4.0	60
Flavicine	5.0*	75*
Formatropin	4.0–8.0	60–120
Formin	0.3–1.0	5–15
Formohydrion	4.0	60
Gonosan	2 cap.	
Helmitol	0.6–1.0	10–15
Hexa-Chloride Compound	4.0–8.0	60–120
Hexalet	1.0	15
Hexaloid	0.3–1.0	5–15
Kavacaps	2 tab.	
Mallophene	2–4 tab.	
Mandechlor Elixir	16.0	240
Mandelamine	3–4 tab.	
Mandelasor Elixir with Chlor-Etha-mine	8.0	120
Mandelix	8.0	120
Mandoket	8.0	120
Murimine	4.0–8.0	60–120
Posta-Cole	1–2 tab.	
Prohydrion	4–6 tab.	
Pyridium	2 tab.	
Salihexin	0.3–0.6	5–10
Santyl	4–8 cap.	
Serenium	1 tab.	
Solurea	1–3 cap.	
Sulamyd	1–2 tab.	
Uraseptine	4.0–8.0	60–120
Uriform	4.0–8.0	60–120
Urised	2 tab.	
Uritone	0.3–1.0	5–15
Urogenine	4.0–8.0	60–120
Urolax	4.0–8.0	60–120
Urolithia	16.0	240
Uro-Phosphate	2 tab.	
Urotropin	1.0	15
Uroxyl Compound	4.0–8.0	60–120
Vera Perles	1–2 cap.	

READY REFERENCE GUIDES

CALCULATION OF DOSAGES FOR INFANTS, CHILDREN, AND AGED PATIENTS

There is no rule, applicable in all cases, for determining the dosage of a given drug for children. The difference between the weight of the child and that of the adult, disproportions between weight and age in the child, and the difference in susceptibility to drugs of certain tissues of the child from those of the adult, make a careful adjustment of dosage in children necessary. In the average case, Young's and Cowling's rules have been considered sufficiently accurate, except for opium and other powerful narcotics to which infants are especially susceptible and of which a relatively smaller dose must be given. On the other hand, relatively larger doses are required for arsenic, bromide, belladonna, and purgatives. To determine the dose for children according to Young's rule, divide the age by the age plus 12; the result represents the fraction of the adult dose suitable for the child. For example, a child three years old will require $\dfrac{3}{3 + 12} = \dfrac{1}{5}$ of the adult dose. Cowling's rule divides the number of the next birthday by 24. For example, in the case of a child five years old, the dose is $\frac{6}{24}$ or $\frac{1}{4}$.

Old age is tolerant to alcohol, but old and debilitated patients are often more sensitive to the depressant effects of morphine. There may be no response from nitrites in elderly people with arteriosclerosis, or from digitalis and other drugs, in heart disease. Sclerotic kidneys may not respond to diuretics.

WEIGHTS, MEASURES, AND EQUIVALENTS

APOTHECARIES' SYSTEM

Weight	Volume
1 scruple (℈) = 20 grains (gr.)	1 fluid dram (ℨ) = 60 minims (℥)
1 dram (ℨ) = 60 grains	1 fluid ounce (℥) = 480 minims
	= 8 fluid drams
1 ounce (℥) = 480 grains	1 pint (pt.) = 7,680 minims
= 8 drams	= 16 fluid ounces
1 pound (lb.) = 5,760 grains	1 quart (qt.) = 2 pints
= 12 ounces	1 gallon (gal.) = 4 quarts

METRIC SYSTEM

Weight	Volume
1 microgram (γ) = 1,000,000 micromicrograms ($\gamma\gamma$) 1 milligram (mg.) = 1,000 micrograms 1 gram. (Gm.) = 1,000 milligrams 1 kilogram (Kg.) = 1,000 grams	1 cubic centimeter (cc.) = 1,000 cubic millimeters (cu. mm.) 1 liter (L.) = 1,000 cubic centimeters

EQUIVALENTS (ALL APPROXIMATE)

LIQUID MEASURE

Metric	Apothecaries'	Metric	Apothecaries'
0.06 cc. =	1 minim	30 cc. =	1 fl. ounce
0.5 cc. =	8 minims	250 cc. =	8 fl. ounces+
1.0 cc. =	15 minims	500 cc. =	1 pint+
4.0 cc. =	1 fl. dram	1,000 cc. =	1 quart+
		(1 liter)	

WEIGHTS

Metric	Apothecaries'	Metric	Apothecaries'
0.2 mg. =	$^1/_{300}$ grain	60.0 mg. =	1 grain
0.3 mg. =	$^1/_{200}$ grain	0.12 Gm. =	2 grains
0.4 mg. =	$^1/_{150}$ grain	0.2 Gm. =	3 grains
0.5 mg. =	$^1/_{120}$ grain	0.3 Gm. =	5 grains
0.6 mg. =	$^1/_{100}$ grain	0.5 Gm. =	7½ grains
1.0 mg. =	$^1/_{60}$ grain	0.6 Gm. =	10 grains
3.0 mg. =	$^1/_{20}$ grain	1.0 Gm. =	15 grains
6.0 mg. =	$^1/_{10}$ grain	4.0 Gm. =	60 grains (1 dram
10.0 mg. =	⅙ grain	6.0 Gm. =	90 grains
15.0 mg. =	¼ grain	10.0 Gm. =	2½ drams
25.0 mg. =	⅜ grain	15.0 Gm. =	4 drams
30.0 mg. =	½ grain	30.0 Gm. =	1 ounce

HOUSEHOLD MEASURES
(with approximate equivalents)

1 teaspoon (tsp.)	=	4 cc. =	1 fl. dr.
1 dessertspoon	=	8 cc. =	2 fl. dr.
1 tablespoon (tbsp.)	=	15 cc. =	½ fl. oz.
1 wineglass	=	60 cc. =	2 fl. oz.
1 teacup	=	120 cc. =	4 fl. oz.
1 tumbler	=	240 cc. =	8 fl. oz. = ½ pt.

COMPARATIVE APPROXIMATE LINEAR MEASURES

1 millimeter (mm.) =	0.04 inch (in.)
1 centimeter (cm.) =	0.4 inch
1 decimeter (dm.) =	4.0 inches
1 meter (M.) =	39.37 inches

CONVERSION FORMULAS

Gallons into Pounds: Multiply the specific gravity of the liquid by 8.33 (weight in pounds of 1 gallon of water); then multiply this result by the number of gallons, to obtain the weight in pounds.

Pounds into Gallons: Multiply the specific gravity of the liquid by 8.33 (weight in pounds of 1 gallon of water); then divide the number of pounds by the result, to obtain the volume in gallons.

Cubic Centimeters into Grams: Multiply the specific gravity of the substance by the number of cubic centimeters, to obtain the weight in grams.

Grams into Cubic Centimeters: Divide the number of grams by the specific gravity of the substance, to obtain its volume in cubic centimeters.

Cubic Centimeters into Pounds: Multiply the number of cubic centimeters by the specific gravity of the substance; then divide the product by 453.59 (equivalent in grams of 1 avoirdupois pound), to obtain its weight in pounds.

Pounds into Cubic Centimeters: Multiply the number of pounds by 453.59 (equivalent in grams of 1 avoirdupois pound); then divide the product by the specific gravity of the substance, to obtain the volume in cubic centimeters.

Cubic Centimeters into Ounces: Multiply the number of cubic centimeters by the specific gravity of the substance; then divide the product by 28.35 (equivalent in grams of 1 avoirdupois ounce), to obtain its volume in ounces.

Ounces into Cubic Centimeters: Multiply the number of ounces by 28.35 (equivalent in grams of 1 avoirdupois ounce); then divide the product by the specific gravity of the substance, to obtain its volume in cubic centimeters.

Grains, Drams, and Ounces into Grams (or cc.): (1) Divide the number of grains by 15; or (2) multiply the number of drams by 4; or (3) multiply the number of ounces by 30. The result in each case = the approximate number of grams (or cc.).

CENTIGRADE-FAHRENHEIT EQUIVALENTS

Conversion:

To reduce degrees F. to degrees C., subtract 32, then multiply by 5/9.		To reduce degrees C. to degrees F., multiply by 9/5, then add 32.	
Centigrade°	Fahrenheit°	Centigrade°	Fahrenheit°
−40	−40	40.5	104.9
		41.0	105.8
Freezing (water at sea level):		41.5	106.7
0	32	42.0	107.6
Clinical Range:			
36.0	96.8		
36.5	97.7	Pasteurization (Holding), 30 min. at:	
37.0	98.6	61.6	143.0
37.5	99.5		
38.0	100.4	Pasteurization (Flash), 15 sec. at:	
38.5	101.3	71.1	160.0
39.0	102.2		
39.5	103.1	Boiling (water at sea level):	
40.0	104.0	100.0	212.0

AVERAGE WEIGHTS OF VARIOUS ORGANS
(in Grams)

ORGAN	CHILDREN			
	NEWBORN	1 YEAR	6 YEARS	12 YEARS
Brain & Meninges	335–380	910–925	1,200–1,250	1,050–1,400
Thyroid	1.6–3	3	8.5	12–20
Thymus	9–14	17–25	20–26	20–38
Heart	17–24	37–44	90–94	124–160
Lung (Right)	21–32	64–75	121–145	200–250
Lung (Left)	18–35	57–75	112–145	190–250
Liver	78–150	280–300	450–640	900–960
Spleen	7.2–11	20–26	52–60	88–93
Kidney	11.5–14	35	55–70	80–95
Adrenal	3–4	1–2	3.3	3.5–5

ORGAN	ADULTS		
	MALE	FEMALE	ADULT RANGE
Brain & Meninges	1,375	1,260	1,100–1,600
Thyroid	30	34	11–60
Thymus	14	14	25–1
Heart			
(Greatest at Age 50)	300	250	240–360
Lung (Right)	550	400	350–370
Lung (Left)	450	350	325–480
Liver	1,600	1,500	1,200–1,700
Spleen	165	150	80–300
Kidney	160	140	120–180
Adrenal	6	6	4–10

ATOMIC WEIGHTS
1948
J. Am. Chem. Soc. (November 1948)

	Symbol	Atomic number	Atomic weight		Symbol	Atomic number	Atomic weight
Aluminum....	Al	13	26.97	Molybdenum.	Mo	42	95.95
Antimony.....	Sb	51	121.76	Neodymium..	Nd	60	144.27
Argon........	A	18	39.944	Neon........	Ne	10	20.183
Arsenic.......	As	33	74.91	Nickel.......	Ni	28	58.69
Barium.......	Ba	56	137.36	Nitrogen.....	N	7	14.008
Beryllium....	Be	4	9.02	Osmium......	Os	76	190.2
Bismuth.....	Bi	83	209.00	Oxygen......	O	8	16.0000
Boron........	B	5	10.82	Palladium....	Pd	46	106.7
Bromine......	Br	35	79.916	Phosphorus...	P	15	30.98
Cadmium.....	Cd	48	112.41	Platinum.....	Pt	78	195.23
Calcium......	Ca	20	40.08	Potassium....	K	19	39.096
Carbon.......	C	6	12.010	Praseodymium	Pr	59	140.92
Cerium.......	Ce	58	140.13	Protactinium.	Pa	91	231
Cesium.......	Cs	55	132.91	Radium......	Ra	88	226.05
Chlorine.....	Cl	17	35.457	Radon.......	Rn	86	222
Chromium....	Cr	24	52.01	Rhenium.....	Re	75	186.31
Cobalt.......	Co	27	58.94	Rhodium.....	Rh	45	102.91
Columbium...	Cb	41	92.91	Rubidium....	Rb	37	85.48
Copper.......	Cu	29	63.54	Ruthenium...	Ru	44	101.7
Dysprosium..	Dy	66	162.46	Samarium....	Sm	62	150.43
Erbium.......	Er	68	167.2	Scandium....	Sc	21	45.10
Europium....	Eu	63	152.0	Selenium.....	Se	34	78.96
Fluorine......	F	9	19.00	Silicon.......	Si	14	28.06
Gadolinium...	Gd	64	156.9	Silver........	Ag	47	107.880
Gallium.......	Ga	31	69.72	Sodium......	Na	11	22.997
Germanium...	Ge	32	72.60	Strontium....	Sr	38	87.63
Gold.........	Au	79	197.2	Sulfur.......	S	16	32.066
Hafnium......	Hf	72	178.6	Tantalum....	Ta	73	180.88
Helium.......	He	2	4.003	Tellurium....	Te	52	127.61
Holmium.....	Ho	67	164.94	Terbium.....	Tb	65	159.2
Hydrogen....	H	1	1.0080	Thallium.....	Tl	81	204.39
Indium.......	In	49	114.76	Thorium.....	Th	90	232.12
Iodine........	I	53	126.92	Thulium.....	Tm	69	169.4
Iridium.......	Ir	77	193.1	Tin..........	Sn	50	118.70
Iron.........	Fe	26	55.85	Titanium....	Ti	22	47.90
Krypton......	Kr	36	83.7	Tungsten....	W	74	183.92
Lanthanum...	La	57	138.92	Uranium.....	U	92	238.07
Lead.........	Pb	82	207.21	Vanadium....	V	23	50.95
Lithium......	Li	3	6.940	Xenon.......	Xe	54	131.3
Lutecium.....	Lu	71	174.99	Ytterbium....	Yb	70	173.04
Magnesium...	Mg	12	24.32	Yttrium......	Y	39	88.92
Manganese...	Mn	25	54.93	Zinc.........	Zn	30	65.38
Mercury......	Hg	80	200.61	Zirconium....	Zr	40	91.22

INDEX

A

Abortion, 634
  complete, 636
  habitual, 637
  imminent, 635
  incomplete, 636
  induced, 634
  inevitable, 636
  missed, 636
  septic, 637
  spontaneous, 634
  therapeutic, 637
  threatened, 635
Abrasions, 1130
Abscess (*see* organ or disease)
Achromia, acquired, 1312
Achylia gastrica, 461
Acid-base and allied disorders, 283
Acidosis, 283, 284
  diabetic, 270, 278
Acne, 1313
  erythematosa, 1317
  frontalis, 1319
  necrotica, 1319
  rodens, 1319
  rosacea, 1317
  varioliformis, 1319
  vulgaris, 1313
Acromegaly, 378
Actinomycosis, 808
Adams-Stokes syndrome, 168
Addiction, drug, 1099
Addison's disease, 388
Adenoiditis, 348
Adenoma, chromophobe, 382
  parathyroid, 376
  thyroid, colloid type, 371
    fetal type, 371
Adiposogenitalism, 382
Adrenal, 388
  cortical insufficiency, chronic, 388
  cortical tumors, 393, 555
  crisis, 389
  hemorrhage, postpartum, 391
Adrenocortical, related therapy, 930
Aeroembolism, 1120
Aero-otitis, 1128
Agalactia, 652, 653
Agranulocytosis, 63
Air sickness, 1129
Alcoholic paranoia, 1095
  trance, automatism, 1094
Alcoholism, 1091
Alkalosis, 283, 286, 292
Allergy, (section), 1
  gastrointestinal, 18
  general considerations, 1
  physical, 23
Allergic reactions—transfusion, infusion, 1136

Allergic, (*cont'd*)
  rhinitis, 7
  shock, 21
Alopecia, 1309
Alphos, 1360
Alternative proprietaries, 1559
Amblyopia, toxic, 442
Amebic abscess, 751, 875
  colitis, 749
  dysentery, 749, 750
  hepatitis, 751, 875
Amebiasis, 749
Amenorrhea, 609
Ametropia, 444
Amyloid disease, 877
Amyloidosis, 289
Amyotonia congenita, 1016
Amyotrophic lateral sclerosis, 1014
Anal fissure, 524
  fistula, 526
  (*see also* Anorectal)
Anaphylaxis, in allergy, 1
  in serum sickness, 21
Anasarca, 129
Anemia, 30
  Addisonian, 39
  aplastic, 45
  Biermer's, 39
  of chronic blood loss, 34, 43
  classification, 31
  congenital, of newborn, 51, 52
  drepanocytic, 36
  hemolytic, 35, 85
    primary, 35
    secondary, 37
  "hyperchromic," 31
  hypochromic, 31
    microcytic, "nutritional," 43
  leuko-erythroblastic, 46
  macrocytic, 39, 42
  microcytic, hypochromic, 43
  myelophthisic, 46
  "nutritional" hypochromic, 43
  osteosclerotic, 46
  pernicious, 39
  posthemorrhagic, acute, 33
  primary refractory, 45
  sickle cell, 36
  spherocytic, 35
  splenic, 82
Anesthesia, local, 1474
Aneurysm, 192
  aortic, abdominal, 193
    dissecting, 193
  arteriovenous, 194
  circoid, 192
  intracranial, 193
  intrathoracic, 193
  mycotic, 192
  racemose, 192